The Clinical Practice of
Neurological and Neurosurgical Nursing

Joanne V. Hickey

R.N., M.S.N., M.A., CNRN

The Clinical Practice of
Neurological and Neurosurgical Nursing

second edition

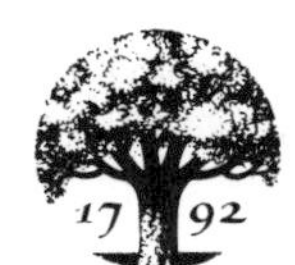

J. B. LIPPINCOTT COMPANY
PHILADELPHIA
LONDON MEXICO CITY NEW YORK ST. LOUIS
SÃO PAULO SYDNEY

The author and publisher have exerted every effort to ensure that drug selection and dosage set forth in this text are in accord with current recommendations and practice at the time of publication. However, in view of ongoing research, changes in government regulations, and the constant flow of information relating to drug therapy and drug reactions, the reader is urged to check the package insert for each drug for any change in indications and dosage and for added warnings and precautions. This is particularly important when the recommended agent is a new or infrequently employed drug.

Sponsoring Editor: Diana Intenzo
Manuscript Editor: Elizabeth P. Lowe
Indexer: Alexandra Weir
Designer: Maria S. Karkucinski
Production Supervisor: J. Corey Gray
Production Coordinator: Barney Fernandes
Compositor: Progressive Typographers
Printer and Binder: The Murray Printing Company
Cover Printer: Waldman Graphics, Inc.

Second Edition

6 5 4

Library of Congress Cataloging in Publication Data

Hickey, Joanne V.
The clinical practice of neurological and neurosurgical nursing.

Includes bibliographies and index.
1. Neurological nursing. I. Title. [DNLM: 1. Nervous System Diseases—nursing. 2. Neurosurgery—nursing. WY 160 H628c]
RC350.5.H52 1986 610.73′68 85-108
ISBN 0-397-54478-2

As always . . . to my dear family — my husband Jim, daughter Kathan, and son Christopher — for their continued love, support, encouragement, understanding, and help, particularly during the writing of the second edition. Without their precious support, I could not have completed this project.

Preface

Since the first edition of *The Clinical Practice of Neurological and Neurosurgical Nursing* was written, the knowledge in the field of neuroscience nursing has continued to grow at an explosive rate. In revising the text I was conscious of this great body of new information and endeavored to include the major developments in the various areas covered in the first edition. In addition, a number of topics were not included in the first edition due to space limitations that I believed should be included in this revision. The considerable expansion of the text has allowed the inclusion of these topics. Finally, my continuous review and use of the first edition, together with the many suggestions from colleagues who have used the text, have led to various changes in the format and the presentation of certain material that were made in order to emphasize nursing diagnosis as a basic approach to nursing management. My overall purpose continues to be to disseminate information about neurological–neurosurgical nursing management of the adult patient to nurses and others through a reliable, well-documented text that incorporates the current accepted standards of patient care.

My goals for the revised text have not changed appreciably from those stated in the preface to the first edition. They remain (1) to contribute to the resource literature available in neurological–neurosurgical nursing; (2) to incorporate current and accepted theoretical and technological knowledge pertinent to the practice of neurological–neurosurgical nursing; (3) to provide a comprehensive and in-depth presentation covering neurological–neurosurgical nursing of the adult patient with special emphasis on the specific points of nursing management in the clinical setting; and (4) to present the information in a well-organized format designed to provide the reader with ready access to information through the judicious use of headings, illustrations, tables, and charts.

Although this text is intended to provide comprehensive coverage of major adult neurological–neurosurgical problems, it is not exhaustive. The material presented focuses on the care of the adult patient. The text reflects currently accepted standards of care and does not, for the most part, discuss information still in the research stage.

The text is organized into eight parts, which contain logically unified chapters. These parts are presented sequentially and proceed from general information to specific problems. Part One includes revised and expanded chapters that introduce the reader to significant trends in neurological–neurosurgical nursing and also provides an overview of neuroanatomy and neurophysiology, which serves as a reference for comparing normal and abnormal physiology. Part Two presents expanded information on assessment of the neurological–neurosurgical patient. Chapter 4, Diagnostic Evaluation, has been extensively revised to include information on many new diagnostic modalities, including magnetic resonance imaging, positron emission transaxial tomography, digital subtraction angiography, and brain stem evoked potentials. Three new chapters are included in Part Three to incorporate areas of patient management necessary to consider the patient holistically. This information should be particularly useful for caring for patients who have serious and long-term health problems. Chapter 6, Nutritional Needs of Neurological and Neurosurgical Patients, provides information on basic nutritional needs, changes in nutritional needs associated with the stresses of illness, assessment of nutritional needs, and methods frequently used to provide adequate nutrition to this patient population.

Patients do not progress without attention to adequate nutrition. Chapter 7, Emotional and Behavioral Responses to Neurological Illness, includes common responses to neurological illness and nursing approaches to support the patient. In Chapter 9, Discharge Planning, the interdisciplinary approach to planning for discharge from the acute-care setting is explored to assist the nurse in this very important and complex process.

Part Four, Special Considerations in Neurological and Neurosurgical Nursing, includes two new chapters as well as considerable expansion of chapters found in the first edition. The environment and workplace expose individuals to neurotoxins that can cause significant neurological illness and deficits. It is important for the nurse working with neurologically impaired patients to develop an awareness of and sensitivity to the possibility of their having been exposed to neurotoxins. For this reason, I have included Chapter 10, Environmental and Occupational Factors in Neurological Nursing. The other new chapter is Chapter 13, Water Balance, which focuses on the endocrine, electrolyte, and osmolar abnormalities often encountered with neurological problems such as diabetes insipidus, syndrome of inappropriate secretion of antidiuretic hormone, hyperglycemic hyperosmolar nonketotic coma, and electrolyte imbalance. Expansion of the scope of Chapter 14 provides more information on the preoperative and intraoperative phases of neurological surgery.

The Multi-trauma Patient, Chapter 16, is the one new addition to Part Five. This chapter was added because so many patients admitted to neurological units have sustained multiple trauma requiring a systematic approach to the patient based on priorities of care. Most of the other chapters in the section have undergone major revisions and expansion. Chapter 17 now includes management of the head-injured patient from the prehospital phase through the postacute phase of management. Central nervous system neoplasms are discussed in Part Six. More information on chemotherapeutic drugs and newer treatment protocols have been incorporated. Various cerebrovascular problems are the focus of Part Seven. The chapters of Part Eight were updated and expanded to include discussion of additional neurological diseases.

This book is intended for use by nursing students at various levels, faculty, and nurses engaged in clinical practice with adult neurological–neurosurgical patients. Students enrolled in basic nursing programs, comprehensive neurological–neurosurgical nursing courses, or continuing education courses in neurological–neurosurgical nursing should find *The Clinical Practice of Neurological and Neurosurgical Nursing, Second Edition,* useful as a basic text or as a resource. Professional nurses engaged in practice in intensive care units, emergency care departments, neurological–neurosurgical specialty units, or other units to which patients with neurological problems are admitted should find this text a ready reference. Throughout the text, pathophysiology and nursing management are correlated and a rationale for nursing care based on the nursing process is presented. Summaries of common nursing diagnoses, expected outcomes, and nursing interventions for nursing management of the patient are included.

Caring for the neurologically disabled patient requires special skills and knowledge. This book was written in an effort to respond to the diverse needs of the many committed nurses who provide this care.

Joanne V. Hickey, R.N., M.S.N., M.A., CNRN
Doctoral student in nursing
University of Texas
Austin, Texas

Acknowledgments

I wish to express my appreciation and gratitude for the help and support of so many people during the preparation of the manuscript for the first and second editions of *The Clinical Practice of Neurological and Neurosurgical Nursing*. Although the completion of the second edition was easier in some respects, nevertheless a fair amount of blood, sweat, and tears was expended during the many months of research and writing. My family, friends, and colleagues provided the support to make this undertaking both a positive and a satisfying experience.

I am indebted to the Rhode Island Hospital neurosurgical nursing and medical staff for their suggestions, clarifications, and critiques. As always, they have my sincere respect and admiration for the quality of care they give and for the dedication with which they have cared for our patients.

To my husband, Jim Hickey, for both helping me to clarify my ideas and assisting with the editing of my writing, I give sincere thanks. Jim, who is a certified industrial hygienist, is also the co-author of Chapter 10, Environmental and Occupational Factors in Neurological Nursing.

To my nursing faculty colleagues who were in some of the photographs—Marly Loebig, Mary Flynn, Elsie Lewis, and Betsy Nield—I extend my appreciation. The photographs in which my colleagues appear were taken by M. F. Logan and E. M. Collins, who provided me with prints of excellent quality. I also wish to acknowledge the gracious assistance of the many medical supply companies that provided photographs for inclusion in this text.

For my many neurosurgical nursing students and participants in workshops that I have given—who stimulated me to expand and clarify this text by asking questions and offering fresh insights into patient care—I am thankful. I hope that the second edition, with its many additions and its expansion of material, will provide a valuable resource for you and all others interested in this fascinating area of nursing practice.

A special thanks to my editor, Diana Intenzo, who continues to guide me through the maze of authorship. Her knowledge, ability, and sense of humor sustained me through the many hills and valleys of this project.

Finally, my research was conducted at the Brown University Libraries and the Rhode Island Hospital Library. The resources available at these libraries afforded me the opportunity to thoroughly review the literature.

Contents

Part Six/Nursing Care of Patients With Tumors of the Neurological System 459

Part Seven/Nursing Care of Patients With Cerebrovascular Problems 493

Part Eight/Special Problems of the Neurological System 541

part one

Overview

chapter 1

Trends in Neurological and Neurosurgical Nursing Practice

Neurological and neurosurgical nursing is a specialized area of practice that falls under the major heading of medical–surgical nursing. The patient population served by this speciality has suffered some degree of physiological and psychosocial alteration because of nervous system dysfunction. The neurological deficits involved usually affect some facet of the patient's intellectual processes, emotional responses, sensory perceptions, autonomic and motor activity, communication systems, and special senses such as vision, hearing, smell, taste, and touch. To provide nursing care for these patients, one must have a thorough knowledge of medical–surgical nursing as well as neuropathophysiology and the elements of patient management and rehabilitation, with special application of the nursing process. The goal of neurological and neurosurgical nursing is to provide quality care, which is directed at assisting the patient to return to as productive and independent a life as possible.

THE DEVELOPMENT AND ORGANIZATION OF NURSING AND NURSING THEORY

Within the last few decades the nursing profession has undergone phenomenal growth and development in the areas of nursing theory, nursing research, and nursing education. The needs of society and the development of the health care system have fostered the emergence of nursing as a true profession, which is reflected in the expanded roles, functions, and responsibilities that nurses now assume.

The development of a body of knowledge called "nursing" has affected all areas of nursing practice including that of neuroscience nursing; accordingly, a greater variety of skills and a broader base of knowledge are now required to deliver safe nursing care. In addition, the development of sophisticated medical and surgical management protocols, as well as complex monitoring, diagnostic, and assessment equipment and procedures, makes it imperative that the nurse acquire appropriate knowledge and develop skills to assume the responsibilities for patient management within the contemporary practice setting.

Every professional group has the responsibility of being accountable for standards of practice. To provide accountability to both the consumer and the profession, the Standards of Neurological and Neurosurgical Nursing Practice was published in 1977 under the auspices of the Division on Medical–Surgical Nursing Practice of the American Nurses' Association and the American Association of Neurosurgical Nurses (the professional organization for nurses involved in the care of patients with neurological dysfunction and disease).[1] The Standards were revised in 1984 to reflect the application of the nursing process to selected phenomena unique to neuroscience nursing. The phenomena initially addressed include consciousness/cognition, communication, mobility, protective reflexes, rest and sleep, sensation, and sexuality. Other phenomena would be added as the development of theory and practice progressed. The format used for the presentation of each phenomenon includes nursing diagnoses, planning/nursing interventions, and outcome criteria.

By developing, approving, and disseminating standards of practice for neuroscience nursing, the organization has adopted a means of evaluating the nursing care administered to the patients and the competence of its members as neuroscience practitioners. This contribution to the development of nursing theory and specialty nursing practice enhances the growth and development of the entire profession.

Another major contribution of the American Association of Neuroscience Nurses (AANN), which was called the American Association of Neurosurgical Nurses until 1983, was the development in 1983 of the AANN Conceptual Framework.[2] The purpose of this project was to construct a framework of related, scientifically based concepts that reflect integral relationships, beliefs, and thoughts about the practice of neuroscience nursing.

THE NURSING PROCESS

Nursing care is implemented through the use of the nursing process, which is a logical, systematic, problem-solving approach. The steps of the nursing process include assessment and analysis, planning, implementation, and evaluation.[3] See Figure 1–1.

ASSESSMENT

Assessment is the data-gathering phase in which the nurse uses all available sources of information to collect data systematically on the biophysical, psychological, and emotional needs of the patient to establish a data base for the analysis and identification of nursing diagnoses. Usual sources of information include the nursing history, interviews with the patient and his family, clinical inspection of the patient, review of the clinical chart, and nursing observations. The perceptions, observations, and communication skills of the nurse, combined with a knowledge base, enable her to collect and analyze data, identify patient problems, and formulate nursing diagnoses. The nursing diagnoses focus on actual or potential problems that may interfere with the patient's ability to achieve the highest level of wellness possible. Through nursing diagnoses, the nurse identifies areas in which nursing intervention can assist in the management or alleviation of these health-related problems.

FIG. 1–1. Diagram of the nursing process, which can be viewed as an ongoing, integrated approach to patient care.

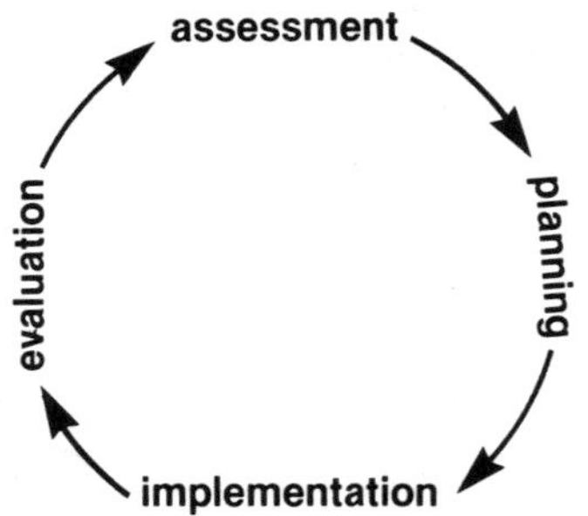

PLANNING

Once the various nursing diagnoses are established, planning begins. *Planning* is the step in the nursing process in which the elements of nursing care necessary to assist the patient in meeting his needs are determined. The planning process focuses on the following points:

- Goals of the care proposed
- Specific nursing protocols to be followed to achieve the goals
- A time frame (deadlines or check dates) by which the identified goals are to be achieved or assessed to determine progress toward meeting the goals
- Priorities of care

IMPLEMENTATION

The third step in the nursing process is implementation. The nursing interventions that have been selected to meet the needs of the patient are put in effect in this phase of the nursing process.

EVALUATION

Evaluation is the fourth step of the nursing process. It requires that a critical appraisal be made to determine to what degree the nursing care has assisted the patient in meeting his health needs. The criteria for evaluation reflect how well the patient has become and whether the identified goals have been achieved. If the evaluation indicates that the goals of care have not been met completely, then the nursing process is once again employed to find a better approach to the patient.

SUMMARY

Although the nursing process has been subdivided into four steps, in actual practice each step is continuously carried out to varying degrees so that the overall process is an ongoing one. Similarly, new assessment data are constantly being integrated, validated, or clarified. Figure 1–1 illustrates the continuity of the nursing process.

FACTORS INFLUENCING CHANGE AND TRENDS IN NEUROLOGICAL AND NEUROSURGICAL NURSING

The delivery of health care and the practice of neurological and neurosurgical nursing are affected by several factors, including scientific developments, changes in the structure of the health care system, and social forces and trends. The most significant of these factors include the following:

1. Changing trends in life expectancy and morbidity
2. Proliferation of scientific knowledge
3. Support of research in the public and private sectors
4. Development of sophisticated diagnostic and monitoring equipment and procedures

5. Development and use of innovative medical and surgical protocols for patient management
6. Changes in the organization, structure, and management of the health care system
7. Changes in financing of health care and reimbursement practices
8. Increased specialization in medical and nursing practice
9. Development and use of regional trauma management networks, neurological intensive care units, and community resources
10. Increased emphasis on rehabilitation
11. Increased awareness of the legal and ethical considerations of health care delivery

Although each of these trends will be discussed separately, they are, in fact, interrelated concepts. The political, economic, legislative/legal, demographic, educational, research, cultural, scientific, and technological developments of society shape the health professions and, subsequently, their roles in providing health care.

CHANGING TRENDS IN LIFE EXPECTANCY AND MORBIDITY

The increase in life expectancy for Americans has been a positive result of the advances and improvements made in several health-related areas. However, since people now live to an older age, a greater number of elderly patients are entering the health care system with age-related disorders such as cardiovascular diseases (stroke, arteriosclerosis) and degenerative conditions (Parkinson's disease). Conditions such as these either directly or indirectly affect the nervous system. As the incidence of such diseases increases, new demands for comprehensive care are placed on the health care system.

At the same time, more people are showing the effects of occupational diseases because of long-term exposure to various chemicals in the workplace. Although exposure to certain chemicals can result in sudden illness, numerous chemical substances do not cause any detectable signs and symptoms of disease until many years (10–30 years) have passed. The highly sensitive cells of the nervous system are particularly vulnerable to this kind of subtle risk. The result is the slow process of cell degeneration and development of irreversible damage, which subsequently lead to neurological deficits. As people live longer and have a greater opportunity to work in high-risk industries for longer periods, there is greater potential for the development of degenerative neurological conditions.

In addition, the greater incidence of alcohol and drug abuse in our society is having its effect on long-term degenerative neurological changes. Both categories of patients are becoming more prevalent in health care facilities.

Finally, trauma caused by vehicular and sports injuries and acts of violence continues to take its toll in increasing numbers among the population at-large. Catastrophic injuries of this type more often than not affect the neurological system as well as other body systems. The needs of these patients create a demand for high-level medical and nursing management.

As a result of these changes in life expectancy and mortality, there is a greater need to develop new nursing skills, knowledge, and approaches to meet the needs of these populations.

PROLIFERATION OF SCIENTIFIC KNOWLEDGE

Proliferation of new scientific knowledge in the physical, biological, and behavioral sciences continues to enrich the knowledge base for application to the health and health-related professions. Knowledge of the nervous system is still relatively meager when compared to our understanding of other body systems; however, new developments in laboratory equipment, techniques, and computer technology are providing the means to explore and uncover the mysteries of neurophysiology and neuropathophysiology. Leadership in these and other endeavors is spearheaded by the National Institute of Neurological and Communicative Disorders and Stroke (NINCDS), a branch of the National Institutes of Health (NIH).[4] The role of this federal agency in relationship to neurological problems is reflected in its mission statement. According to the agency, "the mission of NINCDS is to conduct and support research and research training on the causes, prevention, diagnosis, and treatment of neurological and communicative disorders and stroke. The Institute carries out its mission in the following ways. It

- Awards grants of three types: research project, program project, and center grants
- Enters into contracts for research and research support
- Provides training support to institutions, and fellowships to individuals, to increase academic and research manpower in neurological and communicative fields
- Conducts intramural and collaborative research in its own laboratories and clinics
- Collects and disseminates research information."

NINCDS is organized according to seven program areas: stroke and trauma; communicative disorders; fundamental neurosciences; convulsive, developmental, and neuromuscular disorders; demyelinating, atrophic, and dementing disorders; intramural research (conducting laboratory and clinical research in NIH laboratories); and extramural activities (providing administrative support and coordination).

The proliferation of scientific knowledge is both exciting and mind-boggling as one begins to contemplate its application to neurological problems. Although new knowledge is generated from various scientific disciplines and sources, some of the most exciting information comes from the fields of neurochemistry and neurophysiology. The alterations in neurotransmitters and neuronal cellular activity, as well as the various metabolic functions necessary for cell metabolism, continue to be studied. The ultimate goal of research is to learn how to reverse the effects of apparently permanent injury to the central nervous system through a greater understanding of cellular dynamics and physiology. The accepted premise, up to a few years ago, was that no regeneration in the central nervous system was possible. However, laboratory and clinical findings challenge this formerly dismal outlook for patients. Breakthroughs in understanding central nervous system regeneration have already been made, and more developments can be expected as research continues.

Closely related to research in neurophysiology is the study of the effects of drugs on the nervous system. Although many drugs are recognized for their therapeutic value in the treatment of other body systems, these drugs have proven to be ineffective in treating nervous system disorders because of their inability to cross the blood–brain barrier or to be maintained in sufficient concentration within the tissue to achieve a therapeutic effect. It is also true that several drugs currently administered for the management of nervous system disorders have side-effects that make their prolonged use dangerous or unsatisfactory. However, as a result of research in neuropharmacology, newer, safer, and more effective drugs with fewer serious side-effects are being introduced.

From the field of neuropsychology has come a better understanding of the function and interrelatedness of cerebral function. This information can be applied to the brain-injured patient who needs cognitive retraining. A detailed assessment of the patient through the mental status examination assists the neuropsychologist in identifying the areas of brain damage. Based on this information, a specific treatment plan for cognitive retraining can be developed to help the patient regain as much function and independence as possible.

Nursing research is an integral part of practice for many nurses. Their contributions to the development of nursing theory and patient management help to support the professional image of nursing as a truly scientific practice discipline. Theorists such as Rogers, Roy, Orem, Neuman, King, Johnson, and others have made significant contributions to the development of the theoretical bases for practice in various practice settings. The classification of nursing diagnoses begun in the late 1970s continues to be developed and refined. Standards of care such as those developed by the AANN apply nursing diagnoses to the areas of specialty practice.

Clinical research in all areas of nursing including neurological and neurosurgical practice lays the groundwork for nursing theory and nursing protocols for specific patient problems. The work of Parsons and Mitchell in intracranial pressure, Rimels and Speilman in head injuries, and many others have made significant contributions to neuroscience nursing practice.

The increased understanding and insight resulting from research of basic sciences and neurosciences as well as clinical research contribute to the ever-expanding knowledge base that must be incorporated into current neurological and neurosurgical nursing practice.

SUPPORT OF RESEARCH

Funding from both public and private sectors has provided support for neurological research projects throughout the country. As discussed in the previous section, much of the federal government's commitment to the study of neurological disease is concentrated in NINCDS. Several university-based research projects throughout the country are funded by NINCDS. Many medical schools and institutes also receive federal funds, as well as private contributions and endowments.

In some instances, the sharing of data from various research and clinical centers has been made possible by advanced computer systems for storing and retrieving data. Data may be made available to the practitioner, thereby directly benefiting the patient. For example, there are centers throughout the country that participate in the study and management of brain tumors. Information about the selection and effectiveness of various treatment protocols is stored in the computer system shared by these centers. A physician wishing to determine the most suitable treatment protocol for a particular patient can submit a patient profile and receive immediate feedback on the treatment most likely to be effective, based on the experience of researchers in the affiliated research centers.

Several research projects support basic research, and clinical trials of various protocols are underway throughout the country. A sampling of research areas is cited to provide an appreciation of the scope and breadth of activities: disorders of early life such as congenital disorders, cerebral palsy, mental retardation, hereditary metabolic disease, autism, and dyslexia; convulsive disorders; degenerative diseases; neuromuscular disorders such as myasthenia gravis and peripheral neuropathies; speech disorders; language disorders (including aphasia related to stroke); disorders of taste and smell; cerebrovascular disease including stroke; nervous system trauma such as head and spinal cord injuries; nervous system tumors; headache; chronic pain; nervous system regeneration; and positron emission transaxial tomography (PETT).

In addition to government support, many private foundations and groups have been established to study specific problems such as multiple sclerosis, Alzheimer's disease, Parkinson's disease, and myasthenia gravis, among others. The purpose of many of these organizations is to provide a combination of basic research, selected services to victims, and education of the patient, family, lay persons, and professionals.

DIAGNOSTIC AND MONITORING EQUIPMENT AND PROCEDURES

In 1973 the computed tomography (CT) scan or computerized axial tomography (CAT) scan revolutionized neurodiagnostic procedures. Since then, third and fourth generation CT scanners have been rapidly developed to provide even more precise visualization of the cerebral tissue. The latest technology includes the positron emission transaxial tomography (PETT) and magnetic resonance imaging (MRI). The PETT technology is currently used in only a few centers in the United States. It is a new noninvasive technique useful for detecting biochemical and physiological abnormalities in the living organism and for studying the complex physiological processes of the nervous system.

Without using radiation, MRI provides images that are unmatched for their sharpness and detailed cross sections of living tissue. Many experts believe that the MRI will render the CT scan obsolete in the next few years.

A cursory glance through Chapter 4 of this text suggests the extent of diagnostic testing considered standard for the neurological and neurosurgical patient. There is a wide and expanding array of monitoring devices and equipment for the critically ill neurological patient. The equipment used for monitoring such functions as intracranial pressure, the electrical activity of the brain and the heart, vital signs, and pulmonary wedge pressure is commonly found on the clinical unit. Mechanical respirators, cooling blankets, food pumps, intravenous pumps, trauma beds, and computerized equipment of various sorts are a part of the nurse's work environment.

The number of assessment tools available for qualitative and quantitative measurement of specific functions, parameters, and skills continues to grow. The Glasgow Coma Scale (GCS) was first discussed in the nursing literature in 1975. This widely used scale attempts to standardize the assessment of a patient's level of consciousness, a most important parameter of neurological assessment. Terms such as obtunded, semicomatose, and lethargic, which are frequently used to label the various levels of consciousness, do not provide clear, consistent descriptions of clinical information observed by different practitioners. Thus, without the clarity and precision of a common system of evaluation, data cannot be accurately conveyed from one observer to another.

Since the Glasgow Coma Scale is based on objective criteria, it has gained wide acceptance in neurological centers in both Europe and the United States in the few years since it was introduced. Studies indicate that it has a high degree of reliability as an objective assessment tool. The GCS has been incorporated into the knowledge base of neuroscience practice.

DEVELOPMENT AND USE OF INNOVATIVE MEDICAL AND SURGICAL TREATMENTS AND PROTOCOLS

Correlation of new knowledge in neurophysiology, neuropathology, and pharmacology has spurred the development of protocols for patient management. Included in the vast array of current therapeutic protocols are barbiturate coma for treatment of intracranial hypertension that has been unresponsive to conventional treatment methods; chemonucleolysis for treatment of some herniated lumbar discs; use of computer technology to program paralyzed limbs of spinal cord-injured patients; phrenic stimulators to trigger respiration in the patient injured in the upper cervical region; hyperbaric oxygenation therapy to improve the oxygen supply to the injured neurological system; and biofeedback for pain control.

Advances in neurosurgery are directly related to the development of neurosurgical instrumentation and other equipment, along with safer anesthetic agents and improved manipulation of vital signs. The advent of neuromicrosurgery has enabled the neurosurgeon to visualize and reach formerly inaccessible areas of the brain as well as perform new surgical procedures. Microsurgery can be used to remove diseased cerebral blood vessels and reanastomose vessels to provide an adequate blood supply to areas that had demonstrated the effects of transient ischemia. Spinal cord procedures for various problems and transsphenoidal hypophysectomy to remove pituitary adenomas are a few other common uses of neuromicrosurgery.

Other examples of innovative neurosurgical management include surgical intervention for pain control; embolization, proton-beam radiation, and surgical resection of arteriovenous malformations; use of lasers; early surgical intervention for spinal cord injuries; improved shunting equipment and procedures for treatment of hydrocephalus; spinal cord cooling procedures to control edema of the spinal cord; and use of the CT-guided stereotactic apparatus for biopsy and removal of brain tumors.

The development and use of new medical and surgical protocols for the management of the neurological–neurosurgical patient have a significant impact on nursing practice. The nurse must understand the purpose and principles of treatment and specific interrelated management protocols to participate as a member of the professional health team. New nursing care protocols must be developed so that the nurse can care for the patient competently.

CHANGES IN THE ORGANIZATION, STRUCTURE, AND MANAGEMENT OF THE HEALTH CARE SYSTEM

Health care is a major industry in the United States. Almost 10% of the gross national product is devoted to health care expenditures. As the complexity of its mission and responsibility grows, the organization, structure, and management of health care grow and change. Health care is provided in varied settings, but the effective organizational structure reflects the needs and functions of the system in which it operates. There is an ever-increasing need for fiscal responsibility and accountability for the cost of quality health care. Many complex organizational structures have been developed to manage the needs of the system. Health care facilities of all types must interface when providing many aspects of the care offered to the client. The need to cooperate and to see a facility as part of the overall system that meets the needs of a large number of people fosters the development of organizational patterns. Trauma centers, head injury centers, spinal cord injury centers, various general acute-care hospitals, and rehabilitation facilities share many of the same concerns when providing care for neurologically impaired patients. The issues of triage, rapid stabilization and transportation to the most appropriate facility, discharge planning, and extended care are concerns of all health care providers. The use of community resources, in both the public and private sector, requires mutual planning and the cooperation of the various health care providers to ensure the quality of care for the patient and his family.

The involvement of the federal and state government in

the financing of health care has contributed to the growth and complexity of health care organizational structure and management. Medicare, Medicaid, and quality assurance programs are examples of major federal and state programs that have helped shape the health care system.

CHANGES IN FINANCING OF HEALTH CARE AND REIMBURSEMENT PRACTICES

The cost of health care continues to increase at an alarming rate. Medicare, state funding, private insurance providers, and direct payments to patients provide the money to fuel the ravenous system. The latest attempt to control cost is the institution of diagnostic-related groupings (DRGs); this system was implemented in October 1983 for Medicare patients. The significance of this well-researched and piloted approach is that payment is prospective rather than retrospective. Using a formula that factors in the patient's diagnosis, age, preexisting health problems, complications, and location of the health care facility, the cost that will be paid for the hospitalization is calculated. If the hospital is able to treat the patient for less than the calculated figure, the difference is kept by the hospital. Should the cost of the hospital stay exceed the preset amount, the hospital will absorb the difference.

The innovative DRG reimbursement plan is only in its first stages of implementation. Private health insurance providers are sure to consider prospective payment, if it proves successful, because they face the same problems of escalating cost that governmental agencies confront.

INCREASED SPECIALIZATION IN MEDICAL AND NURSING PRACTICE

Time is known to be a critical factor in determining survival and extent of injury, particularly in instances of neurological trauma when neuronal damage may become irreversible because of oxygen deprivation and changes in hemodynamics. The sooner that aggressive quality health care can be provided, the better the outcome of the patient. By organizing neurotrauma regional networks, the health care delivery system can provide a comprehensive plan for rapid triage so that patients can be transported quickly by ground or air to the most suitable facilities capable of meeting patient needs. Aggressive regional trauma planning has dramatically reduced mortality and complications from neurological injury, as well as decreasing the amount of permanent disability incurred by the patient.

There has also been an increase in the development of neurological intensive units within acute care facilities. These units offer sophisticated equipment and technology as well as highly skilled physicians and nurse specialists who provide expert and intensive management of neurological–neurosurgical patients. Although it is expensive to maintain such a high-caliber unit, the rewards can be measured in improved patient outcome, reduced complications, and higher levels of rehabilitation and independence for the patient.

Because the needs of the neurologically impaired patient are extensive, many community services and resources have been developed to support the patient who is able to live in the community. Such services include physiotherapy, speech therapy, vocational and psychological counseling, and transportation. Some organizations are designed to address the needs of specific populations such as patients with multiple sclerosis, stroke, or epilepsy. When community-based services are made available, patients are given the opportunity to live a life of greater independence and dignity, rather than being confined to an acute-care setting or extended care facility.

Increased specialization has also created new roles and responsibilities for the nurse. Many nurses are now employed in expanded roles with titles such as clinician, clinical nurse specialist, nurse practitioner, or nurse associate. Specialized roles and responsibilities have created new concerns about credentialing. Certification programs have been instituted by many specialty nursing organizations. In some work settings, certification in specialty practice has been necessary for career advancement.

DEVELOPMENT AND USE OF REGIONAL TRAUMA MANAGEMENT NETWORKS, NEUROLOGICAL INTENSIVE CARE UNITS, AND COMMUNITY RESOURCES

The cost of special units and facilities is high. This is especially true of high technology units and facilities. Such resources as regional trauma centers, specialty units such as neurological intensive care units, and other community resources can be valuable in saving lives, preventing more extensive disabilities, and improving the quality of life for the patient and his family. Specialty units are often cost-effective because by managing the patient aggressively, more costly management and treatment of complications can be eliminated or at least limited.

To effectively plan for such complex health care, it is necessary to view the overall needs of the country. National and regional planning is imperative to consider all aspects of making a system operational, such as providing transportation, avoiding duplication of effort and resources, placing equipment and personnel, planning educational programs, and locating populations. Regionalization of health planning has proven to be both effective and cost-effective.

INCREASED EMPHASIS ON REHABILITATION

Improved treatment protocols result in the survival of more patients with multiple and complex rehabilitative needs. The degree of independence and productivity achieved by the patient is directly proportional to the achievement of specific rehabilitative goals. Consistently integrating an aggressive philosophy of rehabilitation throughout the course of health care delivery ensures the possibility of reaching optimal rehabilitative goals. By a comprehensive, collaborative team approach, the expertise of the health professionals is directed toward the goals of prevention, maintenance, and restoration of function. Within the framework of rehabilitation, the physical, psychosocial, emotional, and vocational needs of the patient are addressed.

Incorporating a philosophy of rehabilitation into nursing practice enables the nurse to develop priorities of nursing care that are consistent with a strong commitment to rehabilitation. This is particularly important when caring for neurological–neurosurgical patients who often have complex and long-term rehabilitative needs.

LEGAL AND ETHICAL CONSIDERATIONS

An increased awareness of the legal and ethical considerations of health care has emerged in all areas of practice, including nursing.

Although nursing care must be carried out within the definition and legal bounds provided by the state licensing board, certain issues are confronted by all nurses involved in neurological and neurosurgical nursing, regardless of the state in which they practice. Such issues include implementation of the patient's bill of rights, the criteria used in determining brain death, and the use of resuscitative and heroic measures.

Patient's Bill of Rights

The Patient's Bill of Rights is a statement of the patient's rights as a consumer and recipient of health care. Most hospitals inform the patient, usually in writing, of these rights upon admission to the facility. See Chart 1–1.

When endeavoring to meet standards of nursing care, the nurse may sometimes encounter a conflict in upholding the Patient's Bill of Rights. This is especially likely when caring for the neurological or neurosurgical patient whose level of consciousness or intellectual abilities have been altered. At times, patients will object to certain aspects of their care, such as frequent turning, passive range-of-motion exercises, or the use of restraints.

The decisions relating to the standards of care will de-

CHART 1–1. AHA'S PATIENT'S BILL OF RIGHTS

1. The patient has the right to considerate and respectful care.
2. The patient has the right to obtain from his physician complete current information concerning his diagnosis, treatment, and prognosis in terms the patient can be reasonably expected to understand. When it is not medically advisable to give such information to the patient, the information should be made available to an appropriate person in his behalf. He has the right to know, by name, the physician responsible for coordinating his care.
3. The patient has the right to receive from his physician information necessary to give informed consent prior to the start of any procedure and/or treatment. Except in emergencies, such information for informed consent should include, but not necessarily be limited to, the specific procedure and/or treatment, the medically significant risks involved, and the probable duration of incapacitation. Where medically significant alternatives for care or treatment exist, or when the patient requests information concerning medical alternatives, the patient has the right to such information. The patient also has the right to know the name of the person responsible for the procedures and/or treatment.
4. The patient has the right to refuse treatment to the extent permitted by law and to be informed of the medical consequences of his action.
5. The patient has the right to every consideration of his privacy concerning his own medical care program. Case discussion, consultation, examination, and treatment are confidential and should be conducted discreetly. Those not directly involved in his care must have the permission of the patient to be present.
6. The patient has the right to expect that all communications and records pertaining to his care should be treated as confidential.
7. The patient has the right to expect that within its capacity a hospital must make reasonable response to the request of a patient for services. The hospital must provide evaluation, service, and/or referral as indicated by the urgency of the case. When medically permissible, a patient may be transferred to another facility only after he has received complete information and explanation concerning the needs for and alternatives to such a transfer. The institution to which the patient is to be transferred must first have accepted the patient for transfer.
8. The patient has the right to obtain information as to any relationship of his hospital to other health care and educational institutions insofar as his care is concerned. The patient has the right to obtain information as to the existence of any professional relationships among individuals, by name, who are treating him.
9. The patient has the right to be advised if the hospital proposes to engage in or perform human experimentation affecting his care or treatment. The patient has the right to refuse to participate in such research projects.
10. The patient has the right to expect reasonable continuity of care. He has the right to know in advance what appointment times and physicians are available and where. The patient has the right to expect that the hospital will provide a mechanism whereby he is informed by his physician or a delegate of the physician of the patient's continuing health care requirements following discharge.
11. The patient has the right to examine and receive an explanation of his bill regardless of source of payment.
12. The patient has the right to know what hospital rules and regulations apply to his conduct as a patient.

pend upon several factors that include the patient's level of consciousness and his ability to comprehend reality, the management prescribed by the physician, the judgment of the nurse, and specific circumstances concerning health care. It goes without saying that a high standard of care is applied in managing a psychotic patient or one with an altered level of consciousness. These patients must be protected from injuring themselves, and they must receive care considered to be inherent in good nursing management.

Brain Death Criteria

Because of the life-threatening neurological insults encountered by the neurological and neurosurgical patient (whether due to disease or trauma), the nurse is often confronted with the impending death of the patient and the attendant emotional crises. Tragic accidents and assault injuries can, in a matter of seconds, rob healthy, active persons of life, limb, or normal function. It is often difficult to deal with this painful reality when providing nursing care for these victims. When severe brain injury reduces the victim to a vegetative state, the issues become more difficult.

In critical care settings, as well as the courts of the land, the question of irreversible coma and brain death is subject to much controversy. *Cerebral death* is defined as total destruction of the brain resulting in the absence of any evidence of voluntary or reflex responsiveness. In contrast, *irreversible coma* implies a vegetative state, in which all functions attributed to the cerebrum are absent, although basic vital functions such as pulse, blood pressure, respirations, and temperature remain intact.[5] The distinction between the two terms provides a basis for recognizing differences between death and life.

Various definitions and criteria for death have been proposed. The British criteria, the Harvard criteria, the American Neurological Association criteria, and The President's Commission for the Study of Ethical Problems in Medicine and Biomedical and Behavioral Research have all looked carefully at the definition of death and the criteria. The Harvard criteria list was one of the earliest and best known but was found to be unnecessarily restrictive according to Dr. Earl Walker.[6] The President's Commission for the Study of Ethical Problems in Medicine and Biomedical Research has provided a definition of death either on the basis of absence of respirations and heart beat, or by the absence of all brain functions, if mechanical means are being employed to sustain respirations and cardiac function.[7]

Many state legislatures have dealt with the highly emotional and controversial definition of death. A definition of death, once statutory, guides the physician and the hospital in determining the very difficult medical, legal, and ethical concerns of patient management.

Currently, there is no uniform definition of death, but the basic criteria for diagnosing brain death usually include the following points:

- Apnea testing is done by a prescribed method
- Reflexes are absent, including oculocephalic and oculovestibular reflexes; oropharyngeal reflexes; and others (note: some spinal cord reflexes may persist even after death)

The irreversibility of the condition is often documented on the basis of the following criteria:

- The cause of the coma is established and accounts for the loss of brain function, according to current knowledge
- All appropriate diagnostic and therapeutic procedures have been carried out to no avail (there are no positive patient responses)
- The outlook for the patient is grave and reversal of the condition has been excluded
- The loss of all brain function persists for an extended period of time and is well documented by various accepted diagnostic procedures

The existence of a "complicating condition" may invalidate the usual methods of determining brain death. Declaration of brain death cannot be made without special consideration or possible alleviation of the following:[7]

- Drug and metabolic intoxication/overdose
- Hypothermia
- Immaturity, in children 2 years old or younger
- Shock

The specific criteria used will vary depending on the state and physician. As mentioned previously, there are no uniformly accepted criteria. The issue of determining brain death continues to be controversial and worrisome.

The decision to terminate life-support systems for a patient with apparent brain death is usually made after consultation with at least one other physician. The wishes of the family are also taken into account in making the decision. If any organs such as corneas or kidneys are to be donated to benefit others, a very specific donor protocol—outlined by the hospital—must be strictly followed.

The Decision Not to Resuscitate or Use Heroic Measures

Because of a terminal illness or poor prognosis, the patient, family, or physician may believe that it is not reasonable to use extraordinary means to sustain life, such as cardiopulmonary resuscitation, a respirator, or other procedures.

Establishing who has the right to make such a decision is a sensitive ethical–legal question that is unclear in most instances. If the patient is alert, oriented, and able to make rational decisions, he may choose to refuse certain treatments that would prolong his life. However, when the patient is unable to participate in rational decision-making, the situation becomes unclear. The Karen Ann Quinlan case so prominently covered in the news a few years ago raised more questions than answers about the family's right to request the discontinuance of life-support machines.

SUMMARY

Even a cursory review of the trends and issues cited in this chapter conveys some appreciation and respect for the numerous and complex concerns that have had an impact on neurological and neurosurgical nursing. There is a tremendous challenge for potential growth and development in neurological and neurosurgical nursing in the effort to meet society's special health care needs. As one of the few areas of nursing practice that is still in its early developmental stages, this nursing specialty offers the interested and committed nurse the challenge of participating in and contributing to new and dynamic aspects of patient care.

The development of neurological and neurosurgical nursing practice should reflect an understanding and synthesis of current practice, research data, trends, and issues that are applicable to current practice needs. The fundamental goal is to improve the quality of care offered to neurologically impaired clients so that they can live as fruitful and independent a life as possible.

REFERENCES

1. American Nurses' Association Division on Medical–Surgical Nursing Practice and the American Association of Neurosurgical Nurses: Standards of Neurological and Neurosurgical Nursing Practice. Kansas City, MO, American Nurses' Association, 1977
2. The Standards Committee: The AANN conceptual framework. J Neurosurg Nurs 16(2):117, April 1984
3. Yura H, Walsh M: The Nursing Process: Assessing, Planning, Implementing, and Evaluating, 3rd ed. New York, Appleton–Century–Crofts, 1978
4. U.S. Department of Health and Human Services: National Institute of Neurological and Communicative Disorders and Stroke Fact Book. Bethesda, MD, U.S. Department of Health and Human Services, 1982
5. An appraisal of the criteria of cerebral death: A summary statement. JAMA 237(10):982, March 1977
6. Walker AE: Guest editorial: Current concepts of brain death. J Neurosurg Nurs 15(5):261, October 1983
7. Guidelines for the determination of death. Report of the medical consultants on the diagnosis of death to the President's Commission for the Study of Ethical Problems in Medicine and Biomedical and Behavioral Research. Crit Care Med 10(1):62, January 1982

BIBLIOGRAPHY

Books

Ropper AH, Kennedy SK, Zervas NT: Neurological and Neurosurgical Intensive Care, pp 249–263. Baltimore, MD, University Park Press, 1983

Periodicals

Bernstein A: Death with dignity: Is judicial involvement necessary? Hospitals 9:93, May 1982

Black PM: Brain death. N Engl J Med 299:330–344, 393–401, August 1978

Brent NJ: Uniform determination of death act: Implications for nursing practices. J Neurosurg Nurs 15(5):265, October 1983

Daly K: The diagnosis of brain death: Overview of neurosurgical nursing responsibilities. J Neurosurg Nurs 14(2):85, April 1982

Gideon MD, Taylor PB: Kidney donation: Care of the cadaver donor's family. J Neurosurg Nurs 13(5):248, October 1981

Hassett MR: Computers and nursing education in the 1980's. Nurs Outlook 32(1):34, January/February 1984

Joel LA: DRGs and RIMs: Implications for nursing. Nurs Outlook 32(1):42, January/February 1984

Korcok M: Payment by diagnosis: U.S. government proposes new fee system. Can Med Assoc J 128:833, April 1, 1983

Korein J et al: Brain death: I. Angiographic correlation with the radioisotopic bolus technique for evaluation of critical deficit of cerebral blood flow. Ann Neurol 2(3):195, September 1977

Kottke FJ: Philosophic rehabilitation considerations of quality of life for the disabled. Arch Phys Med Rehabil 63:49, February 1982

Lipe HP, Doolittle N: The neuro nurse specialist—Present and future considerations. J Neurosurg Nurs 15(5):317, October 1983

Parisi JE et al: Brain death with prolonged somatic survival. N Engl J Med 306:14–16, January 1982

Parkinson J: Brain death: Medical and legal opinions. J Neurosurg Nurs 15(5):268, October 1983

Pearson J et al: Brain death: II. Neuropathological correlation with the radioisotopic bolus technique for evaluation of critical deficit of cerebral blood flow. Ann Neurol 1(3):206, September 1977

Ropper AH, Kennedy SK, Russell L: Apnea testing in the diagnosis of brain death. J Neurosurg 55:942, December 1982

Rudy E: Brain death. Dimens Crit Care 1:178, May–June 1982

Searle J, Collins CA: Brain death protocol. Lancet 1:641, March 1980

Sterling–Rollheiser EE: How neurosurgical nurses cope with the "no code" patient. J Neurosurg Nurs 15(5):274, October 1983

Walleck CA: Ethical dimensions of nursing practice. J Neurosurg Nurs 15(6):366, December 1983

chapter 2

Review of Neuroanatomy and Neurophysiology

The purpose of this chapter is to provide a review of essential neuroanatomy and neurophysiology to assist the reader in understanding the underlying principles of neurological function and dysfunction and related nursing management.

EMBRYONIC DEVELOPMENT OF THE NERVOUS SYSTEM

The embryonic development of the nervous system begins in the ectodermal layer of the embryo and proceeds systematically. From a simple invagination on the dorsal portion of the ectodermal layer, a neural groove and neural tube form. At one end of the neural tube, called the cranial portion, rapid and unequal growth occurs, giving rise to the rudimentary structures of the brain in the form of three major vesicles. These vesicles, in turn, become five areas: the telencephalon, the diencephalon, the mesencephalon, the metencephalon, and the myelencephalon (Fig. 2–1, Table 2–1).

At the same time, the cells of the neural tube form two types of cells: the spongioblasts, which give rise to the neuroglia (glia) cells, and the neuroblasts, which give rise to the nerve cells (neurons). Processes from the neuroblasts form the white matter of the brain. Some of these processes leave the brain and spinal cord to form the fibers of the cranial and ventral roots of the spinal nerves.

Throughout the prenatal period, there is further growth and refinement of the nervous system. It is said that all of the neurons that a person will ever have are present at birth. The highly specialized cells of the nervous system are not replaced. Maturation of the nervous system continues throughout childhood up to the age of 12 years.

CELLS OF THE NERVOUS SYSTEM

The nervous system is composed of two types of cells: neurons and neuroglia. The neurons are considered the vital part of the conduction system of the nervous system, while the neuroglia are viewed primarily as supportive.

NEUROGLIA CELLS

The term "glia" comes from a Greek word meaning "glue" or "holding together." In this regard, the glia cells provide structural support, nourishment, and protection for the neurons of the nervous system. There are five to ten times more neuroglia cells than there are neurons. About 40% of the brain and spinal cord is composed of neuroglia cells. Because neuroglia cells lack strong intracellular substances such as collagen or elastin, fresh tissue from the brain or spinal cord appears soft and jellylike.

From a clinical viewpoint, neuroglia cells are important because they can divide mitotically and are the most common source of primary tumors in the nervous system.

There are several types of neuroglia cells in the nervous system. Four such cells commonly found are oligodendroglia, astroglia, ependyma, and microglia.

Oligodendroglia

Oligodendroglia cells have few branching processes and are evident chiefly as satellites to the neurons or as rows of cells lying along bundles of fibers in the white matter. The oligodendroglia produce the myelin sheaths of the axonal projections of the neurons in the central nervous system. An individual oligodendroglial cell can maintain the myelin sheaths of several axons.

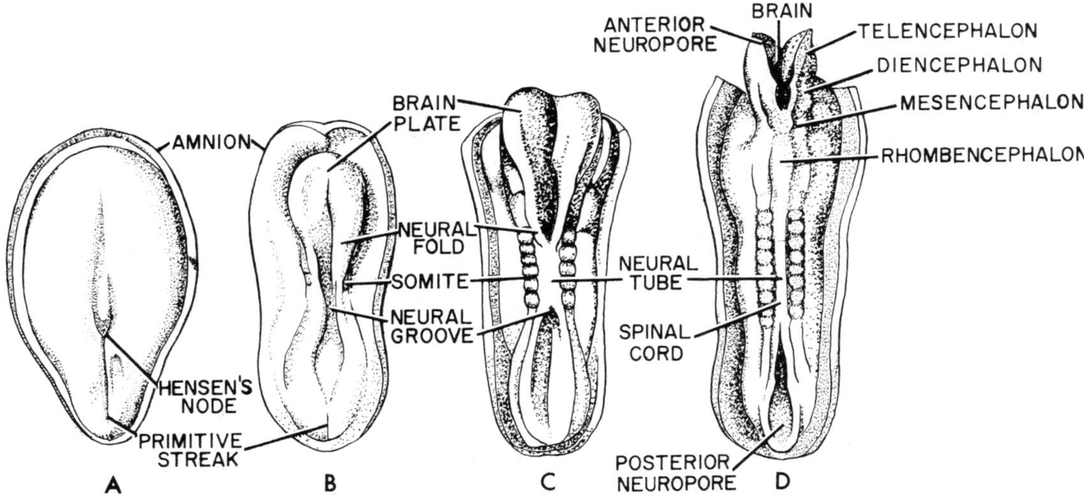

FIG. 2–1. Dorsal view of human embryo. *(A)* Primitive streak stage (16-day, presomite embryo). *(B)* Neural plate stage (20-day, two-somite embryo). *(C)* Beginning of neural tube (22-day, seven-somite embryo). *(D)* Brain vesicle stage (23-day, ten-somite embryo). (Curtis B et al: An Introduction to the Neurosciences. Philadelphia, WB Saunders, 1972)

Astroglia

Astroglia (or astrocyte) is a term derived from the numerous processes extending from the cell body that gives the astroglia a starlike appearance. Functions attributed to the astroglia include (1) providing nutritional needs for neurons, (2) participating as a link between the capillaries and neurons, and (3) providing a protective barrier for neurons.

Ependyma

Ependymal cells line the ventricular system and the choroid plexuses. Ependymal cells aid in the production of cerebrospinal fluid and provide a barrier to prevent foreign substances within the ventricles from entering cerebral tissue.

Microglia

Microglial cells are scattered throughout the central nervous system and have a phagocytic property. When a part of the nervous system is injured, the microglial cells remove and disintegrate the waste products of neurons.

NEURONS

The basic functional and anatomical unit in the nervous system is the neuron, whose special characteristics include conduction of nerve impulses and irritability.

There are three major components of a neuron: a *cell body*, which constitutes the main part of the neuron; a *single axon*, or *axis cylinder*, which consists of a long projection extending from the cell body; and *several dendrites*,

TABLE 2–1. *Development of the Primary Vesicles*

Primary Vesicles	Subdivisions	Structures (that arise)	Ventricular System
Prosencephalon (forebrain)	Telencephalon	Cerebral cortex, corpus callosum, basal ganglia, and rhinencephalon	Lateral ventricle and part of third ventricle
	Diencephalon	Thalamus and hypothalamus	Most of third ventricle
Mesencephalon (midbrain)	Mesencephalon	Midbrain	Cerebral aqueduct (aqueduct of Sylvius)
Rhombencephalon (hindbrain)	Metencephalon	Pons and cerebellum	Fourth ventricle
	Myelencephalon	Medulla oblongata	Fourth ventricle and part of the central canal
Primitive neural tube	Neural tube	Spinal cord	Most of central canal
	Neural crest	Peripheral nerves and ganglia	

which are thin projections extending from the cell body into the immediate surrounding area (Fig. 2–2). The axon carries impulses *away* from the cell body, while the dendrites direct impulses *toward* the cell body.

Neurons are classified as unipolar, bipolar, or multipolar. *Unipolar* neurons possess only one process or pole. This process divides close to the cell body. One branch is called the peripheral process and carries impulses from the periphery toward the cell body. The other branch, called the central process, conducts the impulse toward the spinal cord or the brain stem.

Bipolar neurons are found only in the spinal and vestibular ganglia, the olfactory mucous membrane, and in one layer of the retina. The anatomical structure is peculiar to the organ in which it is found.

Most neurons in the nervous system are *multipolar* cells. These neurons consist of a cell body, one long projection (the axon), and one or more shorter branches (the dendrites).

Components of the Cell Body

The main components of the cell body include the cell membrane, the nucleus, deoxyribonucleic acid (DNA), ribonucleic acid (RNA), endoplasmic reticulum, Nissl bodies, mitochondria, and Golgi apparatus (Fig. 2–3).

The *cell membrane* creates the parameters of the cell body, enclosing the cytoplasm within its border. The main purpose of the cell membrane is to control the interchange of the material between the cell and its environment. The *nucleus* of the cell body is a double-membrane structure that contains DNA. A prominent nucleolus is located within the nucleus and is composed of RNA. *DNA* constitutes the genes that control the overall function of the cell as well as transmission of hereditary data from cell to cell. *RNA*, which permits the synthesis of structural protein and specific catalytic protein regulating cell life, is the "messenger" from the genes of the nucleus.

The *endoplasmic reticulum* of the cytoplasm is a net-

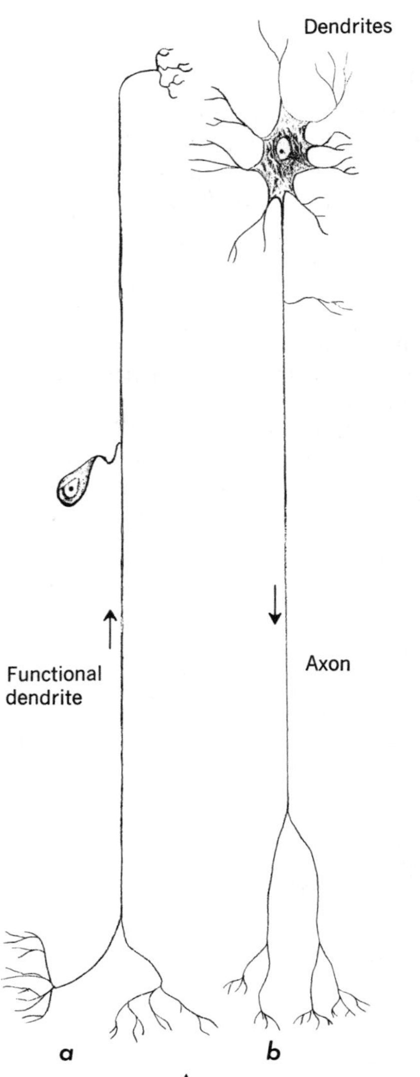

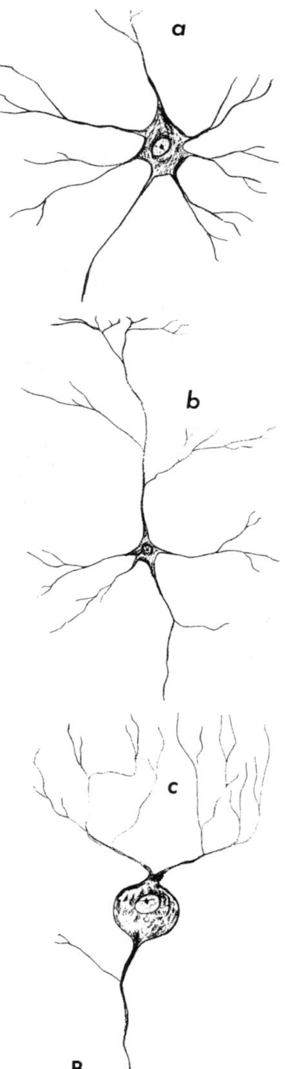

FIG. 2–2. Types of neurons. *(A)* Unipolar neuron *(a)*, multipolar neuron *(b)*. *(B)* Multipolar neurons from spinal cord *(a)*, from cerebral cortex *(b)*, and from cerebellar cortex *(c)*. (Chaffee EE, Lytle IM: Basic Physiology and Anatomy. Philadelphia, JB Lippincott, 1980)

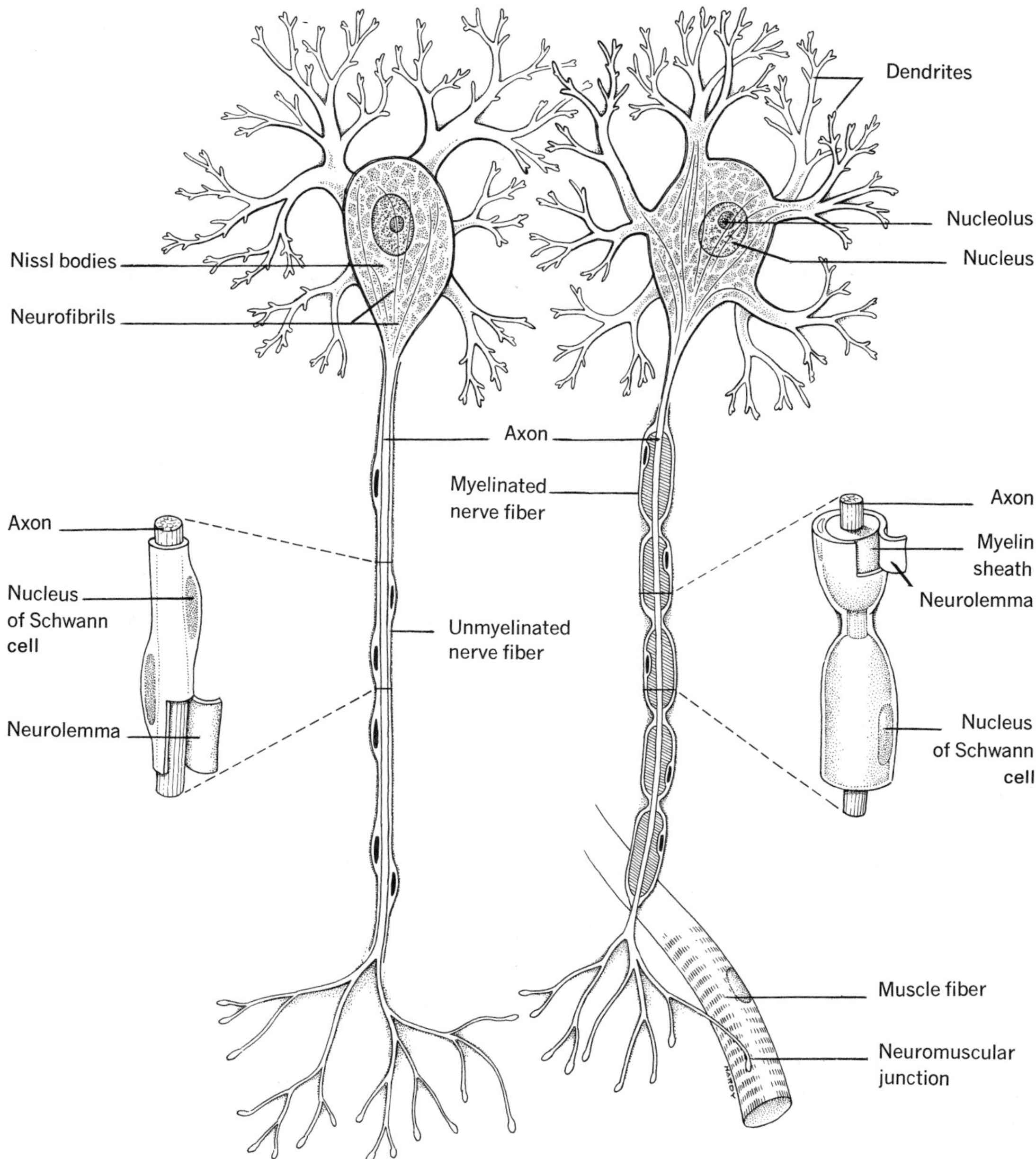

FIG. 2-3. Typical efferent neurons: unmyelinated fiber *(left)*, myelinated fiber *(right)*. (Chaffee EE, Lytle IM: Basic Physiology and Anatomy. Philadelphia, JB Lippincott, 1980)

work of tubular structures consisting of a system of unit membranes. This system connects with the double-membrane nucleus and that portion of the reticulum called the Golgi apparatus. Substances formed in different parts of the cell are transported throughout the cell by means of this system. The *Golgi apparatus* is believed to condense and temporarily store secretory substances and to synthesize carbohydrates and combine them with protein. It is also responsible for the formation of substances important for the digestion of intracellular material.

The *Nissl bodies* are masses of granular endoplasmic reticulum with ribosomes, which are the protein-synthesizing machinery of the neuron. The *mitochondria* are structures that regulate the cell's respiratory metabolism, whereby nutrients of the cell are oxidized to produce carbon dioxide and water. The energy released is used to produce adenosine triphosphate (ATP).

Structures of the Cell Processes

Axons and dendrites constitute the cell processes. Dendrites usually extend only a short distance from the cell body and branch profusely. In contrast, an axon can extend for long distances from the cell body before branching near the end of the projection.

Many axons in the peripheral nervous system are covered by a myelin sheath composed of a white, lipid substance that acts as an insulator for the conduction of impulses. Nerve fibers enclosed in such a sheath are referred to as *myelinated;* those without the myelin sheath are referred to as *unmyelinated* (see Fig. 2–3). As a rule, larger neuron fibers are myelinated, while smaller fibers are unmyelinated.

The myelin sheath is formed by *Schwann cells* that encircle the axons. When several Schwann cells are wrapped around an axon, their outer layer (sheath of Schwann) encloses the myelin sheath. This outer layer is called the *neurolemma* and is said to be necessary for the regeneration of axons. The myelin sheath itself is a segmented, discontinuous layer that is interrupted at intervals by the *nodes of Ranvier.* The distance from one node to the next is called an *internode.* Each internode is formed by, and surrounded by, one Schwann cell. At the junction between each of the two successive Schwann cells along the axon, a small uninsulated area remains where ions can easily flow between the extracellular fluid and the axon. It is this area that is known as the node of Ranvier. In the central nervous system, the oligondendroglial cells provide the myelination of the neurons in a way similar to that of the Schwann cells in the peripheral nervous system.

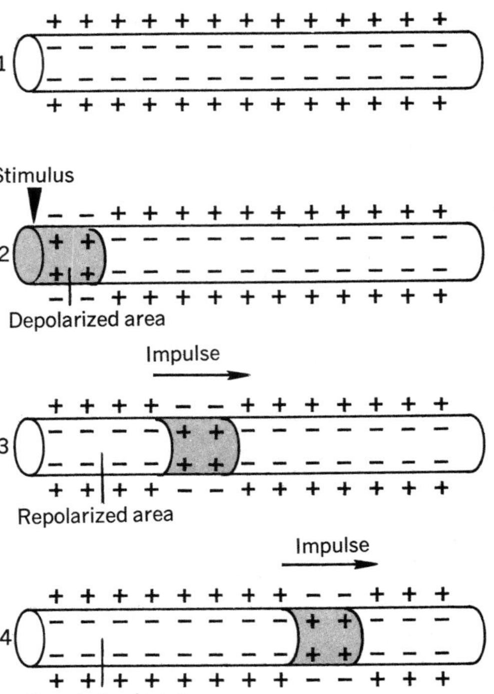

FIG. 2–4. Diagram of membrane potentials. *(1) Resting membrane potential*—outer surface bears a positive charge and inner surface bears a negative charge. *(2) Action potential, first stage*—stimulation of fiber results in depolarization; that is, outer surface becomes negative and inner surface becomes positive. *(3) Action potential, second stage*—repolarization occurs as the resting potential is restored. *(4)* Propagation of impulse continues in direction of arrow. (Chaffee EE, Lytle IM: Basic Physiology and Anatomy. Philadelphia, JB Lippincott, 1980)

Physiology of Nerve Impulses

Resting Membrane Potential of the Neurons. Although a resting neuron is not conducting an impulse, it is considered to be a charged cell. The difference in electrical charge on either side of the membrane is called the *potential difference* and is related to the unequal distribution of potassium and sodium on either side of the membrane. The normal resting potential of −60 to −70 millivolts (depending upon the type of neuron) is maintained by the various concentrations of ions in the fluid on either side of the cell membrane.

The cell membrane is both semipermeable and selectively permeable. The area outside the cell is called the interstitial space; the area inside the cell is called the intracellular space. Sodium ions (Na^+) and chloride ions (Cl^+) are found in much greater concentrations in the interstitial space than in the cell. The sodium ion gradient is caused by the powerful sodium pump that continually pumps sodium out of the cell. The potassium ion (K^+) and organic protein material are found in high concentrations within the cell. Potassium is also pumped back into the cell by the potassium pump, but it is not considered particularly important. This is true because the selective permeability of the cell membrane allows the ion to pass through the pores of the membrane easily.

The Action Potential of the Neuron. The fluid and ions in the intracellular space create a highly conductive solution. The large diameter (10–80 microns [μ]) allows for unrestricted conduction of impulses from one part of the interior of the cell to the other. A variety of stimuli can change the permeability of the cell membrane to certain ions, resulting in alterations in the membrane potential (Fig. 2–4). The stimuli must be of sufficient magnitude to conduct an impulse and thus create an *action potential.* Many simultaneous discharges at the synaptic junction must occur to create a sufficient effect on the cell membrane. The membrane potential must be lowered by 10 to 15 millivolts for an action potential to be created. This means that the membrane potential is changed to approximately −30 to −50 millivolts. When the action potential is realized, there is a sudden reversal of the sodium and potassium relationship across the cell membrane of the axon. This event is called *depolarization.* The neuron receives an influx of sodium and loses potassium to the interstitial space; the time required is only a few milliseconds. With the change in polarity, an impulse is conducted from one neuron to the next, at the same amplitude and speed. The cell repolarizes and returns to its resting membrane potential. This sequence of events occurs during the conduction of an impulse in an unmyelinated nerve.

Saltatory Conduction in Myelinated Fibers. In myelinated nerves, the action potential hops from one node of Ranvier to the next as a means of rapidly conducting an impulse. This is called *saltatory conduction.* Although ions cannot flow out through the myelin sheath of myelinated nerves, the break in the myelin sheath at the nodes of Ranvier provides a perfect route of escape. At this point the membrane is several times more permeable than many unmyelinated nerves. Impulses are conducted from node to node rather than continuing along the entire span of the axon, as is the case in unmyelinated nerves. Saltatory conduction is advantageous because it increases the velocity of an impulse and conserves energy (because only the nodes depolarize). The rate of velocity of an impulse depends on both the thickness of the myelin and the distance between the internodes. As these two factors increase, the velocity of the impulse also increases.

The Synapse. The junction between one neuron and the next where an impulse is transmitted is called the *synapse*. There are three anatomical structures that are necessary for an impulse to be transmitted at a synapse. These include the presynaptic terminals, the synaptic cleft, and the postsynaptic membrane (Fig. 2–5). The *presynaptic terminals* are either excitatory or inhibitory. An excitatory presynaptic terminal secretes an excitatory substance into the synaptic cleft, thereby exciting the effector neuron. The inhibitory presynaptic terminal secretes an inhibitory transmitter, which, when secreted into the synaptic cleft, inhibits the effector neuron. The excitatory or inhibitory transmitter secretions arise from the *synaptic vesicle* in the presynaptic terminal of the axon. Mitochondria in the axon supply the ATP to synthesize new transmitter secretions. The *synaptic cleft* is the microscopic space (200–300 angstroms [Å]) between the presynaptic terminal and the receptor area of the effector cell. The *postsynaptic membrane* is that part of the effector membrane that is proximal to the presynaptic terminal. When an action potential spreads over the presynaptic terminal, the membrane depolarizes, emptying some of the contents of the presynaptic vesicles into the synaptic cleft. The released transmitter changes the permeability of the subsynaptic membrane. This results in either excitation or inhibition of the neuron, depending on the type of transmitter substances spilled into the synaptic cleft.

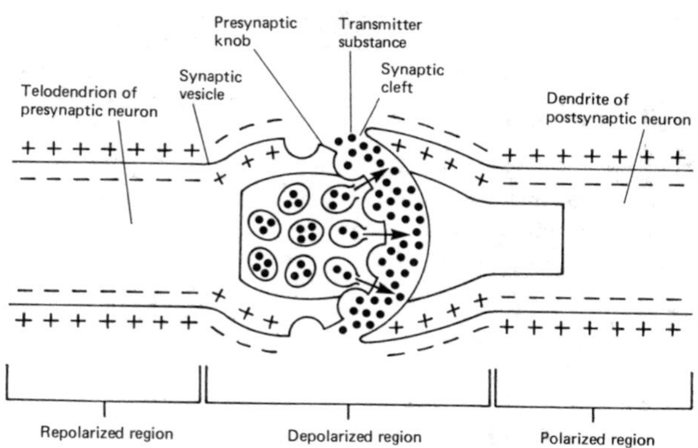

FIG. 2–5. Impulse conduction from a presynaptic knob to a postsynaptic dendrite across a synapse. (Tortora GJ, Anagnostakos NP: Principles of Anatomy and Physiology, 2nd ed. New York, Harper & Row, 1978)

The Neurotransmitters. Neurotransmitters are chemical substances that transfer an electrical impulse from a nerve cell to its target cell. The target cell may be another nerve cell, muscle cell, or gland cell. The neurochemical transmission occurs in the synapse and is unidirectional. Each neuron can secrete only one type of transmitter substance at its terminals. The neurotransmitter acts by changing the membrane permeability so that calcium enters into the nerve terminal, causing the storage apparatus of the neurotransmitter (vesicles) to fuse with the membrane and release the neurotransmitter into the synapse.

Investigation of neurotransmitters has focused on the following substances: acetylcholine, norepinephrine, dopamine, serotonin, and gamma-aminobutyric acid. Table 2–2 summarizes these neurotransmitters. However, it is believed that more neurotransmitters exist, whose importance may become apparent in the future.

The Postsynaptic Membrane—Excitation and Inhibition. The postsynaptic membrane (the dendrite cell body region of the effector neuron) initiates its response to stimuli by decremental conduction through the synapse; that is, the impulse becomes progressively weaker the more prolonged the period of excitation. Stimulation of the effector cell at the dendrite cell body can create an action potential. For the action potential to be fired, however, the intensity of an impulse must be sufficient to fire the intial segment of axon (just distal to the axon hillock), where the action potential is initiated. It is said that any factor that increases the potential inside the cell body at any given point also increases the potential throughout the cell body. Because of differences in the cell membrane and shape of the cell, the intracellular voltage necessary to elicit an action potential will vary at different points on the cell membrane. The most sensitive point is the initial segment of the axon, but the impulse must be of sufficient magnitude to depolarize the axon. *Excitation* is the response of the subsynaptic membrane to the neurotransmitter substance that lowers the membrane potential to form an *excitatory postsynaptic potential (EPSP)* (Fig. 2–6, *top*). The potential is a small depolarization that conducts itself by decrement. The cell membrane is made more permeable to sodium, potassium, and chloride. Sodium ions rush into the neuron, while potassium ions leave the cell through the postsynaptic membrane.

Inhibition acts upon a cell so that it is more difficult for it to fire. The inhibitory neurotransmitters increase permeability to only potassium and chloride ions at the synaptic membrane. The membrane potential is raised to form the *inhibitory postsynaptic potential (IPSP)* (Fig. 2–6, *bottom*).

Presynaptic Inhibition. Another type of inhibition, *presynaptic inhibition*, results from inhibitory knobs being activated on the presynaptic terminal fibrils and synaptic knobs of an axon. When the inhibitory knobs are activated, they secrete a neurotransmitter substance that partially depolarizes the terminal fibrils and excitatory synaptic knobs. As a result, the velocity of the action potential that occurs at the membrane of the excitatory knob is depressed. This action greatly reduces the quantity of excita-

TABLE 2-2. *Summary of the Major Neurotransmitters*

Neurotransmitter	*Synthesis and Degradation*	*Site of Secretion*
Acetylcholine (ACh)		
• First transmitter identified • Chief neurotransmitter of the parasympathetic nervous system • Called cholinergic synapse	• Choline + acetyl-CoA $\xrightarrow{\text{choline acetyltransferase}}$ ACh • ACH $\xrightarrow{\text{acetylcholinesterase (AChE)}}$ acetate + choline	• Autonomic nervous system (ANS) —All preganglionic nerve endings —Parasympathetic postganglionic nerve endings —Sympathetic postganglionic nerve endings of sweat glands • Neuromuscular junctions (voluntary skeletal muscles) • Adrenal medulla
Norepinephrine (NE)		
• Also called noradrenalin • Chief neurotransmitter of the sympathetic nervous system • Causes systemic changes associated with the "fight or flight" response (elevated blood pressure, tachycardia, peripheral vasoconstriction, vasodilation if blood vessels of skeletal muscles) • Adrenergic synapse	• Tyrosine $\xrightarrow{\text{tyrosine hydroxylase}}$ L-dopa $\xrightarrow[\text{(in presence of vitamin } B_6)]{\text{dopa decarboxylase}}$ dopamine $\xrightarrow{\text{dopamine hydroxylase}}$ norepinephrine (NE) • NE $\xrightarrow[\text{catechol-O-methyltransferase (COMT)}]{\text{monamine oxidase (MOA) +}}$ metanephrine/normetanephrine or VMA	• Systemic effect caused by release into bloodstream by adrenal medulla • Sympathetic postganglionic nerve endings (except at sweat glands)
Dopamine (DA)		
• Affects control of fine movement, sensory input integration, and emotional behavior	• Tyrosine $\xrightarrow{\text{tyrosine hydroxylase}}$ L-dopa $\xrightarrow[\text{with pyridoxine}]{\text{decarboxylase}}$ dopamine • Dopamine $\xrightarrow{\text{MAO or COMT}}$ homovanillic acid	• Extrapyramidal system of the basal ganglia • Median eminence and other parts of the hypothalamus • Sympathetic ganglia • Limbic system • Portions of the retina
Serotonin (5-Hydroxytryptamine)		
• Controls heat regulation, sleep, hunger, and behavior and has some effect on consciousness	• Tryptophan $\xrightarrow{\text{trytophan hydroxylase}}$ $\xrightarrow[\text{(in the presence of pyridoxine)}]{\text{5-hydroxytryptophan decarboxylase}}$ serotonin • Serotonin $\xrightarrow{\text{MAO}}$ 5-hydroxyindoleacetic acid	• Hypothalamus, limbic system, cerebellum, and spinal cord
Gamma-aminobutyric acid (GABA)		
• Has an inhibitory effect on the brain, spinal cord, and retina • Present in large amounts in the gray matter of the brain • Regulates portions of available energy	• Glutamic acid* $\xrightarrow{\text{decarboxylase}}$ GABA • GABA $\xrightarrow{\text{GABA aminotransferase}}$ succinic semialdehyde $\xrightarrow{\text{dehydrogenase}}$ succinic acid	• Cerebellum, cerebral cortex, neurons mediating presynaptic inhibitors, retina

* Glutamic acid and its amide, glutamine, are present in the brain in large amounts and comprise almost half of the nonprotein nitrogen.

tory neurotransmitter released by the knob and suppresses the degree of excitation of the neuron.

FUNCTIONS AND DIVISIONS OF THE NERVOUS SYSTEM

In general, the nervous system controls the motor, sensory, and autonomic functions of the body. These general functions can be subdivided into the following areas:

1. Generation of sensory input to be processed (afferent impulse)
2. Generation of efferent impulses that control body action by various voluntary and involuntary motor functions
3. Processing of incoming data
4. Storage of information

The nervous system is divided into a hierarchy with three major functional units: the lowest level of function—the spinal cord level (automatic motor responses as reflexes); the second level of function—the lower brain level (controls for blood pressure, respirations, equilibrium, and primitive emotions); and the highest level of function—the higher brain, or cortical, level (storage of information,

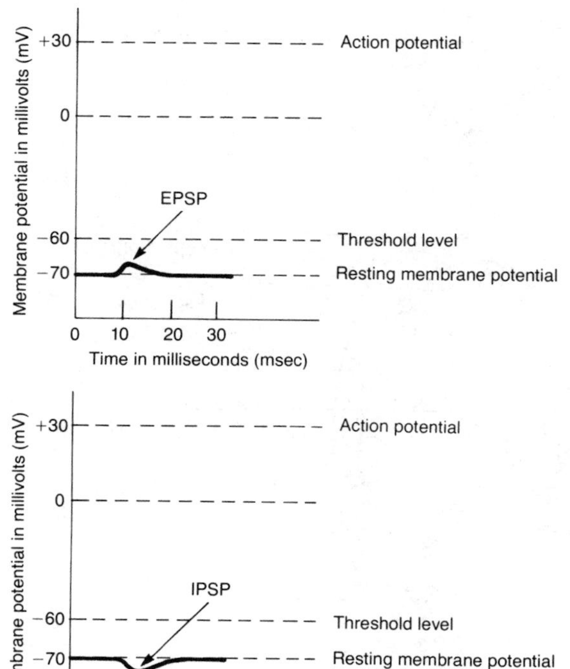

FIG. 2-6. Comparison between excitatory and inhibitory postsynaptic potentials. *(Top)* EPSP. *(Bottom)* IPSP. (Tortora GJ, Anagnostakos NP: Principles of Anatomy and Physiology, 2nd ed. Hagerstown, MD, Harper & Row, 1978)

thinking, abstraction, and patterns of some motor responses).

Divisions of the Nervous System. The nervous system is divided into the central nervous system and the peripheral nervous system. The central nervous system is composed of the brain and spinal cord. The peripheral nervous system includes the following: (1) the 12 pairs of cranial nerves, (2) the 31 pairs of spinal nerves, and (3) the autonomic nervous system, which subdivides into the sympathetic and parasympathetic nervous system.

CRANIAL AND SPINAL BONES

The purpose of the skull and vertebral column is to protect the most vulnerable parts of the nervous system—the brain and spinal cord.

THE SKULL

The *skull* is the bony framework of the head; it is composed of the eight bones of the cranium and the fourteen bones of the face. Knowledge of the anatomy of both the external and internal surfaces of the bones (Figs. 2-7, 2-8) is helpful in understanding the pathophysiology of craniocerebral trauma.

FIG. 2-7. Lateral view of the skull.

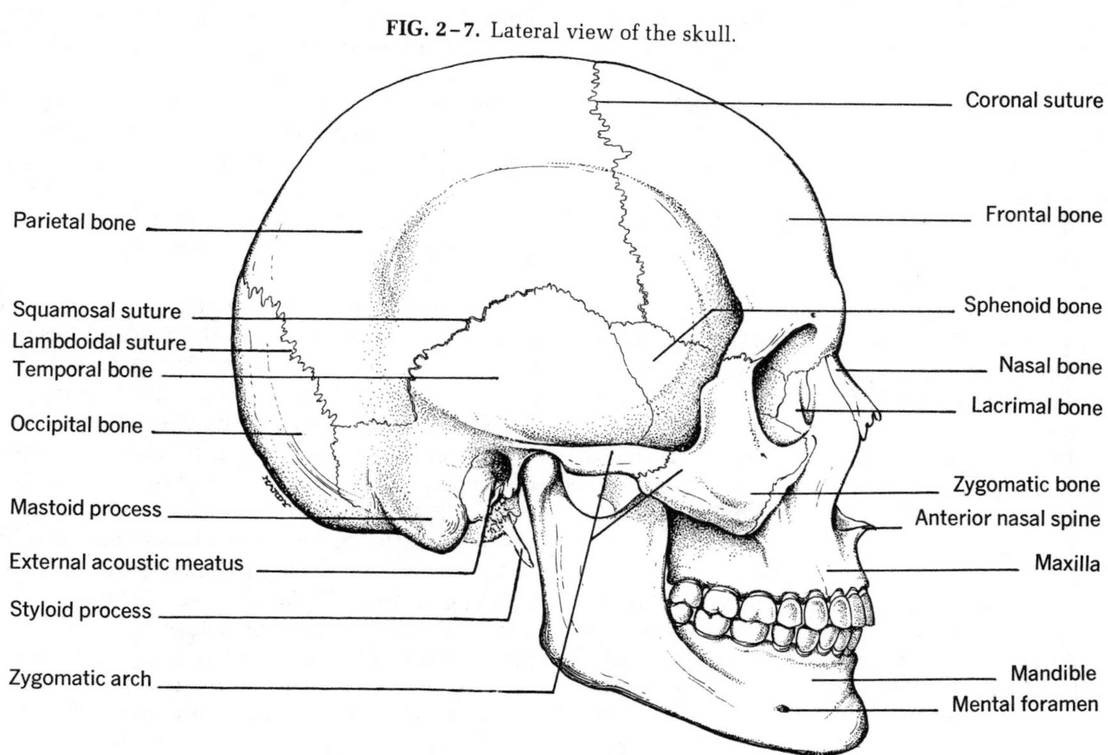

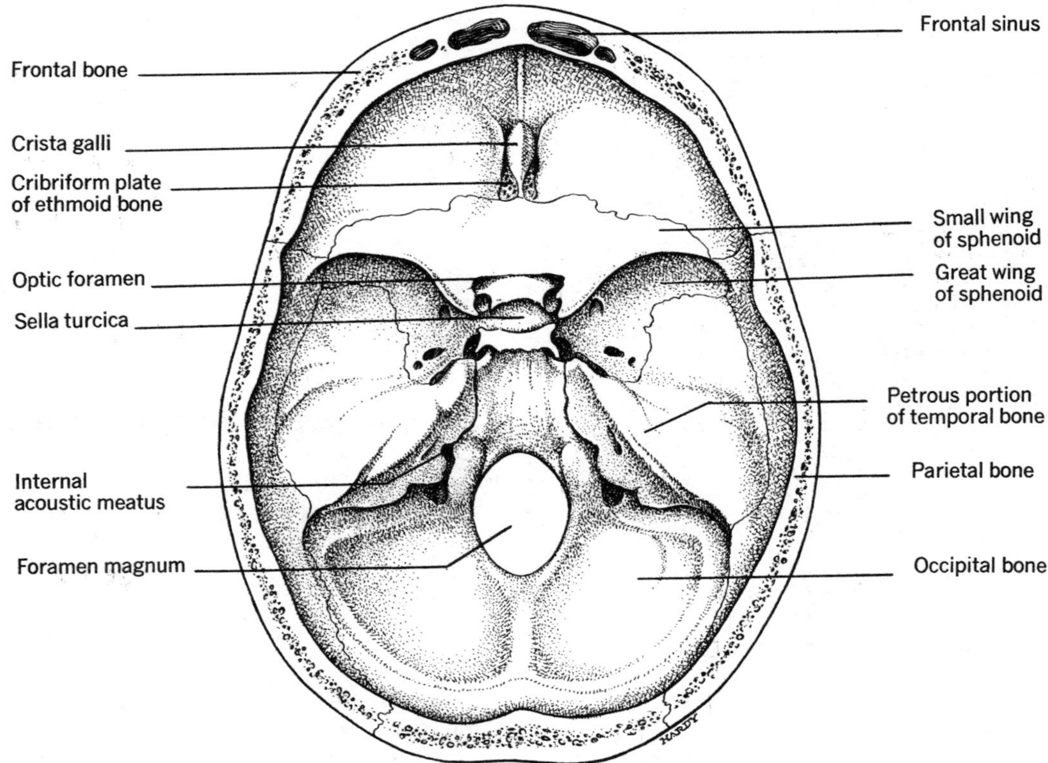

FIG. 2-8. View of base of skull from above showing the internal surfaces of some of the cranial bones.

The *cranium* is defined as that part of the skull that encloses the brain and provides a protective vault for this vital organ. The bones that compose the cranium are the frontal, occipital, sphenoid, and ethmoid, as well as the two parietal and temporal bones.

The *frontal bone* forms the forehead and the front (anterior) part of the top of the skull. The supraorbital arches form the roofs of the two orbits. Frontal sinuses are also located in this bone.

The *occipital bone* is the large bone at the back (posterior) of the skull that curves into the base of the skull. The significant markings include (1) the large hole (foramen magnum) in the base of the skull and (2) the occipital condyles located on either side of the foramen magnum that fit into depressions on the first cervical vertebra.

The *sphenoid bone* is a wedge-shaped bone alleged to resemble a bat's wings. The significant bone markings include a body, lesser wings, greater wings, pterygoid process and the sella turcica (also known as "the Turk's saddle"). The hypophysis (pituitary gland) is located in the region of the sella turcica.

The *ethmoid bone,* largely hidden between the two orbits, contains both a perpendicular and horizontal plate, as well as two lateral masses. The horizontal plate, also called the cribriform plate, forms part of the base of the skull through which the olfactory nerves (first cranial nerves) travel. The perpendicular plate forms part of the nasal septum, while the lateral masses are part of the ethmoid sinuses.

The *temporal bones* are situated at the sides and base of the skull and consist of three anatomical divisions: the squamous, mastoid, and petrous portions. The temporal bone is highly irregular both on the internal and external surfaces.

The *squamous* portion is very thin just above the auditory meatus. It contains the zygomatic process externally; internally, there are numerous eminences and depressions to accommodate the contour of the cerebrum. Two well-marked internal grooves are evident for the branches of the middle meningeal artery, a common point of trauma with head injury.

The *mastoid* portion is perforated by many foramina, including a larger foramen, the mastoid foramen, which contains a vein that innervates the lateral sinus, and a small artery to supply the dura mater. The mastoid process is also contained in this portion of the temporal bone.

The *petrous* portion is so named because it is extremely dense and stonelike in its hardness. There is a pyramidal process that is directed inward and wedged at the base of the skull between the sphenoid and occipital bones. The petrous portion of the temporal bone contains the essential branches of the middle meningeal artery.

The *parietal bones,* which fuse on the top of the skull, form the sides of the skull. Externally, they are smooth and convex; internally, the surface is concave with some depressions to accommodate the convolutions of the cerebrum and the grooves for the middle meningeal artery. With these exceptions, the bone has a regular surface.

Sutures of the Skull

The bones of the skull join at various places, known as suture lines. The four major sutures of the skull are the following (see Fig. 2–7):

1. The *sagittal suture*—the midline suture formed by the two parietal bones joining on the top of the skull
2. The *coronal suture* (frontoparietal)—connecting the frontal and parietal bones transversely
3. The *lambdoidal suture* (occipitoparietal)—connecting the occipital and parietal bones
4. The *basilar suture*—created by the junction of the basilar surface of the occipital bone with the posterior surface of the sphenoid bone

THE SPINE

The spine is a flexible column formed by a series of bones called *vertebrae*, each stacked one upon another to support the head and trunk. The vertebral column is made up of 33 vertebrae: 7 cervical vertebrae, 12 thoracic or dorsal vertebrae, 5 lumbar vertebrae, 5 sacral vertebrae (fused into one), and 4 coccygeal vertebrae (fused into one) (Fig. 2–9). Each vertebra consists of two essential parts, an anterior solid segment or *body*, and a posterior segment or *arch*. Two *pedicles* and two *laminae* supporting seven processes (four articular, two transverse, and one spinous) make up the arch (Fig. 2–10).

The cervical vertebrae are smaller than those in any other region of the spine. The first cervical vertebra is called the *atlas*; the second cervical vertebra, the *axis*. Each of these two vertebrae is unique in appearance. The axis has a perpendicular projection called the *odontoid process* upon which the atlas sits (Fig. 2–11).

The thoracic or dorsal vertebrae are intermediate in size, becoming larger as they descend the vertebral column. The lumbar vertebrae are the largest segments in the spine (see Fig. 2–10).

The vertebral bodies are the largest part of the vertebrae, above and below which flattened surfaces are found for attachment of fibrocartilages. There are apertures for spinal nerves, veins, and arteries. The vertebrae are connected by means of the articular processes and the intervertebral fibrocartilages.

The arch of the vertebrae is composed of two pedicles, two laminae, a spinous process, four articular processes, and two transverse processes. The two *pedicles* are short, thick pieces of bone. The concavity above and below the pedicles creates the intervertebral notches from which the spinal nerves emanate. The two *laminae* are broad plates of bone. They complete the neural arch by fusing in the midline and enclose the spinal foramen, which protects the spinal cord. The upper and lower borders are rough in order to allow for the attachment of the ligamenta subflava. The *spinous process* projects backward from the laminae and serves as the attachment for muscles and ligaments. The four *articular processes* (two on either side) provide stability for the spine. The two *transverse processes* provide stability for the spine and serve as points of attachment for muscles and ligaments.

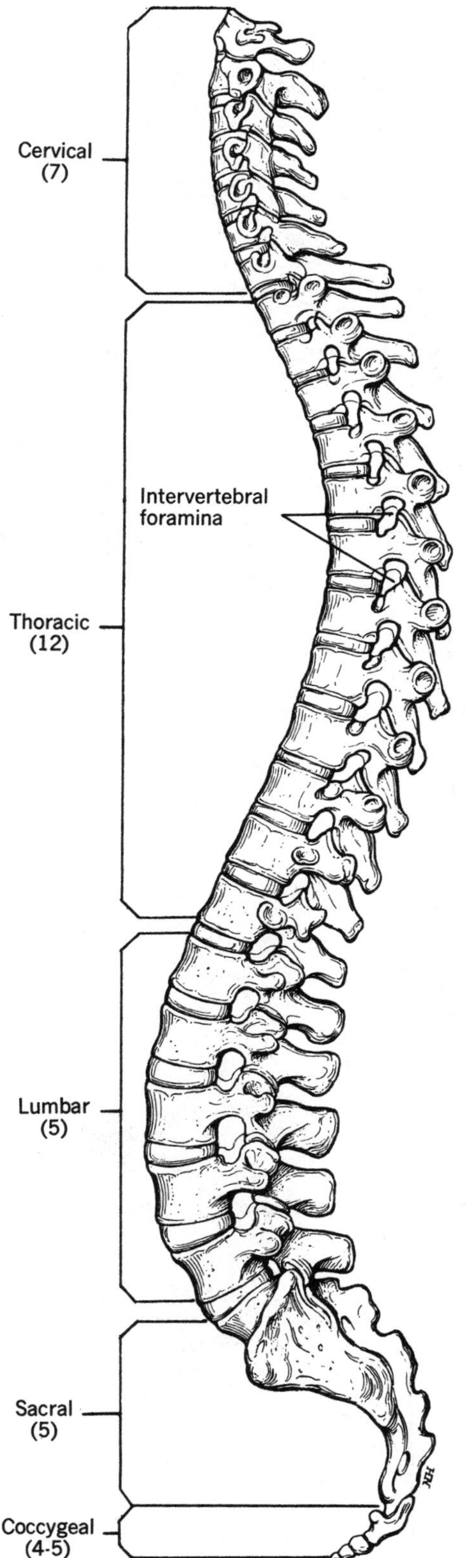

FIG. 2–9. Lateral view of adult vertebral column showing curves.

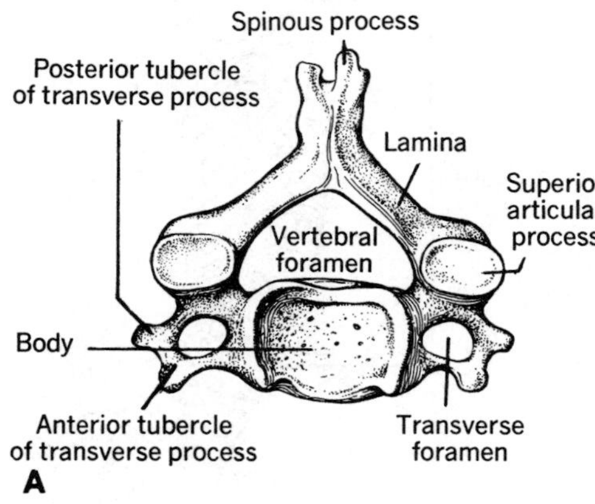

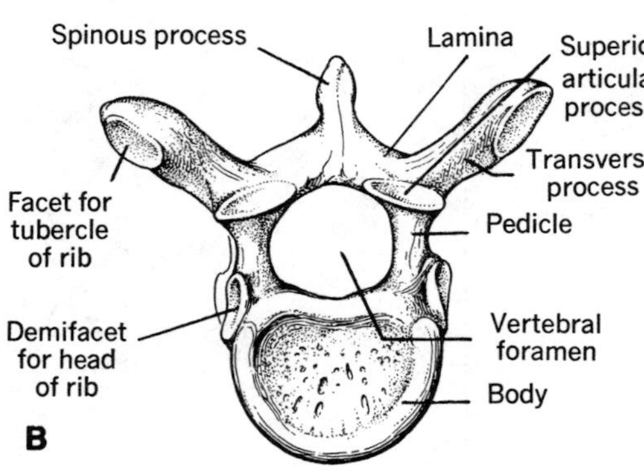

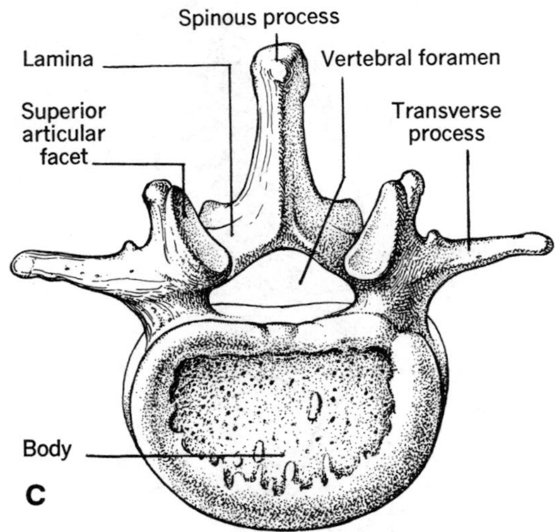

FIG. 2-10. Views of three types of vertebrae. *(A)* Fourth cervical vertebra, superior aspect. *(B)* Sixth thoracic vertebra, superior aspect. *(C)* Third lumbar vertebra, superior aspect.

Ligaments of the Spine

The most important ligaments of the vertebral column are the anterior and posterior longitudinal ligaments and the ligamenta flava. The *anterior longitudinal ligament* consists of longitudinal fibers firmly attached to the anterior surface of the vertebral bodies and intervertebral discs.

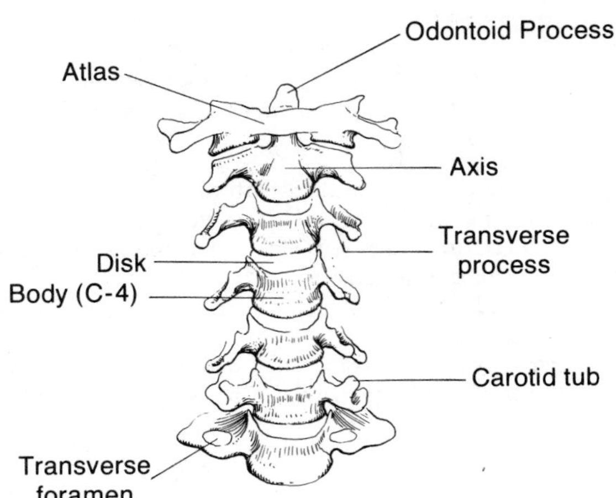

FIG. 2-11. The cervical spine. (Hoppenfeld S: Orthopaedic Neurology. Philadelphia, JB Lippincott, 1977)

The *posterior longitudinal ligament* is attached to the posterior surface of the vertebral bodies within the spinal canal. The *ligamenta flava* consists of yellow elastic fibers that connect the laminae of adjacent vertebrae. The attachment pattern is unique in that the attachment is from the lower margin of the anterior surface of the superior lamina to the posterior surface of the upper margin of the inferior margin. Such an arrangement controls vertebral movement to prevent excessive flexion. If violent force in any direction occurs, these ligaments can be ruptured, possibly causing injury to the vertebrae and spinal cord.

Intervertebral Discs

The intervertebral discs are fibrocartilaginous discs located between the vertebral bodies from the second cervical vertebra to the sacrum. They vary in size, thickness, and shape at different levels of the spine. The purpose of the intervertebral disc is to cushion movement. The central core, the *nucleus pulposus,* is surrounded by a fibrous capsule called the *annulus fibrosus.*

THE MENINGES

Meninges cover both the brain and spinal cord. The layers, from the outermost layer inward, are called the *dura mater,* the *arachnoid,* and the *pia mater* (Figs. 2-12, 2-13).

DURA MATER

The *dura mater* is a double-layered, whitish, inelastic, fibrous membrane that lines the interior of the skull. The outer layer of the dura is actually the periosteum of the bone. The inner layer is the thick membrane that extends throughout the skull and creates compartments. The dura lines various foramina that exit at the base of the skull.

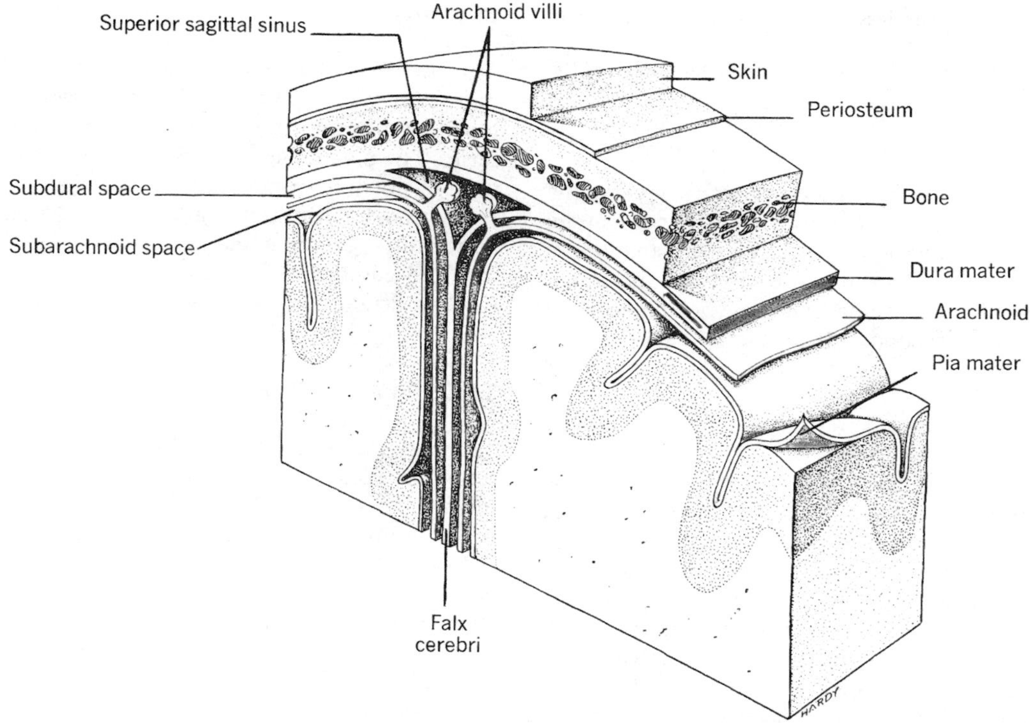

FIG. 2-12. The cranial meninges. Arachnoid villi shown within superior sagittal sinus are one site of passage of cerebrospinal fluid into the blood. (Chaffee EE, Lytle IM: Basic Physiology and Anatomy. Philadelphia, JB Lippincott, 1980)

Sheaths for the nerves passing through these foramina are also formed by the dura.

Four folds of dura are situated within the skull cavity to support and protect the brain. These are the following:

1. The *falx cerebri* descends vertically into the longitudinal fissure between the two hemispheres of the brain.
2. The *tentorium cerebelli* is a double fold of dura, tentlike in shape, that covers the upper surface of the cerebellum, supports the occipital lobes, and prevents them from pressing upon the cerebellum. The falx cerebri attaches midline to the tentorium. (The tentorium is an important anatomical point to note. Surgery above the tentorium is termed *supratentorial*, while surgery below it is called *infratentorial*. The nursing care given

FIG. 2-13. Cranial dura mater. Skull opened to show the falx cerebri and the right and left portions of the tentorium cerebelli, as well as some of the cranial venous sinuses. (Chaffee EE, Lytle IM: Basic Physiology and Anatomy. Philadelphia, JB Lippincott, 1980)

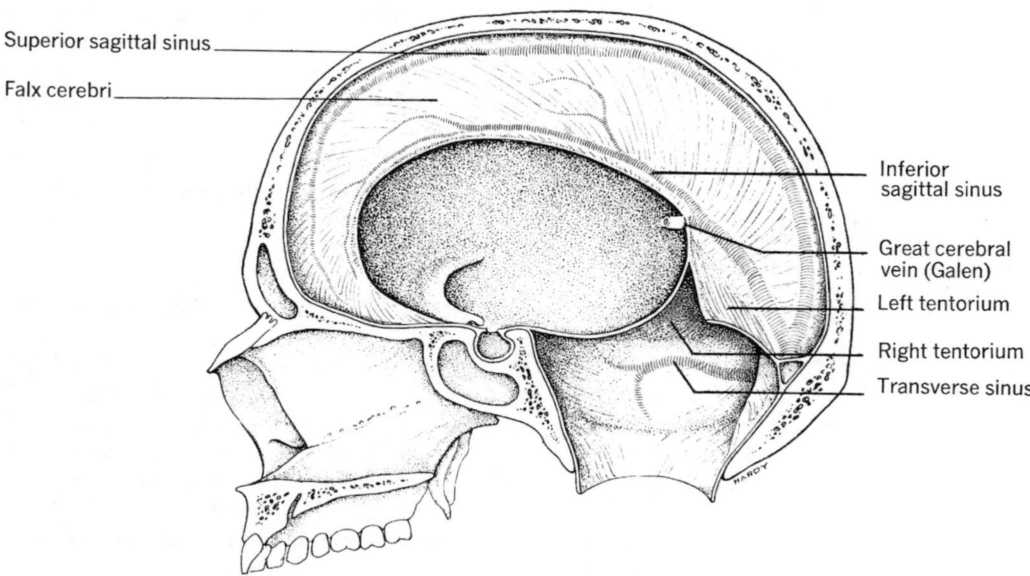

differs based on these two classifications, as will be discussed in a later chapter.)

3. The *falx cerebelli* is found between the two lateral lobes of the cerebellum.
4. The *diaphragma sellae* is a horizontal process that forms a small circular fold, thus creating a roof for the sella turcica.

The spinal dura is a continuation of the inner layer of the cerebral dura. The outer layer of the dura terminates at the foramen magnum, being replaced by the periosteal lining of the vertebral canal. The spinal dura encases the spinal roots, spinal ganglia, and spinal nerves. The spinal dural sac terminates at the second or third sacral level.

ARACHNOID

The second meningeal layer, the *arachnoid membrane*, is an extremely thin and delicate layer that loosely encloses the brain. The subdural space separates the dura mater from the arachnoid layer. Bleeding within this space (subdural hemorrhage) can occur with head injury. The subarachnoid space is not really a clear space because there is much spongy, delicate connective tissue between the arachnoid and pia mater layer. Cerebrospinal fluid flows in the subarachnoid space. The cisterna magnum is a space between the hemispheres of the cerebellum and the medulla oblongata. The arachnoid layer of the spinal meninges is a continuation of the cerebral arachnoid (Fig. 2-14). The arachnoid is a delicate, gossamer network of fine, elastic, fibrous tissue and also contains blood vessels of varying sizes, which may be damaged by lumbar or cisternal puncture, resulting in hemorrhage.

FIG. 2-14. Spinal cord and meninges. (Chaffee EE, Lytle IM: Basic Physiology and Anatomy. Philadelphia, JB Lippincott, 1980)

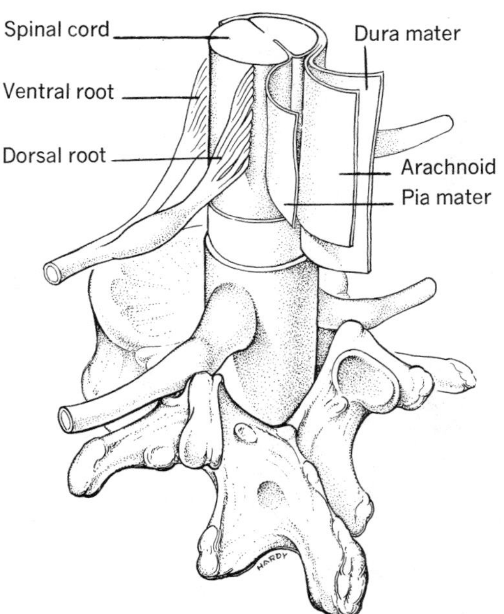

PIA MATER

The innermost layer of the meninges is called the *pia mater*. It is a meshlike vascular membrane that derives its blood supply from the internal carotid and vertebral arteries. The pia mater covers the entire surface of the brain, dipping down between the convolutions of the surface. As the pia covers the gray matter, the vascularity increases and minute perpendicular vessels extend for some distance into the cerebrum. The pia mater of the spinal cord is thicker, firmer, and less vascular than that of the brain.

THE "SPACES" OF THE MENINGES

Three spaces located within the meninges are important to note. The *epidural* or *extradural space* is a potential space located between the skull and outer layer of the dura layer of the brain. In the vertebral column the epidural space is between the periosteum and the single dural layer. The *subdural space* is between the inner dura mater and arachnoid layer. This is a narrow space and the site of subdural hemorrhage with certain injuries. The third layer is the *subarachnoid space*, which is between the arachnoid and pia mater layers and contains cerebrospinal fluid.

CEREBROSPINAL FLUID (CSF)

Cerebrospinal fluid is normally a clear, colorless, odorless solution that fills the ventricles of the brain and the subarachnoid space of the brain and spinal cord. The purpose of the cerebrospinal fluid is to act as a shock absorber and to cushion the brain and spinal cord against injury caused by movement. The specific gravity of cerebrospinal fluid is 1.007. The cerebrospinal fluid differs from other extracellular fluids in the percentage of composition of various factors. It is composed of water, a small amount of protein, oxygen, and carbon dioxide. The electrolytes—sodium, potassium, and chloride—and glucose, an important cerebral nutrient, are also present. An occasional lymphocyte may be present. The normal cerebrospinal fluid pressure is in the range of 60 mm to 180 mm of water pressure in the lateral recumbent position, which is the position assumed for a lumbar puncture. In the sitting position a normal lumbar puncture will register 200 mm to 350 mm of water pressure. Fluctuation in pressure occurs in response to the cardiac cycle and respirations. There are 125 ml to 150 ml of cerebrospinal fluid in the adult.

FORMATION OF CEREBROSPINAL FLUID

Cerebrospinal fluid, produced by active transport and diffusion, is thought to be formed from three different sources. The major source of cerebrospinal fluid is the secretions from the choroid plexus, a cauliflowerlike structure located in portions of the lateral, third, and fourth ventricles (Fig. 2-15). The *choroid plexus* is described as a collection of blood vessels covered by a thin coating of ependymal

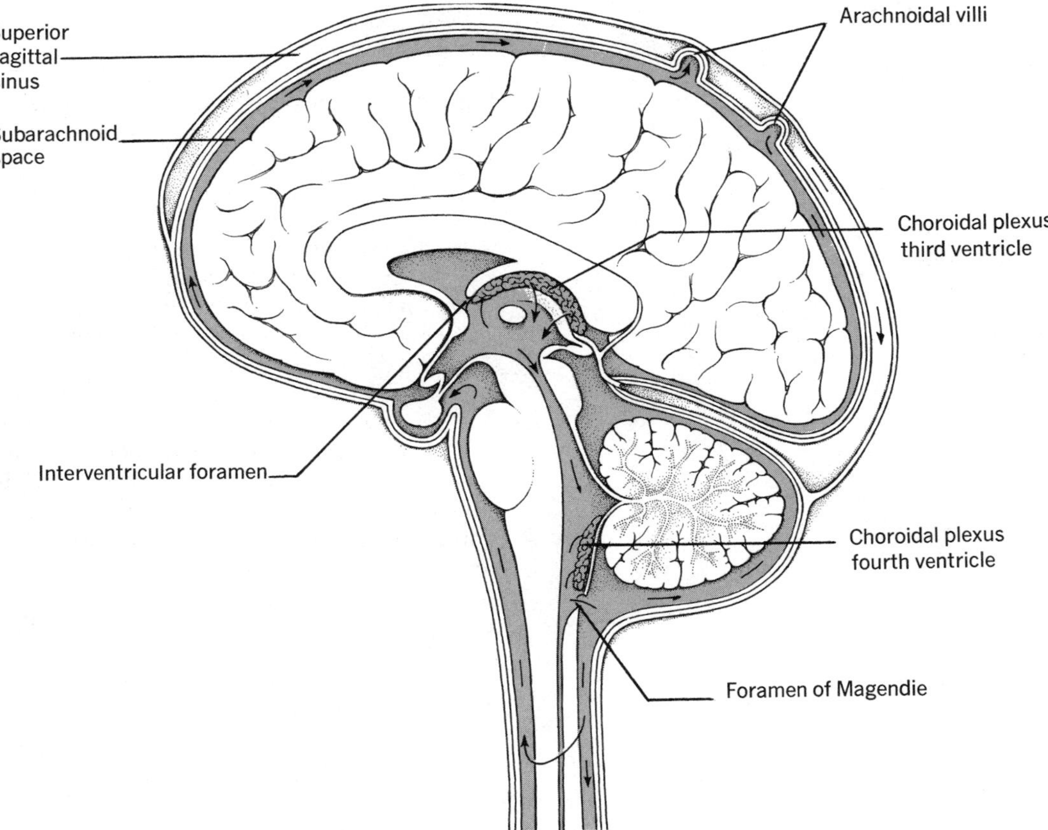

FIG. 2–15. Diagram of the flow of cerebrospinal fluid from the time of its formation from blood in the choroid plexuses until its return to the blood in the superior sagittal sinus. (*Note:* Plexuses in the lateral ventricles are not illustrated.) (Chaffee EE, Lytle IM: Basic Physiology and Anatomy. Philadelphia, JB Lippincott, 1980)

cells. The cerebrospinal fluid is constantly secreted from these surfaces. It is estimated that the amount of cerebrospinal fluid daily produced by the choroid plexus is about 500 ml. A lesser proportion of cerebrospinal fluid is secreted from the second source, the ependymal cells, which line the ventricles and blood vessels of the meninges. The last source of cerebrospinal production is the blood vessels of the brain and spinal cord. The amount produced from this source is very small.

CEREBROSPINAL FLUID ABSORPTION

Most of the cerebrospinal fluid produced daily is reabsorbed into the *arachnoid villi,* which are projections from the subarachnoid space into the venous sinuses of the brain (see Fig. 2–15). Cerebrospinal fluid drains into the superior sagittal sinus. Arachnoid villi are very permeable and allow cerebrospinal fluid, including protein molecules, to exit easily from the subarachnoid space into venous sinuses. Cerebrospinal fluid flows in one direction through the arachnoid villi (most of which are located in the subarachnoid space of the cerebrum), which have been compared to pressure-sensitive valves. When cerebrospinal fluid pressure is greater than venous pressure, cerebrospinal fluid leaves the subarachnoid space. As pressures are equalized, the valves close.

FLOW OF CEREBROSPINAL FLUID

Cerebrospinal fluid circulation has been termed the "third circulation." It is a closed system. Fluid formed in the two lateral ventricles passes into the third ventricle by way of the two foramina of Munro. The single cerebral aqueduct or aqueduct of Sylvius connects the third and fourth ventricle. Cerebrospinal fluid flows through the two lateral foramina of Luschka and midline through the one foramen of Magendie to the cisternal magnum. At this point the cerebrospinal fluid enters the subarachnoid space. The foramen of Magendie allows cerebrospinal fluid to circulate around the cord, while the foramen of Luschka directs the cerebrospinal fluid around the brain (Fig. 2–16).

Expanded areas of the subarachnoid space are called *cisterns.* Cerebrospinal fluid may be aspirated from some of these areas for analysis. The major cisterns are the cisterna magnum, located between the medulla and cerebellar region (see Fig. 4–7) and the lumbar cistern, located between vertebrae L–2 and S–2.

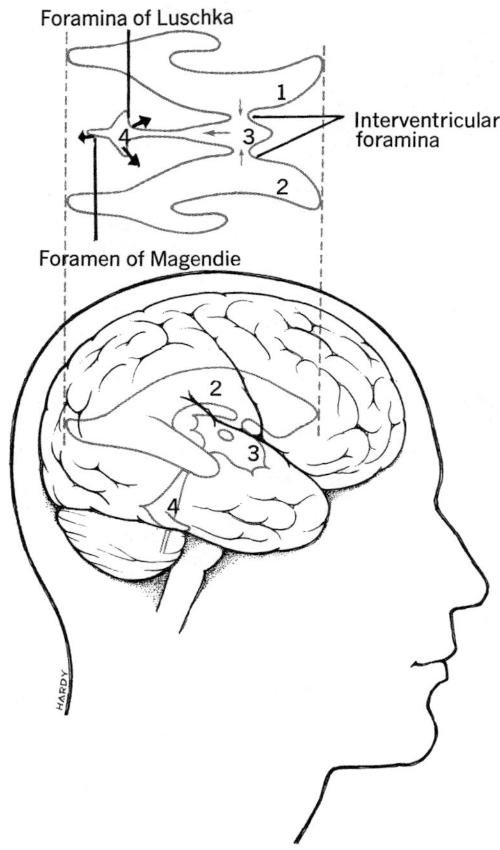

FIG. 2-16. The ventricles of the brain—ventricles are outlined and arrows indicate the direction of flow of cerebrospinal fluid *(above)* and relation to brain as a whole *(below)*. (Chaffee EE, Lytle IM: Basic Physiology and Anatomy. Philadelphia, JB Lippincott, 1980)

CEREBRAL CIRCULATION

The blood vessels that supply the nervous system form an extensive capillary bed, particularly in the gray matter of the brain. About 20% of the oxygen consumed by the body is used for the oxidation of glucose to provide energy. The brain is totally dependent on glucose for its metabolism. A lack of oxygen to the brain for 2 to 5 minutes can result in irreversible brain damage.

The brain receives approximately 750 ml/minute of blood, or 15% of the total resting cardiac output. These figures remain relatively constant because of various control systems affecting the brain. Blood flow rates to specific areas of the brain correlate directly to the metabolism of the cerebral tissue. The brain is supplied by two pairs of arteries: the two vertebral arteries and the two internal carotid arteries (Fig. 2-17).

THE VERTEBRAL ARTERIES

The vertebral arteries, originating from the subclavian arteries, enter the skull through the foramen magnum, ventrolateral to the spinal cord. The vertebral arteries unite at the level of the pons to become the *basilar artery* (Fig. 2-18). The basilar artery subdivides into the posterior cerebral arteries that supply part of the cerebrum:

Two vertebral arteries → basilar artery →
two posterior cerebral arteries

In general, the vertebral arteries and their branches supply the cerebellum, the brain stem, the spinal cord, the occipital lobes, the medial and inferior surfaces of the temporal lobes, and the posterior diencephalon.

Before they begin to supply blood to the brain, the vertebral arteries give off recurrent branches that anastomose with the anterior and posterior spinal arteries, and a posterior meningeal branch. In its intracranial course, the vertebral arteries give rise to direct bulbar arteries to the medulla, the anterior spinal artery, the posterior inferior cerebellar artery, sometimes the posterior spinal artery, and small branches to the basal meninges. The basilar artery is the origin of the pontine arteries, the internal auditory arteries, the anterior inferior cerebellar arteries, the superior cerebellar arteries, and the posterior cerebral arteries. Table 2-3 summarizes the major branches of the vertebral arteries and the areas supplied.

THE INTERNAL CAROTID ARTERIES

The internal carotid arteries originate from two different vessels: the *left common carotid,* which originates directly from the aorta; and the *right common carotid,* which arises from the *innominate artery* also originating from the aorta. The common carotids branch to form the external and internal carotid arteries. The internal carotid artery enters the cranial vault through the foramen lacerum. Most of the hemispheres, excluding the occipitals, the basal ganglia, and the upper two thirds of the diencephalon, are supplied by the internal carotid arteries. As the internal carotid passes through the bone and dura at the base of the skull and approaches the upper brain, it curves sharply several times and roughly forms an S, called the *carotid siphon.*

Before the internal carotids begin to supply blood to the brain they give rise to the tympanic and ophthalmic arteries. The terminal branches of each carotid include the posterior communicating artery, the anterior cerebral artery, and the middle cerebral artery (Fig. 2-19). Table 2-4 summarizes the major branches of the carotid arteries and the areas supplied.

Communication Among Arterial Vessels

The three cerebellar arteries communicate, as do the three cerebral arteries, although the latter communicate even more freely by means of branches anastomosing over the margins of the hemisphere. There is more anastomosing among the vessels than was originally thought.

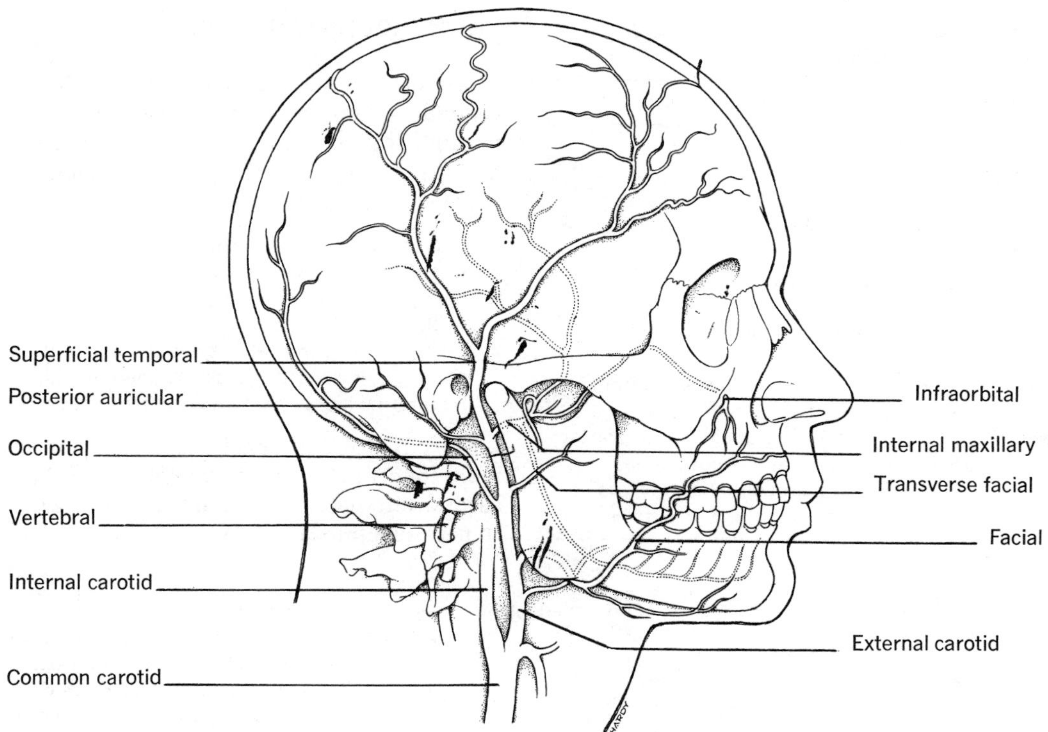

FIG. 2–17. Branches of the right external carotid artery. The internal carotid artery ascends to the base of the brain. The right vertebral artery also is shown as it ascends through the transverse foramina of the cervical vertebrae. (Chaffee EE, Lytle IM: Basic Physiology and Anatomy. Philadelphia, JB Lippincott, 1980)

Peculiarities of the Cerebral Circulation

The following is a list of the outstanding characteristics of cerebral circulation:

1. Cerebral arteries, in general, have very thin walls, comparable to those of veins of similar size in other parts of the body. Cerebral arteries have an internal elastic tissue and scanty smooth muscle.
2. The veins (other than sinuses) have even thinner walls in proportion to their size and lack a muscle layer.
3. The veins and sinuses have *no* valves.
4. The venous return does not retrace the course of corresponding arteries but follows a pattern of its own.
5. The dural sinuses are unique to cerebral circulation.
6. The distribution of the arteries with rich surfaces (arteries anastomose by localized "end-artery" distribution of branches penetrating the nervous tissue) is distinctive.

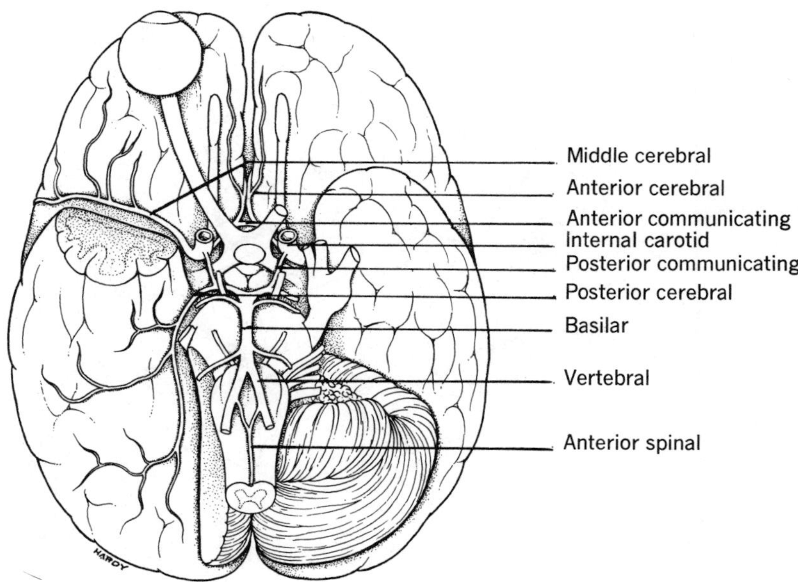

FIG. 2–18. The circle of Willis as seen at the base of a brain that has been removed from the skull. (Chaffee EE, Lytle IM: Basic Physiology and Anatomy. Philadelphia, JB Lippincott, 1980)

TABLE 2-3. ***Summary of the Vertebral Circulation, Its Branches, and the Areas of the Brain Supplied***

Name of Artery	*Area Supplied*
• Anterior and posterior spinal	• Spinal cord
• Posterior inferior cerebellar	• Under surface of the cerebellum, medulla oblongata, choroid plexus of fourth ventricle
• Pontine	• Pons and adjacent areas
• Internal auditory	• Inner ear
• Anterior inferior cerebellar	• Under surface of the cerebellum
• Superior cerebellar	• Upper surface of the cerebellum, and midbrain
• Posterior cerebral	• Occipital lobes, medial and inferior surfaces of the temporal lobes, midbrain, and choroid plexuses of the third and lateral ventricles

THE CIRCLE OF WILLIS

The circle of Willis, which is located at the base of the skull, is divided (for purposes of discussion) into anterior (carotid portion) and posterior (vertebral-basilar portion) circulation (Fig. 2-20). The composition of each portion includes these elements:

1. Two anterior cerebral arteries, whose longest sides are connected by the one anterior communicating artery (essentially, when the two anterior cerebral arteries are connected, internal carotids are connected).
2. Two posterior cerebral arteries and a pair of posterior communicating arteries (the posterior communicating arteries unite the internal carotid system with the vertebral-basilar system).

The circle of Willis encloses a very small area that is little more than 1 in^2 or approximately 6 cm^2. Functionally, the carotid circulation and the posterior circulation usually remain separate. The circle of Willis was thought to have

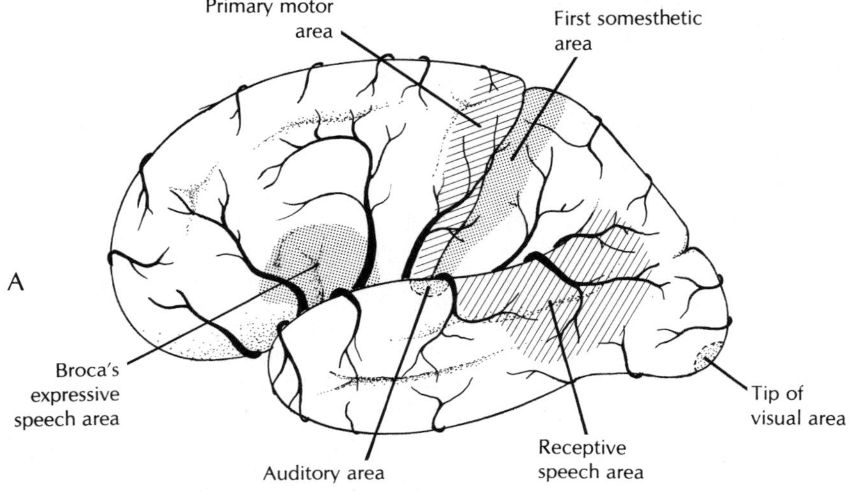

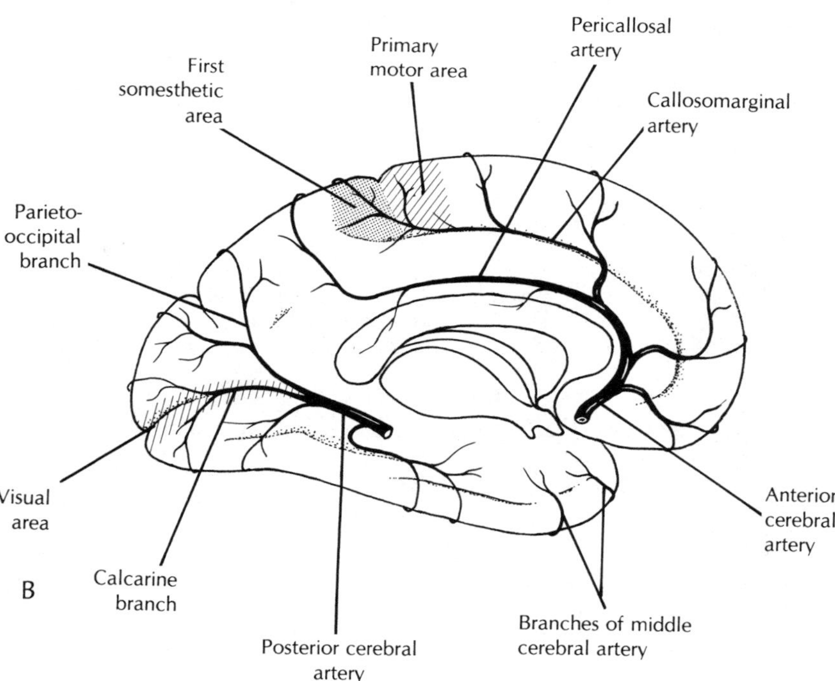

FIG. 2-19. *(A)* Distribution of the middle cerebral artery on the lateral surface of the cerebral hemisphere. *(B)* Distribution of the anterior and posterior cerebral arteries on the medial surface of the cerebral hemisphere. (Barr ML, Kiernan JA: The Nervous System, 4th ed. Philadelphia, Harper & Row, 1983)

TABLE 2-4. ***Summary of the Internal Carotid Circulation, Its Branches, and the Areas of the Brain Supplied***

Name of Artery	*Area Supplied*
• Tympanic	• Middle ear
• Ophthalmic	• Optic nerve, the orbits, and some nasal sinuses
• Anterior choroidal	• Part of choroid plexuses of the lateral ventricles, optic tract, cerebral peduncles, globus pallidus, posterior internal capsule, and lateral geniculate body
• Lenticulostriate	• Basal ganglia and part of the internal capsule
• Anterior cerebral	• Medial frontal and parietal lobes, adjacent cortex, and parts of the corpus callosum
• Middle cerebral	• Lateral surfaces of the four cerebral lobes
• Posterior communicating	• Connects the internal carotid circulation with the posterior cerebral artery

been a protective mechanism by which blood was shunted to compensate for alterations in cerebral blood flow or pressure. However, collateral circulation through the circle depends on the patency of its components. The vessels of the circle of Willis, particularly the communicating arteries, are frequently anomalous. In one study 50% of the cases reviewed varied in one or more important features in vascular structure in the circle of Willis region. Nevertheless, in *favorable instances* the circle does permit an adequate blood supply to reach all parts of the brain even after one or more of the four supplying vessels has been ligated.

VENOUS DRAINAGE

Unlike venous drainage in other parts of the body which closely follows the arterial pattern, the cerebral venous drainage is chiefly managed by vascular channels created by the two dural layers called *dural sinuses*. There are no valves in dural sinuses. A few dural sinuses deserve mention and are included in Table 2-5 along with the areas they supply. See also Figure 2-21. *Emissary veins* join extracranial veins with the venous sinuses. *Bridging veins* connect the brain and dural sinuses and are often the cause of subdural hemorrhage. Cerebral veins empty into the dural sinuses which, in turn, empty into the *jugular veins*, which return the blood to the heart.

MENINGEAL BLOOD SUPPLY

The meninges are supplied with a rich arterial blood supply by the anterior, middle, and posterior meningeal arteries. The main route for the arterial supply of the dura mater is through the middle meningeal branches of the external carotid artery. Each vessel ascends through a foramen in the base of the skull and is then situated between the dura mater and the skull. These vessels may be torn as a result of a head injury, thereby causing an epidural hematoma, which requires immediate attention.

BLOOD SUPPLY TO THE SPINAL CORD, SPINAL ROOTS, AND SPINAL NERVES

The spinal cord receives its arterial blood supply, in part, from the anterior spinal artery and the two posterior spinal arteries, which arise from the vertebral arteries. The *anterior spinal artery* runs the full length of the cord midventrally, while the two *posterior spinal arteries* run full length

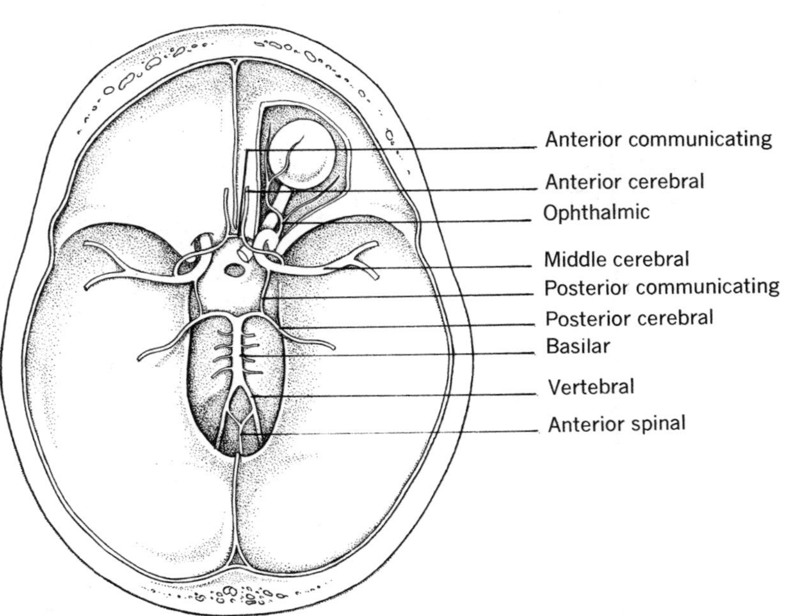

FIG. 2-20. Blood supply to the brain (circle of Willis) and to the eyeball shown in relation to the base of the skull. The brain has been removed; the right orbital cavity has been opened. (Chaffee EE, Lytle IM: Basic Physiology and Anatomy. Philadelphia, JB Lippincott, 1980)

TABLE 2-5. ***Summary of the Major Sources of Venous Drainage of the Cerebral Circulation Including Areas Drained***

Venous Structure	*Area Drained*
• Superior longitudinal (sagittal)	• Drains superior cortical veins of the convexity of the brain; drains cerebrospinal fluid
• Inferior longitudinal sinus	• Drains medial surface of brain
• Straight sinus	• Joins the superior longitudinal sinus; the vein of Galen drains into the straight sinus
• Transverse sinus	• Drains area of the ears; collects blood from superior longitudinal and straight sinuses and drains it into the internal jugular vein
• Cavernous sinus (contains several cranial nerves and internal carotid artery)	• Drains blood from the inferior surface of the brain including the orbits

along each row of the dorsal roots. As these three vessels pass down the cord, they receive feeders from deep cervical, intercostal, lumbar, and sacral arteries. Additional blood supply comes from the *lateral spinal arteries,* which are located at each segment of the cord.

The venous system of the spine includes an intradural and extradural supply: the intradural veins follow the pattern of the arteries and the extradural intravertebral veins form a plexus extending from the cranium to the pelvis and having many communications along the way with veins of the neck, thorax, and abdomen.

THE BLOOD-BRAIN BARRIER AND THE BLOOD-CEREBROSPINAL FLUID BARRIER

For the central nervous system to function normally, a very stable environment must exist within that body system. The so-called blood-brain barrier and blood-cerebrospinal fluid barrier provide that stability for the nervous system. The *blood-brain barrier* is a descriptive term for the network of capillary endothelial cells and the astroglial membranes located in close approximation to the neuron. The tight junctions between the endothelial cells and the astroglial cells are largely responsible for the barrier. The barrier provides selectivity to the substances that cross the neuronal membrane and gain entrance into the neuron. Because of this barrier, most drugs are prevented from affecting the brain and spinal cord.

The movement of substances into the brain depends on particle size, lipid solubility, chemical dissociation, and the

FIG. 2-21. The cranial venous sinuses. The sigmoid portion of the transverse sinus continues as the internal jugular vein. (Chaffee EE, Lytle IM: Basic Physiology and Anatomy. Philadelphia, JB Lippincott, 1980)

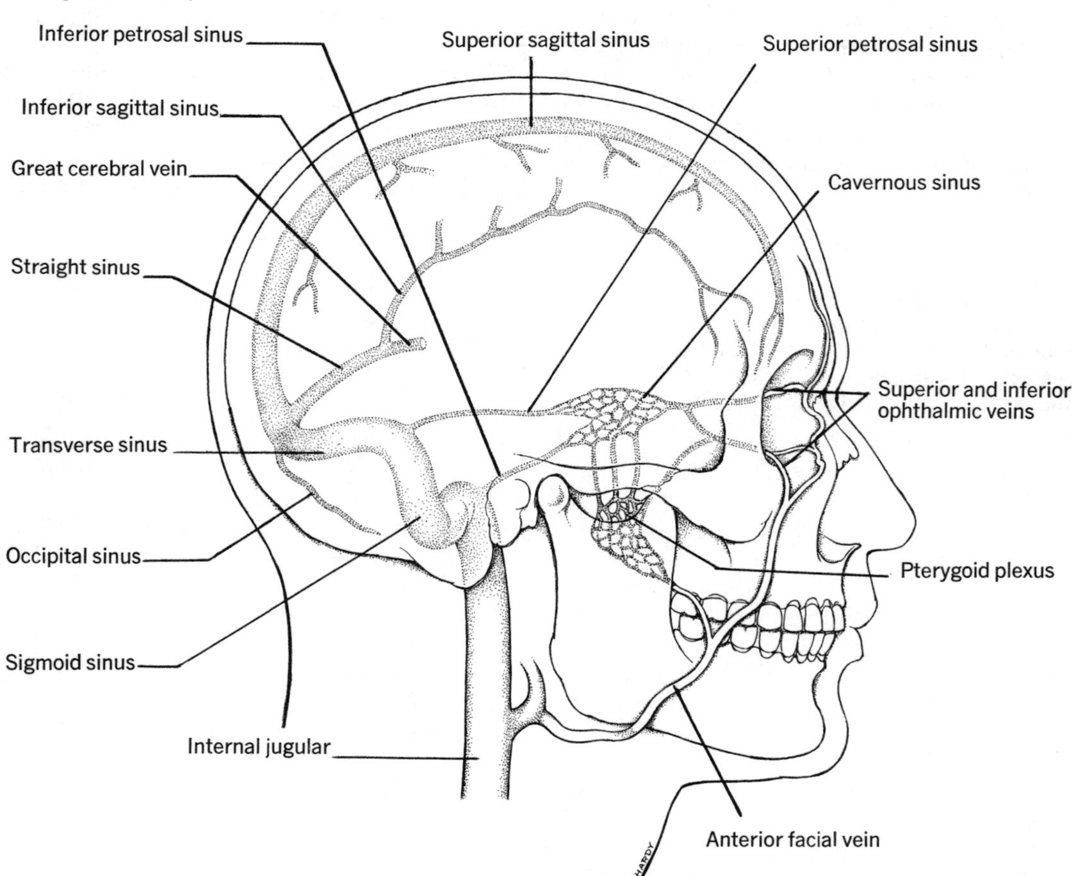

protein-binding potential of the drug. In general, drugs that are lipid-soluble and undissociated at body pH will rapidly enter both the brain and cerebrospinal fluid. When compared with other body organs, the central nervous system is very slow in its uptake of dyes and both organic and inorganic anions and cations (e.g., sodium, potassium, glutamic acid) from the circulating blood. The barrier is very permeable to water, oxygen, carbon dioxide, other gases, glucose, and lipid-soluble compounds.

The *blood–cerebrospinal fluid barrier* is similar to the blood–brain barrier. Its anatomical structures are found in the choroid plexuses.

THE BRAIN (ENCEPHALON)

The brain constitutes approximately 2% of body weight. The average weight of the brain of a young adult male is about 1400 gm. Since women tend to weigh less than men, their brains are lighter. The brains of older people weigh less, with the average being about 1200 mg.

Subdivisions of the Brain

The brain is divided into three major areas: the cerebrum, the brain stem, and the cerebellum (Fig. 2–22). The *cerebrum* is composed of the cerebral hemispheres, thalamus, hypothalamus, and the basal ganglia. In addition, the olfactory and optic nerves (cranial nerves I and II) are located in the cerebrum. The *brain stem* includes the midbrain, pons, and medulla. The midbrain, which contains the cerebral peduncles and corpus quadrigemina, is a short segment between the thalamus, hypothalamus, and the pons.

Another method used to subdivide the brain is by fossae. The *anterior fossa* contains the frontal lobes, the *middle fossa* contains the temporal, parietal, and occipital lobes, and the *posterior fossa* contains the brain stem and cerebellum.

THE CEREBRUM

The cerebrum comprises two cerebral hemispheres that are incompletely separated by the great longitudinal fissure. A *fissure,* also called a *sulcus,* is a large, predictable separation in the cerebral hemisphere. The following are some important fissures that are landmarks in studying the gross anatomy of the brain. The *great longitudinal fissure* is a midsagittal fissure that separates the cerebral hemispheres into a left and right side. The hemispheres are joined at the bottom of the fissure by the corpus callosum. The *lateral fissure of Sylvius* separates the temporal lobe from the frontal and parietal lobes. The *central fissure of Rolando* separates the frontal lobe from the parietal lobe. The last major fissure is the *parieto-occipital fissure,* which separates the occipital lobe from the parietal and temporal lobes (Fig. 2–23).

The surface of the hemispheres consists of numerous "wrinkles," or *gyri* (also called *convolutions*). The gyri fold in upon one another, thereby substantially increasing the surface area of the brain. Each hemisphere is covered by a cerebral cortex of gray matter that is 2 mm to 5 mm thick and contains billions of neurons.

Under the cerebral cortex is white matter, which serves as an association and projection pathway. The white matter of the cerebral hemispheres contains nerve fibers and neuroglia of various sizes. Three types of myelinated nerve fibers comprise the center of the hemisphere. They are the transverse fibers, the projection fibers, and the association fibers (Fig. 2–24).

FIG. 2–22. Midsagittal section of the brain. (Chaffee EE, Lytle IM: Basic Physiology and Anatomy. Philadelphia, JB Lippincott, 1980)

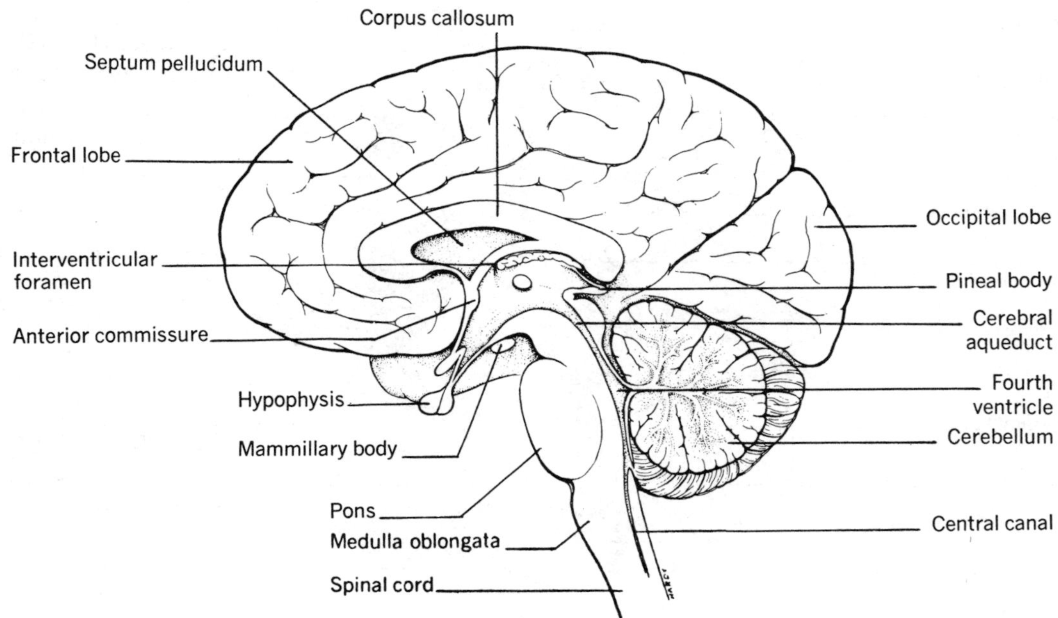

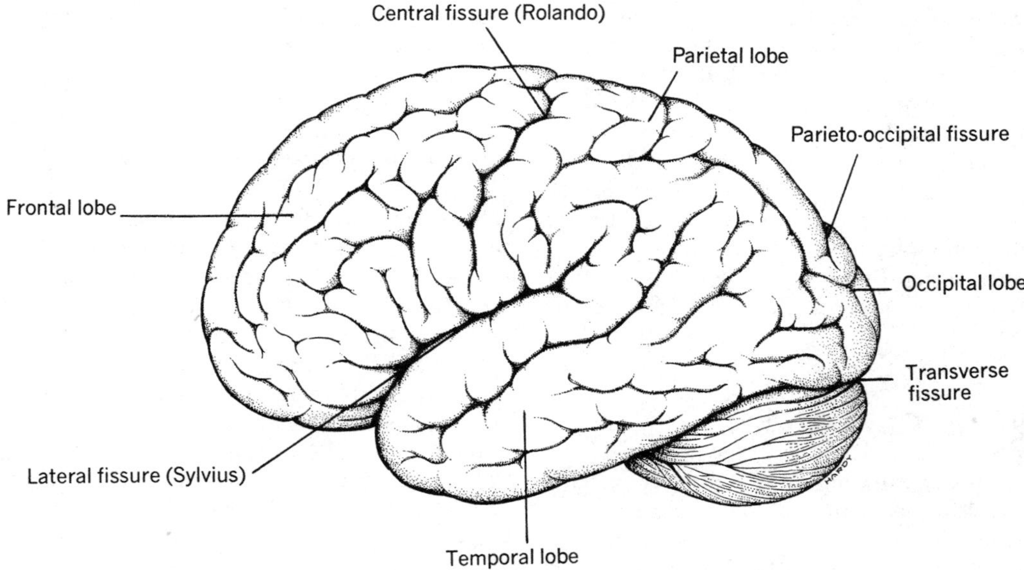

FIG. 2-23. Lateral aspect of the left cerebral and cerebellar hemispheres.

- *Transverse (commissural) fibers* are tracts of fibers that interconnect corresponding parts of the *two* hemispheres. The *corpus callosum* is the largest commissure. It is an arch-shaped structure that crosses the great longitudinal fissure.
- *Projection fibers* connect the cerebral cortex with lower portions of the brain and spinal cord.
- *Association fibers* connect various areas within the *same* hemisphere.

The cerebral hemispheres of the cerebrum are composed of pairs of frontal, parietal, temporal, and occipital lobes. Brodmann is credited with classifying the cortical areas of

FIG. 2-24. Oblique coronal section through the cerebrum and brain stem. Commissural and projection fibers shown in black. (Chaffee EE, Lytle IM: Basic Physiology and Anatomy. Philadelphia, JB Lippincott, 1980)

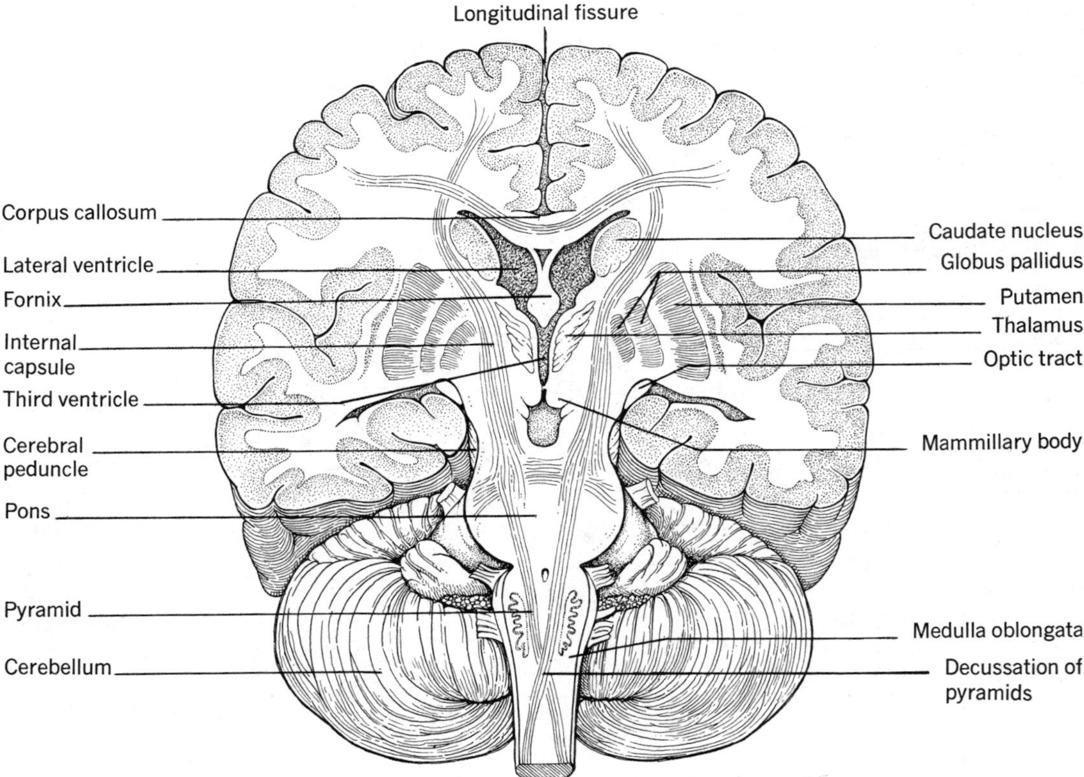

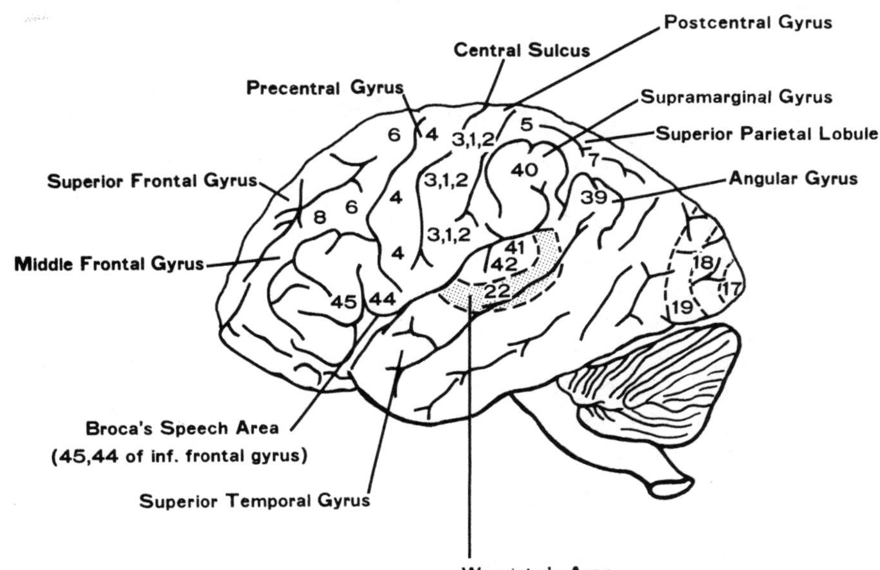

FIG. 2-25. Lateral view of the brain depicting the most significant areas of Brodmann. (Clark R: Manter and Gatz's Essentials of Clinical Neuroanatomy and Neurophysiology, 5th ed. Philadelphia, FA Davis, 1975)

the brain based on slight histological differences of the cells. There are almost 100 different areas of the cerebral cortex that have been identified. This method of classification provides a basis for the discussion of functional areas of the brain (Fig. 2-25). Brodmann's area 4 is the primary motor strip or primary motor cortex; areas 1, 2, and 3 are the primary somatic sensory areas; areas 41 and 42 are primary receptive areas for sound; and area 17 is the primary receptive area for vision (Fig. 2-26). The primary sensory and motor areas perform highly specialized functions.

Other areas of the brain that do not perform primary functions are called *association areas*. Functions of the association areas are more general but nonetheless important. Functional loss of a sensory association area greatly reduces the ability of the brain to analyze characteristics of sensory experience. It should be mentioned that the cerebral cortex is closely associated, both anatomically and functionally, with the thalamus. Many afferent and efferent pathways connect with specific parts of the thalamus to perform various complex functions.

General Functions of the Cerebral Cortex by Lobes

The Frontal Lobes. The prefrontal areas of the frontal lobe (areas 9 through 12 [see Fig. 2-25]) are those areas that lie anterior to the motor regions of the lobe. The major functions of the prefrontal areas are

1. To provide added cortical area for cerebration to take place
2. To control, with the help of the thalamus and hypothalamus, some of the autonomic functions such as respirations, gastrointestinal activity, and blood pressure
3. To provide for the ability to concentrate on a problem without becoming distracted
4. To increase depth and ability of abstractness in thought
5. To provide for storage of information (memory)

The motor cortex (area 4), which is located anterior to the central fissure, contains giant Betz cells or pyramidal cells that control muscle motor function. The various muscles are spatially arranged on the strip so that the feet are located in the area of the longitudinal fissure and the muscles

FIG. 2-26. Diagram of the localization of function in the cerebral hemisphere. Various functional areas are shown in relation to the lobes and fissures—lateral view *(left)* and medial view *(right)*.

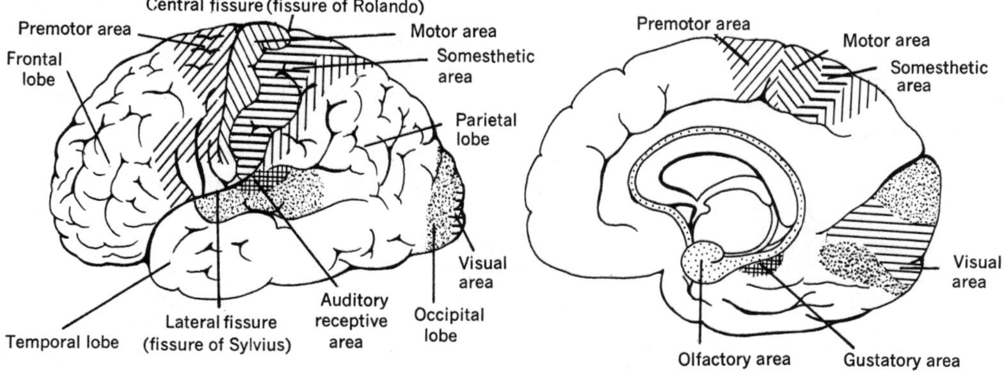

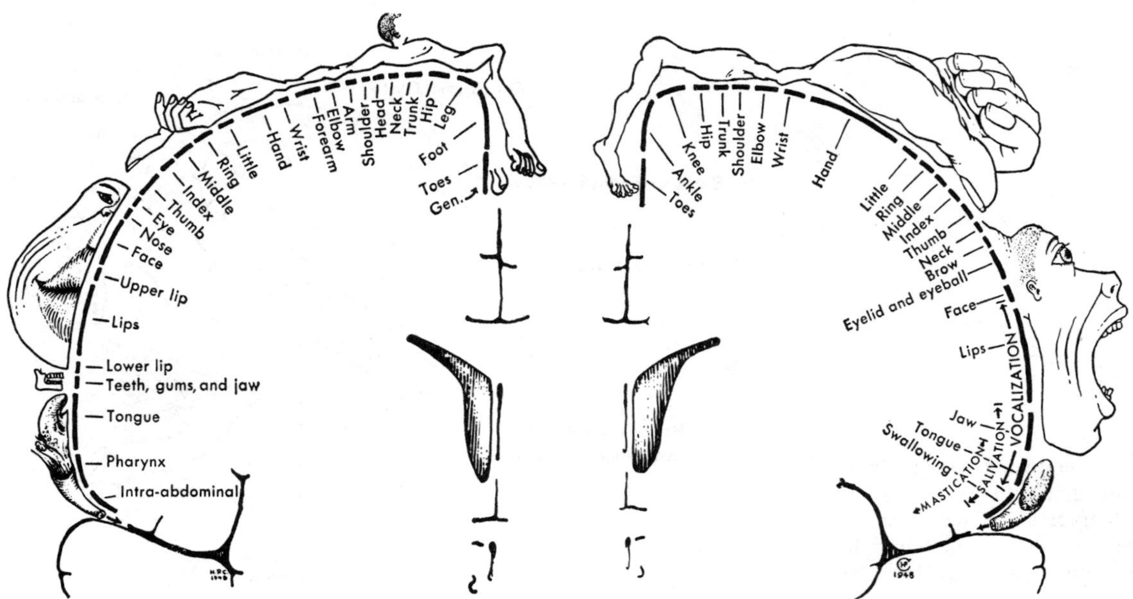

FIG. 2-27. Sensory *(left)* and motor *(right)* representations as determined by stimulation studies on the human cortex at surgery. Compare the sensory homunculus *(left)* to the motor homunculus *(right)*. Note the relatively large area devoted to the lips, thumb, and fingers. (Penfield E, Rasmussen T: The Cerebral Cortex of Man. New York, Macmillan, 1955. Copyright © by Macmillan Publishing Co., Inc., renewed 1978 by Theodore Rasmussen)

of chewing are located at the opposite end of the motor strip. Note the large area allocated to the hand (Fig. 2-27).

Areas 6 and 8 of the cortex are called motor association areas or the premotor cortex. There is a connection between these areas and the following cranial nerves: oculomotor, trochlear, abducens, glossopharyngeal, vagus, and spinal accessory. Stimulation of the lateral portion of area 6 results in massive generalized movements such as the turning of the eyes and head, movement of the trunk, and flexion and extension of the extremities, particularly the hands. Area 8 is concerned with the eye field and results in coordinated eye movement.

Another area of the frontal lobe to be mentioned is Broca's area (areas 44 and 45), located at the inferior frontal gyrus. Although it has been referred to as the speech area, Broca's area is classified as an association area because it aids in the formulation of words. Damage to this area in the dominant hemisphere results in the inability of the patient to speak in sentences. His vocabulary is limited to "yes" and "no" (expressive aphasia).

The Parietal Lobes. Posterior to the central fissure is the primary sensory cortex (areas 1, 2, and 3), which is arranged in the same topographic scheme as the motor strip; that is, the feet located in the area of the longitudinal fissure, and the muscles of chewing located in the temporal region. Area 1 receives fibers responsible for cutaneous and deep sensibility sensations. The fibers in area 2 are concerned with deep sensibility, while those in area 3 deal with the cutaneous sensations of touch, position, pressure, and vibration.

Input from the thalamus also reaches the primary sensory cortex. The purpose of the primary sensory cortex is to analyze only gross aspects of sensation and send the results of its interpretation to the thalamus and other cortical areas. It is the function of the sensory association areas (areas 5 and 7) to analyze the specific characteristics of sensory input.

In summary, in the parietal lobes sensory input is interpreted to define size, shape, weight, texture, and consistency. Sensation is localized and modalities of touch, pressure, and position are identified. In addition, the parietal lobe is essential to a person's awareness of the parts of his body, orientation in space, and discernment of spatial relationships in his immediate environment.

The Temporal Lobes. The primary auditory receptive areas (areas 41 and 42) are located in the temporal lobes. The auditory association area occupies a part of the superior temporal gyrus (area 22) and is also known as *Wernicke's area*. This area is usually larger in the dominant hemisphere. If Wernicke's area is damaged in the patient's dominant hemisphere, words are heard, but they are meaningless (receptive aphasia). A person would be able to verbalize but would unknowingly make many errors in the content because of failure to comprehend what has been said by others or by himself.

A very important area, called the *interpretive area*, is located in the supramarginal and angular gyri of the temporal lobe. This area is at the junction of the lateral fissure where the temporal, parietal, and occipital lobes meet. It provides an integration of the somatic, auditory, and visual association areas and plays the *greatest* role of any area of the cerebral cortex in cerebration. Types of thoughts that might be experienced are greatly detailed memories of past experiences, conversations, artwork, music, and taste. Memory that requires more than one sensory modality is stored, in part, in the angular gyrus of the temporal lobe. Any destruction of the *dominant temporal lobe* and angular gyrus in an adult will result in great impairment of intellectual ability. The patient with such an injury appears to be demented, and although he may develop the nondominant temporal lobe to a slight degree over time, his condition appears to be unchanged. In a child under 6 years of age, damage to a dominant temporal lobe will usually result in complete development of the opposite lobe. The child will be normal in intellectual ability.

The Occipital Lobes. The primary receptive area for vision is area 17 of the occipital lobe. The visual association areas are 18 and 19. Destruction of the visual association areas will not cause blindness; however, though the person can clearly see objects, he will not be able to recognize or identify them (visual agnosia).

The Limbic Lobes. Some texts refer to the limbic lobes. Anatomically, they are considered to be part of the temporal region, although functionally they can be separated. The limbic lobe consists of the cortex and subcortical structures that form the border of the lateral ventricles on the medial surface of each cerebral hemisphere. The limbic lobe consists of the hippocampal and cingulate gyri connected by minor convolutions to form a closed loop. This area includes the isthmus, uncas, primary olfactory cortex, cingulate and septal nuclei, the hippocampal formation, and the amygdala (a part of the basal ganglia). These structures are connected with the mamillary bodies, olfactory tract, the diencephalon, and the upper reticular formation of the midbrain. Together, these structures are referred to as the limbic system (Fig. 2–28).

The function of the limbic system is related to primitive behavior, feeling states, moods, instincts, and self-preservation. Stimulating specific anatomical parts of this system will result in specific responses diverse from those elicited by stimulating other areas of the system. These emotional responses are expressed through endocrine, visceral, and somatic reactions. The neural pathways connect (1) the hypothalamus, brain stem, and spinal cord by way of autonomic responses and (2) the hypophysis and endocrine system.

Dominancy of a Cerebral Hemisphere

As each of the four lobes of the cerebral cortex has been reviewed functionally, the issue of dominancy of one hemisphere has been raised. It is generally accepted that most people do have one cerebral hemisphere that has become more highly developed than the other. At birth, both hemispheres have an equal capacity for development. As a child develops, the attention of the mind is directed to one specific hemisphere, which develops rapidly in relation to the other side. Ninety percent of the population has a highly developed left hemisphere. These are the right-handed people. It is interesting to note that most, but not all, left-handed people also have as their dominant hemisphere the left side of the brain.

If the dominant hemisphere is destroyed in the child younger than 6 years of age, the opposite hemisphere will develop; destruction of the dominant hemisphere in the

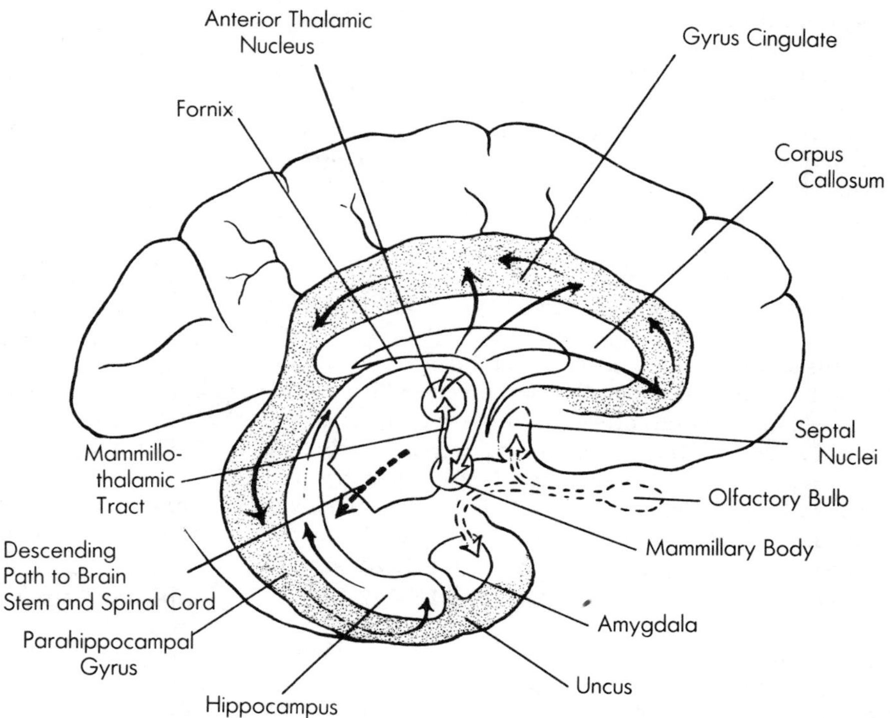

FIG. 2–28. Main connections between the hypothalamus and the cerebral cortex. The limbic lobe is shaded. Solid arrows show the hypothetical circulation of impulses during the experiencing of emotion. The thick dotted arrow indicates the descending path to the brain stem and spinal cord for expressing emotion. Olfactory afferent fibers are lightly dotted. (Clark R: Manter and Gatz's Essentials of Clinical Neuroanatomy and Neurophysiology, 5th ed. Philadelphia, FA Davis, 1975)

adult, however, leaves the person with a severely diminished intellectual capacity.

Many "split brain" studies have been conducted on the left and right hemispheres of the brain. The left side of the brain controls language while the right side is the nonverbal perceptual hemisphere.

Corpus Callosum

The corpus callosum, as mentioned previously, is a thick area of nerve fibers directed transversely, through which every part of one hemisphere is connected with the corresponding part of the other hemisphere. When the fibers of one hemisphere pass into the opposite hemisphere, they permeate the hemisphere in all directions and terminate in the gray matter of the periphery. As a result of this connective process, the two hemispheres are intricately connected.

Basal Ganglia

Basal ganglia are the several masses of subcortical nuclei located deep in the cerebral hemispheres. The anatomical parts include the lenticular nucleus (composed of the globus pallidus and putamen), the caudate nucleus, the amygdaloid body and the claustrum. The lenticular nucleus and the caudate nuclei are collectively called the *corpus striatum*. The lenticular nuclei and the caudate nucleus are closely related functionally to the thalamus, subthalamus, substantia nigra, and red nucleus. These structures compose the basal ganglia system for motor control of fine body movements, particularly of the hands and lower extremities.

Diencephalon

The diencephalon, a major division of the cerebrum, is divided into four regions: the thalamus, hypothalamus, subthalamus, and epithalamus (Fig. 2–29). The thalamus and hypothalamus are the major areas of importance. These four areas will be discussed along with the internal capsule and hypophysis (pituitary gland), which are located in this region.

Thalamus. The thalamus is a pair of egg-shaped masses of gray matter located in the ventromedial part of the hemispheres and connected to the midbrain. The thalamus is the last station where impulses are processed before they ascend to the cerebral cortex. There is a very intimate relationship between the thalamus and cerebral cortex. All sensory pathways (with the exception of olfactory pathways) have direct afferent and efferent connections with the thalamic nuclei. The thalamus plays a role in the conscious awareness of pain, in the focusing of attention, in the reticular activating system, and in the limbic system.

Epithalamus. The epithalamus is the most dorsal portion of the diencephalon. It is composed of the pineal body, which is thought to have a role in growth and development.

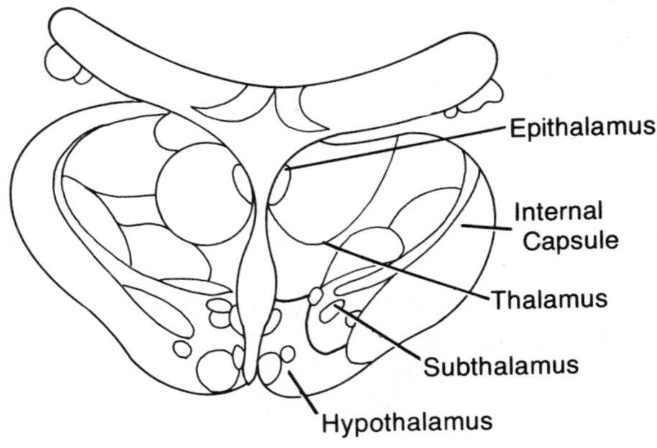

FIG. 2–29. Cross section of the brain stem at the diencephalic level. (Curtis B et al: An Introduction to the Neurosciences. Philadelphia, WB Saunders, 1972)

The epithalamus is also involved in the regulation of the primitive "food-getting" reflex.

Hypothalamus. The hypothalamus is located in the basal region of the diencephalon, forming part of the walls of the third ventricles. The hypothalamus includes several structures of importance:

1. The optic chiasma, the point at which the two optic tracts cross, which is located at the rostral area of the hypothalamic floor
2. The stalk of the pituitary, which connects the hypophysis with the hypothalamus
3. The mamillary bodies, which relay cortically originating limbic data to the thalamus

The general functions of the hypothalamus include

1. Temperature control by monitoring the blood temperature that flows through the hypothalamus and then sending afferent impulses to the sweat glands, peripheral vessels, and muscles (for shivering)
2. Water metabolism through the regulation of the antidiuretic hormone (ADH)
3. Control of other secretions of the hypophysis (growth hormone, follicle-stimulating hormone, and so forth)
4. Chief subcortical center for the regulation of visceral and somatic activities by an excitatory–inhibitory role in the autonomic nervous system (heart rate, motility of peristalsis, dilation and constriction of pupil, and so forth)
5. Mechanism to control appetite
6. Mechanisms to mediate visible physical expressions in response to emotions such as blushing, dryness of mouth, clammy hands, and so forth
7. Part of the sleep–wakefulness cycle

Subthalamus. The subthalamus is located below the thalamus and is closely related to the basal ganglia in function.

Internal Capsule

The internal capsule is part of the white matter of the cerebrum and contains both radiation and projection fibers. Many nerve fibers coming from various parts of the cerebral cortex converge at the brain stem, forming the corona radiata. As the fibers enter the thalamus–hypothalamus region, they are collectively termed the *internal capsule.* The internal capsule is defined as a massive bundle of efferent and afferent fibers connecting the various subdivisions of the brain and spinal cord.

All afferent sensory fibers going to the cortex pass through the internal capsule in the following succession: brain stem → thalamus → internal capsule → cerebral cortex. All efferent motor fibers leaving the cortex for the brain stem pass through the internal capsule in the following schemata: cerebral cortex → internal capsule → brain stem.

Hypophysis (Pituitary Gland)

The hypophysis is a small gland that is located in the sella turcica at the base of the brain and is connected to the hypothalamus by the hypophyseal stalk. The hypothalamus controls pituitary secretions. The hypophysis is divided into two lobes, the anterior and the posterior. The anterior lobe secretes six major hormones related to metabolic function of the body: (1) growth hormone, (2) adrenal-stimulating hormone (adrenocorticotropin), (3) thyroid-stimulating hormone, (4) prolactin, (5) follicle-stimulating hormone, and (6) luteinizing hormone. The posterior lobe produces ADH and oxytocin. The ADH controls the rate of water secretion into the urine, thereby controlling the water content of the body. With respect to intracranial surgery, pituitary adenoma, or cerebral trauma, it is not uncommon to find an abnormal secretion of ADH with observable clinical symptoms.

Relationship Between the Hypothalamus and Hypophysis in Neuroendocrine Control. The control center for the autonomic nervous system and the neuroendocrine system is the hypothalamus. The following two pathways of hypothalamic connection to the hypophysis (pituitary gland) enable hypothalamic influence of the endocrine glands: (1) nerve fibers that travel from the supraoptic paraventricular nuclei to the posterior lobe of the hypophysis (hypothalamohypophyseal tract); and (2) long and short portal blood vessels that connect sinusoids in the median eminence (portion of the hypophysis) and infundibulum with capillary plexuses in the anterior lobe of the hypophysis (hypophyseal portal system). See Figure 2–30.

Hypothalamohypophyseal Tract. The precursors of the hormones vasopressin and oxytocin are synthesized in the nerve cells of the supraoptic and paraventricular nuclei. The precursor material then passes along the axons and is released at the axon terminals where it is absorbed into the capillaries of the posterior hypophyseal lobe. Vasopressin is produced mainly in the nerve cells of the supraoptic nucleus. The functions of vasopressin, also called ADH, are to increase water absorption in the kidney's distal convoluted tubules and to initiate vasoconstriction. The other hormone produced in the posterior hypophyseal lobe is oxytocin. This hormone is produced mainly in the paraventricular nucleus and is responsible for uterine contraction and for stimulating the growth of those cells of the mammary glands responsible for milk production.

Hypophyseal Portal System. The hypophyseal portal system is derived from the superior hypophyseal artery. Upon entering the median eminence and dividing into capillaries, the capillaries drain into long and short descending vessels that terminate in the anterior lobe of the hypophysis. The release-stimulating hormones and release-inhibiting hormones are delivered to cells of the anterior hypophysis so that the appropriate releasing or inhibiting hormone is synthesized and secreted (e.g., thyroid-stimulating hormone, follicle-stimulating hormone). Feedback systems from afferent fibers in the hypothalamus as well as the target organ help to regulate the level of the various hormones.

BRAIN STEM (MIDBRAIN, PONS, AND MEDULLA)

The second major subdivision of the brain is the brain stem. Many significant anatomical parts are noted in the brain stem and will be discussed in relationship to the three major divisions.

Midbrain

The midbrain is a small segment lying between the diencephalon and the pons (Fig. 2–31). Cranial nerves III and IV emanate from the midbrain. The *corpus quadrigemina* (roof of the midbrain) is composed of the superior colliculi (optic system) and the inferior colliculi (auditory system). The crus cerebri and tegmentum are collectively called the *cerebral peduncle* and are made up of the corticospinal and corticopontine tracts. The *substantia nigra* is gray matter located between the peduncles and tegmentum. The superior cerebellar peduncles form the point of decussation. The red nuclei are part of the tegmentum. The tectospinal and rubrospinal tracts arise from the midbrain. On the lateral surface of the midbrain are the medial geniculate bodies, which are the auditory–sensory relay centers. Functionally, the midbrain serves as the nerve pathway of the cerebral hemispheres and the lower brain and as the center for auditory and visual reflexes.

Pons

The pons is located between the midbrain and medulla. Cranial nerves V through VIII connect to the brain in the pons. The inferior, middle, and superior cerebellar peduncles are pathways for the corticospinal tract, and they also connect to the cerebellum. Many other pathways pass through this region as they connect higher cerebral regions with the lower levels of the nervous system. Portions of the pons control respiratory function.

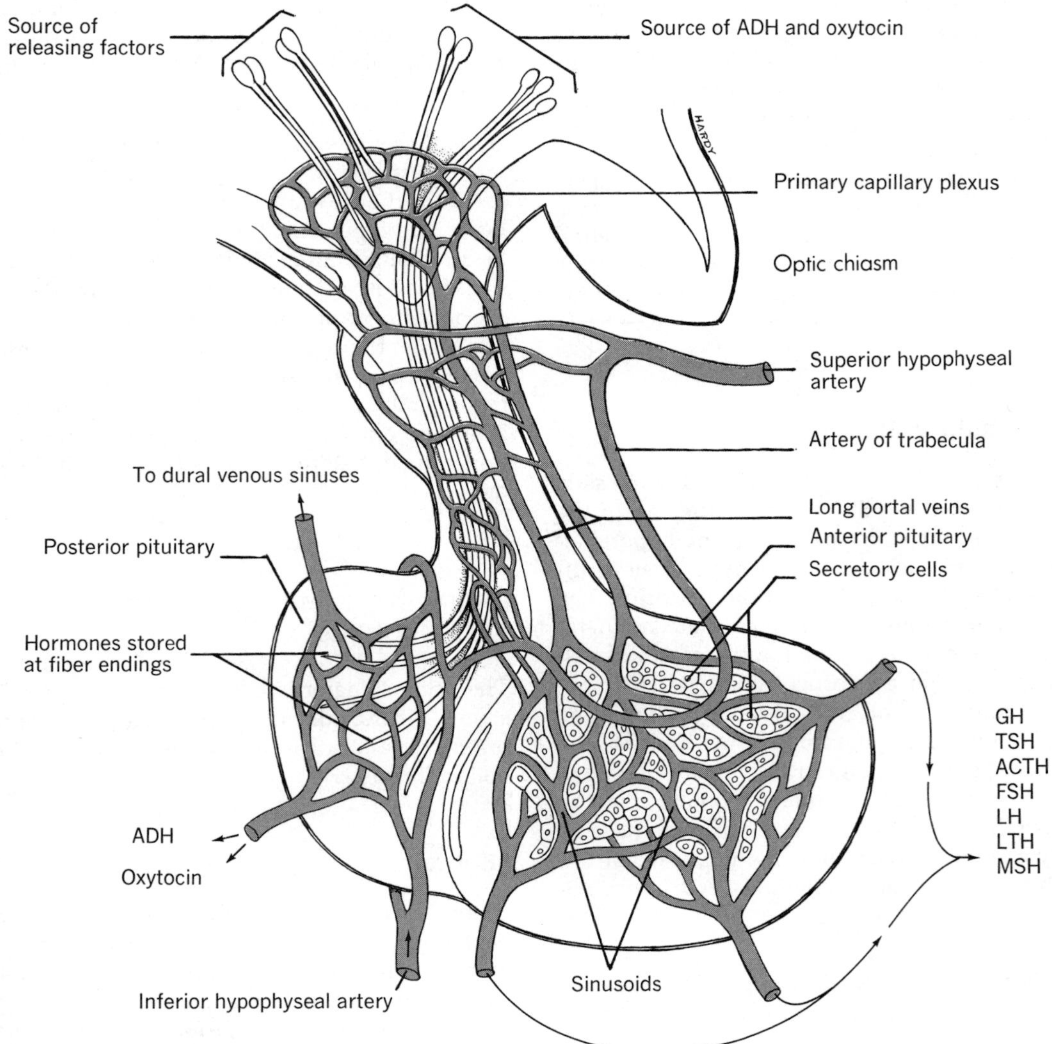

FIG. 2-30. Highly diagrammatic and schematic representation of hypophyseal nerve fiber tracts and portal system. Releasing factors produced by cell bodies in hypothalamus trickle down axons to proximal part of stalk where they enter the primary capillary plexus and are transported via portal vessels to sinusoids in adenohypophysis for control of secretions. ADH and oxytocin, produced by other cell bodies in hypothalamus, trickle down axons for storage in neurohypophysis until needed. (Chaffee EE, Lytle IM: Basic Physiology and Anatomy. Philadelphia, JB Lippincott, 1980)

Medulla

The medulla oblongata is continuous with the spinal cord at the foramen magnum and connects with the pons rostrally. Cranial nerves IX through XII connect to the brain in the medulla. The point of decussation of the pyramidal or corticospinal tract forms a ridge on either side of the median fissure. Many tracts find their way through the medulla.

Summary of Brain Stem Function

In general, the brain stem is important for the following reasons:

1. It acts as the point of attachment for cranial nerves III through XII
2. It contains ascending pathways
3. It contains descending pathways
4. It connects with the cerebellum
5. It contains part of the reticular formation

CEREBELLUM

The cerebellum, located in the posterior fossa, is attached to the pons, medulla, and midbrain by the three paired cerebellar peduncles. The cerebellum consists of three major parts: (1) the cortex, which is the outer gray covering; (2) the white matter, which forms the connecting pathways for efferent and afferent impulses joining the cerebellum with other parts of the central nervous system; and (3) four pairs of deep cerebellar nuclei. The cerebellar peduncles

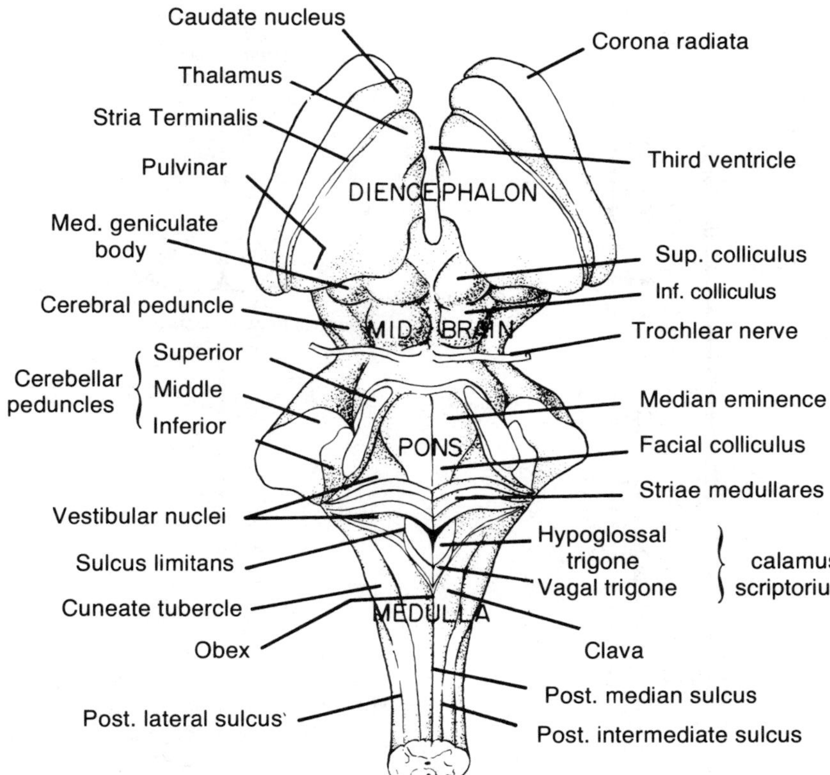

FIG. 2–31. Dorsal view of the brain stem. (Clark R: Manter and Gatz's Essentials of Clinical Neuroanatomy and Neurophysiology, 5th ed. Philadelphia, FA Davis, 1975)

receive direct input from the spinal cord and brain stem and convey it to the deep cerebellar nuclei and cerebellar cortex. The result is both an excitatory and inhibitory influence on the cerebellar nuclei, with the excitatory influences predominating. An excitatory effect on the brain stem and thalamic nuclei maintains a tonic discharge to the motor system.

The cerebellum is integrated into many connective efferent and afferent pathways throughout the brain thus providing muscle synergy throughout the body. All sensory modalities are circuited through the cerebellum, which provides information of muscle activity. Impulses to provide "corrections" are sent after sensory data are evaluated. In other words, there are many feedback loops in which cerebellar function is the center of the circuit receiving and sending impulses to maintain muscle activity. In summary, the cerebellum is responsible for the following functions:

1. Coordination of the action of muscle groups such as the agonist and antagonist muscles
2. Control of fine movement
3. Control of coordination of movement
4. Control of balance
5. Maintenance of feedback loops to correct movement

SPECIAL SYSTEMS WITHIN THE BRAIN

Two systems that entail anatomical structures throughout the various levels of the brain should be mentioned. These include the reticular formation and the reticular activating system.

The Reticular Formation

The brain stem and portions of the diencephalon have areas of diffuse neurons collectively known as the reticular formation. There are motor and sensory neurons scattered throughout the system that provide information concerning muscle activity. As a result of the analysis of this data, both facilitory and inhibitory impulses from the reticular formation affect the bulboreticular facilitory and inhibitory area. The function of the reticular formation is to provide continuous impulses to the muscles to support the body against gravity.

Reticular Activating System (RAS)

The RAS is a diffuse system that extends from the lower brain stem to the cerebral cortex, from which it disperses. The purpose of the RAS is to control the sleep–wakefulness cycle, consciousness, the ability to direct attention to a specific task, and the perception of sensory input that might alter behavior. The brain stem and thalamic portion of the RAS have different functions. Stimulation of the brain stem portion results in activation of the entire brain. It is thought that normal wakefulness of the brain is controlled by the brain stem. Stimulation of the thalamic portion relays facilitory impulses, causing generalized activation of the cerebrum only. Stimulation of selective areas of the thalamus activates specific areas of the cerebral cortex. It is thought

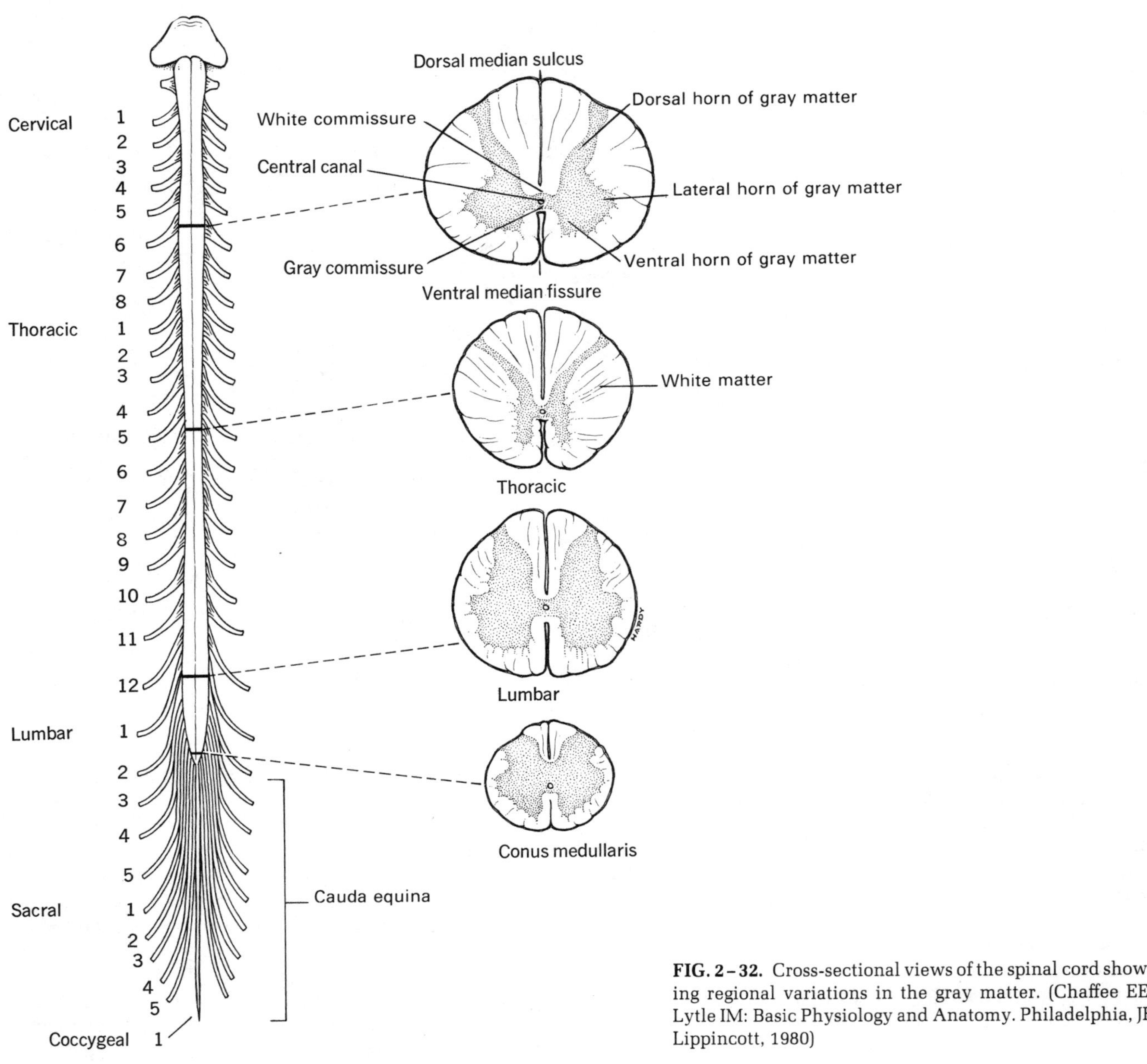

FIG. 2-32. Cross-sectional views of the spinal cord showing regional variations in the gray matter. (Chaffee EE, Lytle IM: Basic Physiology and Anatomy. Philadelphia, JB Lippincott, 1980)

that this selective stimulation plays a role in directing one's attention to certain mental activities.

THE SPINAL CORD

The spinal cord is an elongated mass of nerve tissue that occupies the upper two thirds of the vertebral canal and usually measures 42 cm to 45 cm in length in the adult. The spinal cord extends from the upper borders of the atlas (first cervical vertebra) to the lower border of the first lumbar vertebra (Fig. 2-32). As the cord reaches the lower two levels of the thoracic region, the cord becomes tapered and is called the *conus medullaris*. A nonneural filament called the *filum terminale* continues caudally until it attaches to the second segment of the coccyx. The three meninges surround the spinal cord for protection.

THE SPINAL ROOTS

There are 31 pairs of spinal nerves exiting from the spinal cord (Fig. 2-33), including 8 cervical, 12 thoracic, 5 lumbar, 5 sacral, and 1 coccygeal. Each spinal nerve has a dorsal root by which afferent impulses enter the cord, and a ventral root by which efferent impulses leave the spinal cord. The first pair of cervical spinal nerves leaves the cord above the C-1 vertebra, and C-2 through C-7 spinal nerves leave by way of the intervertebral foramina, above their corresponding vertebrae. Since there are seven vertebrae and eight pairs of spinal nerves, the C-8 spinal nerve

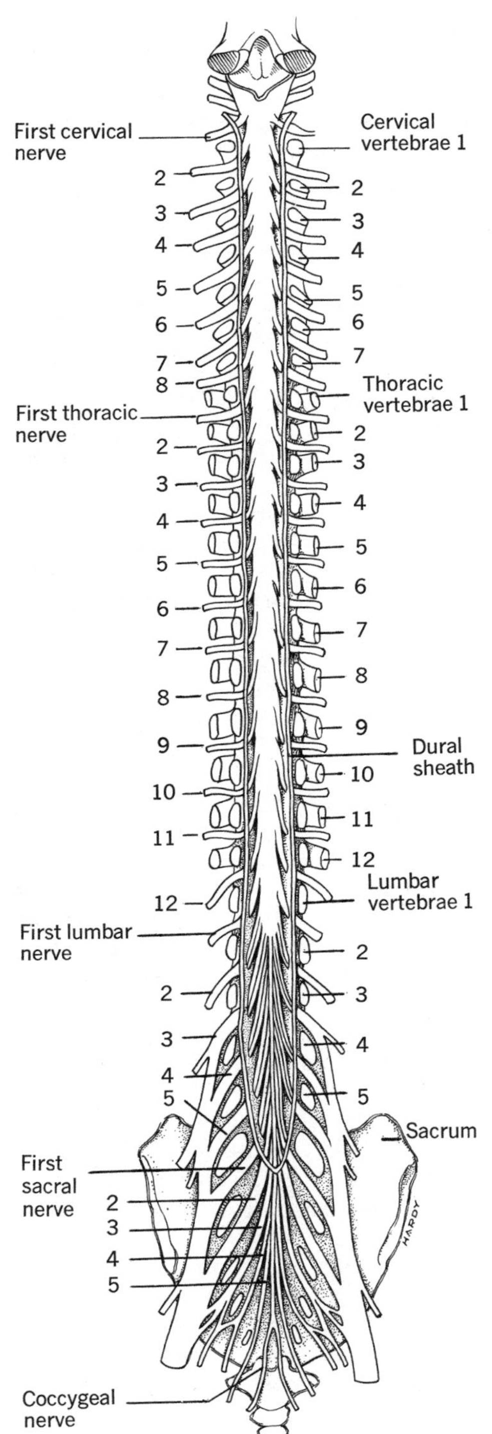

FIG. 2-33. Spinal cord lying within the vertebral canal. Spinal nerves are numbered on the left side; vertebrae are numbered on the right side. (Chaffee EE, Lytle IM: Basic Physiology and Anatomy. Philadelphia, JB Lippincott, 1980)

leaves the cord by way of the intervertebral foramina below the C-7 vertebra. All spinal nerves from T-1 to the caudal end of the cord leave by way of the foramina immediately below the corresponding vertebrae.

In the cervical region, the spinal nerves are almost on a horizontal plane with the corresponding vertebra; however, since the spinal cord is shorter than the vertebral column, the spinal nerves become increasingly oblique as they descend the spinal cord. The lumbar and sacral spinal nerves develop long roots, collectively referred to as the *cauda equina*.

There are two enlargements in the spinal cord to accommodate innervation to the extremities. The cervical (brachial) enlargement innervates the upper extremities and extends from the C-5 to the T-1 spinal levels. The lower extremities are innervated by the lumbosacral enlargement, which extends from L-3 to the S-2 level.

The Dorsal Roots (Posterior Roots)

The dorsal roots convey sensory input (afferent impulses) from skin segments that represent specific areas of the body known as *dermatomes*. There is considerable peripheral overlap between one dermatome and another so that no demonstrable sensory deficit will be found unless the sensory component of two or more spinal nerves is interrupted. Interruption of one sensory nerve root may result in paresthesia or pain in that dermatomal area. Afferent impulses are directed from the dermatomal area by way of the dorsal root to the dorsal root ganglia, in which the cell bodies of the sensory component are located. The sensory fibers are of two types: (1) *general somatic afferent* fibers (GSA), which carry sensory impulses for pain, temperature, touch, and proprioception from the body wall, tendons, and joints; and (2) *general visceral afferent* fibers (GVA), which carry sensory impulses from the organs within the body. See Table 2-6.

The Ventral Roots (Anterior Roots)

The ventral roots convey motor impulses (efferent impulses) from the spinal cord to the body. The motor fibers are of two types: (1) *general somatic efferent* fibers (GSE), which innervate voluntary striated muscles and have axons originating from the alpha and gamma motor neurons of lamina IX; and (2) *general visceral efferent* fibers (GVE), which innervate smooth and cardiac muscle and

TABLE 2-6. *Sensory Nerve Roots and Area Innervated*

Dorsal (Sensory) Spinal Root	*Area of the Body Innervated*
C-2	Back of the head
C-4	Around lower neck and upper thorax in the form of a collar
C-6	Radial aspect of lower arm and thumb
T-1	Upper chest and lower arm on side of small finger (includes small finger)
T-4	Nipple line
T-10	Umbilical region
L-1	Groin region
L-3	Knee cap
L-5	Anterior lower leg and anterior foot
S-3	Medial thigh
S-4, S-5	Perianal region

TABLE 2–7. *Motor Nerve Roots and Muscle Action*

Ventral (Motor Nerve Roots)	*Action of Muscles Innervated*
C–5, C–6	Moves shoulders and flexes elbow
T–1 through T–7	Controls intercostal muscles
T–6 through T–12	Controls abdominal muscles
L–1 through L–3	Flexes hip
L–5, S–1	Everts foot
S–1, S–2	Plantar flexes foot
S–3 through S–5	Controls perianal muscles

also regulate glandular secretion. Impulses to the motor end-plate of voluntary muscle fibers are conveyed by alpha motor neurons; impulses to the motor end-plates of intrafusal muscle cells of the neuromuscular spindles are conveyed by gamma motor neurons. These motor neurons (alpha, gamma) are called lower motor neurons. The preganglionic fibers of the autonomic nervous system are GVE fibers. The following is a list that indicates motor innervation to specific muscle groups. See Table 2–7.

Classification of Nerve Fibers

Nerve fibers can be classified by various criteria, including the diameter of the fiber, thickness of the myelin sheath, and speed of conduction of the impulse. Large fibers conduct impulses quickly, and the thicker the myelin sheath, the faster the speed of the impulse conductivity.

Sensory fibers are classified into group I through group IV, depending on their conduction velocities. Group I fibers most quickly conduct impulses, while group IV fibers have the slowest velocity. Group I is further divided to include I_a fibers (primary sensory endings of the neuromuscular spindles) and I_b fibers (from Golgi tendon organs). Group II conveys sensation from the myelinated skin and joint receptors. Groups III and IV convey impulses from nonmyelinated fibers. Another system uses the capital letters A, B, and C to classify both sensory and motor fibers. Type A is either a small, lightly myelinated sensory fiber for touch, pressure, pain, and temperature, or alpha or gamma motor neurons of lamina IX. The greatest diameter and velocity are characteristic of Type A fibers. Type B has a smaller diameter and is a lightly myelinated preganglionic motor fiber. Type C has a small diameter and is unmyelinated. They include motor postganglionic fibers and sensory fibers for pain and temperature.

PLEXUSES

A *plexus* is a network of interlacing nerves. Sometimes a plexus is formed by the primary branches of the nerves as the cervical, brachial, lumbar, and sacral plexuses (Fig. 2–34). Other plexuses are formed by the terminal funiculi at the periphery. There are four major plexuses noted in most texts. They include the following:

1. The *cervical plexus* is formed from the ventral branches of the first four cervical nerves of the spine. The resulting branches innervate the muscles of the neck and shoulders. This plexus also gives rise to the phrenic nerve, which supplies the diaphragm.
2. The *brachial plexus* is composed of the ventral branches of the lower four cervical and first thoracic spinal nerves. Important nerves that emerge from this plexus are the radial and ulnar nerves.
3. The *lumbar plexus* originates from the ventral branches of the twelfth thoracic and the first four lumbar nerves of the spine. The femoral nerve arises from this plexus.
4. The *sacral plexus* arises from the ventral branches of the last two lumbar and first four sacral nerves of the spine. The sciatic nerve arises from this plexus.

THE SPINAL CORD IN CROSS SECTION

When a cross section is viewed, the spinal cord appears to be a gray H surrounded by white matter. The *gray matter* consists of cell bodies, neuron projections (axons and dendrites), and glial cells. *White matter* includes longitudinal nerve projections, some of which are myelinated. Each funiculus (column) contains ascending and descending tracts (Fig. 2–35). There are two midline sulci, the anterior median sulcus and the posterior median sulcus. The lateral surface contains both a posterolateral and anterolateral sulcus that serve to divide the white matter into the anterior, lateral, and posterior funiculi.

Cross sections of the cord at various levels show striking differences in the shape and extent of gray and white matter. The gray matter of the cord contains the posterior (dorsal) and anterior (ventral) horns. Lateral horns are smaller in the thoracic and upper lumbar segments because the muscle mass of the trunk is less than that of the extremities, and these horns are made up largely of cell bodies of neurons that innervate skeletal muscles. In the lumbosacral region, the anterior horns are larger than those of the cervical area because of the greater muscle mass in the lower extremities. There is more white matter, as compared with gray matter, in the cervical region than in the lumbosacral region. This difference exists because the white matter in the cervical region is made up of connecting fibers that span the entire spinal cord and the brain, while the white matter of the lumbosacral cord contains only fibers serving the caudal end of the cord.

On cross section the gray matter of the spinal cord has been divided into sections I through X, called the *laminae of Rexed* (Fig. 2–36). Each lamina extends the length of the cord. Numbering of the laminae begins at the most dorsal point of the posterior horn while lamina IX is located at the most ventral point of the anterior horn. Therefore, the posterior horn contains laminae I through VI. Cells receive and send information about sensory input from the spinal nerve. Lamina VII is located in the intermediate gray zone and extends into the anterior horn. Within this area is the nucleus dorsalis and the intermediolateral gray columns. The anterior horn contains laminae VIII and IX. Lamina VIII contains neurons that send commissural axons to the opposite side of the cord. Lamina IX contains alpha and gamma motor neurons that innervate skeletal muscles. The area surrounding the central canal is the site of lamina X.

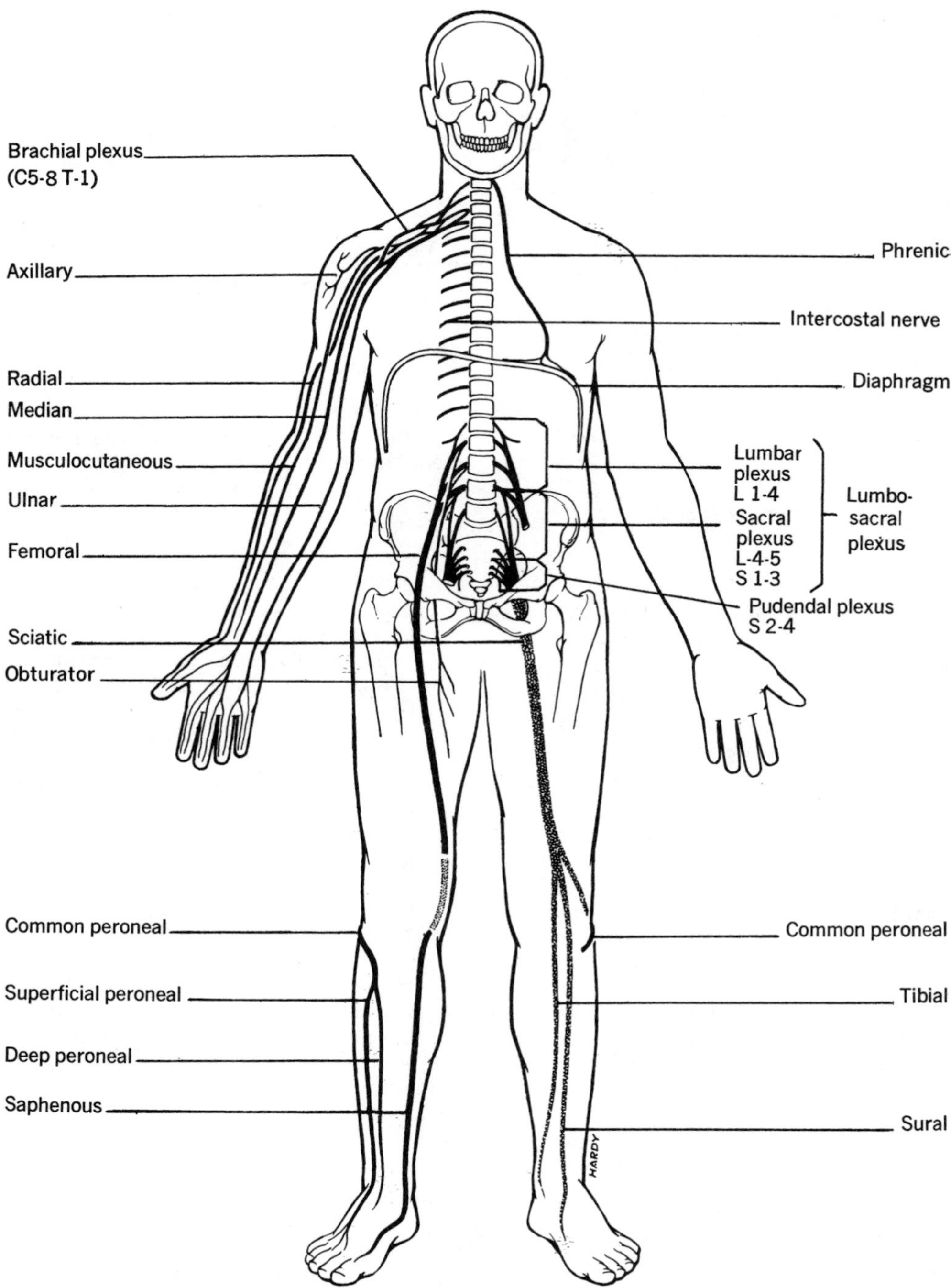

FIG. 2–34. Distribution of certain peripheral nerves, anterior aspect. (Chaffee EE, Lytle IM: Basic Physiology and Anatomy. Philadelphia, JB Lippincott, 1980)

THE MOTOR SYSTEM

The primary motor, premotor, and prefrontal areas of the brain have already been briefly discussed. The motor system consists of descending fibers (Fig. 2–37). Voluntary muscle activity is the sum of neural responses upon the alpha and gamma motor neurons of the spinal cord and upon the motor portions of the cranial nerve nuclei. These neurons make the final connection with the muscle by way of the myoneural junction. These neurons are called the *lower motor neuron* or the *anterior horn motor neuron* (cell bodies located in the anterior horn of the spinal cord). Lower motor neurons are simultaneously located in both the central and peripheral nervous systems. The lower motor neurons are general somatic efferent (GSE) components of the spinal nerves and of cranial nerves III, IV, VI, and XII, and the special visceral efferent (SVE) components of cranial nerves V, VII, IX, X, and XI.

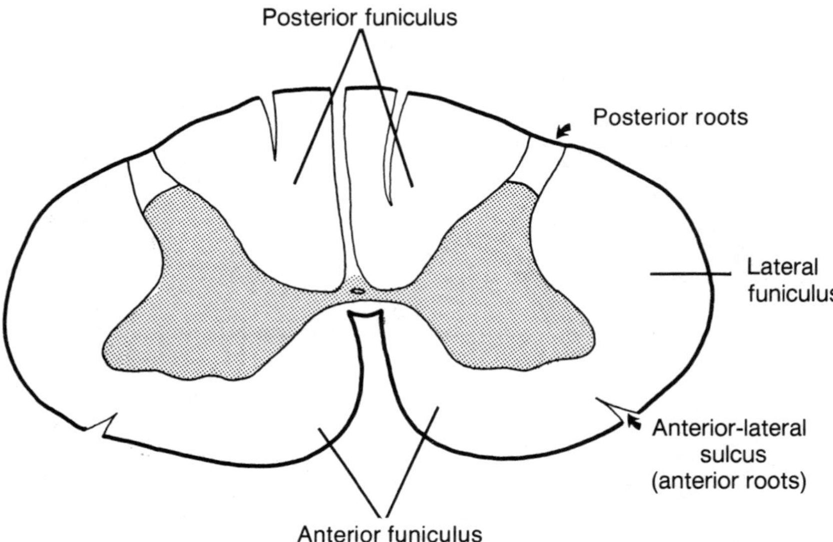

FIG. 2-35. The three funiculi of the spinal cord. (Curtis B et al: An Introduction to the Neurosciences. Philadelphia, WB Saunders, 1972)

There are many descending pathways located in the cerebral cortex, cerebellum, and basal ganglia that have inhibitory or facilitory influences on the lower motor neurons. The cells of these pathways act directly or indirectly upon both the alpha and gamma motor neurons, and motor components of the cranial nerve nuclei through internuncial neurons. These neurons, called *upper motor neurons*, are totally contained in the central nervous system. The following is a list and explanation of some major descending pathways originating from the cerebral cortex:

1. *The corticospinal (pyramidal) tract.* The corticospinal tracts originate in the cerebral cortex and descend through the posterior limb of the internal capsule, middle portion of the crus cerebri, midbrain, pons, and pyramids of the medulla. At the lower level of the medulla, the corticospinal tract crosses (decussates) to the opposite side. About 90% of the fibers cross at this level and become the *lateral corticospinal tract*. The lateral corticospinal tract is the most important upper motor neuron tract. The fibers of this tract terminate at all spinal levels in laminae IV through VII, and IX. The remaining 10% of the fibers do not cross but continue downward into the anterior funiculus of the cervical and upper thoracic cord levels as the *anterior corticospinal tract*. Decussation of the fibers occurs through the anterior white commissure before they enter and synapse with cells of lamina VIII.
2. *The corticobulbar tract.* The corticobulbar tract takes a route similar to the corticospinal tracts to the midbrain. The pathway terminates in the brain stem with the motor nuclei of the following cranial nerves: V (trigeminal), VII (facial), IX (glossopharyngeal), X (vagus), XI (accessory), and XII (hypoglossal). Only nuclei that innervate skeletal muscles are affected.
3. *The corticorubrospinal system.* The corticorubrospinal system gives rise to both the corticorubral and rubrospinal tracts. The tracts descend on the opposite side of the cord, synapsing with the anterior gray column. The rubrospinal tract facilitates flexor alpha and gamma motor neurons and inhibits extensor motor neurons. It also influences muscle tone and synergy.
4. *The corticoreticulospinal system.* The corticoreticulospinal sys-

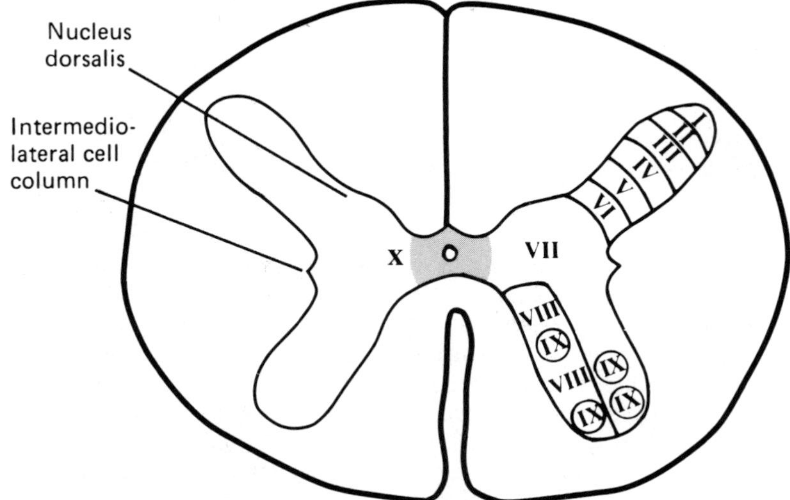

FIG. 2-36. Rexed's laminae of the spinal cord gray matter. (Adapted from Clark R: Manter and Gatz's Essentials of Clinical Neuroanatomy and Neurophysiology, 5th ed. Philadelphia, FA Davis, 1975)

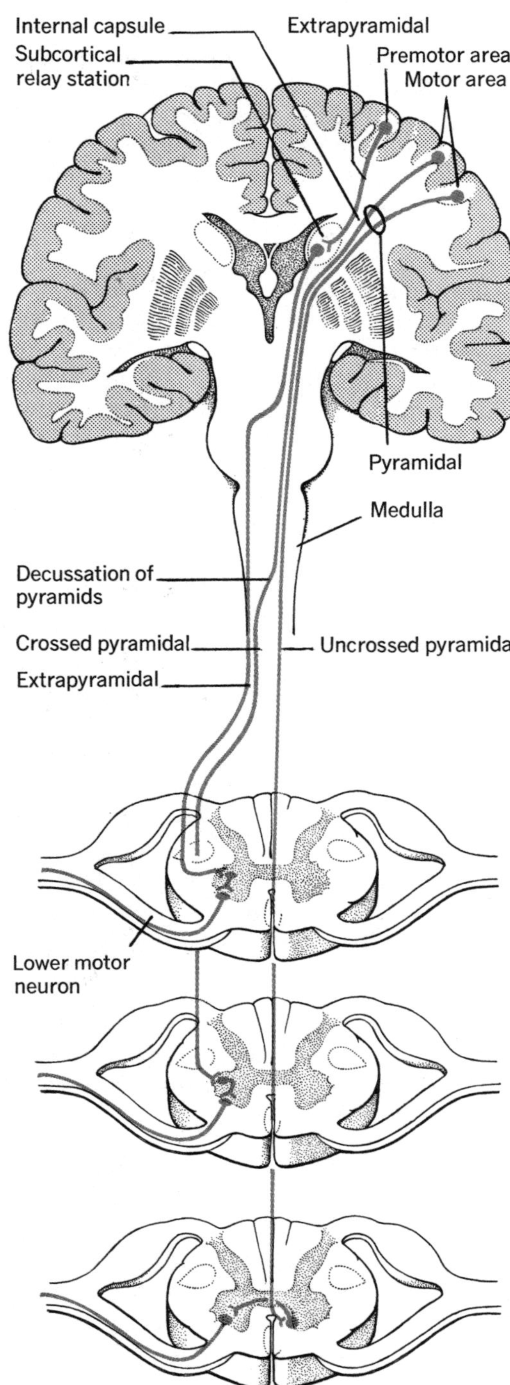

FIG. 2-37. Diagram of motor pathways between the cerebral cortex, one of the subcortical relay stations, and lower motor neurons in the spinal cord. Decussation (crossing) of fibers means that each side of the brain controls skeletal muscles on the opposite side of the body. (Chaffee EE, Lytle IM: Basic Physiology and Anatomy. Philadelphia, JB Lippincott, 1980)

tem, which originates in the pons and medulla, subdivides into the lateral (medullary) reticulospinal tract and the medial (pontine) reticulospinal tract. Collectively, these tracts influence the alpha and gamma motor neurons. The lateral reticulospinal tract exerts an inhibitory influence on the extensor myotactic reflexes and muscle tone, while the medial reticulospinal tract exerts a facilitory influence. The lateral tract also affects the intermediolateral cell column to influence respirations, circulation, sweating, and pupil dilation.

5. *The vestibulospinal system.* The vestibulospinal tract and medial vestibulospinal tract originate in the brain stem. The vestibulospinal tract is concerned with postural control, while the medial tract influences cranial nuclei III, IV, and VI for extraocular movement and visual reflexes. (The tectospinal tract also mediates visual reflexes.)

THE SENSORY SYSTEM

Sensory receptors are located throughout the body and convey afferent impulses for interpretation of stimuli. Sensory input may be integrated into spinal reflexes or it may be relayed to the higher centers of the brain by way of ascending pathways. The impulses are analyzed and can influence unconscious or conscious activities by way of efferent responses. There are various types of receptors that convey specific types of stimuli: *Exteroceptors* are stimulated by touch, light pressure, pain, temperature, odor, sound, and light; *proprioceptors* convey a sense of position, movement, and muscle coordination; *interoceptors* provide visceral information concerning pain, cramping, and fullness; *chemoreceptors* are stimulated by chemicals.

The pain and temperature pathways are so closely related throughout the body that they are treated collectively as one system. The *anterolateral system* is made up of the anterior spinothalamic, lateral spinothalamic, and spinoreticulothalamic tracts. These are the major tracts that convey pain and temperature sensation. The afferent impulse enters the cord by way of the posterolateral tract of Lissauer and crosses to the opposite side of the spinal cord. Impulses ascend the cord to terminate in the thalamus, with synapsing occurring within the reticular formation of the brain stem.

The posterior funiculus is totally enveloped by two ascending tracts—the fasciculus gracilis and fasciculus cuneatus. These tracts ascend the cord uncrossed until they reach the area of decussation in the medulla. After the fibers decussate in this area, they proceed initially to the thalamus and then to areas 1 through 3 of the cerebral cortex. These are the major tracts that convey the sensation of *proprioception*, which includes position and movement, vibration, two-point discrimination, deep pressure, and touch.

The anterior and posterior spinocerebellar tracts convey impulses of proprioception for the coordination of locomotion in the lower extremities. The cuneo- and rostrocerebellar tracts convey similar information from the upper half of the body.

THE AUTONOMIC NERVOUS SYSTEM

The autonomic nervous system—part of the peripheral nervous system—is made up of only motor neurons, collectively called the general visceral efferent (GVE) system. The autonomic nervous system regulates the activities of the viscera, which includes all smooth (involuntary) muscles, cardiac muscles, and glands (Fig. 2–38). The purpose of the autonomic system is to maintain a relatively stable internal environment for the body. The two major subdivisions of the autonomic nervous system are the sympathetic and parasympathetic systems.

The *sympathetic system* is activated during stress situations such as fright, fight, or flight phenomena. During these stressful periods, the heart rate and blood pressure increase, and there is vasoconstriction of the peripheral blood vessels.

The *parasympathetic system* stimulates those visceral activities associated with conservation, restoration, and maintenance of a normal functional level. The parasympathetic system would decrease heart rate and increase gastrointestinal activity.

Both divisions of the autonomic nervous system, which function in an antagonistic relationship, innervate most body organs. The autonomic nervous system is activated primarily by centers located in the spinal cord, brain stem, and hypothalamus. A two-neuron chain is characteristic of the autonomic nervous system. The cell bodies and their fibers are classified into the following two categories: (1) the *preganglionic neuron,* which is the primary neuron and is located in the brain stem or cord (intermediolateral gray column in the thoracic cord); and (2) the *postganglionic neuron,* which is the postsynaptic or secondary neuron located in the ganglia and innervating the end-organ.

THE SYMPATHETIC NERVOUS SYSTEM

The sympathetic system is also called the *thoracolumbar system* because its preganglionic fibers emerge from cell bodies in the intermediolateral nucleus of lamina VII, which extends through the thoracic and upper two lumbar levels (T–1 through L–2). These preganglionic fibers leave the spinal cord with the motor fibers of the ventral roots. After traveling less than 1 cm, the sympathetic fibers pass into the white rami communicantes—a branch of the spinal nerve—which, in turn, enters the sympathetic chain or trunk. (The sympathetic chain consists of a chain of ganglia located on either side of the spinal cord that extends from the base of the skull to the coccyx. These ganglia are all interconnected by longitudinal fibers, thus forming a continuous chain.) In the sympathetic chain, the fibers may synapse immediately with postganglionic fibers located in the chain at the level of entry (paravertebral ganglia); travel up or down the trunk to synapse in one of the chain ganglia above or below the point of entry; or pass on to synapse with a postganglionic neuron in an outlying sympathetic ganglion (prevertebral ganglion).

Some fibers from the postganglionic neuron in the sympathetic chain return to the spinal nerve by way of the gray rami communicantes at all levels of the spinal cord. Each spinal nerve receives a gray ramus, which controls the blood vessels, sweat glands, and piloerector muscles of the hairs.

Sympathetic fibers leave the spinal cord to enter the sympathetic chain in only the thoracic and upper lumbar regions; none enters the chain in the cervical, lower lumbar, or sacral regions. Sympathetic innervation to the head is supplied by sympathetic fibers extending from the thoracic chain. In this way, the neck and all structures of the head are innervated. Sympathetic fibers also pass downward from the sympathetic chain into the lower abdomen and legs.

The sympathetic outflow is distributed in the following way: T–1 to T–5 innervate the head, creating three ganglia (superior cervical, middle cervical, and cervicothoracic stellate); of those sympathetic fibers directed to the head, those from T–1 and T–2 innervate the eye for pupillary dilation; T–2 through T–6 innervate the heart and lungs; and T–6 through L–2 innervate the abdominal viscera through the thoracic and lumbar splanchnic nerves. The thoracic splanchnic nerves carry the preganglionic fibers to the prevertebral ganglia of the abdomen. The celiac, superior mesenteric, and aorticorenal ganglia arise in this area. The lumbar splanchnic nerves terminate in the inferior mesenteric and hypogastric ganglia.

The preganglionic sympathetic nerve fibers pass directly to the adrenal medulla without synapsing. These fibers are cholinergic and end directly on the special cells of the medulla that secrete epinephrine and norepinephrine.

Sympathetic Neurotransmitter

The neurotransmitter released by the postganglionic fibers is norepinephrine (noradrenalin). This is why the sympathetic system is termed *adrenergic.* Acetylcholine is secreted at the preganglionic terminal and quickly deactivated by cholinesterase. (There are few exceptions in the postganglionic neurons in the sympathetic nervous system.) Some blood vessels in skeletal muscles and most sweat glands in the palms of the hands have adrenergic postganglionic neurons.

THE PARASYMPATHETIC NERVOUS SYSTEM

The parasympathetic system is also called the *craniosacral system* because its preganglionic fibers emerge with cranial nerves III, VII, IX, and X. The specific parasympathetic innervation to these cranial nerves includes the following:

1. Oculomotor (III)—supplies the ciliary muscles for accommodation and constrictor sphincter muscles of the pupil
2. Facial (VII)—innervates many glands of the head such as lacrimal, submandibular, sublingual, nasal, oral, and pharyngeal
3. Glossopharyngeal (IX)—innervates the parotid glands
4. Vagus (X)—synapses with terminal ganglia located adjacent to, or within, the various viscera throughout the body

The sacral portion of the parasympathetic system arises from cell bodies in the intermediate gray matter of sacral segments S–2 through S–4. These fibers pass through the pelvic splanchnic nerve to synapse in the terminal ganglia with the postganglionic neurons, which innervate the descending colon, rectum, bladder, lower ureters, and external genitalia. The parasympathetic system is involved with

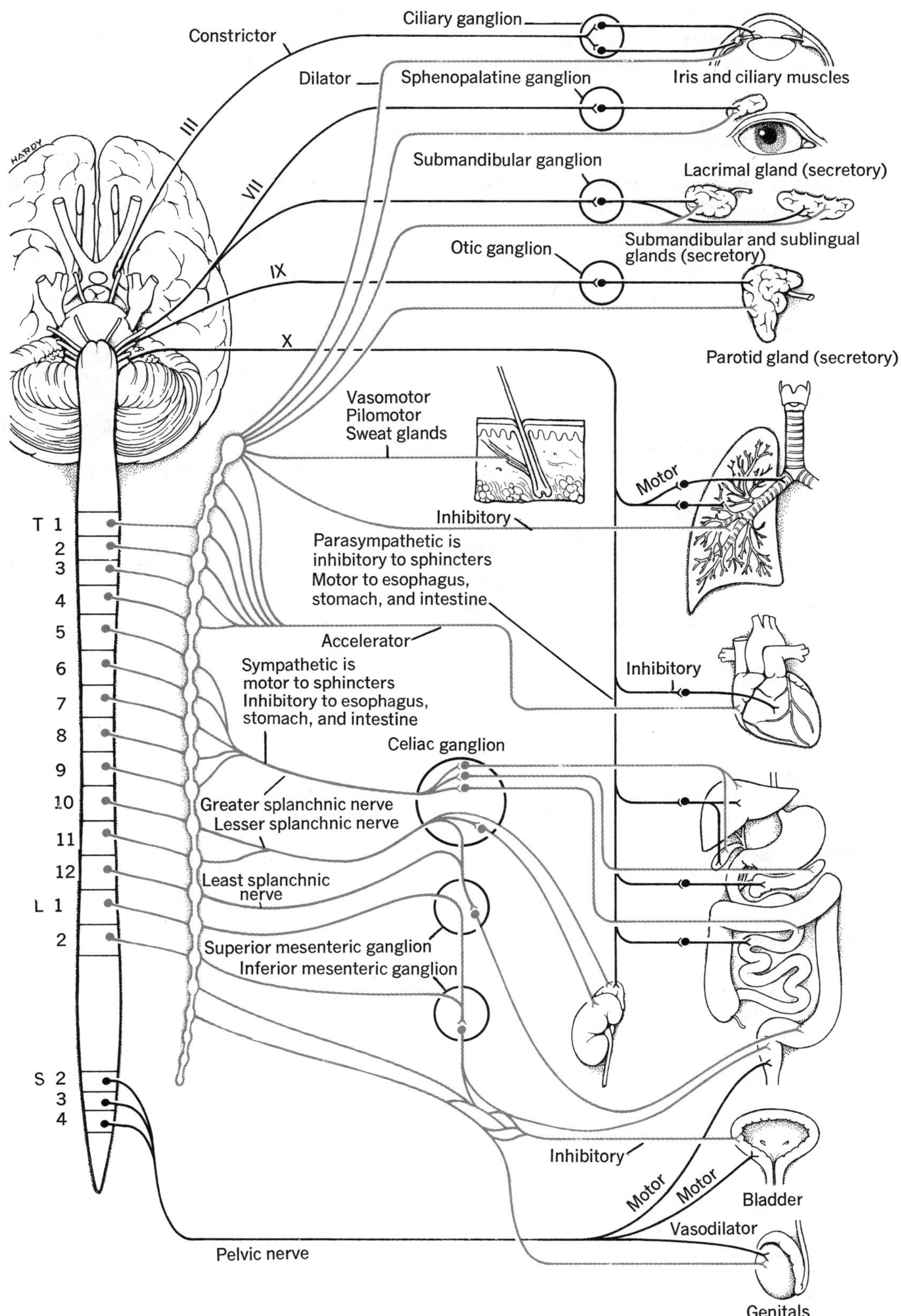

FIG. 2-38. Diagram of the autonomic nervous system, including parasympathetic or craniosacral fibers and sympathetic or thoracolumbar fibers. Note that most organs have a double nerve supply. (Chaffee EE, Lytle IM: Basic Physiology and Anatomy. Philadelphia, JB Lippincott, 1980)

the mechanisms of bladder and bowel evacuation and, unlike the sympathetic system, is designed to respond to a specific stimulus in a localized area for a short period of time.

Parasympathetic Neurotransmitters

The parasympathetic system secretes acetylcholine at the postganglionic neuron. This is why the parasympathetic system is termed *cholinergic*. Acetylcholine is also secreted at the preganglionic neuron and is quickly deactivated by cholinesterase.

Table 2–8 summarizes the effects of the sympathetic and parasympathetic systems on specific structures.

SPINAL REFLEXES

A *reflex* is a stereotypic response, mediated by the nervous system, to a particular stimulus of sufficient magnitude. A *reflex arc* refers to the afferent and efferent limbs involved in the completion of a reflex loop (see Fig. 2–38). Reflexes can be classified by the extent of the regional involvement of the spinal cord. This classification includes segmental, intersegmental, and suprasegmental reflexes.

A reflex whose arc passes through only one anatomical segment is called a *segmental reflex*. A knee-jerk reflex is an example of both a segmental and simple or monosynaptic reflex. A monosynaptic reflex includes an afferent limb that synapses directly with an efferent limb. Most reflexes, however, are more complex and polysynaptic.

An *intersegmental reflex* involves several spinal segments. A flexor or withdrawal reflex is an example of an intersegmental reflex.

A *suprasegmental reflex* involves interaction between the brain centers that regulate cord activity and the segments of the cord itself. An example of a suprasegmental reflex is extension of the legs in response to movement of the head.

Another classification of reflexes that has been useful for

TABLE 2–8. *Autonomic Effects of the Nervous System*

Structure or Activity	*Parasympathetic Effects*	*Sympathetic Effects*
Pupil of the Eye	Constricted	Dilated
The Circulatory System		
Rate and force of heartbeat	Decreased	Increased
Blood vessels:		
In heart muscle	Constricted	Dilated
In skeletal muscle	*	Dilated
In abdominal viscera and the skin	*	Constricted
Blood pressure	Decreased	Increased
The Respiratory System		
Branchioles	Constricted	Dilated
Rate of breathing	Decreased	Increased
The Digestive System		
Peristaltic movements of digestive tube	Increased	Decreased
Muscular sphincters of digestive tube	Relaxed	Contracted
Secretion of salivary glands	Thin, watery saliva	Thick, viscid saliva
Secretions of stomach, intestine, and pancreas	Increased	*
Conversion of liver glycogen to glucose	*	Increased
The Genitourinary System		
Urinary bladder:		
Muscular walls	Contracted	Relaxed
Sphincters	Relaxed	Contracted
Muscles of the uterus	Relaxed; variable	Contracted under some conditions; varies with menstrual cycle and pregnancy
Blood vessels of external genitalia	Dilated	*
The Integument		
Secretion of sweat	*	Increased
Pilomotor muscles	*	Contracted (gooseflesh)
Medullae of Adrenal Glands	*	Secretion of epinephrine and norepinephrine

* No direct effect

(Chaffee EE, Lytle IM: Basic Physiology and Anatomy, 3rd ed. Philadelphia, JB Lippincott, 1980) clinical investigation divides reflexes into stretch, cutaneous and pathological reflexes.

A muscle *stretch reflex* is elicited by striking a tendon that stretches the neuromuscular spindles of the muscle group. The knee-jerk reflex, a stretch reflex, results in contraction of the quadriceps and extension of the leg in response to tapping the patellar tendon. Other common stretch reflexes involve the biceps, the triceps, and ankle. (Muscle stretch reflexes are also termed deep tendon and extensor reflexes.)

Cutaneous reflexes, also termed superficial reflexes, result when the skin is stimulated and a response is observed in a related muscle group. The withdrawal reflex, which is a flexor reflex, is an example of a cutaneous reflex that is protective in nature. In response to a noxious stimulus to the skin on the fingers, the hand is flexed and removed (Fig. 2–39). Another cutaneous reflex is contraction of the superficial abdominal muscles in response to light, rapid stroking of the skin on the abdomen.

The last classification consists of the pathological reflexes, found only when neurological disease is present. A Babinski reflex is a common pathological reflex.

MUSCLE TONE

A muscle normally possesses a minimal amount of residual tension even though it appears to be relaxed. By palpation, some resiliency, rather than complete flabbiness, can be felt. During passive movement of a joint, some resistance is encountered. This is termed *muscle tone.* It is believed that skeletal muscle tone results from nerve impulses from the spinal cord. Muscle spindles, sensory stretch receptors in the muscles, and cortical impulses contribute to the spinal response for tone. Neurological disease can alter the muscle tone that is so vital for normal motor function.

MICTURITION

Micturition is the process of evacuating the bladder when it has collected a certain amount of urine. In the infant bladder, evacuation is a purely reflex act, but early in childhood the motor control of the urinary bladder is brought under voluntary control.

The urinary bladder is composed of smooth muscle.

FIG. 2–39. Diagram of a flexor reflex *(above)* and a stretch reflex *(below).* (Chaffee EE, Lytle IM: Basic Physiology and Anatomy. Philadelphia, JB Lippincott, 1980)

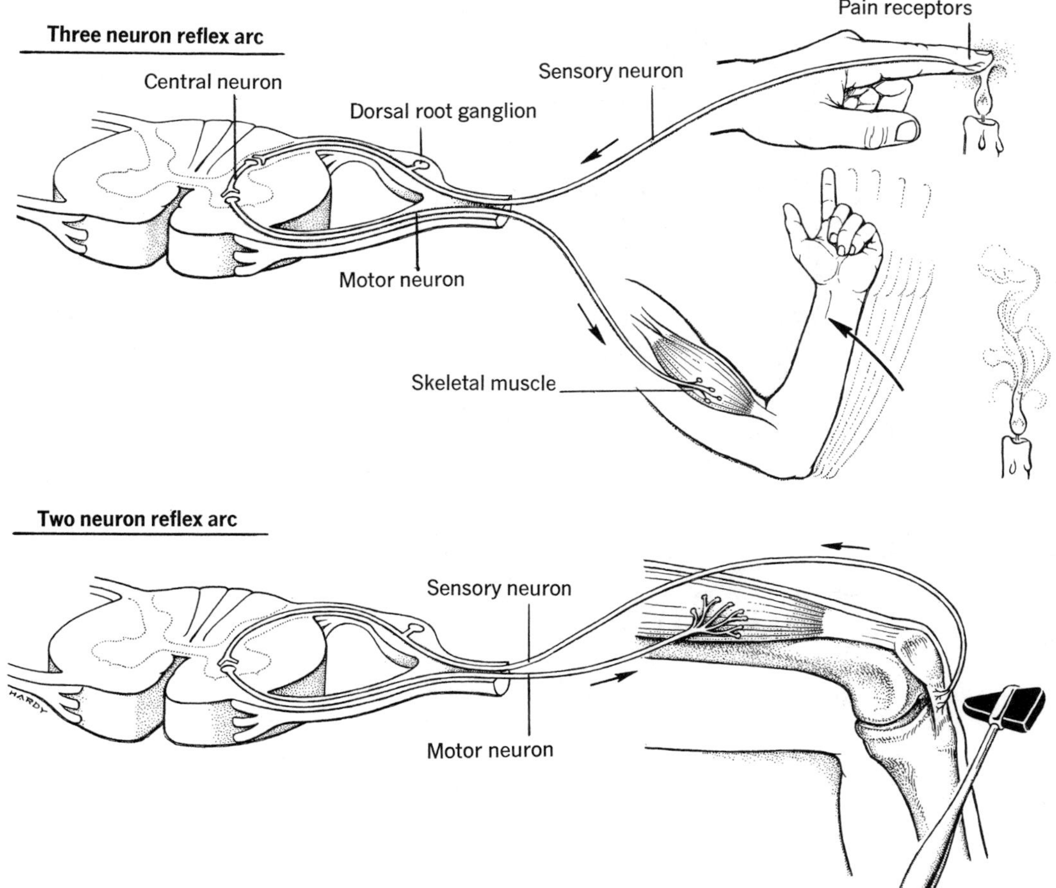

There are two main anatomical parts to the bladder: (1) the body, which is the *detrusor muscle;* and (2) the *trigone,* a small triangular area at the base of the bladder that contains the bladder–ureter junction and the urethra. It also contains the internal sphincter of the bladder, which is an involuntary muscle. An external sphincter (a voluntary skeletal muscle) is located at the opening of the bladder and is normally contracted to prevent dribbling.

The micturition center is located in S–2, S–3, and S–4 spinal segments, from which the preganglionic parasympathetic fibers synapse within the ganglia located in the bladder wall by way of the pelvic splanchnic nerves (Fig. 2–40). Short postganglionic parasympathetic fibers innervate both the detrusor muscle and internal sphincter. Parasympathetic stimulation that is caused by the stretching of the bladder wall results in contraction of the detrusor muscle and relaxation of the internal sphincter. Although there is some sympathetic innervation to the bladder, its role is not certain. Micturition is primarily a parasympathetic function.

The external sphincter is under voluntary control and is mediated by the pudendal nerve. It can be voluntarily contracted, but it relaxes by reflex action when urine is released from the internal sphincter.

DEFECATION

The act of evacuating the bowel is called *defecation.* During infancy it is a purely reflex action; however, in early childhood voluntary control of the lower bowel is learned so that defecation can be postponed until the person is in a socially acceptable place to evacuate his bowel. Two sphincters that are normally contracted control the anus: the internal anal sphincter, which is composed of smooth muscle and situated inside the anus; and the external anal sphincter, a voluntary striated muscle that is located slightly more caudal.

The defecation reflex evacuates the lower bowel. Feces in the rectum stimulate stretch receptors that send afferent impulses to initiate peristaltic waves in the descending colon, sigmoid, and rectum, thereby propelling feces toward the anus. The peristaltic waves relax the internal sphincter. If the external sphincter is relaxed, bowel evac-

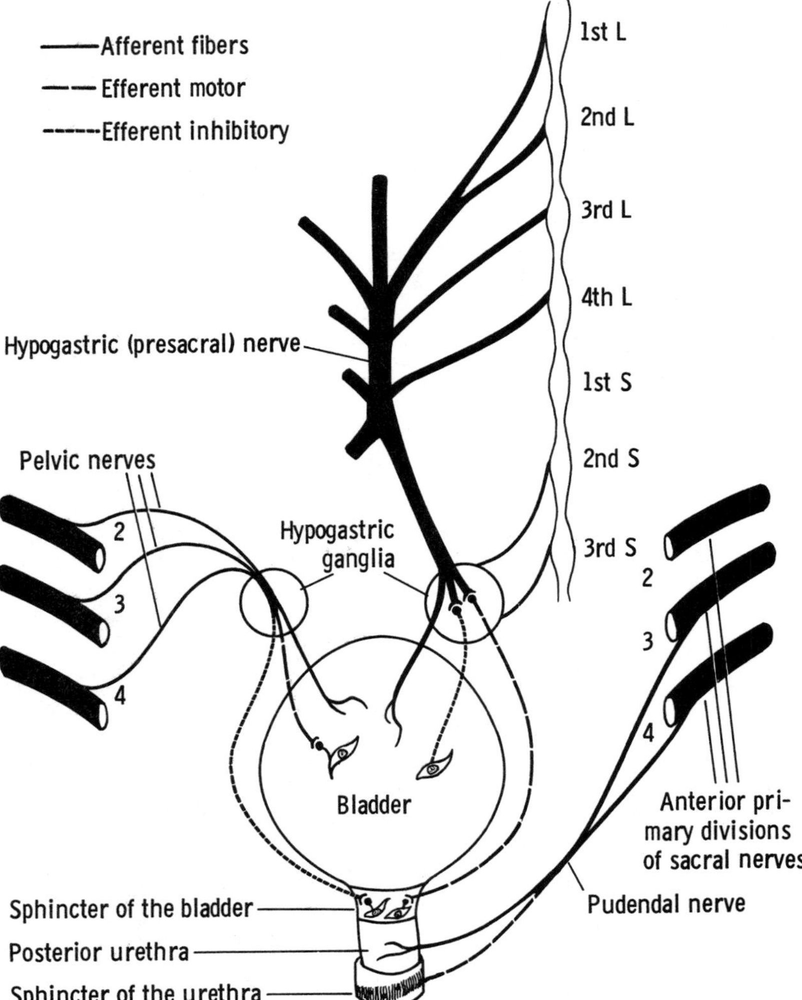

FIG. 2–40. Diagrammatic representation of innervation of the bladder and urethra. (Chaffee EE, Lytle IM: Basic Physiology and Anatomy. Philadelphia, JB Lippincott, 1980)

uation will occur. The defecation reflex is a weak reflex and requires other neural stimulation for effective defecation.

When afferent impulses are created in response to stimulated stretch receptors, the impulse ascends the cord and reflexly involves S–3, S–4, and S–5. The parasympathetic response greatly intensifies the peristaltic waves in the descending colon, sigmoid, and rectum, causing a powerful bowel evacuation if the person relaxes the external sphincter.

THE CRANIAL NERVES

There are 12 pairs of cranial nerves that are considered to be part of the peripheral nervous system. The cranial nerves are numbered by Roman numerals, the first cranial nerve being located most anteriorly in the frontal lobe, and the twelfth being located most posteriorly in the medulla (Fig. 2–41). Cranial nerves are classified as sensory (S), motor (M), or autonomic (A). Some nerves have fibers that are mentioned in more than one classification (Table 2–9).

OLFACTORY (I) NERVE (SENSORY)

The olfactory nerve deals with the sense of smell, a poorly understood sense. The olfactory membrane is located in the superior part of each nostril. The bipolar chemoreceptor cells, called olfactory cells, are composed of hairlike filaments that terminate in the olfactory bulb. From the bulb, the olfactory tract continues backward to the base of the frontal lobes where the two principal areas, the medial olfactory area and the lateral olfactory area, are located. The medial olfactory area is located anteriorly and superiorly to the hypothalamus (septum pellucidum, gyrus subcallosus, para-olfactory area, olfactory trigone, and medial part of the anterior perforated substance). The lateral olfactory area is composed of the prepyriform area, the uncus, the lateral part of the anterior perforated substance, and part of the amygdaloid nucleus. Tumors in the uncal–amygdaloid area result in an abnormal perception of smell.

OPTIC (II) NERVE (SENSORY)

The optic nerve arises from the retina of the eyeball. The retina and anterior optic nerve head are called the *fundus* or *optic disc.* The fundus can be visualized by using the ophthalmoscope (it is the only cranial nerve that can be visualized).

The optic nerve runs posteriorly until it meets another optic nerve at the optic chiasma. The optic nerves deal with the complex process of vision. Vision is considered complex not only because many steps are involved in the process but also because the tracts are dispersed throughout the many anatomical parts of the cerebral hemisphere. The visual system is presented to provide a basic understanding because many patients with neurological problems have visual impairment.

The Visual Pathways

The rods and cones of the retina are the photoreceptors that are stimulated by light, thereby initiating nerve impulses that are conducted to the cerebral cortex (Fig. 2–42). The visual pathways posterior to the retina include the following:

1. The optic nerves come together at the optic chiasma, which is located anterior to the sella turcica. A partial decussation takes place at the chiasma whereby the nasal half of each optic nerve crosses to the other side.

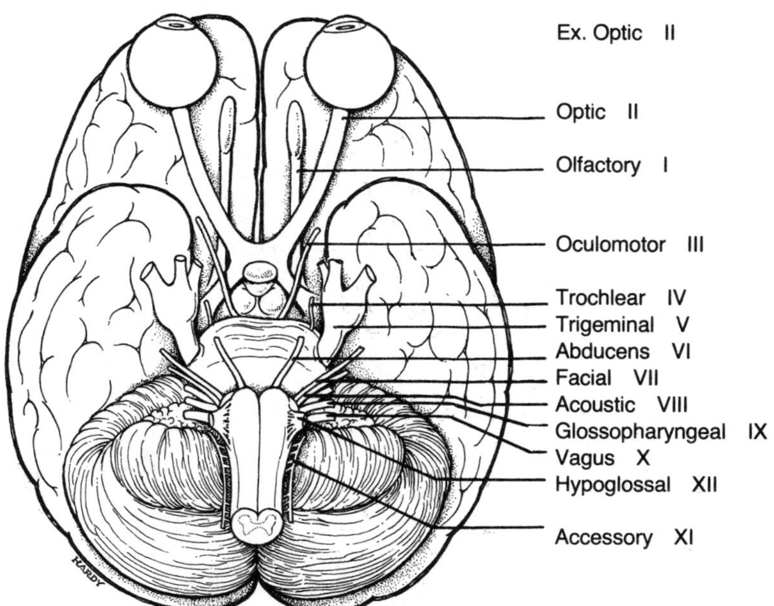

FIG. 2–41. Base of brain showing entrance or exit of cranial nerves. The eyeballs are shown schematically in relation to the optic nerves.

TABLE 2-9. *Functions of Cranial Nerves*

Number	Name	Structures Innervated by Efferent Components	Structures Innervated by Afferent Components	Functions
I	Olfactory	None	Olfactory mucous membrane	Nerve of smell
II	Optic	None	Retina of eye	Nerve of vision
III	Oculomotor	Superior, medial, inferior recti; inferior oblique; levator palpebrae superioris; ciliary; sphincter of iris	Same muscles (muscle sense)	Motor and muscle sense to various muscles listed; accommodation to different distances; regulates the amount of light reaching retina; most important nerve in eye movements
IV	Trochlear	Superior oblique	Same muscle	Motor and muscle sense to superior oblique; eye movements
V	Trigeminal	Muscles of mastication	Skin and mucous membranes in head; teeth; same muscles	Nerve of pain, touch, heat, cold to skin and mucous membranes listed; same for teeth; movements of mastication and muscle sense
VI	Abducens	Lateral rectus	Same muscle	Motor and muscle sense to lateral rectus; eye movements
VII	Facial	Submaxillary and sublingual glands; muscles of face, scalp, and a few others	Same muscles; taste buds of anterior two thirds of tongue	Taste to anterior two thirds of tongue; secretory and vasodilator to two salivary glands; motor and muscle sense to facial and a few other muscles
VIII	Acoustic (cochlear and vestibular portions)	None	Cochlear organ of Corti. Vestibular-semicircular canals, utricle, and saccule	Cochlear division is nerve of hearing; vestibular division is concerned with registering movement of the body through space and with the position of the head
IX	Glossopharyngeal	Superior pharyngeal constrictor; stylopharyngeus muscle; parotid gland	Taste buds of posterior one third of tongue; parts of pharynx; carotid sinus and body; stylopharyngeus muscle	Taste to posterior one third of tongue and adjacent regions; secretory and vasodilator to parotid gland; motor and muscle sense to stylopharyngeus; pain, touch, heat, and cold to pharynx; afferent in circulatory and respiratory reflexes.
X	Vagus	Muscles of pharynx, larynx, esophagus, thoracic and abdominal viscera; coronary arteries; walls of bronchi; pancreas; gastric glands	Same muscles; skin of external ear; mucous membranes of larynx, trachea, esophagus; thoracic and abdominal viscera; arch of aorta; atria; great veins	Secretory to gastric glands and pancreas; inhibitory to heart; motor to alimentary tract; motor and muscle sense to muscles of larynx and pharynx; constrictor to coronaries; motor to muscle in walls of bronchi; important in respiratory, cardiac, and circulatory reflexes
XI	Accessory	Sternocleidomastoid and trapezius muscles; muscles of larynx	Same muscles	Motor and muscle sense to muscles listed; shares certain function of vagus
XII	Hypoglossal	Muscles of tongue	Same muscles	Motor and muscle sense to muscles of tongue; important in speech, mastication, and deglutition

(Chaffee EE, Lytle IM: Basic Physiology and Anatomy, 3rd ed. Philadelphia, JB Lippincott, 1980)

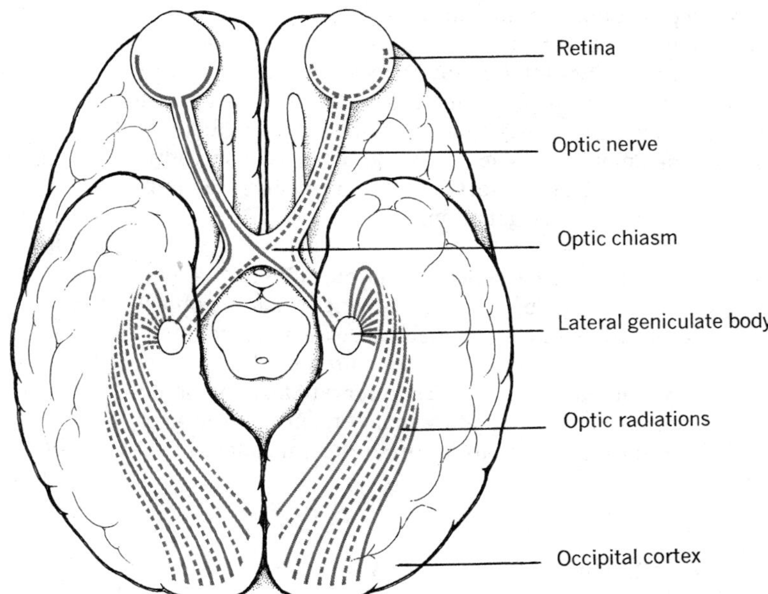

FIG. 2-42. Diagram of optic pathways. Note the crossing of fibers from the medial half of each retina. (Chaffee EE, Lytle IM: Basic Physiology and Anatomy. Philadelphia, JB Lippincott, 1980)

2. The optic tracts project backward from the chiasma and terminate in the lateral geniculate of the thalamus.
3. Fibers of the geniculocalcarine tract (optic radiation) originate from the cells of the geniculate bodies.
4. The geniculocalcarine tract fans backward to the primary optic cortex of area 17 of the occipital lobe.
5. Fibers also project into the visual association areas (18 and 19) of the occipital lobe. Visual reflexes also originate in the visual association area.

Terminology

Several terms help to identify anatomical areas and concepts and make the visual process easier to understand. The following is a list of helpful definitions for the reader:

1. Visual field—the field of vision
2. Macula lutea—a 3-mm circular area on the retina located near the posterior pole of the orbit that is the point of clearest vision
3. Hemiretina—identifies one half of the retina when a vertical line divides the retina into temporal (lateral) and nasal (medial) portions. The hemiretina can be further divided by the use of a horizontal line that divides the retina into four equal quadrants.
4. Optic disc—a natural blind spot because it does not contain any rods or cones. It also is called the *fundus* and is the point at which the optic nerve joins the retina. The optic disc is examined with an ophthalmoscope.
5. Scotoma—a blind spot on the retina. There is an expected blind spot at the optic disc because of lack of rods and cones located 15 degrees lateral to the central point of vision.
6. Bitemporal heteronymous hemianopsia—blindness in each temporal part of the retina
7. Homonymous hemianopsia—loss of vision on the same side of both visual fields
8. Homonymous—the same side of the visual field is affected
9. Heteronymous—the temporal or nasal portions are affected in each visual field

Visual Reflexes

There are a few visual reflexes important in the evaluation of visual function. They are included in this section even though other cranial nerves are involved in the reflex.

The Light Reflex. The light reflex refers to the constriction of the pupil when a light is shone into that pupil. The response in the stimulated pupil is termed the *direct reflex*. There is also a somewhat weaker constriction of the unstimulated pupil, called the *consensual light reflex*. The receptors for this reflex are the rods and cones of the retina. The impulse follows the normal visual pathway as far as the lateral geniculate bodies. The reflex fibers do not enter the geniculate body but rather enter the pretectum area (near the superior colliculus). Connecting neurons send their axons around the aqueduct of Sylvius to the oculomotor nucleus (Edinger-Westphal nucleus) located in the midbrain. In this nucleus, parasympathetic fibers proceed to the ciliary ganglion. Postganglionic parasympathetic fibers supply the constrictor muscles of the iris, resulting in constriction of the pupil. The consensual response is due to the fibers that cross both the optic chiasma and the posterior commissure of the midbrain.

Pupillary Dilation. Pupillary dilation is the result of sympathetic innervation of the pupil, originating in the intermediolateral horn cells that pass to the superior cervical ganglion. There is synapsing with the postganglionic sympathetic fibers that innervate the pupillary dilator fibers of the iris, resulting in dilation of the pupil.

Accommodation Reflex. The thickening or elongation of the lens by the contraction or relaxation of the ciliary mucles in response to focusing on a nearby or distant object is termed *accommodation*. Impulses follow the visual pathway to the visual cortex (area 17). Neurons from the visual cortex connect with the midbrain and the oculomotor nucleus (Edinger–Westphal nucleus). Neurons in the nucleus synapse with the postganglionic fiber of the ciliary ganglion. The smooth muscles of the ciliary body controlling the lens tension are innervated by the parasympathetic neurons of the ciliary ganglion.

Near-Point or Convergence Reaction. When the eyes focus on a nearby object after viewing a distant object, there is a rapid reflex adjustment necessary to accommodate this change. The lens thickens to properly focus on the image, the medial recti muscles innervated by the oculomotor nerves contract to allow convergence of the eyes, and the pupils constrict to increase the sharpness of the image.

THE OCULOMOTOR (III) NERVE (MOTOR, AUTONOMIC)

The oculomotor nerve innervates four of the six muscles responsible for movement of the eyeball. These muscles are the medial, superior and inferior recti and inferior oblique. The eyeballs are rotated by these muscles in the following manner: the medial recti, inward (medially); the superior recti, upward; the inferior recti, downward; and the inferior oblique, upward and outward.

In addition, the oculomotor nerve innervates the levator palpebrae superioris, which elevates the upper eyelid, and the muscles that constrict the pupils in response to light or to convergence and accommodation. Pupillary constriction, convergence, and accommodation have been discussed above.

TROCHLEAR (IV) NERVE (MOTOR)

The trochlear nerve supplies the superior oblique muscle of the eyeball, allowing for the rotation of the eyeball downward and inward.

TRIGEMINAL (V) NERVE (MOTOR, SENSORY)

The sensory components of the trigeminal nerve convey the sensations of pain, temperature, and touch for the supratentorial cranial cavity, the entire face and scalp to the vertex, the paranasal sinuses, and the nasal and oral cavities. The motor component supplies the muscles of mastication and the corneal reflex, a very important protective reflex. The jaw reflex is also controlled by the trigeminal motor component. The trigeminal nerve is divided into three branches: the ophthalmic, maxillary, and mandibular. The area of innervation for each branch is noted in Table 2–9.

The corneal reflex can be elicited by stroking the cornea lightly with a wisp of cotton. The normal response is a bilateral blink. The jaw reflex is a muscle stretch reflex observed by tapping the mandible of the partially open relaxed mouth. The normal response is a slight elevation of the mandible or no response at all.

ABDUCENS (VI) NERVE (MOTOR)

The abducens nerve innervates the lateral rectus muscle, which rotates the eyeball outward. The abducens nerve arises from the nucleus that is located beneath the fourth ventricle of the pons.

FACIAL (VII) NERVE (SENSORY, MOTOR)

The facial nerve, with its nuclei located in the pons, innervates all of the muscles involved in facial expression such as smiling, whistling, showing the teeth, wrinkling the nose and brow, closing the eyes, grimacing, and many other variations. The sensory component of the facial nerve innervates the anterior two thirds of the tongue and certain salivary and lacrimal glands. The lacrimal glands account for tearing and crying.

ACOUSTIC (VIII) NERVE (SENSORY)

The acoustic nerve is divided into two branches: the cochlear, which is concerned with hearing; and the vestibular, which influences balance, maintenance of body position, and orientation in space. Each system will be discussed briefly.

Auditory System

Vibrations proceed through the tympanic membrane and activate the three small bones of the middle ear (malleus, incus, and stapes). These vibrations then continue to the cochlea of the inner ear where the basilar membrane with the organs of Corti (hairlike mechanoreceptors) send fibers to the spiral ganglion. The spiral ganglion contains the bipolar cells of the cochlea that connect to the brain stem. The primary auditory receptive areas of the cortex are 41 and 42. From here, the impulses proceed to the auditory association area where recognition of the particular sound takes place.

Vestibular System

The vestibular receptor end-organs in the vestibular system include the three cristae ampullares, one located in each of the semicircular canals, and the maculae of the utricle and saccule. All of these structures are sensitive to movement in a particular direction. The vestibular ganglion of the vestibular nerve receives input from the vestibular receptors and the cerebellum. The vestibular nuclei have projections into the following areas:

1. Spinal cord by way of the lateral and medial vestibular spinal tracts (inhibitory and facilitory influence to extensor muscle tone and spinal reflexes)

2. Cerebellum
3. Brain stem (vestibulomesencephalic fiber for conjugate eye movement reflexes in response to head movement)
4. Medial geniculate body of the temporal cortex

Both the auditory and vestibular systems are anatomically and physiologically complex systems.

GLOSSOPHARYNGEAL (IX) NERVE (SENSORY, MOTOR)

The glossopharyngeal nerve has five branches. It innervates a portion of the pharyngeal muscles, conveys taste from the posterior third of the tongue, innervates the carotid sinus and carotid body, and conveys sensation from the mucous membranes of the tonsils and pharynx. There are also parasympathetic innervations of the parotid glands. The vagus nerve is closely related both anatomically and physiologically to the glossopharyngeal nerve. Both nerves originate from the medulla.

VAGUS (X) NERVE (SENSORY, MOTOR, AUTONOMIC)

The vagus nerve branches into several segments to innervate all of the organs of the thoracic and abdominal cavities and the larynx, pharynx, and palate. The vagus nerve is the efferent branch in the pharyngeal and palatal reflex. Sensation is conveyed from the heart, lungs, digestive tract, carotid sinus, and carotid body. Many parasympathetic fibers are part of the vagus nerve.

SPINAL ACCESSORY (XI) NERVE (MOTOR)

The two roots of the spinal accessory nerve originate in the lower medulla and upper cervical spinal cord. This nerve supplies the sternocleidomastoid and upper portion of the trapezius muscle and allows one to shrug the shoulder and rotate the head.

HYPOGLOSSAL (XII) NERVE (MOTOR)

The hypoglossal nerve innervates the tongue to provide for normal speech and swallowing, and it originates in the medulla.

BIBLIOGRAPHY

Brown D: Neurosciences for Allied Health Therapies. St Louis, CV Mosby, 1980

Chaplin J, Demers A: Primer of Neurology and Neurophysiology. New York, John Wiley & Sons, 1978

Chusid JG: Correlative Neuroanatomy and Functional Neurology, 18th ed. Los Altos, CA, Lange Medical Publications, 1982

Daube J, Sandok B: Medical Neurosciences—An Approach to Anatomy, Pathology, and Physiology by Systems and Levels. Boston, Little, Brown & Co, 1978

DiPalma J: Drill's Pharmacology in Medicine, 4th ed. New York, McGraw-Hill, 1971

Eliasson S, Prensky A, Hardin W: Neurological Pathophysiology, 2nd ed. New York, Oxford University Press, 1978

Gilman S, Winans S: Manter and Gatz's Essentials of Clinical Neuroanatomy and Neurophysiology, 6th ed. Philadelphia, FA Davis, 1982

Goldberg S: Clinical Neuroanatomy Made Ridiculously Simple. Miami, MedMaster, 1979

Goodman L, Gilman A: The Pharmacological Basis of Therapeutics, 5th ed. New York, Macmillan, 1975

Guyton A: Textbook of Medical Physiology, 6th ed. Philadelphia, WB Saunders, 1981

Noback C, Demarest R: The Nervous System—Introduction and Review, 2nd ed. New York, McGraw-Hill, 1977

Pick TP (ed): Gray's Anatomy. Philadelphia, Running Press, 1974

Simpson J, Magee K: Clinical Evaluation of the Nervous System. Boston, Little, Brown & Co, 1973

Snell R: Clinical Neuroanatomy for Medical Students. Boston, Little, Brown & Co, 1980

part two

Assessment and Evaluation

chapter 3

The Neurological Physical Examination

COLLECTING A NURSING HISTORY

PATIENT ASSESSMENT/HISTORY-TAKING

The circumstances surrounding the assessment of a patient can vary greatly. The patient may be ambulatory, alert, and oriented, or he may be experiencing an altered level of consciousness with neurological deficits. A patient may even be admitted by way of an emergency department as a result of trauma.

The history of the neurological problem is collected before the neurological examination is begun. The circumstances of admission will affect the amount of data gathered and the assessment of the patient's needs, all of which are necessary in the formulation of an individualized nursing care plan.

Ideally, upon the patient's admission, the nurse will have an opportunity to interview him and his family or "significant other," noting any potential patient or nursing problems as the interview progresses. However, the interview is not only a mechanism for gathering data or dispensing information. It also serves as a mode of establishing a working relationship with both the patient and family. If the patient is unable to provide the history, a relative or close friend who is familiar with the patient can provide objective data.

Systematic Approach

Some systematic plan of history-taking should be followed to ensure the completeness of data collection. A history-taking guide developed specifically for the neurological patient, or a general guide such as the one shown in Chart 3–1, may be helpful.

Throughout the interview the nurse must be alert for any misconceptions or misunderstandings on the part of the patient or family. Difficulties of this sort should be corrected and clarified, or the family may be referred to the appropriate person for help. It is also helpful to talk privately with the family to learn about the patient's personality prior to the current illness. This information is most useful if surgery is planned, because the patient's behavior during the postoperative period can be compared with what has been described as "normal behavior" for the patient.

A summary of the interview should be entered into the patient's chart. Based on this systematic assessment, a written patient care plan with nursing diagnoses and nursing protocols should be developed. Because the plan is in writing, it can be used by *all* nursing staff members with adjustments, deletions, and additions being written as changes occur.

In the event of an emergency admission, the points of the interview will probably be collected in a piecemeal fashion until the patient is stabilized. As soon as it is feasible, the nurse should interview the patient and family so that a written care plan can be developed based on a systematic assessment.

THE NEUROLOGICAL EXAMINATION

GENERAL CONSIDERATIONS

Purpose

The purpose of the neurological examination is to determine the presence or absence of disease in the nervous system. Since the nervous system includes tissues that perform highly specialized functions, it is sometimes possible to locate, identify, and estimate the extent of a lesion based

CHART 3-1. GUIDE FOR COLLECTING A NURSING HISTORY

GENERAL APPEARANCE

- Physical appearance — neat, clean, shaven, any apparent physical disabilities such as paralysis, ptosis, or muscle atrophy
- Emotional status — tense, relaxed, anxious, hostile
- Cooperativeness throughout interview
- Mobility — came in wheelchair, walked with shuffling gait
- Level of consciousness

HEALTH HISTORY

- Diseases — diabetes, chronic lung diseases, gastric ulcer, and so forth
- Family health history
- Allergies — food, drug, environmental agents
- Any drugs currently being taken and for what reasons — note if there is a possibility of drug interaction with drugs currently being ordered for the patient
- Use of tobacco
- Use of alcohol
- Dietary restrictions, if any
- Description of general health status prior to illness

DISCUSSION WITH THE PATIENT

- Description by the patient, family, or "significant other" of current health problem — onset, signs and symptoms, progression of illness, and events or precipitating factors associated with the problem
- Patient's understanding of his illness
- Patient's understanding of what the physician has recommended and planned for treatment
- Patient's understanding of expected outcome of hospitalization and what he will be like at discharge

PSYCHOSOCIAL HISTORY OF PATIENT AND FAMILY

- What types of family structure and relationships exist?
- How have the patient and family managed family activities during this illness?
- How will the family manage during the patient's hospitalization (*e.g.,* child care, meals, visits to hospital, and so forth?)
- How is the patient coping with this illness and hospitalization?
- How is the family coping with this illness?
- What are the support systems for the patient and family?
- Are there any ethnic or cultural factors that will influence hospitalization?
- Is the clergy an important support system?
- What is the educational background of the patient?
- What is the occupational history of the patient?

INDIVIDUAL CHARACTERISTICS OF THE PATIENT

- General temperament
- Tendency toward dependence or independence
- Sleep and rest patterns in a 24-hour cycle (special routines)
- Elimination patterns
- Dietary preferences
- Mobility
- Senses — vision (need for glasses), hearing (hearing aid)
- Bathing routine — special skin care for dryness, allergies to soap, and so forth
- Use of leisure time — reading, embroidery, and other hobbies
- Special prosthesis, if any
- Expectations of the nursing staff

on careful evaluations. The examination can also assess a patient's rehabilitative potential and help to set realistic goals for a rehabilitation program.

Role of the Nurse

In some instances where the nurse has an extended role in practice, she may be responsible for conducting the neurological examination. In most situations, however, the physician conducts the neurological physical examination of the patient. When the neurological examination is carried out by the physician, the nurse's role is to be supportive of the patient by providing a brief explanation of the steps in the examination or even to give physical support as necessary. Sometimes the physician will prefer to examine the patient alone, particularly if the patient is easily distracted by the presence of another person in the room. Frequently, a patient will reveal more information to the examiner when no one else is present.

Regardless of whether or not the nurse is present during the examination, it is important to review the written findings of the neurological examination, not only to gain insight into the patient's diagnosis but also to draw attention to specific atypical findings that require certain observations to be made and charted relative to these points. Need for specific observations should be noted on the patient's individualized care plan. For example, a patient with ataxia caused by cerebellar dysfunction should be supervised when ambulating because his coordination is poor. Such a notation should be included in the nursing care plan.

Equipment

The usual equipment includes the following:

Ophthalmoscope	Tape measure
Otoscope	Stethoscope
Tongue blade	Reflex hammer
Flashlight	Tuning forks (two)
Wisp of cotton	Pins

Approach to the Examination

Usually, a general physical examination and history will have been conducted prior to the neurological examination. An abstract of the findings should be included in the chart. The neurological examination proceeds in stepwise fashion as do most examinations. Because the nervous system is organized into a hierarchical arrangement of function, the exam proceeds from the highest level of function to the lowest and from the general integrated functions of an area to those that are very specific.

EVALUATION OF CEREBRAL FUNCTION

General Observations

At the outset of the examination, the patient's general appearance and behavior are noted in regard to the following:

1. The appropriateness of appearance and behavior in relation to the setting
2. Predominant attitude, mood, and facial expressions
3. Flow of speech
4. Thought processes, content, and perceptions

The thought processes, content, and perceptions are evaluated as the patient answers questions and elaborates on his responses. The patient's emotional status is also evaluated as it relates to thought content, mannerisms, tone of voice, and mood changes. Based on the observation of emotional status, a psychiatric consultation may be necessary.

Cognitive functions are tested, including the following areas:

- Orientation to time, place, and person
- Attention and concentration
- Memory
- Retention and immediate recall
- Calculations
- General information
- Vocabulary
- Abstract reasoning
- Similarities
- Judgment

Some parts of the evaluation of cerebral function can be incorporated into the history-taking portion of the interview. The use of this mechanism is a natural way of extracting information without creating an artificial test setting that could make the patient uncomfortable and anxious. These emotional factors could distort the accuracy of the data collected.

General Considerations

Appearance and Behavior. The attire, grooming, and personal appearance of the patient should be appropriate for the setting and patient's age. It may be considered appropriate for a gentleman of 65 years to appear at the neurologist's office in bermuda shorts and a bright shirt if he resided in a retirement resort community in Florida; however, similar attire in Philadelphia on a cold November day would appear inappropriate.

A neat and clean appearance would reflect good grooming and good personal hygiene habits. An unkempt appearance, on the other hand, may indicate depression or chronic organic brain disease. A patient with a compulsive personality would be most apt to be meticulous to a fault about his grooming.

Posture and motor function also contribute to a general impression of the patient. A slumped posture coupled with slow movements may indicate depression, whereas a rigid or tense posture with "nervous mannerisms" could indicate anxiety. Slow, deliberate movement may be associated with parkinsonism.

Predominant Attitude, Mood, and Facial Expressions. Listening to the patient and watching his facial expressions and general movements constitute ways of evaluating his general attitude and mood. However, additional information can be elicited by questioning the patient directly; for example, the patient may be asked the following questions:

- How do you behave at home?
- What makes you angry?
- What makes you sad?

The reaction of the patient to the topic being discussed and to the people around him should also be noted. Abnormal responses might include hostility, evasiveness, anger, elation, and tearfulness. Of special concern is any tendency toward suicide. If the patient even hints at contemplating suicide, then special observation, supervision, and further evaluation are warranted.

Flow of Speech. While the substance of the patient's speech is important, the examiner should also listen to the sound and flow of words. Quality, quantity, pace, and spontaneity should be noted. The content should be evaluated with respect to coherence, relevance, and other specific meanings in the message; for example, changing the topic in midsentences, coining words, and sudden silence are noteworthy abnormal findings.

Thought Process and Perceptions. Thought process and perception refer to a person's subjective responses and interpretations to experiences in daily living. Because both areas are part of the affective domain, the examiner must rely on what the patient says as the means of clinical disclosure.

Thought Content. By listening to the patient and reflecting and exploring the answers offered, the examiner can evaluate the presence of any of the following themes or flaws in the thought content:

- Compulsive phenomena—obsessions, phobias, or repetitive thinking about issues
- Doubting or indecision
- Feelings of unreality, depersonalization, persecution, or control by others
- Delusions or illusions
- Hallucinations

The presence of any one of these findings is abnormal and may indicate psychotic or organic disease.

Cognitive Functions

Cognitive functions include several areas of intellectual ability. This discussion proceeds from simple to complex cognitive functions.

Orientation. The three areas to be tested are orientation to *time, place,* and *person.* Included in these categories are

Time—the time of day; the day of the week; the month, season, date, and year; as well as any possible upcoming holiday or one in the immediate past

Place—present location, home address, city, state

Person—ability of the patient to give his own name, the names of family members, or the names of the professional personnel caring for him

Carefully phrased questions, when asked in the context of the interview, can help when evaluating the patient's orientation. For example, asking the patient his name and address, the names of family members, and specific dates of significant events in his life will provide insight into the patient's awareness of time, place, and person. For some patients, however, a more direct approach using specific questions will be indicated. For example, the examiner may have to ask directly, "Do you get confused?" or "What day is it today?"

Attention and Concentration. The patient's ability to concentrate can be tested by reading a series of digits to him and then asking him to repeat them in turn. The series should start with a short list, each digit being enunciated clearly and paced at 1-second intervals. Number series can begin with two digits, then progress to three, four, five, and so forth (e.g., 7, 2; 9, 5, 2; 4, 2, 7, 6; 5, 8, 3, 1, 4). If the patient makes an error while repeating the digits, he should be given a second chance with another series of digits of similar length. It is advisable both to stop after two consecutive failures in a series of any length and to avoid consecutive numbers or digits that easily form recognizable combinations, such as the date 1776.

In the second part of this test (beginning with the shortest list of digits) the patient is asked to repeat a series in reverse order.

Normally, a person should be able to repeat correctly at least five to eight digits in the same order and four to six in reverse order. Poor performance in this test is characteristic of organic brain diseases such as delirium and dementia. (This test would not be a valid indication of organic brain disease if the patient were mentally retarded.)

Another common exercise is to ask the patient to count backward from 100 in decrements of 7. Normally the patient should be able to complete this exercise with few errors in 60 seconds. Patients unable to do the serial of 7s should be instructed to try serial 3s in similar manner. Poor performance in this test is characteristic of chronic brain disorder or mental retardation.

Memory. Memory can be subdivided into remote, intermediate, and recent. Most questions related to memory can be asked in the context of the history-taking interview.

Remote Memory. Some of the following questions may be asked to evaluate remote memory. The information gathered from the patient can be cross-checked with the information provided by significant people in his life. Questions that will help in evaluating remote memory include

- Where and when were you born?
- How old are you?
- When did you graduate from high school? How many years ago was that?
- When were you married? At what age?
- What are the names, ages, and birthdates of your children?
- How old are your parents? (or) At what age did they die?

Intermediate Memory. Intermediate memory can be tested by referring to personal and general events of the last 5 years; for example, the patient should be asked to give a chronological account of his illness including dates. He may also be questioned about current events of the last 5 years.

Recent Memory. Inquiry should be directed toward recent events that can be counterchecked to determine accuracy. "What were the circumstances of your admission to the hospital?" or "How and with whom did you come to the physician's office?" are good questions.

Retention and Immediate Recall. This cognitive skill can be tested by giving the patient a list of words, including objects, dates, titles, addresses, and so forth. The patient should repeat the words at the time the examiner recites them to verify that the words have been heard. Then, later in the neurological examination (approximately 3 to 5 minutes later) the patient should be asked to repeat the words. If the patient's response is incorrect, it is important to note whether he is aware that he is wrong or if he is attempting to contrive answers.

Normally a person should be able to remember the words correctly. Poor recent memory is characteristic of organic brain disease. Poor remote memory may be noted in psychiatric and severe emotional disorders.

Calculations. In addition to counting backward from 100 in decrements of 7, other simple problems requiring mathematical skill should be included, such as the following:

- What is 4 × 12?
- Count from 1 to 25 and then backwards from 25 to 1.
- If a recipe requires 1¾ cups of flour and you are tripling the recipe, how much flour would you measure?

General Information. General information is a good indicator of underlying intelligence. The following questions are designed to evaluate general intellectual ability:

- How many inches are there in a yard?
- What do we commemorate on Thanksgiving Day?
- What is the function of the lungs in the body?
- What is the capital of England?
- Name three large rivers found in the United States.

Intelligence is affected by severe forms of psychiatric disorders or mental retardation.

Vocabulary. Vocabulary is considered a valid indication of intelligence. The patient is asked to define or use in a sentence about 12 to 24 selected words. The difficulty of the words increases gradually, such as in the following list:

1. Orange	7. Veal	13. Crescendo
2. Cow	8. Dye	14. Ambivalence
3. Ruby	9. Epic	15. Bondage
4. Affix	10. Telescope	16. Diverse
5. Leather	11. Metaphor	17. Flourish
6. Yen	12. Deluge	18. Fiduciary

Abstract Reasoning. The ability to reason abstractly is tested by asking the patient to explain a few common proverbs. The answers are then evaluated in terms of their relevance. Common proverbs which may be used are

- All that glitters is not gold.
- The early bird catches the worm.
- Rolling stones gather no moss.

A tendency to interpret these sayings in literal, concrete terms may indicate organic brain disease, schizophrenia, mental retardation, or simply a limited education.

Similarities. The patient is asked to identify how two given objects are alike, such as the following:

- A rose and a carnation
- A cat and a mouse
- A piano and a violin
- Oil and wood
- Silk and linen

Concrete responses are common with the patient who is schizophrenic or has organic brain disease.

Judgment. The questions that are asked to evaluate the patient's ability to make judgments should take into account the patient's life experiences and his mode of living. Such questions should be structured to test how well the patient can perceive the circumstances of the situation described. The following list provides examples:

- What should you do if you lose your credit cards?
- What should you do if you lock your keys in your car?
- Why are children required to go to school until 16 years of age?
- Why is it better to have a child immunized against measles than to let him get the disease?

Judgment is poor in organic brain disease, mental retardation, and psychotic states.

Special Cerebral Functions

Recognition — Agnosia

Specific functions of the cerebral cortex are tested, beginning with the ability to recognize familiar objects by sight, sound, or feeling. The inability to recognize common objects through the senses is referred to as *agnosia*, with specific sensory deficits in this area identified as visual, auditory, and tactile agnosia.

Visual agnosia is the inability to recognize common objects by sight and is due to a lesion in the occipital area of the brain. To test this ability the examiner shows the patient pictures of common objects, or points to objects in the room such as those below:

• Chair	• Desk
• Pencil	• Automobile
• Door	• Telephone
• Tie	• Carpet

Inability to identify these common objects would be characteristic of visual agnosia.

Auditory agnosia is the inability to recognize the meaning of common environmental sounds such as the ringing of a telephone or the squeaking of brakes. Although the patient hears these sounds, he is unable to attach meaning to them; therefore, he would neither answer a ringing telephone nor understand that squeaking of brakes means that a driver of a vehicle is trying to come to a sudden stop. A lesion in a portion of the temporal lobe is the cause of this form of agnosia.

Tactile agnosia is the inability to recognize common objects such as a pencil, comb, or cloth through the sense of touch. The patient is blind-folded or asked to close his eyes. Common objects such as a key or comb are placed in his hand one at a time and he is asked to identify them. Inability to identify these objects by touch would be characteristic of tactile agnosia. A parietal lobe lesion is the cause of tactile agnosia.

A special type of agnosia called *autotopagnosia* refers to the inability to identify body parts or understand the relationships of body parts. A lesion in the posterior inferior region of the parietal lobe is the offender in this case.

Cortical Motor Integration — Apraxia

The second area of review is cortical motor integration. For a person to perform a skilled motor act, he must understand what the act entails, remember the directions long enough to complete the act, and possess normal motor strength. For example, if a patient is handed a comb and told to comb his hair, he must pick up the comb, lift his arm to his head, and pass the comb through the hair from top to bottom. If the patient cannot carry out such a skilled act in the absence of paralysis, the term *apraxia* is applied.

When commands or directions are given, three steps are necessary to successfully execute the purposeful skilled act:

1. The first step requires the development of a concept or idea of what is required. The idea must be remembered long enough to accomplish the act. Inability to comprehend, develop, or remember the concept of the desired action is called *ideational apraxia*. The etiology of this defect is a general suppression of cerebral function rather than a lesion in one specific cerebral area. The patient can give one the impression of being absent-minded.[1]
2. The second step necessitates formulation of an organized plan by which the desired action is accomplished. This requires a knowledge of the location of one's body and body parts in relation to the environment. A mental image of the action to be performed is created. The mental image is then transmitted as a

code for action to the motor mechanism. A defect in transmission or conversion of the idea into an appropriate blueprint for motor action is called *ideokinetic* or *ideomotor apraxia.* This form of apraxia occurs most commonly when there are lesions of the major hemisphere at the junction of the temporal, parietal, and occipital lobes on the connecting pathways with the frontal lobe.[1]

3. The third step is the actual motor execution of the details of the plan. Failure of the muscles to carry out the action is called *kinetic apraxia.* A lesion of the premotor frontal cortex is the cause in this instance. The disability is usually limited to one extremity, or a part of it, without actual weakness or loss of gross motor movement.

A defect in any one of the three steps outlined above is responsible for apraxia. It is apparent that performing a skilled act on demand requires an integrated function of several areas of the cerebral cortex.

Communication—Aphasia

The last major area of cerebral function is the communication system. Inability to communicate is referred to as *aphasia.* (However, the word dysphasia appears to be more accurate since it refers to difficulty in communications.) Normally, a person can understand the written and spoken word. Inability to do so is called *receptive aphasia.* An inability to express one's thoughts appropriately both verbally and in writing is called *expressive aphasia.*

Most neurological patients have some communication function left intact even though certain functions have been greatly diminished because of a disease process. Carefully evaluating the complex communication system can aid in localizing the lesion if a specific area of the brain is involved. The various aphasias or dysphasias can be subdivided into the following categories, which are listed along with the respective areas of involvement:

- Auditory receptive aphasia—lesion at Wernicke's area of the temporal lobe
- Visual receptive aphasia (alexia)—lesion at parietal–occipital area
- Expressive speaking aphasia—lesion at Broca's area of frontal lobe
- Expressive writing aphasia (agraphia)—lesion at posterior frontal area
- Global aphasia (a form of aphasia that involves both expressive and receptive aphasias)—extensive lesions of Broca's area, Wernicke's area, parietal–occipital area, and posterior frontal area

A few simple examples can show how these various skills can be tested.

Ability to Understand the Spoken Word. The patient is first asked to follow a simple instruction, such as "Close your eyes." If he is able to follow simple directions, then the difficulty of the command is gradually increased. An example of a command of intermediate difficulty would be "Touch your left ear with your right index finger." If this skill can be performed successfully, a more complex set of instructions is then given, such as "When I count to three, touch your right elbow with the palm of your left hand and then clap your hands." If the patient can carry out these commands of increased difficulty, this portion of the communication system appears to be intact.

Ability to Understand the Written Word. Commands of increasing difficulty are written legibly on cards that are shown to the patient, who is then asked to follow the instructions. Examples may include

- Open your mouth.
- Stick out your tongue.
- Put your hands on your shoulders.
- Point to your right ear.

Inability to understand the written word is called *alexia.*

Ability to Express Ideas Verbally. Word formation, hesitation, and flow of words and ideas are evaluated. The patient is asked to identify objects and to answer open-ended questions that require more than simple "yes" or "no" responses, such as the following:

- Tell me about the kind of work you do.
- What types of activities do you enjoy in your free time?
- Tell me about your illness.

Ability to Express Oneself in Writing. The patient is given paper and pencil and asked to write his name and address. The complexity of the instruction should be increased as the simpler tasks are accomplished successfully. Examples of increased complexity might be "Describe today's weather" or "Write an account of a major news item." Inability to express oneself in writing is called *agraphia.*

EVALUATION OF THE CRANIAL NERVES

OLFACTORY (I) NERVE

The sense of smell is tested by obstructing one nostril while testing the other. A piece of cotton that has been saturated with a common odoriferous substance is placed under the unobstructed nostril. Camphor, coffee, lemon oil, and peppermint are possible items that patients should be able to identify by their odors, if cranial nerve I is intact.

Abnormalities

Anosmia indicates an inability to smell. There are several causes of anosmia, some of which are due to neuropathology while others are not. Common neurological causes of anosmia include tumors of the base of the frontal lobe or pituitary area, fractures of the anterior fossa, arteriosclerotic/cerebrovascular syndromes, meningitis, hydrocephalus, and posttraumatic brain syndrome. Common nonneurological causes of anosmia include the common cold, inflammation of the nasal cavity, and congenital defects.

The Foster Kennedy syndrome is a special syndrome involving the olfactory nerve that is caused by a tumor or abscess at the base of the frontal lobe. Signs and symptoms include ipsilateral blindness and anosmia, ipsilateral atrophy of the olfactory and optic nerves, and contralateral papilledema. The frontal mass is on the same side as the atrophy.

OPTIC (II) NERVE

Each eye is evaluated individually. The tests include visual acuity, visual fields, and the ophthalmoscopic examination.

Visual Acuity

Visual acuity is evaluated by asking the patient to read from a newspaper or the standard Snellen chart, which is read from a distance of 20 feet. Normal vision is 20/20, meaning that the patient can read the chart from a distance of 20 feet, taking a separate reading with each eye. Visual acuity of 20/30 would mean that the patient could read at 20 feet what the normal eye can read at 30 feet.

The patient should also be questioned about dimness of vision, which would be characteristic of an optic pathway disorder.

Visual Fields

A visual field normally extends 60 degrees to the nasal side, 100 degrees on the temporal side, and 130 degrees vertically. A rough evaluation can be made by using the *confrontation test*. The patient is asked to lightly cover one eye and look at the examiner's eye directly opposite. The examiner should be positioned 2 feet (approximately 60 cm) away from the patient with his face directly opposite the patient's face. To test the patient's visual field, the examiner closes one eye, and introduces a pencil or another small object from the periphery into the patient's field of vision. The patient is asked to indicate when he sees the object. Each quadrant of each visual field is evaluated for slight and gross movement. The procedure is repeated with the other eye. Simultaneous movement in both halves of the visual field should be checked for visual extinction.

The confrontation test reveals only gross defects. If any defect is found in the confrontation test, the fields should be plotted by the standard perimetric tests or on a tangent screen.

Abnormalities. The tests of the visual fields can reveal disturbances in function anywhere along the visual pathway (retina, optic nerve, optic tract, lateral geniculate body, geniculocalcarine tract, or occipital lobe.) The defects noted are found with particular lesions along the visual pathway (see Chart 3–2). Table 3–1 summarizes common visual defects.

Ophthalmoscopic Examination

The ophthalmoscope contains a special lens that is used to visualize the inside of the eye by shining a beam of light directly into the eye. The room must be darkened with the examiner sitting directly opposite the subject. To examine the patient's right eye, the examiner holds the ophthalmoscope in his right hand and looks through the instrument with his right eye while the patient looks straight ahead (Fig. 3–1). All of these instructions must be followed to observe the fundus of the eye.

The fundus includes the optic disc, macula, and blood vessels on the back wall of the internal eyeball (Fig. 3–2). The optic nerve is visible as a tubelike structure emerging from the back of the eyeball.

The optic disc is the most prominent structure visible and represents the termination of the optic nerve. As one views the optic disc, small blood vessels can be visualized as they exit and enter the eye. The normal disc is round or slightly oval with sharply defined margins. Table 3–2 summarizes common optic disc abnormalities.

The four main pairs of blood vessels exiting and entering the optic disc are examined to compare the diameters of the arterioles and venules and to determine if the veins are tortuous. Normally, the venules are about 30% larger than the arterioles; however, tortuous veins are present in certain clinical conditions in which intracranial pressure is increased.

Another area of the retina is the macula, which has the highest density of visual receptors. The center of the macula, called the *fovea*, represents the point of greatest visual acuity. As the retina is examined, any abnormalities such as hemorrhage, swelling, and exudate should be noted.

OCULOMOTOR (III), TROCHLEAR (IV), AND ABDUCENS (VI) NERVES

The cranial nerves III, IV, and VI are usually tested together since they all supply the various muscles that rotate the eyeball. The muscles innervated by these three cranial nerves, as well as the functions of these muscles, are listed in Table 3–3.

Injury to any of the extraocular muscles will compromise the corresponding eye movement. Injury to the oculomotor nerve will result in an inability to focus the eyes inward, upward, downward, and upward and outward; a droopy eyelid (ptosis); and a dilated pupil. There will not be pupillary constriction upon accommodation from a distant to a nearby point. The trochlear nerve, when damaged, will compromise downward and outward movement of the eyeball, while injury to the abducens will cause loss of lateral movement. Trochlear nerve dysfunction is rare. The abducens nerve has the longest intracranial course and is frequently involved in neurological disease.

General Observations

Two important observations are made of the eye. They are the position of the eyeball in the orbit and the position of the upper eyelid.

The Eyeball. The position of the eyeball within the head is noted. This is determined by looking at the position of the eyeball from a frontal and lateral view as well as looking down at the eyeball from above the patient's head. The

CHART 3-2. VISUAL FIELD DEFECTS PRODUCED BY SELECTED LESIONS IN THE VISUAL PATHWAYS

VISUAL PATHWAYS | VISUAL FIELDS | BLACKENED FIELD INDICATES AREA OF NO VISION

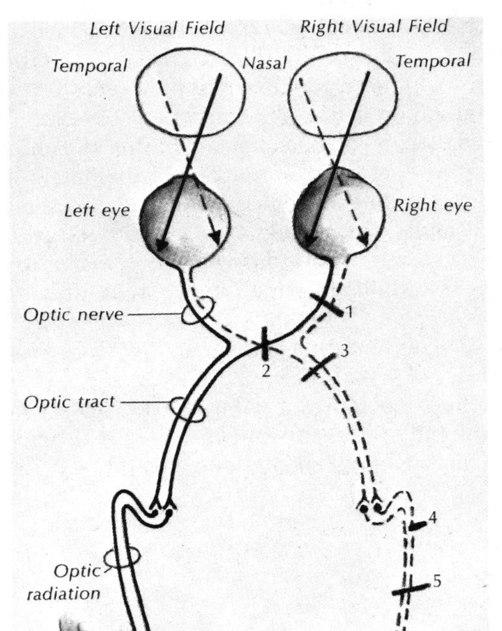

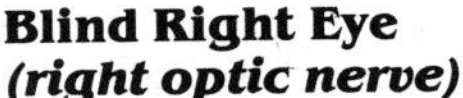

Blind Right Eye
(right optic nerve)

A lesion of the optic nerve, and of course of the eye itself, produces unilateral blindness.

1 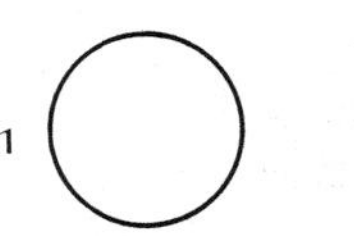 

Bitemporal Hemianopsia
(optic chiasm)

A lesion at the optic chiasm may involve only those fibers that are crossing over to the opposite side. Since these fibers originate in the nasal half of each retina, visual loss involves the temporal half of each field.

2 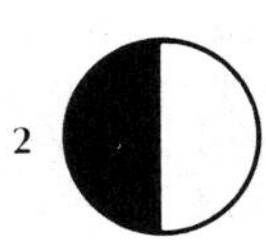 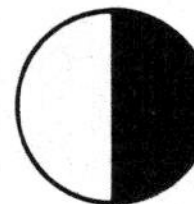

Left Homonymous Hemianopsia
(right optic tract)

A lesion of the optic tract interrupts fibers originating on the same side of both eyes. Visual loss in the eyes is therefore similar (homonymous) and involves half of each field (hemianopsia).

3 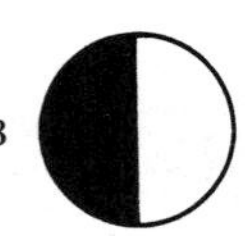 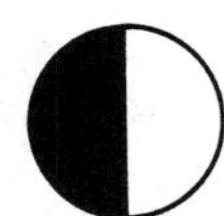

Homonymous Left Upper Quadrantic Defect
(optic radiation, partial)

A partial lesion of the optic radiation may involve only a portion of the nerve fibers, producing, for example, a homonymous quadrantic defect.

4 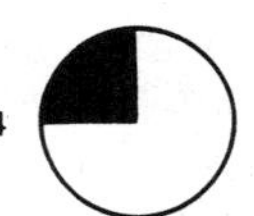 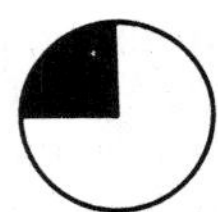

Left Homonymous Hemianopsia
(right optic radiation)

A complete interruption of fibers in the optic radiation produces a visual defect similar to that produced by a lesion of the optic tract.

5 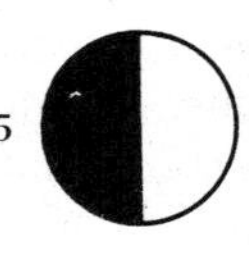 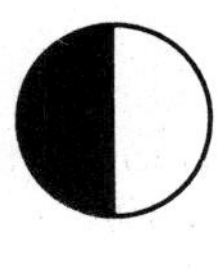

LEFT RIGHT

(Bates B: A Guide to Physical Examination. Philadelphia, JB Lippincott, 1983)

TABLE 3-1. *Common Visual Defects*

Type	*Description*	*Causes*
Scotomas	Abnormal blind spots on the visual fields	Localized lesions, hemorrhage, glaucoma, or neuritis
Amblyopia	Dim vision that results in compromised visual acuity	Hereditary or acquired
Amaurosis	Complete blindness in an eye	Cerebral lesion, retinal or optic nerve disease, or heredity
Photophobia	Sensitivity of the eyes to light; often seen in meningitis and subarachnoid hemorrhage	Etiology is unclear
Diplopia	Commonly known as double vision; special testing of diplopia can be done by using red glass or a Maddox rod	Paralysis of movement of the eyeball in a particular direction; involves extraocular muscles

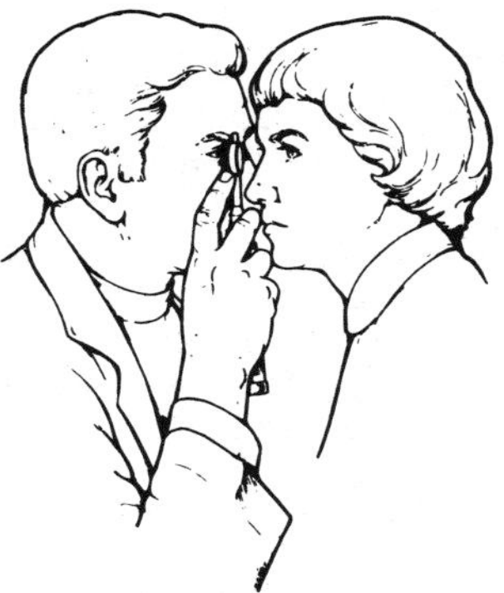

FIG. 3–1. Technique for the proper use of the ophthalmoscope. The examiner's right eye looks into the patient's right eye. The index finger is used to adjust the lens for proper focus.

position of the eyeballs should also be compared for any differences. Abnormal protrusion of one or both eyeballs is termed *proptosis* or *exophthalmos*. Abnormal recession of an eyeball within the orbit is termed *enophthalmos*.

The Upper Lid. To assess the upper lid, ask the patient to look straight ahead. Note the width of the palpebral fissure in each eye and compare them. The *palpebral fissure* is defined as the space between the upper and lower eyelid that extends from the outer to the inner canthus.[3] Next, note the position of the eyelids in relation to the pupil and the iris in each eye and compare. The term for a drooping upper eyelid is *ptosis*. Ptosis is seen in Horner's syndrome and is often seen in myasthenia gravis if the ocular muscles are affected. Edema of the eyelid, if present, should be recorded. Edema can result from trauma to the orbit and may occur in the upper, lower, or both eyelids.

Movement of the Eyes

Extraocular movements are evaluated by asking the patient to follow a finger or a pencil through the six cardinal areas of vision (Fig. 3–3). Normally both eyes move simultaneously in the same direction; this is called *conjugate movement*. If there is a lack of parallelism between the two visual axes, then *strabismus* or *dysconjugate movement* is said to be present. If the deviation is limited to specific fields, then paralysis of the extraocular muscles and the nerves innervating them is involved. *Double vision (diplopia)* may be present if the patient cannot move the eyeball in a particular direction.

The loss of normal function of any of the muscles responsible for extraocular movement may be due to damage to the muscles themselves or injury to the cranial nerve nuclei located in the midbrain and pons. *Ophthalmoplegia* is the term used to describe paralysis of one or more eye muscles. Table 3–4 summarizes the common ophthalmoplegias.

In conducting a neurological examination on the unconscious patient, the oculocephalic reflex (doll's eye response) and the oculovestibular reflex (cold calorics) are evaluated for reflex movement of the eyeball. The presence of these reflexes indicates that the brain stem is intact. See Chapter 5 for further discussion and description of these reflexes.

Severe injury to the peripheral portion of a cranial nerve results in nerve fiber degeneration followed by unpredictable regeneration. Because of the proximity of other cranial nerves, the regenerating fibers from one nerve can be misdirected, resulting in innervation of other adjacent nerves. Such atypical regeneration is called the *misdirection syndrome*. Frequently the oculomotor nerve is misdirected toward cranial nerve IV or V. Examples of this misdirectional syndrome are the pseudo-Graefe lid sign and the Marcus Gunn jaw–winking phenomenon.

The *pseudo-Graefe lid sign* is an example of an atypical connection between cranial nerves III and IV. Any attempt to look downward is followed by upper lid retraction. The *Marcus Gunn jaw–winking phenomenon* involves cranial nerves III and V. As the mouth is opened and the jaw moves to one side, a ptosis of the eyelid will change to lid retraction.

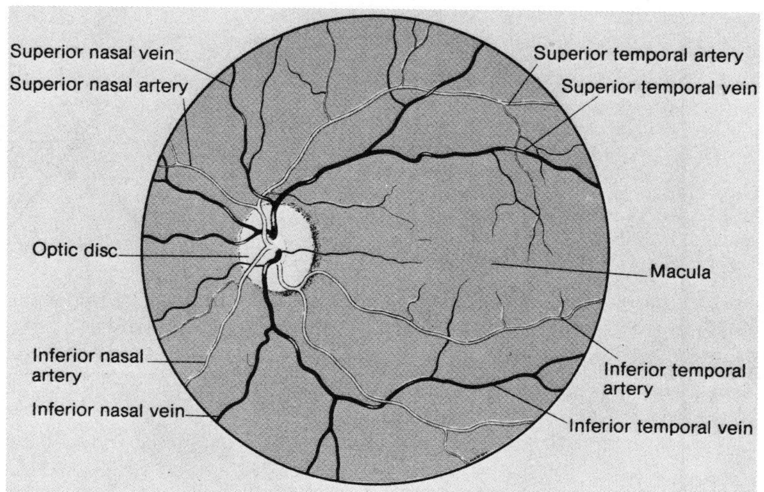

FIG. 3–2. Display of the retina as seen through the ophthalmoscope. The ophthalmoscope is capable of visualizing only a portion of the retina at any one time. It is best to identify the disc, ascertain the sharpness of disc margins, and then follow each vessel that emerges from the disc at least three disc diameters along its course. The macular area should then be identified for any lesion that may be present.

TABLE 3-2. *Common Optic Disc Abnormalities*

Type	*Description*	*Cause(s)*
Papilledema (choked disc)	Margin of the disc is swollen and the entire disc has a reddish hue because of congestion	Increased intracranial pressure
Optic atrophy	Paleness (the disc is light pink, white, or gray due to decreased blood supply to the area); visual acuity is decreased	Primary causes: tabes dorsalis and multiple sclerosis Secondary causes: neuritis or prolonged increased intracranial pressure
Retrobulbar neuritis	Inflammatory lesion of the posterior portion of the optic nerve; no swelling of disc	Hemorrhage, diabetes, or retinitis
Optic neuritis	Inflammation of the disc; associated with loss of vision due to a central scotoma	Inflammatory process

Anatomical and Physiological Basis of Eye Movement

Conjugate eye movement is a composite of integrated functions from various parts of the brain including the cortex and the brain stem. The two areas of the cortex are the following:

- "Frontal gaze center" (located in Brodmann's area 8)
  - —Descending fibers from this area pass through the anterior portion of the internal capsule to the pons and connect with the lower centers for conjugate movement
  - —This area controls rapid voluntary eye movement
- "Occipital gaze center" (located in Brodmann's areas 18 and 19)
  - —Descending fibers from this area pass medially to the optic radiations, down through the posterior portion of the internal capsule, and connect with conjugate eye movement centers in the midbrain and pons
  - —This area controls slow-tracking eye movement (automatic fixation)

The *medial longitudinal fasciculus (MLF)* is the other area important for conjugate gaze. It extends from the thalamic–midbrain region to the anterior horn cells of the spinal cord and serves to coordinate eye and neck movement pathways. The MLF connects and integrates fibers from the following areas of eye movement:

- Oculomotor, trochlear, and abducens nuclei
- Fibers that result from the synapse of cerebellar nuclei and the semicircular canals
- Horizontal gaze center of the pons

Perlia's nucleus mediates convergence of the eyes. It is thought that divergence is controlled by centers located near the abducens nuclei.

Because eye movement is a complex process relying on

TABLE 3-3. *Cranial Nerve Function Relative to Eye Movement*

Cranial Nerve	*Muscle*	*Movement of Eyeball*
Oculomotor (III)*	Medial rectus	Inward or medially on the horizontal plane
	Superior rectus	Upward when looking outward
	Inferior rectus	Downward when looking outward
	Inferior oblique	Upward when looking inward
Trochlear (IV)	Superior oblique	Downward when looking inward
Abducens (VI)	Lateral rectus	Outward or laterally on the horizontal plane

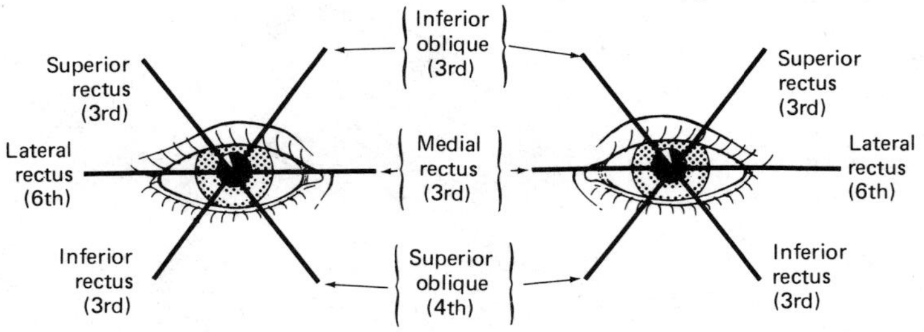

Note that the eye muscles function in pairs: the superior and inferior recti turn the eye upward and downward when the eye is looking out (temporally); the inferior and superior obliques turn the eye upward and downward when the eye is looking in (nasally); and the medial and lateral recti turn the eye inward (nasally) and outwardly (temporally) on the horizontal plane.

* The oculomotor nerve also innervates the levator palpebrae muscle, which elevates the eyelid and the muscles that control the iris and ciliary body.

(Figure from Bates B: A Guide to Physical Examination. Philadelphia, JB Lippincott, 1980)

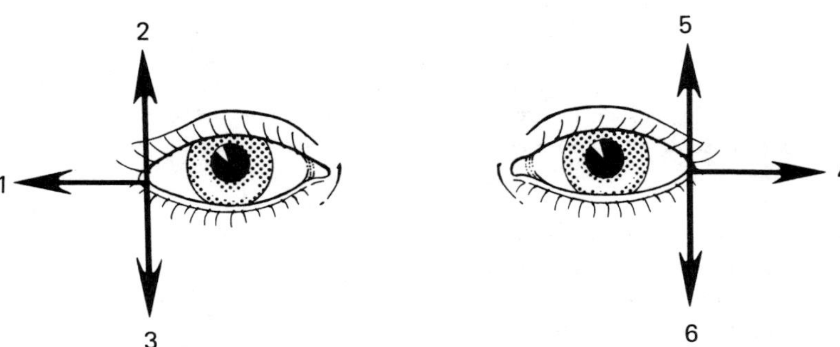

FIG. 3-3. Sequence of eye movement. (*Note:* Numbers indicate sequence of movement.)

the integration of several different areas of the brain, it is obvious that abnormal eye movements can result from injury at several levels of the brain.

Abnormalities in Gaze

The following outline should be helpful in identifying and explaining abnormalities in gaze.

Horizontal Gaze

- In a destructive hemispheric lesion, both eyes deviate *toward* the side of the lesion.
- In an irritative hemispheric lesion such as that which occurs with hemorrhage, both eyes deviate *away from* the side of the irritation. This lasts only minutes or hours and is replaced by paralysis of conjugate gaze.
- Unilateral destructive lesions in the pontine center for conjugate horizontal gaze result in deviations *away from* the lesion.
- A lesion in the lateral midbrain tegmentum will cause a horizontal gaze palsy to the side *opposite* the lesion by interrupting the cerebral pathways for conjugate gaze before their decussation.

Vertical Gaze

- Abnormalities of upward gaze imply an upper brain stem lesion, with one exception: some senior citizens have been observed to have abnormalities with upward gaze with no apparent disease process present. Paralysis of upward gaze is most often caused by destruction at the pretectal and posterior commissural area at the midbrain-diencephalic junction.
- Bilateral lesions of the medial longitudinal fasciculus produce abnormalities in upward gaze, particularly if the reticular formation is involved. (The MLF is located in the brain stem.)
- See also Parinaud's syndrome, Table 3-4.

Medial Longitudinal Fasciculus (MLF)

- A lesion between the pons and midbrain in the MLF of the brain stem produces internuclear ophthalmoplegia. The medial rectus muscle is involved, resulting in dysconjugate gaze. The lesion is very small and is usually caused by an area of demyelinization from multiple sclerosis or a small vascular lesion from diabetes mellitus. The signs and symptoms of internuclear ophthalmoplegia include deficit in adduction of the ipsilateral eye, dissociated nystagmus (more pronounced in the abducted eye), and retention or loss of convergence.
- As mentioned under vertical gaze abnormalities, bilateral lesions of the MLF produce abnormalities in upward gaze.

Other Abnormalities

- *Skewed deviation* (Hertwig-Magendie vertical divergence ocular position) is that condition evidenced by one eye looking downward and the other looking upward. The cause is a lesion in the pons on the same side as the eye that is directed downward. It will be recalled that the MLF receives cerebellar innervation. Skewed deviation can also be a symptom of posterior fossa or cerebellar disease. Skewed deviation is one of four cardinal symptoms of cerebellar disease, the other three being nystagmus, ocular dysmetria, and flutterlike oscillation.[2]
- *Roving-eye movement* is spontaneous, slow, and random deviation. It is seen in comatose patients with intact brain stem oculomotor function. Absence of roving-eye movement indicates brain stem dysfunction.

TABLE 3-4. ***Summary of Ophthalmoplegias***

Type	*Description*
External ophthalmoplegia	• Paralysis of one or more of the extraocular muscles
Internal ophthalmoplegia	• Paralysis of one or more intraocular muscles
Nuclear ophthalmoplegia	• Paralysis caused by a lesion of the nuclei of the motor nerves of the eye (III, IV, or VI)
Internuclear ophthalmoplegia	• Paralysis caused by injury or a lesion of the medial longitudinal fasciculus located within the brain stem
Supranuclear ophthalmoplegia	• Paralysis caused by injury or a lesion to the conjugate eye movement center(s) located in the frontal occipital lobes
Parinaud's syndrome	• A type of supranuclear ophthalmoplegia; conjugate upward gaze paralysis; caused by a lesion or compression around the pineal body; often caused by a pineal tumor

- *Ocular bobbing* is characterized by episodic, intermittent, usually conjugate, downward, brisk eye movement followed by a return to the resting position by a "bobbing action." This is seen in severe destructive lower pontine lesions, such as those seen with pontine hemorrhage or infection.

Nystagmus. Another common abnormality frequently noted with eye movement is called *nystagmus*. It is an involuntary movement of the eyes that may be horizontal, vertical, rotary, or mixed in direction. The tempo of the movements can be regular, rhythmical, pendular, or jerky with a fast and slow component to the movement.

In normal eye activity, there may be some minor oscillations, which should not be classified as true nystagmus. True nystagmus is a pathological finding caused by a lesion along the peripheral or central apparatus. This elaborate apparatus includes the visual perceptual pathways, vestibular system of the inner ear, and portions of the proprioceptive system and their connections with the brain stem and cerebellum. This complex system normally keeps the eyes in a constant relationship with their environment. Specific types of nystagmus can be caused by lesions in particular areas of the system. Therefore, it is important to describe the characteristics of the nystagmus in the patient's chart. There are a few specific types of nystagmus that are noteworthy when evaluating the neurological patient:

- Retractory nystagmus—irregular jerks of the eyes backward into the orbit, precipitated by upward gaze and indicative of midbrain tegmental damage
- Convergence nystagmus—slow, spontaneous, drifting, ocular divergence with a final quick, convergent jerk, indicative of a midbrain lesion
- "Seesaw" nystagmus—rapid, pendular, dysconjugate seesaw movement accompanied by severe visual field defect and loss of visual activity, indicative of a lesion around the optic chiasma
- "Downbeat" nystagmus—irregular jerks precipitated by downward gaze, indicative of lower medullary damage
- Optokinetic nystagmus—normally induced by looking at a moving object but lost with some lesions of the posterior half of the cerebral hemisphere
- Vestibular nystagmus—a mixed nystagmus that can be horizontal, rotational, or both, resulting from vestibular disease
- Toxic nystagmus—associated with treatment using certain drugs such as phenytoin (Dilantin), barbiturates, and bromides

Pupils

To assess the pupils, the patient should be directed to focus on a distant object located straight ahead. In the instance of a comatose patient, the pupils are tested as they are found. The pupils are examined for size, shape, and equality. The size of the normal pupil is 2 mm to 6 mm, with an average diameter of 3.5 mm. When the pupils are compared with each other, their sizes should be equal; however, about 17% of the normal population has discernible unequal pupil size without the presence of pathology (*anisocoria*).

The shape of the pupils is also noted and compared. Normally the pupils are round; however, in patients who have had cataract surgery the pupils assume a *keyhole shape*. An *ovoid* pupil indicates pupillary dysfunction and is sometimes seen in early herniation across the tentorium.

The pupils are next tested for reaction to light (*direct light reflex*). A light is directed into each pupil and then withdrawn. When the light is directed into the pupil, constriction normally occurs as a result of parasympathetic stimulation, which contracts the pupilloconstrictor fibers (Fig. 3-4). When the light is withdrawn, the pupil normally dilates because sympathetic stimulation contracts the pupillodilator muscles. The reaction should occur quickly in the pupil being tested; however, a similar, less pronounced response should occur in the untested pupil (*consensual light reflex*).

The pupil reactions should occur briskly, although age may affect the degree of reaction. In younger people, pupils tend to be larger and more responsive, while in older people they are smaller and less responsive.

Next, observe the pupils for the presence of accommodation. The *accommodation reflex* is assessed by asking the patient to focus on an object, such as the examiner's finger, positioned 2 or 3 feet directly ahead of him and to follow it with his eyes as it is rapidly moved closer to the patient's face. If the accommodation reflex is intact, the pupils will constrict when the patient looks at a nearby object.

Sensitivity to light or *photophobia* may be noted when checking the pupils, or the patient may complain of this

FIG. 3-4. Light and accommodation reflexes. (*Top*) The pupil is constricted, as when exposed to light or when looking at an object that is nearby. (*Bottom*) The pupil is dilated, as when light is withdrawn or when looking at an object from a distance. (Chaffee EE, Lytle IM: Basic Physiology and Anatomy. Philadelphia, JB Lippincott, 1980)

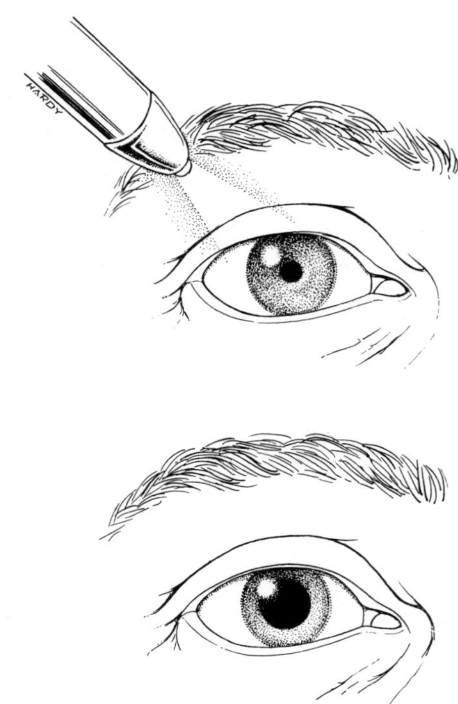

problem. The etiology is not clear but is usually associated with increased intracranial pressure.

Certain abnormal pupillary responses are related to specific cerebral injuries or lesion. Table 3–5 presents a summary of some of these abnormal findings.

Abnormal Pupillary Reactions

Amaurotic Pupil (Blind Eye). Blindness in one eye would be evidenced by (Fig. 3–5).

- No direct pupillary response to light in the blind eye
- No consensual response to light in opposite eye
- Intact, direct pupillary response to light in the normal eye
- Intact consensual response in the blind eye to light shone into normal eye
- The near pupillary response intact in both eyes.

Marcus Gunn Pupillary Response (Swinging Flashlight Sign). A defect in the afferent limb of the pupillary light reflex resulting from a lesion anterior to the optic chiasma in the optic nerve can be confirmed by the Marcus Gunn pupillary response. Minimal visual loss from an optic nerve lesion, or severe retinal dysfunction can be identified with this test.

With the eyes fixated on a distant object, a bright light is shone into the normal pupil. A brisk bilateral contraction occurs. When the light is swung quickly to the affected pupil, a slight dilation occurs and continues for a short time while the light continues and a slight contraction is noted. Moving the light quickly to the intact pupil will produce a brisk bilateral contraction.

Oculosympathetic Paresis (Horner's Syndrome). Horner's syndrome (Fig. 3–6) is due to a unilateral interruption or complete loss of sympathetic innervation to the pupil. The site of the interruption is usually in the neck. The pupil is small (miotic) and round in shape, as would normally be expected. An associated ptosis of the eyelid, often accompanied by loss of sweating on the face is noted on the same side of the face as the miotic pupil. The pupil reacts both to direct light and accommodation.

Tonic Pupil (Adie's Pupil). Adie's pupil (Fig. 3–6*B*) is due to a postganglionic denervation of the parasympathetic supply to the pupil. Although Adie's pupil may be present following a viral infection, the cause is not known. It occurs most often in females in the 20- to 30-year age group. In 80% of the patients there is unilateral pupillary dilation. The direct light reflex is almost abolished, but pupils will contract slowly upon prolonged stimulation with light. The pupil will also dilate slowly in response to darkness. Pupillary constriction occurs in response to accommodation and may even be pronounced; however, dilation after accommodation is slow. No abnormal neurological findings, other than absence of knee and ankle deep tendon reflexes, are found in these patients. The pupil responds normally to

TABLE 3–5. ***Abnormal Pupillary Responses Due to Injury to Selected Cerebral Structures***

Oculomotor Nerve Compression	The ipsilateral pupil is dilated and fixed as a result of uncal herniation compressing the oculomotor nerve (parasympathetic fibers for pupillary constriction) against the tentorium or posterior cerebral artery.
Diencephalic Bilateral Damage	Small, equal, and reactive pupils are usually the result of a supratentorial lesion or metabolic coma.
Hypothalamic Damage	A unilateral Horner's syndrome (small pupil, partial ptosis of the eyelid and loss of sweating on the same side can result from transtentorial herniation, involvement of descending sympathetic fibers in the ipsilateral brain stem or upper cord, or in the ascending sympathetic fibers in the neck or head).
Midbrain Damage	Midposition, nonreactive pupils may be caused by a lesion in the dorsal portion of the midbrain or a nuclear midbrain lesion; in the former instance, the pupils are round and regular, while in the latter instance, they may be irregular and unequal; causes of midposition pupils include midbrain damage from transtentorial herniation, tumors, infarction, or hemorrhage.
Pontine Damage	Small, bilateral, nonreactive pupils may result from the loss of sympathetic innervation. Pupils are called *pinpoint*. The cause is usually pontine hemorrhage, but this condition can also occur with the administration of opiate drugs.
Severe Anoxia or Ischemia; Death	Bilateral, fixed, and dilated pupils are the clinical signs that are seen in the terminal state (they can also result from atropinelike drugs). An intact ciliospinal reflex can produce momentary bilateral dilation.

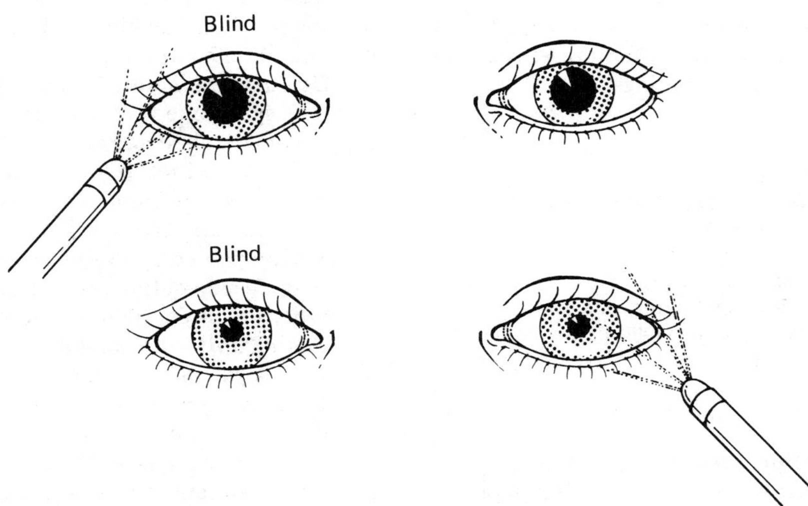

FIG. 3-5. When one eye is blind because of disease in the retina or optic nerve, the sensory limb of the light reflex arc is lost. A light shining into the blind eye produces no pupillary response in either eye. As long as the oculomotor nerve (the motor limb of the arc) is intact, however, a light directed into the sound eye produces normal responses in both eyes (normal direct and consensual reactions).

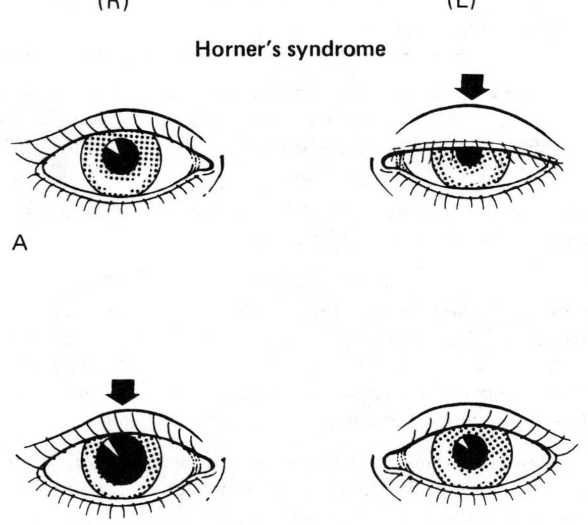

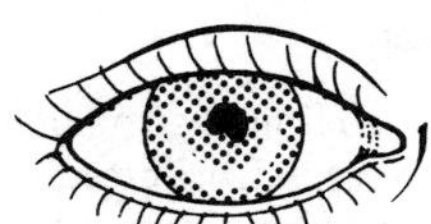

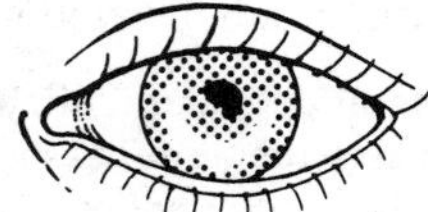

FIG. 3-6. Abnormal pupillary reactions. *(A)* Horner's syndrome. This pupil is small, regular, and unilateral. It is associated with ptosis of the eyelid and often with loss of sweating on the forehead of the involved side. Because of the ptosis, the eye may look small. Horner's syndrome is caused by interruption of the sympathetic nerve supply, most often in the neck. The pupil reacts to light and accommodation. *(B)* Adie's pupil (tonic pupil). This is a large, quite regular pupil usually confined to one side. The involved pupil reacts very slowly to light and accommodation. The disorder is benign and may be accompanied by diminished deep tendon reflexes. *(C)* Argyll-Robertson pupil. Argyll-Robertson pupils are small, irregular, and bilateral. They react to accommodation but not to light. They are often, but not necessarily, related to central nervous system syphilis (tabes dorsalis). (Bates B: Guide to Physical Examination. Philadelphia, JB Lippincott, 1974)

mydriatics. To diagnose an Adie's pupil, 2.5% methacholine (Mecholyl) is instilled into the affected pupil, which promptly contracts. This does not occur in the normal pupil.

Argyll–Robertson Pupil. An Argyll–Robertson pupil (Fig. 3–6, C) is often due to neurosyphilis (tabes dorsalis). The pupils do not react to light, but they react to accommodation. Patients are also observed to have small, irregularly shaped, bilateral pupils.

Miotic Pupils. *Miosis* is a term denoting constriction of the pupil. The most common causes of miosis are ophthalmic miotic drugs (acetylcholine chloride, carbachol, demecarium bromide, echothiophate iodide, isoflurophate, physostigmine, pilocarpine, and others), opiates (heroin, morphine sulfate, hydromorphone), and pontine hemorrhage. Pathophysiology causing miosis can be due to destruction of the sympathetic innervation and interruption of the inhibitory pathways to the third cranial nuclei (Edinger–Westphal nucleus). See also note on orbital injuries.*

Mydriatic Pupils. The term *mydriasis* refers to a dilated pupil. Mydriatic pupils are most often due to amphetamines, glutethimide (Doriden), ophthalmic mydriatics, and cycloplegic agents (atropine sulfate, cyclopentolate hydrochloride, homatropine hydrobromide, scopolamine hydrobromide, tropicamide). See also note on orbital injuries.*

Traumatic Miosis or Mydriasis. Traumatic miosis or mydriasis is due to direct injury to the eye and is often associated with orbital trauma. Miosis after trauma usually results from intraocular inflammation. Mydriasis is the usual result of local sphincter paralysis or tears in the sphincter muscle. In this instance, the pupil will appear irregular in shape as a result of the tearing.

Hippus Phenomenon. With uniform illumination of the pupil exhibiting the hippus phenomenon, there is alternation of dilation and contraction. This may be considered normal if the pupil is being observed under high magnification. The hippus phenomenon is also observed in patients who have beginning pressure on the third cranial nerve. This is often associated with early uncal herniation.

Hutchinsonian Pupil (Oculomotor Paralysis, Unilateral). Hutchinsonian pupil is a pupillary abnormality often seen in the presence of rapidly rising intracranial pressure: The pupil is widely dilated and fixed because of the direct compression of the oculomotor nerve. The affected pupil is on the same side as the intracranial lesion.

TRIGEMINAL (V) NERVE

Sensory Component

The sensory component of the fifth cranial nerve is tested with the patient's eyes closed. Test tubes of warm and cold water are placed at random on the skin of the face to check temperature perception. Touching the face in a similar manner with a wisp of cotton checks perception of light touch. Pain perception can be evaluated either by applying pressure with the wooden end of an applicator or by using the pinprick method. Comparison of responses on each side of the face should be made because one would expect sensation to be the same on both sides. Superficial sensation to the cornea, mucosa of the mouth and nose, and skin of the face and forehead are innervated by the fifth cranial nerve.

Motor Component

The motor components of the trigeminal nerve are those used for chewing. The strength of the masseter and temporal muscles is evaluated by palpating them when the jaws are tightly clamped together. Differences in muscle tone and atrophy should be noted along with the jaw reflex, which is tested by tapping the middle of the chin with a reflex hammer when the jaws are slightly ajar. Although the jaw reflex is relatively weak, tapping the chin in this manner should cause the mouth to close.

The ophthalmic branch of the trigeminal nerve controls the sensory portion of the corneal reflex, a very important protective reflex. (The motor portion is controlled by the facial nerve.) When the cornea is lightly stroked with a wisp of cotton, the patient automatically blinks if the corneal reflex is intact.

FACIAL (VII) NERVE

Sensory Component

The sense of taste in the anterior two thirds of the tongue is controlled by the seventh cranial nerve. Each side of the tongue is tested separately (on the protruding tongue). The patient is asked to identify the taste of sugar, after which a sip of water is given. The same procedure using a salty, sour, and bitter substance should follow.

Motor Component

The motor component is tested by observing the symmetry of the face at rest and during deliberate facial movements such as smiling, closing the eyes tightly, showing the teeth, whistling, pursing the lips, blowing air into the cheeks, wrinkling the nose and forehead, and raising the eyebrows. The facial nerve also controls tearing, salivation, and the motor limb of the corneal reflex. When weakness is noted, it is probably most important to observe whether the entire side of the face or just the lower face (from below the eyes) is affected. If the lower portion of one side of the face is involved, the lesion is said to be central; that is, the lesion involves the central nervous system. In this instance, the contralateral corticobulbar tract is involved. The patient would be unable to retract the corner of his mouth in a smile. Getting the patient to try to smile is important when assessing the patient. If the whole side of the face is involved, the lesion is said to be peripheral, that is, involving the peripheral nervous system. Spasms, atrophy, or tremors of the facial muscles should also be noted.

* A pupil may be abnormally large or small because of orbital trauma. When pupillary asymmetry is noted without any impairment of neurological signs such as consciousness, the possibility of orbital trauma should be explored.

ACOUSTIC (VIII) NERVE

The acoustic nerve, a pure sensory cranial nerve, is divided into two branches, the *cochlear* (hearing) and the *vestibular* (balance). Unless the patient gives a history of vertigo, tinnitus, or disturbed balance, the vestibular branch is not tested. If the above symptoms are present, the caloric tests are conducted (see Chapter 4). The ear canal is examined with an otoscope to determine if there are any visible abnormalities.

To test hearing, a ticking watch can be used and moved to various distances from the ear. Hearing in both the left and right ears should be compared; for example, if the patient hears the ticking watch at 2 feet in the left ear and 6 inches in the right ear, an obvious deficit is apparent. Whispering can also be used to test hearing.

A tuning fork is used to check lateralization. The vibrating tuning fork is placed on the vertex of the head and the patient is asked if its location is central or lateral (Weber test). See Figure 3–7. Air and bone conduction are tested by placing a vibrating fork on the mastoid process until the patient can no longer hear the sound. The vibrating fork is then placed by the ear canal to determine whether or not the patient can still hear the sound. Since air conduction is usually better than bone conduction, the vibrations should be heard for a longer period when the tuning fork is placed next to the ear (Rinne test). See Figure 3–7.

GLOSSOPHARYNGEAL (IX) AND VAGUS (X) NERVES

The glossopharyngeal and vagus nerves are usually tested together because of their innervation overlaps in the pharynx.

The glossopharyngeal nerve supplies sensory components to the pharynx, tonsils, soft palate, and posterior third of the tongue. It also supplies motor fibers to the stylopharyngeus muscle of the pharynx, whose role is to elevate the pharynx. The patient is asked to open his mouth and say "ah." The upward movement of the soft palate and uvula should be noted. He should also be able to feel light touch on the posterior third of the tongue when it is stimulated with the wooden end of a throat swab.

The *pharyngeal (gag) reflex* is innervated by both the ninth and tenth cranial nerves. The reflex is elicited by stroking each side of the mucous membrane of the posterior pharynx with a tongue blade. The normal response is

FIG. 3–7. Weber test and Rinne test. Note placement of tuning fork for each test. (Bates B: A Guide to Physical Examination, 3rd ed. Philadelphia, JB Lippincott, 1983)

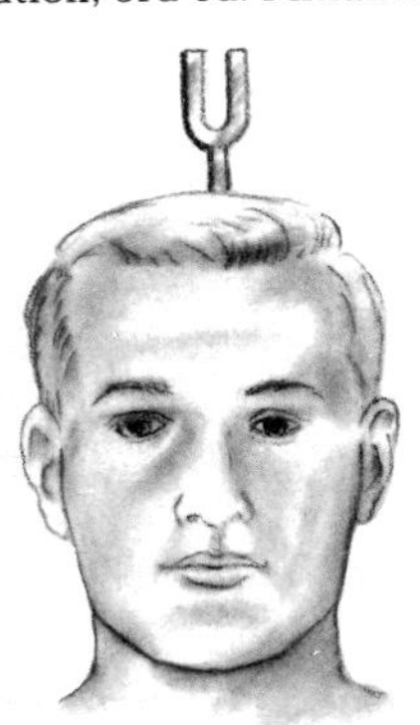

1. *Test for lateralization (Weber test).* Place the base of the lightly vibrating tuning fork firmly on the top of the patient's head or in the middle of his forehead. Ask where he hears it: on one or both sides. Normally the sound is perceived in the midline or equally in both ears. Sometimes the normal patient perceives the sound only vaguely. If he hears nothing, press the fork more firmly on his head.

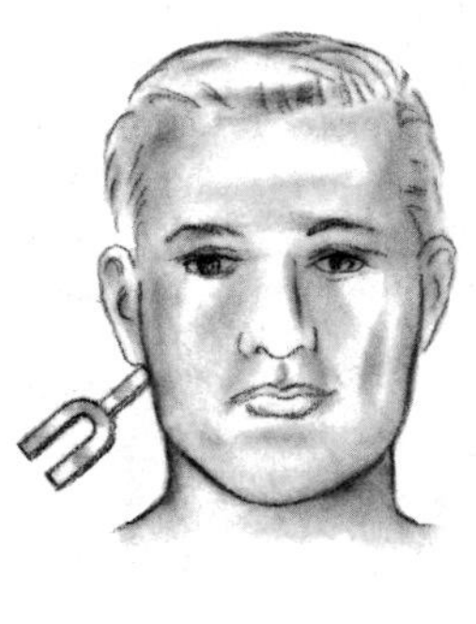

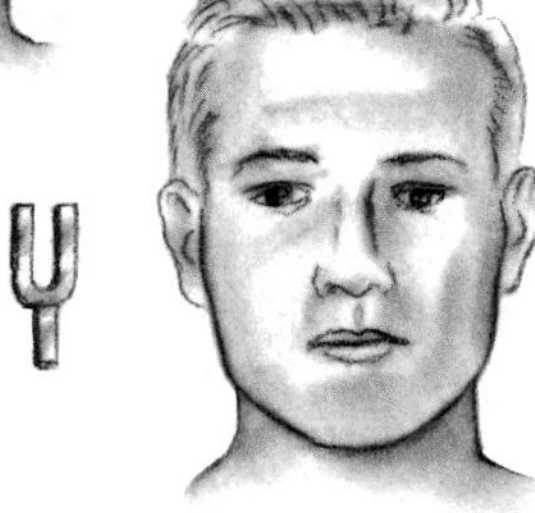

2. *Compare air conduction (AC) and bone conduction (BC) (Rinne test).* Place the base of a lightly vibrating tuning fork on the mastoid process until the patient can no longer hear the sound. Then quickly place the vibrating fork near the ear canal, with one side toward the ear as shown. Ascertain whether he can hear it. Normally the sound can be heard longer through air than through bone (AC > BC).

elevation and constriction of the pharynx along with retraction of the tongue.

The vagus nerve controls swallowing and speaking (the vocal cords) by the innervation of the soft palate, larynx, and pharynx. The soft palate is examined with the patient's mouth open. The palate should elevate when the patient says "ah." The uvula should be checked to see if it deviates to one side or the other (Fig. 3–8). The *palatal (swallowing) reflex* is tested by stroking each side of the mucous membrane of the uvula. Normally, the uvula should rise and deviate to the stimulated side. The quality of the voice is evaluated for hoarseness or dysarthria. If either is present, the vocal cords are examined for evidence of paralysis.

FIG. 3–8. Observing the palate. *(A)* Normal palate with mouth open and at rest. *(B)* Right unilateral vagus paralysis with mouth at rest. *(C)* Right unilateral vagus paralysis on pronation. (Kintzel KC: Advanced Concepts in Clinical Nursing, 2nd ed. Philadelphia, JB Lippincott, 1977)

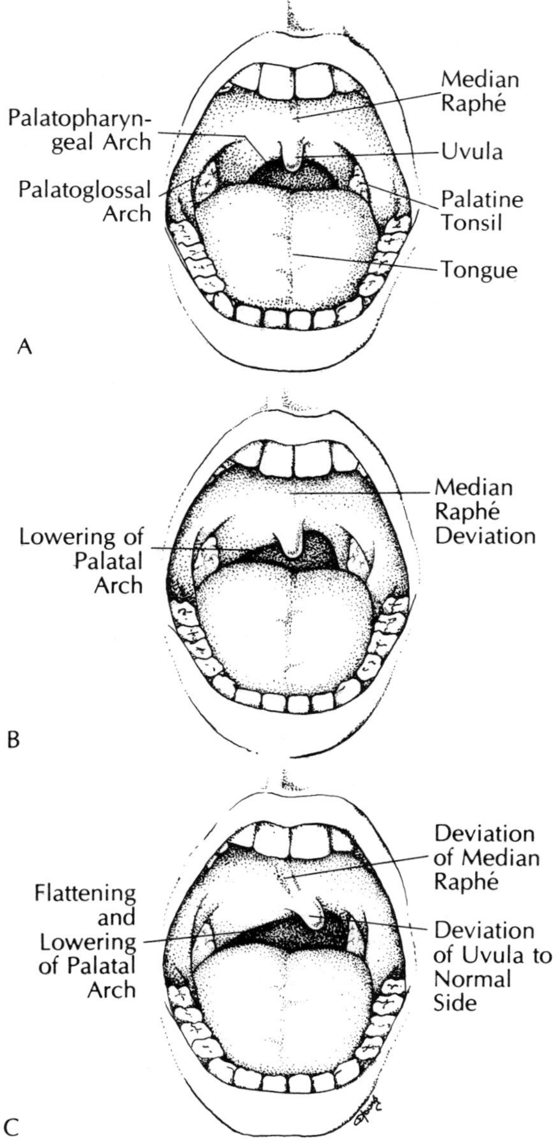

Aphonia or dysphonia is due to disease of the larynx or its innervation. Vocal quality is tested by listening to the patient speak. A difficulty in speaking such as hoarseness is termed *dysphonia;* a difficulty while speaking in a whisper is called *aphonia.* Paralysis of the soft palate *(palatal paralysis)* can result in "nasal" speech. *Dysarthria* refers to defective articulation caused by a motor deficit of tongue or speech muscles. Slurred speech is noted along with difficulty pronouncing the letters m, b, p, t, and d, and the number 1.

The autonomic functions of the vagus nerve throughout the body are many and are usually evaluated as part of the general physical examination.

SPINAL ACCESSORY (XI) NERVE

The accessory nerve, as it is sometimes called, is tested in two segments: first, the trapezius muscle is palpated and its strength evaluated while the patient shrugs his shoulders against resistance provided by the examiner's hands; second, the patient is asked to turn his head to one side and push his chin against the examiner's hand, thereby allowing the sternocleidomastoid muscle to be palpated and its strength evaluated (followed by performing the same procedure for the other side). The symmetry of the trapezius and sternocleidomastoid muscles is noted, along with any wasting or spasm.

HYPOGLOSSAL (XII) NERVE

The patient's tongue is first elevated (in the opened mouth) to determine lateral deviation, atrophy, fibrillations (or fasciculation), or spasticity. *Fibrillations* are the slight muscle flickerings seen in true atrophy that suggest lower motor neuron disease. Next, the patient is asked to stick out his tongue and push it laterally against a tongue blade. The examiner moves the blade first to one side and then to the other. In this way the strength of the tongue can be evaluated, and any deviation to one side or the other can be noted.

EVALUATION OF MOTOR FUNCTION

GAIT EVALUATION

The third step in the neurological examination is the examination of motor function. The first observation is that of a patient's gait. The patient is asked to walk back and forth naturally in the room. Points to observe are posture, movement of body parts, and the type of steps taken. The following is a list of the more common disturbances in gait that are seen with neurological problems. (See Chart 3–3.)

Steppage Gait. Steppage gait is associated with flaccidity of the leg and footdrop. To compensate for the dropped foot, the patient lifts the thigh and leg high to clear the dropped foot from the ground. As a result, the foot slaps against the floor. Steppage gait can be unilateral when caused by a

CHART 3–3. GAIT CHANGES IN NEUROLOGICAL DISEASE

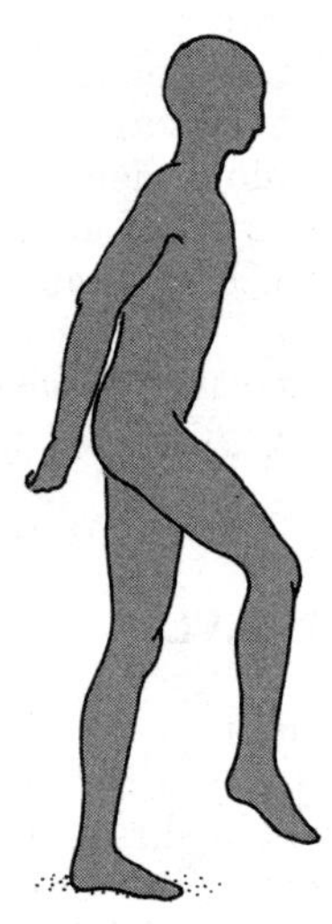

Steppage gait is associated with footdrop, usually secondary to lower motor neuron disease. The feet are lifted high, with knees flexed, and then brought down with a slap on the floor. The patient looks as if he were walking up stairs.

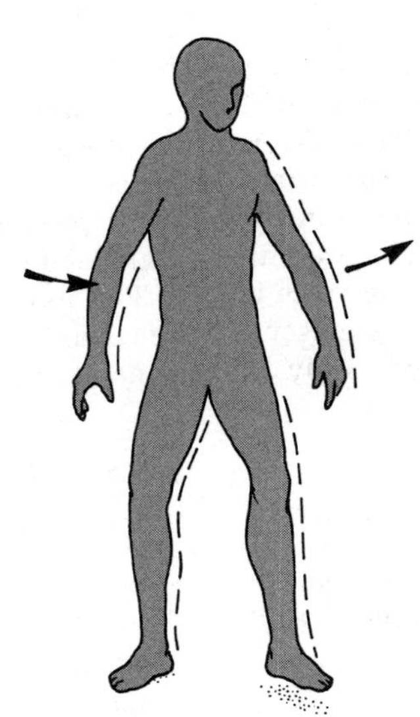

Cerebellar ataxia is associated with disease of the cerebellum or associated tracts. The gait is staggering, unsteady, and wide-based, with exaggerated difficulty on the turns. The patient cannot stand steadily with feet together, whether eyes are open or closed.

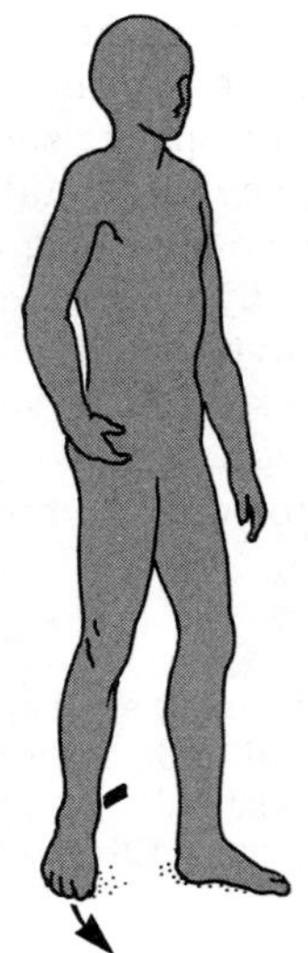

Spastic hemiparesis is associated with unilateral upper motor neuron disease. One arm is flexed, close to the side, and immobile; the leg is circled stiffly outward and forward (circumducted), often with dragging of the toe.

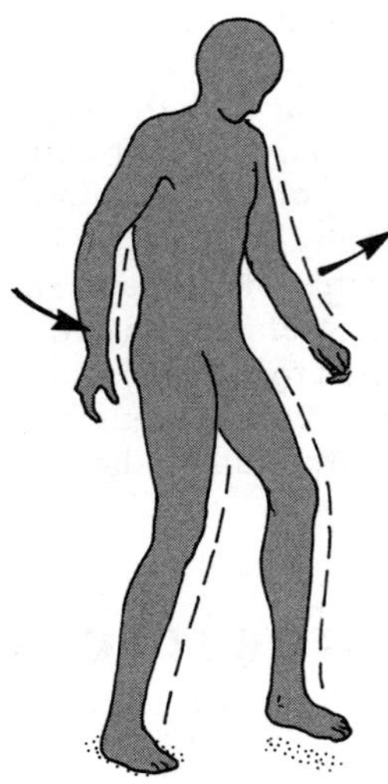

Sensory ataxia is associated with loss of position sense in the legs. The gait is unsteady and wide-based (the feet are far apart). The feet are lifted high and brought down with a slap. The patient watches the ground to guide his steps. He cannot stand steadily with feet together when his eyes are closed (positive Romberg test).

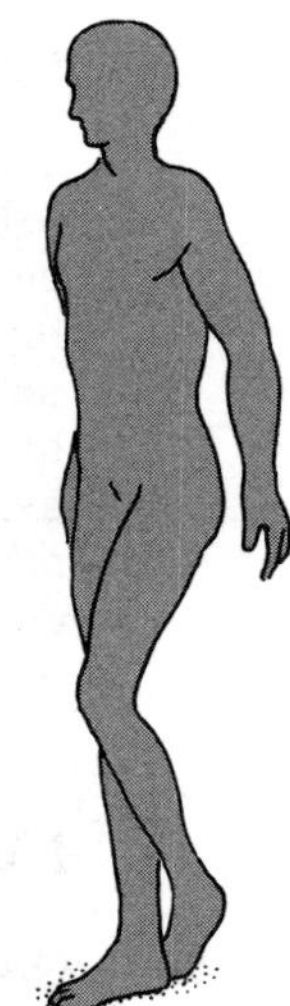

Scissors gait is associated with bilateral spastic paresis of the legs. Each leg is advanced slowly and the thighs tend to cross forward on each other at each step. The steps are short. The patient looks as if he were walking through water.

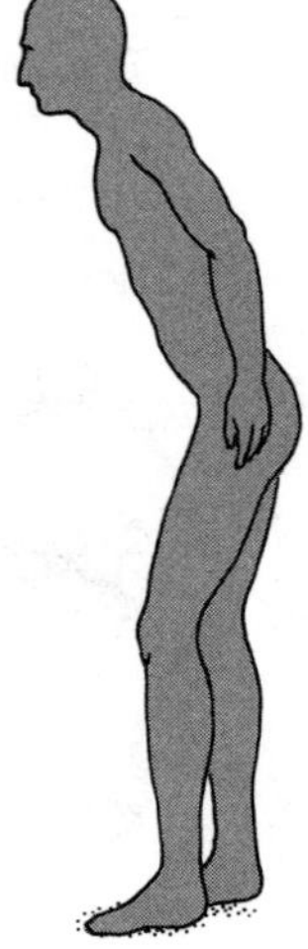

Parkinsonian gait is associated with the basal ganglia defects of Parkinson's disease. The posture is stooped, the hips and knees slightly flexed. Steps are short and often shuffling. Arm swings are decreased and the patient turns around stiffly—"all in one piece."

(Adapted from Bates B: A Guide to Physical Examination. Philadelphia, JB Lippincott, 1983) lesion of the external popliteal nerve, bilateral as in peroneal muscular atrophy (Charcot–Marie–Tooth disease), or bilateral when spinal cord segments L–5 to S–1 are involved, as in poliomyelitis and certain advanced polyneuropathies.

Waddling Gait. A waddling gait is characterized by a broad base lordosis and a lateral jerking movement of the hips and the trunk. The cause is weakness of the gluteal, psoas, and truncal muscles.

Hypotonic (Tabetic) Gait. Hyperextension of the knees, wide-based flaillike movements of the legs with high steps terminating in the heel being brought down, and a slap on the floor as the toes touch are the major characteristics of tabetic gait. Degeneration of the posterior columns with a loss of the proprioception reflex is usually due to tabes dorsalis. The patient must watch his limb to ascertain position. The gait is much exaggerated in the dark or when the eyes are closed.

Cerebellar (Ataxic) Gait. The cerebellar gait is wide-based, staggering, lurching, and uncoordinated. A similar gait is seen in a severely intoxicated person. The cause is any type of disease of the cerebellum such as a tumor, multiple sclerosis affecting the cerebellum, or Friedreich's ataxia.

Spastic Corticospinal Gaits. Diseases of the corticospinal tract that result in spasticity produce hemiplegic, spastic, and scissor gaits.

The *hemiplegic gait* is unilateral and includes

- Semiflexed arm, with the elbow held close to the waist
- Flexed fingers with wristdrop
- Extended, spastic, stiff leg, which is swung semicircularly in walking
- Inverted foot with footdrop

The *spastic gait* is the result of bilateral involvement of the corticospinal tract. The gait is characterized by

- Shuffling with the legs stiffly moving over the floor without being lifted
- Extension of legs

The *scissor gait* is a bilateral condition caused by severe spasticity of the adductor muscles of the legs and includes

- Legs crossed over, one in front of the other with each step
- Knees brought inward
- Patient often walking on his toes because of the swaying motion

Basal Ganglia Gaits. There are two major gaits of importance, the parkinsonian gait, as seen in Parkinson's disease, and the athetoid gait, seen in other basal ganglion disease disorders.

The *parkinsonian gait* is manifested by a loss of automatic arm swinging while walking, which is noted in the early stage of the disease. As the condition becomes more advanced, the patient walks in the following fashion:

- Head and body flexed forward
- Arms semiflexed and adducted
- Legs rigid and flexed
- Slow, shuffling gait

The initiation of the act of walking is slow and deliberate, but once walking begins the patient may propel himself forward with increasing momentum.

The *athetoid gait* is characterized by sudden, wormlike movement of the arms, head, and legs, which makes forward progress difficult.

MUSCLE EVALUATION

The motor examination proceeds from upper limbs to the neck, trunk, and, finally, the lower extremities. The symmetry of each side of the body is compared, as is each muscle or muscle group. Four points are considered in the evaluation: (1) muscle size, (2) muscle tone, (3) muscle strength, and (4) involuntary movement.

Muscle Size. Each of the muscles to be evaluated is first inspected and palpated. A tape measure can be used to obtain accurate data if visual inspection raises questions of differences in muscle size. The muscle on the left side of the body is compared with the same muscle on the right side of the body. Palpating the bulk of the muscle may help to detect any wasting or atrophy.

Muscle Tone. Palpation of the muscle is conducted while it is at rest and during passive movement. With the patient relaxed, the joints are put through the normal range of motion (flexion and extension) by the examiner. The systematic evaluation proceeds from the fingers, wrist, elbow, and shoulder in the upper extremities to the ankle, knee, and hip in the lower extremities. The left side and the right side are then compared.

Abnormalities in muscle tone are checked in terms of spasticity, rigidity, and flaccidity. *Spasticity* refers to undue resistance of the muscles to passive lengthening because of injury to the corticospinal system. *True spasticity* is described as an increase in resistance to passive movement followed by a sudden or gradual release of resistance.

Rigidity is a more constant state of resistance that involves the extrapyramidal motor system. Initially, rigidity includes tremors *(cogwheel rigidity)*. As the involved muscle is passively manipulated, a series of small, regular jerks is felt. As the rigidity becomes more fixed, the term *dystonia* is used to describe the muscle tone.

Flaccidity refers to decreased muscle tone or *hypotonia*. The muscle is weak, soft, and flabby. Muscle fatigability is also noted.

Unconscious patients with motor tract interruption can exhibit abnormal muscle tone or inappropriate motor responses that appear as characteristic movements or postures and are initiated by noxious stimuli. The particular posture or stereotypical movement assumed by the patient varies according to the anatomical level of injury. *Decortication* is characterized by flexion of the arm, wrist, and fingers, with adduction in the upper extremity, and extension, internal rotation, and plantar flexion of the lower extremity. Simply stated, there is hyperflexion of the upper extremities and hyperextension of the lower extremities. Lesions of the frontal hemispheres or internal capsule cause decortication by interrupting the corticospinal pathways (see Chap. 5, Fig. 5–6).

Another abnormal motor response is *decerebration*. When fully developed, decerebration includes opisthotonus (tetanic spasms that arch the back with backward flexion of the head and feet), adducted, extended, and hyperpronated arms, and stiffly extended legs with plantar flexion of the feet. Stated simply, there is hyperextension of both upper and lower extremities. This response results from rostral-to-caudal deterioration, which can occur when a diencephalic lesion extends into the midbrain or when a midbrain or upper pons lesion is present (Fig. 5–6).

It should be mentioned that intermittent decortication and decerebration may be observed. The intermittency is due to the obscure division line between deep cerebral hemispheric structures and the upper brain stem tissue of the midbrain. The shifting from one posture to the other occurs because of alterations in the blood supply to the cerebral tissue involved. Such changes in posture can be complete or partial. The patient can change from complete decerebration to decortication, or changes can occur in only one side of the body, one side being decorticate while the other is decerebrate.

Of the two abnormal postures presented, decerebration is considered to be a sign of greater cerebral dysfunction than decortication. If there is change from decorticate to decerebrate posture, it is an ominous sign. In the unconscious patient, muscle tone can be assessed by guiding the extremities through a passive range of motion. Rigidity, flaccidity, and spasticity can be noted through these simple movements.

The "Locked-In Syndrome." The "locked-in syndrome" is a term coined by Plum and Posner, representing a clinical picture of paralysis of motor function to all four extremities and the lower cranial nerves, so that all movement and ability to verbalize are lost. The only intact voluntary functions are vertical eye movement and blinking. The patient can be fully conscious of himself and his environment—he has been "locked into" the paralyzed body without a change in his level of consciousness.

Muscle Strength. The muscles of the major joints being tested are put through their normal range of motion. Muscle strength is evaluated by using passive range of motion and by testing strength first against gravity and then against the active resistance of the examiner.

Upper Extremities

To check for mild hemiparesis, the patient is asked to close his eyes and extend his arms straight out in front of him, palms up, for 20 to 30 seconds (Fig. 3–9, *A*). Downward drifting of the arms or pronation of the palms on one side would suggest mild hemiparesis.

With the patient's arms outstretched in front of him, the examiner tries to depress one outstretched arm against the resistance provided by the patient (Fig. 3–9, *B*). The movement of the scapula and the strength it exerts on that side should be noted for increased prominence of the scapular tip accompanied by displacement inward and upward. Such movement is suggestive of serratus anterior muscle weakness. This test should then be repeated with the other arm.

The patient is asked to raise his arms over his head, palms forward, for 20 to 30 seconds (Fig. 3–9, *C*), while the examiner tries to force the arms downward. Drifting or weakness on one side suggests mild hemiparesis or disease of the shoulder girdle. The patient is asked to grasp the examiner's hands. The examiner pulls the forearms downward and upward to test extension and flexion of the elbows, respectively.

With the patient's hands flexed into fists, the examiner attempts to push the wrists downward against resistance exerted by the patient (Fig. 3–9, *D*). If the examiner is successful, there is an indication of wristdrop, which is associated with an ulnar nerve disorder.

The examiner extends his index and middle fingers to the patient with the instructions, "Squeeze my fingers as hard as you can." Normally there should be some difficulty pulling the fingers out of the patient's grip (Fig. 3–9, *E*). A weak grip in either hand would indicate weakness of the forearm muscles, such as is seen with a hemiparesis or disorder of the hand. The left and right grips are compared for strength and equality.

The patient is instructed to spread his fingers so that the examiner can attempt to force them together (Fig. 3–9, *F*). If the fingers can be forced together, then there is possible ulnar nerve disorder. Flexion and adduction of the fingers, along with thumb opposition, are tested by instructing the patient to hold his fingertips and thumb together. The examiner's thumb is then placed into the palm of the patient's hand and attempts are made to pull it out of the patient's grasp. If this can be easily accomplished, there is weakness of these muscles.

In the unconscious patient, noxious stimuli are applied to elicit a motor response. Withdrawal of the stimulated extremity will occur if the motor system is intact. To assess the patient's arms for the presence of paralysis (paresis), the nurse should place the patient in neutral position on his back, lift the extended arms by the hands or wrists to the same height, and simultaneously release them. The weaker or paralyzed arm will fall more quickly and in a flaillike motion. The normal arm will fall more slowly. An alternative method is to position the elbows perpendicular to the bed while holding the arms by the patient's hands or

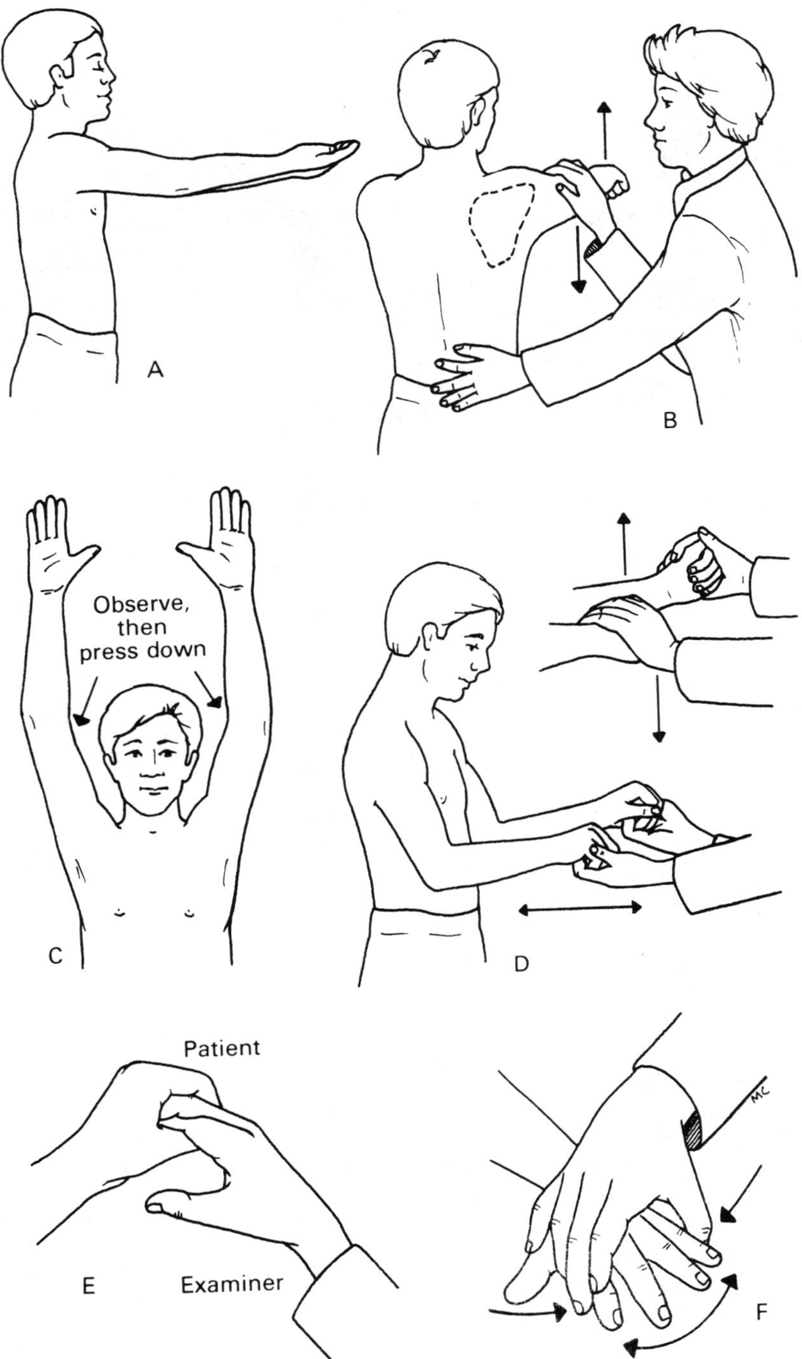

FIG. 3–9. Testing muscle strength of upper extremity. *(A)* Ask the patient to close his eyes and for 20 to 30 seconds to hold his arms straight in front of him, with palms up. Watch how well he maintains this position. (Tendency to pronation suggests mild hemiparesis; downward drift of arm with flexion at the elbow may also occur.) *(B)* On each side try to depress his outstretched arms against his resistance. Note his strength and watch the scapula on that side for winging or displacement. (Increased prominence of the scapular tip [winging] with displacement in and up suggests a weak serratus anterior muscle.) *(C)* Ask the patient to raise his arms over his head with palms forward for 20 to 30 seconds. Again observe the maintenance of this position. Try to force his arms down against his resistance. Note any weakness. (Drifting or weakness on one side suggests hemiparesis or shoulder girdle disease.) *(D)* Test flexion and extension at the elbow by having the patient pull and push against your hands. Test dorsiflexion at the wrist by asking the patient to make a fist and resist your pushing it down. (There will be wristdrop in radial nerve disorders.) *(E)* Test the grip by asking him to squeeze your fingers as hard as he can. You can avoid painful, hard gripping by offering the patient only your index and middle fingers, with the middle finger on top of the index. You should normally have difficulty removing your fingers from the patient's grip. (Grip may be affected by forearm muscle weakness and painful disorders of the hands.) *(F)* Ask the patient to spread his fingers. Check abduction by trying to force them together. (There will be weak abduction in ulnar nerve disorders.)

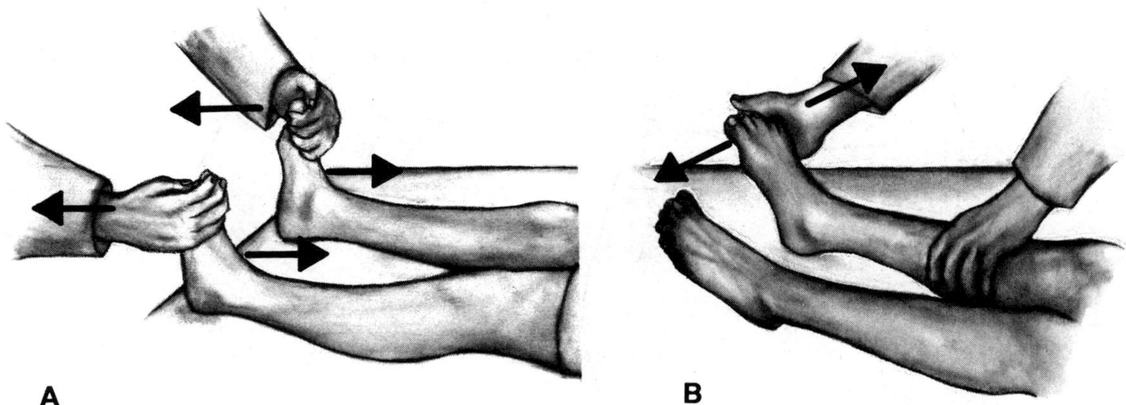

FIG. 3-10. Testing for dorsiflexion (*A*) and plantar flexion (*B*). Test dorsiflexion and plantar flexion at the ankle by asking the patient to push down and pull up against your hands.

wrists. Observe the movement of both arms while releasing the extremities simultaneously. The paralyzed arm will fall more quickly, possibly striking the face.

Lower Extremities

While lying on the bed, the patient is asked to separate his legs. This movement tests hip abduction. He is then asked to place his legs together again. Hip adduction should be noted. Knee flexion and extension are tested by positioning the patient on the desired section of the bed and applying active resistance to see if the resistance exerted by the patient can be overcome. Plantar flexion and dorsiflexion of the foot are tested by instructing the patient first to push down and then up against the examiner's hand, which is positioned on the foot (Fig. 3-10).

Throughout the examination it is most important for the examiner to compare the responses elicited on the left and right sides of the body.

Muscle function can be assessed using a scale of 0 (complete paralysis) to 5 (normal muscle strength). These numbers can be used as follows when recording muscle function: a stick figure is drawn and numerical values are placed at various points along the figure to indicate motor response. This approach is depicted in Figure 3-11.

In the unconscious patient, noxious stimuli are applied to elicit a motor response that would be observed as withdrawal if the motor system were intact. The legs can be assessed for paralysis or paresis by positioning the patient in the neutral position on his back and flexing the knees so that both feet are flat on the bed. The knees are simultaneously released and the movement of the legs is observed. The paralyzed or paretic leg will fall to an extended position with the hip outwardly rotated. The normal leg will maintain the flexed position for a few moments and then gradually assume its previous position. The extended legs may also be lifted to the same height and simultaneously released. The weaker limb will fall more quickly than the unaffected leg.

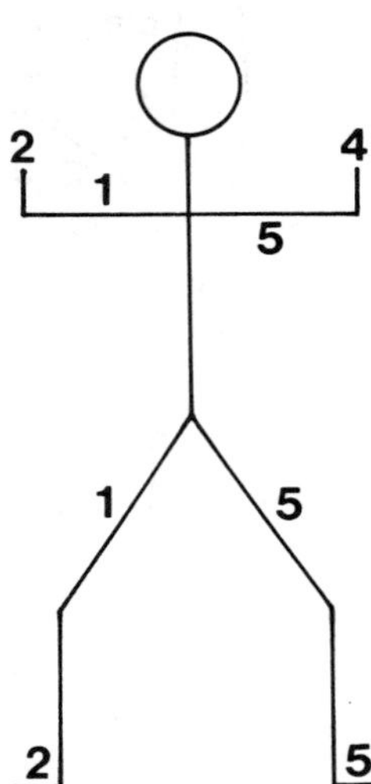

FIG. 3-11. Assessment of muscle strength: 5 = normal muscle strength; 4 = although the muscle can go through its normal range of motion, it can be overcome by increased resistance; 3 = the muscle is able to move through the normal range of motion against gravity only (it cannot tolerate any other external resistance at all); 2 = a weak contraction is noted, but not of a sufficient magnitude to overcome gravity; 1 = although there is a visible or palpable flicker of muscle contraction, no movement results; 0 = complete paralysis. Note that there are other grading systems that may be used.

INVOLUNTARY MOVEMENT

Any involuntary movements are noted. In observing involuntary movement, consideration is given to rate (cycles per second), distribution (proximal muscles, distal muscles), and relationship to movement (increase or decrease with movement). Common abnormalities of movement include tremors, choreiform movements, myoclonus, athetosis, tics, spasms, and ballism. Table 3-6 summarizes involuntary movements.

TABLE 3-6. *Involuntary and Abnormal Movement Patterns*

Type	*Description*	*Comments*
I. Tremors	• Involuntary trembling movement of the body or limbs resulting from contraction of opposing muscles; tremors are characterized by rate, distribution, and relationship to movement	• Seen with certain organic diseases; some forms of tremors are due to psychogenic causes
A. Specific types of tremors		
• Physiological	• Occasional tremors seen in healthy people precipitated by extreme fatigue or stress	
• Essential (familial, senile)	• Tremors occur when muscles are brought into action to support or move an extremity; also affect the jaw, lips, and head (head nods from side to side or to and fro) • Absent at rest • Tremor has characteristics similar to those of parkinsonian tremors	• Improvement usually noted with alcohol, sedatives, and propranolol
• Toxic	• Tremors are due to toxic states (e.g., uremia) or ingestion of toxic substances (e.g., drug withdrawal)	
• Cerebellar	• Tremors during movement that increase toward the end of the purposeful act	• Due to cerebellar lesions • May be seen in multiple sclerosis
• Parkinsonian	• Regular rhythmic tremors that are described as "pill-rolling tremors" (alternating flexion–extension of the fingers and adduction–abduction of the thumb) • Observed at rest • Associated with increased muscle tone	• Basal ganglia disorder seen in Parkinson's disease
B. Classification of tremors as related to rest and purposeful activity		• Vague, ambiguous classification that is used infrequently
• Resting tremors	• Tremor occurs when the patient is at rest; diminished by purposeful activity	
• Intentional tremors	• Increased or precipitated by purposeful activity	
II. Choreiform movements	• Characterized by irregular, jerky, uncoordinated movements and abnormal posture • Represent a more generalized condition than tremors • May be evidenced by grimacing and difficulty in chewing, speaking, and swallowing • Increase with purposeful activity making it difficult to complete the simplest of motor functions	
III. Myoclonus	• Sudden, brief, jerking contraction of a muscle or muscle group	
IV. Athetosis	• Involuntary, repetitive, slow, gross movements, particularly of posture • Arms tend to swing from a widely abducted base	• Movements described as snakelike
V. Tics	• Involuntary compulsive stereotyped movements • Described as "nervous habits" • Repeated at irregular intervals • Often involve the face	• Often associated with psychogenic origins
VI. Spasms	• Involuntary contraction of large muscle groups (arms, legs, neck)	• Oculogyric spasms, as seen in Parkinson's disease, are an example; oculogyric spasms are characterized by fixed upward gaze of extraocular muscles
VII. Ballism	• More or less continuous gross abrupt contractions of the axial and proximal muscles of the extremities • Violent flaillike movements	• Usually involves one side of the body (hemiballismus) • Caused by a destructive lesion in or near the contralateral subthalamic nucleus

TABLE 3-7. *Sensory System Evaluation*

Sensory Modalities	Description/Technique
I. Primary sensory modalities	
A. Superficial sensations	
• Superficial tactile (light touch) sensation	• A wisp of cotton is used as the stimuli. The patient is asked to close his eyes and signify with a word, such as "yes," when he feels a light touch. The examiner lightly touches the skin with the cotton wisp beginning at the head and working downward. Each side of the body must be assessed. • Light touch sensation is often preserved while other sensory modalities are compromised in lesions of the spinal cord. This is true because there is an overlap of innervation to areas.
• Superficial pain Within a few segments after entering the cord, fibers conveying pain and temperature synapse and cross the midline through the ventral commissure to the opposite lateral spinothalamic tract. This is important to note because there may be dissociation of pain and temperature loss while the ability to feel light touch is preserved.	• A pin or other sharp object is used as a stimuli. Care must be taken to prevent injury to the patient. • The same systematic procedure is followed as for light touch.
• Temperature sensation Note that the tracts conveying pain and temperature both cross to the opposite side of the spinal cord.	• Two test tubes, one filled with cold water and the other filled with warm water, are used for the stimuli. • Following the same procedure as for light touch and pain, the patient is systematically touched and his response noted.
B. Deep sensation	
• Sense of motion and position	• Passive motion is tested in upper extremities on the fingers and in the lower extremities on the toes. The sides of the toes and fingers are lightly grasped by the examiner's index finger and thumb. • Note that the digits and toes should be touched lightly so that the pressure needed to move the appendage is not apparent to the patient. • As the examiner moves the fingers and toes, the patient is asked to identify the direction of movement and the final position of the digit.
• Deep pain	• The Achilles tendon, calf, and forearm muscle are squeezed on each side of the body. Note the patient's sensitivity to the stimuli.
• Vibration sensation	• Using a vibrating tuning fork, place the instrument on bony prominences (wrist, elbow, shoulder, hip, knee, ankle). • The patient should be instructed to say when he feels vibration and when it is no longer present. • Compare the sensitivity from side to side as well as from proximal to distal portions of the same extremity.
II. Cortical and discriminatory forms of sensation (complex somatic sensory impressions that require cerebral cortex interpretation)	
• Two-point discrimination Note that various regions of the body differ greatly in their ability to discriminate simultaneous-point stimulation.	• A small pair of calipers or a drafting compass is used to provide the stimulus. • The patient, with eyes closed, is simultaneously touched with the sharp object. He is asked to identify if he is being touched by one or two objects. This testing procedure continues over the surface of the body.
• Point localization	• The patient's skin is lightly touched at a particular point while his eyes are closed. He is asked to identify where he was touched. Compare each side of the body for response.
• Stereognosis	• With the patient's eyes closed, common objects such as a pencil, comb, jackknife, and ball are placed in his hand. He is asked to identify the object.
• Texture discrimination	• With eyes closed, the patient is asked to differentiate between various textures of materials. Each side of the body is tested and compared.
• Traced-figure identification Note that if the normal superficial sensation is tested and present but this skill is absent, there is usually a lesion on the contralateral side of the parietal lobe.	• The examiner traces a number or letter on the patient's palm, back, or other part of the body with his finger, a blunt pencil, or an applicator stick. Each side of the body is tested.
• Double simultaneous stimulation (extinction)	• Simultaneously touch two corresponding body parts. • Ask the patient to identify area touched. Note whether he is aware that he was touched on both sides.

EVALUATION OF SENSORY FUNCTION

In evaluating the sensory system, the examiner determines the patient's ability to perceive various types of sensations with his *eyes closed*. Each side of the body is compared with the other, as are sensory perceptions at the distal and proximal portions of each extremity. The testing proceeds in an orderly fashion. The usual body areas used for evaluation include hands, forearms, upper arms, trunk, thighs, lower legs, feet, and the perineal and perianal areas. The following is a listing of sensory modalities tested and methods of evaluation:

- Superficial touch—A wisp of cotton is used to lightly stroke the various areas of the skin.
- Superficial pain—Various areas of the skin are pricked with a pin or other instrument.
- Sensitivity to heat and cold—A tube of hot water and one of cold water are applied to the same areas used in other tests.
- Sensitivity to vibration—A tuning fork is placed on bony prominences of the wrist, elbow, shoulder, hip, knee, shin, and ankle.
- Deep pressure pain—Achilles tendon and gastrocnemius and forearm muscles are squeezed.
- Sensitivity to position—Extremities, fingers, and toes are moved in various directions, which should then be identified by the patient.

Discriminative sensation is tested for the following modalities:

- Two-point discrimination—A part of the body is touched simultaneously with a sharp object to determine if the patient can feel one or two pricks. (The presence of receptors varies in different parts of the body.)
- Point discrimination—The patient is asked to name the location at which he has been touched with the wooden end of an applicator.
- Recognition of shape and form—The patient is asked to identify familiar objects that are placed in his hand. An inability to recognize objects in this manner is called *astereognosis*.
- Texture discrimination—The patient is asked to differentiate among various textures (e.g., silk, polyester, and wool).
- Graphesthesia—The patient is asked to identify letters written on palms, back, or other body parts.
- Extension phenomenon—The patient is touched on the skin on the two sides of the body simultaneously. He should feel both stimuli. See Table 3-7.

EVALUATION OF CEREBELLAR FUNCTION

The following list outlines the most common methods used to evaluate the patient's balance and coordination.

1. Starting with his arms outstretched, the patient is asked to touch his nose, first with eyes open, and then with his eyes closed.
2. The patient is asked to touch the examiner's finger with his finger (examiner moves his own finger to change position).
3. Sitting on a chair, the patient is asked to alternately pat his knee with his left and right hand as rapidly as possible; he is also asked to rapidly pronate and supinate his hands and forearms.

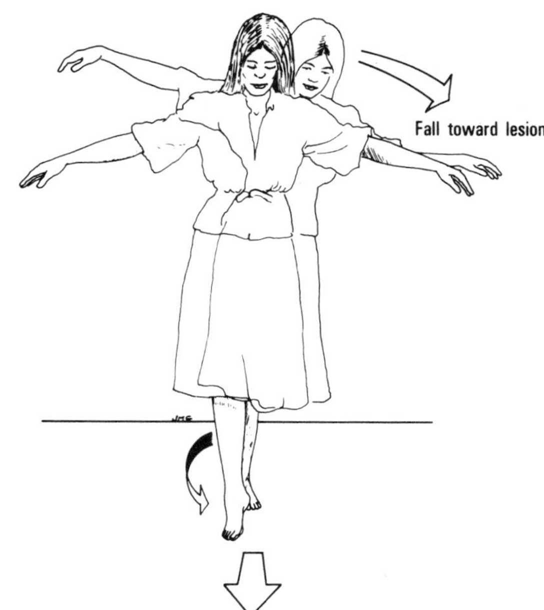

FIG. 3-12. The integrity of the cerebellum can be tested by having the patient walk heel to toe along a line (tandem gait). In cerebellar hemispheric involvement, the patient often falls toward the side of the lesion and there is ataxia. In midline cerebellar dysfunction, the gait is wide based and tandem gait walking cannot be performed. (Smith R: Essentials of Neurosurgery. Philadelphia, JB Lippincott, 1980)

4. Lying on his back, the patient is asked to move one foot down the shin of the opposite leg; the action is then repeated with the other foot.
5. The patient is asked to draw the number "8" with his foot in the air. This action is then repeated with other foot.
6. The patient is asked to stand erect with his feet together, first with his eyes open, then with them closed. This is called Romberg's test. After opening his eyes, he is asked to walk naturally. If the patient can stand with the eyes open but loses his balance when the eyes are closed, he is said to have a positive *Romberg's sign*. A positive Romberg's sign is indicative of dorsal column damage (Fig. 3-12).

Throughout the cerebellar evaluation, the accuracy of the action is assessed, and staggering gait, uncoordinated movements, and tremors are noted as abnormal findings. *Ataxia* is defined as uncoordination of voluntary muscle action, particularly of the muscle groups used in activities such as walking or reaching for objects.

EVALUATION OF REFLEXES

Testing the reflexes provides an important indication of the status of the central nervous system in both the conscious and unconscious patient. A stimulus is mediated by a definite pathway through the receptor organ, afferent limb, spinal cord or brain stem, efferent limb, and effector organ. The reflex is modified by the simultaneous activity of other pathways, particularly the corticospinal tract. Alterations in reflexes may be the earliest signs of pathology involving

CHART 3-4. IMPORTANT MUSCLE-STRETCH REFLEXES (DEEP TENDON REFLEXES)

In assessing deep tendon reflexes (DTR), proper technique must be used to elicit an optimal response. The *briskness* of the response is noted. To remember the major DTRs, recall the ascending sequential order of ½—¾—⅚—⅞.[3]

REFLEX	DESCRIPTION OF TESTING METHOD
Achilles reflex (S-1, S-2) (ankle jerk) 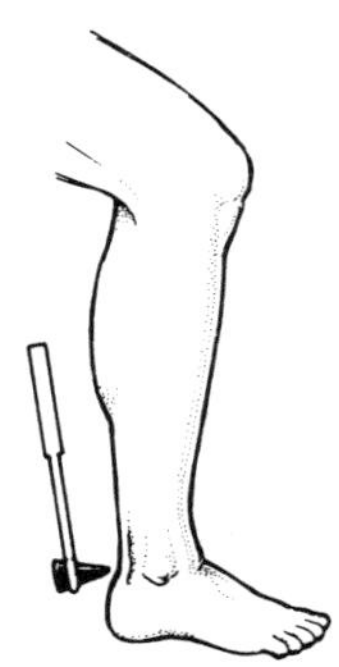	With the knee flexed, the Achilles tendon is struck; the foot should plantar flex.
Quadriceps reflex (L-3, L-4) (knee jerk) 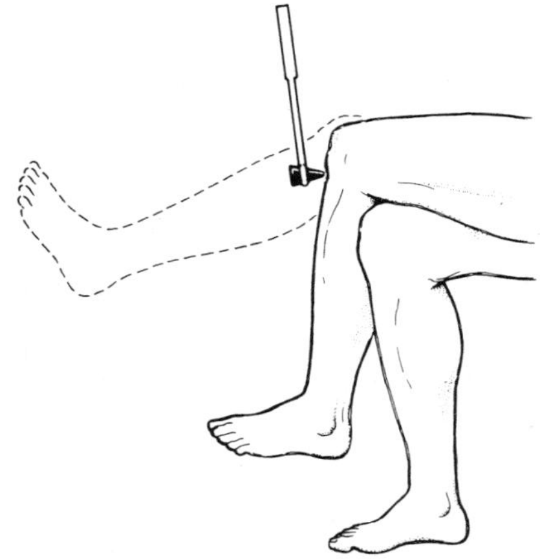	With the knee flexed, the patellar tendon is struck; the knee should extend.
Biceps reflex (C-5, C-6) 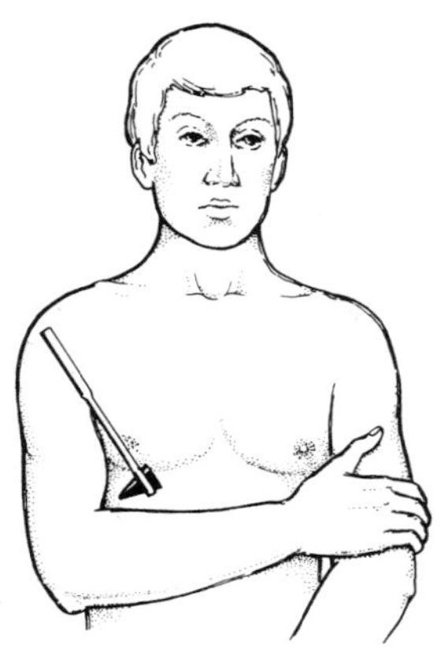	With arm partially flexed at the elbow with palm down, the examiner's finger is placed on the biceps tendon; the examiner's finger is struck and the stimuli is conveyed to the biceps; the elbow should flex.

CHART 3–4 (continued)

Triceps reflex (C–7, C–8)	With the arm partially flexed at the elbow with the palm directed toward the body, the triceps tendon is struck above the elbow; the elbow should extend.

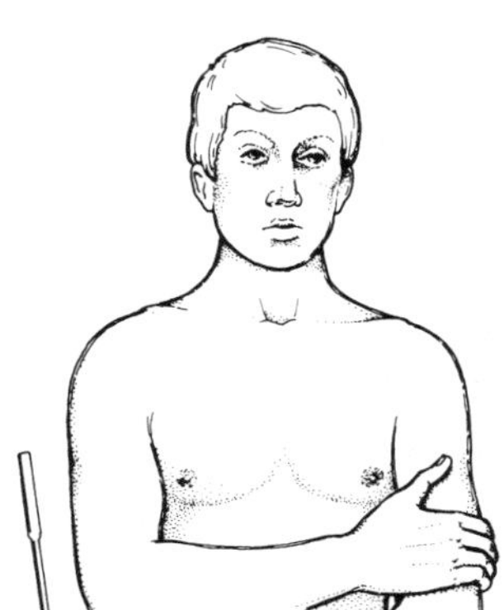

the corticospinal pathways (upper motor neuron disease), anterior horn cells or their axonal projection (lower motor neuron disease), or the afferent sensory components of the muscles. In clinical evaluation, reflexes are classified into three categories: (1) muscle-stretch reflexes (also known as deep tendon reflexes or DTR); (2) superficial or cutaneous reflexes; and (3) pathological reflexes.

The *muscle-stretch reflexes* are evaluated first. These reflexes occur in response to a sudden stimuli such as the percussion hammer that causes the muscle to stretch. Chart 3–4 lists the major muscle-stretch reflexes tested. It is important to use the proper technique to elicit a reflex. With the muscle relaxed and the joint at midposition, the tendon is tapped directly, using a percussion or reflex hammer. Normally, there is contraction of the muscle with a quick movement of the limb or structure innervated by the muscle. Test both sides of the body and compare. Note the briskness of the response.

(Text continued on page 88.)

TABLE 3–8. ***Important Superficial Reflexes***

Reflex	*Description*
Corneal reflex (cranial nerves 5 and 7)	The cornea is touched lightly with a wisp of cotton; the eye should quickly close.
Pharyngeal reflex (cranial nerves 9 and 10)	Also called the gag reflex; the pharynx is stimulated with a tongue depressor; there should be retching or gagging; each side of the pharynx should be tested.
Palatal or uvular reflex (cranial nerves 9 and 10)	The uvula is stimulated with a cotton-tipped applicator; there should be elevation of the uvula; each side of the uvula should be tested.
Abdominal reflexes (T_8, T_9, T_{10}) and (T_{10}, T_{11}, T_{12})	Each side of the abdomen is stroked as indicated in Figure 3-13; the umbilicus should move in the direction of the skin stimulated; note that the upper and lower quadrants are tested and that the mediation of each is innervated by different areas; a tongue blade can be used to provide the stimuli.
Perineal reflexes: anal reflex (S_3, S_4, S_5) and bulbocavernous reflex (S_3, S_4)	The *anal reflex* is elicited by scratching the skin at the side of the anus (perianal area) with a blunt instrument or pin; there should be puckering of the anus; also, if a gloved finger is inserted into the rectum, contraction is felt. The *bulbocavernous reflex* is elicited by the examiner applying direct pressure over the bulbocavernous muscle behind the scrotum and pinching the glans penis; the muscle should contract.
Cremasteric reflex (L_1, L_2)	The inner aspect of the thigh or lower abdomen is lightly stroked in the male; there should be elevation of the ipsilateral testicle or both testicles (see Fig. 3-13).

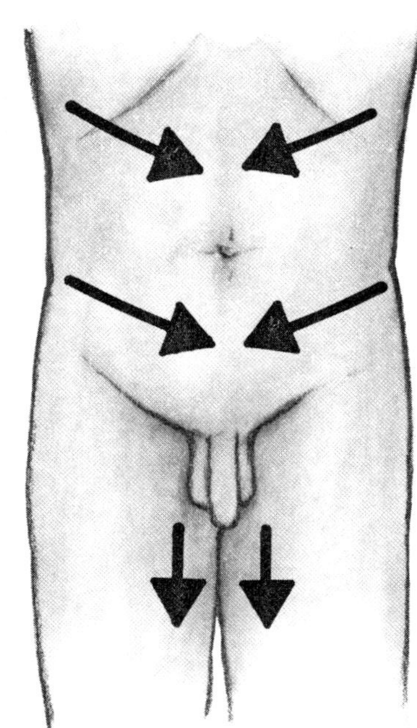

FIG. 3-13. The abdominal and cremasteric reflexes. Test the abdominal reflexes by lightly but briskly stroking each side of the abdomen, above (T-8, T-9, T-10) and below (T-10, T-11, T-12) the umbilicus, in the direction illustrated. Use a key or tongue blade, twisted so that it is split longitudinally. Note the contraction of the abdominal muscles and deviation of the umbilicus toward the stimulus. Obesity may mask an abdominal reflex. In this situation, use your finger to retract the patient's umbilicus away from the side to be stimulated. Feel with your retracting finger for the muscular contraction. Test the cremasteric reflexes (L-1, L-2) by lightly scratching the inner aspect of the upper thigh. Note elevation of the testicle on that side. Abdominal and cremasteric reflexes may be absent in both upper and lower motor neuron disorders.

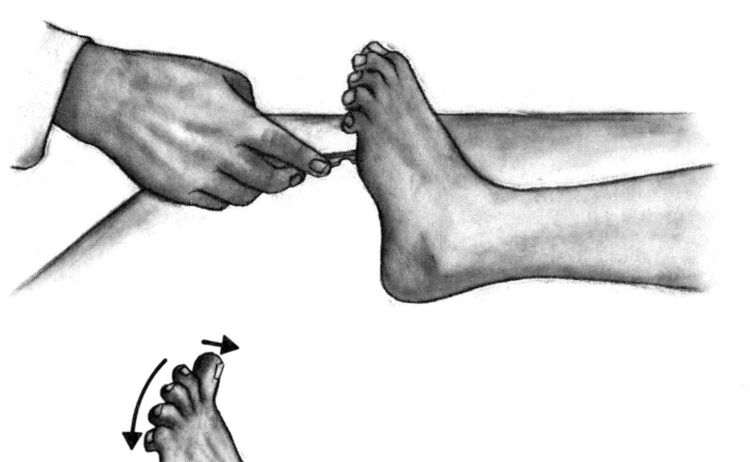

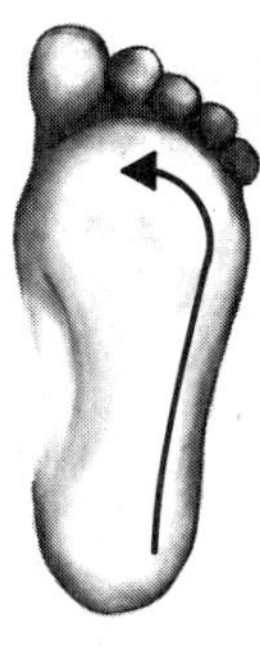

FIG. 3-14. Babinski reflex. With a moderately sharp object such as a key, stroke the lateral aspect of the sole from the heel to the ball of the foot, curving medially across the ball. Use the lightest stimulus that will provoke a response. Note movement of the toes, normally flexion. (Dorsiflexion of the great toe with fanning of the other toes indicates upper motor neuron disease.) (Bates B: Guide to Physical Examination, 3rd ed. Philadelphia, JB Lippincott, 1983)

CHART 3–5. PATHOLOGICAL (PRIMITIVE) REFLEXES

REFLEX	ASSOCIATED CONDITIONS[3]
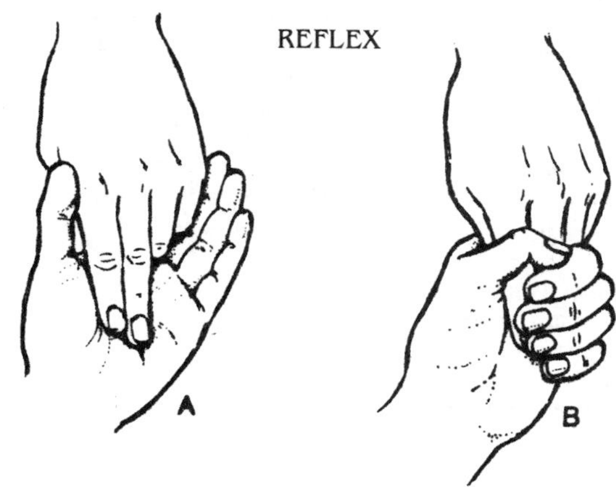 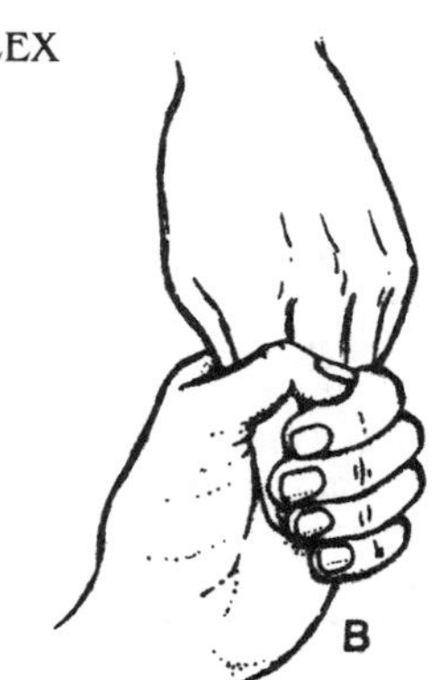 Grasp reflex. (*A*) Palmar stimulation; (*B*) grasp response	• Mostly frontal lobe disease • Sometimes occipital lobe disease • Bilateral cerebral atrophic disease (*e.g.,* Alzheimer's disease) • Bilateral thalamic degeneration • Advanced age and dementia *Note:* The reflex may be interpreted by family members and others as a voluntary act.
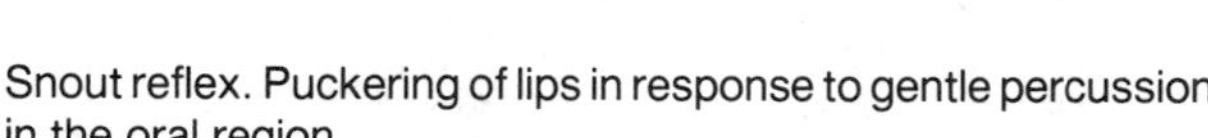 Snout reflex. Puckering of lips in response to gentle percussion in the oral region	• Cerebral degenerative diseases (*e.g.,* Alzheimer's disease) *Note:* In late stages of dementia some patients demonstrate continuous mouth and licking movements along with pursing of the lips.[4]
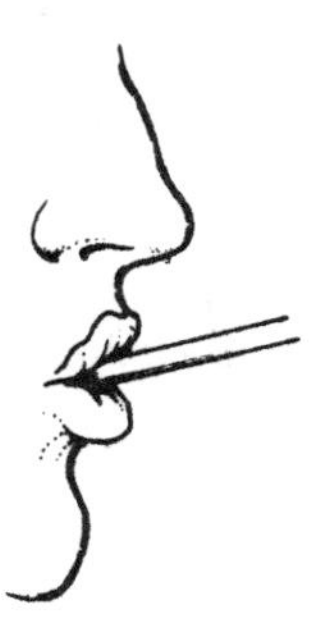 Sucking reflex. Sucking movement of the lips in response to tactile stimulation in oral region	• Same as for snout reflex *Note:* The reflex may be noted when the patient is suctioned or when mouth care is administered.

TABLE 3-9. *Plantar Responses — Pathological Reflexes*

Name	*Description*
Plantar response	When a designated area is stimulated, the response of the toes is observed. Normally, plantar flexion of the toes is observed. In the presence of pyramidal tract disease, extension or dorsiflexion of the big toe with fanning of the other toes is observed. Therefore, a plantar response is considered normal, while an extensor response is indicative of pyramidal tract disease. Babinski's, Chaddock's, and other signs listed are just variations of the plantar response. The response of the toes indicates the presence or absence of pyramidal tract disease.
Babinski's sign	The lateral aspect of the sole of the foot is rapidly stroked with a key from the heel to the ball of the foot. If a plantar response occurs, it is considered negative for a Babinski's sign (normal). An extensor response indicates a positive Babinski's sign (abnormal). See Figure 3-14.
Oppenheim's sign	An extensor response is elicited by stroking the anterior medial tibial muscle.
Gordon's sign	An extensor response is elicited by firmly squeezing the gastrocnemius muscle.
Hoffmann's sign	When the distal phalanx of the index or middle finger is snapped, there is sudden clawing of the fingers and thumb; presence of this sign indicates pyramidal tract disease.

The grading of muscle-stretch reflexes ranges from zero (0) to four (4):

- 4+ Very brisk, hyperactive; muscle undergoes repeated contractions or clonus; often indicative of disease
- 3+ More brisk than average; may be normal for that person or indicative of disease
- 2+ Average or normal
- 1+ Minimal or diminished response
- 0 No response

Superficial reflexes are elicited by light, rapid stroking or scratching (depending on the tissue being tested) of the skin, the cornea, or mucous membrane in a particular area. Table 3-8 lists the most common superficial reflexes tested. These reflexes are initiated by cutaneous receptors that are stimulated by stroking. The grading of superficial reflexes is different from that used with muscle-stretch reflexes. Superficial reflexes are graded as either present (+) or absent (0). See Figure 3-13.

Of the *pathological reflexes*, the *Babinski reflex* is the most important. Table 3-9 lists the most common pathological reflexes. The grading of pathological reflexes is that of presence or absence of the pathological sign. The presence of a pathological sign (+) is abnormal. Absence of a pathological sign (−) is normal. See Figure 3-14.

Other pathological reflexes are associated with damage to the cortical levels and are termed primitive. The term primitive is used because the reflexes were seen in early stages of development and then disappeared. See Chart 3-5.

REFERENCES

1. Members of the Department of Neurology and the Department of Physiology and Biophysics, Mayo Clinic and Mayo Foundation for Medical Education and Research, Graduate School, University of Minnesota, Rochester, MN: Clinical Examinations in Neurology, 5th ed. Philadelphia, WB Saunders, 1981
2. Bates B: A Guide to Physical Examination, 3rd ed. Philadelphia, JB Lippincott, 1983
3. Rosenfield DB: A practical neurological screening examination. Hosp Med 32A, June 1982
4. Wells CE (ed): Dementia. Philadelphia, FA Davis, 1977

BIBLIOGRAPHY

Books

Alpers B, Mancall E: Essentials of the Neurological Examination. Philadelphia, FA Davis, 1971

Ashworth B, Isherwood I: Clinical Neuro-Ophthalmology, 2nd ed. Oxford, Blackwell Scientific Publications, 1981

Bannister R: Brain's Clinical Neurology, 5th ed. New York, Oxford University Press, 1978

Chusid JG: Correlative Neuroanatomy and Functional Neurology, 18th ed. Los Altos, CA, Lange Medical Publications, 1982

Cogan DG: Neurology of the Ocular Muscles, 2nd ed. Springfield, IL, Charles C Thomas, 1975

Denny-Brown D: Handbook of Neurological Examination and Case Recording, rev. ed. Cambridge, MA, Harvard University Press, 1974

Eliasson S, Prensky A, Hardin W: Neurological Pathophysiology, 2nd ed. New York, Oxford University Press, 1978

Gilman S, Winans S: Manter and Gatz's Essentials of Clinical Neuroanatomy and Neurophysiology, 6th ed. Philadelphia, FA Davis, 1982

Plum F, Posner J: The Diagnosis of Stupor and Coma, 3rd ed. Philadelphia, FA Davis, 1980

Strub R, Black FW: The Mental Status Examination in Neurology. Philadelphia, FA Davis, 1977

Vaughn D, Ashbury T: General Ophthalmology, 9th ed. Los Altos, CA, Lange Medical Publications, 1980

Periodicals

Alexander MM, Brown MS: Physical examination, part 17: Neurological examination. Nurs76 6:38, June 1976

Alexander MM, Brown MS: Physical examination, part 18: Neurological examination. Nurs76 6:50, July 1976

Campbell WW: Periodic alternating nystagmus in phenytoin intoxication. Arch Neurol 37:178, March 1980

Condi J: Types and causes of nystagmus in the neurological patient. J Neurosurg Nurs 15(2):56, April 1983

Johnson J, Cryan M: Homonymous hemianopsia: Assessment and nursing management. Am J Nurs 79:2131, December 1979

Kupersmith M, Ransohoff J: Identifying Horner's syndrome. Hosp Med 38, March 1980

Lawyer T: Diagnosis: External neurological examination of the eye. Hosp Med 35, June 1980

Malasanos L: Tremors: Associations and assessment. J Neurosurg Nurs 14(6):290, December 1982
Mechner F: Patient assessment: Neurological examination, part I: Programmed instruction. Am J Nurs 75(9):1, September 1975
Mechner F: Patient assessment: Neurological examination, part II: Programmed instruction. Am J Nurs 75(11):1, November 1975
Mechner F: Patient assessment: Neurological examination, part III: Programmed instruction. Am J Nurs 76(4):1, April 1976
Medical Programs Incorporated: Patient assessment: Taking a patient's history. Am J Nurs 74(2):293, February 1974
Melamed M: Identifying Adie's syndrome. Hosp Med 65, February 1982
Mitchell P, Irvin N: Neurological examination: Nursing assessment for nursing purposes. J Neurosurg Nurs 9(1):23, March 1977
Thomas S: Guide to reflexes in neurologic diagnosis. Hosp Med 88, April 1977
Walleck D: Neurological assessment for nurses: A part of the nursing process. J Neurosurg Nurs 10(1):13, March 1978

chapter 4

Diagnostic Evaluation

At a time when refined, sensitive laboratory tests and diagnostic protocols have been developed to facilitate accurate and very specific diagnosis in other areas of medicine, the diagnostic tools of neurology remain crude by comparison. Most neurological diagnostic tests provide general information on the presence of an abnormality but do not indicate the specific nature of the causative lesion. For example, an echoencephalogram can confirm the presence of a space-occupying lesion, but it does not indicate whether the lesion is a tumor, a hematoma, or an abscess. It is true that the technology associated with the newer computed tomography (CT) scanners provides more specific pathological data; however, the specificity of most neurological tests cannot compare with the specific diagnostic tools available to specialists in other areas of practice. The development of technology such as positron emission transaxial tomography (PETT) and magnetic resonance imaging (MRI) will ensure advanced diagnostic capability for neurology and neurosurgery in the near future.

PATIENT TEACHING

Patient preparation or teaching is part of the supportive and teaching role of the nurse. With the exception of the neurological examination and lumbar puncture, most neurological diagnostic procedures are performed in such places as the operating room, radiology department, or special procedure areas rather than in the clinical nursing unit. If at all possible the nurse caring for the patient should accompany the patient to a diagnostic procedure. Sometimes this is an absolute necessity—for example, if the patient needs frequent suctioning or respiratory assistance. For the patient with impaired cognitive function or a high anxiety level, the nurse may make the difference between success and failure of the diagnostic procedure. It is often necessary for the patient to cooperate, lie quietly, or follow instructions. The familiar nurse from the nursing unit is often able to gain the patient's cooperation.

Other times, only the preprocedural preparation is completed in the clinical unit by the nurse. The patient is then taken to the designated area by someone responsible solely for the transportation of patients. Once the patient arrives at the procedure site, technicians and/or the physician are the personnel principally involved. It is therefore most important that a proper explanation of the procedure be provided to the patient beforehand.

A patient undergoing a diagnostic procedure needs a general explanation of the procedure with special emphasis on his participation in it. For example, a patient about to undergo a CT (brain) scan should be told that he must remain very still while the scan is being taken to ensure accuracy and quality graphics. For a more thorough briefing, information can be expanded to provide an explanation based on the patient's level of understanding and his desire for more information. He should know where the procedure will take place and where he will be taken after the test is completed.

If a patient's level of consciousness has been altered so much that it affects his understanding of what is being said, the nurse should provide a simple explanation. The following nursing diagnoses, if applicable to the patient, will require special consideration by the nurse when she prepares and teaches the patient for a scheduled diagnostic procedure. The nursing diagnoses include the following:

1. Cognitive impairment, potential or actual, related to
   - Hearing and/or visual deficit
   - Decreased level of consciousness
   - Effects of drug therapy
   - Neuropathological processes
2. Knowledge deficit related to
   - Anxiety state

- Cognitive (intellectual) limitations
- Memory deficits
- Decreased level of consciousness

3. Sensory deficits (hearing, visual, touch, agnosias) related to neuropathological processes
4. Short-term memory deficits related to
   - Neuropathological processes
   - Anxiety
5. Thought processes, impaired, related to
   - Neuropathological processes
   - Cognitive limitations
   - Limited attention span
   - Anxiety/fear

The nurse may need to repeat information about the diagnostic procedures several times. This information often must be reinforced over and over again because the patient has difficulty comprehending and remembering what is said. Neurologically impaired patients with cerebral dysfunction may have short attention spans and difficulty in making cause and effect associations with basic information. Therefore, the nurse must explain even simple points to allay the patient's fears. An example of such a situation may be telling the patient that he will be returning to his room after the procedure is over.

Written consent is required for many of the neurological diagnostic procedures. If the patient has an altered level of consciousness, cognitive deficits, or other impairments that will affect his ability to give consent knowingly, a family member must give written consent. It is the physician's responsibility to obtain written consent after explaining the procedure to the patient and family and answering their questions.

SKULL FILMS

Skull films generally include anteroposterior and lateral radiographic views (Fig. 4-1). Other angles may be included in the series to provide specific diagnostic information, but the anteroposterior and lateral views are the most common. Skull films are taken to furnish information about (1) the presence of skull fracture, (2) the position of the pineal body, (3) unusual calcification, (4) the size and shape of skull bones, (5) bone erosion, particularly of the sella turcica, and (6) abnormal vascularity.

When skull films are reviewed, certain landmarks are sought to determine the presence of pathology. For example, the pineal body, which is normally calcified in the adult, is the midline structure. If it appears to be skewed to one side, it is indicative of the fact that pressure from a space-occupying lesion is responsible for the deviation from the midline. Calcification that is noted in an area where it is not normally present would raise the suspicion of a calcified component located within a tumor. The appearance of bone erosion can suggest the presence of an intracranial lesion.

One of the most frequent reasons for ordering skull films

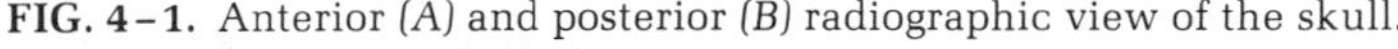
FIG. 4-1. Anterior *(A)* and posterior *(B)* radiographic view of the skull.

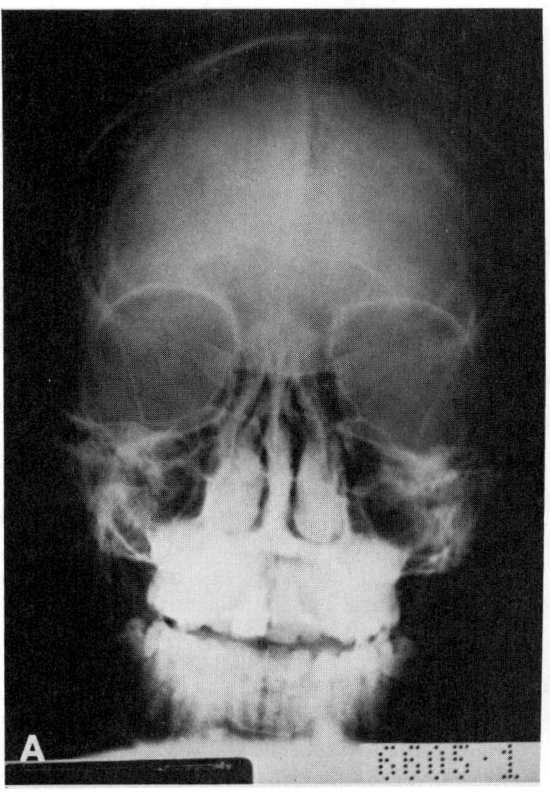

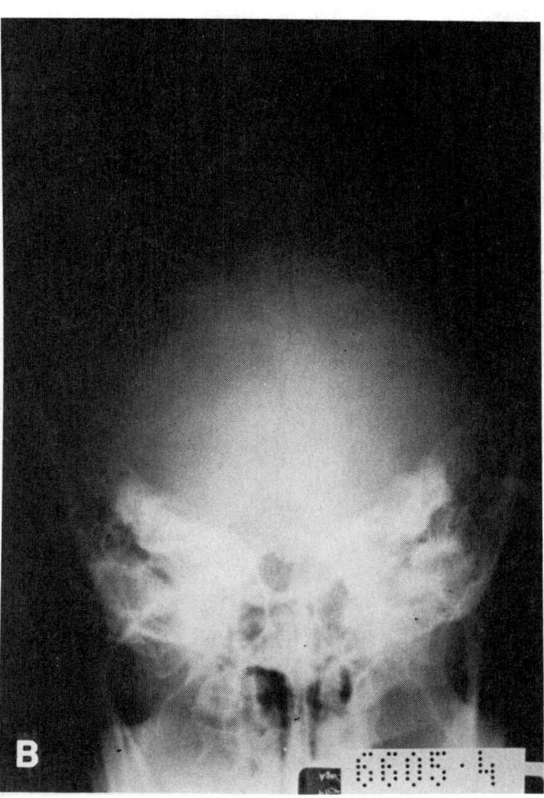

is to determine whether a skull fracture is present. If a patient has sustained trauma to his head, skull films will be ordered to rule out such a fracture.

SPINE FILMS

Spinal films are simple radiographs of various regions of the spine: cervical (Fig. 4–2), thoracic, lumbar, or sacral. The anterior, posterior, and lateral views are those commonly taken. Various abnormal findings may include (1) wedging of a collapsed vertebra, (2) erosion of bone caused by a neoplasm, (3) irregular calcification as a result of an inflammatory process, (4) narrowing of the vertebral canal because of obstruction by a neoplasm or protruding disc, (5) vertebral fractures and/or dislocations, (6) spondylosis, and (7) spurs.

Indications for spinal films include any trauma to the back or vertebral column, or conditions in which the patient experiences pain or motor or sensory impairment. Because the vertebrae are such highly irregular anatomical structures, it is easy to overlook fractures of these bones. This is why lateral films along with anterior and posterior views are necessary in many cases to rule out the possibility of fracture.

FIG. 4–2. Radiograph showing abnormality of cervical spine.

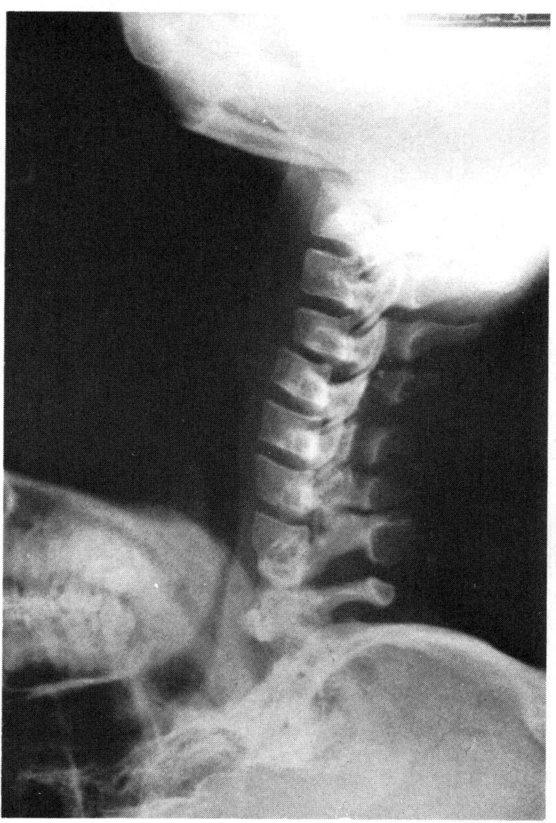

COMPUTED AXIAL TOMOGRAPHY OR COMPUTED TOMOGRAPHY

Computed axial tomography (CAT) or computed tomography (CT) was introduced as a clinical diagnostic tool by Hounsfield in England in 1972. The noninvasive diagnostic technology has been accepted for its accuracy and safety and has significantly altered the methods of diagnosis, especially in neurology and neurosurgery. Although the CT scan was originally used to examine the brain, the technology has since been applied to all parts of the body. In the 4 short years after the first CT scanner was introduced, the technology was significantly refined, and the first generation scanners had been replaced by fourth generation scanners. The refinements to the various generations of scanners include reduction in scan time (from 5 minutes to 1.5 seconds); better control of patient movement; reduction in computations of images by the computer; and improvement in the quality of the image. Further refinement of CT scanning is certain to occur (Fig. 4–3).

THEORETICAL BASIS

The basic components of the CT unit are one or more x-ray tubes and scintillation crystal detectors (scanner); one or more computers; a data display system; and a mechanism for making prints of the images. The head is scanned in successive layers by narrow x-ray beams that pass through the head and are absorbed and/or transmitted, depending on the density of tissue. The thickness of a scanner layer, called a slice, can vary from 2.0 mm to 15.0 mm. The radiation transmitted from the tissue is detected by an array of scintillation crystals (scanner), which convert the transmitted x-ray (radiation) into light photons in proportion to the energy and intensity of the transmitted radiation. The photons are, in turn, converted to electrical signals that are digitized and stored in a computer. The digitized information can then be manipulated by specialized computer programs to reproduce images representing the various slices of the cranium/brain in various orientations (coronal, sagittal, horizontal) on a display monitor. The display image may be photographed with a standard x-ray film or Polaroid film. Different types of equipment use varying numbers of detectors in various geometric arrays to improve image quality and reduce scan time. Each arrangement has its own special advantages.

In the digitized conversion of the image, the denser structures such as bone are assigned higher numbers so that bone appears as a whiter area on the display image. Cerebrospinal fluid (CSF) is less dense so its digitized numbers are lower; it appears as a black area on the monitor display. The brain appears as various shades of gray. The information provided by the CT scan is most helpful in determining whether a substance is composed of air, cerebrospinal fluid, blood, white or gray matter, congealed blood, bone, or calcification. The visualization (in gray tones) correlates to tissue density.

When the radiologist reviews a CT scan, changes in tis-

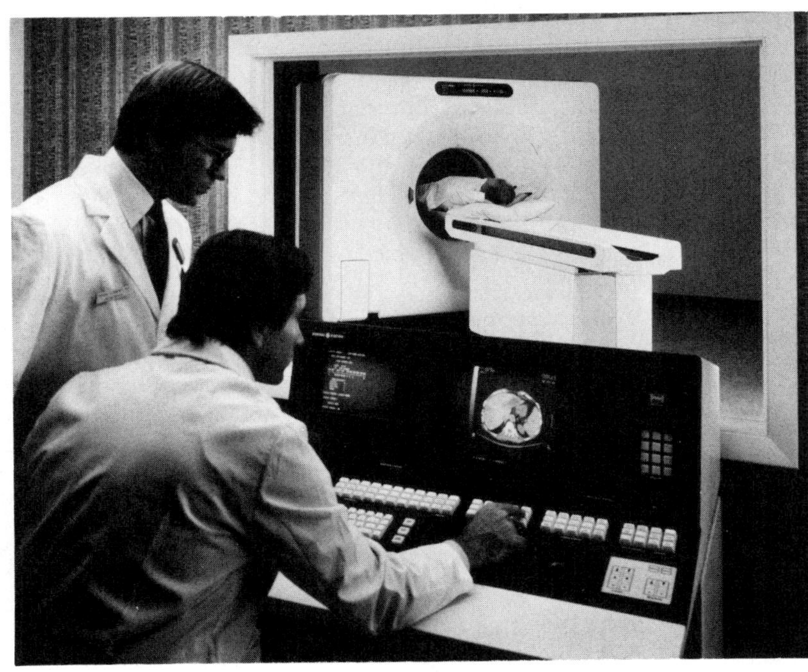

FIG. 4-3. General Electric CT 9800 Computed Tomography System. (General Electric Company, Medical Systems Operations, Milwaukee, WI)

sue density, displacement of structures, and abnormalities in size, shape, or location of structures are considered (Fig. 4-4).

PROCEDURE

The patient lies on an x-ray table, with his face uncovered and his head immobilized. His head is moved into the scanner. A movable circular frame (gantry) encircles the head and revolves around it making a clacking sound while taking radiographic readings. Slight adjustments to the machine are made periodically. The head is scanned numerous times at different angles (180 times at 1-degree intervals on an arc) to collect the data.

If contrast medium is injected to enhance certain areas, more pictures are taken after a short delay. The entire procedure takes from 15 to 30 minutes. The critical concern when collecting data is for the patient to remain motionless. Movement will cause artifacts within the image that

FIG. 4-4. Computed tomography (CT) scan of the brain. *(A)* Normal scan. *(B)* Scan showing a large mass in the left frontal lobe.

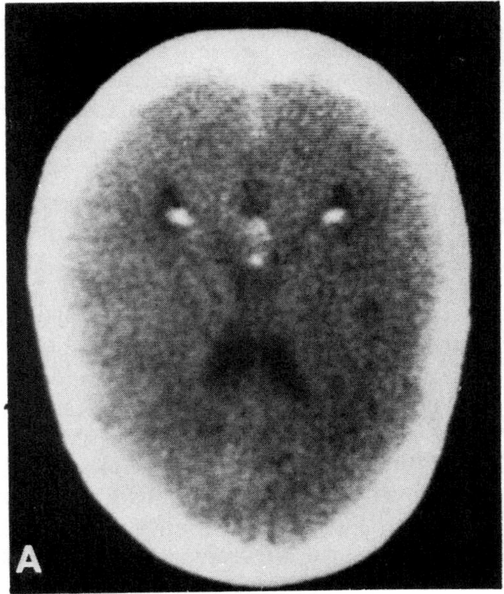

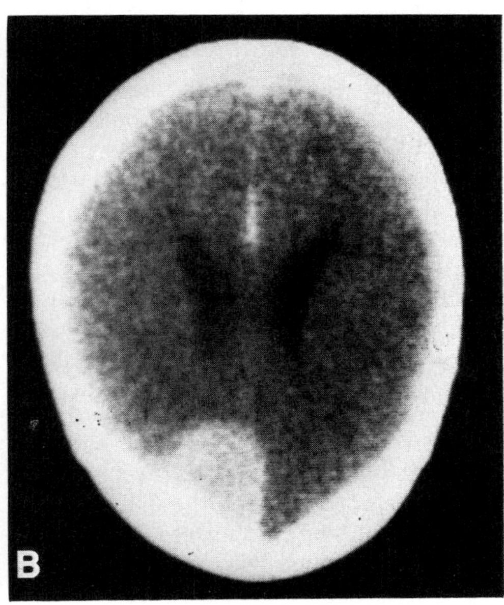

will affect the clarity of the pictures. If the patient is confused, agitated, or uncooperative, sedation or anesthesia will be necessary to ensure the quality of the pictures.

CONTRAST

If contrast enhancement is desired, iodinated radiopaque material will be administered intravenously. Precontrast scanning may be done before the contrast medium is injected. The purpose of the enhancement is to improve the clarity of the images for more accurate diagnosis.

DIAGNOSTIC APPLICATION

The CT scan is extremely useful in locating and diagnosing various cranial lesions such as abscesses, cysts, infarctions, hematomas, arteriovenous malformations, aneurysms, contusions, hydrocephalus, and primary and metastatic tumors.

Several advantages are cited for the use of the CT scan: (1) much information can be collected when a problem is still in its early stages; (2) it is painless and safe and can be done on an outpatient basis; (3) it has drastically reduced the need for more dangerous diagnostic tests such as pneumoencephalogram and cerebral angiogram; (4) serial CT scans can be taken to follow the resolution of cerebral disorders (e.g., hemorrhage, edema); (5) the amount of radiation exposure is relatively low (depending on the scanner, the radiation exposure is between 2 rad and 10 rad) and is similar to skull films; and (6) the scan can be performed on conscious and unconscious patients who can remain still while it is being taken.

PREPROCEDURAL PREPARATION

The hair should be clean and free of hair pins. No special attire is required; the outpatient can wear regular street clothes. All jewelry and metal objects should be removed from the head and neck. Unless contrast medium will be administered, there are usually no dietary restrictions on the patient before the procedure. However, some physicians prefer to restrict the patient's intake to clear liquids. The specific routine of the physician and the hospital should be followed.

Before a contrast radiopaque medium is administered, a skin test should be performed to check for an allergic reaction. Most protocols require that when a contrast medium is used, the patient not be given anything by mouth for 4 to 8 hours before the test. Some patients experience flushing or a feeling of warmth, transient headache, a salty taste in the mouth, nausea, or vomiting when the contrast medium is administered. Patients who will receive contrast medium should be prepared for these possible reactions.

For the adult patient who will require sedation to prevent motion, the drug should be administered shortly before the procedure is scheduled to begin. A drug frequently chosen for sedation is diazepam (Valium), which is administered intravenously.

The procedure and equipment used are described to the patient. Reassure him that the procedure is painless. No motion will be felt, and the clacking sound of the machine is to be expected. He should know that even though the technician and radiologist are outside the room, they can see and hear the patient at all times. The need to remain perfectly still should be emphasized.

POSTPROCEDURAL CARE

There is no special aftercare for the patient who has not been given contrast medium. The patient who has received enhancement medium should be observed for signs and symptoms of a delayed reaction to the medium. Hives, skin rash, itching, nausea, or headache are common findings. If symptoms are severe, antihistamines may be administered.

MAGNETIC RESONANCE IMAGING

An exciting new technology that is expected to revolutionize medical diagnosis in the near future is magnetic resonance imaging (MRI). The new name, magnetic resonance imaging, is preferred to the older term, nuclear magnetic resonance (NMR), because some people associate the word "nuclear" with negative connotations. Magnetic resonance images are unmatched for showing sharp and detailed cross sections of living tissue, which provide not only anatomical information but also information about the chemistry and physiology of living tissue.

Many experts predicted that the MRI technology would be available at major teaching and research centers by 1985 and that once the technology became established, it would render CT scans obsolete! The CT scan uses radiation exposure to image cross sections of body tissue to demonstrate anatomical structures, while MRI is based on a new method for image production that does not use radiation, therefore eliminating the hazards of radiation exposure to the human body. The procedure for MRI is noninvasive and painless and has no known risk to the patient. While lying on a table, the patient is placed in a strong magnetic field and is then subjected to precise, computer-programmed bursts of radio pulse waves. The patient feels nothing and hears only a soft humming sound and on–off pulses of the radio waves (Fig. 4–5).

A brief overview is presented to give the reader a basic understanding of the MRI technology. MRI was discovered in 1946 by scientists working independently at Harvard and Stanford universities. Since then, the technology has been refined for use as a diagnostic tool. Initially, researchers found that atoms with an odd number of nuclei protons (protons are positively charged particles) spin naturally like tiny tops so that their axes point in random directions. When a strong magnetic field is applied, the nuclei will line up in a uniform manner (like small bar magnets) in a north–south magnetic field orientation. If

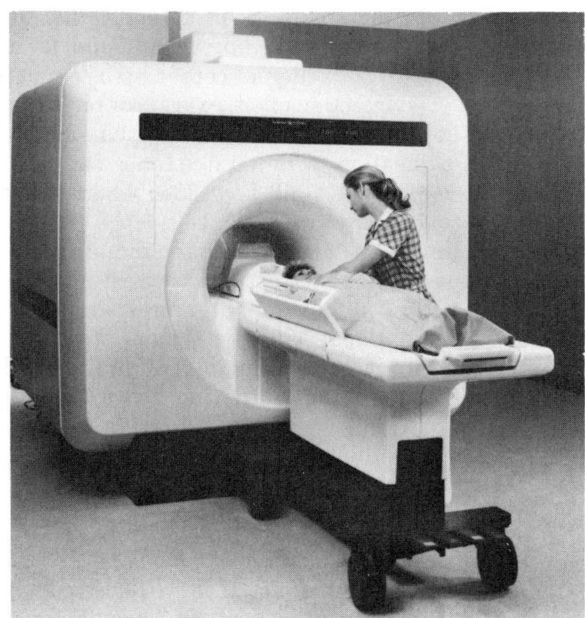

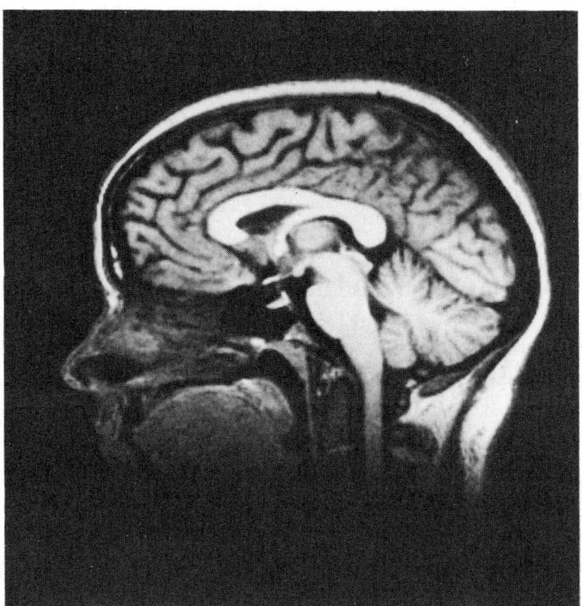

FIG. 4-5. *(Top)* General Electric SIGNA magnetic resonance system. *(Bottom)* Sagittal image of normal head acquired on a GE 1.5T research system.

additional energy is applied in the form of radio pulse waves, the nuclei can be predictably tipped out of alignment. The radio waves are introduced into the magnetic field at right angles and cause uniform gyrations or resonance of the nuclei. When the radio pulse waves are terminated, the resonating nuclei will "relax back" and return to their previous magnetic state. Momentary, tiny radio frequency signals are emitted as the nuclei relax. These signals can be monitored. By programming the computer to create a nonuniform magnetic field, the protons in different parts of the magnetic field would resonate differently, and varying the radio pulse waves would cause differences in radio frequency emissions. The computer could collect all of the data and construct an image of the tissue.

Magnetic resonance images of the human body are images of the hydrogen distribution of the body because hydrogen (1) has a single proton (odd number) in its nucleus; (2) resonates under specific conditions; and (3) is the most abundant atom in human tissue. By providing different radio pulse wave patterns that "tickle" the hydrogen ions, different images are produced. Some images depict the amount of time that it takes for the hydrogen protons to relax to their prior magnetic state after they have been turned 90 or 180 degrees by the radio wave pulses. This parameter is called T1, and it reflects the hydrogen-tissue density and its relative liquidity or solidity. The T1 time can differ greatly in various tissues. One important breakthrough in NMR technology is the ability to differentiate between gray and white matter. Although white and gray matter differ in water content by only 10%, their T1 times differ by 150%. This difference allows for selective imaging of gray matter so that multiple sclerosis and other degenerative diseases can be diagnosed early and their progress followed.

Another relaxation parameter that is based on the relationship of hydrogen atoms to each other is called T2. This radio wave pulse pattern causes hydrogen protons to gyrate in unison initially, so that each proton generates its own tiny magnetic field. Because of complex interactions among the magnetic fields, some protons accelerate while others decelerate. Various types of tissue have characteristic differences in their T2 relaxation pattern. The slight differences in tissue biochemistry, which can be correlated to the inception of disease processes, can be detected long before any structural changes have occurred. This knowledge could provide a major breakthrough in early diagnosis of illness.

DIAGNOSTIC APPLICATION TO CENTRAL NERVOUS SYSTEM DISEASE

Although MRI technology has diagnostic application to several body systems, let us consider its application to the nervous system. MRI is said to be particularly effective in detecting necrotic tissue, oxygen-deprived tissue, small malignancies, and degenerative diseases within the central nervous system. This means that MRI should be efficient in identifying cerebral and spinal cord edema; central nervous system ischemic-infarcted areas; hemorrhage; arteriovenous malformations; tumors, particularly in the difficult-to-visualize areas of the brain stem, basal skull, and spinal cord; degenerative diseases (e.g., multiple sclerosis, Alzheimer's disease); and congential anomalies. The sharpness and detail of the images produced are expected to allow MRI to serve as a "knifeless biopsy" for diagnostic purposes and to provide for identification of abnormalities very early, even before structural changes have occurred.

CURRENT PROBLEMS

Metallic equipment such as artificial pacemakers, prosthetic devices (e.g., metallic hip replacements, orthopedic pins), artificial limbs, respirators, and other equipment can be affected by the strong magnetic field. Patients with intracranial aneurysm clips or metal bullet fragments in the brain should *not* be exposed to MRI because the magnetic field has been known to move the metal objects. Therefore, patients with metallic equipment cannot be exposed to MRI. These limitations must be overcome to provide MRI technology to all people.

POSITRON EMISSION TRANSAXIAL TOMOGRAPHY (PETT)

Positron emission transaxial tomography is a new noninvasive technique that appears to be useful in detecting biochemical and physiological abnormalities in a living organism. The subject inhales or is injected with a compound (often carbon 11) that has been specially treated with a positron-emitting nuclide, which acts as a tag on the compound. Once inside the body, the tag or positron-emitting nuclide leaves the compound and reacts with an electron, producing two gamma ray photons. A special scanner detects the gamma rays and codes this data into a computer. The computer then reconstructs cross sectional images of "tags" distributed in the tissue being studied.[1]

PETT is a new and developing technology used on a very limited basis in a handful of centers in the United States. The technology will be used to study complex physiological processes in various body systems, including the central nervous system. It is expected to provide a better understanding of diseases such as epilepsy, Alzheimer's disease, dementia, cerebrovascular disease, mental illness, and cerebral injuries. There is much interest in the investigation of cerebral oxygen and glucose metabolism, the blood–brain barrier, and cerebral blood flow. Some studies using the PETT scans have been funded by the National Institutes of Health.

The PETT scan has the potential to make a major impact on central nervous system research and clinical practice. However, this new technology is only beginning to develop so it is too soon to tell if it will fulfill its proposed role.

LUMBAR PUNCTURE (LP)

A lumbar puncture consists of introducing a hollow needle with a stylet into the lumbar subarachnoid space of the spinal canal under strict aseptic technique. In the adult, the needle is placed between lumbar vertebrae three and four or four and five. This location is a safe distance from the end of the spinal cord, which terminates at L–1.

The indications for lumbar puncture can be divided into diagnostic and therapeutic purposes. The diagnostic indications include (1) measurement of cerebrospinal fluid pressure; (2) examination of cerebrospinal fluid for the presence of blood; (3) collection of cerebrospinal fluid for laboratory study; (4) injection of air, oxygen, or radiopaque material to visualize parts of the nervous system radiologically; and (5) evaluation of spinal dynamics for signs of blockage of cerebrospinal fluid flow. (See Chart 4–1 for characteristics of cerebrospinal fluid.)

The therapeutic indications of lumbar puncture include (1) introduction of spinal anesthesia for surgery and (2) intrathecal injection of antibacterial or other drugs.

The purpose of a lumbar puncture is to aid in the diagnosis of tumors, subarachnoid hemorrhage, multiple sclerosis, meningitis, and other central nervous system processes.

CONTRAINDICATIONS

Contraindications for lumbar puncture are relative and require careful medical judgment, weighing benefits against risks. When clinical evidence indicates a substantial increase in intracranial pressure, caution is advised. Increased intracranial pressure can be found in patients with any space-occupying lesions such as brain tumors.

- Performing a lumbar puncture in the presence of drastically increased intracranial pressure may result in brain stem compression, herniation or "coning" through the foramen magnum, and death.

Any cutaneous or osseous infection at the site of the lumbar puncture is an absolute contraindication for lumbar puncture. A patient who is receiving anticoagulation therapy should also be carefully considered because of the added risk of hemorrhage.

PROCEDURE

The lumbar puncture is usually done at the patient's bedside or in an outpatient facility. A lumbar puncture set is prepared by the nurse for the physician. The patient assumes the lateral recumbent position along the edge of the bed and arches his back so that his knees are flexed on his chest with his chin touching his knees (Fig. 4–6). In this position there is maximum separation of the vertebrae so that insertion of the lumbar needle is easier and less traumatic. The nurse may be called upon to assist the patient if he cannot assume this position independently.

Before any attempt is made to insert the lumbar needle, the lumbar site is aseptically prepped, draped, and locally anesthesized with an intradermal injection of procaine (Novocain). Aseptic technique is emphasized to prevent the introduction of organisms that might cause infection. After the lumbar needle is successfully introduced into the subarachnoid space, the stylet is removed and a monometer is affixed to measure entrance pressure of cerebrospinal fluid. After this is recorded, the monometer is re-

CHART 4-1. CHARACTERISTICS OF CEREBROSPINAL FLUID (CSF)

Volume

The volume of CSF increases with hydrocephalus and decreases with space-occupying lesions. The normal range is 135 ml to 150 ml.

Specific Gravity

The normal value is 1.007.

Color

Xanthochromia is the term used to describe discoloration of the CSF. It is most often due to blood in the CSF. This discoloration may be yellow, orange, or brown and is due to the red blood cell (RBC) breakdown and the liberation of bilirubin.

Turbidity or Cloudiness of the CSF

Turbidity usually indicates an increased number of white blood cells (WBCs) in the CSF. A high protein content or microorganisms in the CSF can cause clouding. An infection process would increase the WBC and microorganism count. Elevated protein levels occur with brain tumors.

Cell Count

Blood can appear in the CSF as soon as 3 hours after the blood enters the CSF from a subarachnoid hemorrhage. The discoloration of the CSF can continue for up to 28 days after the initial bleeding. There are no RBCs normally present in CSF.

White Blood Cells (WBCs)

The range of 0 to 5 cells/mm³ is considered normal as long as these cells are agranulocytes. If there are 5 to 10 cells/mm³, it is highly suspicious of abnormality. More than 10 cells/mm³ indicates disease of the central nervous system. Leukocytosis in the CSF can result from an inflammatory process within the ventricular system of the brain or the meninges. The most common cause of such an inflammatory process is meningitis. Inadequately treated open head injuries, brain abscess, sinusitis, or mastoiditis can be the underlying cause by which invading microorganisms enter the meninges, thereby causing inflammation. Intracranial tumors, spinal tumors, and multiple sclerosis also elevate the whole blood count of the CSF.

Protein Content

The protein count is elevated with tumors, infections, and hemorrhages. The normal range is 15 mg to 45 mg/100 ml.

Glucose

Normally 60 mg to 80 mg/100 ml (approximately 80%) of the blood glucose level is found. An elevated CSF glucose level has no specific significance; however, a decreased glucose level indicates the presence of glycolytic substances such as bacteria in the CSF.

Electrolytes in CSF

The following is a list of values for four electrolytes:

- Sodium: 141 mEq/liter (= to blood: 135–145)
- Potassium: 3.3 mEq/liter (< than in blood: 3.5–5.0)
- Chloride: 118–132 mEq/liter (> than in blood: 96–105)
- Calcium: 2.5 mEq/liter (< than in blood: 5.0)

Colloidal Gold Curve

The colloidal gold curve is a test that indicates alterations in the albumin–globulin ratio in CSF. Reactions in this test are sometimes seen in neurosyphilis, multiple sclerosis and purulent meningitis. This is an unreliable test with many false positives and false negatives; therefore, a diagnosis is never made solely on the basis of this test.

Culture and Sensitivity

CSF can be cultured to identify the invading organism within the fluid. Sensitivity can also be determined to identify what drug therapy will be the most effective.

Smears

Smears for Gram stain are essential in diagnosing specific meningitis, such as tubercular meningitis.

Serology

Serology testing of CSF can be performed to diagnose neurosyphilis.

moved and samples of the cerebrospinal fluid are collected into sterile test tubes for visual and laboratory examination. The physician may choose to record the exit pressure, for which the monometer would once again be necessary. If the lumbar puncture was done solely for purposes of instilling a contrast medium or medication, it would not be necessary to either record the cerebrospinal fluid pressure or collect cerebrospinal fluid specimens.

When the procedure is completed, the lumbar needle is removed and a bandage is applied over the puncture site.

TRAUMATIC TAP *VERSUS* CENTRAL NERVOUS SYSTEM (CNS) HEMORRHAGE

It is important to know when a lumbar puncture has resulted in trauma. A traumatic tap causes trauma to the tissue at the lumbar puncture site with subsequent bleeding. In this instance, the initial sample of cerebrospinal fluid would contain blood. Such bleeding could be misinterpreted as occurring from subarachnoid hemorrhage. However, in the case of a traumatic tap, the cerebrospinal

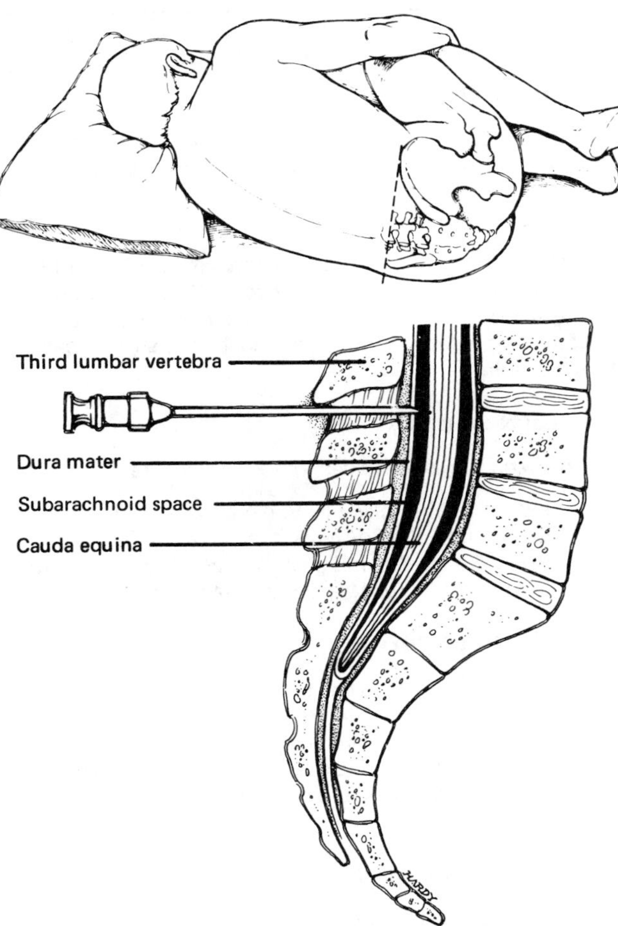

FIG. 4-6. Technique of lumbar puncture. The interspaces between the spines of L-3 and L-5 are just below the line joining the anterosuperior iliac spines. (Brunner LS, Suddarth DS: Textbook of Medical-Surgical Nursing, 5th ed. Philadelphia, JB Lippincott, 1984)

fluid clears progressively in successive samples. If there has been hemorrhage into the subarachnoid space from intracranial bleeding, successive samples of cerebrospinal fluid would continue to be just as bloody as the first specimen. Other characteristics that differentiate a traumatic bloody tap from a cerebral nervous system hemorrhage are summarized in Table 4-1.

PREPROCEDURAL PREPARATION

Ask the patient to empty his bladder immediately before the procedure. There is usually no dietary restriction or preprocedural medication.

POSTPROCEDURAL CARE

The care following a lumbar puncture includes the following:

1. The patient is to lie flat in bed from 6 to 24 hours depending on physician preference, hospital policy, and continued signs of headache.
2. Neurological and vital signs are monitored frequently.
3. Fluids are forced.
4. An analgesic is given as needed.

Headache, which can be caused by leakage of cerebrospinal fluid at the puncture site or irritation of the meninges, can be mild to severe in nature. Acetaminophen

TABLE 4-1. *Traumatic Bloody Tap* **Versus** *Central Nervous System (CNS) Hemorrhage*

Characteristics	*Traumatic Bloody Tap*	*CNS Hemorrhage*
Color	Clears with successive sampling	Same in all samples
Coagulation	Often clots	Rarely clots
Supernatant fluid after centrifuge	Clear	Xanthochromic
RBC's appearance	Normal	Crenated

(Tylenol) or acetylsalicylic acid (aspirin), 650 mg, given orally every 4 hours is used for milder headaches, while propoxyphene (Darvon), 32 to 65 mg, is given orally for moderately severe headaches. In some instances, methylmorphine (codeine phosphate), 30 mg (taken orally), may be ordered for severe headaches. Because headaches are aggravated by the upright position, the patient is advised to lie flat in bed to relieve the pain.

Other possible symptoms that can occur after lumbar puncture include

- Backache or spasms in the lower back or thighs
- Transient voiding problems
- Nuchal rigidity
- Slight rise in temperature

QUECKENSTEDT'S TEST

The Queckenstedt's test or maneuver is sometimes performed as part of the lumbar puncture if an obstruction of the spinal subarachnoid space is suspected. Complete or partial obstruction of the spinal subarachnoid space may be caused by a herniated intervertebral disc or spinal cord tumor.

CONTRAINDICATIONS

Queckenstedt's testing can be very dangerous and is therefore contraindicated in a patient with increased intracranial pressure or cerebral hemorrhage because brain stem herniation or rebleeding can occur.

PROCEDURE

After insertion of the lumbar puncture needle and notation of the cerebrospinal fluid pressure by the examiner, an assistant is asked to manually compress both jugular veins for 10 seconds. (Each jugular vein may also be compressed separately.) The pressure is read and recorded every 5 seconds. After 10 seconds, the jugular pressure is released, and the cerebrospinal fluid pressure is read and recorded every 5 seconds for 30 seconds, or until the pressure returns to baseline.

FINDINGS

In the patient who does not have a subarachnoid blockage, this procedure will cause obstruction of the cerebral blood from the brain, an increase in intracranial pressure, and a sharp immediate increase in cerebrospinal fluid pressure. A patient who has a partial subarachnoid block will exhibit a slow and slight to moderate increase in pressure. Finally, a complete blockage to the flow of cerebrospinal fluid will be noted as no increase in pressure.

Abnormal findings on this procedure indicate the need for further diagnostic studies such as a myelogram.

PNEUMOENCEPHALOGRAM (PNEUMOENCEPHALOGRAPHY)

Most authorities now state that the development of the CT scan has rendered the pneumoencephalogram (PEG) obsolete since more and better information can be ascertained by use of the CT scan. The other major advantage of the CT scan over the pneumoencephalogram is safety. The CT scan is much safer and causes no discomfort to the patient.

A lumbar puncture is performed according to the outlined procedure, but the patient stays in the sitting position. There is alternate withdrawal of cerebrospinal fluid (about 5 ml each time), and replacement with an equal amount of air or oxygen by means of a syringe attached to the lumbar needle. Enough cerebrospinal fluid is removed so that the ventricles can be filled with air. No standardized amount of gas is suggested because the size of an individual's ventricles can vary greatly. The injection of air serves as a contrast medium to outline the ventricles. Radiological studies are taken for visualization of the ventricles. When the procedure is completed, a sterile dressing is applied to the puncture site.

INDICATIONS

A pneumoencephalogram may be ordered to detect small tumors within or proximal to the ventricular system or base of the skull.

CONTRAINDICATIONS

The pneumoencephalogram is contraindicated when a great increase in intracranial pressure is suspected.

PREPROCEDURAL PREPARATION

To conduct this procedure, the cooperation of the patient is mandatory. He should also be told that the insertion of the air into the subarachnoid space will produce the sensation of bubbles moving up his back and into his head.

Most physicians order a hypnotic at bedtime on the evening before the procedure. The patient is allowed nothing by mouth after midnight. In the morning, usual preoperative medications are given. The patient is prepared in the same manner as the surgical patient (e.g., dentures and nail polish are removed). Hospital pajama bottoms (with a slit in the back) and a hospital gown (open in the back) are worn. This attire prevents needless exposure. The patient should be informed about the procedure and should be prepared for the sensation of air insertion as it rises to the ventricles.

POSTPROCEDURAL CARE

Frequent monitoring of vital and neurological signs is most important. The patient is kept flat in bed for at least 24 to 48 hours. An ice cap can be applied for comfort if the patient experiences a severe headache. Fluids are encouraged (up to 3000 ml in 24 hours). If the patient is unable to take fluids orally because of nausea or vomiting, the intravenous route should be used. An accurate intake and output record is kept. Analgesics and antiemetics are given for headache and nausea (with or without vomiting), respectively. If the patient is able to take oral fluids, citrus fruit juices are eliminated for the first 24 hours, since they tend to increase the likelihood of nausea and vomiting. A darkened, quiet room helps to control the headache. Seizure precautions are also instituted.

The patient should be carefully observed for changes in vital and neurological signs that herald deterioration. Hemorrhage, shock, air embolism, and seizures are other possible occurrences.

CISTERNAL PUNCTURE

A cisternal puncture consists of the introduction of a short, beveled needle with a stylet into the cisterna magnum. The needle is passed upward toward the base of the skull and proceeds under the posterior margin of the foramen magnum into the cisterna magnum (Fig. 4-7). This procedure requires a great deal of skill in order to avoid serious consequences such as injury to the medulla. The indications for this procedure include (1) withdrawal of cerebrospinal fluid for laboratory study, and (2) introduction of air or a radiopaque medium to demonstrate lesions of the upper cord, abnormalities of the cervical vertebrae, or subarachnoid blockage.

The patient sits with his head tilted slightly forward. The needle follows the tract outlined to a depth of about 5 cm to 6 cm. When the procedure is completed, the puncture site is sterilely dressed.

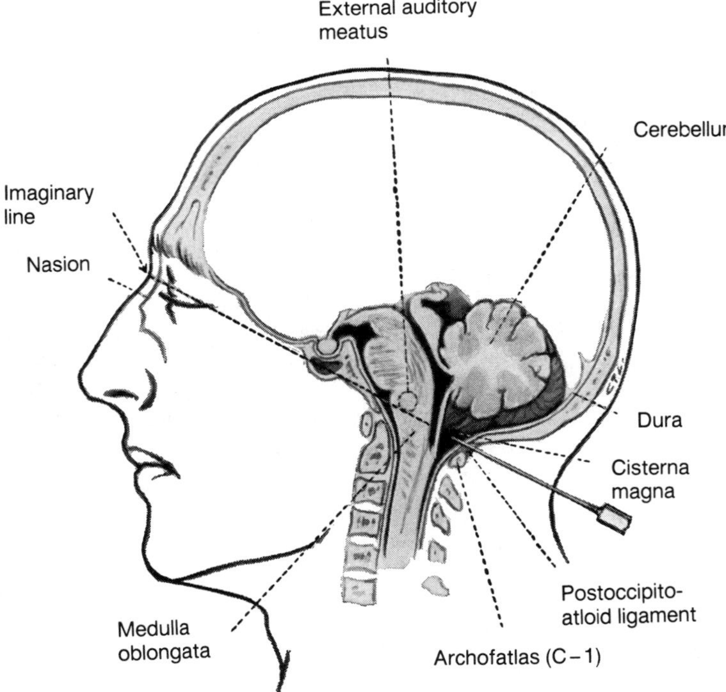

FIG. 4-7. Cisternal puncture. An imaginary line is constructed between the external auditory meatus and the nasion. The needle enters above the spinous process of the first cervical vertebra, parallels this line, and enters the cisterna magna. The medulla is about 2.5 cm anterior to the posterior occipitoatloid ligament. (Thorek P: Surgical Diagnosis, 3rd ed. Philadelphia, JB Lippincott, 1977)

PREPROCEDURAL PREPARATION

The nape of the neck is shaved and, depending on the physician, some preliminary medication such as secobarbital (Seconal) or pentobarbital (Nembutal) may be ordered.

POSTPROCEDURAL CARE

Vital and neurological signs should be assessed frequently, and the patient should be observed for cyanosis, dyspnea, hemorrhage, and shock. There should be no pain apart from that related to the striking of bone during the procedure. Pain indicates deviation from the midline and possible penetration of cerebral tissue. Chills, fever, and nuchal rigidity may indicate meningeal irritation or infection.

As with lumbar puncture, the patient is kept flat in bed for 6 to 8 hours. Fluid intake is encouraged and an accurate intake and output record is maintained.

CISTERNOGRAM (RADIOISOTOPE CISTERNOGRAPHY)

A cisternogram consists of the injection of a radioisotope into the subarachnoid space by means of a lumbar or cisternal puncture. The radioisotope becomes dispersed into the cerebrospinal fluid, which is then scanned periodically. Since cerebrospinal fluid is normally absorbed by the arachnoid villi, it can be determined how long it takes for the radioisotope to be cleared from the circulating fluid. Following administration of the radioisotope, scans are taken at regular intervals, such as 3, 6, 12, 24, 48, and 72 hours.

Indications for a cisternogram include the diagnosis of

(1) hydrocephalus, (2) blockage to the flow of cerebrospinal fluid in the vertebral column from spinal cord compression, (3) blockage caused by adhesions, and (4) tearing of the meninges with subsequent otorrhea or rhinorrhea of cerebrospinal fluid.

MYELOGRAM (MYELOGRAPHY)

A myelogram is a radiograph of the spinal cord and vertebral column (Fig. 4–8) taken after injection of a contrast medium into the subarachnoid space. A myelogram may show the lumbar, thoracic, or cervical area or the whole spinal column. The contrast media most often used are Pantopaque, an oil-based medium, and, more recently, Amipaque, a water-soluble substance. Gas has been used as a negative contrast medium more extensively in parts of Europe than in the United States. The gas technique is highly sophisticated but yields excellent results when used by an expert clinician.

In performing a myelogram, a subarachnoid puncture is performed, most often in the lumbar area, and approximately 10 ml of cerebrospinal fluid are removed. The contrast medium is injected and radiographs of the suspect area are taken (see page 102 for description of the two types of contrast medium). Any partial or complete obstruction that hinders the flow of the contrast medium will be visualized on the film.

FIG. 4–8. Myelogram.

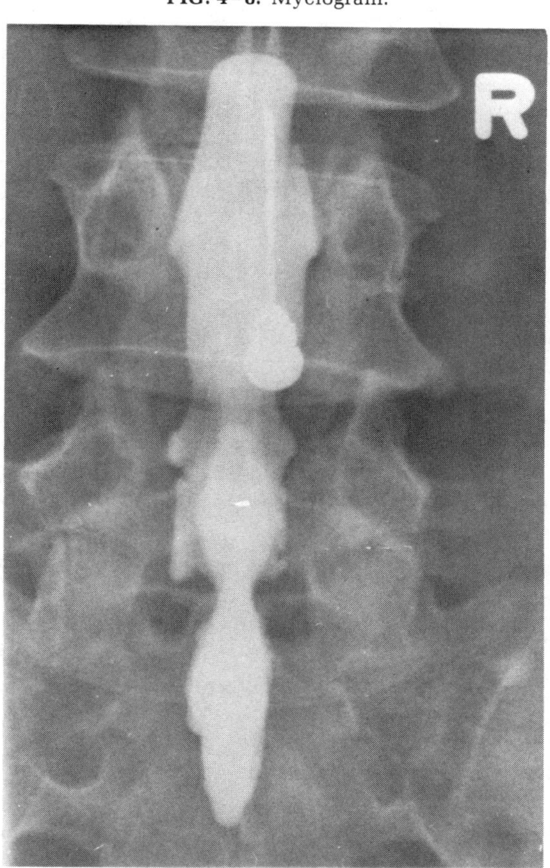

A myelogram is ordered as a diagnostic tool when a spinal cord tumor, a herniated intravertebral disc, or a ruptured disc is suspected.

PREPROCEDURAL PREPARATION AND POSTPROCEDURAL CARE

Differences in patient management must be observed depending on whether Pantopaque, the oil-based medium, or Amipaque, the water-soluble material, was used for the patient's myelogram.

Nursing Management Before Myelogram Using Pantopaque

The patient should not eat or drink for approximately 4 hours preceding the test. A light breakfast may be given if the procedure is scheduled after lunchtime. Most physicians order that a medication such as 50 mg to 100 mg pentobarbital (Nembutal), 50 mg to 100 mg meperidine (Demerol), or 0.4 mg atropine be given intramuscularly half an hour prior to the procedure. The patient should also empty his bladder before the procedure is begun.

Nursing Management After Myelogram Using Pantopaque

The patient is kept flat in bed for 6 to 24 hours, depending on the physician's orders. The most common postprocedure problem is headache, which is relieved by the horizontal position and aggravated by the upright position. Analgesics are given, with acetaminophen (Tylenol), aspirin, Darvon, or codeine being the usual choices, depending on the severity of the pain.

Nursing actions include

1. Frequently assessing neurological and vital signs
2. Keeping the patient in the flat position
3. Forcing fluids
4. Recording intake and output
5. Observing for untoward signs and symptoms, such as back pain, spasms, elevated temperature, voiding difficulty, nuchal rigidity, nausea, and vomiting

Nursing Management Before Myelogram Using Amipaque

The patient may have a regular diet up to 2 hours before the procedure. Encourage the intake of fluids up to the time of the myelogram. The following drugs are discontinued 48 hours before the procedure: all neuroleptic drugs (or major tranquilizers); MAO inhibitors; psycho-stimulants; and phenothiazines. Patients receiving *minor* tranquilizers or anticonvulsants should continue to take their medication. The physician may choose to give the patient analgesics before the procedure to maintain comfort. (See Nursing

Management Before Myelogram Using Pantopaque, above, for frequently ordered drugs.) The patient should also empty his bladder before he reports for the procedure.

Nursing Management After Myelogram Using Amipaque

The patient is kept supine with his head elevated 30 to 60 degrees for the first 8 to 24 hours following the procedure. The manufacturer's instructions and routine of the physician should be carefully followed to prevent seizures. Unlike the oil-based Pantopaque, which is aspirated with a needle and syringe after the procedure is complete, water-soluble Amipaque remains in the cerebrospinal fluid. The head is kept elevated at all times and the patient kept quiet to reduce the rate of upward dispersion of the contrast medium (Amipaque). Upward dispersion would cause irritation of the cervical nerve roots and the cranial structures, and this could result in seizures or other untoward reactions. (See Chart 4-2.) Therefore, the patient who has received Amipaque should not be allowed to lie flat or have his head lower than the designated height under any circumstance.

In the radiology department, the head of the stretcher should be raised at least 15 to 30 degrees before the patient is moved onto it. Once the patient is on the stretcher, the head of the stretcher should be elevated immediately. Movement on and off the stretcher and into the bed should be executed slowly with the patient being completely passive. Before moving the patient onto the bed, raise the head of the bed to the designated height (30 to 45 degrees).

Nursing actions include

1. Frequently assessing neurological and vital signs
2. Keeping the patient supine with his head elevated 15 to 30 degrees for the first 8 hours postprocedure
3. Maintaining the patient in the horizontal position for the next 16 hours
4. Keeping activity to a minimum for the first few hours; a quiet restful environment should be maintained
5. Encouraging intake of fluids and food as tolerated
6. Avoiding administration of phenothiazines
7. Recording intake and output
8. Observing for untoward signs and symptoms, such as back pain, spasms, elevated temperature, nuchal rigidity, nausea and vomiting, and seizure activity
9. Not administering phenothiazine antiemetics if nausea or vomiting occurs. If nausea and vomiting persist, dehydration will result. Therefore, prompt consideration of intravenous fluid replacement is recommended
10. Using standard analgesics to treat headache, which is safe

CHART 4-2. PROPERTIES OF PANTOPAQUE AND AMIPAQUE

Iodophenylundecylic Acid (Pantopaque)

Pantopaque is an iodine compound suspended in an oil base used as a contrast medium in myelography. Since Pantopaque is hyperbaric, it must be manipulated into position. A tilt table is maneuvered to help the oily content medium to flow, and films are taken. As much Pantopaque as possible is removed upon completion of the procedure because the medium is very irritating to the neural tissue.

Adverse Reactions

In addition to the local tissue irritation, possible effects include meningeal irritation with possible aseptic meningitis, local root irritation with prolonged radicular pain, and rarely, arachnoiditis.

Metrizamide (Amipaque)

Amipaque is a water-soluble contrast medium that is injected into the subarachnoid space. It is used for myelography as well as for CT scanning requiring contrast medium. Following administration by the subarachnoid route, Amipaque diffuses upward via the cerebrospinal fluid, *regardless of the position maintained by the patient.* Since Amipaque is a completely diffusable contrast medium, it is not necessary to alter the patient's position by means of a tilt table or some other method to obtain very satisfactory views of the entire circumference of the spinal cord. Amipaque is particularly useful when a myelogram of the cervical region is desired. In this instance, entrance to the subarachnoid space can be gained by way of the lateral cervical-one (C-1) approach. Amipaque is absorbed from the cerebrospinal fluid into the blood, and approximately 60% of the drug is excreted by the kidneys within 48 hours. Amipaque should be administered very cautiously to patients with a history of epilepsy, severe cardiovascular disease, chronic alcoholism, multiple sclerosis, bronchial asthma, or any allergic reactions.

Adverse Reactions

In addition to the usual milder adverse reactions to subarachnoid injection such as headache, nausea, backache, and neck stiffness, other serious signs and symptoms, including seizures, may occur. Seizures are particularly likely in patients in whom the Amipaque has ascended to the intracranial vault. In addition, hallucinations, depression, hyperesthesia, confusion, disorientation, visual and/or speech disorientation, chest pain, and arrhythmias can develop.

DISCOGRAM (DISCOGRAPHY)

A discogram is a radiograph of an intervertebral disc(s) that has been directly injected with a radiopaque material. Anteroposterior and lateral films of the spine are taken. The indication for the procedure is diagnosis of intervertebral disc herniation that has not been apparent on myelography.

Since there would be danger of cord injury in higher vertebral areas, discography is limited to the L-3, L-4, and L-5 disc areas. Because the procedure is very painful and can be dangerous, it is infrequently used.

PREPROCEDURAL PREPARATION

Common preprocedural medication given includes pentobarbital (Nembutal), 100 mg, or meperidine (Demerol), 75 mg with 0.4 mg atropine.

POSTPROCEDURAL CARE

The usual monitoring of vital and neurological signs is included, and the patient must be carefully observed for any untoward reaction from the procedure. Analgesic drugs are also ordered.

CEREBRAL ANGIOGRAPHY

A cerebral angiogram consists of injecting a radiopaque contrast medium into an artery for radiological visualization of the intracranial and extracranial blood vessels (Fig. 4–9). The method of approach is either by direct injection into the carotid or vertebral arteries, or by the indirect route through catheterization or injection of the carotid or vertebral arteries by way of the femoral, brachial, subclavian, or axillary artery. Radiographic films are taken at various intervals after injection.

Cerebral angiography is used to diagnose intracranial lesions. The lumen of the blood vessels can be visualized to indicate patency, narrowing or stenosis, thrombosis, and occlusions. Abnormalities of cerebral blood vessels such as aneurysms and arteriovenous malformations are also visible. Displacement of cerebral vessels can be noted. Reasons for displacement include any space-occupying lesions such as hematomas, cysts, tumors, and abscesses. Herniation and cerebral edema can also affect the position of cerebral blood vessels. Cerebral angiography can be performed under local anesthesia or as part of a surgical procedure if the patient has undergone general anesthesia. For example, cerebral angiography can be conducted during an aneurysm clipping to check the position and integrity of the clip.

During the preparation for the examination in the special procedure area, emergency equipment must be available on a standby basis. This equipment includes suction devices and a resuscitation apparatus. The patient is placed in a supine position on the examination table. A wide area around the puncture site is shaved. If a local anesthetic is to be administered, procaine (Novocain) is the usual choice. The puncture site is aseptically cleansed. After injection of the Novocain, the contrast medium is either directly injected, or a catheter is inserted through which the contrast medium is injected. When the examination is completed, direct manual pressure is applied to the puncture site for 5 to 10 minutes to prevent bleeding into the subcutaneous space.

PREPROCEDURE PREPARATION

A skin shave at the puncture site may be ordered on the evening preceding the procedure. The patient should be told that during injection a burning sensation may be felt for a few (4–6) seconds behind the eyes, or in the jaw, teeth, tongue, and lips. Even the fillings in the teeth may feel warm. The physician also explains the possibility that the procedure may precipitate a stroke, although this is unlikely. If the carotid artery in the neck is to be directly injected, the patient should know that he may feel the needle close to the trachea, and it may cause some difficulty in breathing. Emphasis on the need to lie still without talking or coughing is discussed.

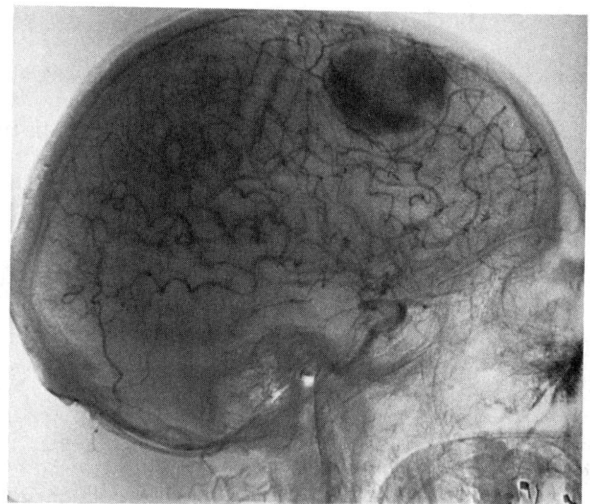

FIG. 4–9. Cerebral angiogram showing an abnormal, large space-occupying lesion at one o'clock.

Preoperative medication is usually administered half an hour before the procedure. The choice of drugs used varies from physician to physician and may include any of the following drugs: pentobarbital (Nembutal); atropine sulfate to protect against the effect upon the carotid sinus; diazepam (Valium); and meperidine (Demerol).

Preparation for the examination is similar to any preoperative preparation. Dentures and eyeglasses are removed. Most physicians prefer that the patient not have anything by mouth for 6 to 8 hours before the examination. Baseline vital and neurological signs are recorded.

POSTPROCEDURAL CARE

When the procedure is completed, the patient is returned to his room and placed on bed rest. Vital and neurological signs are assessed and recorded frequently for a 24-hour period. An accurate intake and output record is maintained. The pressure dressing at the puncture site is checked for bleeding, and an ice bag is applied to the site to control edema and discomfort and to decrease the possibility of bleeding. The head is usually elevated. The puncture site is immobilized for 6 to 8 hours to prevent the recurrence of bleeding. If an extremity, or an area proximal to an extremity, was used for the puncture site, the extremity should be checked for color, temperature, and presence of a pulse. In the case of a femoral puncture, the pedal pulses would be checked. It is necessary to assess the adjacent extremity because vasospasms, thrombosis, or formation of a hematoma can occur, thereby obstructing a normal blood supply distal to the puncture site.

COMPLICATIONS

Possible complications that can occur following cerebral angiography include (1) allergic reactions to the contrast media, (2) seizures, (3) stroke, (4) hemiparesis, (5) pulmonary emboli, (6) thrombosis, (7) symptoms of carotid sinus sensitivity (hypotension, syncope, and bradycardia), (8) dyphasia, and (9) visual difficulty.

DIGITAL SUBTRACTION ANGIOGRAPHY (DSA)

Digital subtraction angiography is a computer-assisted radiographic procedure for visualization of extracranial or intracranial vessels as well as other vascular conditions within other body systems. The image produced is made more distinct by the elimination of surrounding and interfering anatomical structures. This is accomplished by taking images before and after injection of contrast medium and subtracting the first image from the second.

PURPOSE

The procedure is considered to be safer than cerebral or femoral angiography and can be used to aid in the diagnosis of the following conditions:

- Arteriosclerotic disease (stenosis, occlusions, ulcerations)
- Vascular lesions (arteriovenous malformations, aneurysms, carotid cavernous fistulas)
- Tumors and other space-occupying lesions
- Postoperative evaluation of endarterectomy, anastomoses, aneurysms, clipping, arteriovenous malformation repair, and anastomosis

PROCEDURE

The antecubital area, usually of the right arm, is cleansed and lidocaine injected locally so that the antecubital vein (usual approach) or brachial artery can be incised. A catheter is advanced into the superior vena cava, and a contrast medium is injected. Selected vessels are visualized with an image-intensifier video system that displays vessels on a TV monitor. Pictures are taken and stored on magnetic tape. The images are received by the computer, and the images are collected before contrast injection; these images are subtracted from those taken after injection so that the image of the desired area is enhanced. The remaining contrast-enhanced images can be manipulated by the computer to focus on specific problems that may otherwise not be visualized.

On completion of the procedure, which takes from 30 to 45 minutes, the catheter is removed. Pressure is applied to the puncture site for several minutes, and a sterile dressing is applied.

PREPROCEDURAL PREPARATION

Oral intake is withheld for 2 hours before the procedure. The procedure is explained to the patient. He will be required to hold his breath on command, remain motionless, and lie in the supine position on the x-ray table. The patient should be questioned for evidence of allergic reaction to iodine or contrast medium.

POSTPROCEDURAL CARE

Vital signs should be checked. Observe for the unlikely occurrence of stroke, allergic reaction, or hemorrhage/hematoma at the injection site. Fluids should be forced, with up to 2000 ml being given in the next 24 hours to facilitate excretion of the contrast medium. Other possible rare complications are venous thrombosis and infection.

DURA SINOGRAPHY

The superior sagittal sinus is directly injected with contrast medium at surgery to determine the patency of the sinus that may have been damaged by a space-occupying lesion such as a tumor. Immediately upon injection of the sinus, lateral radiographic films are taken. These films are then read to determine the patency of the sinus.

CEREBRAL BLOOD FLOW STUDIES

Regional blood flow studies have been developed and refined over the last 30 years. The current approach is to use a noninvasive inhalation technique using xenon 133. The inhaled tracer is carried to the brain by way of the bloodstream and is monitored by extracranial probes that have been placed on the scalp (older models used 16 probes while the new ones use 32). Each probe collects information about the clearance of xenon gas from particular regions of the brain. The information is stored in a computer, and a computer printout depicts the regional distribution of blood flow across both hemispheres. By assessing the data it can be determined whether blood flow is within normal limits, increased, or decreased. Values for blood flow are calculated for gray matter and white matter. The xenon in the blood is returned to the lungs and exhaled. A value for clearance of the tracer gas from the airway is also calculated.

NORMAL BLOOD FLOW VALUES

The mean blood flow in normal persons is 50 ml to 55 ml/minute/100-gm brain. The blood flow in gray matter is considered fast, having a mean value of 74 ml/minute/100-gm brain. White matter is considered to have a slow flow of blood. Regional blood flow changes dramatically when the person is engaged in various types of activities.

For example, a patient at rest with his eyes closed will normally have a 20% increase in blood flow to the frontal lobes.

PURPOSES

Blood flow studies have been helpful in diagnosing blood flow changes caused by intracranial tumor, subarachnoid hemorrhage, vasospasms, and cerebrovascular disease. It can provide helpful data for predicting patient outcomes and has also been used a part of brain death criteria in some institutions.

In addition to its use in the diagnosis of disease, blood flow studies have been of value in various types of clinical research, including clinical investigations of the effects of specific drugs on cerebral tissue and the neurophysiology of autoregulation of cerebral arteries.

PREPROCEDURAL PREPARATION

Blood must be drawn to determine the hemoglobin level. This information is necessary for calculating cerebral blood flow. Notation should be made of respiratory problems (such as chronic obstructive lung disease, asthma, or dyspnea) and cardiac problems (such as hypertension or congestive heart failure). Problems in either system can result in altered data on the blood flow studies because of abnormal transport of the tracer gas to the brain and back to the lungs.

The procedure should be explained to the patient. The blood pressure will be taken and recorded. There is no postprocedural care of the patient.

DOPPLER IMAGING

Doppler imaging is a noninvasive diagnostic test in which a Doppler ultrasonic probe (which sends high frequency sound waves) is placed on the skin over the carotid artery and slowly moved from the common carotid artery to the bifurcation to the internal carotid artery to the external carotid artery. The sound waves strike the moving red blood cells within the lumen of the blood vessel, and the sound reflected back to the Doppler probe represents the velocity of the blood flow. These data are amplified, and a graphic recording and sound recording of the blood flow are produced.

The test is safe and about 95% accurate. It takes about 5 to 10 minutes to complete.

PURPOSE

Doppler imaging is used to diagnose abnormalities of carotid blood flow, ulcerative plaques within the carotid arteries, and carotid artery occlusive disease.

PREPROCEDURAL PREPARATION

Explain the procedure to the patient. Tell him that he will lie on an examining table for the procedure. His blood pressure will be taken. This is a painless procedure. There is no special postprocedural care necessary.

B-MODE IMAGING (REAL-TIME ULTRASOUND ANGIOGRAPHY)

B-mode imaging ultrasound is a noninvasive procedure for the visualization of soft-tissue structures by recording the reflection of ultrasonic waves that have been directed into soft body tissue. The B-mode (brightness-modulated) scan provides two-dimensional images of pulsating blood vessels in longitudinal and transverse sections, allowing most of the vessel's circumference to be visualized. The image is reflected on a display screen in tones of gray. Photographs of the images may be taken to provide a permanent record.

PURPOSE

The purposes of the procedure are many and it can be applied to many body systems. In neurological or neurosurgical practice, the procedure is applied to cerebrovascular extracranial and intracranial vessels. B-mode ultrasound can detect minimal plaque formation and stenosed cerebral vessels.

PREPROCEDURAL PREPARATION

The procedure should be explained to the patient. He should know that the procedure is painless. It will take approximately 35 to 45 minutes to complete, and the patient will be asked to remain motionless during portions of the scan. Fasting is usually not required.

POSTPROCEDURAL CARE

Other than removing any gel that may have been used as a conductor of the sound waves, there is no specific aftercare of the patient.

CAROTID PHONOANGIOGRAPHY

Carotid phonoangiography is a noninvasive technique that uses a transducer to record carotid bruit during systole and diastole. Information about the presence, location, and severity of carotid artery occlusive disease and carotid bruit is collected. The soundings are transmitted as graphic images on an oscilloscope, and a Polaroid picture is taken for evaluation.

The patient lies supine on the examining table and is asked to hold his breath while the probe is placed over various areas along the carotid vessels. No special preprocedural preparation or postprocedural care is necessary, with the exception of explaining the procedure to the patient.

OCULOPLETHYSMOGRAPHY AND OCULAR PNEUMOPLETHYSMOGRAPHY

Oculoplethysmography (OPG) and ocular pneumoplethysmography are discussed together because there are some similarities in the procedures. Often, both tests are ordered in the diagnostic work-up of a patient.

OCULOPLETHYSMOGRAPHY

OPG is a diagnostic procedure for indirectly measuring the ophthalmic blood flow. The ophthalmic artery is the first major arterial branch coming off the internal carotid artery and therefore is an accurate indicator of carotid artery blood flow.

Contraindications

OPG and ocular pneumoplethysmography are both contraindicated for patients receiving anticoagulation therapy. They are also contraindicated for patients who have had

- Allergic reactions to anesthetic eyedrops
- Lens implants
- Eye surgery within the last 6 months
- Enucleation
- Retinal detachment

Procedure

Anesthetic eyedrops are instilled into each eye to minimize any discomfort associated with the procedure. Photoelectric probes are attached to each earlobe to detect blood flow to the ear by way of the external carotid artery. Tracings of the blood flow to both ear lobes are taken and compared (they should be the same). The tracing from the right ear is used for comparison with tracings from the eyes.

An eye cup (similar to a contact lens) with a recording device is applied to each cornea. It is kept on the cornea with slight suction (40 mm Hg–50 mm Hg). Tracings of the pulsations within each eye are taken and graphically recorded. The eye tracings are compared to each other and also to the tracing of the right ear.

PURPOSE

The OPG test is one procedure used in making the diagnosis of partial or complete stenosis of one or both ophthalmic arteries.

* * *

The following preprocedural preparation and postprocedural care apply to both OPG and ocular pneumoplethysmography.

Preprocedural Preparation

The procedure should be explained to the patient. A history of allergic drug reactions, particularly to anesthetic eyedrops, should be reviewed.

Postprocedural Care

The patient should be cautioned against rubbing his eyes to prevent abrasions. The effects of the eyedrops will wear off within a few hours. The nurse should inspect the eyes for signs of corneal abrasions, irritation, or scleral hematoma. Complaints of eye pain are reported to the physician. Patients who wear contact lenses should not reinsert the lenses for at least 2 hours after completion of the procedure.

OCULAR PNEUMOPLETHYSMOGRAPHY

Ocular pneumoplethysmography is a diagnostic procedure to indirectly measure the intraocular ophthalmic arterial pressures. These readings are compared to each other and to the brachial artery pressures. Ocular pneumoplethysmography is often conducted along with OPG.

Procedure

As with OPG, the anesthetic eyedrops are instilled into each eye. An eye cup, also similar to that used in OPG, is applied to the eye. In this instance, the eye cups are applied to the sclera of each eye. Suction of approximately 300 mm Hg is applied to each eye cup; this pressure corresponds to a mean pressure of 100 mm Hg in the ophthalmic artery.[2] This pressure obliterates the ophthalmic pulses. The pressure is then reduced, and the point at which ocular pulsation reappears is noted. This point represents the systolic pressure of the ophthalmic artery. (Both ophthalmic pulses should reappear simultaneously.) The numerical values collected for each eye are compared. A difference between the two readings of more than 5 mm is indicative of occlusive disease in, or proximal to, the ophthalmic artery on the side of the lower reading. The blood pressure from each brachial artery is also recorded because there is a direct relationship between the concurrent ophthalmic and brachial arterial pressures. The bilateral brachial artery pressures and ophthalmic pressures are compared. If there are significant differences between these two values, bilateral carotid occlusive disease is suspected.

Purpose

Ocular pneumoplethysmography is helpful in diagnosing bilateral carotid occlusive disease and in screening candidates for carotid ligation or carotid endarterectomy. Patients who have transient ischemic attacks or carotid bruits should be considered for both OPG and ocular pneumoplethysmography.

Preprocedural Preparation, Postprocedural Care, and Contraindications

Preprocedural preparation, postprocedural care, and contraindications are the same as for OPG.

TEMPORAL ARTERY BIOPSY

Under local anesthesia, a small incision is made over the superficial temporal artery. A small piece of temporal artery is removed for biopsy. The specimen is examined for evidence of temporal arteritis.

RADIONUCLIDE SCAN (BRAIN SCAN)

A radionuclide scan or a brain scan is a diagnostic procedure in which a small amount of radioisotope is administered to measure the tissue uptake of the isotope. The gamma rays emitted by the radioisotope tracers are measured by a scanning device, and a graph indicating the degree of concentration throughout the brain is made. Although all tissue, both normal and abnormal, will take up the isotope, in areas of cerebral lesions the isotope will accumulate and be retained in greater concentration (Fig. 4–10). This is due to a defect in the blood–brain barrier that will allow increased access to the abnormal tissue.

A brain scan is indicated to detect the presence of a space-occupying intracranial lesion. The general size and location of the lesion can be determined from the scan. Although the brain scan cannot indicate specifically whether the lesion is a tumor, hematoma, abscess, or arteriovenous malformation, it does indicate the presence of an abnormality.

The procedure for a brain scan requires the administration of the radioisotope. The usual route of administration is intravenously, although oral and intra-arterial routes can also be used. The patient's history of allergies is reviewed to determine if any allergies, particularly to iodine, exist. Skin testing may be done before the isotope is administered. Once the isotope is administered, the patient is observed for any untoward reaction. Time is allowed for the isotope to circulate throughout the body, and the patient lies on a table while a large scanner moves overhead.

PREPROCEDURAL PREPARATION

The patient should be aware that the scanning will be done by a large overhanging machine and that a ticking sound will be heard as the machine moves. The patient should also be instructed to lie quietly while the test is in progress.

There are no dietary or dress restrictions. Other than the venipuncture for administration of the isotope, the procedure is painless.

ECHOENCEPHALOGRAPHY (ECHOENCEPHALOGRAM)

An echoencephalogram (ECHO) is a simple diagnostic test that uses pulsating ultrasonic waves to indicate deviation of the midline structures. A probe is placed on the midaxis, which is on the temporal bones of the skull.

The probe contains a transducer and also emits an ultrasonic beam that travels through the patient's skull. Because certain structures such as bone reflect some of the ultrasonic waves back to the source, the waves are recorded and projected on an oscilloscope screen (Fig. 4–11). This represents a graphic interpretation of the distance from the reflecting surface to the source of the ultrasonic beam. Echoencephalography is based on the fact that bones of the skull are reflectors and the distance between them can be gauged. Since midline structures also serve as reflectors, any deviation from the midline can be projected on the oscilloscope.

A Polaroid picture is taken of the waves on the oscilloscope, and measurements are calculated. The information obtained is based on the two midaxes of the inner surfaces of the temporal bones and the third ventricle. The third ventricle should be halfway between the temporal bones. Abnormal shifts are recorded in millimeters. A shift of 3 mm or more is considered abnormal in the adult.

If the ECHO shifts because of an abnormal focus, this indicates a space-occupying lesion. It does not indicate the

FIG. 4–10. Brain scan.

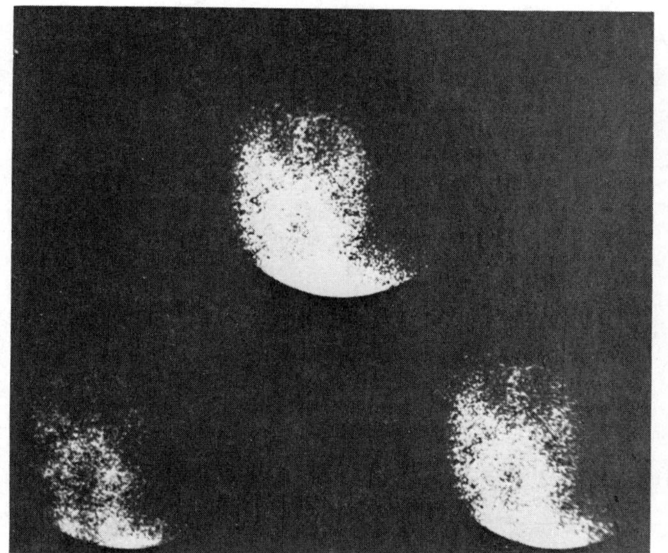

FIG. 4–11. Abnormal echoencephalogram.

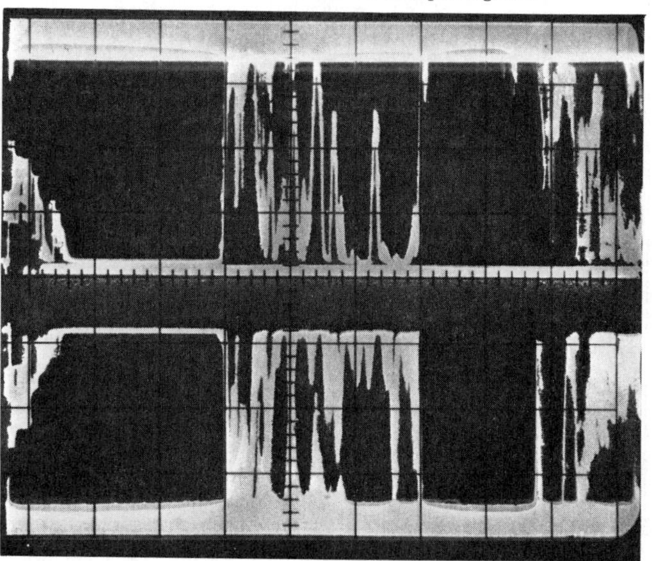

particular type of lesion creating the deviation. The reliability of the ECHO depends on the skill of the technician who is taking the recording. The procedure takes from 1 to 3 minutes. The report indicates in what direction, left-to-right or right-to-left, the deviation has occurred.

Since the advent of CT scans, ECHOs are rarely ordered.

ELECTROENCEPHALOGRAPHY (ELECTROENCEPHALOGRAM)

An electroencephalogram (EEG) is a recording of the electrical activity of the brain (brain waves) (Fig. 4–12). Ordinarily, 17 to 21 surface electrodes are attached to the scalp with a pastelike substance. A few hospitals use subdermal needle electrodes that are inserted into the scalp and are therefore uncomfortable. Brain waves are recorded (1) at rest, (2) after hyperventilation, (3) with photic stimulation, and (4) during sleep. The type of waves varies with activity and specific stimulation.

The electrical signals received from the brain are about 1% as strong as those from the heart. Brain signals are picked up from the neurons on the surface of the cerebral cortex and must be amplified one million times for an acceptable recording to be made.

The following list outlines the outstanding features of an EEG in the normal awake adult (Fig. 4–13).

1. *Alpha rhythm* occurs at 8 to 13 cycles/second in the adult. These waves, which are most prominent in the occipital leads, have an amplitude of 1 to 100 microvolts, with an average of 25 to 50 microvolts. Alpha activity responds to environmental stimuli and can be blocked when the eyes are open, when there

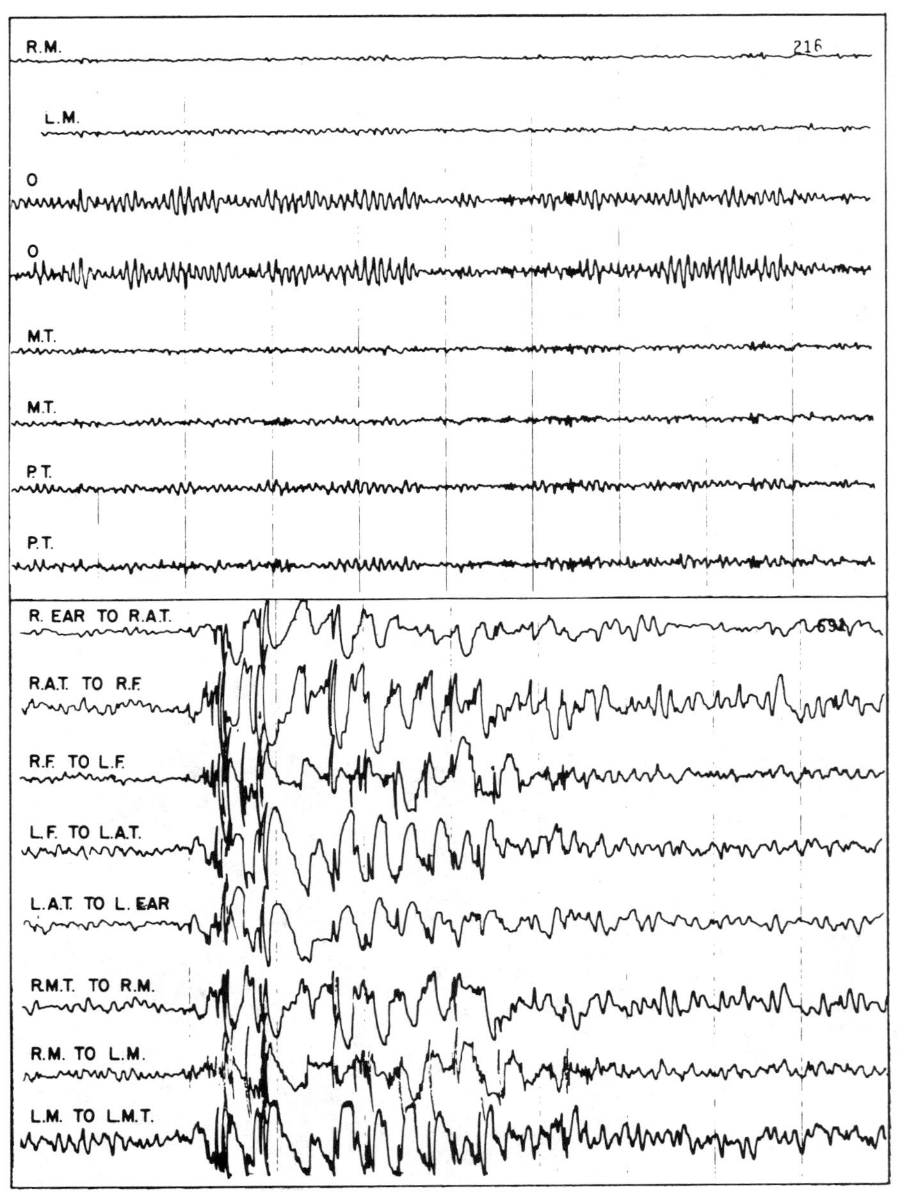

FIG. 4–12. Contrast of a normal electroencephalogram (EEG) *(top)* with that of an epileptic patient during a grand mal seizure *(bottom)*. Note the sharp, spiky waves recorded during the seizure.

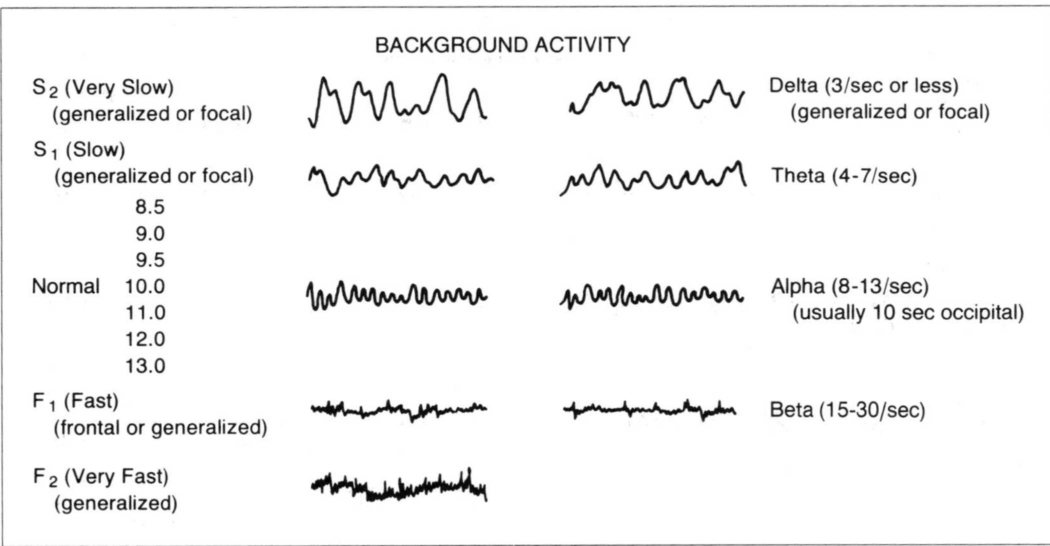

FIG. 4-13. EEG classifications.

is mental effort, and when a sudden noise or touch occurs. Anxiety and apprehension can decrease the number of alpha waves.

2. *Beta rhythm* occurs in excess of 13 cycles/second and is most prominent in the frontal and central areas. The amplitude is lower than alpha rhythm, averaging less than 20 microvolts. Beta waves can be elicited by opening the eyes, mental activity, anxiety, or apprehension.
3. *Theta rhythms* occur at the rate of 4 to 7 cycles/second, largely from the temporal and adjacent parietal areas. The amplitude is less than 20 microvolts. These waves are common in children but occupy about 5% of a tracing in the adult. Theta rhythm is normal for drowsiness.
4. *Delta rhythms* are slower than 4 cycles/second and are normally seen in early sleep. They do not normally occur in the adult who is awake.

With supratentorial lesions there are usually focal abnormalities in the EEG because the lesions either directly involve the cerebral cortex or interrupt the thalamocortical projection pathways. Hemorrhage, infarction, tumor, or abscess can cause unilateral or focal slowness of activity; however, as the lesion increases in size and affects the diencephalon, this slowness of activity can become bilateral.

In infratentorial lesions that involve the reticular formation of the midbrain, the EEG slows bilaterally. Infratentorial caudal lesions demonstrate a poor correlation of the EEG changes and the state of consciousness.

An EEG is particularly useful for differentiating functional from organic brain disorders and in identifying specific types of seizure activity. An EEG can aid in the diagnosis of head injury, stroke, metabolic disorders, retardation, drug overdose, and brain death.

The actual recording requires the patient to sit in a comfortable armchair in a relaxed manner, while a baseline recording is made. The cooperation of the patient is paramount, since he is asked to hyperventilate through his mouth for about 3 to 5 minutes. This raises the serum pH to 7.8 from the normal 7.35 to 7.45. The excitability of the nerve cells is increased, triggering seizure activity in a susceptible patient. After the hyperventilation phase, the recording is continued to determine how long it takes to reestablish baseline readings.

The photic stimulation is produced by focusing a flickering light on the patient while his eyes are closed. A recording is taken, during which seizure activity may be noted. The last recording phase is that of drowsiness and sleep. The patient is asked to sleep; however, if this is not possible, a hypnotic drug is given. The recordings are much more valuable if drugs are not necessary. The entire EEG takes from 40 to 60 minutes and covers about 100 pages of recording paper.

PREPROCEDURAL PREPARATION

Preparation is very important. The patient should know that an EEG is painless, presents no possibility of electrical shock because the patient's electrical brain activity is being recorded, does not determine intelligence quotient (IQ) or the presence of mental illness, and is not a form of therapy. The patient should be allowed to express his fears and anxieties about the procedure, although it must be emphasized that unless he is calm the recording will not produce worthwhile data. Anxiety can block alpha rhythms and produce tension in the head and neck muscles, resulting in artifacts on the recordings.

Since medications such as anticonvulsants, stimulants, tranquilizers, and depressants can alter the brain waves and mask or suppress abnormal brain waves, most physicians withhold these drugs for 24 to 48 hours prior to the EEG. It is best if the patient goes to sleep late and arises early. The patient should not be allowed to nap prior to the recording. This is done to promote the possibility of sleep when it is required for the tracings. Sleep deprivation may evoke abnormal brain waves.

The hair is washed well prior to the EEG. Oils, sprays, or

lotions should not be applied. Normal meals are served, but coffee, tea, and cola drinks are withheld because of their stimulant component.

POSTPROCEDURAL CARE

The hair is washed to remove the paste used to affix the electrodes. Anticonvulsant drugs are resumed and vital and neurological signs are checked.

ELECTROMYOGRAPHY (EMG)

The recording of the electrical activity of the muscle and peripheral nerve is called electromyography. The indications for the test are to detect the presence and type of neuromuscular disorders that affect the lower motor neuron, the neuromuscular junctions, skeletal muscle fibers, the primary sensory neuron, and the voluntary and reflex activity of muscles. The electromyogram can detect minimal denervation of a muscle. A single muscle, which had been obscured because it functioned synergistically with other muscles of a group, can be tested.

The actual examination procedure consists of insertion of needle electrodes into the muscle to be examined. There will be an uncomfortable sensation upon insertion. Recordings are made of the electrical activity of the muscle at rest and during contraction.

The accuracy and value as a diagnostic tool of the electromyogram greatly depend on the training, experience, and knowledge of neurological problems possessed by the person conducting the examination.

In the normal muscle, there is no electrical activity when the muscle is at rest. During a slight voluntary muscle concentration, a single motor unit may be activated with an action potential of 4 to 10 times per second. During a strong contraction, so many units are activated that one action potential is indistinguishable from the other.

In lower motor nerve disease, fibrillations are seen. These are small potentials produced by single contractions in muscle fibers at the rate of 1 to 5 per second. When reinnervation occurs, the potentials are large but polyphasic because of the small size and slow conduction of some of the regenerated nerve branches to a unit. Fasciculations seen in lower motor neuron disease are large, but normal potentials are repeated at long intervals (2 to 10 seconds) in muscle relaxation.

With muscle disease there is decreased amplitude and decreased duration of muscle contraction. Fewer muscle fibers are functional because of the presence of disease.

PREPROCEDURAL PREPARATION

The patient should be informed that momentary discomfort will accompany insertion of the electrode needles and that he will be asked to contract and relax particular muscles during the test.

NERVE CONDUCTION TIMES

Nerve conduction time records the speed of the conduction of motor and sensory fibers in the peripheral nerves. The motor conduction rate is measured by first determining the latency period of the compound action potential of an innervated muscle by distal and proximal stimulation. The latency period can be determined from these recordings. The distance between the two stimulations is measured in meters and divided by the difference in latency to give the speed of conduction in meters per second.

Normal motor conduction speeds are 50 m to 60 m/second for the ulnar and median nerves and 45 m to 55 m/second for the lateral popliteal nerve. Values below 40 m/second are found in neuropathy. A delay in conduction time can persist long after evidence of clinical recovery exists. Motor conduction studies are helpful when nerve damage is doubtful, but slight symptoms of motor weakness or atrophy exist. The delay in motor conduction can help to clarify and confirm the findings.

Sensory fiber conduction rates can also be calculated. The sensory volley of impulses is slight. A single electric stimuli is applied to the tip of a finger and the action potential is recorded by a well-placed electrode on the skin where the nerve is near the surface.

Conduction studies are helpful in the diagnosis of neuropathy of diabetic, alcoholic, metabolic, and nutritional disorders. It is also helpful in identifying compression or trauma to nerves.

ELECTRONYSTAGMOGRAPHY (ENG)

Electronystagmography is a sensitive diagnostic test that measures and records the electrical potentials emitted by the eye movements of spontaneous, positional, or calorically evoked nystagmus. The graphic data collected includes the frequency, intensity, and maximum speed of the slow and fast components of the nystagmus. The basic principle on which the procedure is based is the difference in voltage in the eye between two dipole structures. The cornea is considered to be the positive pole and the retina the negative pole, with at least a 1-millivolt difference in potential normally existing between the two poles. When the eyeball moves or rotates, field changes are produced that are picked up by electrodes placed on adjacent periorbital skin. The field changes or potentials are then amplified and recorded. A baseline recording is obtained by asking the patient to look straight ahead with eyes in midposition. Horizontal eye movement to the right is recorded as an upward pen deflection and horizontal eye movement to the left as a downward deflection. On the vertical plane, upward pen deflection records upward eye movement while downward deflection denotes downward movement. Data is collected through the use of various stimulations such as fixation points on the horizontal and vertical planes, a moving object for tracking, and others. An advantage of electronystagmography is that it enables nystagmus to be recorded behind closed eyelids as well as in the dark.

CONTRAINDICATIONS

Electronystagmography is contraindicated in patients with pacemakers. The equipment used for electronystagmography may interfere with the operation of the pacemaker.

PROCEDURE

Various maneuvers are followed to collect data on nystagmus. The patient is seated on a table and placed in a reclining position with his head hanging over the table at prescribed times. The examiner supports the patient's head while directing the patient to focus on his finger. The patient is observed for nystagmus, which may appear within 15 seconds. He is then raised to the sitting position. Other similar maneuvers are undertaken. The patient should be cautioned not to be alarmed if vertigo occurs.

PURPOSE

Electronystagmography is indicated when diagnosing the cause of nystagmus and vertigo. These problems may be associated with head injuries and lesions involving the vestibular branch of the eighth cranial nerve.

PREPROCEDURAL PREPARATION

The procedure should be explained to the patient, and he should be assured that the examiner will support him through the various positions assumed. Nothing is given by mouth for at least 8 hours before the test. Antivertigo drugs, tranquilizers, depressant drugs, alcohol, and stimulant drugs and foods (cola, coffee, and so forth) are usually withheld for 24 to 48 hours. The physician should be consulted about withholding any drug therapy.

POSTPROCEDURAL CARE

The patient should lie down until any vertigo, dizziness, nausea, or vomiting has subsided. An antiemetic may be given as necessary. The diet is resumed when the patient is able to tolerate it.

CALORIC TESTING FOR VESTIBULAR FUNCTION

Caloric testing is a diagnostic procedure designed to evaluate the vestibular portion of the eighth cranial nerve. The underlying principle of the procedure is that thermal stimulation of the vestibular end organs with warm and cold water will elicit the oculovestibular reflex. The oculovestibular reflex, if intact, results in induced nystagmus and eye movement in response to cold or warm water irrigation of the external auditory canal.

Caloric testing is usually conducted by the physician, who first must confirm that the tympanic membrane is intact. A ruptured tympanic membrane is a contraindication for testing. Active labyrinth diseases, such as Ménière's disease, are another contraindication.

A baseline assessment of Romberg's sign and the presence of nystagmus is established. The patient and physician are seated facing each other. The nurse assists in the procedure and is usually responsible for observing the patient and recording the time interval between the beginning of the irrigations and the onset of nystagmus or other untoward symptoms. The patient is directed to keep his eyes open and focused straight ahead. He is also told to report any unusual symptoms or discomfort.

Certain positions of the vertical and horizontal canals optimize their responsiveness to testing. To test the vertical canals, the patient's head is tilted forward 30 degrees. The head is tilted backward 60 degrees to test the horizontal canals. Cold water used for irrigations is 86° F (30° C) and hot water is 110° F (44° C). The external meatus is irrigated for 30 seconds to 3 minutes with each temperature, with a pause of at least 5 minutes between irrigations. Irrigations are discontinued when nystagmus or other symptoms appear, and the time interval from initiation of the irrigation to this point is recorded.

TESTING HORIZONTAL EYE MOVEMENT

If the oculovestibular reflex is intact, there is initial conjugate eye movement toward the side being irrigated with the cold water. Unilateral cold water irrigations result in slow nystagmic movement on the same side, followed shortly by rapid nystagmus to the opposite side (which begins in 20 to 30 seconds). Irrigation with warm water produces rapid nystagmus on the same side of the irrigation. The mnemonic "COWS" is used to remember the direction of the *fast* component: Cold, Opposite; Warm, Same.

Note that when describing nystagmus, there are two components identified: the fast component and the slow component. The fast component refers to rapid nystagmic movement while the slow component refers to slow nystagmic movement.

If the oculovestibular reflex is absent, there will be no movement of the eyes. If the reflex is diminished, there will be dysconjugate movement. Oculovestibular responses may be abnormal or absent with brain stem lesions involving the vestibular nerve (Fig. 4–14).

TESTING VERTICAL EYE MOVEMENT

To test vertical eye movement, simultaneous irrigation of both canals with cold water normally causes the fast component nystagmus to occur in a downward direction. When warm water is used for irrigation of both canals, the fast component of nystagmus is noted in an upward direction.

UNTOWARD EFFECTS OF CALORIC TESTING

Nausea, vomiting, or dizziness can be precipitated by caloric testing. Patients with diseases involving the vestibular branch of the eighth cranial nerve, such as an acoustic

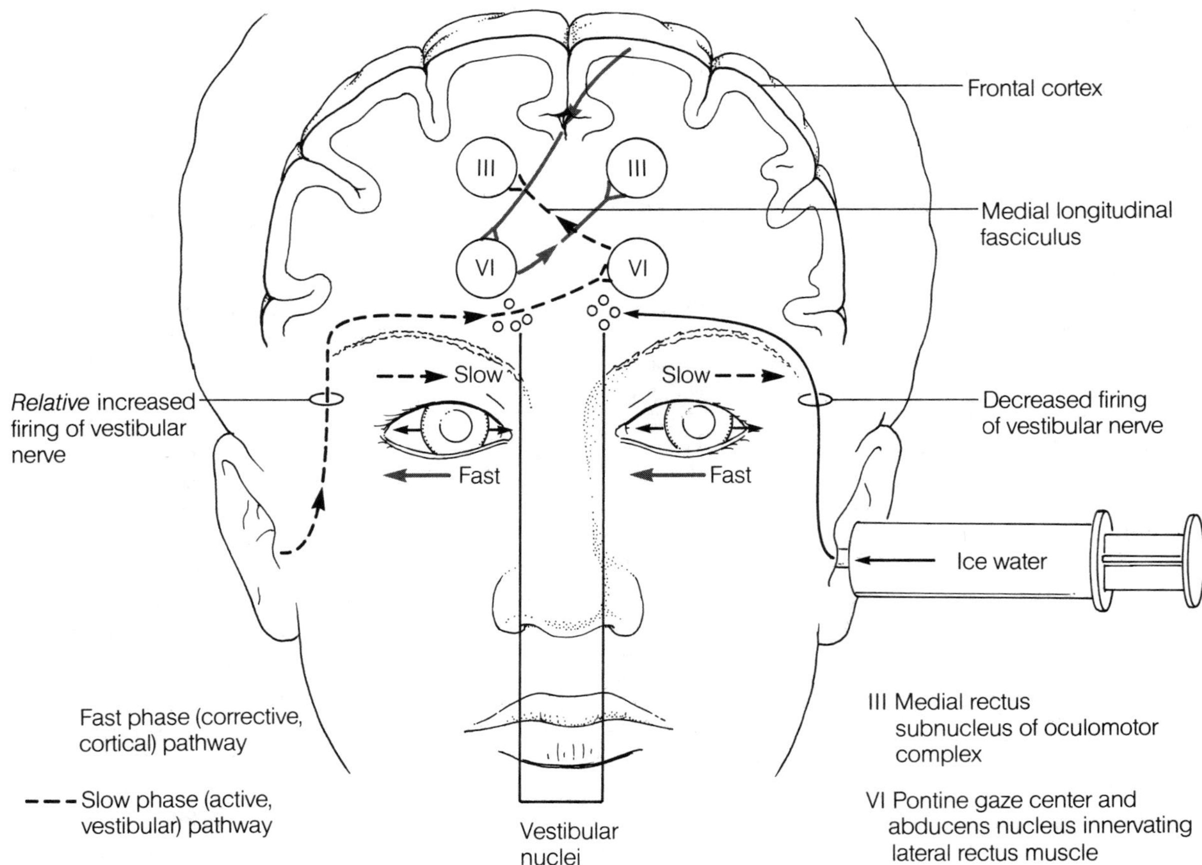

FIG. 4-14. Physiology of the oculovestibular reflex (vestibulo-ocular reflex, cold calorics). Ice-water infusion in the ear of a comatose patient will elicit the oculovestibular reflex if both the cerebral hemisphere and brain stem are intact. With an intact brain stem, a signal passes through pathways from the medulla to the midbrain, generating a slow movement of the eyes to the side of the ice-water infusion. This is followed by a rapid corrective movement of the eyes, generated by an intact ipsilateral side of the cerebral hemisphere. The ice-water infusion test can be repeated in the other ear of the comatose patient to test the integrity of the other side of the brain and brain stem. (Redrawn from *Patient Care* magazine. Copyright © 1981, Patient Care Communications, Inc., Darien, CT. All rights reserved.)

neuroma or Ménière's disease, will not have the eye movements normally associated with caloric testing; instead, the movements will be diminished or absent.

HALLPIKE CALORIC TESTING

The Hallpike caloric test is a variation of the caloric testing technique previously described. The patient is placed in a supine position on an examining table or bed with its head elevated 30 degrees. The same baseline parameters are recorded (Romberg's sign, nystagmus). With the patient focusing straight ahead, the external auditory canal (in which an intact tympanic membrane is present) is irrigated with 250 ml to 500 ml of warm or cold water for 40 seconds. The patient is observed for tonic eye movement and nystagmus.

Preprocedural Preparation

The procedure should be explained to the patient. Nothing should be given by mouth for 6 to 8 hours before the procedure.

Postprocedural Care

The patient should lie down until all untoward effects such as nausea, vertigo, or dizziness have passed. Diet can be resumed when the patient feels ready.

USE OF COLD CALORIC TESTING TO DETERMINE BRAIN STEM FUNCTION

In some instances, such as when a comatose patient has just been admitted to the emergency department, it may be helpful in initially assessing the patient to establish if brain stem function is intact. After inspecting the tympanic membrane to ensure that it is intact, cold water irrigations are initiated. If there is tonic deviation of the eyes toward the side being irrigated, brain stem function is intact. This is considered a positive prognostic sign. With a brain stem lesion, the caloric reflex will be absent or the ocular movement will be dysconjugate. Absence of the reflex is associated with a poor prognosis.

AUDIOMETRIC STUDIES

Hearing loss and complete deafness caused by injury of the auditory branch of the eighth cranial nerve is seen in all age groups. Loss of hearing is frequently seen in the elderly and is often associated with various aspects of aging. Otosclerosis is the chief cause of deafness in adults. Children may sustain hearing loss as a result of birth trauma or ear infections. All age groups may incur hearing loss as a result of head injury, meningitis, acoustic tumors, and certain drug toxicity. To assess the type and cause of hearing loss, it may be necessary to conduct a battery of tests that are collectively referred to as audiometric studies. The tests use the voice, tuning forks, a ticking watch, and an electronic audiometer to assess the hearing loss. Once a specific diagnosis is established, a treatment plan can be developed.

BRAIN STEM EVOKED POTENTIALS

Evoked potentials are minute voltage changes that occur in response to a brief sensory stimuli. Recorded from scalp electrodes, evoked potentials are very weak (0.5–5 microvolts) as compared to the amplitude of the spontaneous random activity (50–100 microvolts) of the brain recorded on an EEG. The evoked potentials are time-related to a sensory stimuli while the activity on the EEG is random. To study the evoked potentials, a method for enhancing evoked potentials as compared to the EEG was developed by a computer averaging process. In this method, a stimulus is repeated several times; the brain is allowed to return to a resting state between stimuli. Each transient evoked response is measured by a computerized instrument, and the data are stored. When several (100–200) potentials have been stored, the computer calculates the average curve. The EEG background activity does not directly relate to the stimulus but varies randomly, and the background distraction collects much less rapidly than the summed evoked potentials.[3]

The diagnostic value of evoked potential studies is that it reflects neural activity of the peripheral and central nervous system that can be recorded and evaluated for evidence of dysfunction and disease. The procedure is noninvasive and safe for the patient.

Evoked potentials are classified into three categories based on the type of stimulus provided and the sensory system stimulated. Each system stimulated produces a characteristic wave formation. The three sensory systems are the visual, auditory, and somatosensory pathways.

VISUAL EVOKED POTENTIALS (VEP)

In visual evoked potentials, the stimuli are provided by patterned stimuli, usually checkerboards, and unpatterned flashing lights. With repeated stimuli, the retina is stimulated and the pathways to the occipital cerebral cortex can be evaluated. To collect valid data, the patient must be able to follow directions and cooperate.

Visual evoked potentials testing is helpful in evaluating optic neuropathies and optic nerve lesions (tumors).

BRAIN STEM AUDITORY EVOKED RESPONSES (BAER)

In brain stem evoked responses the stimuli provided are clicks and tone pips. This test can be conducted on an alert and oriented patient as well as one in a coma. The potentials created are correlated to specific areas along the auditory pathway. This test can be helpful in diagnosing demyelinating disease, posterior fossa tumors such as acoustic neuromas and cerebellar pontine angle tumors, stroke, and conduction hearing loss.

SOMATOSENSORY EVOKED POTENTIALS

The development of somatosensory evoked potentials has not been as rapid as the development of auditory and visual evoked potentials. The stimulus applied to peripheral nerves is usually electrical, which is unpleasant. In some instances mechanical stimuli can be applied. Spinal cord function has been the major focus for the use of somatosensory evoked potential.

NEUROPSYCHOLOGICAL TESTING

Neuropsychological testing or assessment is defined as an objective comprehensive assessment of a wide range of cognitive, adaptive, and emotional behaviors that reflect the adequacy or inadequacy of cortical function.[4] Neuropsychological testing assesses a wider range of performance skills in greater depth and detail than other tests. Performance tests are the major tests used to evaluate organic brain damage. (Projective tests and personality inventories have been of little value in the study of brain damage.) The extent of assessment is reflected in the time necessary for testing, which is approximately 6 to 10 hours. The tests included in the assessment have been standardized on normal and brain-injured populations. The data collected from testing is objective, quantifiable, and comparable with values obtained from the normal population. Another benefit of the extensive testing is that subtle changes may be uncovered that would not be detected with less refined testing methods.

Neuropsychological testing is conducted by a clinical neuropsychologist who has earned a doctorate and participated in a clinical internship. The clinical internship included practice in the use and method of administering and interpreting standard psychological tests and specialized neuropsychological techniques to evaluate patients with organic brain disease. The neuropsychologist correlates the test data from the neuropsychological assessment with information about the type of neurological insult, premorbid function and personality, and findings on other diagnostic tests. The neuropsychological evaluation is an integral part of the neurological examination and must be viewed in that context. When the findings of the neurological examination are unclear or inconclusive, the physician may wish to request a neuropsychological examination to provide more information.

PURPOSES OF THE NEUROPSYCHOLOGICAL EVALUATION

The purposes of neuropsychological testing include (1) assistance in diagnosing the presence or absence of an organic brain lesion; (2) assistance in determining whether the brain dysfunction is localized (focal) or diffuse; (3) description of the effects of an identified lesion on cognition and behavior in a particular patient; (4) assistance in planning and evaluating an individualized rehabilitation program; and (5) assistance in identifying a realistic prognosis.

COMPONENTS OF THE NEUROPSYCHOLOGICAL EVALUATION

The specific tests included in a neuropsychological evaluation will vary depending on the age of the patient, nature of the problem, deficits present, specific questions asked by the physician in the referral note, and the ability of the person conducting the testing. However, all test batteries will include the following assessment:

- Attention: vigilance (the ability to sustain attention over a period of time, concentration), self-regulation, and screening out of distracting environmental stimuli
- Memory: recent, immediate, remote; new learning such as remembering word lists; and verbal and nonverbal memory
- Language: understanding single words and sentences; reading; speaking; and auditory discrimination
- General intelligence: verbal and nonverbal
- Constructional ability: draw to command; draw to copy; block designs; visual organization of a picture and its parts; right–left orientation; clock setting
- Map orientation
- Conceptualization: metaphors; proverbs
- Abstraction: verbal and nonverbal abstract reasoning
- Perceptual motor speed: ability to plan ahead and shift from one concept to the other

COMMON DEFICITS WITH ORGANIC BRAIN DYSFUNCTION

Many patients with organic brain dysfunction develop cognitive and behavioral deficits as a result of head trauma, stroke, central nervous system degenerative disorders (e.g., Alzheimer's disease), and central nervous system infectious diseases (e.g., encephalitis, meningitis). Common deficits include decreased ability to concentrate, increased irritability, emotional lability, decreased ability to screen out irrelevant information, decreased ability to solve problems, inability to correctly sequence complex actions, inability to learn new tasks, deficits in memory, deficits in logical reasoning, perceptual deficits, and general slowing of all cognitive functions. These cognitive and behavioral deficits cause serious difficulty in the social readjustment of the patient into the family, community, and work setting.

IMPORTANCE OF THE PROBLEM

Managing and rehabilitating the neurologically impaired patient has always focused on physical disabilities. Although cognitive and behavioral deficits have been recognized, it was usually believed that nothing could be done to overcome these deficits or that these deficits would improve with time without treatment. This philosophy is gradually changing. Many health professionals now recognize that the most significant long-term problems are cognitive, behavioral, and emotional, rather than physical. Research has also proven that cognitive functions continue to improve for several years after cerebral insult, especially if proper stimulation and management are provided. As a result, cognitive, behavioral, social, and adaptive daily living skills retraining programs are being developed in many facilities throughout the country and are becoming an integral part of the overall rehabilitation program offered the patient and family. Such programs can greatly help the patient reestablish his place in his home and community without the frustration, disequilibrium to family structure, humiliation, and depression that were often observed in the past.

REFERENCES

1. Dagani R: Radiochemicals key to new diagnostic tool. Chemical & Engineering News 59(45):30, November 9, 1981
2. Nursing '82 Books: Diagnostics. Springhouse, PA, Intermed Communications, 1982
3. Regan D: Electrical responses evoked from the human brain. Sci Am 241(12):134, December 1979
4. Strub R, Black FW: The Mental Examination in Neurology, p 137. Philadelphia, FA Davis, 1977

BIBLIOGRAPHY

Books

Chusid JG: Correlative Neuroanatomy and Functional Neurology, 18th ed. Los Altos, CA, Lange Medical Publications, 1982

Davis DO, Kobrine A: Computed tomography. In Youmans JR (ed): Neurological Surgery, 2nd ed, vol 1, pp 111–142. Philadelphia, WB Saunders, 1982

Fischbach FT: A Manual of Laboratory Diagnostic Tests, 2nd ed. Philadelphia, JB Lippincott, 1984

Hendee WR: The Physical Principles of Computed Tomography, pp 21–33. Boston, Little, Brown, & Co, 1983

Jennett B, Teasdale G: Management of Head Injuries. Philadelphia, FA Davis, 1981

Mayo Clinic and Mayo Foundation: Clinical Examinations in Neurology, 5th ed. Philadelphia, WB Saunders, 1981

Pincus J, Tucker G: Behavioral Neurology, 2nd ed. New York, Oxford University Press, 1978

Price RR et al (eds): Digital Radiography: A Focus on Clinical Utility. New York, Grune & Stratton, 1982

Walsh K: Neuropsychology—A Clinical Approach, pp 282–331. New York, Churchill Livingstone, 1978

Periodicals

Bydder G: Nuclear magnetic resonance of the brain. Appl Radiol 27, January/February 1983

Byers V, Gendell H: Using metrizamide for lumbar myelography: Adverse reactions and nursing implications. J Neurosurg Nurs 14(6):315, December 1982

Chambers A: How to read skull x-rays. Hosp Med 32AA, December 1982

Christenson PC et al: Intravenous cervicocerebrovascular angiography. Am J Radiol 135:1145, 1980

Cochran R: Determining cerebral death with radiologic diagnostic procedures. Radiol Technol 51:779, May–June 1980

Couvillon LA, Brenkus LM: The commercial systems for digital radiology. Diagn Imaging 1:4, January 1982

Gilmor R: Computerized axial tomography in head trauma. Crit Care 2(1):61, June 1979

Hall J et al: Auditory evoked responses in acute severe head injury. J Neurosurg Nurs 14(5):225, October 1982

Haughey CW: What to say . . . and do . . . when your patient asks about CT scans. Nurs81 11:72, December 1981

Kattan K: Reading cervical spine films. Hosp Med 32E, January 1983

Knox R: A diagnostic dream machine. Boston Globe Sunday Magazine 59, April 10, 1983

Lassen N et al: Brain function and blood flow. Sci Am 239(20):62, October 1978

Lee B: CT scans of the head: Basic interpretation. Hosp Med 21, January 1982

Long N: How to see your patient safely through an angiogram. RN 60, October 1978

Lyons M, Wilson D: Regional cerebral blood flow—A newer non-invasive neurodiagnostic test. J Neurosurg Nurs 13(6):286, December 1981

Maida M: Regional cerebral blood flow: Patient correlation. J Neurosurg Nurs 14(5):309, October 1982

McManus J, Hausman K: Deciphering diagnostic studies: Cerebrospinal fluid analysis. Nurs82 12:43, August 1982

O'Reilly B: Preparing the patient for computerized tomography. J Neurosurg Nurs 11(1):41, March 1979

Pykett I: NMR imaging in medicine. Sci Am 246(5):78, May 1982

Warren JB, Goethe KE, Peck EA: Neuropsychological abnormalities associated with severe head injury. J Neurosurg Nurs 16(1):30, February 1984

Zawadzki M et al: Applications of NMR to CNS disease. Appl Radiol 25, March/April 1983

chapter

5

Assessment of Neurological Signs

PURPOSES OF ASSESSMENT

Nursing care of the neurological patient depends on highly developed skills of observation. To be a skilled observer, one must know both what to observe and how to interpret the observations to decide what action, if any, should be taken. Inherent in this skill is the ability to detect changes, both obvious and subtle, in the patient's condition. A baseline assessment of the neurological signs is made so that deviations from this data base can be noted. Continuous comparisons between present findings and preceding assessments are essential, since the degree of change in the patient's neurological status can be rapid and dramatic or very subtle and innocuous, developing over a period of days, weeks, or even months.

Information on a patient's health history and current health status is available from a variety of sources, including the patient's chart, the Kardex, and the nursing care plan, as well as the intershift report from the nursing staff who provided care during the previous time period. The family, too, can contribute a wealth of information about the precipitating factors, the course of the illness, and the patient's behavior before admission and/or illness.

The patient himself can provide both objective and subjective data that can be obtained by listening to him and observing his behavior; in fact, the most valuable method of assessment is clinical observation of the patient.

When the patient's neurological signs are assessed, it is important to check the following:

1. Level of consciousness
2. Pupillary observations
3. Ocular movements
4. Motor function
5. Sensory function
6. Vital signs (particularly the respiratory pattern)

LEVEL OF CONSCIOUSNESS

The level of consciousness is the most important factor in the neurological assessment of the patient. It is the earliest and most sensitive of indicators, providing valid information about changes in neurological status. Change can occur very slowly over the course of many hours, days, or even weeks, or it can occur very rapidly in a few minutes or a few hours. The rapidity of change is an indicator of the acuity of the neurological problem. Alteration in consciousness is the hallmark of cerebral injury.

PHYSIOLOGY OF CONSCIOUSNESS

The reticular activating system (RAS) is the portion of the nervous system that controls the degree of central nervous system activity, including wakefulness.

Anatomically the RAS is a very diffuse system. The nuclei that compose the system begin in the lower brain stem (medulla) and proceed through the pons, midbrain, and thalamus to be finally dispersed throughout the cerebral cortex. Studies indicate that the brain stem and thalamic portions function differently; the former is believed to be responsible for wakefulness or arousal, while the latter appears to control the sum of mental activity or the content of consciousness.

Although consciousness has been defined as a state of

general awareness of oneself and the environment, this definition is not an altogether satisfactory one because it is based on a subjective evaluation of the patient's appearance and behavior. Based on physiological function, consciousness has been divided into two components: (1) the *content* of consciousness, which includes the sum of cerebral mental functions that are controlled by the cerebral hemispheres; and (2) *arousal*, which is concerned with the patient's appearance of wakefulness. Because content and arousal are independent components, each has numerous possible states that can be affected by different types of cerebral lesions.

Consciousness, however, is difficult to estimate with any degree of accuracy because the patient's behavior merely provides an estimate of his arousability at *a given time*. If the patient can hear and verbalize, then thought content should be evaluated for appropriateness and accuracy; however, content may be influenced by many variables, such as whether a patient is hard-of-hearing, has a language barrier, is aphasic, or is experiencing extreme psychological stress.

Impairment of consciousness can vary in severity from slight to complete. Impaired consciousness indicates brain dysfunction or brain failure. The longer the duration and more severe the dysfunction, the less chance of complete recovery. Consciousness is a dynamic state that is subject to change. The change can occur very rapidly, as in the instance of an epidural hematoma in which the patient can move from complete consciousness to coma in a matter of hours, or it can occur so slowly that it is discernible only with the passage of weeks or months, such as may occur in a patient with a chronic subdural hematoma.

MAJOR CAUSES OF ALTERATIONS IN CONSCIOUSNESS (STUPOR OR COMA)

The major causes of altered levels of consciousness (stupor or coma) are summarized by Plum and Posner and include[1]

1. *Supratentorial lesions*
   To produce stupor or coma, a lesion must affect the cerebral hemispheres *directly and widely* to cause diffuse bilateral cerebral hemispheric dysfunction and subsequent coma.
   Common lesions that can have diffuse effects on the brain include
   - Subcortical destructive lesions such as thalamic lesions
   - Hemorrhagic lesions (intracerebral, epidural, subdural hematomas)
   - Tumors
   - Abscesses
   - Closed head injury
2. *Subtentorial (infratentorial) lesions*
   These lesions *directly compress or destroy* the neurons of the RAS that lie in the central gray matter of the diencephalon, midbrain, and upper pons.
   Common compression lesions include
   - Basilar artery aneurysms
   - Posterior fossa subdural or epidural hemorrhage
   - Cerebellar hemorrhage, abscess, tumor, or infarction

   Common destructive lesions include
   - Pontine hemorrhage
   - Brain stem infarction

ASSESSING LEVELS OF CONSCIOUSNESS

The patient's level of consciousness is evaluated by providing stimuli and observing his response. Pain and sound are the major stimuli used. When any kind of stimulation is provided, it is best to start with the minimal amount necessary to evoke a response; then, the stimuli can be increased as necessary. Speaking to the patient is the most common method of applying auditory stimuli, whether he is alert and oriented or in a coma. The response to auditory stimuli is evaluated with all patients. Painful stimuli are reserved for unconscious patients or those with obviously decreased levels of consciousness.

Auditory Stimuli

When the fully conscious patient is addressed in a normal tone of voice, he should reply with an appropriate verbal response. A person with a decreased level of consciousness can respond to auditory stimuli in a variety of ways. He may respond with an appropriate simple reply, he may respond in a puzzled manner, or he may not respond at all, not even wincing when someone speaks directly into his ear.

Painful Stimuli

Withdrawal from pain is considered a noteworthy finding in the unconscious patient. Painful tactile stimuli can be provided by exerting firm pressure to the following areas: the Achilles tendon, the gastrocnemius or trapezius muscles, or the fingernails (Fig. 5–1). Pressing a key on the skin or running it over the skin is another possible technique. Although some writers suggest applying sternal massage or pressure, it should be noted that many people bruise easily in this area. Applying supraorbital pressure is another form of stimulus that has been suggested; however, it is a questionable practice to apply pressure to a possibly injured head when other methods of evaluating consciousness can elicit valid data.

Response to painful stimuli can be classified into the following categories:

- Purposeful
- Nonpurposeful (with or without withdrawal from the source of pain)
- Unresponsive

A *purposeful response* is one in which the patient winces, pushes the examiner away, and withdraws the affected body part simultaneously in response to the painful stimulus.

In a *nonpurposeful response*, removal from the noxious stimulus is incomplete. The patient may attempt to withdraw only the stimulated part of the body, or the patient may move the stimulated part only slightly, without any attempt to withdraw the part. In some unconscious patients, application of painful stimuli will cause an extensor response only, that is, a contraction of muscles, such as the quadriceps muscles of the thigh, which extend the joints.

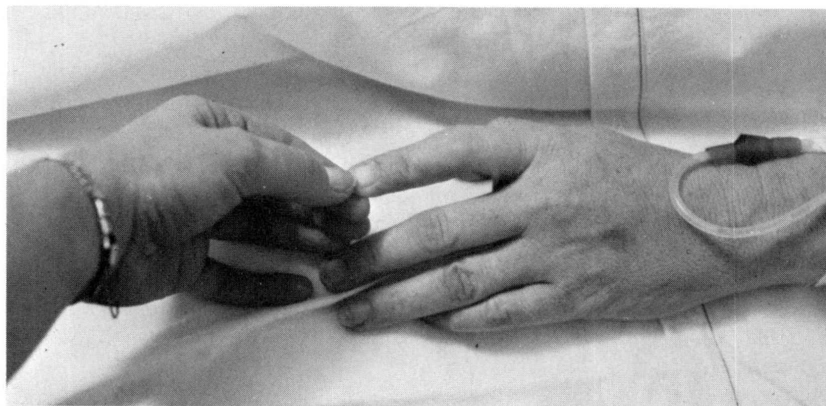

FIG. 5-1. Applying pressure to fingernail is one kind of stimuli to use in assessing the patient's level of consciousness.

An *unresponsive* patient would show no signs of reacting to painful stimuli. Such an absence of response is noted in a patient in a deep coma.

IDENTIFYING THE LEVEL OF CONSCIOUSNESS

Labeling the levels of consciousness can create a great deal of confusion because no uniform, precise definitions have been accepted. An accurate description of the patient's behavior and response to stimuli is of greater importance than the use of labels. (See Chart 5-1, Nursing Assessment of the Levels of Consciousness.) The following terms appear quite often in the literature and are frequently used for clinical assessment although they are subject to varied interpretation:

1. ***Full Consciousness***
   The patient is awake, alert, and fully able to maintain an appropriate conversation. He comprehends spoken and written words and is aware of time, place, and identity.
   - The fully conscious patient should be capable of assuming some responsibility for independent self-care.
2. ***Confusion***
   The patient may misinterpret stimuli and demonstrates a shortened attention span. He first becomes disoriented to time, then to place, and finally to his own person and that of others. Confused patients become bewildered easily, have poor memories, and have difficulty following commands. Daytime drowsiness can alternate with nighttime agitation.
   - The confused patient requires special nursing management to prevent injury. Side rails, and possibly a jacket restraint, may be necessary to prevent the patient from falling or getting out of bed unattended.
3. ***Delirium***
   A delirious state is characterized by restlessness, agitation, irritability, disorientation, and possible hallucinations. The patient is frequently boisterous, offensive, suspicious, and combative, and thrashes about in his bed. He can be overcome by fear of personal harm because of misinterpretation of environmental stimuli, as well as delirium and hallucinations.
   - Special nursing precautions should be taken to prevent injury to the delirious patient. If the threat of injury to the patient or the moving about of vital equipment persists, restraints may be necessary.
4. ***Obtundation***
   The patient can be readily aroused when stimulated. He can speak and respond to the spoken word if the communication is simple and responds appropriately when stimulated; otherwise, he appears drowsy. Lethargy, somnolence, and drowsiness are synonymous with obtundation.
   - Side rails should be raised and the patient should be observed frequently because he is unable to assume any responsibility.
5. ***Stupor***
   The patient is in a very drowsy and lethargic state and is generally unresponsive. He can be briefly aroused only by repeated, vigorous, painful stimuli from which he withdraws purposefully.
   - Side rails should be raised and the patient should be observed frequently.
6. ***Coma***
   A patient who appears to be asleep but does not respond appropriately to body or environmental stimuli is said to be in a coma.

   Some confusion exists in describing the comatose state because of variations in the definition of coma. Some authors subdivide coma into gradients of depth by correlating certain alterations in motor function with deterioration of the patient's level of consciousness. Such motor alterations include purposeful withdrawal from painful stimuli, nonpurposeful withdrawal from stimuli, unresponsiveness to painful stimuli, and loss of the gag reflex. Others disagree with these correlations, claiming that the neural regulation of consciousness and that of motor function are physiologically independent. Despite the acceptance of the physiological uniqueness of each system, most clinicians, based on current knowledge, will attest to the validity of applying painful stimuli and observing the patient's response as a means of collecting data on the level of consciousness.

   Coma can be divided into semicoma, coma, and deep coma. The differentiation among these three levels can be useful in assessing the presence of slight improvement or deterioration in the patient's condition.

   The *semicomatose* patient does not move spontaneously in bed and is unresponsive to stimuli, although shaking the patient, speaking loudly to him, shouting, or applying painful stimuli to the skin (pinching or pricking) may result in stirring or moaning. The patient will also attempt to completely withdraw either the stimulated body part or himself from the source of noxious stimuli. Unlike a stuporous patient who can be aroused briefly in response to loud talking, the semicomatose patient will only stir and moan under a similar stimulus.

   In the semicomatose patient most reflexes such as the cor-

CHART 5-1. NURSING ASSESSMENT OF THE LEVELS OF CONSCIOUSNESS

In assessing a patient's level of consciousness, start by calling the patient's name as you move into his view. Raise your voice gradually and repeat the patient's name as necessary. If need be, apply painful stimuli to elicit a reaction. To avoid confusion in terminology, record the patient's response to terms of his behavior.

Responses	Chart Information
1. An *alert* patient will respond immediately when first approached. The response will include • Appropriate acknowledgment of your presence • Movement of the head and/or body in your direction unless motor impairment negates this possibility • Patient's attention focused upon you	**1.** "Alert and oriented to time, place, and person . . . able to carry on appropriate conversation and follow directions." (Full consciousness)
2. A *confused* patient may need some repetition before his attention is directed toward the speaker.	**2.** "Patient appears confused. He fluctuates between stating that he is at his daughter's home and stating that he is in the hospital. He responds to his name after a few repeated calls. The same questions are asked repeatedly by the patient." (Confusion)
3. A *delirious, obtunded,* or *stuporous* patient will require repeated, loud, verbal stimulation and physical shaking. The arousal, particularly of the stuporous patient, may be momentary. Many stuporous patients require painful stimuli for arousal.	**3.** "Thrashes about in bed, banging on side rails, and screams periodically; appears to be having auditory hallucinations at times. Has lucid periods when he responds momentarily to his name." (Delirium) "Readily arousable when called by name and when hands are rubbed. Answers simple questions appropriately. Without constant stimulation, he is very lethargic." (Obtundation) "Very drowsy, lethargic, and generally unresponsive. Arousable momentarily to repeated loud stimuli." (Stupor)
4. The *semicomatose* patient is unresponsive unless superficial noxious stimuli are used.	**4.** "Withdraws hand when noxious stimulus is applied to fingers; otherwise unresponsive to loud verbal stimuli." (Semicoma)
5. The *comatose* patient may or may not react to an increased degree of noxious stimuli.	**5.** "Unarousable and unresponsive." (Coma)
6. The *deeply comatose* patient does not respond at all to any type of stimuli, including pain.	**6.** "Unarousable and unresponsive to all stimuli." (Deep coma)

neal, pupillary, pharyngeal, and tendon are intact. The Babinski sign may or may not be present.

The patient in a *comatose* state is unarousable and will neither stir nor moan regardless of the kind or amount of stimuli applied. Response to painful stimuli is nonpurposeful in that there may be a slight movement of the area stimulated, but there is *no attempt to withdraw* the body part from the stimuli. Most brain stem reflexes such as the corneal, pupillary, and pharyngeal are intact. Extensor rigidity, decerebration, or decortication may or may not be present.

The patient who is in a *deep coma* is completely unarousable and unresponsive to any kind of stimulus, including pain. The brain stem reflexes, corneal, pupillary and pharyngeal reflexes, and the tendon and plantar reflexes are all absent.

- Special nursing care for the comatose patient must be implemented. Maintenance of a patient airway is top priority.

CHANGES IN LEVEL OF CONSCIOUSNESS

Changes in the level of consciousness are, to some extent, predictable in that a patient who has been in a coma and now is arousable with repeated stimulation is described as displaying improvement in his level of consciousness. Clinicians frequently say, "The patient appears to be lighter." What they are actually implying is that the deteriorated level of consciousness appears to have improved from the last examination.

The various stages of consciousness are arranged on a crude continuum that aids the clinician in assessing changes in the patient's condition. It is possible, and indeed probable, that all of the levels of consciousness are not observable in particular patients as they recover from injury.

A few final points concerning the level of consciousness should be kept in mind:

1. When a patient with a head injury is evaluated during the posttraumatic period, he may arrive at an extended plateau of consciousness in the recovery process. For example, a patient can be in a coma for 6 to 8 weeks and then become restless, agitated, and delirious. He may stay in this state for 4 to 6 weeks and then one day become fully conscious. Each patient has his own unique pattern of recovery based on the type, extent, and site of injury.
2. It is most important to record the time of observation of postoperative patients who have undergone intracranial surgery. It makes a great difference whether there is a 1-hour or 4-hour interval between observations that indicate how rapidly the

neurological status of the patient might be changing following surgery.

3. Recovery from an altered level of consciousness is influenced by age, type of injury, and premorbid health status. Patients under 20 years of age have a much better prognosis of recovery than older patients.
4. The longer the coma, the worse the outcome. Absence of pupillary and/or oculocephalic responses initially or during the course of illness indicates a poor outcome. Decortication, decerebration, or flaccidity of the motor system denotes a poor prognosis.

METABOLIC CAUSES OF DELIRIUM, STUPOR, AND COMA

Structural lesions of the central nervous system are not always the cause of a decreased level of consciousness. Delirium, stupor, and coma may be due to metabolic causes such as[2]

1. Deprivation of oxygen and other key metabolic necessities (hypoxia, ischemia, hypoglycemia, or vitamin deficiency)
2. Disease of organs excluding the brain
   - Nonendocrine organs: kidney — uremic coma; liver — hepatic coma; lungs — carbon dioxide narcosis; and pancreas — exocrine pancreatic encephalopathy
   - Endocrine organs, hypofunction and hyperfunction: thyroid — myxedema and thyrotoxicosis; parathyroid — hypoparathyroidism and hyperparathyroidism; adrenals — Addison's disease, Cushing's disease, pheochromocytoma; pancreas — diabetes mellitus and hypoglycemia
3. Pharmacological agents
   - Sedatives: barbiturates and nonbarbiturates; hypnotics; tranquilizers; ethanol; opiates; and bromides
   - Acidic toxins: paraldehyde; methyl alcohol; ethylene glycol; and ammonium chloride
   - Psychotropic drugs: amphetamines; lithium; tricyclic antidepressants; and others
   - Other drugs: steroids; cimetidine; salicylates; anticonvulsants; and others
4. Electrolyte and acid-base imbalance

The most common metabolic causes of delirium, stupor, and coma seen in the general hospital are said to be cerebral ischemia, hypoglycemia, and sedative drug overdose. It is routine practice in most emergency departments to draw blood from newly admitted comatose patients to test for blood gases and glucose level and to screen for drugs.

In assessing a comatose patient, the nurse should be aware that several problems outside the central nervous system can cause a decreased level of consciousness. It may be helpful for the nurse to consider a comparison of coma caused by metabolic and nervous system structural lesions (Table 5-1).

PROBLEMS OF ASSESSING THE LEVEL OF CONSCIOUSNESS

The level of consciousness has been described as the earliest and most sensitive indicator of neurological change, thus making it very critical information in neurological assessment. To be considered valid and reliable, most data must provide an understandable, objective, qualitative, or quantitative means of classifying the information being studied. The level of consciousness, however, is not amenable to the collection of standardized, objective data that can be quantified or qualitatively grouped in the same way as blood pressure or intracranial pressure. Information about the level of consciousness is collected by a trained assessor, thus introducing subjectivity into the assessment process. To further add to the confusion, there is no internationally accepted system of precise definitions with which to label levels of consciousness; therefore, no precise understanding of terminology exists from one clinician to another.

The Glasgow Coma Scale (GCS)

In assessing levels of consciousness, the validity and reliability of data depend on the assessor's ability to accurately describe the patient's behavior in response to stimuli. In an attempt to refine and standardize observations for objective assessment of the level of consciousness, the GCS was developed in 1974 at the University of Glasgow. The scale was designed to assess the level of consciousness in head injury patients. Since its introduction, the GCS has been employed in a variety of settings in Europe and the United States. The GCS has gained increasing acceptance as an accurate and effective means of evaluating levels of consciousness. Since it appears to have significant impact on

TABLE 5-1. *Comparison of Coma Caused by Metabolic and Central Nervous System (CNS) Structural Lesions*

Observation	*Metabolic Coma*	*CNS Structural Coma*
Motor system	*Diffuse* abnormal motor signs (tremors, myoclonus, and especially asterixis); symmetrical	*Focal* abnormal signs that are unilateral; asymmetrical
Motor abnormalities	Coma *precedes* motor abnormalities	Coma *follows* motor abnormalities
Pupils	Bilaterally *reactive*	Unilateral or later, bilaterally *nonreactive*
Progression of neurological deterioration	*Partial* dysfunction affects many levels of the CNS while other functions are retained	*Orderly* rostral-caudal deterioration with supratentorial lesions
EEG	*Diffusely* but not locally slow	May be slow but will also show abnormal *focal* areas

neurological assessment, an example is presented in Figure 5-2.

The scale is divided into three areas of focus: eye opening, best verbal response, and best motor response.[3] A rating scale exists for each area. The information collected is plotted on graph paper to provide a visual perspective of deterioration, improvement, or stabilization. In interpreting the GCS, one can add the numerical values of each of the three areas.

Based on this figure, certain deductions can be made about the level of consciousness. For example, the high score of 15 would reflect a fully alert, well-oriented person, while a score of 3, the lowest possible score, is indicative of deep coma. A score of 7 or less can be considered to be a generally accepted level for coma and indicates the need for a standard of nursing care conducive to the requirements of the comatose patient.

SPECIAL STATES OF ALTERED CONSCIOUSNESS

Plum and Posner state that nearly all patients in coma begin to awaken from their comatose state within 2 to 4 weeks after injury regardless of the severity of brain damage if they survive at all. Once a sleep-wakefulness cycle

FIG. 5-2. Glasgow Coma Scale. How to Score Responses on the Glasgow Coma Scale.
Scoring of Eye Opening: 4 = if the patient opens his eyes spontaneously when the nurse approaches; 3 = if the patient opens his eyes in response to speech (spoken or shouted); 2 = if the patient opens his eyes only in response to painful stimuli such as digital squeezing around nail beds of fingers; 1 = if the patient does not open his eyes in response to painful stimuli.
Scoring of Best Motor Response: 6 = if the patient can obey a simple command such as "Lift your left hand off the bed"; 5 = if the patient moves a limb to locate the painful stimuli applied to the head or trunk and attempts to remove the source; 4 = if the patient attempts to withdraw from the source of pain; 3 = if the patient flexes only his arms at the elbows and wrist in response to painful stimuli to the nail beds (decorticate rigidity); 2 = if the patient extends his arms (straightens his elbows) in response to painful stimuli (decerebrate rigidity); 1 = if the patient has no motor response to pain on any limb.
Scoring of Best Verbal Response: 5 = if the patient is oriented to time, place, and person; 4 = if the patient is able to converse although not oriented to time, place, or person (e.g., "Where am I?"); 3 = if the patient speaks only in words or phrases that make little or no sense (e.g., "B—H, N—K"); 2 = if the patient responds with incomprehensible sounds such as groans; 1 = if the patient does not respond verbally at all.

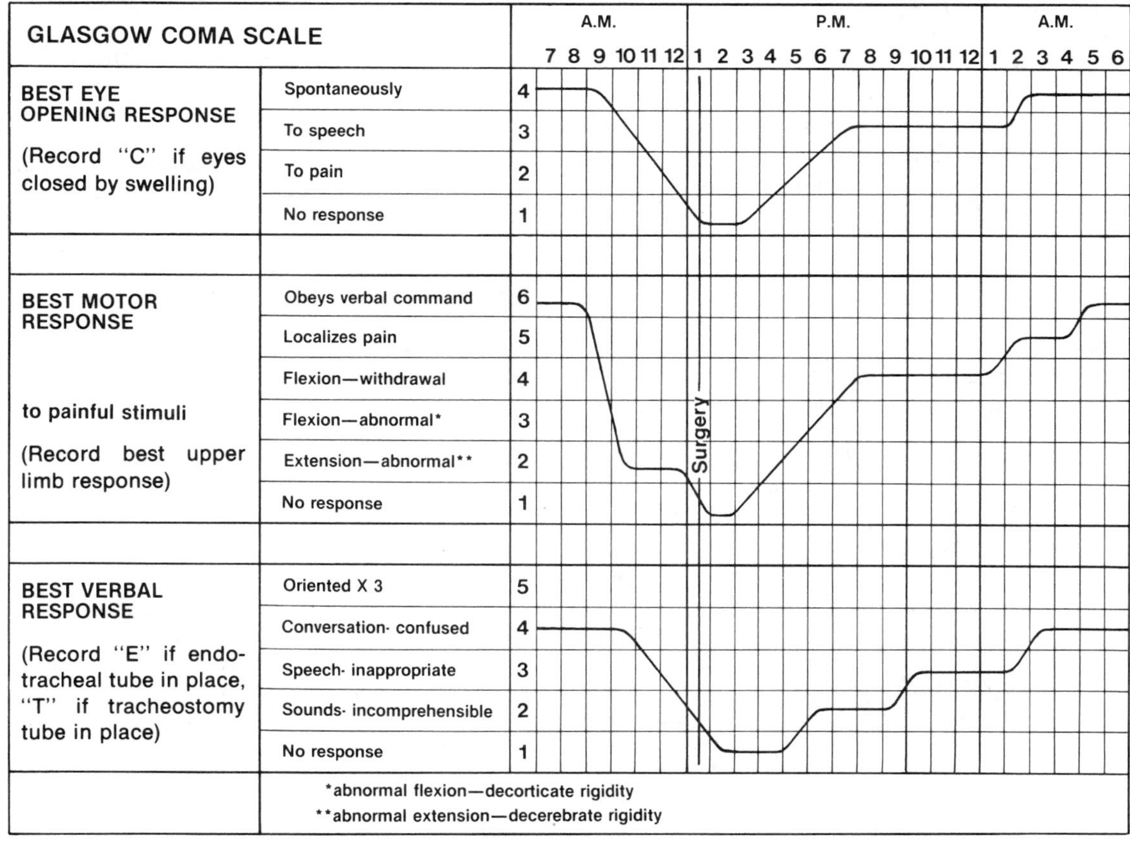

has been reestablished, Plum and Posner state that it is inaccurate to say that the patient is in a coma even though there is no apparent awareness of or interaction with the environment.[4]

A few special states of altered consciousness should be mentioned because they are seen and discussed in the clinical setting and in the literature. These special states include dementia, vegetative state, akinetic mutism, locked-in syndrome, and brain death.

Dementia

Dementia is an extended or permanent decline in the overall cognitive functions without any reduction in arousal. The causes of dementia are primary organic disorders of the cerebral cortex or hemisphere due to traumatic injuries, tumors, or degenerative disorders. On occasion, the condition may be partially reversed as in the case of normal pressure hydrocephalus or vitamin deficiency. However, dementia usually implies an irreversible disorder in which the person is not able to independently assume responsibility for himself.

Vegetative State

Vegetative state is the term suggested by Jennett and Plum to describe a subacute or chronic condition, usually occurring after severe cerebral injury and characterized by (1) intact autonomic functions, including those that maintain vital signs; (2) intact reflexes, especially the brain stem reflexes (e.g., pupillary response and swallowing); (3) presence of a sleep–wakefulness cycle; (4) spontaneous eye opening to verbal stimuli; (5) no localizing motor responses to stimuli; and (6) no intact cognitive functions or awareness of self or of the environment.[5] The vegetative state usually follows a period of sleeplike coma. Other terms that have been proposed to describe the vegetative state include coma vigil, the apallic syndrome, and irreversible coma. If the vegetative state lasts for an extended period of time it is called *persistent* or *chronic vegetative state.*

Akinetic Mutism

Akinetic mutism is a subacute or chronic state of altered consciousness characterized by (1) periods of appearing to be alert although there is no evidence of cognitive function or awareness of self or the environment; (2) eyes that are usually closed although at times the patient may focus and appears to follow an object; and (3) the existence of a sleep–wakefulness cycle. The specific etiology is unclear although this condition is seen with various cerebral conditions such as lesions of the medial basal region of the frontal lobes, lesions of the paramedian reticular region of the upper brain stem and diencephalon, and advanced subacute communicating hydrocephalus.

Locked-In Syndrome

Locked-in syndrome is a term coined by Plum and Posner. The signs and symptoms include (1) complete paralysis of all four extremities and lower cranial nerves so that the patient loses the ability to move and speak; (2) the only intact voluntary functions being vertical eye movement and blinking; and (3) full consciousness being maintained.[6] This syndrome is seen in such conditions as poliomyelitis, myasthenia gravis, and certain cerebral vascular diseases. The cause of the locked-in syndrome is interruption of the brain stem corticospinal tract and the corticobulbar fibers of the lower cranial nerves while the RAS and cerebral cortices are intact.

Brain Death

Brain death is a state of irreversible severe brain damage that is characterized by (1) absence of cognitive functions and awareness of self and the environment; (2) inability to maintain vital functions (e.g., cardiovascular, respiratory); (3) absence of isoelectric activity on EEG; and (4) a heart that will fail in a few hours or weeks even with mechanical support. The criteria by which a patient is declared brain dead is a serious, controversial, legal, ethical, and medical dilemma. Brain death criteria are discussed in Chapter 1.

NURSING INTERVENTION FOR THE PATIENT WITH AN ALTERED LEVEL OF CONSCIOUSNESS

1. Maintaining a patent airway is a top priority in a patient with an altered level of consciousness. The patient should not be left on his back because of the possibility of aspiration. A position should be selected that allows oral secretions to be drained.
2. Change in the level of consciousness is the most sensitive indicator of neurological change and, therefore, the first neurological sign to change when there is alteration in the neurological status. The level of consciousness should be assessed periodically by the nurse (as often as every 5 to 10 minutes in the acute unstable patient to as seldom as every 4 hours in the apparently stable patient). Regardless of all the technological advances in medicine, the observant nurse who knows her patient is still the *most sensitive "sensor" of neurological changes.* The nurse who is well acquainted with the personality and behavioral characteristics of her patient can best evaluate whether behavioral changes are caused by psychological stress, pain, fatigue, or neurological deterioration. The nurse has the responsibility of advising the physician of changes in the patient's level of consciousness.
3. When managing a patient whose level of consciousness has deteriorated, the nurse should talk to the patient in a calm, normal voice explaining, in simple terms, what she is doing and orienting him to his environment. If the patient normally wears glasses or a hearing aid, he should wear them.
4. When talking to the patient, try to screen out external environmental stimuli that can confuse the patient. Also, a group of people entering the room and talking to the patient can be overwhelming and confusing. In essence, it creates a sensory overload for the fragile recovering neurological circuits and causes confusion and misinterpretation of stimuli.
5. Once patients begin to awaken and verbalize, they often begin to recognize a void of time for which they canot account. This can be very frightening to the patient. The nurse should fill the gaps of time by briefly recounting what has happened during the lapse. Also, when the patient begins to verbalize facts that are incorrect, the nurse should matter-of-factly correct any misconceptions.

6. The nurse is responsible for protecting the patient from injury. As the patient's level of consciousness deteriorates, the nurse must assume total responsibility for his safety. The methods employed depend on the availability of staff (usually less staff on evenings and nights), patient's degree of agitation and impulsive behavior, location of the patient's room in relationship to the nurse's station, and use of support equipment for the patient (respirator, central venous pressure line, intravenous lines, intracranial pressure monitoring device, and others). Regardless of the circumstances, the standards of care for the patient require much more nursing time and intervention than that required for an alert oriented patient. The nurse should observe the patient frequently; talk to him in a calm manner; be sure that the bed is kept low, unless contraindicated, and that both bottom and top siderails are up; and apply restraints such as a jacket restraint, arm restraints, and so forth, as necessary, according to the standing orders of the physician and hospital policy.
7. Nighttime and darkness often lead the patient to misinterpret the environment and other stimuli. A night light and periodic visits by the nurse can help to control confusion, fear, and hallucinations.
8. The family and other visitors need help to learn how to visit a patient whose level of consciousness has deteriorated and who has cognitive deficits. The guidelines suggested will depend on the particular patient. The nurse should be available to intervene if problems occur during the visit as well as to evaluate the effects of the visit on the patient and visitors afterwards. If the patient is upset, the reasons for his reaction should be pursued. Family members may also need support after the visit to express their concerns and fears.

NURSING DIAGNOSES FREQUENTLY IDENTIFIED FOR PATIENTS WITH AN ALTERED LEVEL OF CONSCIOUSNESS

The following nursing diagnoses are frequently identified for the patient with an altered level of consciousness caused by neurological dysfunction:

- Health management deficit, total or specific, depending on the specific level of consciousness
- Physical injury, potential for
- Noncompliance, potential for
- Fluid volume deficit, potential for
- Nutrition, alterations in: less than body requires
- Urinary elimination, impairment of: incontinence
- Activity tolerance, decreased
- Home maintenance management, impaired
- Self-care deficit, total or in specific areas depending on level of consciousness
- Cognitive deficit
- Knowledge deficit
- Memory deficit
- Thought processes, impaired
- Coping, ineffective
- Fear, potential of (depends on the level of consciousness)
- Socialization, alterations in

See Nursing Diagnoses Frequently Identified for Patients With an Altered Level of Consciousness.

COGNITIVE ASSESSMENT

Assessing the level of consciousness for orientation to time, place, and person provides little information about cognitive function. The nurse who works closely with the patient becomes aware of cognitive deficits. It is often the nurse who must convince the physician that the patient does indeed have cognitive deficits that need to be identified by cognitive testing (see Chapter 4) and that a cognitive retraining program should be planned based on the test results.

As nurses, we are all too familiar with the quick visit of the busy physician to a head injury patient who is recovering. The patient may be sitting in a chair looking so much better than he did just a few weeks ago. The physician glances at the parameter and flow sheets, pleased that all is going well. He speaks to the patient and says, "Good morning, Mr. Jones." The patient replies, "Good morning, doctor." The physician now asks the patient how he is doing. To this the patient replies, "Fine." The physician now tells the patient to keep up the good work, and he is off to see another patient. Meanwhile, the patient repeats over and over again, "Good morning, doctor, I'm fine." This is an example of perseveration, a common behavior seen in patients with cognitive deficits.

Perseveration is defined as persistence of one reply or one idea in response to various questions or as continuance of an activity after cessation of the causative stimuli. The nurse working with this patient knows that he is not able to retain new information from minute to minute, is very distractible, is very slow, and has difficulty in putting on his clothes (he buttons the shirt before he puts it on and then can't understand why he is unable to put his arm into the sleeve). It is very apparent that he will have great difficulty managing at home even though he has excellent muscle function.

The nurse should be aware that the common cognitive deficits include problems in attention, concentration, memory, sequencing activities, logical reasoning, and perception and general slowing. She should assess the patient's ability in these areas and document her findings in the patient's record. Her next responsibility is to make the physician aware of the deficits and urge him to follow through on the problem (e.g., cognitive testing to identify the specific areas of deficit, cognitive retraining therapy to begin to rehabilitate the patient).

Cognitive retraining is a new area in patient management. Nurses and physicians alike must be educated about this kind of treatment so that patients can be rehabilitated in all areas, not just motor deficits. The most significant long-term problems with head injuries are cognitive, behavioral, and emotional deficits rather than physical deficits. This is important to remember to ensure the highest quality of life to the patient and his family. See Nursing Diagnoses Frequently Identified for Patients With Cognitive Deficits.

NURSING DIAGNOSES FREQUENTLY IDENTIFIED FOR PATIENTS WITH COGNITIVE DEFICITS

The following nursing diagnoses are frequently identified for the patient with cognitive deficits related to neurological dysfunction:

- Cognitive impairment, actual (specify)
- Comfort, alteration in: pain
- Knowledge deficit (specify)
- Sensory-perceptual alterations: input deficit or sensory deprivation
- Memory deficit, specify type (short- or long-term)
- Thought processes, impaired
- Socialization, alterations in

PUPILLARY OBSERVATIONS

ASSESSMENT

Evaluating the pupils is an extremely important part of patient assessment that provides vital information about central nervous system function or dysfunction. The general points to note when assessing the pupils include their (1) size, (2) shape, and (3) reaction to light. The finding in one pupil is always compared with the finding in the other pupil. Differences between the two pupils should be noted and recorded.

Size

Normally, the pupils are equal in size, measuring about 2 mm to 6 mm in diameter with an average diameter of 3.5 mm. Two methods are commonly used to record pupillary size: the millimeter scale and descriptive terms.

If the millimeter scale is used, the examiner, using a diagrammatic gauge, estimates the size of each pupil by comparing the gauge with the patient's pupils. This assessment is carried out for each pupil. The examiner then records a numerical value from 2 mm to 9 mm to signify the size of each pupil. See Fig. 5-3 for the pupil gauge.

If descriptive terms are used to evaluate the size of the pupils, the following terms are used: pinpoint, small, midposition, large, and dilated (see Chart 5-2).

FIG. 5-3. Pupil gauge in millimeters.

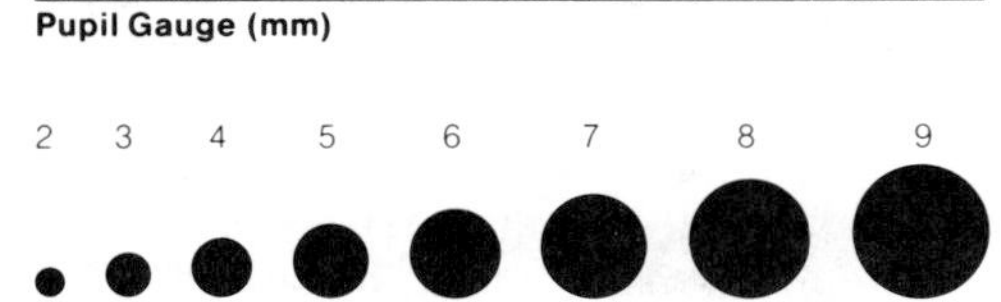

Shape

Normally, both pupils are round. Shape is assessed simply by looking at the contour of the pupils. Abnormal pupil shapes may be described as ovoid, keyhole, or irregular (see Chart 5-3).

Reaction to Light

When light is shone into the eye, the pupil should immediately constrict. Withdrawal of the light should produce an immediate and brisk dilation of the pupil. This is called the *direct light reflex* (Fig. 5-4). Introducing the light into one pupil should cause similar constriction to occur simultaneously in the other pupil. When the light is withdrawn from one eye, the opposite pupil should dilate simultaneously. This response is called the *consensual light reaction*.

Pupillary reaction to light is recorded with descriptive terms or symbols (see Chart 5-4). The descriptive terms that are used include brisk, sluggish, and nonreactive or fixed. Plus and minus signs are recorded if a symbol recording system is used. (Common abnormal pupillary responses and findings are found in Chart 5-5. Refer also to Chapter 3 for more information on pupils).

Accommodation

Accommodation of the pupil from a distant to a nearby point can only be assessed on a conscious cooperative patient. The patient is instructed to focus his eyes on a point such as the examiner's finger that has been positioned about 4 or 5 feet directly in front of the patient. The examiner directs the patient to follow the movement of the finger with his eyes as the examiner rapidly moves his finger within an inch or two of the patient's nose. The examiner should observe pupillary constriction in the patient's eyes as he accommodates from a distant to a nearby point.

The accommodation response is noted once or twice a shift in the conscious cooperative patient.

ABNORMAL PUPILLARY OBSERVATIONS

Nursing Assessment

Assessing the size and shape of the pupils and the direct light reaction are ways of gathering data about the condition of important selected intracranial structures that are known to respond in particular ways owing to brain dysfunction. The nurse must interpret what is observed to decide what action, if any, should be taken. The pupil size and reaction to light are indicative of the patient's condition. As these signs are checked, the following should be asked:

- What do I see?
- What does it mean?
- How does it relate to previous assessments?
- How am I going to proceed?

The third question, How does it relate to previous assess-

(Text continued on page 128.)

CHART 5-2. NURSING ASSESSMENT OF PUPILLARY SIZE

In assessing pupillary size using either descriptive terms or a gauge, each pupil is assessed individually and then the findings for each pupil are *compared.* This is very important because pupils are normally equal (See note on anisocoria).

DESCRIPTIVE TERM	DEFINITION	FINDINGS
Pinpoint 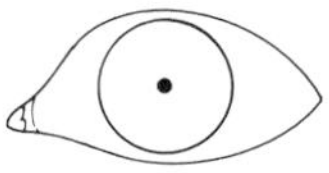	Pupil is so small that it is barely visible or appears as small as a pinpoint	Seen with opiate overdose and pontine hemorrhage
Small 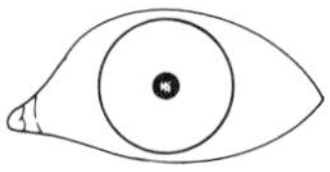	The pupil appears smaller than average but larger than pinpoint	Seen normally if person is in bright room; also seen with miotic ophthalmic drops, opiates, pontine hemorrage, Horner's syndrome, bilateral diencephalic lesions, and metabolic coma
Midposition 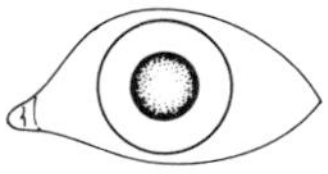	When the pupil and iris are observed, about half of their diameter is iris and half is pupil	Seen normally; if pupils are midposition and nonreactive, midbrain damage is the cause
Large 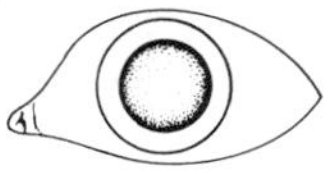	Pupils are larger than average, but there is still an appreciable amount of Iris visible	Seen normally if room is darkened; may be seen with some drugs such as amphetamines, glutethimide (Doriden) overdose, mydriatics, cycloplegic agents, and some orbital injuries
Dilated 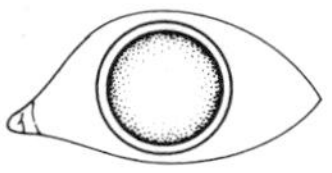	When the pupil and iris are observed, one is struck by the largeness of the pupil with only the slightest ring of iris, which is barely visible	Abnormal finding; bilateral, fixed, and dilated pupils are seen in the terminal stage of severe anoxia–ischemia or at death

Note: Anisocoria is the term used to describe inequality in size between the pupils. About 17% of the population has slight anisocoria without any related pathology. It is therefore important to make a baseline assessment of pupillary size and compare subsequent assessments with the baseline. If pupillary inequality is a new finding, it should be reported. On the other hand, if the patient was admitted with slight pupillary inequality and had no other abnormalities detected on the neurological assessment, the pupil inequality may not be significant.

CHART 5-3. NURSING ASSESSMENT OF PUPILLARY SHAPE

DESCRIPTIVE TERM	DEFINITION	FINDINGS
Round 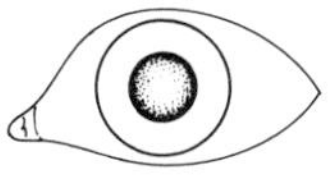	Like a circle	• Normal finding
Ovoid 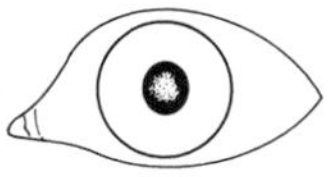	Slightly oval	• Almost always indicates intracranial hypertension and represents an intermediate phase between a normal pupil (round) and a fully dilated fixed pupil; an early sign of transtentorial herniation
Keyhole 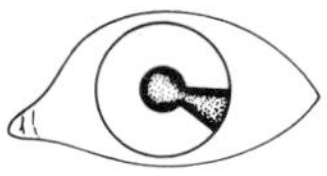	Like a keyhole	• Seen in patients who have had an iridectomy (excision of part of the iris). An iridectomy is often part of cataract surgery, a common procedure in the elderly population. (The reaction to light is very slight.)
Irregular 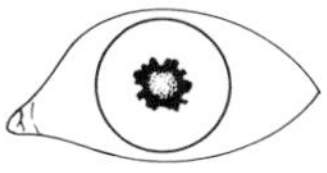	Jagged	• Seen in Argyll–Robertson pupils and with traumatic orbital injuries

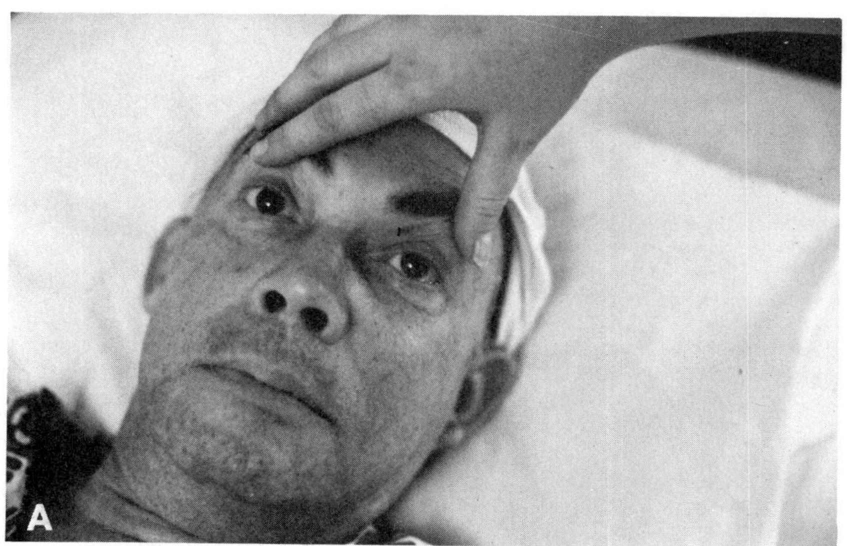

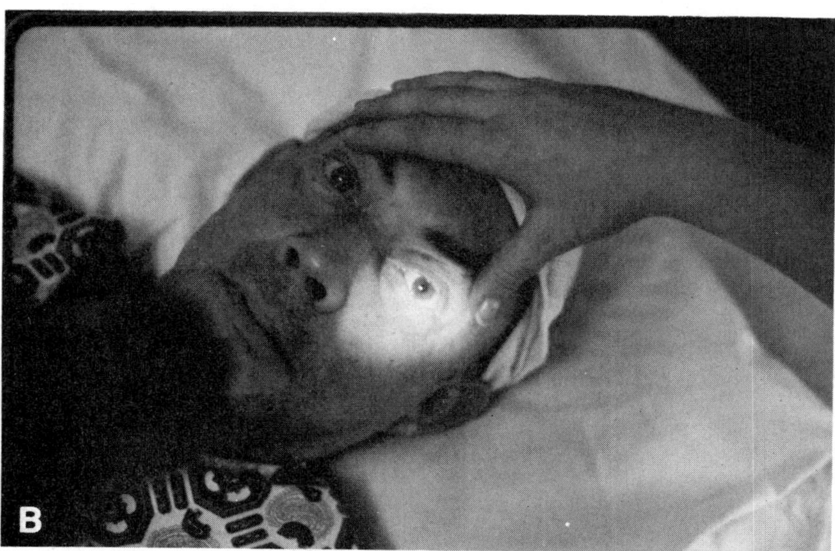

FIG. 5-4. Evaluating pupillary reactions by checking pupil size *(A)* and reaction to light *(B)*.

CHART 5-4. NURSING ASSESSMENT OF PUPILLARY LIGHT RESPONSES

DESCRIPTIVE TERM	SYMBOL	FINDINGS
Brisk	++	Normal finding
Sluggish	+	Found in conditions that cause some compression of the oculomotor (III) nerve; seen in early transtentorial herniation, cerebral edema, and Adie's pupil
Nonreactive or fixed	−	Found in conditions that include compression of the oculomotor nerve; seen with transtentorial herniation syndromes and in severe hypoxia and ischemia (terminal stage just before death)
Swollen closed	c	One or both eyes are tightly closed because of severe edema of the eyelid; the pupillary light reflex could not be assessed

One other response is included, the Hippus phenomenon, which does not usually appear on assessment sheets, but may be observed in the clinical area

Hippus phenomenon	None	With uniform illumination of the pupil, dilation and contraction are noted. This may be considered normal if pupils are observed under high magnification. The Hippus phenomenon is also observed in patients who are beginning to have pressure on the third cranial nerve. This is often associated with early transtentorial herniation.

Note: On some pupillary assessment sheets, symbols are used rather than descriptive terms.

CHART 5-5. COMMON ABNORMAL PUPILLARY RESPONSES

Oculomotor Nerve Compression

Observation

One pupil (R) is larger than the other (L), which is of normal size. The dilated pupil (R) does not react to light, although the (L) pupil reacts normally.

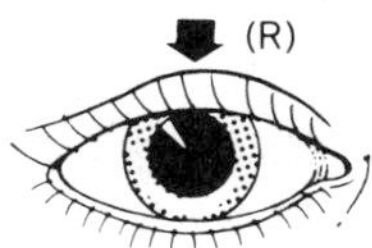

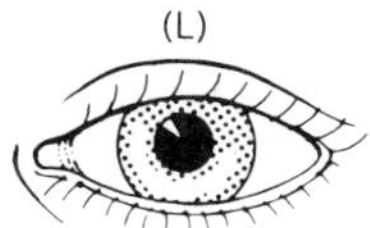

Meaning

The dilated, unreactive (fixed) pupil indicates that the controls for pupillary constriction are not functioning. The parasympathetic fibers of the oculomotor nerve control pupillary constriction. The most common cause of interruption of this function is compression of the oculomotor nerve usually against the tentorium or posterior cerebral artery.

The compression of the oculomotor nerve against these structures is caused by a lesion such as a hematoma, tumor, or cerebral edema on the same side of the brain as the dilated pupil. This causes downward pressure so that the uncus of the temporal lobe herniates, trapping the oculomotor nerve between it and the tentorium.

Action

The nurse will need to check previous assessments to determine what the pupil size and reaction to light have been. If the dilated pupil is a new finding, it should immediately be reported to the physician because the process of rostral–caudal downward pressure must be treated without delay. It would be expected that changes would also be apparent in the level of consciousness, motor function, and other areas of the neurological assessment.

Bilateral Diencephalic Damage

Observation

Upon examination, the pupils appear small but equal in size, and both react briskly to direct light, contracting when light is introduced and dilating when light is withdrawn.

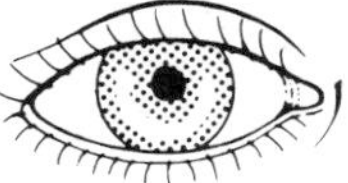

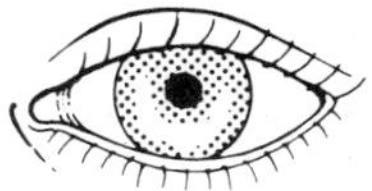

Meaning

The sympathetic pathway that begins in the hypothalamus is affected. Since both pupils are equal in size and respond equally to light, the damage is bilateral. Therefore, the pupils are indicating that there is bilateral injury in the diencephalon (thalamus and hypothalamus).

Since metabolic coma can also result in bilaterally small pupils that react to light, the possibility of metabolic coma must be ruled out.

Action

These findings should be compared to previous assessments to determine whether this is a new development. The possibility of metabolic coma should be considered by reviewing blood electrolyte and blood sugar levels. For example, diabetic acidosis may result in a metabolic coma because of an excessive amount of glucose in the blood. The abnormal glucose level would be evident by checking the blood glucose level.

Reviewing blood chemistry is particularly important if the patient was a recent emergency admission, which indicates that an adequate history was not collected. If the small, reactive pupils are a new finding, this information should be reported.

Horner's Syndrome

Observation

One pupil (L) is smaller than the other (R), although both pupils react to light. The eyelid on the same side as the small pupil droops (ptosis). There may be deficiency of sweat (anhidrosis) on the same side of the face as the ptosis. The symptoms of a small reactive pupil, ptosis, and anhidrosis are called *Horner's syndrome.*

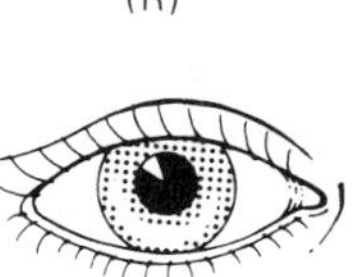

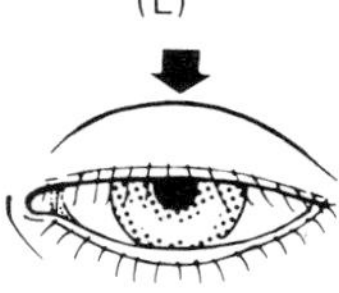

(continued)

CHART 5–5. (continued)

Meaning

There is an interruption of the ipsilateral sympathetic innervation to the pupil that can be caused by hypothalamic damage (posterior or ventrolateral portion), lesion of the lateral medulla, lesion of the ventrolateral cervical spinal cord, and sometimes occlusion of the internal carotid artery. Downward displacement of the hypothalamus along with a unilateral Horner's syndrome may be an early sign of transtentorial herniation.

Action

If this is a new finding, it should be reported.

Midbrain Damage

Observation

Both pupils are at midposition and are nonreactive to light.

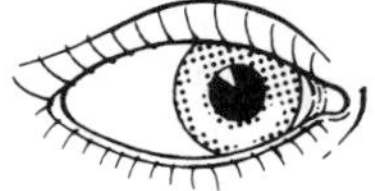
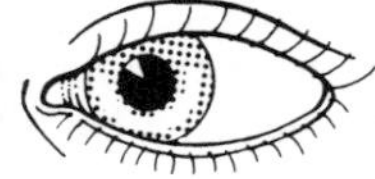

Meaning

Because the pupils are midposition in size and are nonreactive, there is indication that neither the sympathetic nor parasympathetic innervation is operational. This finding is often associated with midbrain infarction or transtentorial herniation.

Action

Evaluate the pupils in conjunction with other neurological assessments. Report the change in pupil size and reaction if this is a new finding.

Pontine Damage

Observation

Very small (pinpoint), nonreactive pupils are seen.

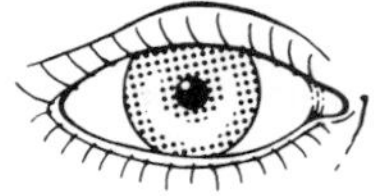
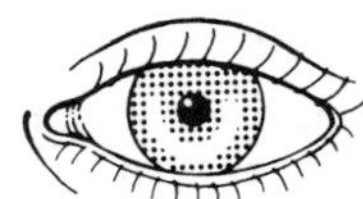

Meaning

Most often this finding indicates hemorrhage into the pons, a very grave occurrence since the pons controls many motor pathways and vital functions. Bilateral pinpoint pupils are also found with opiate drug overdose, so this possibility should be ruled out.

Action

Report this finding if it is new. The prognosis is grave with pontine damage. Other changes in the neurological assessment, such as a decreased level of consciousness and respiratory abnormalities, would also be expected.

Dilated Unreactive Pupils

Observation

Both pupils are dilated and nonreactive (fixed).

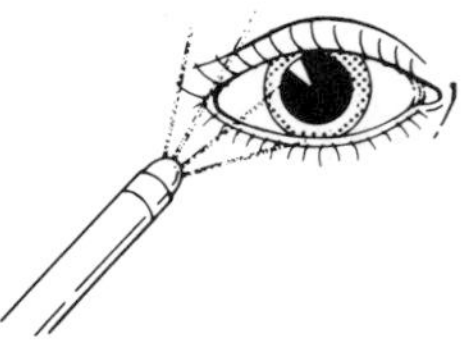
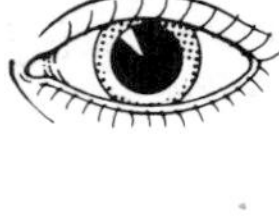

Meaning

This finding is found in the terminal stages of severe anoxia, ischemia, and death. Since atropinelike drugs will cause dilated pupils, this possibility must be ruled out. In addition, an intact ciliospinal reflex can produce momentary bilateral dilation.

Action

Emergency action is necessary to reverse the anoxic state to prevent death. Oxygen therapy at high concentrations and a patent airway must be ensured to provide oxygen for the ischemic cerebral cells.

ments?, is important because data are compared with the previous baseline assessments to denote change. The assessment can reveal no change, subtle change, or dramatic change from previous findings. Generally, a change of any kind is important to note because it is indicative of an intracranial change.

Any change in a particular finding of the neurological assessment must be considered in conjunction with changes in other areas evaluated in the assessment. A rapidly developing hematoma or cerebral edema would affect other aspects of the assessment such as the level of consciousness and motor and sensory function. On the other hand, if the pupil appears dilated and fixed (a new finding from the last assessment) and the patient continues to be well oriented and maintains motor and sensory function, then the pupillary signs should be rechecked. See Nursing Diagnoses Frequently Made for Patients With Pupillary Dysfunction.

NURSING DIAGNOSES FREQUENTLY MADE FOR PATIENTS WITH PUPILLARY DYSFUNCTION

The following nursing diagnoses are frequently made for the patient with pupillary deficits caused by neurological dysfunction:

- Sensory deficit (visual)
- Sensory–perceptual alterations: input deficit or sensory deprivation
- Physical injury, potential of

OCULAR MOVEMENT

Ocular movement and the position of the eyeballs are assessed. In the normal healthy person one would expect to observe the following:

- The eyes move conjugately in the orbital sockets
- The eyes blink periodically
- No nystagmus or abnormal eye movement is noted
- The eyeball neither protrudes nor is sunken in the orbits
- The upper eyelid does not droop and the palpebral fissures in both eyes are equal

This are the established normal criteria that will guide the assessment of ocular movement in the patient.

ASSESSMENT OF THE CONSCIOUS COOPERATIVE PATIENT

Position of the Eyeballs

The position of the eyeballs is assessed by observing the eyeballs from a frontal and lateral view (observe the patient's profile) as well as by looking downward from above the patient's head. The position of each eyeball is noted and then the two are compared.

- Abnormal protrusion of one or both eyeballs is termed *proptosis* or *exophthalmos.*
- Abnormal recession of one or both eyeballs is termed *enophthalmos.*

Position of the Upper Eyelids

Ask the patient to look straight ahead and note the width of the palpebral fissure in each eye and compare them. The palpebral fissure is the space between the upper and lower eyelid, extending from the outer to the inner canthus. Next, assess the position of the eyelid in relation to the pupil and iris in each eye and compare. Normally, the lid slightly covers the outer margin of the iris.

- A narrowed palpebral fissure usually indicates a droopy eyelid, which is also known as *ptosis.* Ptosis is seen in Horner's syndrome and conditions that affect the oculomotor nerve (e.g., transtentorial herniation syndromes, myasthenia gravis if the ocular muscles are involved).

Edema of the Eyelids

Note the presence of edema of the eyelids. Edema can result from trauma to the orbit and may occur in the upper, the lower, or both eyelids.

Movement of the Eyeballs

Extraocular movement is assessed by asking the patient to follow a pencil or the examiner's finger through the six cardinal movements of vision with the eyes (see Chart 5–6, *A*). Note the specific movement(s) that the patient cannot complete and record this finding.

- A lack of parallelism between the two visual axes or movement in opposite directions is called *dysconjugate movement.*

See Nursing Diagnoses Frequently Made for Patients with Pupillary Dysfunction.

- If the dysfunction is limited to a specific movement or movements, an ophthalmoplegia is present. *Ophthalmoplegia* is defined as paralysis of one or more eye muscles (see Chapter 3, Table 3–4, for a summary of common ophthalmoplegias).

Ask the patient if he is experiencing double vision (diplopia) when he focuses in a particular direction. If the patient with ophthalmoplegia moves the eyeball in a certain direction, visual images will fall on the retina in different locations rather than in the same location on each retina. This lack of parallelism can cause double vision when the patient focuses in a particular direction.

Abnormal Movements

When the patient focused straight ahead and then followed the examiner's finger through the six cardinal eye movements, were any abnormal eye movements noted? *Nystagmus* is defined as involuntary movement of an eye, which may be horizontal, vertical, rotary, or mixed in direction. The tempo of the movements can be regular, rhythmical, pendular, or jerky, with the movement having a fast and slow component. Nystagmus can result from several different problems. If nystagmus is present, the nurse should document the characteristics of the movement and include any information on precipitating circumstances that seem to cause the nystagmus (e.g., focusing the eye in a certain direction). Specific types of nystagmus are discussed in Chapter 3.

Periodic Blinking

As mentioned earlier, periodic blinking is normally expected. The nurse should assess blinking by observing the patient. In some conditions, such as Parkinson's disease, blinking is decreased.

CHART 5–6. NURSING ASSESSMENT OF EYE MOVEMENT

A. Conscious Patient

Assessment Technique

If the patient can follow instructions, ask him to follow your finger (or a pencil) through the six cardinal positions of ocular mobility (upward, downward, inward medially, upward and outward, downward and outward, and outward).

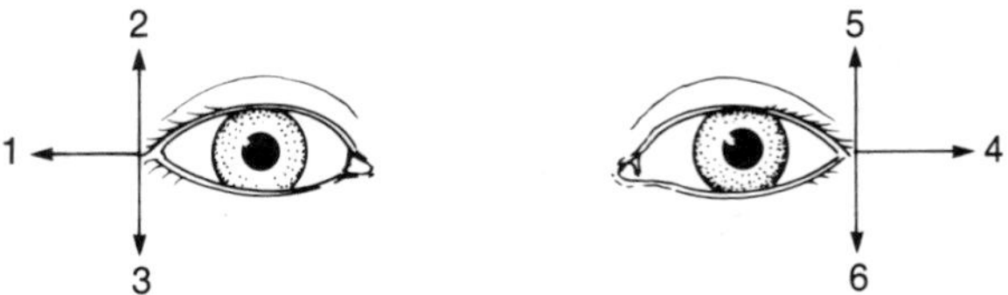

Findings

Normally the eyes move conjugately in the orbital sockets with periodic blinking. No nystagmus or abnormal eye movement should be apparent.

B. Unconscious Patient

In the comatose patient, eye movement is generally absent (the eyes assume a prolonged stare) or the eyes move slowly from side to side. Eye movement in the unconscious patient can be assessed by means of the oculocephalic response (doll's eye phenomenon). *Contraindication:* Presence or suspicion of a cervical fracture or dislocation

Assessment Technique

1. Briskly rotate the head from side to side, or
2. Briskly flex and extend the neck

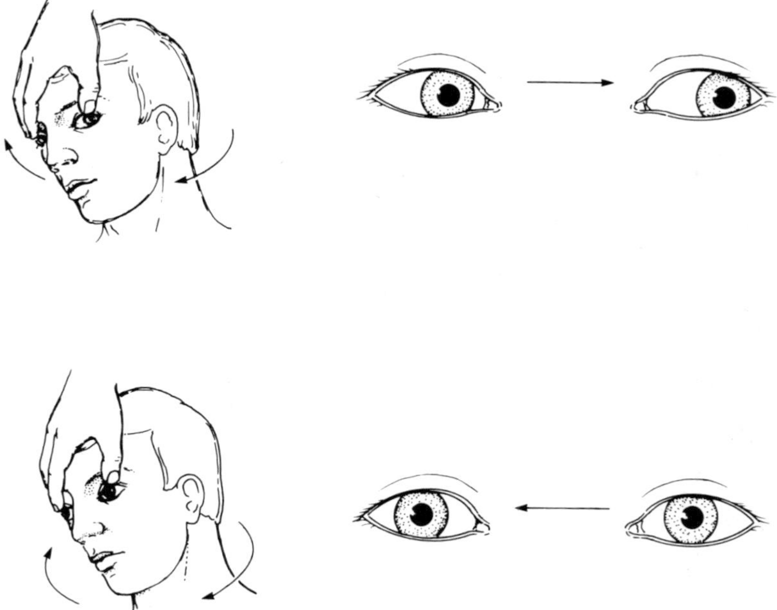

Findings

1. When the head is rotated, the eyes should move in the direction opposite to the head movement. (If the head is rotated to the left, the eyes appear to move to the right.)
2. When the neck is flexed, the eyes appear to look upward; when the neck is extended, the eyes look downward.
3. When the doll's eye reflex is absent, the eyes do not move in the sockets and thus follow the direction of passive rotation.

Loss of the oculocephalic reflex in the comatose patient indicates a severe lesion at the pontine–midbrain level of the brain stem. *Note:* To determine whether the oculocephalic reflex is intact, the oculovestibular reflex (cold calorics) can be tested (see chapter 3).

ASSESSMENT OF THE COMATOSE PATIENT

General Observations

The comatose patient usually appears to be in a sleeplike state, with or without his eyes being closed. If the eyes are closed, the eyelids can be gently raised to inspect the position and movement of the eyes. The eyes may assume a prolonged stare without any movement being discernible, or they may move slowly from side to side. Absence of any movement usually indicates that the eye movement center in the brain stem is not functioning. This is a poor prognostic sign. Conversely, slow movement from side to side usually indicates an intact brain stem.

The Eyelids

After the eyes are inspected, the eyelids are released. Notice whether the lids slowly cover the eyes. This point is noteworthy when a hysterical patient is examined. In true coma, the eyelids close gradually once they are released, but in the hysterical patient, the eyes will close quickly.

Eye Movement

Because the patient is not conscious and cooperative, eye movement cannot be assessed. However, to determine whether the brain stem center for eye movement is intact, the oculocephalic response can be assessed (see Chart 5–6, *B*). If the oculocephalic response is inconclusive, the oculovestibular reflex (cold calorics) can be assessed by the physician. This is a more sensitive test of brain stem function.

Frequency of Assessing Ocular Movement

Ocular movement parameters do not change as rapidly as other portions of the neurological assessment. The nurse should assess ocular movements once during a shift and more often if indicated. See Nursing Diagnoses Frequently Made for Patients With Ocular Deficits.

NURSING DIAGNOSES FREQUENTLY MADE FOR PATIENTS WITH OCULAR MOVEMENT DEFICITS

The following nursing diagnoses are frequently made for the patient with ocular movement dysfunction caused by neurological dysfunction:

- Body image disturbance, potential of
- Sensory deficit (visual)
- Physical injury, potential of

MOTOR FUNCTION

ASSESSMENT

The motor examination is conducted in an orderly fashion, beginning with the neck, and proceeding to the upper extremities, trunk, and finally, the lower extremities (see Chapter 3 and Figs. 3–8, 3–9, and 3–10). Some cranial nerves have motor components. These motor functions can be assessed as part of the complete assessment of the cranial nerves, or the examiner may choose to assess these components with motor function assessment (see Chapter 3 for assessment techniques).

The purposes of the neurological assessment are different from those of the neurological physical examination, which includes a detailed examination of the motor system. The neurological assessment provides a baseline from which to denote change. When the nurse assesses motor function as part of the ongoing neurological assessment, she is looking for significant changes from the established baseline. Motor function examination in the neurological assessment usually focuses on the arms and legs. The identification of significant changes is important for denoting deterioration, improvement, or stabilization in condition. Changes in function are also helpful for the nurse to note when assessing a patient's independence in activities of daily living. Deficits in motor function might indicate the need for adaptation of activities to meet the patient's individual needs.

The techniques used to evaluate motor function depend on the patient's level of consciousness. In the conscious and alert patient, the assessment can be conducted by observing responses to directions and questioning the patient. In an unconscious patient or one who is not able to provide accurate responses to questions, the nurse must rely on neurological testing and observation skills as a source of information.

The basic approach to assessment of motor function is included in Chart 5–7. A few additional points will help to guide the assessment process. In assessing motor function consider (1) muscle size, (2) muscle tone, (3) muscle strength, (4) presence of involuntary movement, and (5) posture and gait. When one muscle or muscle group is assessed, it is always compared with the same muscle or group on the opposite side of the body. Normally, function should be about the same on both sides of the body.

Muscle Size

Observe the muscle or muscles. A tape measure may be used if a difference in size seems to exist.

Muscle Tone

Palpate the muscle at rest and then during passive movement. Common abnormal findings follow:

- *Spasticity* is the undue resistance of the muscle to passive lengthening caused by upper motor neuron disease. In examining the patient, there is increased resistance to passive movement followed by sudden or gradual release of resistance.
- *Flaccidity* is decreased muscle tone caused by lower motor neuron disease; it is also evident early in spinal cord injuries.
- *Rigidity* is a constant state of resistance because of involvement of the extrapyramidal system.
- Decortication and decerebration are special states of rigidity that require more detailed explanation.

CHART 5-7. NURSING ASSESSMENT OF MOTOR FUNCTION

Motor Function: Conscious Patient

Assessment

- Ask patient to move his arms and legs, checking to see if movement is symmetrical or if there are any signs of unilateral paresis or paralysis.
- Check the facial muscles by asking the patient to smile and wrinkle his brow.
- Test muscle strength and the patient's ability to follow commands by extending the index and middle fingers of both of your hands and asking the patient to squeeze (Fig. 5-5). Note the patient's grasp, the strength of the squeeze, and how the grasp of one hand compares with the other. (The grasp should be strong, firm, and equal.)
- To test muscle strength in another way, ask the patient to extend his arms with palms upward and eyes closed. A weak arm will drift downward and pronate.
- Assess posture by observing the patient as he lies in bed and also as he stands if he is able to bear weight.
- If the patient is able to ambulate, assess the patient's gait (see Chapter 3, Chart 3-2).

Motor Function: Comatose Patient

Assessment

- Apply painful stimulus and note if patient withdraws the stimulated part. (If withdrawal does not occur, more specific neurological testing should be carried out.)
- Evaluate the presence of paralysis of the arms by lifting both arms and releasing them simultaneously. (If the descent of one arm is more rapid and flaillike, it indicates paralysis or paresis of that limb.)
- To evaluate motor function of the legs, flex the patient's legs so that both heels are on the bed. When the legs are released, the normal limb will hold the present position for a few moments and then gradually return to the position assumed before testing. The weak or paralyzed limb slumps to a position of extension with outward hip rotation.
- To test the facial muscles, apply firm pressure over the eyeballs or supraorbital notches. Note the muscle reaction of the face to see if both sides respond when the patient grimaces or moves. If one side of the face does not react, paralysis of the facial muscles is present.
- Gross abnormalities of motor function may be detected by observing the patient's body for the manner in which his arms and legs are positioned on the left and right sides. Flaccidity, or the loss of muscle tone, contractures, and spasticity, as well as abnormal posturing of decorticate or decerebrate position, may be noted and require further evaluation.

Decortication and Decerebration. Noxious stimuli can initiate rigidity and abnormal posture if the motor tracts are interrupted at specific cerebral levels. These abnormal postures are called decortication and decerebration. In some instances, either posture may be apparent without the application of noxious stimuli.

- Decortication and decerebration are indicative of cerebral damage at a certain level as well as a change in the patient's condition. The particular posture or stereotypic movement assumed by the patient differs depending on the anatomical level of injury.

Decortication is characterized by flexion of the arms, wrists, and fingers, with adduction in the upper extremities and extension, internal rotation, and plantar flexion of the lower extremities (Fig. 5-6, *A*). Simply stated, decortication is hyperflexion of the upper extremities and hyperextension of the lower extremities.

Lesions of the cerebral hemispheres or internal capsule cause decorticate posturing by interrupting the corticospinal pathways.

Decerebration, when fully developed, includes opisthotonus (tetanic spasms that arch the back with backward flexion of the head and feet), adduction and hyperpronated arms, and stiffly extended legs with plantar flexion of the feet (Fig. 5-6, *B*). Stated simply, decerebration is hyperextension of both upper and lower extremities.

This response results from rostral-to-caudal deterioration, which can occur when a diencephalic lesion of the hemisphere extends, thereby causing midbrain or upper pontine damage. (Both the midbrain and pons are brain stem structures.)

Intermittent decortication or decerebration may be observed in the patient because of variations in the blood supply to the involved cerebral area, if the line of demarcation between the deep cerebral hemispheric structures and upper brain stem tissue is obscure. The variations in posturing can be complete or partial. The patient can change from bilateral decerebration to decortication (or vice versa) or from unilateral decerebration to unilateral decortication (or vice versa), or one side can be decorticate while the other side of the body is decerebrate.

Nursing Implication. Of the two abnormal postures, decerebration is considered a sign of greater cerebral dysfunction than decortication. Presence of either position should be reported at once. Also, a change from decorticate to decerebrate posture must be reported immediately because this is an ominous sign of extension of the lesion into the upper brain stem.

Muscle Strength

Muscle strength is assessed by testing active, passive, and active resistive movements. The various techniques for assessing these functions in the upper and lower extremities of the conscious and comatose patient are included in Chart 5-7.

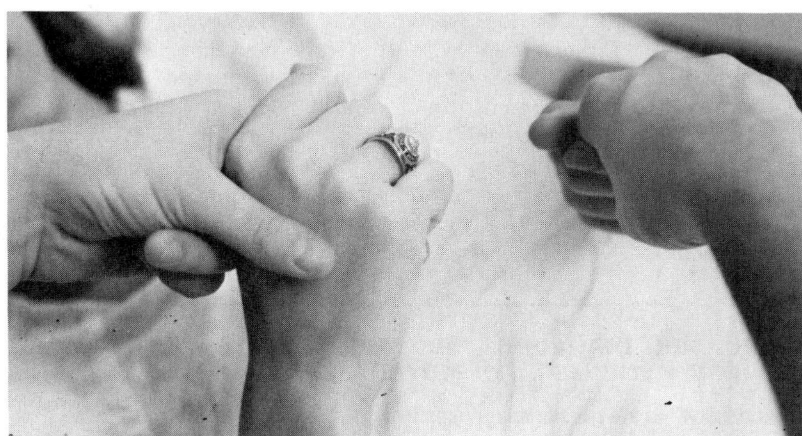

FIG. 5-5. Testing motor strength by noting patient's ability to squeeze nurse's hands.

Involuntary Movement

The presence of involuntary movement such as tremors, choreiform movements, myoclonus, athetosis, tics, spasms, or ballism is noted (see Chapter 3, Chart 3-6 for information on involuntary movement).

Posture and Gait

Posture is defined as the attitude of the body. First, observe the patient's posture while he lies in bed. Next, if the patient is able to bear weight, the nurse should observe the patient's posture while he is standing still and then while

FIG. 5-6. *(A)* Decorticate rigidity. In decorticate rigidity the upper arms are held tightly to the sides, with elbows, wrists, and fingers flexed. The legs are extended and internally rotated. The feet are plantar flexed. This posture implies a destructive lesion of the corticospinal tracts within or very near the cerebral hemispheres. When rigidity is unilateral, this is the posture of chronic spastic hemiplegia. *(B)* Decerebrate rigidity. In decerebrate rigidity the jaws are clenched and the neck extended. The arms are adducted and stiffly extended at the elbows, with forearms pronated, wrists and fingers flexed. The legs are stiffly extended at the knees, with the feet plantar flexed. This posture may occur spontaneously or only in response to external stimuli such as light, noise, or pain. It is caused by a lesion in the diencephalon, midbrain, or pons, although severe metabolic disorders such as hypoxia or hypoglycemia may also produce it. (Bates B: Guide to Physical Examination, 3rd ed. Philadelphia, JB Lippincott, 1983)

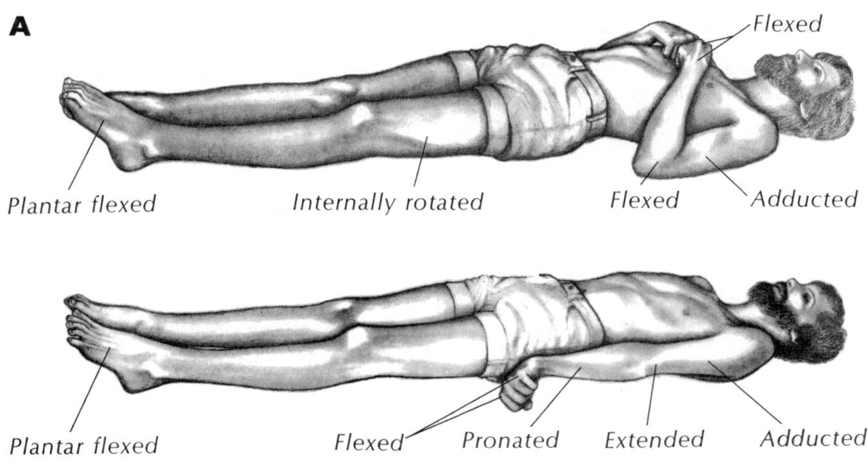

he is walking. *Gait* refers to the manner of progression in walking. Observe the patient while he walks and note these characteristics: whether he is erect or stooped or leans toward one side; the posture of his arms in relationship to his body; how much and what kind of movement is seen in the lower extremities). A description of common gait abnormalities appears in Chapter 3, Chart 3–3. See Nursing Diagnoses Frequently Made for Patients With Motor Deficits.

NURSING DIAGNOSES FREQUENTLY MADE FOR PATIENTS WITH MOTOR DEFICITS

The following are nursing diagnoses frequently made in patients with motor deficits caused by neurological dysfunction:

- Physical injury, potential of
- Decubitus ulcer, potential of
- Skin integrity, potential of impairment
- Activity tolerance, decreased
- Diversional activity deficit
- Home maintenance management, impaired
- Mobility, impaired physical
- Joint contractures, potential
- Self-care deficit, total or specific depending on the level of deficit by the patient
- Body image disturbance
- Depression, reactive to mobility deficit
- Fear

SENSORY FUNCTION

ASSESSMENT

A detailed sensory examination of all sensory modalities was included in the neurological physical examination. In the neurological assessment, the sensory portion of the assessment focuses on the patient's responsiveness to light touch and painful stimuli. The specific assessment parameters are often adapted to meet the needs of the particular patient. For example, if the nurse is assessing the sensory level of a patient with a spinal cord injury, greater emphasis would be placed on a detailed sensory assessment. In the case of a patient with a head injury, it probably would not be necessary to include as much detail.

The techniques used in assessing the patient will depend on the patient's level of consciousness. The basic assessment approaches for both the conscious and comatose patient are included in Chart 5–8.

CHART 5–8. NURSING ASSESSMENT OF SENSORY FUNCTION

Sensory Function: Conscious Patient

In the conscious and alert patient, sensory stimuli are provided with a cotton-tipped applicator or pin and tactile stimulation from the examiner.

Assessment Technique

1. Ask the patient to close his eyes.
2. The same areas on opposite sides of the body are assessed and compared.
3. Brush the patient's skin with the cotton applicator or lightly prick the skin with the pin (Fig. 5–7 *A*).
4. Compare the response on one side of the body with that on the other.

Sensory Function: Comatose, But Not Deeply

Apply a noxious stimulus in one of several ways:

- Pinch the patient's skin.
- Firmly grasp a muscle of tendon.
- Press on a bony prominence (Fig. 5–7, *B*).
- Use a sharp instrument such as a pin or wooden end of an applicator.

Findings for Both the Conscious and Comatose Patient

If the sensory innervation is functional, the patient should demonstrate a facial response such as wincing or grimacing. If the motor function is also intact, the patient might withdraw the body part stimulated.

Both sides of the body should be evaluated for sensory as well as motor function, because unilateral functional loss is a problem commonly observed in neurological patients.

Frequency of Assessment

The nurse should assess sensory function once per shift or more often if necessary. Examples of situations that would probably require more frequent assessment of sensory function include acute spinal cord injury, acute transverse myelitis, and Guillain–Barré syndrome. The sensory function can often be assessed during the administration of basic care to the patient. See Nursing Diagnoses Frequently Made for Patients With Sensory Deficits.

NURSING DIAGNOSES FREQUENTLY MADE FOR PATIENTS WITH SENSORY DEFICITS

The following are frequently made nursing diagnoses for the patient with sensory deficits caused by neurological impairment:

- Sensory–perceptual alterations: input deficit or sensory deprivation
- Physical injury, potential of
- Home maintenance management, impaired

VITAL SIGNS

The vital signs provide qualitative and quantitative data concerning vital functions of the body. (For nursing assessment measures see Chart 5–9.) The frequency with which

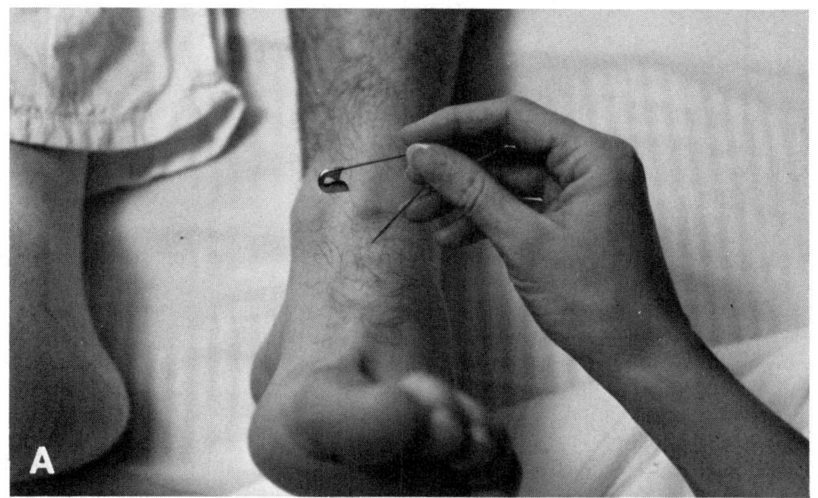

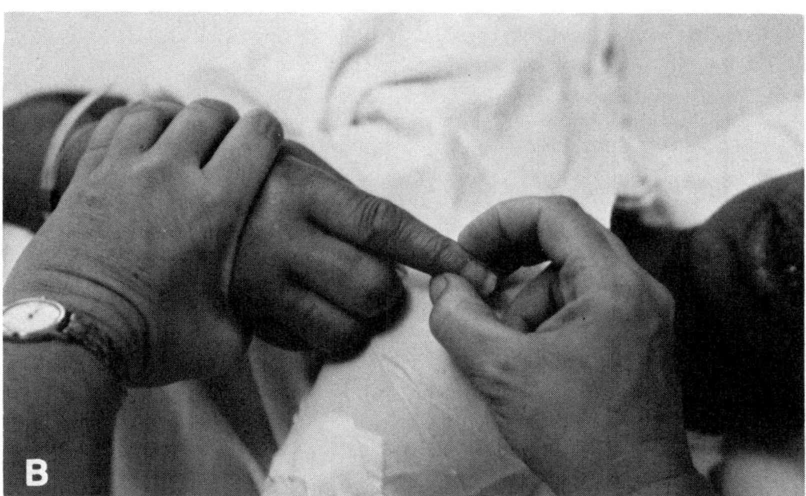

FIG. 5-7. Assessing sensory function by applying pinprick *(A)* and pressing on finger *(B)*.

vital signs are recorded will depend on the stability of the patient's condition. In an acute trauma victim or early post-operative patient, vital signs may be ordered every 15 minutes. Once the patient is stable, the order may be changed to hourly, or longer, intervals.

In a conscious patient verbal cues of subjective symptoms may be elicited to help to evaluate the patient's condition so that a correlation of symptoms with the characteristics and readings of vital functions can be made. In the comatose patient the nurse must rely on observations and evaluation of the vital signs as indicators of changes in the patient's condition. Vital signs are not only considered individually, but also in relationship to each other. However, there are limitations; the nurse should not rely too heavily on vital signs as an early index of neurological deterioration.

RELATIONSHIP OF VITAL SIGNS TO INCREASED INTRACRANIAL PRESSURE

There is some confusion in the literature about the relationship of changes in vital signs and increased intracranial pressure. A few terms should be defined for clarification:

- *Cushing's response or reflex (also called Kocher–Cushing response)* results from pressure in the cerebrospinal fluid increasing to the level of the arterial blood pressure. When the pressure within the cerebrospinal fluid and the arterial pressure are equal, the arteries within the intracranial space become compressed, thus compromising the blood supply to the brain. As a result, a special type of central nervous system ischemic response (Cushing's response) is initiated, thereby causing the arterial pressure to rise slightly above the cerebrospinal fluid pressure so that the arterial blood supply continues to flow. The clinical signs that may be observed in this process include a rising systolic pressure, a widening pulse pressure, and bradycardia.[7]
- *Cushing's triad (also called Kocher–Cushing triad)* refers to three signs/symptoms—bradycardia, hypertension, and bradypnea—that are often irregular. These findings are due to beginning pressure on the medullary centers of the brain as a result of intracranial hypertension and rostral–caudal herniation. In examining these conditions, Cushing's triad appears to be the further development of Cushing's response when intracranial pressure continues to rise unchecked.

For many years nursing literature emphasized the close correlation between increased intracranial pressure and Cushing's response and the triad. It is now established that although there may be a correlation in some instances,

CHART 5-9. NURSING ASSESSMENT OF VITAL SIGNS

Respiratory Function

Nursing Assessment

Respirations may be assessed as follows:

- Record the rate, depth, and rhythm of the respirations.
- Observe for the presence of cyanosis or pallor in the perioral area, the ear lobes, or nail beds.
- Notice the movement of the chest in the respiratory cycle to see if the entire chest is involved in respirations.
- Observe the abdominal movements during inspiration and expiration for excessive motion, which would denote abdominal breathing. (This would indicate possible respiratory obstruction or paralysis of respiratory muscles.)
- Listen (with the ear) to detect gross abnormalities of the respiratory system such as wheezing or partial obstruction of the airway with mucus.
- Auscultate the chest with a stethoscope to evaluate complete lung expansion and the presence of any mucus in the respiratory tract.
- Draw blood gases periodically in the comatose patient or the patient with respiratory dysfunction.
- Check pulmonary vital capacity periodically.

Nursing Implementation/Responsibilities

Maintenance of Patent Airway

Conscious Patient:
Encourage coughing and deep breathing every hour; perform chest percussion, as needed

Unconscious Patient or Patient at Risk:
Suction periodically

- Follow strict aseptic technique. Use disposable catheters each time the patient is suctioned.
- Check suction equipment at the beginning of each shift.
- Keep equipment ready for emergency use.
- Never suction nasally if there is a possible basal skull fracture or if there are signs of cerebrospinal fluid drainage from the nose.
- Limit suctioning to 15 seconds to prevent hypoxia or hypercapnia.
- Prior to and following suctioning, hyperaerate patient with 100% oxygen *with approval of physician.*

Positioning

- Place patient in lateral recumbent position to allow for the drainage of mucus and to prevent the tongue from slipping back and obstructing the airway. Keep the neck in neutral position.
- Turn the patient from side to side every 2 hours.
- Make sure that the patient is positioned properly in the bed. If he is too close to the foot of the bed and the head of the bed is elevated, he will not achieve optimal lung expansion.

Expansion of the lungs

- Ambu the patient every 1 to 2 hours to prevent atelectasis.
- Administer chest percussion as necessary. This helps the lungs to expand and stimulates the patient to take deeper respirations.

Tracheostomy care

- Administer every 4 hours.
- Remove inner cannula, soak it in solution, and clean it with a tracheostomy brush or pipe cleaners to remove exudate.
- Rinse inner cannula in normal saline, shake cannula to remove excess liquid, and reinsert.
- Remove sterile dressing and clean the skin with sterile cotton-tipped applicator and sterile saline.
- Replace with new, dry sterile tracheostomy dressing around tracheostomy tube and surgical site.

Observe for pulmonary complications

- Observe the patient for the development of pulmonary insufficiency and pulmonary complications such as atelectasis, pneumonia, mechanical insufficiency, adult respiratory distress syndrome, and neurogenic pulmonary edema.

CHART 5–9. (continued)

Pulse

Nursing Assessment

- Note and record the rate, rhythm, and quality of the pulse (full, bounding, thready, and so forth).
- Record whether the pulse has been derived apically or radically.
- If the patient is receiving any medications, consider whether the drug has had any effect on the pulse rate.
- Report any evidence of tachycardia, bradycardia, and other cardiac arrhythmias:
  - Tachycardia indicates
    - Hypoxia/hypoxemia
    - Terminal stage of disease
    - Possible internal bleeding
  - Bradycardia indicates
    - Later stages of increased intracranial pressure
    - Early stage after acute spinal cord injury

Blood Pressure

Nursing Assessment

- Record the blood pressure on a flow sheet.
- Indicate which arm was used to measure the pressure.
- Compare the current findings with previous findings to identify any trends or changes.

Elevated pressure: Late sign of advancing increased intracranial pressure
Low pressure: Inadequate cerebral profusion, general neurological deterioration; terminal stages

Temperature

Subnormal

- Spinal shock
- Metabolic or toxic coma
- Drug overdose
- Destructive brain stem or hypothalamic lesion
- Terminal stage of some neurological diseases

Management

- Hyperthermia blanket
- Extra blankets (preferrably ones that have been warmed)

Elevated

- Central nervous system infection
- Subarachnoid hemorrhage
- Lesion of hypothalamus
- Petechial hemorrhage of hypothalamus or brain stem
- Traction on the hypothalamus or brain stem
- Bacterial endocarditis
- Pneumonia, and so forth

Management

- Aspirin or acetaminophen (Tylenol) suppositories
- Alcohol sponge baths
- Hypothermia blanket
- Special attention to fluid balance, urinary output, skin breakdown

Nursing Assessment

- If a tracheostomy or Levin tube is in place, or if the patient is receiving oxygen, take his temperature using the rectal route.
- Use the rectal route in an unconscious patient.
- Stay with the patient while the thermometer is in place.
- Record the temperature, including route, on a flow sheet.
- Indicate whether a continuous monitoring device is being used.

Cushing's response and the triad are *late* clinical findings, which may not develop at all with certain kinds of lesions such as certain ones located in the supratentorial area. Therefore, the nurse is cautioned *not to wait* for Cushing's response or triad to develop before taking action to control increasing intracranial pressure, or it may be *too late* to prevent irreversible neurological damage or even death.

RESPIRATORY FUNCTION

Many studies indicate that of the data collected when monitoring vital signs, perhaps the most valuable information is that of the respiratory pattern, because it provides *early* information about malfunction in a specific area of the brain. The respiratory pattern can be correlated with the

CHART 5-10. TYPES OF ABNORMAL RESPIRATORY PATTERNS

Cheyne-Stokes Respirations (CSR)

Description

There is a rhythmic waxing and waning in the depth of the respiration followed by apnea. The abnormal respiratory pattern is due to two factors: (1) increased sensitivity to carbon dioxide, which results in the abnormal increase in the depth and rate of respirations; and (2) decreased stimulation from the cerebral hemispheres resulting in the apneic phase.

Level of Lesion

Lesions are most often located deep in the cerebral hemispheres and basal ganglia, with damage to the internal capsule or bilateral damage to the diencephalon (thalamus and/or hypothalamus).

Possible causative lesions include

- Bilateral cerebral infarction
- Encephalopathy caused by hypertension
- Metabolic diseases (*e.g.,* uremia, diabetic coma)

Central Neurogenic Hyperventilation (CNH)

Description

There are continual, rapid, regular respirations with somewhat of an increase in depth of the respiration; the rate is 24 or more per minute. This respiratory pattern cannot be attributed to neurogenic origin unless arterial blood oxygen is 70 mm Hg to 80 mm Hg or greater for 24 hours.

Level of Lesion

The lesion destroys part of the reticular formation located in front of the fourth ventricle in the lower midbrain to the middle of the pons.

Possible causative lesions include

- Midbrain or pontine infarction
- Anoxia
- Ischemia and/or decrease in glucose to midbrain/pontine region
- Tumors of midbrain region

Apneustic Breathing

Description

There is prolonged inspiration with a pause at the point where the respiration is full blown and lasts for 2 to 3 seconds. This may alternate with an expiratory pause.

Level of Lesion

Injury has occurred to the respiratory control center located in the middle to lower third of the pons.

Possible causative lesions include

- Extensive brain stem lesion as an infarction of the pons
- Severe meningitis

Cluster Breathing

Description

There are clusters of irregular breathing with periods of apnea at irregular intervals. (Gasping breathing occurs at a slow rate and has features similar to those of cluster breathing.)

Level of Lesion

The lesion in the area of the upper medulla can be relatively small with a poor prognosis.

Possible causative lesions include

- Tumor of medulla
- Infarction of medulla

CHART 5–10. (Continued)

Ataxic Breathing

Description

There is a completely irregular, unpredictable breathing pattern with deep and shallow random breaths and pauses.

Level of Lesion

Medulla

Ataxic breathing involves the major center for respiration, the medulla, which controls the to-and-fro rhythmicity of breathing and has a poor prognosis.

Possible causative lesions include

- Cerebellar bleeding
- Pontine bleeding
- Compressing supratentorial tumors
- Severe meningitis

anatomical level of dysfunction, since specific respiratory patterns are evident when a certain anatomical area is not functioning properly.

Physiology

The respiratory centers of the brain make up a widely dispersed system composed of neurons situated in three areas of the reticular substance of the medulla and pons. The pons contains the apneustic and pneumotaxic areas, while the medulla contains the rhythmicity area. The most important of the three areas, the medullary rhythmicity area, is also called the medullary respiratory center because it sets the basic rhythm of the inspiratory and expiratory pattern. Adjustments of respiratory rate and rhythm are regulated by many neurological mechanisms so that constant blood levels of oxygen and carbon dioxide can be maintained. With injury to the respiratory centers of the brain, changes occur in the respiratory patterns that provide valuable information about the level of injury (see Chart 5–10 and Fig. 5–8).

FIG. 5–8. Abnormal respiratory patterns associated with coma. (Gifford RRM, Plaut MR: Abnormal respiratory patterns in the comatose patient caused by intracranial dysfunction. J Neurosurg Nurs 7[1]:58, July 1975)

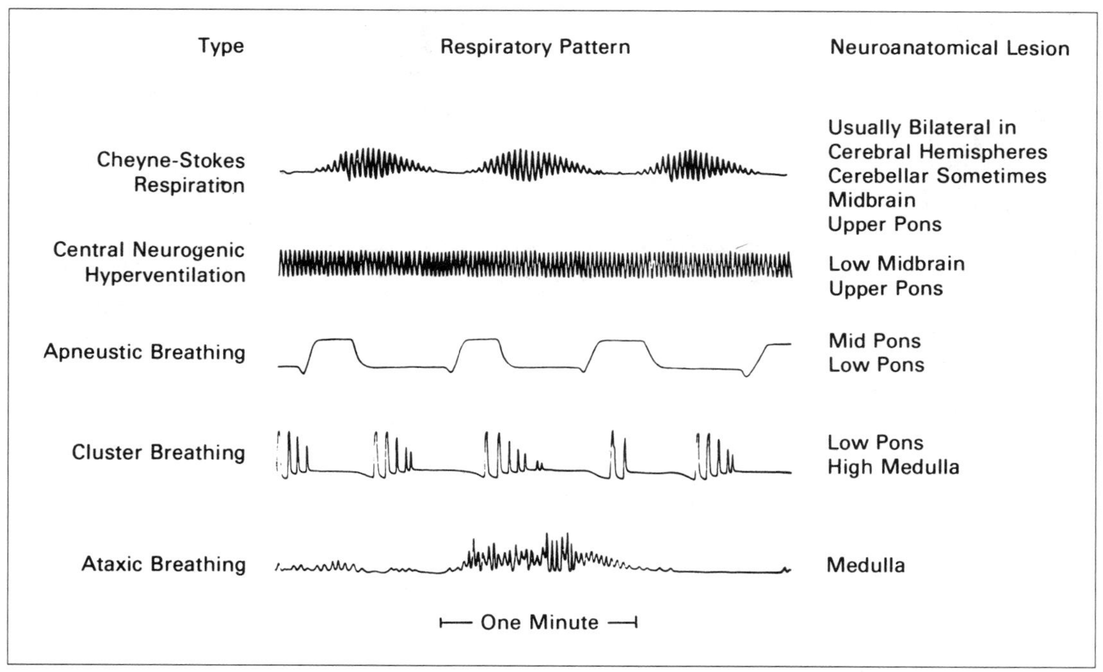

Because a human being is a complex physiological and psychosocial entity, abnormal respiratory patterns in the neurological patient can be initiated by conditions in other body systems. Acidosis, respiratory alkalosis, electrolyte imbalance, congestive heart failure, anxiety, and respiratory complications from prolonged immobility or infections such as atelectasis, pneumonia, and pulmonary edema should be considered.

Drugs—particularly narcotics and anesthetic agents—that have a depressant effect can also affect the respiratory system. Morphine sulfate depresses the rate of respirations as well as causing constriction of the pupils. Because of the effect of respiratory depression and the masking of the neurological sign of the pupillary response, *morphine sulfate is contraindicated in the neurological patient.*

Changes in Respiratory Rate

Cerebral injury produces several types of abnormal respiratory patterns. Several are included in Figure 5–8. A few more points should be made. Initially, an acute rise in intracranial pressure is reflected by a slowing of the respiratory rate. As the intracranial pressure continues to rise, the rate becomes rapid. These respirations are almost always noisy. Keep in mind that metabolic disorders can also trigger changes in respiratory patterns. Trauma to the cervical spine may produce respiratory embarrassment or, if above the phrenic segment (C–4), total arrest.

Whatever the reason for changes in the rate and rhythm of respirations, such changes should be reported to the physician at once.

- In general, the role of the nurse in relation to respiratory function is to (1) periodically record the rate and rhythm of the respirations and notify the physician of changes, (2) implement nursing measures to maintain a patent airway and promote respiratory function, and (3) assess the patient for respiratory complications or insufficiency.

Nursing Measures to Ensure Adequate Respiratory Function

The most basic of all nursing responsibilities for any patient is to ensure a patent airway. This means that the nose, mouth, and respiratory passages are clear, allowing adequate oxygen–carbon dioxide gas exchange.

A patient who is *conscious* enough to follow instructions should be directed to take deep breaths hourly and to cough and expectorate mucus frequently.

The *unconscious patient* is defenseless against threats to a patent airway, particularly if the cough reflex is absent. The same is true of the incapacitated patient who cannot change positions or cough or breathe freely. In these instances the maintenance of a patent airway becomes a major nursing responsibility.

- Suctioning the patient periodically and frequently changing his position constitute effective nursing interventions for clearing the airway in an unconscious patient

Positioning. Placing the unconscious or incapacitated patient in the lateral recumbent position facilitates respirations, promotes drainage of secretions, and prevents the tongue from falling back and obstructing the airway (Fig. 5–9). The patient should be turned from side to side every 2 hours to prevent the pooling of secretions in the lungs.

Suctioning. In some instances, exudate from the nose may be managed with sterile cotton-tipped swabs; however, in other instances suctioning may be necessary, as is the case for removing drainage from the oronasopharynx and mouth (Fig. 5–10).

- *Never* suction a patient *nasally* if there is a possibility of a basal skull fracture or cerebrospinal drainage from the nose.

When the patient is suctioned, strict aseptic technique should be followed. Disposable sterile catheters should be used each time the patient is suctioned to prevent the growth of microorganisms such as *Pseudomonas* and *Staphylococcus*. Suction equipment should be checked at the beginning of every shift and maintained in a ready state so that suctioning can be instituted immediately should aspiration occur.

Each suctioning of a neurological or neurosurgical patient should be limited to 15 seconds to prevent hypoxia and hypercapnia, which would increase an already elevated intracranial pressure. Each time, before and after suctioning, it is recommended that the patient be hyperaerated with 100% oxygen for 60 seconds, *with the approval of the physician*. Certain conditions such as chronic lung disease would contraindicate the use of pure oxygen; therefore, prior approval from the physician must be obtained before hyperaeration is implemented. The limitation both of suctioning time and hyperaeration with oxygen is employed to prevent hypoxia and hypercapnia, which are so detrimental to the patient with an increase in intracranial pressure.

Tracheostomy and Suctioning. Maintaining a patent airway is often possible only with a tracheostomy. Most tracheostomy tubes used today have a cuff attachment, which provides special benefits. The inflated cuff forms a seal between the patient's trachea and the tracheostomy tube, providing for better control of oxygen delivery by a mechanical respirator or intermittent positive pressure treatments. The inflated cuff can also be helpful in preventing the aspiration of tube feeding if it is inflated before the feeding is begun. Should the patient regurgitate his feeding, the inflated cuff will prevent aspiration into the lungs, which could result in instant pneumonia. If a cuffed tracheostomy tube is used, it must be deflated hourly to prevent tracheal ischemia.

Suctioning is much easier if a tracheostomy is present. Strict aseptic technique must be followed, using a sterile catheter each time the patient is suctioned as a precaution against infection. Periodic tracheostomy care is given at least every 4 hours, at which times the inner cannula of the tracheostomy tube is removed, soaked in a hydrogen peroxide/normal saline solution, and cleaned with a tracheostomy brush (or pipe cleaner) to remove the exudate.

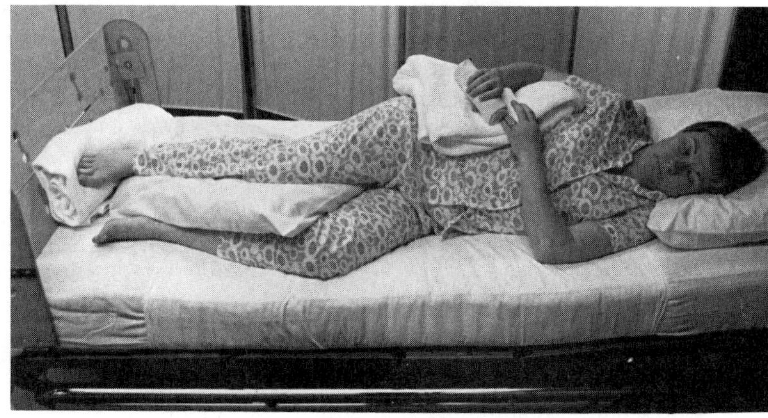

FIG. 5-9. Positioning the unconscious patient.

After the inner cannula is rinsed in normal saline, the excess saline is shaken off and the cannula is reinserted into the tracheostomy. In addition, the sterile dressing around the tracheostomy incision is removed and the skin is cleansed of mucus and drainage with sterile cotton-tipped applicators and sterile normal saline. A new and dry sterile tracheostomy dressing is fitted around the tracheostomy tube and surgical site.

Patients on Respirators. Inflate the cuff on the tracheostomy tube or endotracheal tube to create a proper seal between the tracheal wall and the tube. Deflate the cuff of the tracheostomy tube periodically (every 1 to 2 hours for 5 minutes) to improve the circulation to the tracheal wall. Be sure that the cuff is inflated when giving a tube feeding to prevent possible aspiration. Ambu the patient every 1 to 2 hours for a few minutes to fully expand the lungs (expand dead air space). This helps to prevent atelectasis and pneumonia. Periodically assess the patient's blood gases. Be sure that the respirator alarm is left in the "on" position at all times.

Respiratory Insufficiency and Respiratory Complications

Assessment. In assessing the respiratory function of a neurological patient, the nurse should be aware of the common problems of respiratory insufficiency and respiratory complications that may develop in the patient. These conditions affect the vital signs and, very often, the level of consciousness. Since respiratory compromise will affect the oxygen supply to the cerebral cells, the neurological status of the patient will soon deteriorate unless the nurse recognizes the early signs and symptoms of respiratory insufficiency and intervenes appropriately. The problems to be considered include (1) mechanical insufficiency, (2) neurological metabolic dysfunction, (3) neurogenic pulmonary edema, (4) adult respiratory distress syndrome, and (5) disseminated intravascular coagulation.

Mechanical Insufficiency. The most commonly seen clinical respiratory problem is a partially obstructed airway. This can occur because of improper positioning of the head

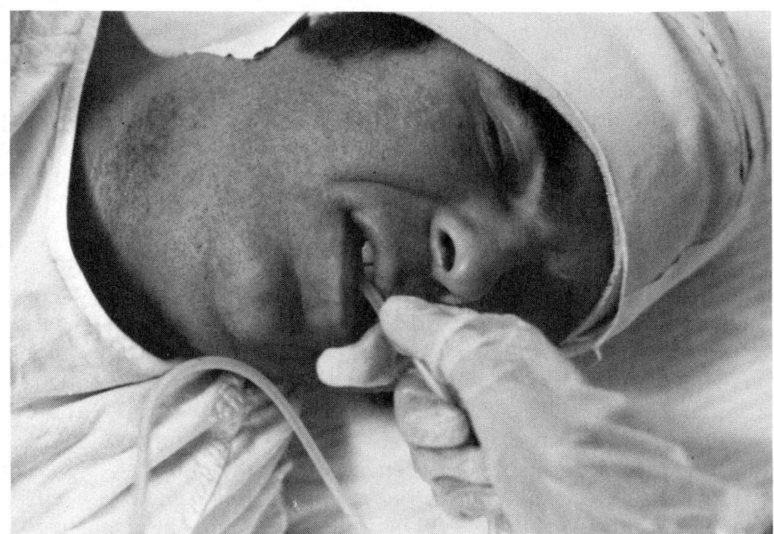

FIG. 5-10. Suctioning the unconscious patient.

and neck of the unconscious patient. Other mechanical deficits in the structures that comprise the respiratory tract include postanesthesia recovery phase insufficiency, aspiration, airway edema after extubation, muscle paralysis (diaphragm or intercostals) from spinal cord injury or other neuromuscular diseases, and airway obstruction from mucus or other foreign material.

The nurse will observe the following:

- Respirations that are shallow and sound like snoring
- Increased secretion from the mouth
- Restlessness

The results of mechanical insufficiency include alveolar hypoventilation; hypoxemia; atelectasis; hypostatic, aspiration, or bacterial pneumonia; and pulmonary emboli.

Neurological Metabolic Dysfunction. Various types of intracranial disease processes cause metabolic changes in the cerebral tissues as a result of inadequate cerebral oxygenation. The metabolic by-products of cell metabolism are largely acidotic. The acidic material enters the cerebrospinal fluid and influences the respiratory center in the medulla as it circulates in the ventricular system. The medulla responds by increasing the respiratory rate. However, the tidal volume either remains the same or is diminished. These conditions, accelerated by immobility, cause small airways to close, with the subsequent development of atelectasis and shunting of pulmonary blood flow.

Neurogenic Pulmonary Edema. Neurogenic pulmonary edema in humans was first described in 1918. The exact mechanism responsible for this acute condition is unclear, but it is accepted that there is a neurological pathway responsible for neurogenic pulmonary edema following central nervous system injury. The most widely accepted explanation was proposed by Theodore and Robin, who identified two primary physiological events: (1) a shift of blood volume from the systemic to the pulmonary circulation and (2) damage to the pulmonary capillaries (Fig. 5–11).[8] The sequence of pathophysiology that results in a shift of the blood volume is accomplished in the following steps. At the moment of trauma, a massive sympathetic discharge that is mediated by the hypothalamus causes generalized transient vasoconstriction. The blood shifts from the high-resistance systemic circulation to the low-resistance pulmonary circulation. The increased amount of blood in the pulmonary vascular beds causes an increase in the pulmonary capillary pressure. The net result is pulmonary edema because of hydrostatic pressures produced by the pulmonary hypertension.

In the second state of neurogenic pulmonary edema, the transient pulmonary hypervolemia damages the pulmonary capillary membranes. The pulmonary capillary permeability is altered so that a plasmalike fluid leaks into the alveolar spaces. Because of the defect in the pulmonary capillary membranes' permeability, the pulmonary edema persists even after normal hemodynamic and cardiac function have been reestablished. Because the patient has a plasmalike fluid in his alveoli rather than air, the blood from the right side of the heart is shunted to the left side of the heart without the usual gas exchange of carbon dioxide for oxygen. The resultant hypoxemia is a serious form of oxygenation deficit that affects the entire body, including the brain.

Neurogenic pulmonary edema is frequently seen after massive head injury and also after abrupt elevations in intracranial pressure. The signs and symptoms of neurogenic pulmonary edema are the same as those seen with the conventional acute pulmonary edema, that is, dyspnea; severe restlessness and anxiety; confusion; diaphoresis; cyanosis; distention of the neck veins; moist, rapid, shallow respirations; rales and rhonchi; elevated blood pressure; and a rapid thready pulse. The patient may cough up frothy blood-tinged fluid.

The nurse should be aware that neurogenic pulmonary edema is possible in acute head injury patients and those with grossly elevated intracranial pressure. She should also know the signs and symptoms that she would see clinically in the patient and be prepared to act quickly if the problem begins to develop.

The usual management includes propping the patient to an upright position with his legs and feet down, if at all possible; administration of oxygen, diuretics, and possibly aminophylline (if wheezing and bronchospasms are severe); rotating tourniquets; and intermittent positive pressure breathing (IPPB) therapy or positive end expiratory pressure breathing (PEEP) therapy to keep the alveoli from collapsing.

Adult Respiratory Distress Syndrome (ARDS). Adult respiratory distress syndrome, previously called shock lung syndrome, is a less acute syndrome than pulmonary edema, and it develops at a slower rate. It is a type of pulmonary insufficiency sometimes seen after a major insult or shock to the body such as head or abdominal injury, hemorrhage, aspiration of gastric contents, or sepsis. There is compromise of the alveolar capillary membranes so that a plasmalike fluid seeps into the alveoli. This interferes with gaseous exchange at the alveoli and causes loss of lung compliance and loss of lung volume. Hypoxemia and, later, hypocapnia develop as the patient blows off more carbon dioxide.

The nurse will observe the following signs and symptoms: dyspnea, hyperventilation, tachypnea, rising blood pressure, and anxiety. Later, the dyspnea will become more pronounced, and grunting respirations, intercostal and substernal retractions, cyanosis, rhonchi and rales, diaphoresis, tachycardia, and confusion will be evident. When tested, the arterial blood gases will show a decrease in oxygen and carbon dioxide, which is indicative of respiratory alkalosis.

The management of the patient includes oxygen therapy, ventilation assistance as indicated (PEEP), bronchodilators, diuretics, supporting carbon dioxide retention, and bed rest. A medical–surgical textbook should be consulted for other specifics of care.

Disseminated Intravascular Coagulation (DIC). A recently recognized pathophysiological response of the body's hemostatic mechanism to disease and injury is

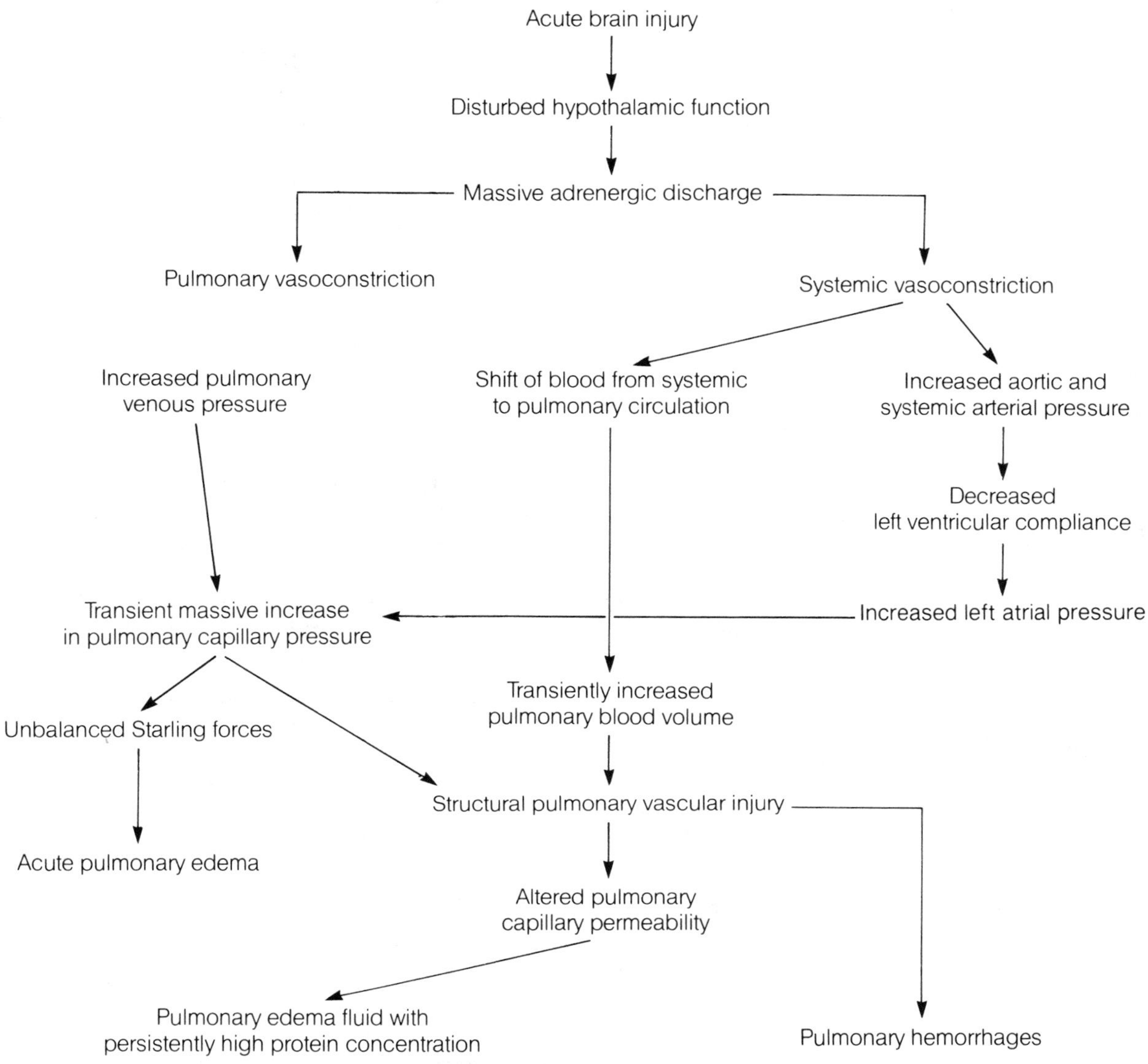

FIG. 5–11. Sequence of events leading to pulmonary dysfunction following acute brain injury. (After Theodore J, Robin ED: Editorial: Speculations on neurogenic pulmonary edema. Am Rev Respir Dis 113:405, 1976)

called disseminated intravascular coagulation or DIC. Although the cause is unknown, it is always associated with a primary disease process of injury. In the neurological patient, the syndrome can be triggered by conditions associated with thrombus formation (e.g., hypotensive states) as well as conditions associated with massive tissue injury or neoplasms (e.g., multi-trauma, brain tumor). The syndrome is usually associated with severe respiratory distress and hypoxia because of clots in the lungs followed by probable bleeding. The condition is potentially lethal.

The pathophysiology of disseminated intravascular coagulation is characterized by two phases: an initial clotting phase and a secondary hemorrhage phase. The primary disease triggers the initiation of the clotting mechanism throughout the vascular system. In this initial phase there is free thrombin in the blood, fibrin deposits in the capillary beds, and platelet aggregates. As a result, microthrombi are formed that obstruct blood flow to organs, and the fibrin causes changes in the red blood cells. Common clinical manifestations may include respiratory failure, renal failure, and adrenal insufficiency. Purpural lesions may be noted on the patient's chest and abdomen.

In the second phase, clotting factors are depleted and fibrin-degrading products from fibrinolysis are present in large amounts. These products act as anticoagulation agents and result in bleeding at many sites. If a tube of blood is drawn at the patient's bedside, clotting time will be prolonged. Laboratory examination of blood will show the presence of thrombocytopenia, low levels of fibrinogen, and prolonged prothrombin and partial thromboplastin times.

Management of the patient with disseminated intravascular coagulation is directed at treating the underlying primary cause, then at controlling bleeding and restoring normal levels of clotting factors. Fresh frozen platelets, whole blood, and possibly heparin may be given. The use of heparin is controversial. Heparin is administered to inhibit the formation of thrombin and allow fibrinogen and platelet levels to increase, yet heparin is an anticoagulation drug and can increase bleeding. The decision to use heparin will depend on the condition of the patient and the presence of bleeding.

The nurse's responsibility includes an awareness of the possibility of disseminated intravascular coagulation in the patient at risk. Early recognition of purpural lesions, increased bleeding from chest tubes or nasogastric tubes, bleeding on dry sterile dressings, or bleeding from the gums should be noted, recorded, and brought to the attention of the physician. The patient must be closely monitored for fractional urinary output, occult and frank bleeding, respiratory distress, and vital signs. Laboratory data on blood coagulation should be carefully noted. The patient with disseminated intravascular coagulation is critically ill and requires excellent monitoring and management by the nurse to survive. See Nursing Diagnoses Frequently Made for Patients With Respiratory Deficits.

NURSING DIAGNOSES FREQUENTLY MADE FOR PATIENTS WITH RESPIRATORY DEFICITS

The following are frequently made nursing diagnoses for the patient with respiratory deficits caused by neurological dysfunction:

- Infection, potential of
- Fluid volume deficit, potential of
- Urinary elimination pattern, altered
- Airway clearance, ineffective
- Breathing pattern, ineffective
- Cardiac output, alteration in: decreased
- Gas exchange, impaired
- Tissue perfusion, alteration in
- Activity tolerance, decreased
- Anxiety (specify severity of)

PULSE

Assessment

The rate, rhythm, and quality of the pulse should be recorded, using either the radial or apical pulse sites. Any abnormalities such as tachycardia, bradycardia, or cardiac arrhythmias should be noted.

Tachycardia

Tachycardia in a neurological patient can indicate that (1) a patient is reaching the terminal stages of the disease process or (2) a patient with neurological injury caused by multiple injuries is experiencing internal bleeding (most often intra-abdominal).

Bradycardia

Bradycardia can occur in the later stages of progressive increased intracranial pressure. In this condition, blood is pumped to the edematous brain against great pressure, so that the pulse is decreased in rate (40–60/minute) and bounding. Hypotension and bradycardia may be secondary to cervical spinal cord injury with interruption of descending sympathetic pathways.

Cardiac Arrhythmias

Cardiac arrhythmias are not uncommon symptoms. In specific neurological conditions, patients with blood in the cerebrospinal fluid appear to have an increased incidence of cardiac arrhythmias (subarachnoid hemorrhage, ruptured cerebral aneurysm, severe head injury). Patients who have undergone posterior fossa surgery also have a high incidence of abnormal rhythms.

If there is evidence of abnormalities in rate or rhythm, a rhythm strip should be taken immediately to document and identify the problem. Continuous cardiac monitoring may be ordered. See Nursing Diagnoses Frequently Made for Patients With Cardiac (Pulse) Deficits.

NURSING DIAGNOSES FREQUENTLY MADE FOR PATIENTS WITH CARDIAC (PULSE) DEFICITS

The following nursing diagnoses are frequently made for the patient with cardiac (pulse) deficits caused by neurological dysfunction:

- Urinary elimination pattern, altered
- Activity tolerance, decreased
- Cardiac output, alteration in: decreased
- Tissue perfusion, alterations
- Anxiety (specify severity)

BLOOD PRESSURE

Physiology

The vasomotor center of the medulla is responsible for regulating blood pressure. This area receives input from the *chemoreceptors*, which determine blood levels of carbon dioxide, and *pressor receptors*, which are sensors for blood pressure.

Changes in Blood Pressure

- Hypertension
  - An elevated blood pressure in the neurological patient is usually associated with a severely rising intracranial pressure. An elevated systolic blood pressure, widening pulse pressure, and bradycardia are seen in the advancing stages of increased intracranial pressure. This is known as Cushing's response.
- Hypotension
  - Hypotension is rarely due to cerebral injury. When it is seen

with severe injury, it occurs only as a terminal event and is seen with tachycardia. Inadequate cerebral perfusion denies the cerebral tissue of an adequate oxygen supply and the regulatory mechanisms no longer function. In this stage of decompensation, deterioration is rapid and death results.

- The suspicion of occult internal hemorrhage (intrathoracic, intra-abdominal, pelvic, or long bone) should be raised when hypotension and tachycardia are seen together. This is especially true when assessing the trauma patient.
- Hypotension and bradycardia may be seen in the patient with a cervical spinal injury. In this case, the altered signs would be due to interruption of the descending sympathetic pathways.

See Nursing Diagnoses Frequently Made for Patients With Blood Pressure Alterations.

NURSING DIAGNOSES FREQUENTLY MADE FOR PATIENTS WITH BLOOD PRESSURE ALTERATIONS

The following nursing diagnoses are frequently made for the patient with blood pressure alterations caused by neurological dysfunction:

- Breathing pattern, ineffective
- Cardiac output, alteration in: decreased
- Gas exchange, impaired
- Tissue perfusion, alteration in

TEMPERATURE

Physiology

The hypothalamus is the center for the regulation of body heat and acts by monitoring the temperature of blood. Regulation of heat is accomplished by afferent impulses to the sweat glands, peripheral vessels, and skeletal muscles for shivering. Through these structures the body can conserve or divest itself of body heat.

Hypothermia. The temperature can be subnormal (hypothermia) in conditions such as spinal shock when autonomic innervation is lost; metabolic or toxic coma of any cause; drug overdose, especially from depressant drugs (barbiturate overdose); destructive brain stem or hypothalamic lesions, and in the terminal stages of certain neurological disease processes.

Hyperthermia. The temperature can be elevated (hyperthermia) in conditions such as central nervous system infection, subarachnoid hemorrhage, lesions of the hypothalamus, petechial hemorrhage of the hypothalamus or brain stem, traction on the hypothalamus or brain stem, heat stroke, bacterial endocarditis, pneumonia, overdose of phenothiazine or anticholinergic drugs, and other infections outside the central nervous system.

Nursing Assessment

The following situations indicate a need to take the temperature by the rectal route: a patient with a tracheostomy or nasogastric tube; a patient receiving oxygen; a combative, confused, or disoriented patient; and an unconscious patient. The nurse should stay with the patient while the thermometer is in place. The temperature and the route by which it was taken should be recorded on the flow sheets. If a continuous monitoring device has been used to monitor the temperature, this should be noted on the flow sheets. If the temperature is elevated and the patient has been placed on a hypothermia blanket, the temperature should be monitored every half hour until it begins to drop to an acceptable level.

Treatment and Nursing Management

In the neurological patient temperature elevations can exceed 106° F (41° C) in a short time. An elevated temperature is treated vigorously in the neurological patient because it results in increased cell metabolism, which in turn produces an increase in carbon dioxide, a by-product of cell metabolism. Carbon dioxide, a potent cerebral vasodilator, will cause an increase in intracranial pressure in a patient who may already have high intracranial pressure. If the oxygen supply to the cerebral tissue is insufficient, cerebral ischemia develops. Therefore, aggressive treatment of hyperthermia to prevent neurological deterioration is important and necessary in a neurological patient.

Hyperthermia is managed with acetylsalicylic acid (aspirin) or acetaminophen (Tylenol) suppositories, alcohol sponge baths and massage, a hypothermia blanket, and removal of excessive bed-clothing. The patient must be observed for shivering, which would counteract attempts to cool the patient and could also interfere with respiratory function. Special attention should be paid to fluid balance, urinary output, and skin breakdown.

Consider the reason for the elevated temperature. Listen to the chest for breath sounds and rales. Culture the urine and the sputum. Assess the dressing and drainage, if present.

The Effects of Steroids on Temperature

The neurological and neurosurgical patient may at times be treated with large doses of steroids. A frequently ordered steroid is dexamethasone (Decadron). One action of steroids should be remembered, that is, that steroids are anti-inflammatory agents that tend to mask the classical signs of infections such as an elevated temperature. Therefore, a neurological patient receiving large doses of steroids can have an infection without exhibiting an elevated temperature. It is important to order a routine urinalysis on a weekly basis or more frequently, if necessary. Urine cultures and sputum cultures should also be monitored if there are any indications of infection such as foul-smelling urine or yellowish, foul-smelling sputum. See Nursing Diagnoses Frequently Made for Patients With Altered Body Temperature.

ST. FRANCIS MEDICAL CENTER
La Crosse, Wisconsin
Neurological Flow Sheet

92-626 Nurse's Signature and Initials

Pt. Name Plate

COMA SCALE		Date and Time														
	EYES OPEN	Spontaneously	4													C = Eyes Closed by Swelling
		To Command	3													
		To Pain	2													
		No Response	1													
	BEST MOTOR RESPONSE	Obeys Commands	6													Record Best Arm Response
		Localizes Pain	5													
		Flexion-Withdrawal	4													
		Flexion (abnormal)	3													
		Extension (abnormal)	2													
		No Response	1													
	BEST VERBAL RESPONSE	Oriented	5													T = Endotracheal Tube or Tracheostomy A = Aphasia
		Confused	4													
		Inappropriate Words	3													
		Incomprehensible Sounds	2													
		No Response	1													
	TOTAL SCORE															
PUPILS	Size		R													B = Brisk S = Sluggish N = No Reaction C = Closed
	Reaction															
	Size		L													
	Reaction															
LIMB MOVEMENT	Grade Limb Movement Spontaneous or to Command, Do Not Rate Reflex Movement		RA													Use Limb Movement Scale To Grade
			RL													
			LA													
			LL													
VITALS	Blood Pressure			/	/	/	/	/	/	/	/	/	/	/	/	Respiration Type N = Normal CS = Cheyne Stokes SH = Sustained Hyperventilation U = Uncoordinated
	Pulse															
	Temperature															
	Respiratory Rate															
	Respiratory Type															
	Nurse's Initial															

Limb Movement Scale
0 - No Response
1 - Flicker of Trace of Contraction
2 - Active Movement with Gravity Eliminated
3 - Active Movement Against Gravity
4 - Active Movement Against Gravity and Resistance

1MM 2MM 3MM 4MM 5MM 6MM 7MM 8MM 9MM

FIG. 5-12. Neurological flow sheet developed at St. Francis Medical Center, La Crosse, WI. (Chief authors: LR Dunnum, P Davenport-Fortune)

NURSING DIAGNOSES FREQUENTLY MADE FOR PATIENTS WITH ALTERED BODY TEMPERATURE

The following nursing diagnoses are frequently made for the patient with altered body temperature caused by neurological dysfunction:

Hyperthermia

- Fluid volume deficit, potential of
- Nutrition, alteration in: less than body requires
- Urinary elimination, impairment of: retention
- Bowel elimination, alterations in: constipation
- Tissue perfusion, alterations in
- Gas exchange, impairment of
- Breathing pattern, ineffective, potential of
- Anxiety

Hypothermia

- Tissue perfusion, alterations in
- Urinary elimination, alterations in
- Comfort, alterations in

SUMMARY

In this chapter, the assessment of neurological signs has been discussed in detail, yet one might still wonder how often the assessment should be conducted and how much detail is necessary. The answer to these questions depends on several points: the acuity and stability of the patient's condition; the purpose of the assessment; and the particular circumstances surrounding the patient.

A patient admitted with a serious head injury will be monitored every 5 to 15 minutes. This may be necessary because there is suspicion that intracranial bleeding such as a epidural or subdural hematoma will develop. In this instance, the patient has sustained an acute injury and his condition is unstable. Once the patient is stabilized, the frequency of the assessment can be decreased to every 1 to 2 hours and then to every 4 hours, with the consent of the physician. If the condition of a patient who has been stable begins to deteriorate, it will be necessary to exercise prudent judgment and assess the patient more frequently.

The detail included in a neurological assessment will also vary depending on the circumstances. In conducting an initial neurological assessment on the newly admitted patient who is a planned admission, the nurse will need to conduct a detailed assessment. An example of this situation is a patient admitted by his physician for a neurological work-up. Once a baseline assessment has been established and the patient is stable, the nurse may assess the level of consciousness, pupillary signs, motor function, and vital signs every 4 hours and the sensory and ocular signs every 8 hours. There may be other specific areas to be assessed, such as the highest level of sensation in a patient admitted with a spinal cord tumor. The need for special assessment should be noted on the nursing care plan and on the assessment parameter sheets.

Data from a neurological assessment can be recorded in several ways. Information about the initial neurological assessment is summarized in the nursing history and admission assessment. Subsequent assessments are recorded in the manner established by the facility. Many hospitals use special neurological assessment flow sheets that provide space for recording the neurological parameters on one sheet (Fig. 5-12). This is helpful because it provides a composite of all information on one sheet, making it easier to identify trends and make correlations of the various parameters. Another advantage of the standardized assessment sheet is that all assessors using the sheet will assess the same parameters on the patient and record the information in the same prescribed manner.

The neurological assessment is a basic tool for the nurse to use in making nursing diagnoses and planning nursing intervention for the patient. She must develop the skills and knowledge to conduct this assessment competently.

REFERENCES

1. Plum F, Posner J: The Diagnosis of Stupor and Coma, 3rd ed, p 2. Philadelphia, FA Davis, 1980
2. Plum, pp 178-180
3. Teasdale G, Jennett W: Assessment of coma and impaired consciousness. Lancet 2:81, July 1974
4. Plum, p 3
5. Jennett B, Plum F: The persistent vegetative state: A syndrome in search of a name. Lancet 1:734, April 1972
6. Plum, p 9
7. Guyton A: Textbook of Medical Physiology, 5th ed, p 272. Philadelphia, WB Saunders, 1981
8. Theodore J, Robin ED: Editorial: Speculation on neurogenic pulmonary edema. Am Rev Respir Dis 113:405, 1976

BIBLIOGRAPHY

Books

Bates B: A Guide to Physical Examination, 2nd ed. Philadelphia, JB Lippincott, 1979

Burton G et al (eds): Respiratory Care: A Guide to Clinical Practice. Philadelphia, JB Lippincott, 1977

Cogan D: Neurology of the Ocular Muscles. Springfield, Charles C Thomas, 1975

Eliasson S et al: Neurological Pathophysiology, 2nd ed. New York, Oxford University Press, 1978

Kintzel K (ed): Advanced Concepts in Clinical Nursing, 2nd ed. Philadelphia, JB Lippincott, 1977

Periodicals

Bakow E: Respiratory care of the critically ill patient with head trauma. Crit Care Q 2(1):81, June 1979

Cline B, Fisher M: A.R.D.S. means emergency. Nurs82 12:62, February 1982

Eggleston C: Clinical correlation of neurogenic pulmonary edema to increased intracranial pressure. J Neurosurg Nurs 14(5):245, October 1982

Fuller E: Coma—evaluating depth of consciousness. Patient Care 15(16):127, September 30, 1981

Habermann B: Cognitive dysfunction and social rehabilitation in the severely head-injured patient. J Neurosurg Nurs 14(5):220, October 1982

Haerer A: Coma: Some differential considerations in the diagnosis and management. Hosp Med 68, April 1976

Hinterbuchner L: Evaluation of the unconscious patient. Hosp Med 83, February 1977

Jennett B, Teasdale G: Predicting outcome in individual patients after severe head injury. Lancet 1:1031, May 15, 1976

Jones C: Glasgow coma scale. Am J Nurs 79(9):1551, September 1979

Jones C: Asepsis in pulmonary care: Improving old traditions. J Neurosurg Nurs 11(2):76, June 1979

Jones C: Monitoring recovery after head injury: Translating research into practice. J Neurosurg Nurs 11(4):192, December 1975

Kupersmith M, Rasonhoff J: Identifying Horner's syndrome. Hosp Med 38, March 1980

Mahoney E: Alterations in cognitive functioning in the brain damaged patient. Nurs Clin North Am 15(2):283, June 1980

March K: "Look into my eyes." J Neurosurg Nurs 15(4):213, August 1983

Mechner F: Patient assessment: Neurological examination, part I. Am J Nurs 75(9):1, September 1975

Mechner F: Patient assessment: Neurological examination, part II. Am J Nurs 75(11):1, November 1975

Mechner F: Patient assessment: Neurological examination, part III. Am J Nurs 76(4):1, April 1976

Mechner F: Patient assessment: Examination of the eye, part II. Am J Nurs 75(1):1, January 1975

Melamed M: Identifying Adie's syndrome. Hosp Med 65, February 1982

Miller L: Neurological assessment: A practical approach for the critical care nurse. J Neurosurg Nurs 11(1):2, March 1979

Minnick A: Locked-in syndrome. J Neurosurg Nurs 15(2):77, April 1983

Mitchell P, Irvin N: Neurological examination: Nursing assessment for nursing purposes. J Neurosurg Nurs 9(1):23, March 1977

Mitchell P, Mauss N: Intracranial pressure: Fact and fancy. Nurs76 16:53, June 1976

Nelson C, Miner M: Brain injury disseminated intravascular coagulation and fibrinolysis syndrome in children. J Neurosurg Nurs 15(2):72, April 1983

Neumann D, Bailey L: An overview of neurogenic pulmonary edema. J Neurosurg Nurs 12(4):206, December 1980

Norman S: The pupil check. Am J Nurs 82(4):588, April 1982

Shafer T: Nursing care of the patient with ARDS. Crit Care Nurs March/April 1981

Stephens G, Parsons M: A delicate balance: Managing chronic airway obstruction in a neurological patient. Am J Nurs 75(9):1492, September 1975

Teasdale G: Assessing "conscious level." Nurs Times 914, June 12, 1975

Wachter–Shikora N: Chemoreceptors of respiration: Physiology and nursing implications. J Neurosurg Nurs 10(2):68, June 1978

Walleck C: A neurological assessment procedure that won't make you nervous. Nurs 82 12:50, December 1982

Walleck C: Pulmonary complications in the neurosurgical patient. J Neurosurg Nurs 9(3):102, June 1977

Zegeer L: The patient in the persistent vegetative state. J Neurosurg Nurs 13(5):243, October 1981

part three

General Considerations in Neurological and Neurosurgical Nursing

chapter 6

Nutritional Needs of Neurological and Neurosurgical Patients

Providing for the nutritional needs of the neurological–neurosurgical patient is a critical component in the healing and recovery process. Injury, physiological dysfunction, and stress often change the nutritional requirements and utilization of nutrients and water necessary for meeting basic requirements of energy and cell function and for repairing injured tissue. Reparative tissue consumes more protein, carbohydrate, lipid, water, and oxygen than normal tissue. Dietary and nutritional modifications imposed by illness also have a direct effect on adequate nutrition and normal body function. The patient with neurological dysfunction may have deficits such as an altered level of consciousness or paresis/paralysis of the muscles needed for chewing and swallowing that further complicate ingestion of an adequate dietary intake. Consideration of these factors plus the effect of illness on other body systems creates special complexities in meeting the nutritional needs of the neurological–neurosurgical patient. In managing the patient holistically, nutritional needs cannot be overlooked because no patient will recover from illness without adequate nutritional support.

BASIC NUTRITIONAL REQUIREMENTS

CALORIC INTAKE

The caloric intake necessary for a person depends on the person's age, sex, body size, activity level, and body temperature and the environment's ambient temperature. The range of calories required for a woman is 1700 to 2500 calories per day while a man will need between 2300 and 3100 calories per day. The caloric intake needed increases in any stressful situation such as physiological trauma, emotional stress, surgery, fever, seizure activity, decorticate or decerebrate rigidity, restlessness, agitation, hypermetabolic states, and sepsis. Caloric requirements can be increased two to three times for a patient with ongoing stress or serious injury such as multi-trauma or septic states. Patients with serious head injuries can require 4000 to 5000 calories per day.

Caloric intake of 40 kcal to 80 kcal/kg of body weight is generally required. In determining the amount of calories required, the basal energy expenditure (BEE) is calculated using the Harris–Benedict formula.[1] This formula considers weight, sex, height, and age in the calculations.

PROTEINS

Proteins are organic substances composed of amino acids. Although carbohydrate, fat, and protein all contain carbon, hydrogen, and oxygen, only protein contains nitrogen. Nitrogen is a component of every cell in the body. When 6.25 gm of protein are metabolized, 1 gm of nitrogen results. By weight, 1 gm of protein is 16% nitrogen. The primary function of protein is to build and repair body tissue. One gram of protein yields 4 calories when metabolized.

Essential and Nonessential Amino Acids

Amino acids are classified as essential and nonessential. *Essential amino acids* are necessary for normal growth and development and cannot be manufactured by the body. *Nonessential amino acids* are defined as amino acids not necessary for normal growth and development that can be manufactured by the body. Table 6–1 lists both essential and nonessential amino acids.

TABLE 6-1. *Essential and Nonessential Amino Acids*

Essential Amino Acids	*Nonessential Amino Acids*
Histidine	Alanine
Isoleucine	Arginine
Leucine	Aspartic acid
Lysine	Cysteine
Methionine	Cystine
Phenylalanine	Glutamic acid*
Threonine	Glycine
Tryptophan	Hydroxylysine
Valine	Hydroxyproline
	Proline
	Serine
	Tyrosine*

* Classified as semiessential because the need for these amino acids depends on the supply of the essential amino acids from which they are made.

Complete and Incomplete Proteins

Protein can also be classified into complete and incomplete protein. A *complete protein* is one that contains all of the essential amino acids in sufficient quantity and appropriate proportions to supply the body's needs. Proteins of animal origin such as milk, meat, cheese, and eggs are examples of complete proteins. An *incomplete protein* is defined as one that is deficient in one or more essential amino acids. Incomplete amino acids are of plant origin and include grains, legumes, and nuts.

Daily Protein Requirements

The healthy adult requires 0.8 gm/kg of protein per day. The protein requirement for the adult is approximately 45 gm to 65 gm per day. Patients with major injuries or wounds will require a daily intake of protein that is two to four times the normal daily requirement.

Nitrogen Balance

Nitrogen is the major component of protein. Almost all of the nitrogen ingested comes from protein, and most of the nitrogen lost from the body is in the form of nitrogenous end products found in the urine as urea, creatinine, uric acid, and ammonium salts. A small amount of nitrogen loss occurs through the stool and skin. Nitrogen balance indicates whether the patient is anabolic (has a positive nitrogen balance) or catabolic (has a negative nitrogen balance). The normal healthy adult who is not growing, who consumes an adequate diet, and whose lean body mass remains the same is said to be in nitrogen balance. Nitrogen balance is calculated as follows:

- Nitrogen balance equals nitrogen intake/24 hours minus nitrogen output/24 hours
- Nitrogen intake is calculated from the protein intake in 24 hours
- Nitrogen output is calculated from a 24-hour urine urea nitrogen (UUN) excretion study[2]

Positive Nitrogen Balance. When the nitrogen intake is greater than the nitrogen output, the patient is said to be in positive nitrogen balance or an anabolic state. Anabolism is a constructive metabolic building process that is responsible for growth or repair of body tissues. A positive nitrogen balance of 4 gm to 6 gm indicates anabolism.[2] Anabolism is the opposite of catabolism.

Negative Nitrogen Balance. When the nitrogenous output exceeds the nitrogen intake, a state of negative nitrogen balance exists. In this state, the lean body mass is being metabolized and decreases in quantity. Negative nitrogen balance occurs in states of inadequate essential amino acid intake and use, immobilization for any reason (e.g., unconsciousness, paralysis, spinal cord injury), and exposure to stress (e.g., trauma, surgery, disease processes). Catabolism is a destructive phase of metabolism in which complex substances are broken down and energy released. The opposite of catabolism is anabolism. Any patient who is in a negative nitrogen balance will not recover from surgery, trauma, sepsis, or a disease process until an anabolic state (positive nitrogen balance) is created.

CARBOHYDRATES

Carbohydrates (CHO) are defined as starches and sugars that are used by the body for energy. One gram of carbohydrate yields 4 calories when metabolized. Carbohydrates are classified as monosaccharides, disaccharides, or polysaccharides. Table 6-2 describes the categories, types, and sources of carbohydrates. For carbohydrates to be used by the body, they must be broken down into glucose. Glucose is the simplest form of sugar that circulates in the bloodstream, is oxidized to release energy, and is the source of energy for cerebral cell metabolism. Glucose may be used in the body in any of the three following ways:

- Glucose is oxidized in the body for energy.
- Glucose is stored as a reserve in the liver (and in muscle tissue to a lesser degree) in the form of glycogen through a process called *glucogenesis*. Hydrolysis of glycogen to glucose is called *glycolysis*.
- Excess glucose can be converted into fat and stored in the body as adipose tissue.

FATS

Fats occurring as organic substances in the body are called lipids. Fatty acids are the basic unit of structure in lipids; they can be divided into essential fatty acids and nonessential fatty acids. An *essential fatty acid* cannot be manufactured in the body and will cause a specific deficiency disorder if not ingested in an adequate amount. There is one essential fatty acid called linoleic acid that is important in the maintenance of the skin, hair, nerve linings, and cell membranes and is also a component of prostaglandins and other body chemicals. It is also necessary for forming other acids such as arachidonic acid. Nonessential fatty acids do

TABLE 6–2. *Types of Carbohydrates*

Category	Type	Sources
Monosaccharides (simplest form of carbohydrates)	Glucose (dextrose)	Natural glucose found in food or formed in the body from starch digestion
	Fructose (levulose) (converts to glucose for energy)	Sugar found in fruits and honey
	Galactose (not found free in food); changed to glucose for energy	Produced from lactose (milk sugar)
	Alcohol derivatives	
	Mannitol	From mannose
	Sorbitol	From glucose
Disaccharides (more complex sugars made up of two monosaccharides)	Sucrose = glucose + fructose	Table sugar, brown sugar, molasses, maple sugar
	Lactose = glucose + galactose	Sugar in milk
	Maltose = glucose + glucose	Malt products and germinating cereals
Polysaccharides (very complex carbohydrates)	Starch	Potatoes, cereal grains including rice, root vegetables, legumes
	Cellulose	Dietary fiber

not cause specific deficiency disorders if not ingested in sufficient amounts because they can be manufactured in the body.

The purpose of fat in the diet is primarily to produce energy, although it is also important in relationship to fat-related compounds in the body such as cholesterol, triglycerides, phospholipids, and lecithin. The major sources of fat in the normal diet are butter, margarine, oil, bacon, meat, fats, egg yolks, nuts, and legumes. When one gm of fat is oxidized, 9 calories are yielded.

TABLE 6–3. *Vitamins and Their Functions*

Vitamins	Functions
Fat-Soluble Vitamins	
Vitamin A	• Growth and maintenance of epithelial tissue • Bone development • Visual acuity in dim light
Vitamin D	• Assists in the absorption and utilization of calcium in bone and tooth development
Vitamin E	• Cellular antioxidant
Vitamin K	• Essential in prothrombin formation and blood clotting
Water-Soluble Vitamins	
Thiamine	• Key role in carbohydrate oxidation • Participates in the Krebs' cycle • A component of enzymes
Riboflavin	• Involved in amino acid and purine metabolism • Necessary for generation of adenosine triphosphate (ATP)
Niacin	• Essential in protein utilization • Necessary in the synthesis of fatty acids and cholesterol
Pyridoxine	• Essential for protein metabolism
Pantothenic acid	• Involved in synthesis of acetylcholine, cholesterol, fatty acids, and steroids • Involved in oxidation of energy nutrients
Biotin	• Important in the synthesis of fatty acids, utilization of glucose, and metabolism of protein
Folic acid	• Essential in amino acid metabolism • Important in maturation of red blood cells
Cobalamin	• Involved in the manufacture of enzymes necessary for the metabolism of nutrients and synthesis of deoxyribonucleic acid (DNA)
Vitamin C	• Production of collagen • Involved in hormonal synthesis, amino acid metabolism, integrity of capillary walls, and red blood formation • Important in wound healing

VITAMINS, MINERALS, AND WATER

In addition to proteins, carbohydrates, and fats that are necessary for proper nutrition, vitamins, minerals, and water are also requisites. Certain vitamins and minerals cannot be stored in the body, so the patient will quickly become deficient if an adequate diet is not consumed daily. Other vitamins can be stored in the body so that deficiencies will not be apparent until after a month or two of inadequate vitamin intake.

Vitamins

Vitamins are classified as either water-soluble or fat-soluble vitamins. Water-soluble vitamins are vitamin C and the B-complex vitamins, which include thiamine, riboflavin, niacin (nicotinic acid), pyridoxine, pantothenic acid, biotin, folic acid, and cobalamin. The fat-soluble vitamins are A, D, E, and K. (See Table 6–3 for description.)

Minerals

Minerals can be divided into major minerals and trace minerals. Major minerals include calcium, chloride, magnesium, phosphorus, potassium, and sodium. The trace minerals include cadmium, chromium, copper, fluoride, iodide, iron, manganese, molybdenum, nickel, selenium, silicon, tin, vanadium, and zinc. (See Table 6–4 for description.)

Water

The amount of water necessary for adequate nutrition depends on the weather, amount of perspiration, activity, endocrine function, urinary output, and other factors. Under normal conditions, the average person requires approximately 2600 ml of water a day. This can be subdivided into intake from three sources:

- In the form of liquids—1200 ml to 1500 ml/day
- Within foods—700 ml to 1000 ml/day
- From oxidation of food—200 ml to 300 ml/day

Hypermetabolic states, fever, profuse perspiration, significant drainage from wounds, and excessive urinary output (e.g., from diabetes insipidus) are a few situations that warrant a higher fluid intake.

METABOLIC CHANGES FOLLOWING INJURY AND STARVATION

Significant differences accompany the body's response to injury (trauma, surgery, sepsis) and to fasting/starvation. The major differences are listed in Table 6–5.

RESPONSE TO INJURY

Acute Phase

Any type of injury is a form of stress that triggers the stress response and arouses the central nervous system to activate the sympathetic nervous system. The body's response to stress/injury is to *survive* by meeting increased metabolic needs to preserve vital functions. The sympathetic nervous system immediately stimulates the adrenal medulla to release catecholamines (epinephrine, norepinephrine), corticosteroids (glucocorticosteroids, mineralosteroids), glucagon, and insulin.[3] Catecholamines act on the liver and muscles to convert stored glycogen into glucose by a process called glycogenolysis so that the glucose can be released into the bloodstream. At the same time, insulin secretion from the pancreas is suppressed so that hyperglycemia exists to meet the increased demand for energy. In addition, catecholamines increase lipolysis and gluconeogenesis. Lipolysis is a process by which fatty acids are released from fat stores and are then converted into glucose as another source of energy. Gluconeogenesis is the process of converting amino acids from skeletal muscles into glucose.[4]

Glucocorticosteroids stimulate the pancreas to secrete glucagon. Cortisol acts by increasing the breakdown of lipids. At the same time, aldosterone, a mineralocorticoid, increases water and sodium retention. There is a decrease in serum potassium that may last for several days because, initially, the excretion of potassium through the urine is increased while the excretion of sodium through the urine is decreased. The sodium retention phase is followed by diuresis. In the acute phase, fluid retention is also enhanced by an increased secretion of antidiuretic hormone (ADH) that is prompted by the hypothalamus.

Glucagon has a major effect on the liver—it causes the liver to convert amino acids into glucose (gluoneogenesis). It also suppresses the anabolic effect of insulin in protein synthesis (proteolysis).[2] As mentioned previously, the initial response to stress is suppression of insulin secretion so that hyperglycemia and gluconeogenesis result, creating ready sources for increased energy demands.

Summary. In the acute phase, the blood glucose level is elevated. There is rapid utilization of glycogen, amino acids, and fatty acids for energy. Within a few days or a week, the body enters an adaptation phase.

Later Response (Adaptation Phase)

In the adaptation phase, there is a decrease in the blood glucose and blood urea nitrogen levels. At the same time, ketosis and ketosuria appear. In some instances of prolonged stress, such as that seen in neurosurgical patients, the body does not develop starvation ketosis of the adaptation phase but continues to break down body protein mass.[5,6] There are about 6 kg of protein in the average adult. Between 25 gm and 75 gm will be metabolized daily, yielding 100 to 300 calories daily.[7] In the catabolic phase, the patient can lose 10 gm to 30 gm of nitrogen daily as the

TABLE 6-4. *Mineral Requirements and Their Functions*

Name	Functions
Major Minerals (relatively large amounts necessary for health)	
Calcium	• Necessary for bone formation, teeth, blood clotting • Involved in muscle contraction and relaxation, cardiac function, and transmission of nerve impulses • Activates enzymes • Affects the permeability of the cell membrane
Chloride	• Regulates osmotic pressure and acid-base balance • Activates the enzyme amylase in saliva
Magnesium	• Important cation within the cell • Involved in the function of B vitamins • Necessary for the utilization of potassium, calcium, and protein • Assists in the maintenance of electrical activity in muscles and nerves
Phosphorus	• Involved in bone formation and nerve and muscle action • Involved in carbohydrate metabolism, fatty acid transport, and energy metabolism
Potassium	• Maintenance of intracellular osmotic pressure and acid-base balance • Involved in glycogen formation, contraction of muscle fibers, and transmission of electrical impulses within the heart
Sodium	• Maintenance of extracellular osmotic pressure and acid-base balance • Involved in cell permeability, absorption of glucose, muscle irritability, and muscle contraction
Trace Minerals (small amounts necessary for health)	
Cadmium	• Function not clear but appears to be involved in basic biological systems
Chromium	• Associated with glucose metabolism
Copper	• Component of certain enzymes and elastin • Involved in the formation of myelin, melanin pigment formation, and synthesis of hemoglobin • Involved in the maintenance of bones and neurological function
Fluoride	• Involved in the mineralization of bones and teeth and helps prevent the development of dental caries and osteoporosis
Iodine	• Necessary for skin integrity, thyroid function, and neuromuscular function
Iron	• Component of hemoglobin, myoglobin, and certain enzymes • Involved in normal blood platelet production, oxygen transport and utilization, and integrity of the mucous membrane
Manganese	• Activates several enzymes • Involved in formation of urea, central nervous system function, carbohydrate and fat metabolism, and synthesis of cartilage
Molybdenum	• Component of certain enzymes • Involved in fatty acid utilization and bone formation
Nickel	• Associated with thyroid hormone and ribonucleic acid (RNA)
Selenium	• Associated with fat metabolism • Component of the enzyme that protects red blood cells from damage
Silicon	• Necessary in bone, cartilage, and connective tissue formation
Tin	• Involved in protein synthesis and enzyme systems
Vanadium	• Thought to be involved in bone and teeth formation
Zinc	• Associated with skin integrity and wound healing • Involved with normal sense of taste and smell, bone growth and strength, and sexual maturation • Component of several enzymes

TABLE 6-5. *Differences in Early Metabolic Responses to Fasting and Injury*

Metabolic Activity	Fasting	After Injury
Glucose levels	Low	High (hallmark of stress response)
Protein catabolism	Low	High
Fat catabolism	High	Low/none
Ketosis	Present	Absent
Ketosuria	Present	Absent
Basal metabolism rate	Low	High

result of protein breakdown. The excessive amount of nitrogenous waste challenges the ability of the kidneys to excrete the urea. The increase in urea also has an effect on the osmotic pressure in the tubules, causing an increased amount of water to be excreted. Unless a high-protein diet is given, wound healing and recovery will be seriously hampered.

RESPONSE TO STARVATION

Early Phase

After several hours without food intake, the body responds to frank starvation by *conservation*. Initially, the lowered glucose level causes a drop in the circulating insulin. The level of glucagon increases and activates glycogenolysis (glucose produced from glycogen liver stores for 24 to 36 hours). The liver now metabolizes amino acids for energy, which causes a gradual increase in the blood urea nitrogen (BUN) level for 2 to 4 days. Protein catabolism provides energy for the glucose-dependent brain.[7] The decreased level of insulin appears to be the major control in lipolysis. Lipolysis produces free fatty acids and glycerol.[8] Utilization of body fat gradually increases over the next 20 to 40 days, so that the blood urea nitrogen level gradually decreases.[9]

In brief starvation, the following characteristics are noted: there is an increase in urine nitrogen and urinary output; rapid weight loss occurs; and there is a decrease in muscle mass, serum glucose, and circulating insulin.

Later Developments (Keto-Adaptation Phase)

The body now enters the keto-adaptation phase as more body fat is metabolized. This period of prolonged starvation can last for several months. There is an increase in ketosis and ketosuria, both of which are related to the by-products of fat metabolism. Ketone bodies contribute to the conservation of muscle protein. Another important adaptive change noted at this time is that the brain utilizes ketone bodies as its major source of energy.

The characteristic changes noted in prolonged starvation can be summarized as the following:[8]

- Increased fat catabolism
- Slow weight loss
- Slow loss of muscle mass
- Increased urinary ammonia levels
- Decreased urinary urea and nitrogen levels
- Metabolic acidosis that is usually compensated for by respiratory alkalosis
- Decreased basal metabolism rate and body temperature
- Increased extracellular fluid and peripheral edema (late finding)

Premorbid Starvation Phase

When the fat stores of the body are exhausted, the patient enters a premorbid state of starvation. Protein muscle mass is utilized for energy so that decreased muscle mass and rapid weight loss ensue. Death will result unless aggressive nutritional support is given.

EFFECTS OF MALNUTRITION

A short period (less than 1 week) of catabolism can be tolerated by the well-nourished patient without negative effects. However, for patients who were poorly nourished before the injury or who are unable to establish a normal eating pattern within a week of injury, serious problems will develop. The depletion of protein from the body produces a catabolic state of malnutrition with the following consequences:

- Compromised wound healing
- Predisposition to development of decubiti ulcers
- Decreased immunological response to infection
- Increased susceptibility to development of complications
- Increased mortality

MALNUTRITION SYNDROMES

Two types of malnutrition syndromes may be found in hospitalized patients:

1. *Marasmus*. The patient appears malnourished as a result of rapid loss of fat and muscle mass because of improper protein and caloric intake. The visceral protein is maintained until the muscle mass is severely depleted. Clinically, the patient appears grossly underweight with loss of both muscle mass and subcutaneous fat. Diarrhea is common. Metabolic activity is decreased and prostration is seen.
2. *Protein deficiency state*. This condition is found in the normal or obese patient who has undergone stress. The patient has an above-standard fat store and muscle mass, but the visceral protein store is depleted. The disorder is similar to kwashiorkor syndrome in children. Clinical evidence of protein deficiency includes edema, muscular wasting, depigmentation of hair and skin, scaly and flaky skin, hypoalbuminemia, moderate anemia, and diarrhea.

Other clinical signs and symptoms that are associated with malnutrition are hair loss, dull looking hair, seborrhea, swelling of the tongue, and bleeding from the gums.

NUTRITIONAL ASSESSMENT

Various nutritional assessment protocols have been developed to determine the patient's nutritional status, identify specific nutritional deficits, and develop appropriate nutritional therapy to meet the patient's needs. A team approach that includes the physician, nurse, and clinical dietician is helpful. If there is a nutritional services department in the facility, a multidisciplinary team may be asked to provide nutritional consultation for the patient. In other organizational structures, the physician and the nurse may be solely responsible for nutritional assessment. Patients should be screened for nutritional support very soon after they have been hospitalized (within the first 24 hours). Nutritional assessment can easily be forgotten when life-threatening events occur. However, without sufficient nutritional support, wound healing will be delayed, the patient will have increased susceptibility to infections, and overall recovery will be seriously hampered.

In assessing the nutritional status of a patient, the following data are collected:

1. Physical inspection of the patient includes the following: skin for turgor, dryness, edema, or easy bruising; mucous membranes for dryness, color, bruising, or bleeding (especially gums for easy bleeding); tongue for swelling and papillary atrophy; eyes for pale or dry conjunctiva or sunken eyeballs; and muscles for atrophy or wasting.
2. The dietary and weight loss history is documented. An involuntary weight loss of 10% or more in 1 year is considered significant. Information on recent dietary changes and what constitutes a normal daily dietary intake is noted.
3. Anthropometric measurements are considered, including weight, height, triceps skinfold (TSF), arm muscle circumference (AMC), and mid-upper-arm circumference (MUAC). These data provide information about growth, development, and body composition (they measure body fat and lean body muscle). Abnormally low values indicate that protein stores have been depleted. Data can be distorted if the patient is obese or edematous.

   The triceps skinfold is calculated by lifting the skin of the posterior arm away from the triceps muscle and measuring the skinfold thickness with standard calipers. The measurement is made midway between the posterior aspect of the top of the shoulder and the bony projection of the elbow. If the patient can stand, the arm should hang freely. The bedridden patient should be positioned flat in bed and then his arm raised upright. Mid-upper-arm circumference is measured at the same point as the triceps skinfold. The mid-upper-arm circumference indicates the fat and protein stores available. The arm muscle circumference is a good indicator of protein nutrition and can be calculated from the other two arm measurements:

   $$\text{AMC (cm)} = \text{MUAC (cm)} - (3.14 \times \text{TSF cm})$$

4. Laboratory studies include
   - Serum creatinine (0.6 mg–1.2 mg/dl), which is an end product of protein metabolism; indicates depletion of muscle mass
   - Serum albumin (3.3 gm–4.5 gm/dl); estimates visceral protein stores
   - Serum total protein (6.6 gm–7.9 gm/dl); estimates visceral protein stores
   - Blood urea nitrogen (8 mg–20 mg/dl); indicates rate of protein metabolism
   - Blood glucose (70 mg–100 mg/dl); indicates a prime energy source
   - Serum transferrin (250 mcg–390 mcg/dl); indicates iron-transporting capacity and excess protein loss
   - Total iron-binding capacity (300 mcg–400 mcg/dl for men and 300 mcg–450 mcg/dl for women); estimates visceral protein stores
   - Serum osmolality; estimates water balance
   - Serum free fatty acids; estimates fat breakdown
   - Liver function studies
   - Kidney function studies
   - 24-hour urine urea nitrogen (maximal clearance: 64 ml–99 ml/minute); measures nitrogen balance
   - 24-hour creatinine height index (84 ml–90 ml/minute); indicates degree of muscle depletion
   - Serum sodium, chloride, potassium, calcium, phosphorus, magnesium, and cholesterol; indicate electrolyte balance and nutritional status
   - Total white blood cell count, total lymphocyte count, hemoglobin and hematocrit; indicate immune response, anemia, and fluid balance
5. Immune function is assessed by examining the total white blood cell count and the total lymphocyte count. When protein malnutrition exists, there is a decrease in peripheral lymphocytes (also a decreased ability to fight infection).
6. Cellular immunity response, in the malnourished patient, shows a decrease in the synthesis of antibodies and the antibody response. Tests used to assess this response may include purified protein derivative skin test, mumps skin test, and others. In the malnourished patient there is a delay (greater than 24 hours) in response. In the normal person, a response is noted within 24 hours.

ONGOING ASSESSMENT

The nurse can determine the patient's nutritional status by following these steps:

- Weighing the patient twice a week and noting trends in stability of the weight
- Observing skin turgor, condition of the tongue, muscle tone, and muscle bulk on a daily bases
- Assessing the intake and output record daily
- Noting the patient's energy level (if he is conscious)
- Monitoring appropriate laboratory data

COMMON NEUROLOGICAL PROBLEMS THAT INTERFERE WITH NUTRITION

For a patient to consume a normal oral diet that will then be digested and supply the necessary nutrients for the body, several functions must be intact. The patient must be alert and oriented and have an attention span sufficient for concentrating on the task at hand; he must be able to feed himself, chew, and swallow; and he must be able to digest and utilize the nutrients through a functional gastrointestinal tract. Many patients with neurological and neurosurgical problems have deficits that interfere with adequate nutrition. Common deficits that interfere with adequate nutrition in these patients are as follows:

- Altered levels of consciousness (e.g., confusion, stupor, restlessness, coma)
- Alterations in mentation (e.g., short attention span, distractibility, refusal to eat)
- Diminished or absent swallowing or gag reflex
- Paresis or paralysis of arms necessary for feeding self
- Paresis or paralysis of muscles of mastication and/or the tongue
- Irradiation or chemotherapy for nervous system neoplasms, which results in anorexia, nausea, vomiting, and excessive weight loss

Special protocols and alternative methods of providing nutrition are necessary to support the nutritional needs of the patient.

SPECIAL NEUROLOGICAL DISORDERS AND THEIR EFFECTS ON THE PATIENT'S NUTRITION

A number of common neurological disorders affect the nutritional needs of the patient. Several of these disorders and the interventions used in addressing these problems are presented in Table 6–6.

Dexamethasone (Decadron) is a drug frequently ordered for neurological and neurosurgical problems. Several metabolic changes are associated with the use of the drug; these are particularly significant for the patient undergoing the stress response to injury or early starvation. If a steroid such as dexamethasone is ordered for the patient, it is usually ordered on admission with a course of therapy to last several days. This time period coincides with the early responses to stress. The specific points of steroid therapy that relate to the patient's nutritional status include the following:

- Increased salt and water retention and increased excretion of potassium
- Increased calcium excretion
- Decreased carbohydrate tolerance
- Development of negative nitrogen balance because of increased protein catabolism
- Possible development of hypercholesterolemia and hypertriglyceridemia
- Electrolyte imbalance
- Impaired wound healing
- Modification of the body's immune response

The nurse should keep these effects of glucocorticosteroid therapy in mind when considering the nutritional effects of illness on the patient.

METHODS OF PROVIDING NUTRITION FOR NEUROLOGICAL AND NEUROSURGICAL PATIENTS

Initially, the hospitalized neurological or neurosurgical patient may be given intravenous fluid if he is unable to consume a diet orally. For a patient who is well nourished, a few days of intravenous therapy will not be harmful to his nutritional status. However, few calories can be administered by the peripheral intravenous route, and the patient must rely on body stores to provide necessary nutrients and calories. In a liter of 5% dextrose and water, there are only

TABLE 6–6. *Nutritional Implications in Specific Neurological Disorders*

Disorders	Nutritional Effects	Correction

Epilepsy (drugs used in treating the various types of epilepsies cause nutritional deficits)	• Primidone, phenobarbitol, and phenytoin can cause decreased serum levels of several B-complex vitamins.
	• Phenytoin can cause
	  • Megaloblastic anemia
	  • Carbohydrate intolerance (rarely) that can lead to hyperosmolar coma
		• Supplement with B-complex vitamins.
		• Provide supplemental folic acid.
		• Monitor serum glucose levels.

Parkinson's disease	• Levodopa is not as effective if patient is on a high-protein diet and taking pyridoxine	• Avoid a high-protein diet. • Avoid multivitamins that include pyridoxine
Spinal cord injuries	• Loss of calcium from bones from not bearing weight (increased possibility of urinary tract calculi) • Negative nitrogen balance (loss of protein from muscles)	• Provide fluid intake of at least 3000 ml/day to "flush" the urinary tract to prevent infection and calculi. • Increase protein intake to about 125 gm/day. • Administer supplemental vitamins.
Head injuries and comatose state	• Negative nitrogen balance due to nothing being taken by mouth and limited coloric intake by intravenous route • Dehydration from altered osmotic gradient due to drugs that increase excretion of water (during catabolic phase) • Loss of calcium from bones if not weight bearing	• Administer high protein 1.5 gm to 2.0 gm/kg/day. • Administer sufficient water. • Give supplemental vitamins and minerals. • Provide 2000 to 5000 calories/day.
Infectious processes that increase body temperature (meningitis, encephalitis, abscess)	• Elevated temperature increases metabolic rate • Loss of fluid through perspiration with fever	• Increase caloric intake to 2000 to 5000 calories/day • Increase fluid intake to compensate for fluid loss.
Increased activity states such as seen with decortication/decerebration, restlessness, agitation, seizure activity, delirium tremors, chorea	• Need additional calories to compensate for energy expended	• Increase caloric intake to 2000 to 5000 calories/day; a nutritional consultation should be conducted

200 calories. If the patient is unable to consume an adequate diet by the oral route within a few days, then a nasogastric tube, other enteral tube, or total parenteral nutrition will be necessary to nourish the patient. An assessment of the patient will be necessary to determine his nutritional needs and the best method to meet those needs.

Alternative methods of providing adequate nutrition (tube feeding, total parenteral nutrition) as well as special procedures for oral feeding will be discussed in the following sections.

FEEDING TUBES

Feeding tubes have been employed to provide nutrition on a temporary basis to patients who are unable to ingest food by the normal oral route. The feeding tube is inserted through the nose and into the stomach or upper small bowel. The type and the size of feeding tube chosen vary, with obvious advantages and disadvantages with each choice. Large, hard feeding tubes can cause erosion of the nose, nasal passages, esophagus, and stomach, but the large bore of the tube ensures better delivery of the feeding without congealing. Smaller, softer tubes are less likely to erode tissue, but the tube is more likely to become occluded by congealed tube feeding.

In certain patients the use of a feeding tube is undesirable or contraindicated. Some of the common reasons that a feeding tube may be avoided follow:

- When long-term nutritional support will be required
- When a basal skull fracture, facial fractures, or leakage of cerebrospinal fluid is present
- When injury has been sustained or there is a disease process affecting the oropharynx, esophagus, or other portions of the gastrointestinal tract

In these situations, a gastrostomy or jejunostomy tube may be inserted.

Beginning Feedings

After the nasogastric, gastrostomy, or jejunostomy tube is inserted, feedings are not begun until bowel sounds have returned. A small amount of water or 5% dextrose and water is often the initial feeding. The following points are observed in beginning feedings:

- Begin with 50 ml by gavage feeding and administer it slowly.
- If a food pump is to be used, begin at a slow rate of about 30 ml/hour.
- If the water is tolerated, begin a commercial or blenderized tube feeding slowly. Some physicians order dilution of the feeding with half water initially to improve the patient's tolerance of the nutrients.
- Observe the patient for intolerance or any untoward effects (e.g., distention, vomiting, diarrhea).
- Maintain an accurate intake and output record.

NURSING RESPONSIBILITIES IN ADMINISTERING NASOGASTRIC FEEDINGS

Nasogastric feedings may be administered in one of two ways: continuously with the use of a food pump or intermittently with the use of a gavage bag. Special nursing protocols are followed to prevent vomiting and aspiration of the feeding. The patient should be observed frequently and suction equipment should be handy and ready should evidence of aspiration develop. The nursing interventions and responsibilities for the patient receiving nasogastric feeding follow:

1. Raise the head of the bed 30 to 45 degrees.
2. Check the position of the tube to be sure that it is in the stomach.
   - Aspirate gastric contents.
   - Inject about 5 cc of air into the tube and listen with a stethoscope just below the xiphoid process for the sound of air entering the stomach.
   - Place the end of the feeding tube into a cup of water; if there are periodic bubbles that synchronize with respirations, the tube is probably in the lung.
3. Aspirate the tube to determine if the previous feeding has been absorbed; if 100 ml or more of residual feeding is aspirated, the feeding should be withheld or the food pump turned off for 2 hours; this information should be reported. It may be necessary to reevaluate the patient's feeding schedule. In 2 hours, aspirate the tube again to reassess the amount of residual feeding present. If there is a minimal amount or no residual feeding remaining, begin the feeding again.
4. If the patient has a tracheostomy tube in place, inflate the cuff; keep it inflated for 1 hour after completion of the feeding. The purpose of this action is to prevent aspiration.
5. Intermittent feedings should be administered over 30 to 60 minutes depending on the amount of the feeding. On completion of the feeding, cleanse the tubing with 50 ml of water and clamp the tube.
6. Record the amount and type of feeding on the intake and output record.
7. Monitor the patient's weight; weighing the patient twice a week is usually adequate.
8. Monitor the following laboratory studies: blood urea nitrogen, serum electrolytes, and serum creatinine.
9. Observe the patient for signs and symptoms of dehydration from hyperosmolar feedings that can lead to hyperosmolar nonketotic coma. Be sure that adequate supplemental water is ordered for the patient especially if hyperosmolar feedings are being administered.
10. Monitor the urine for specific gravity and adequacy of output.
11. Observe the patient for signs and symptoms of abdominal distention, regurgitation, aspiration, nausea/vomiting, diarrhea, or intolerance to the feeding.

INDICATIONS FOR A GASTROSTOMY OR JEJUNOSTOMY

Many serious problems can develop from prolonged nasogastric intubation. Possible problems include erosion and/or necrosis of the nares or nasal septum, peptic esophagitis from gastric reflux along the tube, and gastric erosion or ulcers. The need for prolonged tube feeding is an indication for a simple surgical procedure in which a gastrostomy or jejunostomy tube is sutured into position. After the tube is inserted, it is usually left to gravity drainage for the first 24 to 48 hours. When bowel sounds have returned, a small amount of water or glucose and water, as outlined earlier, is begun. The insertion site is treated as any other surgical wound:

- The incision and tissue around the tube are cleansed daily with normal saline and hydrogen peroxide; other cleansing protocols may be used.
- An aseptic ointment may be applied around the tube.
- A dry sterile dressing is applied over the incision and around the tube.
- The wound and the area around the tube are observed for any signs or symptoms of infection.
- The incision should be dressed and assessed on a daily basis.

Feedings can be administered intermittently a few times a day, or a food pump may be used to provide nutrition on a continual basis.

TYPES OF TUBE FEEDINGS

Tube feedings can be classified into three major categories: elemental, low-residue, and blenderized diets. An *elemental diet* provides nutrients in the simplest chemical form for easy absorption with no residue. Nitrogen and protein are given in the form of amino acids, and the carbohydrate is supplied as simple sugar or glucose. This is best administered by way of tube feeding because it has an unpleasant taste if administered orally. Elemental formulas are prepared commercially and are fortified with vitamins and minerals.

The *low-residue diet* is a variation of the elemental diet and uses albumin as the protein source. It is more palatable than the elemental diet. The *blenderized diet* is prepared from table food by blenderizing the food. It must be fortified with vitamin and mineral supplements, but it is much more economical than the commercially prepared feedings. Examples of commonly used commercially prepared feedings are included in Table 6–7.

TABLE 6–7. *Selected Commercially Prepared Tube Feedings (Calculations/1000 ml)*

Product	*Calories*	*Protein (gm)*	*Carbohydrates (gm)*	*Fat (gm)*	*mOsm/kg**	*Comment*
Ensure	1060	37	143	37	450	Lactose free May be used as a full liquid diet, liquid supplement, or tube feeding
Ensure Plus	1500	54	197	52.5	600	High-calorie liquid diet For tube or supplemental oral feeding
Citrotein	533	32	97	1.4	496	For tube or supplemental oral feedings; lactose free
Flexical	1000	22.5	152	0.34	805	For tube or oral feeding; lactose free
Isocal (regular)	1000	33	125	43	350	Lactose free
Isocal (high calorie and nitrogen)	2000	73.5	221.6	89.6	690	Lactose free For tube feeding only
Magnacal	2000	70	250	80	590	High caloric density Nutritionally complete for oral or tube feeding
Osmolite	1006	37	143	38	300	Tube or oral feeding; lactose free
Sustacal	1000	65	148	24	625	Tube or oral feeding
Vivonex	1000	20.4	225	13	550	Lactose free
Vivonex HN (high nitrogen)	1000	43	210	0.9	844	High nitrogen feeding to restore positive nitrogen balance For tube feeding only Requires no digestion Full-strength Vivonex HN is hypertonic and has an osmolarity of 810 mOsm/kg; vomiting, diarrhea, and dumping syndrome can occur

* Formulas of high osmolarity (more than 450 mOsm) are often associated with the dumping syndrome and diarrhea.

PROBLEMS ASSOCIATED WITH TUBE FEEDINGS

Several potential problems and complications are associated with the use of tube feedings. These potential problems and the appropriate nursing interventions are presented in Table 6–8.

One important consideration with the use of continuous enteral tube feeding for patients who are receiving phenytoin (Dilantin) should be mentioned. It was noted in some studies that patients receiving continuous feedings required larger doses of phenytoin to maintain therapeutic levels. These patients also developed signs and symptoms of phenytoin toxicity when the tube feedings were discontinued.[10] It appears that enteral tube feedings interfere with phenytoin absorption. Many patients receive both continuous enteral feedings and phenytoin therapy simultaneously. Larger doses of phenytoin will be required when the patient is receiving simultaneous tube feedings. The dosage will need to be evaluated and probably decreased when the tube feeding is discontinued. The patient should have phenytoin levels monitored routinely when he is receiving phenytoin therapy, and he should be assessed for signs and symptoms of toxicity.

TOTAL PARENTERAL NUTRITION (TPN)

Total parenteral nutrition, also known as parenteral hyperalimentation, is a method of administering a highly concentrated hypertonic solution of essential nutrients intravenously to provide the total nutritional needs of the patient over an extended period. This method of providing nutrition can be initiated early in the acute stage (within 24 to 48 hours) to maintain the nutritional needs of the patient. Some patients may be able to convert to enteral feedings, but there are those who will need to continue on total parenteral nutrition for various reasons. The usual criteria for the selection of patients to use total parenteral nutrition follow:

- Inability to eat or use the gastrointestinal tract for digestion and absorption of food
- Involuntary loss of 10% of body weight
- Existence of a state of malnutrition
- Existence of a hypermetabolic or a catabolic state

Neurological or neurosurgical patients who are good candidates for total parenteral nutrition include the following:

- Multi-trauma patients with gastrointestinal injuries that interfere with digestion and absorption of nutrients
- Patients with extensive sepsis
- Malnourished patients who are in a severe catabolic state (negative nitrogen balance) associated with such conditions as prolonged coma, spinal cord trauma, and other major injuries

A large-bore catheter is inserted into the subclavian vein or vena cava for administration of the total parenteral nutrition solution. The solution administered is prepared in the pharmacy under strict aseptic conditions. The solution provides the following:

- Carbohydrates: 20% to 25% glucose
- Protein: amino acids as a nitrogen source to counteract the negative nitrogen balance
- Vitamins
- Minerals
- Electrolytes
- Water

The contents of the total parenteral nutrition provide sufficient amounts of nutrients to allow for tissue repair and building and normal physiological activity. Each liter of solution can provide 1000 calories. The usual precautions of administering a hyperosmolar solution should be followed. The patient should be monitored using the following parameters:

- Stable rate of infusion of fluid that is checked at least every hour
- Urine for sugar and acetone checked every 6 hours
- Urine specific gravity checked every 6 hours
- Intake and output record kept
- Weight taken and recorded at least twice a week
- Complete nutritional profile of laboratory studies recorded as discussed earlier

Patients receiving total parenteral nutrition should also receive fat emulsions such as 500 ml of intralipid once or twice weekly by the intravenous route to prevent essential fatty acid deficiency.

More studies are being conducted to address nutritional support and outcome in patients. Results indicate that patients supported with total parenteral nutrition have improved outcomes when compared with those supported with enteral tube feedings. One study indicated better survival rates and improved functional outcomes for head injury patients managed with early parenteral feedings (within 48 hr of hospitalization).[11] This supports other studies that recommend aggressive early parenteral nutritional support of total parenteral nutrition for critically ill patients.

ORAL FEEDINGS

The goal for the nutritional management of the patient is that he may be rehabilitated so that he will be able to consume an adequate diet by the oral route. Before beginning to feed the patient by the oral route, several nursing actions should be initiated:

- Assess the gag and swallowing reflexes. Do *not* initiate oral feedings if the gag or swallowing reflexes are not intact because aspiration is possible.
- Note the presence of any facial weakness. The paresis or paralysis may be confined to only one side of the face.
- Auscultate the abdomen for the presence of bowel sounds. Oral feedings are *not* begun or resumed if bowel sounds are absent.
- Elevate the head of the bed to the sitting position.
- Be certain that suction equipment is readily available and in good working order, should it be needed.

TABLE 6–8. *Potential Problems Encountered With Tube Feedings*

Problem	Possible Cause(s)	Nursing Actions
Diarrhea	• Hyperosmolarity of feeding (usually 450 mOsm/liter or more)	• Begin very slowly and allow patient to adapt to formula. • Dilute feeding or give free water. • If ordered, a few drops of deodorized tincture of opium (DTO) may be added.
	• Rapid rate of infusion	• Give very slowly until gastrointestinal tract adapts to the feeding. • Feeding may have to be discontinued and started again slowly in a diluted form. • If diarrhea is not extensive, paregoric or diphenoxylate (Lomotil) may be given temporarily.
	• Lactose intolerance	• Avoid feeding with lactose unless patient normally drinks milk daily without ill effects.
Constipation	• Diet high in milk content • Inadequate fluid intake	• Change type of feeding. • Give sufficient free water in diet. • Record frequency of bowel movement. • Give stool softeners and mild laxatives if necessary.
Vomiting	• Feeding too soon after intubation or suctioning • Too rapid rate of infusion	• Allow patient a rest period before beginning feeding • Run slowly.
Dumping syndrome	• Too rapid infusion of hyperosmolar solutions	• Run slowly. • Administer free water after intermittent feeding to dilute intake.
Dehydration	• Rapid infusion of hyperosmolar carbohydrates that cause hyperglycemia → osmotic diuretic → dehydration • Excessive protein and electrolytes (have an osmotic effect)	• Administer slowly. • Check sugar and acetone periodically (usually every 6 hours). • May need to administer regular insulin to cover glycosuria. • Adjust formula. • Administer free water. • Monitor serum electrolytes and balance as necessary.
Edema	• Excessive sodium in formula	• Change feeding as necessary. • Monitor serum electrolytes. • Balance electrolytes with drug therapy as ordered.
Aspiration	• Feeding tube not in stomach/jejunum • Vomiting (see vomiting for description) • *Note:* Aspiration can cause pneumonia; every precaution should be taken to prevent aspiration	• Check position of tube *before* beginning feeding. • Position with head of bed elevated 30 to 45 degrees. • Have suction equipment handy.
Plugging of feeding tube	• Coagulation of feeding in tube due to spoilage of feeding • Low pH of gastric secretions causes plugging at the end of the feeding tube	• Place container with feeding into a basin of ice. • Rock salt may be added to ice to keep it from melting as quickly in hot weather. • Flush tubing with water after each feeding. • Change connecting tube daily if it is disposable or washable.
Excessive feeding in stomach upon aspiration	• Malabsorption of feeding	• Give feeding at a slower rate. • Aspirate feeding tube periodically (every 4 to 6 hours; if more than 75 ml to 100 ml are obtained, report it and postpone feeding; check again in 2 hours to see if contents have been absorbed (if patient receiving feeding through a food pump, turn off the machine for 2 hours and then recheck). • May need to change type of feeding.
Other intolerance to feeding	• Renal or hepatic disease (patient may not tolerate even normal levels of amino acids)	• Change feeding. • Monitor kidney and liver blood studies before and during administration of feedings).
Malnutrition	• Inadequate diet (protein, carbohydrate, fats, minerals, or vitamins)	• Check type of feeding; supplement with vitamins, minerals, and other requirements as necessary.
Negative nitrogen balance	• Inadequate intake of nitrogen (protein chief source of nitrogen) • Catabolic state	• Monitor blood urea nitrogen and creatinine levels. • Weigh periodically. • Increase nitrogen intake.

- If the patient has a tracheostomy tube in place, inflate the cuff before beginning to offer oral intake. The cuff is kept inflated for 45 to 60 minutes after the feeding is completed.

Once the preliminary assessment and necessary precautions have been taken to prevent aspiration of oral intake, the nurse can initiate oral nutrition. The following points will guide the process:

- Begin with clear liquids. The patient should be encouraged to take a small sip through a straw, hold it in his mouth, and then swallow it.
- If he cannot manage a straw, offer a gelatine dessert from a spoon. (If the patient has any facial weakness, give the diet on the nonaffected side.)
- Give small feedings, and frequently assess the patient's response to and tolerance of the feeding.
- If the clear liquids are well tolerated, the patient can progress to pureed foods and then to a soft diet. Continue to assess his tolerance of the diet and progress slowly.
- Progress to a regular diet, as tolerated. Encourage a well-balanced diet.
- Assess the patient's ability to feed himself. Cognitive, motor, and coordination deficits may interfere with this activity. Several problems that interfere with eating can be identified. These problems and appropriate nursing actions are described in Table 6–9.
- *Note:* Although it can be time consuming to supervise a patient while he eats, it is an important consideration in the rehabilitation process and achievement of independence. Every effort should be made to assist the patient in achieving this goal.

FLUID-RESTRICTED DIETS

One component of the overall approach to management of increased intracranial pressure and cerebral edema is the fluid-restricted diet. The purpose of the diet is to limit fluid intake so that the patient is kept slightly underhydrated. The resultant hemoconcentration will draw fluid across an osmotic gradient and decrease cerebral edema and intracranial pressure. Overhydration of a patient will contribute to increasing intracranial pressure and cerebral edema.

A fluid-restricted diet is ordered by the physician in the number of milliliters of fluid allowed in a 24-hour period.

TABLE 6–9. ***Problems Encountered With Oral Feeding***

Problem	*Description*	*Nursing Action*
Distractibility	Becomes interested in the activity around him and stops eating	• Screen patient from distraction. • Take excess dishes off his tray. • Redirect his attention to eating.
Inability to concentrate	Forgets what he is doing or forgets what to do with his food once he gets it on his eating utensil	• Screen patient from excessive environmental stimuli. • Break activity of eating into steps and direct the patient in the steps of eating (e.g., pick up the potatoes with your spoon, lift it to your mouth, open your mouth).
Disorientation	• Is not always aware of time, place, his person • May think that the food belongs to someone else or that it is poisoned	• Provide reality orientation and assist patient in feeding himself. • Give many verbal cues for eating. • Correct any misconceptions. • Reassure patient in a calm voice.
Visual deficits such as diplopia, dimness, or hemianopsia		• Be sure patient has glasses on if he normally wears glasses.
	• Double vision	• Apply eye patch to one eye or cover one lens if double vision is present.
	• Loss of vision in half of the visual field (hemianopia)	• If patient eats food on only one side of his dish, turn his dish; remind him to turn his head to scan his dish
	• Vision may be dim or fuzzy	• Good light may be of some help for dimness
Motor deficits (plegia or paresis)		
Muscles of chewing, of the face or tongue	• May be deficits of cranial nerves V, VII, or XII	• Encourage patient to put food on unaffected side.
Arm or hand	• Associated with hemiparesis or hemiplegia; monoplegia of one extremity may be present	• See if patient can eat with other hand. • Use built-up eating utensils. • Use special equipment such as a guard around plate to prevent food from spilling off dish. • Consult with occupational therapist for suggestions. • Prepare patient's tray (e.g., cut up meat, pour milk).

The patient must stay within the fluid restriction. All intake, regardless of the route—oral, enteral, or intravenous—is calculated in the total. For example, a patient may be placed on a 1500-ml fluid-restricted diet. The nurse must now assess the patient's dietary intake, intravenous fluid intake, and need for other fluid intake. Let's assume that the patient is receiving a tray from the dietary department three times a day. An intravenous infusion is maintained as a "keep open" because the patient is receiving an antibiotic by the intravenous route every 8 hours. The drug must be given in 50 ml of fluid and a 10-ml flush is necessary after each administration of the drug. The patient also receives oral medication (tablets) four times a day. The nurse must plan how to allocate the overall fluid allotment. The following calculations are made:

• "Keep open" will provide	400 ml/24 hours
• For intravenous medication	180 ml/24 hours
• For oral medications 60 ml × 4	240 ml/24 hours
• Total for three meals	680 ml/24 hours
	1500 ml/24 hours

The nurse will have to carefully check the patient's trays to be sure that he had no more than 680 ml combined fluid intake for all three meals. For a patient who chooses to have only coffee and orange juice for breakfast for a total of 200 ml, the remaining 480 ml is the total allocation for lunch and dinner. The patient and his family need to understand the purpose of the fluid-restricted diet. An accurate intake and output record must be maintained, and good communication between nurses on all shifts is needed.

Let us further assume that this same patient completes his course of antibiotic therapy and the intravenous infusion is removed. The only sources of intake now are his diet and the fluid needed to swallow his pills; thus, the nurse can redistribute the fluid intake. The nurse and the patient may decide to allocate some of the intake to an afternoon and a bedtime beverage. The distribution of fluid intake for the day is based on the patient's needs and the nurse's judgment, but the overall intake must be within the limits of the fluid restriction.

SUMMARY

The nutritional needs of a patient must be addressed early in his hospitalization to prevent states of malnutrition and negative nitrogen balance. The patient with a severe head injury or other serious neurological dysfunction will often have increased caloric needs that may exceed 4000 or 5000 calories. Unless the nutritional requirements for energy and tissue repair are met, the patient will not recover to his optimum potential.

REFERENCES

1. Rutten P, Blackburn GL: Determination of optimal hyperalimentation infusion rates. J Surg Res 18(5):478, 1975
2. Hoppe MC: Nutritional management of the trauma patient. Crit Care Q 6(1):1, June 1983
3. Wilmore DW: Hormonal responses and their effect on metabolism. Surg Clin North Am 56(5):999, 1976
4. Mequid MM et al: Hormone-substrate interrelationships following trauma. Arch Surg 109:776, 1976
5. Benotti P, Blackburn GL: Protein and caloric or macronutrient metabolic management of the critically ill patient. Crit Care Med 7(12):520, 1979
6. Blackburn GL, Bristrian BR: Curative nutrition. In Schneider HA (ed): Nutritional Support of Medical Practice, pp 80; 91–92. New York, Harper & Row, 1977
7. Taylor T: A comparison of two methods of nasogastric tube feedings. J Neurosurg Nurs 14(1):49, February 1982
8. Stotts NA, Friesen L: Understanding starvation in the critically ill patient. Heart Lung 11(5):471, September–October 1982
9. Behrends EA et al: Nutrition in neuro science. J Neurosurg Nurs 14(1):44, February 1982
10. Bauer LA: Interference of phenytoin absorption by continuous nasogastric feedings. Neurology 32:570, 1982
11. Rapp RP et al: The favorable effect of early parenteral feeding on survival in head-injury patients. J Neurosurg 58:906, 1983

BIBLIOGRAPHY

Books

Ballinger WF et al (eds): Manual of Surgical Nutrition. Philadelphia, WB Saunders, 1975
Bodinski LH: The Nurse's Guide to Diet Therapy. New York, John Wiley & Sons, 1982
Butterworth CE, Weinser RL: Malnutrition in hospital patients: Assessment and treatment. In Goodhart RS, Shils ME (eds): Modern Nutrition in Health and Disease, 6th ed. Philadelphia, Lea & Febiger, 1980
Howe JR: Manual of Patient Care and Neurosurgery, 2nd ed, pp 145–150. Boston, Little, Brown & Co, 1983
Jennett B, Teasdale G: Management of Head Injuries, pp 232–233. Philadelphia, FA Davis, 1981
Physicians' Desk Reference, 37th ed. Oradell, NJ, Medical Economics, 1983
Schneider AH (ed): Nutritional Support of Medical Practice. New York, Harper & Row, 1977
Smith RR: Essentials of Neurosurgery, pp 39–41. Philadelphia, JB Lippincott, 1980
Suitor CW, Hunter MF: Nutrition: Principles and Application in Health Promotion. Philadelphia, JB Lippincott, 1980
Williams SR: Nutrition and Diet Therapy. St Louis, CV Mosby, 1981

Periodicals

Anderson BJ: A theoretical protocol for nutritional maintenance in head-injured patients. J Neurosurg Nurs 16(1):50, February 1984
Borders CR (ed): Aggressive nutrition: Feeding the malnourished patient. Patient Care 50, January 30, 1981
Ensin J: Nutritional assessment of a severely head-injured, multi-trauma patient. J Neurosurg Nurs 14(5):262, October 1982
Hargrove R: Feeding the severely dysphagic patient. J Neurosurg Nurs 12(2):102, June 1980
Hostetler CA, Lipman T: Techniques for providing enteral nutrition. Drug Therap Hosp 12:31, 1980
Hutchison MM: Administration of fat emulsions. Am J Nurs 82(2):275, February 1982
Keithley JK: Infection and the malnourished patient. Heart Lung 12(1):23, January 1983

Koretz RL, Meyer JH: Elemental diets, facts and fantasies. Gastroenterology 78:393, 1980

Lumb PD, Dalton B, Bryan-Brown C, Donnelly C: Aggressive approach to intravenous feeding of the critically ill patient. Heart Lung 8(1):71, January-February 1979

McDonald E et al: A comparison of four holding devices for anchoring nasogastric tubes. J Neurosurg Nurs 14(2):90, April 1982

Salmond SW: How to assess the nutritional status of acutely ill patients. Am J Nurs 80(5):922, May 1980

Vernoski B, Chernow B: Steroids: Use and abuse. Crit Care Q 6(3):28, December 1983

Wieman TJ: Nutritional requirements of the trauma patient. Heart Lung 7(2):278, March-April 1978

Zalago G, Chernow B: Hormones as therapeutic agents in the intensive care unit. Crit Care Q 6(3):75, December 1983

chapter 7

Emotional and Behavioral Responses to Neurological Illness

The purpose of this chapter is to provide a practical approach to patient assessment and nursing interventions for the major emotional and behavioral responses to neurological illness. The emotional needs of the family are considered, as well as the stresses and responses precipitated in the nursing staff who work with neurological and neurosurgical patients.

Injury or disease to the nervous system often has farreaching effects, not only on the neurological–physiological body system, but also on the cognitive and affective functions, personality, and individual characteristics that give the person his uniqueness, individuality, and identity. These compounded deficits and devastating losses create stresses for both the patient and family that tax coping and adaptive skills. Because many neurological conditions alter the person's cognitive abilities, the patient often lacks an awareness of the change in his behavior and cognitive functions. If he recognizes changes in these higher level functions, the patient may not have the insight into the cause, amount or degree, significance, or implications of the behavioral changes in relationship to his lifestyle.

Family members and significant others are better able to accept physiological changes in their loved ones than behavioral, cognitive, or personality changes. Changes in a patient's behavior affect group dynamics and interpersonal relationships. The normal patterns of family interactions are altered, and family structure changes accordingly. Changes in patterns of interaction and family structure also alter methods of problem solving and the use of effective coping mechanisms. These factors contribute additional stresses to the already stressful experience of neurological illness.

STRESS AND THE STRESS RESPONSE

The writings of Selye provide a basic foundation for understanding the physiological and psychological responses to stress. According to Selye, stress is defined as "the nonspecific response of the body to any type of increased demands upon it."[1] The increased demands on an organism are termed *stressors*, and the stressors cause stress. Regardless of whether the stressor is associated with a desirable effect (*eustress*) or an undesirable effect (*distress*), the same physiological responses are precipitated.[2] The interaction and integration of physiological and psychological responses to stress were documented by Selye and other writers who came before him such as Cannon and Jacobsen. Cannon is credited with recognizing that the physiological reactions of the sympathetic system that occur in response to various emotional states are similar to those that occur in response to biological precipitators.[3] Jacobsen noted similar reactions in the sympathetic nervous system and skeletal muscles in response to emotional states.[4]

Selye is credited with the introduction of the term "general adaptation syndrome" (GAS) into the literature. The *general adaptation syndrome* refers to the nonspecific reactions of the hypothalamic–pituitary–adrenocortical system to any type of stress. The general endocrine changes associated with the response are enlargement of the adrenal cortex, shrinkage of the thymus gland, and ulceration of the stomach (stress ulcers). These responses are mediated by the pituitary–adrenocortical axis of the neuroendocrine system and cause a multi-system response. Much interest and research have been devoted to understanding the neuroendocrine influence during stress.

In considering the general adaptation syndrome, three phases can be identified: (1) the alarm reaction, in which the sympathetic system is activated and subsequently activates the neuroendocrine system; (2) resistance to stress, a period of adaptation to the stress; and (3) exhaustion from stress, a time when the coping mechanisms are insufficient or ineffective for continuing to deal with the stress. The degree to which the general adaptation syndrome is implemented and the amount of time for which it is operational depend on the intensity and type of stress experienced. Selye suggested that continued intense stimulation from stress will lead to depletion of the organism's ability to respond at all or to respond effectively to stress.[5]

The concept of stress as a psychological phenomenon has evolved from the work of various theorists.[6–9] The conceptualization model of stress has taken on many diverse configurations. The critical components that contribute to the understanding of stress have been identified as follows: the stimulus (stressor) must be viewed as a threat by the individual; the stimulus, regardless of whether it is positive or negative, must be viewed as being significant or relevant to the individual's welfare; and the organism's capacity for adaptation must have been exceeded.[5] These critical components address the type and intensity of a stimulus, the individual's perception of the stimulus, and the duration of the stimulus that depletes the capacity to cope.

What kinds of stimuli cause activation of the stress response in the neurological patient? Any intense physical or psychological stimuli such as forced immobilization, trauma, pain, fear, threat of loss, lack of control, or anxiety can cause the multi-system stress response. It is also true that there are degrees of intensity of stimuli that cause a proportional stress response. For example, one would expect a much less intense stress response in a patient who has been admitted for an elective cranioplasty for cosmetic purposes long after an injury occurred than in a patient who has been admitted for a craniotomy for removal of a brain tumor of unidentified histological origin.

HUMAN ADAPTATION AND COPING

Adaptation is the process of change undertaken by an organism in response to a change in the internal or external environment for the purpose of maintaining equilibrium. Physiological adaptation supports survival and homeostasis within the organism. Psychological adaptation is directed toward maintaining a psychological homeostasis and supporting the self-concept and the self-esteem of the individual. Adaptation may be positive or negative in that the process either supports or is detrimental to the well-being of the individual. Behaviors that are detrimental to the individual are termed maladaptive behaviors. Those that support the well-being of the individual are called adaptive behaviors.

Much has been written about how individuals adapt to changes in their internal and external environment. The conceptualization of adaptation is central to the practice of nursing because much of the nurse's time and energy is directed at supporting healthy adaptation. Roy's conceptualization of adaptation has significantly influenced nursing since the early 1970s. As a theoretical approach, Roy's adaptation model views adaptation as a dynamic state of equilibrium between the individual and the environment. Roy identified several assumptions underlying the conceptualization of the person and the process of adaptation.[10] The assumptions include the following:

1. The person is a bio-psycho-social being.
2. The person is in constant interaction with a changing environment.
3. To cope with a changing world, the person uses both innate and acquired mechanisms, which are biological, psychological, and social in origin.
4. Health and illness are one inevitable dimension of the person's life.
5. To respond positively to environmental changes, the person must adapt.
6. The person's adaptation is a function of the stimulus he is exposed to and his adaptation level.
7. The person's adaptation level is such that it constitutes a zone indicating the range of stimulation that will lead to a positive response.
8. The person is conceptualized as having four modes of adaptation: physiological needs, self-concept, role function, and interdependence relations.

As Roy's model developed, other assumptions concerning the person evolved. They included[11,12]

1. As an adaptive system, the person functions as a totality. Adaptive behavior is behavior of the whole person.
2. The person has great potential for self-actualization.
3. The person is an active participant in his own destiny.

Roy's adaptation model has continued to develop and be refined over the years and has contributed to nursing theory by viewing the person's adaptation to a changing environment and promotion of health. The person is viewed as not only a biological being but also as a psychological and social being. The model has made a significant contribution by providing an approach to nursing practice. Other conceptual models have also been developed and are being refined and developed so that the approach to professional nursing practice offers options to the practitioner.

COPING

The word *coping* refers to methods, skills, or processes used by an individual in adapting to stresses in the internal or external environment. Coping has been defined in the literature in many different ways to fit the needs of particular models. However, the definition above is broad enough to provide a basic structure for the concept. Coping mechanisms may be effective in dealing with a stress (problem) or they may be ineffective. The choice of coping mechanisms and how they are applied to particular situations will affect the promotion of health in the health care setting. The role of the nurse is to assist and to support the patient so that he can use effective coping skills and mechanisms to deal with the stresses precipitated by illness.

NEUROLOGICAL ILLNESS AND ITS PSYCHOLOGICAL EFFECTS

Illness is a stressor that creates both physiological and psychological stress for the person involved. Stress responses may be viewed on a scale of gradation that varies depending on the amount of noxious stimuli, the patient's perception of the significance of the stimuli, and the length of time the stimuli remain. So far this discussion of stress, adaptation, and coping could be applied to either physiological or psychological stress. The discussion will now focus on the psychological stresses and psychological responses to neurological illness.

In the case of neurological illness, the psychological stressors and stress response can be particularly taxing on the person's ability to cope and adapt to the illness. Common situations, concerns, and losses precipitated by neurological illness may include the following:

- Threat to survival
- Threat to the quality of life as it was known before illness—lifestyle, occupation, social and recreational activities, freedom to make changes, and control over one's being and destiny
- Development of neurological deficits such as
  - Paresis/paralysis (interferes with mobility, swallowing, self-control, speech)
  - Bowel/bladder dysfunction
  - Communication deficits
  - Sexual dysfunction
  - Emotional deficits and responses (emotional lability, aggression, depression, anxiety)
  - Cognitive deficits (difficulty in reasoning, making judgments, memory)
  - Sensory deficits (hearing loss, loss of visual acuity, diplopia, paresthesias, anesthesia)
  - Autonomic deficits (orthostatic hypotension, loss of ability to perspire, difficulty in controlling body temperature)
- Precipitation of important and significant losses such as
  - Independence in the activities of daily living
  - Control over decisions that affect one's destiny
  - Ability to perceive the environment accurately through the senses (stimuli may be perceived as meaningless, confusing, or absent)
  - Ability to understand language and to express oneself verbally and in writing
  - Ability to be responsible for oneself

In assessing the patient's ability to cope and adapt to the emotional and behavioral responses created by the impact of neurological illness, the nurse seeks feedback from the patient to validate perceptions, clarify information, and ascertain whether the patient understands information provided. The feedback collected is both verbal and nonverbal and may be only nonverbal in some patients depending on the type and degree of neurological deficits sustained. For the patient with neurological illness, these interactions may be severely compromised or impossible (e.g., comatose state, aphasia).

Many patients have neurological deficits that compromise normal interpersonal relationships and the ability to express themselves and comprehend information. Such situations create additional stress. Stress will cause various emotional and psychological responses that may require the intervention of the nurse.

GENERAL PRINCIPLES FOR CONSIDERING THE PATIENT'S EMOTIONAL AND BEHAVIORAL RESPONSES TO NEUROLOGICAL ILLNESS

Certain emotional and behavioral responses can be expected in patients with any illness. Although the nurse can anticipate responses, the patient must be carefully assessed to determine how he as an individual has responded to his circumstances. The nurse would expect the person who is alert and well oriented to be fearful of anticipated surgery. However, the specific reasons or perceptions of the planned events that contribute to the fear can vary from patient to patient. For example, for one patient the most terrifying aspect of having a craniotomy may be having his head shaved. If the nurse recognizes that this issue is the source of greatest fear or stress to the patient, discussing his concerns may help to alleviate some of his fear if he is provided with information and encouraged to participate in problem solving to deal with the temporary loss of hair. Although the shaving of the head will still cause a certain amount of fear, much can be done to dispel some of his concerns and thus modify the emotional and behavioral response of the patient.

ASSESSMENT

In assessing the psychological aspects of the patient the nurse should

1. Observe the patient's behavior both when he is alone and as he interacts with others (family members, significant others, staff, other patients); note his facial expressions, body language, tone of voice, and reactions to particular individuals
2. Establish rapport with the patient; give him opportunities to communicate in whatever why he can, depending on what communication skills are intact
3. Focus the communication on the patient by using open-ended questions, if the patient has adequate neurological function to respond
4. Listen to what the patient has to say and how he says it (e.g., how he describes things, his use of analogies)
5. Collect information from the patient and his family/significant others on the following:
   - Previous adjustment patterns and use of coping mechanisms
   - Personality before illness
   - Previous emotional and behavioral responses to stress
   - How he usually deals with stress (e.g., jogging, withdrawal)
   - Support systems
   - Family interactions
6. Validate information collected with the appropriate persons (e.g., family, other health professionals), as necessary
7. Consult with others to broaden the base of information about the patient
8. Validate your perceptions

ONGOING ASSESSMENT AND NURSING DIAGNOSES

Assessment is an ongoing process. The assessment data collected are analyzed and nursing diagnoses made. Once the nursing diagnoses have been made, the nurse plans the nursing interventions.

NURSING INTERVENTIONS

The nursing interventions necessary for dealing with the many emotional and behavioral responses to the stress of neurological illness are directed at helping the patient maintain his identity, a positive self-concept, and self-esteem. General principles that can guide the nurse in dealing with the many emotional and behavioral responses to the stress of neurological illness follow:

1. Provide an open, nonjudgmental environment.
2. Be supportive of the patient.
3. Develop alternate ways of communication if communication deficits exist.
4. Accept the patient's perceptions and behavior.
5. Matter-of-factly correct any inaccurate factual information.
6. Encourage the patient to express his feelings in whatever way he can.
7. Listen empathetically and attentively; reflect his thoughts and apparent feelings to clarify and validate them.
8. Help the patient to use his positive adaptive coping mechanisms.
9. Allow him to make decisions and maintain control over himself, to the degree that he is able.
10. Allow him to be involved in problem solving as much as possible.
11. Provide information as necessary.
12. Make referrals to other health professionals when appropriate.
13. Help the patient set realistic goals.
14. Support a positive self-concept and self-esteem.

COMMON EMOTIONAL AND BEHAVIORAL RESPONSES TO THE STRESS ASSOCIATED WITH NEUROLOGICAL ILLNESS

The general management principles of assessment and nursing intervention discussed in the previous section can be applied to the management of the common emotional and behavioral responses seen in many patients as they face the prospect of acute or chronic neurological disease. The emotional and behavioral responses discussed include anxiety, frustration, anger, hostility, fear, regression, denial, guilt, depression, powerlessness, and stigma. Although common emotional and behavioral responses are discussed as separate entities, several of these responses can occur concurrently in the patient.

ANXIETY

Anxiety is a feeling of uneasiness, apprehension, or dread that is associated with an unrecognized, subjective source of anticipated danger. It results from the real or perceived conflicts and frustrations of living. For patients who are unable to speak because of neurological disability or a tracheostomy, their ability to ventilate feelings of frustration, anger, and hostility is negated. This causes anxiety for the patient, and perhaps for the nurse. Anxiety is often classified as mild, moderate, or severe to convey the notion that the feeling can range from the mild awareness of fear or anticipatory danger to outright panic. Physiological alterations of the autonomic system such as an elevated pulse rate and blood pressure, perspiration, or diarrhea often accompany this mood state. The patient who is anxious will demonstrate various recognizable behaviors associated with the degree of anxiety, including irritability, uneasiness, apprehension, demanding or unreasonable behavior, and often, verbal abusiveness. The patient is described as "very difficult." Occasionally, a patient may be charming and agreeable but does not comply with established treatment protocols. This is his way of dealing with anxiety.

Nursing Intervention

Because anxiety is associated with an unrecognized, subjective source of anticipated danger, some time should be spent in trying to discover what is generating the anxiety. Often there are several concerns that are responsible for anxiety, some of which cannot be identified on the conscious level. For the patient who cannot communicate, the nurse must try to anticipate potential sources of anxiety and provide information. Alternate methods of communication should be developed, and the nurse must become very good at reading body language.

Recognizing potential sources of anxiety must be a major concern in caring for the patient. To alleviate anxiety, the nurse must explain to the patient what she is going to do and keep the patient apprised of what is being done while care is administered. All aspects of care should also be explained to the so-called "unresponsive or unconscious" patient because there is no way to determine whether sensory stimuli are getting through to the brain and being processed. The caregiver must assume that some verbal stimuli will penetrate the barriers of neurological illness to provide information and comfort to the patient.

For patients who are able to cooperate and have intact neurological function that will make it possible for them to follow directions, progressive relaxation therapy may reduce anxiety. This is a systematic approach to tightening and relaxing muscle groups to relieve muscle tension. Another relaxation technique is the use of imagery. The patient is encouraged to select an image that is particularly relaxing and pleasing. The patient is taught to close his eyes, relax, and focus on actually experiencing all of the pleasing sensations of being in this chosen setting. Any type of relaxation technique takes time to learn and must be practiced to achieve optimum results. Appropriate patients must be selected for this therapy.

FRUSTRATION

Frustration is defined as the feeling that occurs when a course of action or activity cannot be carried out or brought to a desirable conclusion. The patient who is frustrated is often irritable and anxious. He may express his frustration by verbal outbursts. The amount of frustration experienced will be proportional to the value and desirability he places on the thwarted action.

Nursing Intervention

The nurse can help the patient to identify the source of his frustration. Once identified, problem solving should be employed to determine why the desired result was not achieved. It may be that the patient had set unrealistic goals. In this instance, realistic goals should be identified. Another possibility may be that an alternate approach is necessary to achieve the desired goal. The patient must be encouraged to realistically examine the situation and select appropriate strategies or alter his goals. Expressing his frustration is helpful in dissipating his feelings.

ANGER

Anger is an intense feeling of displeasure and antagonism in response to mounting frustration, conflict, or anxiety. It connotes strong feelings in response to the actual prevention or threat of prevention of achievement or maintenance of a desired goal or state. Anger that is turned inward is called *depression*. The behavioral manifestations of anger may include aggressive or destructive acts, verbal attacks, silence, or depression.

Nursing Intervention

The patient who is angry needs the same kind of help and support that the anxious or frustrated patient needs. If the angry patient is apt to lose self-control and cause bodily injury to another or himself, or if he is prone to cause property damage, he must be controlled. Drug therapy, restraints, or other forms of therapy may be necessary. The patient must be provided with an appropriate outlet for his feelings of anger. If the source of the anger can be identified, it may be possible to alleviate the situation.

HOSTILITY

Hostility is usually seen in association with anger. It is a feeling of antagonism directed toward another and is associated with a wish to hurt, humiliate, or discredit that person. Hostility is generally thought to be the result of frustrated or unfulfilled needs or wishes. According to Horney, repressed hostility is one of the major sources of anxiety.[13] Kiening describes the development of hostility in the following way:[14]

- A person experiences frustration, loss of self-esteem, or unmet needs for status, prestige, or love.
- Within a given situation, he has certain expectations for himself and others.
- The expectations are not met.
- The person feels inadequate, hurt, or humiliated.
- He experiences anxiety that becomes hostility to which he may react in any of three ways:
  - — He represses the hostility and withdraws
  - — He disowns the feeling and behaves in an extremely polite and compliant manner
  - — He behaves overtly hostile either in a verbal or nonverbal manner

Nursing Intervention

The patient who is hostile needs help to understand the origin of his feelings. He also needs to be able to express his feelings in a safe, nonjudgmental environment. The nurse caring for the hostile patient can manage him in a similar manner as she manages the anxious patient.

FEAR

Fear is a feeling of extreme apprehension or dread associated with a potential or real threat to the well-being of the individual. The fear may be associated with fear of the unknown, mutilation, loss of control, pain, disability, or other specifics. Behavioral manifestations of fear often include excitability, irrational behavior, and irrational and inaccurate beliefs about the feared object. There are also physiological signs and symptoms of the activated sympathetic nervous system (fight or flight response) such as pallor, tachycardia, pupillary dilation, dry mouth, and cold clammy hands.

Nursing Intervention

The nurse should try to identify the source of the patient's fear. Identifying the source of fear will require the nurse to explore concerns with the patient. Once the source of the fear is identified, the nurse may be able to correct misinformation. The need to verify the patient's understanding and perceptions as well as to clarify and amplify information are ongoing, necessary aspects of communication. The nurse may also need to make appropriate referrals to assist the patient in alleviating his fears.

Many studies have documented increased development of intraoperative and postoperative complications in patients who are very anxious or fearful. It is important for patient outcome that fear be addressed and alleviated.

REGRESSION

The person under extreme and continued stress may retreat to the use of behavioral patterns that were appropriate during an earlier developmental stage. This response is called *regression*. On a temporary basis, regression can be a protective mechanism that preserves the person's limited ego strength. Most authorities suggest that a certain amount of regression occurs with all serious illness as part of the response to the illness. The behavioral manifestations vary and cover a wide gamut of behaviors that include helplessness, crying, temper tantrums, withdrawal from responsibilities, preoccupation with self, dependency, giddiness, and stubbornness.

Nursing Intervention

The patient who demonstrates evidence of regression needs a supportive, safe environment. The regression indicates that the patient is overwhelmed by the current stressors and cannot cope effectively. The nurse needs to consider methods of helping the patient to reduce stress and of supporting effective coping mechanisms.

DENIAL

Denial is a defense mechanism, sometimes referred to as a temporary protective mechanism, whereby the person refused to acknowledge the existence or significance of a know fact. The known fact is too painful for the person to deal with so he denies its existence. The degree of denial varies from person to person. Denial can be an effective, temporary method of dealing with a stress-producing situation until the person is able to muster the ego strength to deal with the problem. Continued denial becomes a negative mechanism in that the person does not incorporate the information into reality for problem solving and realistic planning. The characteristic behavior includes a refusal to discuss the denied topic. The patient behaves as if the situation does not exist.

Nursing Intervention

At some point, denial becomes an ineffective coping mechanism for dealing with stress. The seriousness of the illness or the probable outcome can then no longer be denied. An enormous amount of stress is associated with this realization. The patient gradually begins to acknowledge some of the more obvious aspects of his illness. The patient needs the support of the nursing staff to make this adaptation. Questions should be answered honestly and as completely as possible, based on the known facts. The patient gradually faces most of the realities of his illness. Depression and grieving are characteristics of this period. The patient is now able to make realistic decisions based on his altered and realistic self-concept, if positive adaptation has occurred.[15]

GUILT

The feeling that one has done something wrong and is directly responsible for precipitating negative outcomes, pain, or frustration of goals is called *guilt*. The behavioral manifestations of guilt include a feeling of regretful responsibility for negative consequences, self-deprecation, lowered self-esteem, and possibly self-hate.

Nursing Intervention

The patient must identify the source of his guilt. He must deal with the situation realistically and honestly.

DEPRESSION

Depression is a feeling of sadness and self-depreciation accompanied by difficulty in thinking and carrying out usual activities and responsibilities, a lowered energy level, and preoccupation with oneself. The depressed person is unable to express his feelings and internalizes them. Depression has also been defined as anger turned inward. The characteristic behaviors associated with depression are a sad, expressionless face; flat affect; listlessness; lack of interest in others or the environment; possible crying spells; and a sense of hopelessness. Some persons who are depressed see no possible resolution of their situation and may contemplate suicide. Allusion to suicide may be made either directly or indirectly.

Nursing Intervention

There are varying degrees of depression. The person who is severely depressed may need psychiatric consultation and help. Drug therapy may be helpful in treating temporary depression. However, the reason(s) for the depression must be sought, identified, and addressed.

POWERLESSNESS

Powerlessness is defined as a perceived or real lack of control over one's body, mind, environment, or life. The typical behavioral characteristics include a feeling of frustration, anger, hopelessness, depression, and apathy.

Nursing Intervention

The patient who perceives himself as powerless, in the psychological sense, may need to be reminded that he has more power than he believes. Because of illness his power is often altered, but it is not lost. The patient needs to recognize the power that he has, and he should be encouraged to use it appropriately.

Neurological illness may have deprived the patient of power over certain physiological functions. Participating in a rehabilitation program may help the patient to gradually reclaim his altered control and power over body functions. If complete rehabilitation is not possible, the patient may benefit from adaptive devices or altered methods of accomplishing tasks.

STIGMA

The condition in which a person views himself as devalued or unable to meet minimum societal norms is termed *stigma*. The feeling of stigmatization can result from physical or emotional deficits, behavioral abnormalities, or violation of societal laws or codes. The person who feels stigmatized demonstrates characteristic behaviors that include feelings of shame, alienation, or being devalued; a decreased feeling of self-esteem or social worth; isolation from normal relationships; rejection of attempts by others to reach out to him; suspiciousness; paranoid behavior; loneliness; hostility; and anger.

Nursing Intervention

Dealing with the patient who feels stigmatized can be difficult. His feelings are usually based on deep-seated beliefs and values. The patient needs assistance in exploring his feelings so that he can better understand them. The nurse needs to present reality and correct erroneous information that the patient expresses. It is also important to support and build the patient's self-esteem.

EMOTIONAL AND BEHAVIORAL RESPONSES TO SPECIFIC ASPECTS OF ILLNESS: NURSING IMPLICATIONS

Some emotional and behavioral responses associated with certain aspects of neurological illness and hospitalization call for specific nursing interventions in addition to the general nursing approaches discussed previously in this chapter. The following psychological and emotional experiences will be discussed: loss, grief and mourning, immobility, dehumanization, change in body image, sensory deprivation, isolation, sensory overload, the intensive care unit syndrome, and transfer anxiety.

LOSS

Loss is defined as a state in which a person experiences deprivation or the complete lack of something that was previously present and available to him. The person who has sustained a significant loss will demonstrate the behaviors consistent with grieving and mourning. See the section on Grief and Mourning for specific behavioral manifestions.

Loss can be sudden or gradual, predictable or unexpected, or temporary or permanent. Paralysis can be used to illustrate sudden and gradual loss. The patient who sustains a spinal cord injury in a motor vehicle accident may experience sudden loss of motor function below the level of injury. By contrast, a patient with progressive multiple sclerosis often experiences a gradual decline in motor function until he is a complete paraplegic. In the first instance, paralysis occurs in a split second while in the second example, it develops gradually over years.

Some losses are predictable while others are unexpected. The patient diagnosed as having amyotrophic lateral sclerosis is expected to develop severe difficulty with speech and swallowing as the course of his illness progresses. On the other hand, the patient with Parkinson's disease who demonstrates mental deterioration in cognitive functions has experienced symptoms that are not part of the disease process and are unexpected. Some losses are temporary while others are permanent. For example, the patient who has had surgery in the left parietal lobe of the brain may be aphasic postoperatively because of cerebral edema. Given a few days of treatment of the cerebral edema, the speech will gradually return in the next several days. Such a loss is temporary. An example of a permanent loss may be seen with the patient who has had a large acoustic neuroma removed that involved the facial (VII) cranial nerve. All attempts to identify and dissect the tumor from the cranial nerve were unsuccessful, and the nerve was severed. In this instance, the facial paralysis will be permanent unless there is peripheral nerve regeneration and anastomosis of the ends.

Significant losses may include loss of family members or significant others, body parts, life, possessions, and physical, psychological, or cognitive functions. The individual's response to the loss will depend on the value that he places on the lost object or body function, societal and cultural value placed on the loss, and the cultural, economic, and support groups available to assist the individual in dealing with the loss. Each person has a unique value system. How the person values an object, person, or function dictates how he responds to the loss. For example, the person who loses the use of his right arm may be devastated if he is right-handed and enjoys activities that require fine motor control of his hands such as painting. Another patient who is left-handed and retired and spends his leisure time reading or watching television would be inconvenienced by the loss, but it would not alter his lifestyle or self-concept to the same degree as the other patient's.

Certain body functions such as continence of the bladder and bowel and sexual function are functions valued by the adult person. Loss of these functions are viewed as significant losses by the person and society.

Cultural values also dictate an individual's response to his loss. If the culture places a high value on the ability or body part lost, then the impact on the individual as a respected member of the culture is significant. When a person sustains a loss, how he responds and adjusts to the loss will depend on the cultural, economic, and support groups available to him. All societies, regardless of whether they are primitive or highly sophisticated, have customs and rituals that are followed when someone dies. However, no such customs exist when there is loss of body function. Often, the loss of body function (disability) renders the person socially unacceptable because other people feel uncomfortable being around the person. The person who has dysphagia may not be a welcome guest at the dinner table. Even if other people were able to accept the patient's difficulty in managing food, the patient may feel humiliated to be drooling or have food falling from his mouth.

The economic impact resulting from losses is significant. Life insurance is helpful when a family member dies. Various health insurance policies assist with the cost of health care, and some people elect to purchase policies that provide payments if disability occurs. However, disability often results in the inability to participate in one's occupation, resulting in loss of salary. If the person is able to benefit from a rehabilitation program, he may be able to return to work at some job but at a much lower salary than he was receiving. The decreased financial income lowers the patient's economic status and lifestyle. The spouse or other family member may have to seek employment, or in some cases, to leave a job to care for the patient. The decrease in income at a time when extra expenses from loss are incurred has a dramatic effect on the patient's lifestyle and self-concept.

Support groups are available for some patients with particular problems such as head injuries and multiple sclerosis. The purpose of the support group is to assist the patient and often family members with the loss of health and the disabilities incurred from the illness. The particular services offered vary from organization to organization but may include practical information on how to live with the problems of illness, psychological and emotional support, and identification of resources to assist the patient and his family.

Nursing Intervention

The nurse must explore the significance to the patient of the loss. What does the loss of a function mean to the patient within the context of his lifestyle and self-concept? Until the nurse can appreciate the significance of the loss from the patient's point of view, it is difficult to be supportive. Once the nurse understands the significance of the loss, she can provide information and assistance to the patient. Referrals to others may be part of the approach to the patient.

GRIEF AND MOURNING

According to Engel, following the loss of any valued object or function, the person passes through three stages that lead to healthy resolution and include (1) shock and disbelief; (2) development of awareness (recognition) of the loss; and (3) restitution (reconciliation).

The shock phase immediately follows the loss. The patient is stunned, appears to be out of contact with his environment, and is in a state of disbelief. He may be able to intellectualize the loss but not accept it emotionally. He does not believe that this is happening to him and may verbalize that this cannot be true.

In the recognition phase, the patient begins to realize that the loss is real. Characteristic behavior includes anger, blaming himself, and depression. The person is preoccupied with the loss and what it means to him. There is an internalization of the loss. The final stage, restitution, is consistent with a realistic acceptance of what has happened. There is a gradual interest in others and the environment. The patient begins to see himself realistically and to integrate the change in body image into a positive self-concept. He is able to make decisions about himself and the future and to see a realistic future for himself.

Nursing Intervention

In the shock phase, accept the patient's behavior. Denial may be a protective coping mechanism. Allow the patient to deny the loss, if he must. Listen to him in an accepting, nonjudgmental manner. Don't tell him that you understand how he feels unless you have experienced the same loss.

In the recognition phase, accept the patient's anger. Allow him to express his feelings. Correct misinformation. Support him through his depression. Explain the patient's response to his loss to his family. Be supportive of the family. As the period of restitution emerges, encourage the patient to express his views and to plan realistically. Help him to collect necessary information either personally or by making appropriate referrals. Be supportive and help the patient adapt and integrate the altered body image into his self-concept. Allow him to be as independent as possible and assume responsibility for himself.

IMMOBILITY

The prescribed, enforced, or unavoidable limitation of movement that occurs over a prolonged period of time is called *immobility*. Immobility can occur in the physical, psychological, intellectual, or social domains. The person who is physically immobilized may develop psychological immobility. Immobility reduces the quality and quantity of sensory input available to the person. This, in turn, leads to a reduction of the individual's ability to interact with his environment. The behavioral manifestations of immobility include (1) a sense of confinement and limitation of space, resulting in frustration and anxiety; (2) a lack of control, which can lead to anger and depression; and (3) a forced change in body image and self-concept.

The neurological patient may suffer immobility in all domains. Paresis or paralysis can impose an involuntary confinement and immobilization. The patient is not able to move about freely; movement is a means of control that is highly cherished as a requisite for independence. Equipment such as ventilators, food pumps, urinary catheters, intravenous lines, and orthopedic traction enforce varying degrees of immobility upon the patient. Cognitive and psychological deficits precipitated by neurological disease block or severly compromise the psychosocial and intellectual input for the patient so that he will feel confined or immobilized. The patient with an altered level of consciousness may be completely isolated from input in all domains. Social immobility may result because of how people treat him because of physical condition and disabilities.

Nursing Intervention

The goal of the nurse is to draw the patient into the mainstream of life and involve him as much as possible, provided that this is not contraindicated by the therapeutic plan. Provide reality orientation (by using clock, calendar, or radio or telling the patient what is happening around him) so that the patient will be drawn into the environment. Extend the patient's environment, if possible, by taking the him out of his room, moving him near a window, or providing him with a wheelchair. Encourage social interaction and expression of feelings.

DEHUMANIZATION

Viewing the patient as a disease entity and divesting him of human capacities, qualities, and functions so that he is considered an object is called *dehumanization*. When dehumanization exists, the focus of attention is not a person or unique individual who is experiencing illness, but rather signs, symptoms, diagnostic data, and equipment. Since the patient is divested of his humanity, he is not consulted on decisions concerning himself, provided with information, or treated with the respect and consideration normally extended to a person. The caregivers take over the day-to-day decisions affecting the patient.

It is not necessarily the uncaring nurse who treats the patient as less than human. In caring for an unresponsive patient, it is very easy to lose sight of the patient as a person. Human relationships are built on interactions between individuals. If this interchange is not ongoing, it is very easy to lose sight of the humanity of the other individual.

Nursing Intervention

Address the patient by name; think of him by name and as a unique individual rather than as a room number or diagnosis. Treat the patient as the unique individual that he is. Speak to him, and involve him in the environment and in the decisions about his care as much as possible. Allow him to assume as much control and responsibility for himself as possible.

CHANGE IN BODY IMAGE

A concept basic to one's sense of identity, security, self-esteem, and self-concept is body image. *Body image* is defined as the conscious and unconscious perceptions (feelings and attitudes) that one has about his body as a separate and distinct entity. It is a developmental and social creation that is subject to very slow change in adult life. Illness, disability, and loss of function force a change in body image on the patient. If the change can be integrated realistically within the patient's self-concept without altering his self-esteem, then the adaptation and adjustment are positive.

The behavioral manifestations associated with a change in body image often include those discussed with loss, grief, and bereavement. The change is viewed as a threat or significant loss, and the patient passes through the characteristic stages of shock, recognition, and reconciliation.

Nursing Intervention

If the nurse views the change in body image within the conceptual framework of loss, grief, and bereavement, the nursing intervention will follow a similar approach. Accept the patient's perception of himself. Recognize that changing one's body image is a slow process. Support the patient as he begins to recognize the impact of illness on his concept of body image. Help the patient accept and adapt to the change by supporting his self-esteem.

SENSORY DEPRIVATION

Sensory deprivation is defined as a lack of or decreased sensory input from the external or internal environment. There is a lack of or decreased perception of multi-sensory input of various intensities and meanings to the person. The behavioral manifestations of sensory deprivation vary depending on the degree of deprivation and may include abnormalities in feeling states; disorientation; impairment of the ability to think; distortion of perception; and illusions and hallucinations. The patient with neurological illness may experience any number of neurological deficits that contribute to sensory deprivation such as an altered level of consciousness, paresis or paralysis, paresthesias, visual deficits, hearing loss, taste or smell deficits, and cognitive or emotional deficits. Head injury, spinal cord injury, cerebrovascular accident, multiple sclerosis, and any number of other neurological conditions can precipitate sensory deprivation. Therapeutic protocols such as instituting subarachnoid precautions are still another cause of sensory deprivation.

Nursing Intervention

The nurse should be aware of the frequency with which sensory deprivation occurs, especially in neurological patients, and assess the patient for its presence. The nurse must identify the causes and the specific types of sensory deficits present. Once these questions are answered, the nurse can develop an approach to provide multi-sensory stimuli to the patient as a means of compensation. Sensory input can be provided by talking to the patient; playing the radio, television, or tape recordings of family members' voices; reality orientation; touch; and positioning. Reality orientation is a process of actively making the patient aware of his environment (e.g., activities, weather, date, time, place, people, objects). Sensory deprivation may be the cause of a patient's disorientation rather than physiological deficits of the reticular activating system (RAS).

SLEEP DEPRIVATION

Sleep deprivation has been defined as a lack of adequate sleep or dream time in relation to prior or usual sleep patterns.[16] Persons deprived of sleep for prolonged periods of time experience behavioral, psychological, and physiological alterations. Behavioral manifestations are similar to those seen in schizophrenia (alterations in perceptions, cognition, mood, affect). Patients admitted to intensive care units, those requiring constant care and monitoring, those receiving certain medication, and those experiencing extreme stress are prime candidates for sleep deprivation.

The strange environment and constant activity of the hospital predispose patients to this common phenomenom. Because of injuries to the brain and their need for attention, neurological patients often experience sleep deprivation.

Nursing Intervention

The nurse should assess the patient's 24-hour schedule to determine how much sleep time is actually provided. Nursing care should be planned to provide uninterrupted sleep time. Drug therapy can also have an effect on the quality of sleep and dream time. Certain drugs may alter the depth of sleep and the sleep pattern. Deprivation of the various levels of sleep such as rapid eye movement (REM) stage is thought to have a negative effect on the patient. The nurse should be aware of the various factors that influence the patient's ability to sleep and control the environment, as much as possible, to facilitate sleep.

SENSORY OVERLOAD

Sudden, excessive, sustained, multi-sensory experiences that are perceived as confusing, bothersome, meaningless, and extremely stressful to the patient are defined as *sensory overload*. The behavioral manifestations of sensory overload are confusion, disorientation, irritability, restlessness, agitation, anger, panic, and possible hallucinations.

The neurological patient may experience sensory overload from equipment (e.g., respirator, cardiac monitor), conditions that intensify sensory input (meningitis, encephalitis), and the constant stimuli of nursing care, particularly if he is critically ill.

Nursing Intervention

The nurse should identify the various sensory levels and sources of input in the patient's environment. Every effort should be made to control and moderate the intensity of stimuli. Special situations exist such as when subarachnoid precautions are instituted. The purpose of this protocol is to decrease all stimuli so that the patient will not rebleed. In the instance of a patient with meningitis or encephalitis, minimize tactile stimuli and control all other environmental stimuli.

INTENSIVE CARE UNIT SYNDROME

The *intensive care unit syndrome* (ICU syndrome) has been defined as an "acute organic brain syndrome involving impaired intellectual functioning which occurs in patients who are being treated within a critical care unit. When the impairment is of such magnitude that the patient cannot adequately judge reality, the syndrome can be termed an ICU psychosis."[17] The behavioral manifestations include fear, anxiety, depression, and denial, and possibly psychosis and panic. The factors that contribute to the development of ICU syndrome are the noise level, isolation, loss of day–night orientation, immobilization, sleep deprivation, depersonalization, and use of medications.[17,18]

Many neurological–neurosurgical patients are admitted to ICU units for treatment so these patients are prone to the development of ICU syndrome. Neurological patients are frequently admitted to the ICU because of trauma of various types (head injuries, spinal cord injuries, multitrauma), for neurosurgery (craniotomies for various reasons), and for special neurological–neurosurgical procedures.

Nursing Intervention

The ICU syndrome is a variation of sensory overload and is managed in a similar manner as sensory overload.

TRANSFER ANXIETY

The increased anxiety and feelings of insecurity experienced by a patient when he moves from one unit or facility to another is called *transfer anxiety*. The patient may be transferred from the intensive care unit to a regular clinical unit or other site. The neurological patient may also be transferred to a rehabilitation facility, chronic care facility, or nursing home. The patient or family may be concerned that the quality of care and the commitment of the nursing and medical staff will not be as good. There is the underlying feeling that the quality of care will deteriorate and that the person will not be recognized as the unique individual that he is. The unit on which the patient is currently assigned is perceived as one that offers a higher level of nursing, medical, and technological support than the unit to which he is being transferred. The patient experiences fear of the unknown and views the transfer as a threat to his security and well-being.

The major behavioral manifestation is anxiety that may develop into a paniclike state as the day of transfer approaches. The patient may also experience physiological responses (psychosomatic responses) to the stress of an impending transfer. Common signs and symptoms may include elevation of the blood pressure, shortness of breath, tightness in the chest, palpitations, or elevation in body temperature.

Nursing Intervention

Comprehensive discharge planning should include the psychological preparation of the patient and his family for a smooth transition from the acute care setting to another facility or home. The liaison nurse from the new facility may need to visit the patient to help to bridge the transition and provide information about the new facility. Encourage questions and provide complete information to dispel the patient's fear of the unknown facility. A visit to the new unit or facility is desirable so that the patient (if possible) or family members can tour the facilities and meet members of the staff.

If the neurological patient is going home, the physical environment should be evaluated and the delivery of any necessary equipment arranged before the day of discharge. Patient and family teaching should be conducted in plenty of time so that they will feel comfortable. If possible, a weekend visit by the patient to his home should be arranged. In this way problems can be addressed and solved before the actual discharge is made. Every attempt should be made to anticipate potential problems so that a smooth transition can occur.

THE PSYCHOLOGICAL, EMOTIONAL, AND BEHAVIORAL RESPONSES OF THE NEUROLOGICAL PATIENT'S FAMILY OR SIGNIFICANT OTHERS

The impact of neurological illness has serious consequences not only for the patient but also for his family or significant others. The family structure, relationships, and methods of dealing with stress and crisis become important considerations for the nurse. Family members will react to illness individually within the entire gamut of responses of anxiety, anger, depression, denial, grieving, and fear. Neurological illness is often a chronic condition with permanent disabilities or progressive disabilities that evolve and impose dependency on the family to meet the patient's basic needs. The stresses incurred by neurological illness are significant and require the support and assistance of health professionals for the family to make a realistic adjustment. The ability of the family to accept the situation and adapt will directly influence the emotional well-being of every member of the family unit, including the patient.

NURSING INTERVENTION

The role of the nurse in supporting the family includes the following:

- Talk to the family to determine their understanding and perception of the patient's illness.
- Determine the schemata of family interactions and support systems.
- Allow the family members to express their feelings.
- Correct misinformation and provide data, as necessary.
- Make referrals as appropriate.
- Allow the family to become involved in the care of the patient, if they so wish.
- Promote normalcy.
- Support the family in their decision on the patient's care and/or plans for posthospital care.

THE EMOTIONAL AND BEHAVIORAL RESPONSES OF THE NURSE WHO CARES FOR THE PATIENT WITH NEUROLOGICAL ILLNESS

The nurse who cares for neurological–neurosurgical patients works in a very stressful environment and thus becomes a prime target for job-related stress responses and burnout. Common job-related stressors include caring for patients who have

- Sustained neurological injury as a result of trauma (e.g., motor vehicle accidents, assaults, self-inflicted injuries)
- Terminal diagnoses, especially if they are young
- Cognitive and emotional disability
- Sustained neurological deficits that render them completely dependent on the nurse
- Tracheostomy tubes, ventilators, and support equipment
- Significant pain that does not respond to the normal modalities of pain control
- Multiple trauma or are critically ill
- Agreed to donor organ transplant
- Been designated as brain dead
- Been discharged to another facility after a long stay on the unit

There are other job-related stressors in the work environment that are sources of stress such as

- Experiencing interpersonal conflict with co-workers or administration
- Dealing with the family of a dying patient
- Dealing with a disoriented, demanding, noisy, or "difficult" patient
- Having to assume responsibilities that the nurse is not prepared to manage
- Dealing with the physicians, residents, nursing students, and faculty
- Rotating shifts and working double shifts
- Working with insufficient staff
- Working with inadequate supplies or auxilliary staff (e.g., transport services, laboratory services)
- Working without effective leadership
- Earning poor salaries and fringe benefits
- Lacking recognition
- Having to channel communications through the bureaucracy to get results

Unless the nurse takes the time to protect herself from the acute and chronic stresses of her job, her mental and physical health are at risk. Burnout is the result of chronic stress, and it affects the quality of the care administered to the patient as well as the professional and personal life of the nurse. The nurse must learn to recognize the signs and symptoms of stress and do something positive to deal with them before serious problems result. The nurse is encouraged to choose appropriate coping mechanisms to deal with stress and practice good health habits herself (e.g., eat well; participate in an exercise program or recreation).

Recently, many articles and continuing education offerings have addressed the needs of the nurse as a person and professional who is subject to significant stress. The concept of burnout is well documented and discussed in the literature. It is now recognized that nurses as caregivers are very vulnerable to stress and that measures should be taken to protect and support the nurse. Each nurse must assume responsibility for her own mental health and practice appropriate methods of stress control.

REFERENCES

1. Selye H: The Stress of Life. New York, McGraw–Hill, 1956
2. Selye H: Stress Without Distress. Philadelphia, JB Lippincott, 1974

3. Cannon WB: The Wisdom of the Body. New York, WW Norton & Co, 1936
4. Jacobsen E: Anxiety and Tension Control. Philadelphia, JB Lippincott, 1965
5. Phipps WJ, Long BC, Woods NF (eds): Medical-Surgical Nursing Concepts and Clinical Practice, 2nd ed, pp 161-169. St Louis, CV Mosby, 1983
6. Levine S, Scotch NA: Social Stress. Chicago, Aldine Publishing, 1970
7. Coehlo GV, Hamburg DA, Adams JE: Coping and Adaptation. New York, Basic Books, 1974
8. Mason JW: A historical view of the stress field. J Human Stress 1(1):6; 1(2):22, 1975
9. Lazarus RA: Psychological Stress and the Coping Process. New York, McGraw-Hill, 1966
10. Roy C: The Roy adaptation model. In Riehl JP, Roy C: Conceptual Models for Nursing Practice, 2nd ed, pp 180-182. New York, Appleton-Century-Crofts, 1980
11. Roy C: Adaptation model. Presented at the Second Annual Nurse Educator Conference, New York, December 1978 (audio-tape)
12. Fawcett J: Analysis and Evaluation of Conceptual Models of Nursing, pp 247-285. Philadelphia, FA Davis, 1984
13. Horney K: Collected Works of Karen Horney, vol 1, p 63. New York, WW Norton & Co, 1937
14. Kiening MM Sr: Hostility. In Carlson CE, Blackwell B: Behavioral Concepts & Nursing Interventions, 2nd ed, p 131. Philadelphia, JB Lippincott, 1978
15. Kiening Sr MM: Denial of Illness. In Carlson CE, Blackwell B: Behavioral Concepts and Nursing Interventions, 2nd ed, p 217. Philadelphia, JB Lippincott, 1978
16. McFadden E: Sleep deprivation in patients having open heart surgery. Nurs Res 20:249, May-June 1971
17. Eisendrath SJ: ICU syndromes: Their detection, prevention and treatment. Crit Care Update 7(4):5, 1980
18. Kleck HG: ICU syndrome: Onset, manifestations, treatment, stressors, and prevention. Crit Care Q 6(4):21, March 1984

BIBLIOGRAPHY

Books

Borg N (ed): Core Curriculum for Critical Care Nursing, 2nd ed, pp 441-478. Philadelphia, WB Saunders, 1981

Carlson CE, Blackwell B (eds): Behavioral Concepts and Nursing Intervention, 2nd ed. Philadelphia, JB Lippincott, 1978

Christopherson V, Coulter P, Wolanin M: Rehabilitation Nursing Perspectives and Applications. New York, McGraw-Hill, 1974

Edwards BJ, Brilhart JK: Communications in Nursing Practice. St Louis, CV Mosby, 1981

Hoff LA: People in Crisis: Understanding and Helping. London, Addison-Wesley Publishing Co, 1978

Kintzel K (ed): Advanced Concepts in Clinical Nursing, 2nd ed. Philadelphia, JB Lippincott, 1977

Lambert V, Lambert C: The Impact of Physical Illness and Related Mental Health Concepts. Englewood Cliffs, NJ, Prentice-Hall, 1979

Leininger M: Transcultural Nursing: Concepts, Theories, and Practices. New York, John Wiley & Sons, 1978

O'Brien M: Communications and Relationships in Nursing, 2nd ed. St Louis, CV Mosby, 1978

Oswald I: Sleep. Baltimore, Penguin Books, 1968

Potter DO (ed): Practices, pp 426-437. Springhouse, PA, Nursing '84 Books, 1984

Roberts SL: Behavioral Concepts and the Critically Ill Patient. Englewood Cliffs, NJ, Prentice-Hall, 1976

Spector R: Cultural Diversity in Health and Illness. New York, Appleton-Century-Crofts, 1979

Strub R, Black F: The Mental Status Examination in Neurology. Philadelphia, FA Davis, 1977

Sundeen S et al: Nurse-Client Interaction—Implementing the Nursing Process, 2nd ed. St Louis, CV Mosby, 1981

Werner-Beland JA: Grief Responses to Long-Term Illness and Disability. Reston, VA, Reston Publishing Co, 1980

Periodicals

Atkinson JH, Stewart N, Gardner D: The family meeting in critical care settings. J Trauma 20:43, 1980

Baker CF: Sensory overload and noise in the ICU: Sources of environmental stress. Crit Care Q 6(4):66, March 1984

Bayer LM, Bauers CM, Kapp SR: Psychosocial aspects of nutritional support. Nurs Clin North Am 18(1):119, March 1983

Beeken J: Body image changes in plegia. J Neurosurg Nurs 10(1):20, March 1978

Beglinger JE: Coping tasks in critical care . . . patients and families. Dimens Crit Care Nurs 2(2):80, March-April 1983

Bergerson R: Understanding the patient in all his human needs. J Adv Nurs 8(3):185, May 1983

Billings CV: Emotional first aid. Am J Nurs 80:2006, November 1980

Boss B: Acute mood and behavior disturbances of neurological origin: Acute confusional state. J Neurosurg Nurs 14(2):61, April 1982

Braulin JLD, Rook J, Sills GM: Families in crisis: The impact of trauma. Crit Care Q 5(3):38, December 1982

Brodoff AS: Helping your patient live with epilepsy. Patient Care 17(17):24-27; 29-32; 35, September 15, 1983

Carlson CC: Psychological aspects of neurologic disability. Nurs Clin North Am 15(2):309, June 1980

Carnes BA: Concept analysis: Dependence. Crit Care Q 6(4):29, March 1984

Carnevali D, Brueckner S: Immobilization—reassessment of a concept. Am J Nurs 70(7):1502, July 1970

Counte MA et al: Stress and personal attitudes in chronic illness. Arch Phys Med Rehabil 64(6):272, June 1983

Coutant NS: Rage: Implied neurological correlates. J Neurosurg Nurs 14(1):28, February 1982

Deliege D et al: Psycho-social care in hospital. Int Nurs Rev 28:83, May/June 1983

DeVillier B: Physiology of stress: Cellular healing. Crit Care Q 6(4):15, March 1984

Elliott FC: A nursing protocol for anxiety following catastrophic injury. Rehabil Nurs 18, May/June 1983

Gans JS: Depression diagnosis in a rehabilitation hospital. Arch Phys Med Rehabil 62:386, August 1981

Gardner D, Stewart N: Staff involvement with families of patients in critical care units. Heart Lung 7(1):105, 1978

George G: Exercise—coping with stress. Top Clin Nurs 4:13, July 1982

Germain CP: Cultural concepts in critical care. Crit Care Q 5(3):61, December 1982

Hickey JV: Combating burn-out by developing a theoretical framework. J Neurosurg Nurs 14(2):103, April 1982

Jack S: When regression becomes a problem. Can Nurs 77:31, April 1981

Jones C: Outcome following closed head injury. J Neurosurg Nurs 13(4):178, August 1981

Kinzel SL: What's your stress level? Nurs Life 2(2):54, March/April 1982

Kleinman A: Concepts and a model for the comparison of medical systems as cultural systems. Soc Sci Med 12:85, 1978

Kleinman A: Culture, illness, and care: Clinical lessons from anthropological and cross-cultural research. Ann Intern Med 88:251, 1978

Locke AM et al: Managing psychological disturbances in critical care. Dimens Crit Care Nurs 2(5):314, September-October 1983

Lust BL: The patient in the ICU: A family experience. Crit Care Q 6(4):49, March 1984

Mathis M: Personal needs of the family members of critically ill patients with and without acute brain injury. J Neurosurg Nurs 16(1):36, February 1984
Mauss-Clum N, Ryan M: Brain injury and the family. J Neurosurg Nurs 13(4):165, August 1981
Molter N: Needs of relatives of critically ill patients: A descriptive study. Heart Lung 8:332, 1979
Montague MC: Physiology of aggressive behavior. J Neurosurg Nurs 11(1):10, March 1979
Pollack SE: The stress response. Crit Care Q 6(4):1, March 1984
Quinn A et al: Families and feelings: A time for sharing. J Neurosurg Nurs 13(4):217, August 1981
Schwartz L, Brenner Z: Critical care unit transfer: Reducing patient stress through nursing interventions. Heart Lung 8(3):540, May/June 1979
Seremet NK: Needs of the attempted-suicide patient in the ICU. Crit Care Q 6(4):40, March 1984
Shubin S: Nursing patients from different cultures. Nurs80 10(6):78, June 1980
Stanton GM: Spinal cord injury: Psychological adaptation. J Neurosurg Nurs 15(5):306, October 1983
Stensrud R, Stensrud K: Interpersonal stress as a consequence of being disabled. J Rehabil 4(Winter):43, 1981
Storlie FJ: Burnout: The elaboration of a concept. Am J Nurs 79(12):2108, December 1979
Talbert RL: Pharmacotherapeutic modification of the stress response by anxiolytics. Crit Care Q 6(4):58, March 1984
Tanaka HT: Psychosocial rehabilitation: Future trends and directions. Psychosoc Rehabil J 6(4):7, April 1983
Weller DJ, Miller PM: Emotional reactions of patient, family and staff in acute care period of spinal cord injury, part two. Soc Work Health Care 3:7, 1977
Wolcott M: Clear communications and attitude in conflict resolution. J Neurosurg Nurs 15(3):174, June 1983

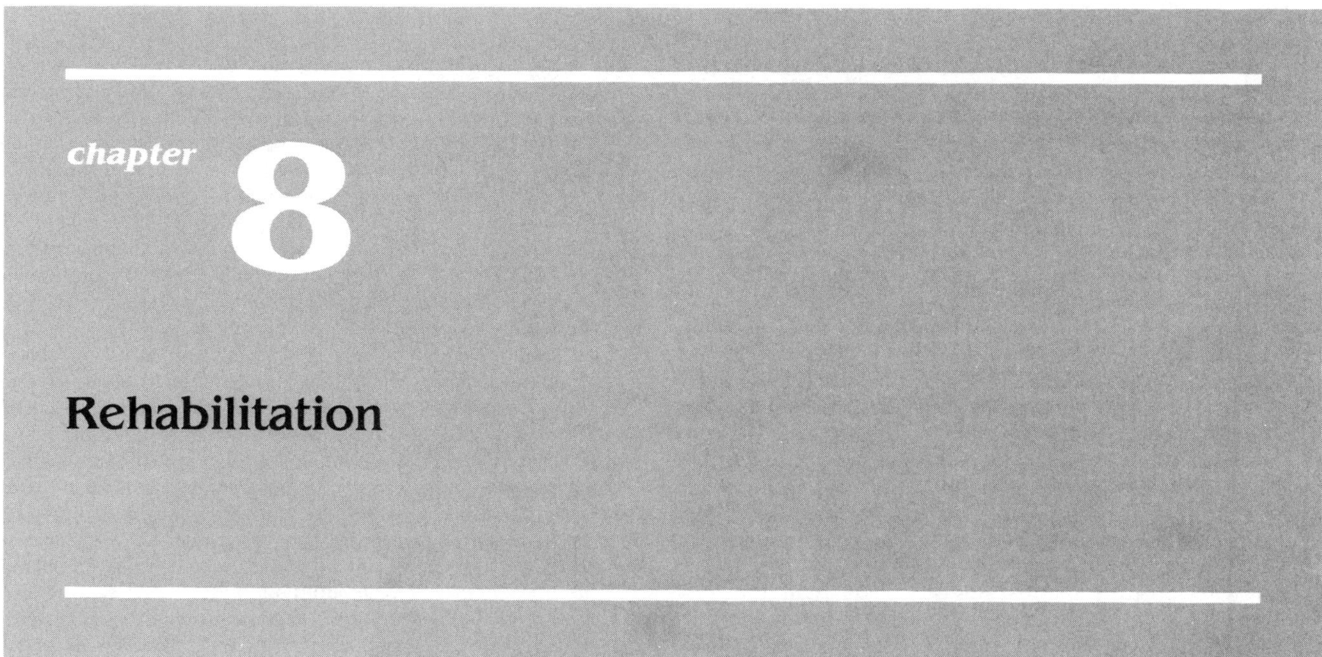

Rehabilitation is a dynamic process in which a disabled person is aided in achieving optimum physical, emotional, psychological, social, or vocational potential to maintain dignity and self-respect in a life that is as independent and self-fulfilling as possible. To be effective, rehabilitation must be a philosophy of care that is an integral part of health care delivery.

Often rehabilitation is defined as the restoration of the person to his former capacity. In some situations complete rehabilitation is possible, such as is the case when a patient sustains a mild concussion. In such an instance, complete recovery is the rule. However, in other situations complete recovery of function is not possible, and the patient faces a permanent disability. This patient must be helped to accept, adjust to, and compensate for the existing deficit to establish an optimum level of function. For example, a paraplegic patient with a severed spinal cord will be permanently paralyzed. Present medical technology cannot restore the severed cord to its premorbid condition. However, a well-designed comprehensive rehabilitation program can help the patient live a useful, relatively independent life from a wheelchair.

Another aspect of rehabilitation addresses itself to chronic health problems and degenerative diseases such as idiopathic seizures and multiple sclerosis. Although there is no cure for either category of illness, a rehabilitative program can improve the quality of life. In the case of chronic conditions, careful medical management and thorough patient education can offer the patient the opportunity to live a near-normal life if proper guidelines are followed. Care is directed toward the maintenance of optimum function and prevention of complications. In the case of degenerating diseases, even though it is known that there is no cure for the disease and that the condition will ultimately result in deterioration of the patient's health, there is a vital need for rehabilitation. In this sense rehabilitation means retaining the greatest amount of function and independence for as long as possible. As the disease process progresses, rehabilitation can offer alternate ways of carrying out the activities of daily living with the help of adaptive devices and alternate methods of performing skilled acts. Regardless of the type of specific problems faced by the patient, the major goal of rehabilitation is to help the patient achieve the highest level of independence possible and maintain a satisfying, productive life.

PHILOSOPHY OF REHABILITATION

A *philosophy* is a broad statement of basic related principles, concepts, and beliefs. A philosophy of rehabilitation offers a framework from which the overall rehabilitation process can be developed. One philosophy of rehabilitation is based upon the following premises:

1. *A well-established tenet of American society and rehabilitation recognizes the worth of the disabled person as a valuable human resource.* The practical objective of preparing the person for productive employment (or restoring him to it) is intertwined with the humanistic concern for the disabled person's transformation from a life of helplessness and dependency to one of dignity, self-respect, and independence. To achieve this end, economic support has come from state, federal, and various private agencies. There is indisputable evidence that rehabilitation, although expensive, is extremely cost-effective in that it is much more economical for the taxpayer to invest money in assisting a patient to become rehabilitated and independent than it is to relegate him to a role in which he is totally dependent on society for survival. One valuable return on the tax investment is the rehabilitated worker who is capable of earning a living and paying taxes.

   Of equal importance is the goal of restoring the individual's capacity to a level sufficient to resume roles not specifically designed for financial gain. These roles offer many social, emotional, and psychological returns to society. For example, the disabled homemaker who can be sufficiently rehabilitated to return to homemaking contributes to society by being able to maintain a viable family unit (e.g., resuming the homemaker role, even in modified form, provides the opportunity to rear the children without the need for foster care and special welfare payments).

2. *Rehabilitation must be a major integral component of all care offered by those involved in health services.* Rehabilitation should not be considered *after* there is a disability but should begin the moment the person seeks health care. In this sense, the element of prevention is incorporated into the rehabilitation process. A major goal in educating members of the health services professions is to prepare them to "think rehab" from initial contact with the patient.

3. *Rehabilitation necessitates the active participation and coordination of the health team members through constant communication to offer a truly comprehensive rehabilitation plan for the patient.* Methods commonly used for team communications are team conferences, informal discussion, written plans of care, and progress notes. To illustrate, optimum restoration of motor function is a goal for any patient. A nurse who does not know that the physiotherapist is "walking" the patient in the physical medicine department may continue to lift the patient from bed to chair rather than assisting him to ambulate on the nursing unit.

   Coordination of treatment extends into scheduling various therapies when they will be of maximum benefit. This concept applies to scheduling specific activities within the daily routine, such as mat work in the physical therapy department, when the patient's energy level is highest and he is well rested. Perhaps this would be most beneficial to the patient early in the morning or in the afternoon after a nap. Since most patients have a diminished energy level, scheduling is very important. Skills are arranged on a hierarchical scheme, and lower level skills must be mastered before a patient is ready to master higher level skills. For example, before a patient can hope to relearn holding a cup, he must be able to bend his forearm and grasp an object in his hand. Until these skills have been mastered, drinking from a cup is unachievable.

   Co-treatment means that various health team members are working at achieving specific identified mutual goals regardless of their professional discipline. For example, the physiotherapist may administer specific exercises to the weakened muscles of the arm when the goal is to strengthen these muscles. Concurrently, the occupational therapist works with the same goals in mind. The dietitian may provide special eating utensils so that the patient can use the affected arm. Using the arm with modified utensils improves muscle strength and also allows the patient a degree of independence not previously enjoyed. The success also generates a positive motivational force for the patient to continue with the prescribed therapies. When interdepartmental co-treatment is initiated, the therapists involved should also try to use the same terminology with the patient to reinforce principles and to clarify them.

4. *Rehabilitation requires the active participation of the patient to achieve optimum rehabilitative potential.* The patient is viewed as a team member. The health team members, and particularly the nurse, must help to motivate the patient to be actively involved in the rehabilitation process, slow as it may be. For example, return of voluntary motion to a paralyzed limb does not occur easily or quickly. The patient must undergo an exercise program and faithfully continue the daily exercise on his own. Unless the patient is encouraged and motivated, he may become discouraged and discontinue the exercises.

5. *Rehabilitation should actively involve the family or other significant people in the patient's life; they should be recognized as a potential support system for the patient.* The family must be reached at their level of understanding, considering their educational, socioeconomic, and cultural backgrounds. The family must understand the rehabilitative goals set for the patient and the methods selected to meet these goals. It is usually the nurse who interprets this information for the family, helping them to understand how they can best participate. For example, family members may be oversolicitous of the patient's every want and need, doing everything for him although the patient can and should do these things for himself. The family must be helped to understand that the greatest kindness for the patient is to allow him to do as much for himself as possible. In addition, the family can be taught to administer range-of-motion or other exercises, thus enabling them to feel that they are helping the patient to get better. As a resource, the family is a rich source of information about the patient's premorbid personality and lifestyle.

6. *Members of the family should be evaluated to determine their ability to help with the rehabilitation process.* All families cannot contribute in the same way or to the same degree. In some family situations, the patient could return home and receive excellent care and help. In other families, while there is a sincere interest in helping, other responsibilities and commitments prevent participation. In still other situations, the family is not willing to help or care for the patient. Perhaps other extended care facilities need to be considered. Since each family and patient present different problems, individual evaluation is necessary.

7. *The patient reacts to illness and disability according to previous adjustment patterns.* The strengths and weaknesses of the patient's personality will essentially be the same. A person who was optimistic and willing to persevere before illness will probably be the same after the initial adjustment to illness. A person who was pessimistic before the illness will probably experience a glum view of prospects for the future.

   The team members should also recognize the social and cultural influences that affect the patient's adjustment pattern. How does the patient perceive his illness, disability, and hospitalization? Does he understand the cause of his illness? What are the patient's fears? Is there reluctance to accept nursing care from the nurses or care from other team members?

8. *Rehabilitation takes place within the context of the patient's whole life space: the sociocultural aspects of his life, his job or vocation, his family, his home, his place in the community, his religion, and his relationship to himself.* When illness strikes, family life is abruptly interrupted and altered. The effects of illness affect not only the patient, but also the family. Therefore, plans for the rehabilitation process should also include the needs of the family. Since rehabilitation is a long and involved process, all aspects of the patient's life should be included in the planning.

9. *It is the goal of rehabilitation to achieve the highest level of independence for the patient.* The patient must be allowed to assume greater and greater responsibility for himself and his needs as he progresses. One way to evaluate the patient's level of independence is by evaluating the activities of daily living or ADL.

   It is recognized that regression is a part of illness. However, if this view is reinforced by the nursing personnel, then they contribute to the development of a "crippled personality." Some patients are inclined to let the nurse do everything for them; however, it is the nurse's responsibility to encourage, motivate, and support the patient to do for himself. While it is actually much easier and faster to do everything for the patient, such an approach will only enforce dependency and be a great disservice to him.

10. *Rehabilitation is a dynamic process in which there is progress, plateaus, and setbacks.* Only through an ongoing, systematic, problem-solving process such as the nursing process is the achievement of patient goals possible. Other occupational groups call the process the scientific method of thinking and problem-solving. Regardless of what term is used to identify this model, the process includes the elements of assessment, planning, implementation, and evaluation. Based on the process of evaluation, changes in the plan of care may be indicated so that the process with its four components is implemented as a continuous process.
11. *Plans for extended care after hospitalization in an acute care facility should be made far in advance of the actual discharge date.* The patient and family need to be presented with alternatives of care and helped to evaluate the implications of each choice. The patient and family must actively participate in the decision-making process of discharge planning to the degree that they are able and willing to participate. In this way, they are helped to realistically plan, anticipate, and deal with problems so that a relatively smooth adjustment is possible.

TERMS COMMONLY USED IN REHABILITATION

Rehabilitative potential – based on a thorough assessment of a patient, the health team can identify those areas of deficits (physical, emotional, psychological, occupational) that can benefit from a rehabilitation program.

Long-range goals – goals projected for completion in the extended future; can be considered the ultimate objectives of the rehabilitation program

Short-range goals – immediate goals to be achieved (frequently the small day-to-day skills to be learned so that mastery of more complex skills is possible); the steps by which long-range goals are achieved

Optimum goals – goals stated in the most optimistic terms concerning those rehabilitative expectations might be achieved by the patient barring any setbacks or complications

Realistic goals – goals set by a realistic appraisal of the patient, reflecting those realistic rehabilitative expectations that can be obtained

Physical disability – the actual, observable physical deficit noted; indicates nothing about the cause or the treatment (e.g., three patients can be dragging their left legs; in one person, the cause can be stroke, in another the cause may be arthritis, while in the third it is multiple sclerosis; treatment will vary depending on the cause).

Chronic disability – an ongoing disability that limits the patient in some way; other terms used are *permanent* and *irreversible*

Acute disability – a disability that becomes completely resolved in a short time (sometimes by death); other terms used are *temporary* and *reversible*

Team approach – various health professionals contributing their expertise and working together to provide total care for the patient

Team rounds – activity in which the various health professionals of the health team visit the patient as a group to quickly assess the patient's current status, problems, and concerns; rounds, usually conducted on a daily or weekly bases; provide a basis for further discussion at a team conference

Family meetings – planned meetings with one or more health professionals and family members to discuss the patient and/or family education; this activity recognizes the importance of the family in rehabilitation of the patient and helps to maintain open communications

HEALTH TEAM MEMBERS

Several health professionals with a unique knowledge base and special skills can participate as team members in providing a comprehensive rehabilitation program. Although all patients will not require the services of every discipline listed, these professionals may be called upon to participate in the assessment, planning, implementation, and evaluation of patients.

- Primary physician—assumes the overall responsibility to direct the patient's plan of care, making appropriate referrals as necessary
- Professional nurse—using the nursing process, the nurse is responsible for the nursing care necessary in the rehabilitation program; plays a major role in patient and family teaching
- Physiatrist—a physician with specialized, formal preparation in physical and rehabilitative medicine
- Physical therapist—provides for the rehabilitation of deficits primarily of the musculoskeletal system
- Speech therapist—works with patients who have deficits or problems in communicating
- Occupational therapist—works with the patient to develop the skills of daily living
- Vocational counselor—tests and evaluates the patient's interests and potential for vocational training
- Dietitian—counsels the patient and family on good nutrition and any dietary modifications necessary as a result of illness
- Social worker—assists the patient and family in the socioeconomic concerns of illness; also makes referrals to extended care and community resources to provide for continuity of care
- Psychologist—assesses the emotional and psychological responses of the patient and family as they deal with the stresses of illness; may provide therapy and/or work with a psychiatrist in selected instances to aid the patient and/or family
- Neuropsychologist—assesses and treats the specific cognitive and emotional problems associated with head injury and neurological disease

REHABILITATIVE NURSING

Rehabilitative nursing is an integral part of all nursing care and includes the major elements of prevention, maintenance, and restoration. For the neurological–neurosurgical patient, much of nursing management is directed toward preventing complications and added disability. Skin care, positioning, turning, and range-of-motion exercises are a few examples of nursing protocols directed at prevention.

The maintenance of intact skills and functions is supported by such activities as deep breathing exercises, eye care, range-of-motion exercises, and support of intact skills associated with activities of daily living. This is particularly vital in the long-term management of comatose patients as the effects of immobilization on all body systems are observed.

The restoration of function can be supported by outlining an exercise program to reestablish independent function in a paralyzed limb. It should be noted that many nursing protocols contain elements of prevention, maintenance, and restoration depending on how they are viewed in relation to a particular patient.

The major goal of rehabilitation nursing is to help the patient achieve the greatest degree of independence possible. In working toward this goal, the nurse acts as the patient's advocate and teaches both the family and the patient. Part of this teaching function includes encouraging and supporting the patient to carry out as many independent activities as possible.

Unlike other aspects of nursing, rehabilitation is often a very slow process requiring continued dedication and effort. However, the long-lasting reward is the knowledge that a human being has been helped to achieve his maximum potential.

Rehabilitation is a cooperative process involving health professionals of various disciplines working together to achieve mutual goals. Because rehabilitation is a responsibility shared by various health disciplines, coordination and communication are critical for achieving the desired goals for the patient. As the member of the rehabilitation team who spends the most time with the patient on a daily basis, and is involved with his care from the moment that he enters the hospital until he is discharged from the acute care setting, the nurse often coordinates the various aspects of care provided by other health team members. The nurse can help coordinate and manipulate the patient's daily schedule so that he will derive optimum benefit from his therapy. As already mentioned, the patient should be at a high energy level for the strenuous activity of mat work or ambulation in his physical therapy program. Scheduling him for these activities when he is tired is counterproductive to the goals of physical therapy.

Because the nurse spends more time with the patient throughout the day than other health care team members, she is able to assess the patient's physical, emotional, and psychological response to various therapies. Based on the assessment, she is able to identify concerns or problems faced by the patient. One common problem is that health professionals use unfamiliar terminology when talking to the patient. Another problem is the lack of consistency in terminology when the various team members describe the same phenomenon to the patient. Such areas of concern can be referred to the health team members so that clarification and consistency of terminology is incorporated into care.

The family often approaches the nurse with questions and concerns about the overall plan of care. In some instances the nurse can provide information and clarification. In other instances it may be necessary to refer questions to other team members or to initiate a family–team meeting. Keeping the lines of communication open is a tedious and difficult job that is compounded by the large number of people involved in the care of the patient. The nurse often becomes the clearinghouse for information, concerns, and confrontations.

Further elucidation of the role of the nurse in rehabilitation is addressed in *Standards of Neurosurgical Nursing Practice* and the *Standards of Rehabilitation Nursing Practice*. Both publications were written and published by the specialty organization and the American Nurses' Association, Division of Medical–Surgical Nursing Practice.

PRINCIPLES OF LEARNING AND TEACHING

An important role of the nurse in the rehabilitation process is that of teaching the patient and family. Effective teaching rests on an understanding of the principles of learning and teaching as applied to the clinical setting.

The following basic principles can serve as a guide in teaching the patient:

- The objectives of the teaching session should be clearly defined; it is wise to write down behavioral objectives in order to identify the knowledge and skills the patient is expected to learn.
- The skills involved in the activity should be limited to small, critical units to facilitate learning.
- People learn best when they are able to perceive a need or value in the learning.
- Readiness to learn is important if the patient is to benefit from the material presented; he must have sufficient physical and mental function to learn successfully.
- The patient should be rested and comfortable before the teaching session begins in order to enhance concentration.
- The nurse should demonstrate the skill and then have the patient perform the skill under supervision; if the skill is not performed correctly, it should be demonstrated again; the patient may need extensive supervision, as well as repetition, to master the skill.
- The more senses involved in learning, the more apt the patient is to learn (e.g., demonstrate and tell him what you are doing; use gestures).
- Reinforcement of learning should be followed through in the same manner by all staff members working with the patient. Such reinforcement should be based on a written teaching plan.
- The patient's age, neurological deficits, educational background, fluency, and intelligence should be considered when individualizing a teaching plan that is appropriate for his needs.
- The patient should be given positive verbal feedback for his accomplishments.
- The patient should be motivated to actively participate in the learning process.
- The patient and family should be encouraged to ask questions.

For the neurological patient it is important to allow for the perceptual, motor, communication, visual, and intellectual deficits that adversely affect the learning–teaching process. An individual assessment of the patient will indicate how the teaching approach can be modified to compensate for the particular deficits the patient has sustained.

TEACHING THE PATIENT WITH A CEREBRAL INJURY

Patients with cerebral injury caused by trauma, stroke, abscess, and other etiologies present special problems in learning and teaching because of cognitive deficits. These deficits include memory loss, inability to think abstractly, easy distractibility, short attention span, poor judgment, and inability to transfer learning from one situation to another.

The following general suggestions may be helpful in teaching the patient with a cerebral injury:

- If a neuropsychological assessment of the patient has been done, review the results and seek suggestions from the neuropsychologist.
- Develop a written teaching plan for use by all personnel.
- For the patient who is easily distracted, it is best to establish an environment that is free from distractions.
- Use simple, specific instructions.
- Proceed systematically, step by step.
- Reinforce learning by constant repetition and reinforcement.
- Praise the patient for any accomplishments made.
- Assume a calm and positive attitude toward the patient's ability to learn.
- Be realistic in your expectations of the patient.

ACTIVITIES OF DAILY LIVING (ADL)

The activities of daily living, often called ADL, refer to those self-care activities that must be independently accomplished each day in order for the patient to assume responsibility for his own needs and to actively participate in society. These activities include

Bathing	Eating
Toileting	Ambulation
Hair grooming	Safety needs
Oral hygiene	Communication
Dressing	Manual tasks

Independence can be measured to the degree that the patient can successfully assume responsibility for those tasks of daily living that are necessary for successful functioning at home, at work, and in social situations.

Helping the patient relearn activities of daily living begins with an assessment of those skills that are intact, those that are lost, or those that cannot be accomplished without some help. The major barriers to relearning ADL skills in the neurological patient are deficits affecting perception, motor activity, communication, vision, and intellectual functions.

The teaching plan devised must be based on the individual needs of the patient and the principles of learning and teaching. The occupational therapist can be very helpful in making suggestions for teaching the patient activities of daily living. If the patient is being seen by the occupational therapist on a regular basis, the nurse should coordinate her activities with that of the therapist so that the patient will not become confused.

Each activity that the patient must relearn must be analyzed to identify the critical components of the activity. The teaching program begins with these basic components so that the patient may learn to accomplish the overall activity. Use of adaptive devices may be necessary to compensate for neurological deficits and to allow the patient to be independent in the activities of daily living. For example, a spoon with a bulky stem may allow the patient with contractures of the hand to grasp the spoon, an act that he could not accomplish if the spoon were of regular size or shape.

MANAGEMENT OF NEUROMUSCULAR DEFICITS

Independence is closely correlated with a person's ability to move his individual body parts or his body as a total unit. Loss of this ability as a result of neurological impairment imposes severe constraints on the individual's freedom and independence, and it is a devastating loss. Unlike patients with disabilities to other body systems, the patient with a cerebral injury may not have the intellectual ability to fully comprehend the extent of implications of his disabilities because of an altered level of consciousness and injury to the cerebral cortex. He may not understand the relationship of prescribed treatment to maintenance of motor function, prevention of functional loss, or restoration of previously intact abilities. The rehabilitative protocols implemented by the nurse are necessary if the patient is to achieve an optimum level of independence.

Several types of activities contribute to the rehabilitation of neuromuscular function. Each complex activity is composed of elementary building blocks that must be mastered before the patient can successfully accomplish the more complex skills. For example, a patient cannot sit on the side of the bed until he has developed the ability to assume the vertical position without the consequence of orthostatic hypotension. In addition, he must be able to hold his head up and balance himself. After mastery of these skills, he is ready to learn the more complex task of sitting.

The following activities require consideration in rehabilitation of neuromuscular function:

- Proper positioning
- Range-of-motion exercises
- Balancing and sitting
- Transfer activities
- Ambulation
- Equipment to aid in ambulation

POSITIONING

Positioning the patient in proper body alignment is necessary to prevent the development of (1) musculoskeletal deformities such as contractures and ankylosis, (2) skin breakdown, including skin irritation, blisters, and pressure necrosis, and (3) decreased vascular supply, thrombosis, and edema.

Positioning the neurological patient may be complicated by spasticity, nuchal rigidity, decortication, decerebration, the presence of a cast, limitation of positioning because of surgery, and multiple skin lacerations or abrasions associated with multiple traumas. These specific problems encountered in positioning change as the muscles undergo the various phases of recovery (see Table 8–1).

A few basic principles can serve as a guide in positioning the patient in bed:

- The position of the unconscious patient should be changed every 1 to 2 hours around the clock. As the patient regains consciousness he must be encouraged to move independently if he can do so and participate in self-care activities to maintain muscle strength and tone. Proper positioning should be taught to the patient.
- If spasticity is present, frequent repositioning will be necessary.
- Any restrictions on position should be conspicuously labeled on 4-inch tape at the head of the bed and included in the nursing care plan.
- The patient should be placed on a firm, supportive mattress preferrably with a bedboard and alternating pressure mattress. A footboard should be attached to the foot of the bed to provide resistance and support to the feet so that footdrop will not develop (Fig. 8–1). Other foot-positioning devices may also be used to prevent abnormal positioning of the foot.
- A bed cradle may be used to prevent pressure from the bedclothes on the body.
- A sufficient number of pillows should be available to maintain body position.
- Trochanter rolls, slings, sand bags, and other positioning devices may also be used.
- If an arm is paralyzed, the arm should be positioned to approximate the joint space of the glenoid cavity; a sling or pillows may be helpful; do not pull on the paralyzed limb.
- The patient's heels should be kept off the bed to prevent bed sores from developing; a pillow should be placed crosswise to elevate the lower legs; heel guards may be applied.
- Wrist–palm splints may be necessary to maintain functional position of the hands.
- A pillow in the axillary region will help to prevent adduction of the shoulder.
- Edema of the extremities, particularly the hands, can be controlled by positioning and elevating the hand higher than the elbow.

Supine Position

An unconscious patient, or one who has a diminished or absent swallowing or gag reflex, should not be positioned directly on his back because his tongue may fall back, occluding the airway. In addition, secretions may be aspirated if the patient is left on his back. Therefore, positioning the patient in the true prone position is reserved only for the conscious patient.

In the instance of a patient who has been on long-term bed rest, it may be necessary to use a modified position halfway between the prone and side-lying position to relieve pressure on body surfaces. This position requires that the patient's head be turned to provide for drainage of oral secretions and patency of the airway (Fig. 8–2).

Prone Position

Positioning the patient on his abdomen may be a welcome relief for him. However, such a position is contraindicated in the presence of a gastrostomy tube or a tracheostomy, or when it is necessary to keep the head of the bed at a 30-degree angle (Fig. 8–3).

Side-Lying Position

The side-lying position (with bed flat to 10 degrees) facilitates drainage of secretions from the mouth. The head should be checked to prevent hyperflexion, which would partially obstruct the airway as well as impede venous drainage from the head. Proper body alignment is maintained through the use of pillows.

TABLE 8–1. *Neurological Patterns of Muscle Recovery in Hemiplegia*

Stage	*Name*	*Onset*	*Description*
I	Flaccidity	Injury to 2 or 3 days	No tendon reflexes or resistance to passive movement
II	Spasticity (late onset of spasticity indicates a poor prognosis)	2 days to 5 weeks	Hyperactive tendon reflexes and exaggerated response to minimal stimuli
III	Synergy (flexion then extension)	2 to 3 weeks	Appearance of simultaneous flexion of muscle groups in response to flexion of a single muscle (attempt to flex elbow results in contraction of fingers, elbow, and shoulder)
IV	Near normal; possible weakness or slight incoordination may still be present (late return of tendon reflexes indicates a poor prognosis)	1 week to 6 months	Control of voluntary movement; recovery occurs predictably from the proximal muscles of the extremity to the distal muscles (voluntary movement of hand and foot is last to recover and tends to be weaker)

EXERCISE PROGRAM

Any voluntary muscle will lose muscle tone and strength if it is not used. Patients with neurological deficits of paresis and paralysis as well as those confined to prolonged bed rest are subject to these deleterious muscle effects (Table 8-2).

Since the flexor and adductor muscles are stronger than the extensors and abductors, contractures of the flexor and adductor muscles will quickly develop if preventive measures are not instituted. An exercise program must be aggressively followed to maintain muscle tone and function, to prevent additional disability, and to aid in restoration of impaired motor function.

Range-of-motion exercises include the full range of movement that each joint of the body can *normally* perform. A patient who cannot carry out independent range-of-motion exercises should be assisted in this activity by the nurse. Once radiographs have proven negative for fractures, and no other medical problems or medical treatment contraindicates movement of a particular body part, range-of-motion exercises should begin.

Exercises can be classified into the following categories:

- *Passive*—motion provided to a body joint by another person or outside force without the voluntary participation of the patient
- *Active*—voluntary motion to a body joint that is independently accomplished by the individual
- *Active assistive*—motion to a body joint accomplished by the patient with the assistance of another person
- *Active resistive*—motion voluntarily provided to a body joint against resistance
- *Isometric* or *muscle-setting*—exercise accomplished by alternately tightening and relaxing the muscle without joint movement

The particular exercise program selected by the physician and physiatrist will depend on the stage of illness and the particular disabilities experienced by the patient. In the acute stages of illness a physical therapist often comes to the nursing unit once or twice daily to administer specific exercises ordered for the patient at bedside. Once the patient's condition improves he will be taken to the physical medicine department where equipment is available for a more sophisticated, aggressive rehabilitation program. An awareness of the objectives of the physical therapy program will enable the nurse to reinforce the rehabilitation skills learned by the patient by integrating them into other aspects of the plan of care. At the same time the patient's family can be taught the method of carrying out the prescribed exercises.

Passive Range-of-Motion Exercises

When passive range-of-motion exercises are administered, two factors must be considered: the joint being exercised and the placement of the hands in carrying out the exercise properly.

- One hand is placed above the joint to provide support against gravity and any unwanted movement.

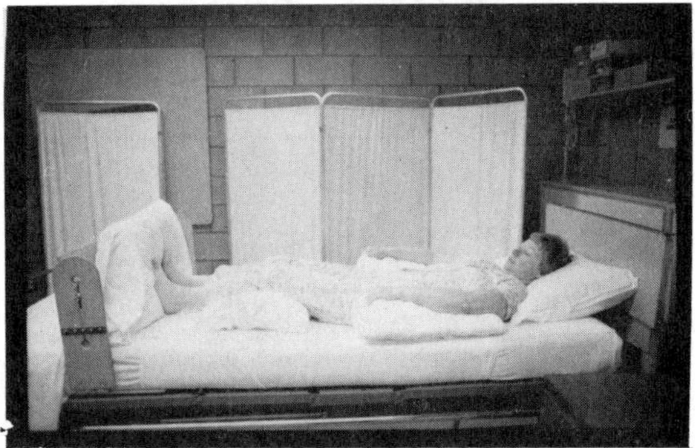

FIG. 8-1. A foot board may be used for proper positioning to prevent footdrop.

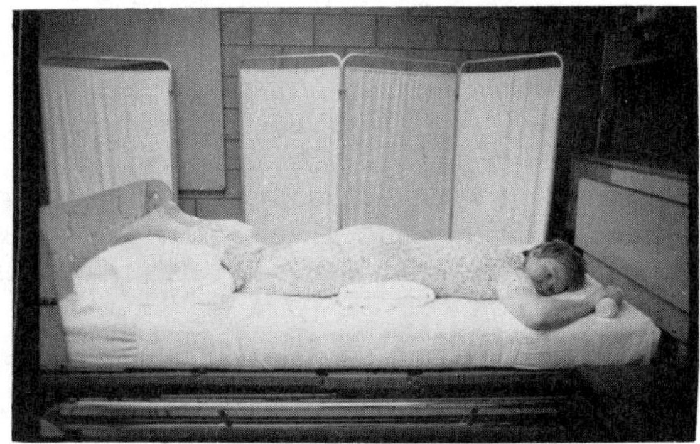

FIG. 8-2. Proper positioning of the patient in supine position.

FIG. 8-3. Proper positioning of the patient in side-lying position.

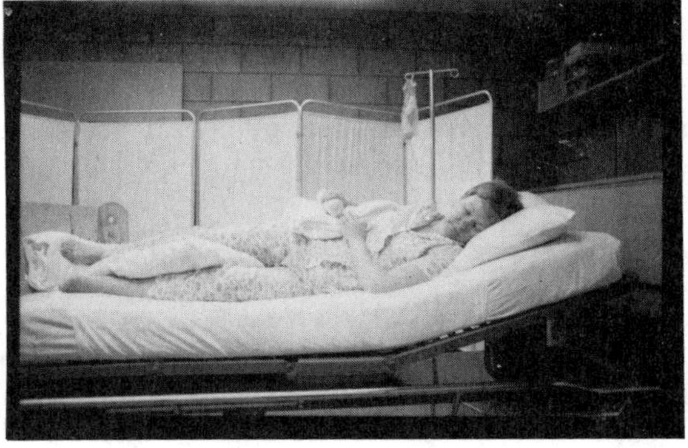

- The other hand gently moves the joint through its normal range of motion.

Passive range-of-motion exercises are usually administered to the patient at least four times daily and may be incorporated, in part, with other procedures such as bathing or repositioning. It is best to choose a time when the patient is rested, comfortable, and pain-free in order to gain his cooperation. An explanation of what is being done should be given to the patient, even if he appears to be unconscious. The patient should be positioned in proper body alignment on the bed and draped to maintain his dignity. Room temperature should be comfortable so that

TABLE 8-2. *The Effects of Prolonged Immobilization on the Musculoskeletal System*

Structure	Initial Changes	Advanced Changes
Bones	Skeletal malalignment; loss of calcium	Skeletal deformities Generalized osteoporosis
Joints	Joint stiffness and limitation of mobility; shortening or stretching of ligaments	Ankylosis
Muscles	Muscle weakening; shortening or stretching of tendons	Muscle atrophy Fibrotic changes and muscle contractures

chilling, shivering, and unwanted muscle contractions do not occur. The door should be closed or the curtains drawn around the bed to provide privacy and exclude environmental stimuli in the instance of an easily distracted patient. The nurse should maintain good posture to ensure efficient body movement and should face the patient, if possible, to observe his reaction to the exercises. The movements of the exercise should be slow, smooth, and rhythmical. The following principles should be observed when administering passive range-of-motion exercises:

- Move body part to the point of resistance and stop.
- Move body part to the point of pain and stop.
- If the patient becomes excessively fatigued, stop the exercises.

Although the physiotherapist may move a body part beyond the point of pain or resistance, this is not within the normal scope of nursing practice and should be avoided unless prescribed by the physician. As the patient's condition improves, self-care should be encouraged for as many activities as possible. Since return of motor function is a very slow process, the patient needs to be encouraged to carry out the exercises and reminded of the need to continue with these activities as part of the rehabilitation program.

Other Exercises

Specific exercises such as lifting hand weights may be ordered to strengthen a weakened arm. In addition to verbally encouraging the patient to engage in these activities, having the necessary equipment at hand serves as an added incentive for the patient. At the same time, activities can be adapted to provide movement for specific muscle groups. For example, providing a ball of yarn for a female patient who enjoys knitting can improve motor function of a weakened hand and also provide sensory stimulation.

Balancing and Sitting Activities

Once the patient's condition has stabilized and range-of-motion exercises have begun to be implemented, the next activity ordered for the patient is balancing and sitting. Most patients are encouraged to walk as soon as possible to prevent the development of the various problems of prolonged bed rest. If the patient is able to get out of bed within 3 or 4 days, he will probably not experience the problems of orthostatic hypotension or have difficulty with balance.

For the patient who has been confined to bed for a long time, it will be necessary to progress slowly. The head of the bed will have to be raised gradually over a period of days to overcome orthostatic hypotension. At the beginning of the procedure, the patient's reactions can be assessed by taking vital signs, checking skin color, and asking the patient if he is experiencing dizziness or lightheadedness. After the head of the bed is raised the prescribed number of degrees, the patient should again be assessed. A drop in blood pressure, a thready but increased pulse rate, pale diaphoretic skin, dizziness, or lightheadedness are untoward signs. If these signs are momentary and quickly pass, no action may be necessary. Severe symptoms that tend to last will require that the head of the bed be lowered slightly until symptoms subside. Since many neurological patients are placed at a 30-degree angle while confined to bed, there may not be too much adjustment necessary for them to tolerate the change to a vertical position. For the patient who has been maintained in a flat position or at a 10-degree angle, the adjustment will take longer. If the patient has great difficulty with orthostatic hypotension, a tilt table can be used. A tilt table can be adjusted to any angle as it is brought to a vertical position. This allows the patient to gradually adjust to the vertical position.

For paraplegic or quadriplegic patients orthostatic hypotension can be a stubborn problem to manage because of the extensive vasomotor paralysis that results in a subsequent drop in blood pressure when the vertical position is assumed. These patients, particularly the quadriplegics, will undoubtedly require use of the tilt table. An abdominal binder and thigh-high elastic stockings are helpful in increasing the tone of the blood vessels.

Balancing. Balancing, that is, the ability to sit or stand erectly, can be achieved for a patient with the use of support devices to steady the patient's center of gravity. The use of a sling on the paralyzed arm of a hemiplegic, or a back or neck brace on a cord-injury patient, can make the difference between success and failure. With a hemiplegic patient, the sling is used to approximate the shoulder joint (glenoid cavity). Thus, the affected arm is used to improve balance and is protected against injury. The hemiplegic patient should be helped to the sitting position and instructed to support himself with his good arm and hand. The hand should be placed flat on the bed slightly behind him or at his side as a means of support. Since there is a tendency to slouch to the affected side, the patient should be reminded to sit straight and erect; a sling is helpful for maintaining proper position.

Some conscious patients who have difficulty balancing while sitting in bed do well when they are helped to sit at the side of the bed or in a chair with their feet flat on the floor.

In the case of the unconscious patient, the same process for overcoming orthostatic hypotension can be used with the exception of collecting information from the appearance of covert symptoms. Ability to balance will not be possible until the level of consciousness improves; however, the patient can be propped in the required position.

Once the patient has mastered balancing in the sitting position, he is ready to begin balancing in the standing position at the bedside.

Sitting. Both the conscious and unconscious patient can sit in a chair, although the unconscious patient would not be positioned in the sitting position on the side of the bed. The conscious patient may sit on the side of the bed and lean on the overbed table for support. The chair selected should provide firm support and have a high back and arms, especially if the patient has motor weakness or paralysis. For the weak, debilitated patient who cannot hold up his head or neck, a high-back chair that extends to the top of the head is most effective. This patient often has a neck brace, which should be applied for sitting.

To position the patient in a chair a vest restraint can be helpful for providing added support. Pillows or rolls should be used to support the arms in the desired position. The feet should be flat on the floor. The pressure from the floor on the bottom of the foot tends to stretch the heel cord, which will lead to footdrop if stretching of the cord is not provided. The head must be positioned carefully so that the airway or tracheostomy is not obstructed. Any equipment such as a Foley catheter or continuous tube feeding that may be attached should be checked carefully to see that they are patent and free from traction.

If the patient has some independent motor function, necessary equipment should be placed near at hand, possibly on an overbed table that has been lowered and placed in front of the patient's chair. The call bell should be close at hand or pinned to the patient's clothing if the patient has neurological deficits that could interfere with his ability to find the cord easily.

The patient should be observed often and his tolerance to being out of bed evaluated. He should not be allowed to become overtired. It is best to plan a schedule that allows for periods of bed rest and out-of-bed activity based on an individual assessment of the patient's tolerance and fatigue.

TRANSFER ACTIVITIES

Once the patient is able to balance and sit he is ready for transfer activities. (Techniques described are adopted from "Up and Around," a booklet distributed by the American Heart Association.) As a rule, transfer toward the unaffected side is easiest.

Transfer Activity: Lying in Bed to Sitting Position

Hemiplegic Patient. For the hemiplegic patient, lying in bed on his back and wishing to assume the sitting position (Fig. 8–4), the ensuing steps are followed:

- The patient moves toward the side of bed upon which he intends to sit.
- The unaffected leg is slipped under the affected leg at the angle so that the unaffected leg becomes a transfer cradle for the affected limb.
- The affected arm is placed on the abdomen or in a sling.
- The patient pushes down on the mattress with the unaffected elbow, raising his upper body, while turning his hips toward the side upon which he will sit; he swings his unaffected leg upon which the affected leg rests over the side of the bed and pushes himself up with the unaffected hand.
- Once in the sitting position the patient leans on the unaffected hand to maintain an erect position.

Initially, the patient will need help in this maneuver, but as he develops skill it will become an independent activity.

Paraplegic or Quadriplegic Patient. Most transfer activities will have to be done for the patient in the acute-care setting. An orthopedic trapeze over the bed can be used to assist the paraplegic and some quadriplegic patients.

Transfer Activity: Sitting on Side of Bed to Back-Lying Position

To return to the back-lying position from a sitting position on the side of the bed involves the following steps (Fig. 8-5):

- The patient should be sitting slightly above the center of the side of the bed so that he will be in the proper position on the mattress once he is lying on the bed.
- The affected arm is placed on the lap.
- The unaffected foot is slipped under the affected ankle.
- The unaffected hand is placed on the edge of the mattress near the unaffected hip.
- The hand presses into the mattress, lowering the body onto the bed while the elbow bends.
- Simultaneously, the unaffected leg swings into the bed as the body is lowered.
- The ankle is uncrossed and the unaffected knee is bent; the body is pushed up or pulled down onto the bed, as necessary, with the bending and pulling action of the knee.

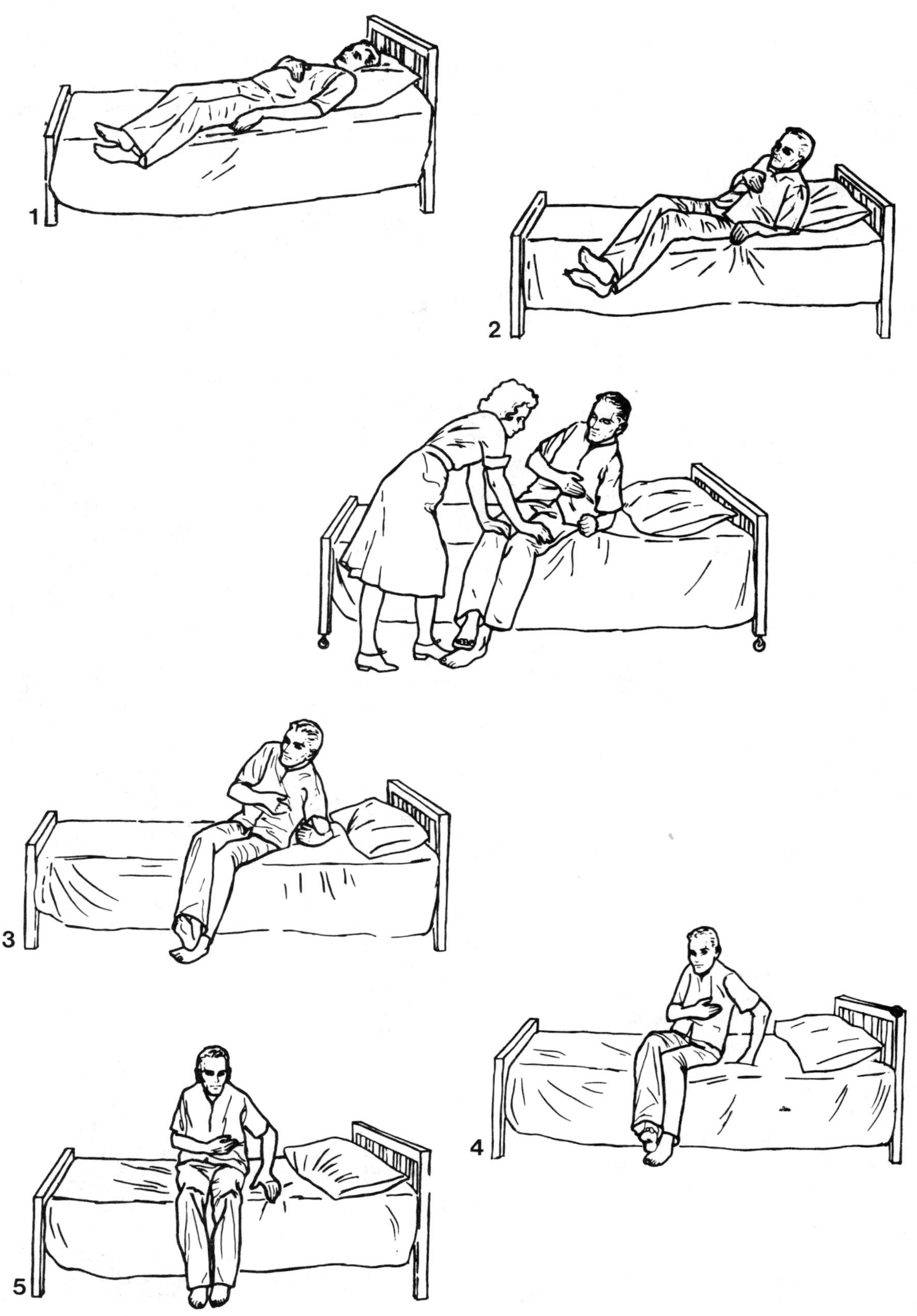
1
2
3
4
5

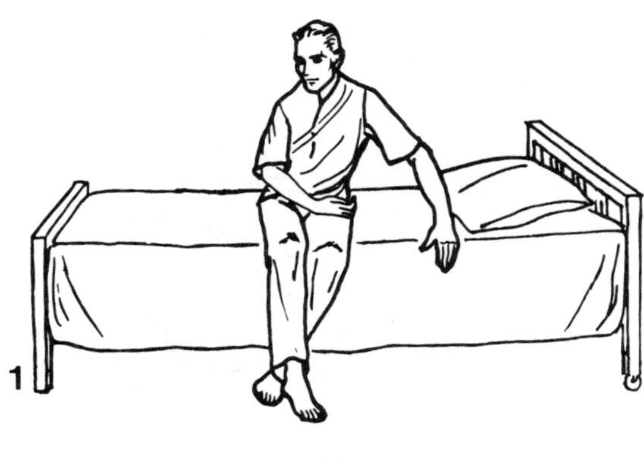

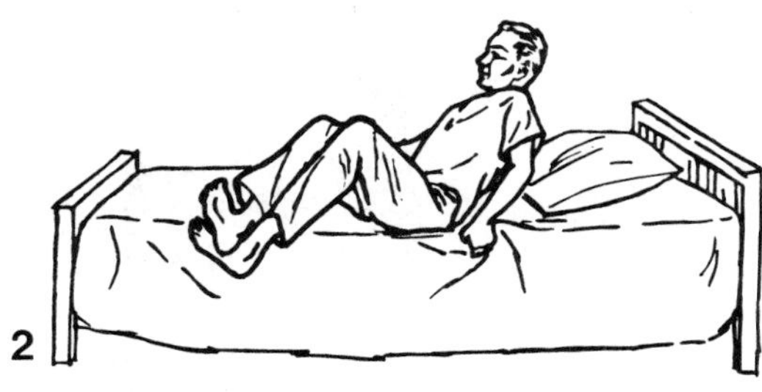

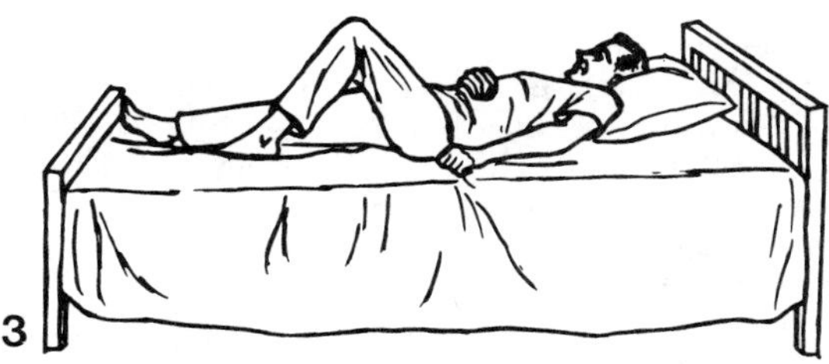

FIG. 8-5. Moving from a sitting position on the edge of the bed to a back-lying position. *(1)* Place weak arm across the lap. Slide strong foot under weak ankle. *(2)* With strong hand grasp edge of mattress near the hips and press against bed, lowering body to bed as elbow bends. At the same time swing legs onto bed. (Note: Patient should be seated in proper spot so that his head will be on the pillow when he lies down.) *(3)* Uncross legs. Bend strong hip and knee and push against bed with heel to move body up or down in bed to proper position. (Up and Around. Reprinted with permission of the American Heart Association)

Transfer Activity: Sitting Position on Bed to Chair

To transfer from the bed into a chair requires planning. If a chair is used, it should provide firm support and have arms. In the case of a wheelchair, the chair should be locked with the footrests up.

Hemiplegic Patient. The following steps should be followed (Fig. 8-6):

- Any catheter or tubes secured to the bed are unpinned.
- The chair is placed at a slight angle as close as possible to the bed on the patient's unaffected side.
- With feet close together, the patient leans forward slightly, puts unaffected hand on the mattress edge, and pushes to a standing position bearing weight on the unaffected side.
- Once balance has been steadily maintained, the patient uses the unaffected arm to grasp the chair arm most distant from the side of the bed.
- The patient pivots himself on the unaffected foot while he continues to lean forward slightly and lowers himself onto the chair.

Paraplegic or Quadriplegic Patient. In the hospital, the paraplegic or quadriplegic patient will need to be lifted into the chair with the aid of two or three people, depending on the patient's height and weight. Some patients can learn to transfer themselves from the bed to a chair with the use of a transfer board.

Transfer Activity: From Chair to Bed

To go from a chair to a sitting position on the bed the following technique is followed (Fig. 8-7):

- The chair should be at a slight angle as close to the bed as possible; the patient's unaffected side should be closest to the bed.
- The patient's feet should be placed firmly on the floor close to the chair with the unaffected heel slightly in back and directly under the edge of the seat.
- The patient moves forward in the chair, placing the unaffected hand on the front portion of the arm of the chair.
- Leaning forward over the unaffected leg, the patient pushes himself to the standing position so that his feet are slightly apart with most of his weight on the unaffected leg.
- After regaining his balance with the support of the armrest he leans slightly forward, reaches for the edge of the mattress, and pivots on his unaffected foot, slowly lowering himself to the sitting position

◀ **FIG. 8-4.** Getting up and sitting on the side of the bed. *(1)* Use strong hand to place weak arm across abdomen. Slide strong foot under weak ankle; move both legs to side of bed on strong side and over the side. *(2)* Grasp edge of mattress as illustrated and push with elbow and forearm against the bed. (Caution: If patient feels dizzy when he first sits up, the nurse should stand in front of him and give support if needed.) *(3)* Come to half-sitting position, supporting body weight on strong forearm. (Note: Assistance can be given in 2 and 3 by the nurse pushing down on patient's knees. If this is not enough, the nurse can place her left hand in back of his shoulders and exert pressure forward and to the strong side. Someone should stand in front of him after he is sitting up in order to steady him. If his balance is very poor, one may sit on his weak side and support him while he tries to support himself with his strong hand. *(4)* Move hand to the rear, pushing to full sitting position. *(5)* Move around until sitting securely on side of bed, uncross legs. (Up and Around. Reprinted with permission of the American Heart Association)

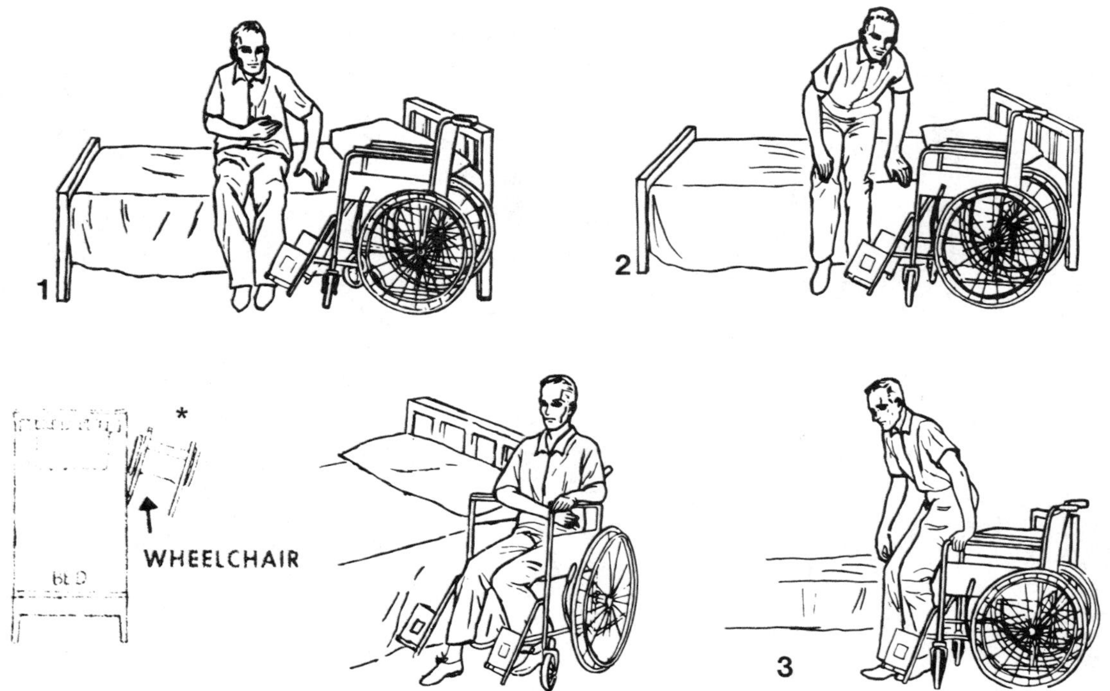

FIG. 8–6. Moving into a wheelchair from the bed. *(1)* Place wheelchair at slight angle to bed on patient's strong side, facing foot of bed. Keep the right front corner of the chair as close to the bed as possible (see *asterisk* in figure). Lock brakes and put up footrests. (Note: An armchair can be used by the bed instead of a wheelchair. A chair that is heavy enough not to slide—with a firm seat that is not too soft or too low—will be suitable. *(2)* Keep feet beneath body, lean forward placing strong hand near edge of bed, and push to standing position keeping weight well over strong foot. *(3)* When standing position is steady enough for momentary release of support by strong hand, move strong hand to farther armrest of wheelchair. Keeping body weight well forward, turn on strong foot and lower to sitting position. (Up and Around. Reprinted with permission of the American Heart Association)

Transfer Activity: Sitting to Standing Position

Hemiplegic Patient. The same technique can be used as outlined for the patient transferring from a sitting position on the bed to a chair (Fig. 8–8). A walker or four-point cane may be used for support. If the patient is unsteady, the nurse should stand on the patient's affected side so that she is in a position to slip a hand under his upper arm, grasp a belt around his waist, or secure the top of his pajama bottom.

If the patient requires even more assistance, the nurse can stand in front of the patient with her feet apart. The patient can be grasped around the waist and pulled to an erect position, while the nurse's knee is pushed against the patient's unaffected knee to lock the knee in position and prevent it from buckling. This action enables the patient to bear some of the weight of his body.

Learning to stand erect is necessary before ambulation training can begin. If the patient has difficulty raising his affected leg, a special shoe with a foot brace may be helpful. In any event, well-fitting, sensible shoes, rather than slippers, should be worn. Most slippers offer little support and tend to slide on the floor.

Other transfer activities that the patient may need to learn, depending on the permanence of the disability, could include transferring from the wheelchair to the toilet or bathtub or automobile.

Ambulation

Hemiplegic Patient. Before a patient can ambulate, he must first learn to stand and balance himself in the upright position. Standing exercises can begin at the bedside and proceed in the parallel bars in the physical therapy department. Standing helps to reinforce a good, positive body image and a feeling of wholeness and improves overall physical fitness.

Once the patient has mastered standing, he is evaluated to determine if any special bracing or support equipment is necessary. If the patient is developing footdrop or has a tendency to drag the foot, a short leg brace with a spring in it can be very helpful. This type of brace is designed to prevent extreme plantar flexion. If the patient is weak, a crutch, four-point cane, or walker may be necessary (Fig. 8–9). A sling may be applied to the affected arm for balance. The sling should be adjusted to approximate the glenoid (shoulder) joint space. Do not pull on the affected arm.

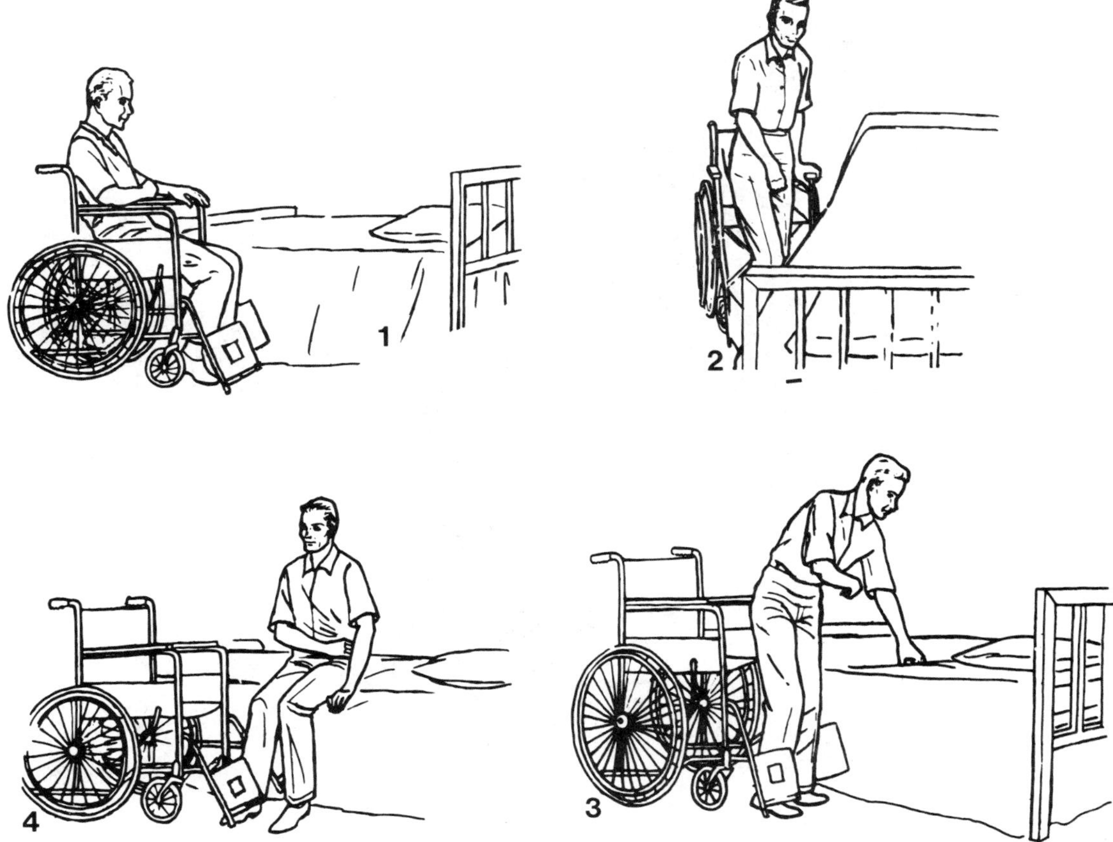

FIG. 8–7. Moving *(clockwise)* from wheelchair to bed. *(1)* Place wheelchair toward head of bed. Keep front corner of chair (on patient's unaffected side) as close to bed as possible (as wheelchair shown in *2*). Position the wheelchair so the patient sits near the center of the bed, or closer to the foot if the person is tall. Lock brakes and lift footrests. *(2)* Assume standing position from wheelchair. *(3)* Move strong hand to edge of bed for support. *(4)* Lean forward, turn on strong foot, and slowly lower to sitting position. (Up and Around. Reprinted with permission of the American Heart Association)

Ambulation or gait training often begins at the parallel bars where the patient learns to bend a knee and then extend it again. This exercise is alternated from one knee to the other. If the affected knee continues to be weak and tends to buckle, a longer leg brace can be designed to compensate for this disability.

In helping the patient to ambulate on the nursing unit, the nurse should walk on his affected side. Added support may be given by grasping the patient's belt or the top of his trousers or by applying a safety belt. The patient may feel more secure walking near the wall with his unaffected side nearest the wall. A handrail in the corridor or room is also another source of support and security. Concurrently, the patient is also learning transfer activities. In the physical therapy department climbing and descending stairs is also taught.

For the patient unable to master ambulation, wheelchair mobility may be achieved using the unaffected extremity to propel the wheelchair on a level surface. This provides a degree of independence. Electric (battery-operated) wheelchairs are still another alternative for providing mobility.

It is impossible to state the intervals when the activities for balancing, sitting, standing, and walking should be introduced and mastered. The patient's age, severity of illness, other neurological deficits, chronic conditions, and complications contribute to the patient's progress. The patient's attitude and motivation are also important factors in the rehabilitation process. Frequent assessment provides systematic evaluation of the patient's needs so that rehabilitation can progress steadily toward the greatest level of independence.

Paraplegic or Quadriplegic Patient. Some paraplegic and a few quadriplegic patients can walk with the help of braces and canes. Others are confined to wheelchairs that they must learn to operate. The process of teaching the patient to adjust to life in a wheelchair is termed *wheelchair rehabilitation*. Rehabilitation of this magnitude is usually conducted in a rehabilitation center after the patient is discharged from an acute-care setting.

Battery-operated wheelchairs that are activated by a breath sensor located near the mouth of the quadriplegic patient provide a degree of independence for the patient. Even a quadriplegic patient with an injury at C–5 can use

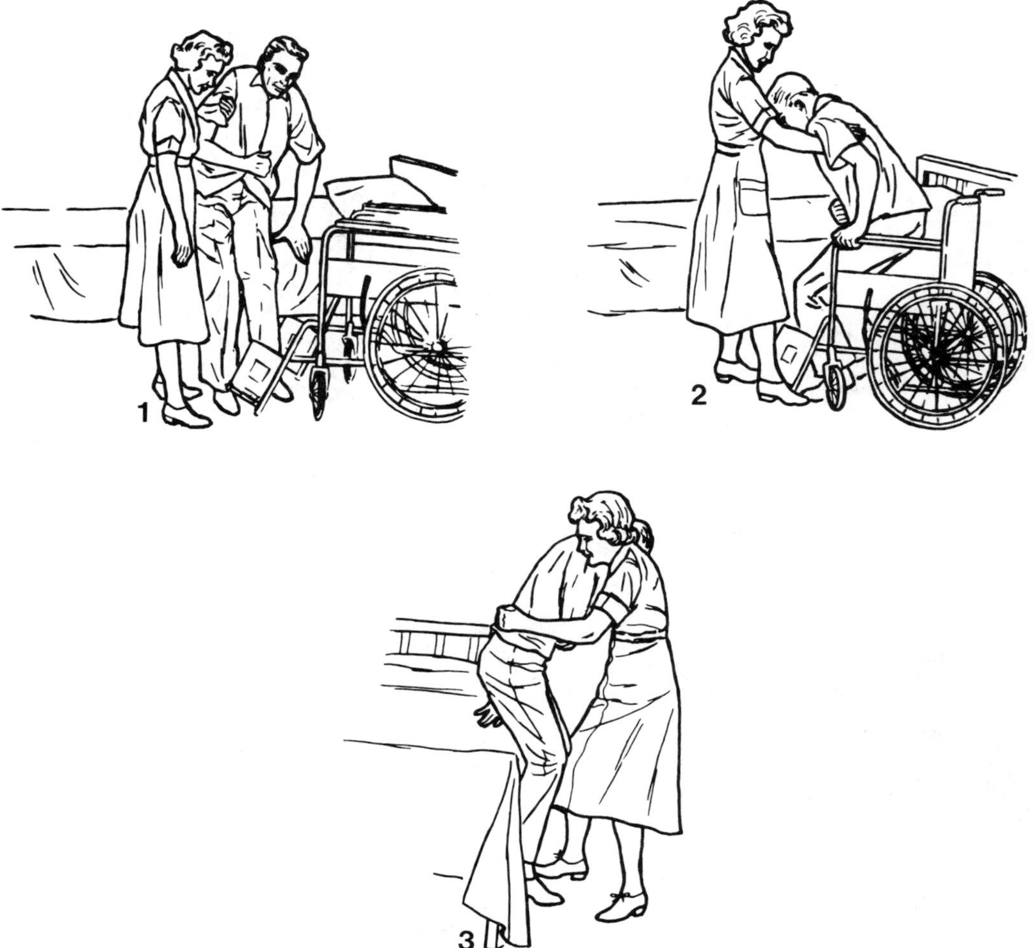

FIG. 8–8. Assisting the patient to a standing position. *(1)* When minimum help is needed, stand on patient's weak side and place your hand under his weak arm. If his shoulder is sore, grasp him by his belt or the top of his pants at the rear. *(2)* For greater assistance, place your arms under both of his armpits with your hands well onto his back. Keep his weight forward. *(3)* When even more help is needed, place your right knee against his strong knee. Grasp patient around the waist with both arms and pull him forward and up, requiring him to take weight on his strong leg by pressure of your knee forcing his knee straight. Using your right leg and his strong leg as a pivot, turn around and lower him into the wheelchair. (Place wheelchair as shown in *1* and *2*.) (Note: The helper should have feet well apart and should lift with the legs rather than the back.) (Up and Around. Reprinted with permission of the American Heart Association)

this wheelchair. The paraplegic patient does well in a standard wheelchair or an electric wheelchair operated by hand controls.

The use of computer-operated equipment programmed to execute many mundane activities such as moving draperies on traverse rods or turning out lights have afforded a greater degree of independence to the disabled person. Computer technology for the disabled person is developing rapidly. As the technology improves, the cost decreases, making the equipment more accessible for the patient.

MANAGEMENT OF THE SKIN

The patient with neurological disease is a prime candidate for the development of pressure sores because of the motor, sensory, and vasomotor deficits resulting from neurological disease. The lack of muscle tone, voluntary movement, and perception of pain can be cited as contributory factors in the development of pressure sores, but the most important factor is the lowered tissue resistance to pressure caused by interruption of the vasomotor pathways. Pressure that exceeds the tissue capillary pressure leads to tissue ischemia from the diminished cellular metabolism because of deficient nutritional and blood supply to the area. Prolonged tissue ischemia results in decubitus ulcers.

Several factors contribute to the development of decubitus or pressure sores:

- Poor nutritional status; emaciation
- Infections
- Debilitated condition (e.g., multiple-trauma patient, elderly)
- Edema
- Anemia

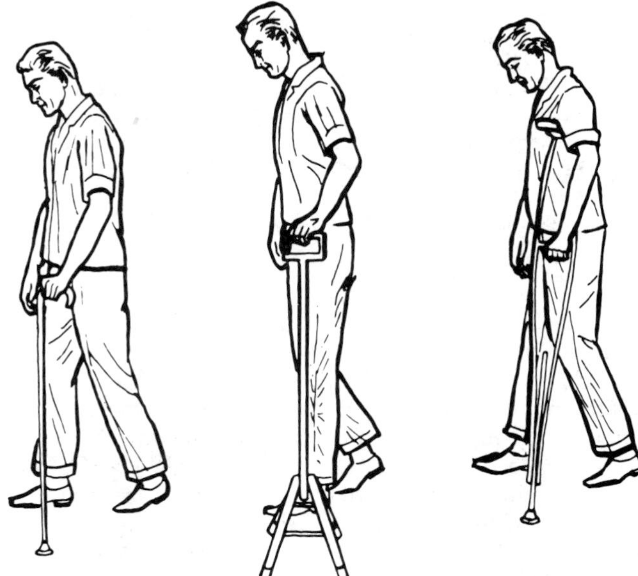

FIG. 8–9. Assistive devices such as a cane, a wide-base cane, or crutches may be necessary for ambulation. (Up and Around. Reprinted with permission of the American Heart Association)

- Prolonged bed rest and immobility
- Tropic skin changes

The aforementioned neurological deficits, coupled with any of these contributing factors, increase the incidence of pressure sores.

The bony prominences that are covered with a small amount of muscle and/or subcutaneous tissue are frequent sites for pressure sores. The sacrum and trochanters in the bedridden patient and the ischial tuberosities in the patient who sits for prolonged periods of time (paraplegics, victims of multiple sclerosis) are examples of thinly covered bony prominences subject to skin breakdown. Other areas include the scapulae, elbows, spine, occiput, knees, malleoli, and heels.

PREVENTION

Nursing care is always directed towards the prevention of pressure sores. Once a broken area develops, it is very difficult for injured tissue to heal. The nurse must assess the skin at frequent intervals to maintain its integrity. An individual assessment of contributing factors that increase the possibility of pressure sores should be compiled and kept up-to-date.

Nursing protocols commonly incorporated into the nursing care plan to prevent skin breakdown include

- Applying an alternating pressure mattress on the bed to temporarily relieve skin areas of continuous pressure
- Turning the patient from one side to the other (or from side to back to side in the conscious patient) to relieve pressure on the skin, especially bony prominences; the patient is turned at least *every 2 hours.*
- Repositioning the patient at least *every 2 hours* to change the areas of skin-bearing weight
- Using sheepskin under the shoulders, back, and buttocks to relieve pressure
- Using special pads to relieve pressure
- Providing skin care every 2 to 4 hours; skin care is directed toward maintaining clean, well-lubricated, moisture-free skin
- Massaging any reddened areas to improve circulation; the patient should be repositioned to prevent any pressure on that area
- Applying tincture of benzoin to persistent reddened areas to form a protective coating against added irritation (the tincture should be well dried to prevent the patient from sticking to other surfaces that can cause the skin to be pulled off once the foreign material is removed)
- Keeping the heels off the bed with proper positioning techniques
- Protecting the skin from excess cold or heat

Skin care entails keeping the skin clean, well lubricated, and dry. The presence of moisture from perspiration, urine, or feces can contribute to rapid skin breakdown. The skin should be washed with mild soap and warm water. If the skin is very dry, adding a lubricating bath preparation or a little baby oil to the bath water will prevent more drying and will lubricate the skin. The skin should be meticulously dried after washing. If a patient is obese and perspires between skin folds, special care should be given to keeping the skin dry. Applying corn starch or powder may be helpful.

Healthy skin is neither oily nor dry. Dry skin can crack, leading to skin breakdown and providing a major entrance for microbial invasion. Extremely dry skin should be lubricated with cream or lanolin–cocoa butter preparations. Trophic changes associated with neurological disease can cause very dry skin, which requires special management.

ASSESSMENT OF THE SKIN

A systematic ongoing assessment can reveal any evidence of skin irritation and breakdown.

The following points should be considered in assessing the skin:

- Every square inch of skin should be visually inspected at least every 24 hours; some areas require inspection as frequently as every 2 hours.
- The heel of the foot must be inspected since pressure sores commonly develop in this area and can easily be overlooked unless the foot is lifted up and checked.
- Bony prominences should be inspected for redness when the patient is turned and repositioned (every 2 hours).
- The ear lobes can crack from irritation caused by the tape used for head dressings and frequent turning; thus these areas must be checked.
- Elbows should be checked for possible irritation from starched bed linen.
- Special skin precautions must be taken for patients suffering from lacerations and contusions associated with multiple injuries.
- Any skin irritation or redness should be reported and documented; a written nursing care plan should be developed to correct the problem.

MANAGEMENT OF A PRESSURE SORE

A pressure sore can range from a reddened area to necrosis of skin, fat, or muscle with bone involvement. The management of the patient will depend on the extent of involvement and the protocols followed by the physician and institution. The more severe pressure sores may require surgical débridement and plastic surgery. Less severe areas require the application of heat, topical drugs, and dressings.

IMPAIRMENT OF PERCEPTION

The major function of the parietal lobe of the nondominant hemisphere is to recognize, interpret, and integrate sensory stimuli from the body, thereby providing accurate information concerning the internal and external environment. The nondominant parietal lobe in most patients is located in the right hemisphere. Injury to this lobe from such conditions as stroke, tumor, or ischemia can result in perceptual deficits, which can be generally classified into the following categories:

- Deficits in perception of self and illness
- Deficits in perception of spatial relationships
- Agnosias
- Apraxias

DEFICITS IN PERCEPTION OF SELF AND ILLNESS

Body image is the concept one has of the relationship of the sum of one's body parts in forming a whole unit in space. Lesions of the parietal lobe can result in a distortion of body image and impaired awareness of disability or illness. The term *anosognosia* is used to describe denial of disability. For example, a hemiplegic patient may neglect the paralyzed portion of his body or deny the presence of illness. The degree of anosognosia can range from inattention to one side of the body to absolute denial of the existence of paralysis or other deficits.

Assessment for Anosognosia

Anosognosia may be reflected in any of the following behaviors:

- Failure to use the involved side of the body without being reminded to do so
- A lack of concern about the disability and failure to understand how the paralysis and other deficits will affect lifestyle
- Lack of awareness or outright denial of the presence of paralysis or other deficits on the involved side

Nursing Management for Anosognosia

For the patient who neglects one side of his body or denies deficits on that side the nurse should

- Accept the patient's perception of himself and provide for the safety and cleanliness of the area.
- Provide tactile stimuli to the affected side by touching or stroking the affected side by itself rather than stimulating both sides simultaneously.
- Teach the patient to position the affected extremity carefully and to check its position by looking at it; if he completely ignores the area, use positioning to improve his perception (*e.g.*, position patient facing his affected side so that he is looking at the area).
- Encourage the patient to handle his affected side.

DEFICITS IN PERCEPTION OF SPATIAL RELATIONSHIPS

Spatial relationships refer to one's awareness of oneself in relationship to the location of environmental objects. A patient with a perception deficit may neglect half of the environment and disregard objects as well as that part of his body located on that side. All sensory input from the affected side is disregarded. One simple test to demonstrate spatial neglect is to ask the patient to draw a clock. A patient with a spatial deficit will draw only that portion of the clock within his unaffected field.

In general, the patient's ability to judge position, distance, movement, form, and the relationship of his body parts to the surrounding environment is impaired. He may have difficulty in any of the following activities:

- Impaired recall of the placement of objects in a familiar environment, such as the location of windows and doors in the room
- Difficulty in learning his way around the hospital unit, such as from the hospital room to the kitchen and back
- Dyslexia in reading and computing figures because of inability to move eyes from left to right on a page or line up numbers accurately to compute the figures
- Inability to identify left or right

Assessment for Spatial Deficits

Observing the patient's behavior is one way to determine if he tends to ignore half of his body or environment. If he ambulates, does he seem to have difficulty moving through doorways, judging distance from one point to another? Does he become lost on the unit, unable to find his room? Does he have difficulty following directions when advised to turn "left" or "right"? Does he wash only half of his body or eat the food on only half of his tray? Does he ignore any stimuli from the affected side of his body?

Nursing Management for Deficits of Spatial Relationships

To aid the patient with spatial relationship deficits the nurse should

- Increase stimulation to the affected side.
- Because the patient tends to be easily distracted, screen him and remove any excess stimuli from the environment when working with him.
- Position the bedside unit and objects the patient will need, such as the bell cord or facial tissues, on his unaffected side.

- Do not allow the patient to wander around the unit alone or be sent anywhere alone because he will get lost.
- Use descriptive terms to identify areas rather than "left" or "right" (e.g., "Lift your unaffected leg").
- Use a mirror to help the patient adjust his position if he has difficulty in maintaining position.

AGNOSIAS

Inability to recognize familiar environmental objects through the senses is called *agnosia*. Agnosia can be subdivided into

- *Visual agnosia*—inability to recognize familiar objects by sight
- *Auditory agnosia*—inability to recognize familiar objects through sound
- *Tactile agnosia (astereognosis)*—inability to recognize familiar objects through the sense of touch

Assessment for Agnosia

Observing and listening to the patient may reveal that he uses incorrect terms when referring to familiar objects, does not respond correctly to a familiar sound (e.g., does not answer the telephone when it rings), or cannot identify familiar objects placed in his hand when his eyes are closed.

Nursing Management of Agnosias

In working with the agnosia patient the nurse should

- Use other senses that are intact to identify environmental stimuli (e.g., if patient has visual agnosia, have him use voices and sounds to identify familiar objects).
- Use the drill method of teaching to help patient to relearn stimuli that he cannot identify.

APRAXIA

Apraxia is the inability to carry out a learned voluntary movement without the presence of paralysis. See page 63 for a discussion of the various types of apraxia.

Assessment for Apraxia

In giving or supervising care the nurse may notice that the patient does not respond appropriately to familiar items or directions. For example, the patient does not know what to do when a comb is placed in his hand with the direction, "Comb your hair." The patient may look bewildered or make a mistake in doing this or other tasks he has done for years.

Nursing Management of Apraxia

In working with the patient the nurse should

- Encourage the patient to participate in the activities of daily living.
- Correct any misuse of equipment or incorrect actions; guide the patient's hand, if necessary.
- Reteach any forgotten skills.

VISUAL DEFICITS

The major visual deficits found in neurological patients include diplopia, decreased acuity, and the hemianopsias. *Diplopia* is a term used to describe double vision. *Decreased acuity* of vision results in fuzzy vision, which makes it difficult to collect information concerning the environment. *Hemianopsia* refers to loss of vision in half of the visual field (see page 66).

ASSESSMENT OF VISUAL DEFICITS

Assessing the patient for visual deficits reveals that the patient

- Does not appear to see stimuli introduced from one particular side
- Complains of seeing double
- Complains about dimness or fuzziness of vision

NURSING MANAGEMENT FOR VISUAL DEFICITS

To assist the patient with visual deficits the nurse should follow the instructions for each type of deficit outlined below:

Diplopia

- Provide an eye patch for the affected eye or tape the lens of the eyeglasses on the affected side.

Decreased Acuity

- Encourage the patient to use other senses to gather information.

Hemianopsia

- Approach the patient from the unaffected side.
- Encourage the patient to turn his head and scan the area to compensate for decreased visual field.

COMMUNICATION DEFICITS

Dysphonia (difficulty in communicating) or *aphasia* (loss of the ability to communicate) are the two major terms used to describe communication deficits.

Aphasia is subdivided into the following major classifications:

- Expressive aphasia, or an inability to express oneself verbally (also called Broca's aphasia)
- Receptive aphasia, or an inability to understand the spoken word (also called Wernicke's aphasia)
- Global aphasia, a combination of both expressive and receptive aphasia

APHASIA

Expressive Aphasia

With expressive aphasia the patient has difficulty expressing his thoughts verbally or in writing. The degree of difficulty can range from mild hesitancy in flow of speech to limitation of expression to "yes" and "no." The ability to understand the written and spoken word remains intact.

In expressive aphasia, injury has occurred to Broca's area, located in the frontal lobe close to the area of the motor cortex that controls the movement of the lips, jaw, tongue, soft palate, and vocal cords.

Broca's area is identified as area 44 according to Brodmann. Broca's area contains the memory for motor patterns of speech.

Receptive Aphasia (Wernicke's Aphasia)

Receptive aphasia results from injury to Wernicke's area located in the temporal lobe flanked by Heschl's gyrus on one side and the angular gyrus on the other. Heschl's gyrus is the primary receptor area for auditory stimuli; the angular gyrus conveys stimuli between the auditory and visual fields. Wernicke's area provides the connection pathways to bridge the primary auditory cortex and the angular gyrus. Although the patient hears the sounds of speech, the parts of the brain that give meaning to the sounds of speech are not activated so that comprehension of speech is impaired. Since the control of the musculature for speech is not impaired, the patient can speak, but he makes many errors when using words. Because he is unaware of his imperfect messages he may talk at great length. The patient's ability to express his words in writing is also compromised.

Global Aphasia

Global aphasia is a combination of both expressive and receptive aphasia whereby the patient is left with little, if any, communication system intact. He neither understands what he hears or reads, nor can he convey his thought in speech or writing. The prognosis is poor. Global aphasia is the result of a massive stroke or lesion involving both Broca's and Wernicke's areas of the brain.

ASSESSMENT OF THE COMMUNICATION SYSTEM

To plan nursing care the nurse will need to assess the patient's communication system to determine what skills are intact so that an alternate means of communication can be developed. Assessment of the patient includes the following areas:

- The ability to speak in response to an open-ended question such as "Tell me about your hobbies" should be assessed.
- The use of vocabulary, grammar, and syntax and the relevance of the answer to the question should be noted along with the flow of words to note spontaneity, hesitancy of pronunciation, and speed of speech.
- The ability to understand the spoken word is checked by giving the patient instructions and evaluating the appropriateness and accuracy of his response; instructions of increasing complexity should be included proceeding from the simple to the complex.
- The ability to understand the written word is evaluated by giving the patient instructions in writing and observing and listening to his response; the instructions should range in complexity from an appropriate response of "yes" or "no" to more complex answers.
- The ability to express ideas in writing is assessed by asking the patient to write a response such as "Write your name" or "Describe this room."

Although a comprehensive evaluation is the responsibility of the speech therapist, the nurse's assessment is carried out to increase the effectiveness of nursing care. Information gained from the evaluation of the speech therapist usually is available only in selected cases and in the later part of the rehabilitation program. Since many patients are never evaluated by a speech therapist, the nurse's assessment can provide an opportunity for identifying those patients who should be evaluated.

Several factors associated with illness can mask an accurate determination of the patient's communication skills, such as

- Deteriorated level of consciousness
- Visual field deficits (hemianopsias)
- Visual deficits (decreased acuity of vision, not wearing prescribed corrective lenses)
- Hearing loss (primary hearing loss caused by injury or not wearing prescribed hearing aid)
- Dysarthria
- Unfamiliarity with the language

In addition, since the use of language is closely associated with attention and concentration, if the patient has difficulty with a short attention span or concentration, his ability to follow verbal or nonverbal cues will be altered. Since concentration and attention seem to vary from day to day or even minute to minute, there can be great differences in the patient's ability to communicate at any given time.

NURSING MANAGEMENT OF THE APHASIC PATIENT

The loss or impairment of the ability to communicate is devastating and frustrating to the patient, resulting in fear and depression. To work effectively with the patient, it is best to assume a calm, reassuring, and supportive manner that conveys a sense of acceptance of the patient's behavior. Spending plenty of time with the patient and assuming an unhurried approach reinforces this message. The following suggestions can serve as guidelines in working with the aphasic patient:

Mild Expressive Aphasia

- Stimulate conversation and ask open-ended questions.
- Allow the patient time to search for the words to express himself.
- Disregard choice of incorrect words.
- Be supportive and accepting of the patient's behavior as he

deals with the frustration of finding the right words to express himself.

- Assure the patient that his speech will gradually improve with time.

Severe Expressive Aphasia

- Accept self-expression by whatever means possible (e.g., pantomime, pointing).
- Do not pressure the patient into self-expression.
- Be supportive of the patient and accept his behavior if he shows frustration (cries, and so forth) because of the difficulty in expressing himself.
- Provide a loose-leaf book with pictures of common objects so that the patient can point to the picture when he cannot say the word.
- Tell the patient that speech skills can be relearned, given time.

Mild Receptive Aphasia

- Stand close to the patient (within his line of vision) so that he can also observe lip movements as an added cue to communication.
- Speak slowly and distinctly, using simple sentences and a common vocabulary.
- Use simple gestures as an added cue in speaking.
- Repeat or rephrase any instructions if they are not understood.
- Speak in a normal speaking voice.

Severe Receptive Aphasia

- Use whatever vocabulary the patient can still understand.
- Use very simple sentences or phrases that express only the critical essence of a thought.
- Divide any tasks in small units, working with the individual units to accomplish the task.
- Use pantomime, pointing, touch, and so forth to express ideas.

PROGNOSIS FOR RECOVERY FROM APHASIA

Generally speaking, the greatest degree of spontaneous functional return occurs in the first 3 to 6 months following injury, although substantial deficits may still occur. Additional improvement can occur for 2 or 3 more years. Each patient must be viewed as an individual in the rehabilitative process. Age, area of injury, presence of other health problems, and motivation are but a few factors having direct bearing on recovery.

BLADDER RETRAINING

Urinary continence is the ability to exercise voluntary control over the urge to void. Patients with neurological disease or injury may be unable to achieve urinary continence either because they do not receive or are unaware of the impulses indicating the need to void, or they are unable to control the urge to void until they are in a socially acceptable place to empty their bladder. *Micturition* is the act of evacuating the urinary bladder when a certain amount of urine has collected. The parasympathetic branch of the autonomic nervous system is primarily responsible for micturition. The center for micturition is controlled by spinal segments S–2, S–3, and S–4. Stretching of the bladder wall stimulates the parasympathetic system to contract the bladder and relax the internal sphincter. The external sphincter can be voluntarily contracted by means of the pudendal nerve. By reflex action, it relaxes when the internal sphincter relaxes.

Bladder control is a learned behavior. In the infant, bladder evacuation is a reflex act. In early childhood, the higher centers of the brain come into play and the child learns to control micturition. Even when bladder fullness is perceived and associated with the need for evacuation, the child learns to consciously control the urge until he is in a socially acceptable place for bladder evacuation.

CAUSES OF BLADDER DYSFUNCTION

Urinary bladder dysfunction is associated with various problems such as urinary tract infection; urinary tract calculi; neurogenic bladder dysfunction caused by head injury, spinal cord injury/lesions, sacral nerve injury, multiple sclerosis, or other neurological conditions; and a diminished level of consciousness. The focus of this discussion is bladder dysfunction caused by neurogenic origin.

NEUROGENIC BLADDER

The term *neurogenic bladder* is used to describe any bladder disturbance that is due to a lesion of the nervous system. Spinal segments S–2, S–3, and S–4 control the bladder and are also under the control of the higher centers in the frontal lobes of the cerebral hemispheres. Neurogenic bladder disorders are usually classified as the following:

- Upper motor neuron bladder
- Lower motor neuron bladder
- Mixed motor neuron bladder

A description of each type of bladder is included in Table 8–3.

The effect of spinal shock on the bladder is that it initially becomes atonic. The atonic bladder gradually converts to a spastic bladder as the spinal shock diminishes over days or weeks. If the spasticity of the bladder is severe, any slight stimulus such as a minimal amount of urine in the bladder (20 ml to 50 ml) or stroking of the abdomen, thigh, or genitals will cause the bladder to empty. For the patient with an atonic bladder, urinary drainage is controlled by inserting an indwelling catheter. The head-injured patient with an altered level of consciousness has an intact sacral segment but has a diminished or absent response to impulses that herald the need to evacuate the bladder. These patients are also initially managed with an indwelling catheter. As soon as possible, the catheter should be removed because unnecessary use of a catheter leads to urinary tract infection. Once the catheter is removed, a bladder retraining program is begun. Chart 8–1 summarizes the methods of managing urinary drainage in patients unable to maintain a normal voiding pattern.

TABLE 8-3. *Bladder Dysfunction*

Name	*Other Names Used*	*Sacral Reflex (S-2, S-3, S-4)*	*Control of Higher Cortical Centers*	*Conditions Seen*	*Description*
Upper motor neuron bladder	Spastic, reflex, automatic, and central	Preserved: sensory and motor pathways to the sacral reflex are intact	Loss of inhibitory influence	Spinal cord injury; cord lesions above the sacral reflex; can occur after spinal shock has resolved	Since the reflex arc is intact, the bladder empties, but without voluntary control. If spasticity is severe, the slightest stimulus such as straining, coughing, or a small amount of urine (15 ml to 25 ml) in the bladder can stimulate emptying of the bladder. If spasticity is minimal to moderate, the patient is instructed in recognizing signs associated with bladder fullness; he may then evacuate it by stimulating the sacral reflex—pressing on bladder (Credé method); stroking thigh).
Lower motor neuron disease	Atonic, flaccid, autonomous, peripheral, areflexic	Damaged: sensory input from the full bladder does not trigger the sacral reflex	Loss of sensation to cortical level	Spinal shock Sacral cord injury	Patient is unaware of bladder fullness and need to void. Bladder overdistends. Overflow incontinence, especially during coughing or transfer, often occurs. Autonomic hyperreflexia may be stimulated in a patient with high cord injury. Bladder is managed initially with an indwelling catheter, then intermittent catheterization. Bladder retraining is begun later.
Mixed motor neuron bladder	Any or all of the above	Diminished	Diminished	Stroke Brain tumor Multiple sclerosis Head injury	Patient often has urgency to void but is unable to control the urgency. Condition is associated with frontal lobe lesion or unconsciousness. Until patient is able and willing to cooperate, continence will not be achieved. Patient is good candidate for continence because perception of fullness and control are diminished, not lost.

CHOOSING THE BEST TIME TO BEGIN BLADDER RETRAINING

The timing of the beginning of the bladder retraining program is critical to the success or failure of the program. The head-injury patient must be conscious, alert, and oriented. He must be able to react to the urge to void either independently or by summoning help from the nurse. A bedpan, bedside commode, or access to the bathroom are necessary. The patient should be stable and free from urinary tract infection. Every attempt must be made to motivate the patient to participate in the program.

A spinal cord injured patient should be stable, free of urinary tract infection, and motivated to participate in the program. Facilities must be available for voiding.

If there is a question about the nervous innervation to the bladder, the physician may order cystometric studies to assess bladder function. In addition, a recent urinalysis, the culture and sensitivity of the urine, and the intake and output record will be evaluated to detect abnormalities in the urine, urinary tract infection, and the hydration level.

CHART 8-1. METHODS OF MANAGING URINARY DRAINAGE

Indwelling Catheter

- Often used with an acute atonic bladder to prevent overdistention of the bladder
- Used for a comatose patient or a patient with a spastic bladder if keeping the patient dry becomes a problem
- Provides for continual drainage of urine

Continuous Bladder Irrigation

- Used with a triple-lumen indwelling catheter
- Often used with the immobile or comatose patient
- Continually bathes the bladder with a bacteriostatic or acidifying solution (Neosporin or acetic acid solution) to prevent infection
- Provides for continual drainage of urine and irrigating solution

Intermittent Catheterization

- May be used during acute or postacute phase of spinal cord or other injury
- Patient is catheterized periodically (4 to 8 hours) with a straight catheter that is removed each time
- If upper extremities function, many patients (both male and female) can be taught self-catheterization
- Believed to reduce incidence of infection

Clamping Indwelling Catheter

- Used to increase bladder tone when an indwelling catheter has been in place for a while
- Plan a clamp-release schedule
- Start with clamping for an hour (if it can be tolerated), then release
- Increase period of clamping until 300 ml to 400 ml can be tolerated in the bladder
- Catheter is then removed and a bladder retraining program begun

Condom Catheter

- Used to manage incontinence in males
- Applied over penis to drain urine into the collection bag and keep the patient dry

Bladder Retraining Program

- Used to attempt to help patient regain continence. Although successful retraining will not be achieved with all patients, an honest effort should be made.

The physician may order cystometric studies on the bladder to evaluate bladder function.

BLADDER RETRAINING PROGRAM

The methods for retraining a patient with an upper motor neuron bladder and one with a lower motor neuron bladder vary although the goals of bladder retraining are the same for all patients. The goals for a bladder retraining pogram include the following:

- To empty the bladder regularly (and with a minimum of residual urine) in a socially acceptable place
- To maintain continence between voidings
- To prevent or control the development of urinary tract infection or calculi

Training for Upper Motor Neuron Bladder

Although the brain of the patient with a complete upper motor neuron bladder does not receive the message of the need to void, there may be other indications associated with a full bladder. Common signs include sweating, restlessness, and abdominal discomfort. The patient must learn to relate the presence of these symptoms to a full bladder.

- Voiding may be induced by actions that stimulate trigger areas. Examples are stroking the inner thigh, abdomen, or genitalia; pulling pubic hair; applying digital stimulation to the anus or rectum (which is very effective); and doing push-ups on the commode.

Most hospitals have established written protocols for bladder training after the catheter has been removed for a trial voiding. The following program is typical:

- Fluids are given between 7 AM and 8 PM.
- The catheter is removed at 7 AM.
- A glass of fluid (240 ml) is given hourly.
- After a few hours (usually 3), the patient tries to void by stimulating a "trigger area."
- If the patient voids, the amount of residual urine in the bladder is checked immediately.

- A residual of less than 100 ml indicates that the training can continue.
- A residual of greater than 100 ml requires reinsertion of the catheter, in which case the training will be rescheduled for trial on another day.

A positive attitude should be maintained by the staff, and the patient should be encouraged to try again. Even in a male patient who has achieved relative bladder control, there may be some dribbling of urine. A condom catheter or external drainage device may be used to avoid "accidents."

Training for Lower Motor Neuron Bladder

Since the sacral reflex arc is not intact, there is no spontaneous evacuation in the lower motor neuron bladder. Bladder evacuation is assisted by the following methods:

1. Application of manual pressure over the suprapubic area (Credé method)
2. Straining against a closed epiglottis (Valsalva's maneuver)
3. Contracting abdominal muscles to cause pressure on the bladder

In a typical bladder training program, time limits (usually between 7 AM and 8 PM) are set for intake to avoid nocturnal incontinence.

- The catheter is removed at 7 AM with fluid given in 240-ml amounts hourly.
- After a few hours, the patient tries to void, using pressure as outlined.
- If the patient voids, the residual is measured immediately.
- The training proceeds if the residual is less than 50 ml.
- Residual amounts greater than 50 ml indicate the need to reinsert the catheter.

A lower amount of residual is expected, since the sphincter is flaccid and the urine can be adequately expressed.

Self-Catheterization. If the patient is not able to gain bladder control, intermittent catheterization may be used. This technique can be employed in the hospital setting when there is an adequate staff skilled in this procedure. If there is a need for intermittent catheterization after discharge, selected patients can be taught this procedure using a "clean technique" rather than the "sterile technique" used in hospitals. By "clean technique" it is meant that the patient starts with a clean catheter rather than sterilized equipment. He should use warm tap water and a bar of soap for washing the perineal area. Hands are meticulously washed with soap and water, but sterile gloves need not be worn. If the patient is not able to self-catheterize, use of an external drainage device or a catheter connected to a leg bag may be used. Continuous drainage during sleep is suggested for these patients.

Training for Mixed Neurogenic Bladder

The chances of successfully bladder training a patient with a mixed neurogenic bladder are good because sensation and ability to void are intact, although somewhat diminished. The procedure for trial voiding is the same as for an upper motor neuron bladder. The patient with a head injury or some form of cerebral dysfunction has a neurogenic bladder.

SUMMARY OF BLADDER RETRAINING

It is correct to state that bladder training is not an easy task. One can expect some setbacks even under ideal circumstances. The plan must be individualized, and active patient participation is necessary for success. Surgical procedures are sometimes elected to deal with specific urinary tract problems that may improve the prospect of continence in selected patients.

BOWEL RETRAINING

The act of bowel evacuation is called *defecation*. The anus, the terminal end of the large bowel, is controlled by two sphincters:

- Involuntary internal anal sphincter (smooth muscle)
- Voluntary external anal sphincter (striated muscle)

Defecation is a coordinated reflex of sacral segments S-3, S-4, and S-5, which is initiated by stimulated stretch receptors located in the anus that initiate peristalic waves. These waves propel fecal matter toward the anus and relax the internal sphincter. If the external sphincter is also relaxed, bowel evacuation will occur.

The sacral reflex for bowel evacuation is a weak one that is aided by parasympathetic responses (peristalsis caused by ingestion of food and inreased pressure within the lower bowel, which relaxes the internal sphincter). Also, contraction of the abdominal wall aids bowel evacuation by increasing pressure on the bowel.

CAUSES OF BOWEL DYSFUNCTION

Bowel dysfunction can result from decreased intake of food, especially roughage; being given "nothing by mouth"; immobility (e.g., because of unconsciousness, fractures, pneumonia); autonomic dysfunction; spinal cord injury; sacral injuries; and dementia.

BOWEL INCONTINENCE CAUSED BY FRONTAL LOBE LESIONS

Patients with dysfunction of the frontal lobes of the brain (the area of the brain concerned with higher level functions such as judgment, social behavior, and learning) caused by primary injury, cerebral edema, or space-occupying lesions may exhibit fecal incontinence. When indifference to the time and the place of defecation is apparent, the patient often demonstrates a lack of other social inhibitions such as:

- He may inform the nurse that he has defecated
- He may "play" with his excreta
- He does not respond to reminders such as "Tell the nurse when you need to move your bowels"

CHART 8-2. EXAMPLE OF A BOWEL RETRAINING PROGRAM

1. Give 30 ml of milk of magnesia orally at bedtime.
2. Administer docusate sodium (Colace), 100 mg orally three times a day.
3. Offer a breakfast that includes hot food; prune juice or any food known to have a laxative effect for the patient should be included.
4. *Day 1*—The patient sits on toilet, if possible, in a comfortable position. He attempts to have a bowel movement by intermittent straining for about 20 minutes. For patients unable to strain, doing "push-ups" on the commode or applying pressure to the abdomen may be helpful.
   If unsuccessful, further efforts are postponed until the next day.
5. *Day 2*—Patient strains again, as on first day; a Glycerine or Bisacodyl (Ducolax) suppository is inserted. After 20 minutes, the patient tries straining again. If not successful, digital stimulation should be tried. If results are poor, then efforts are postponed until the next day.
6. *Day 3*—The Day 2 routine is followed. If results are still poor, then an enema is given.
7. When the patient is successful, he returns to the Day 1 plan on the following day.
8. When a routine has been established for the particular patient (a bowel movement every 2 or 3 days), then that pattern is maintained without the preliminary procedures.

NURSING MANAGEMENT OF THE INCONTINENT PATIENT

In managing the incontinent patient the nurse should

- Continue to try to gain the patient's cooperation.
- Maintain a matter-of-fact attitude.
- Observe any cues in behavior that correlate to the need for defecation; the patient should then be placed on the toilet or bedpan.
- Note the usual time of day of defecation and place the patient on the toilet or bedpan daily at that time.
- Diaper or use other means to protect the patient.
- Provide meticulous skin care.
- Support the patient's self-esteem and a positive self-concept.
- Consider implementing a bowel retraining program (Chart 8-2).

BOWEL INCONTINENCE CAUSED BY SPINAL CORD INJURY

Patients with cord injuries are very prone to constipation and impaction in addition to loss of neurogenic bowel control. A bowel retraining program based on the needs of the patient can be developed. The cooperation of the patient, the physician, and the nurse are necessary to achieve success. See Chart 8-2.

REHABILITATION OF BRAIN-DAMAGED PATIENTS

Rehabilitation of brain-damaged patients tends to focus on the physical, observable deficits. However, the most significant long-term problems incurred in brain injury appear to be cognitive, behavioral, and emotional deficits. Although one may think that these deficits have a grim outlook, various studies show that one can be cautiously optimistic about cognitive functions because they can continue to improve for several years after significant brain damage, particularly if proper stimulation is offered to the patient.

The category of "brain-damaged patients" includes patients with primary head injury, stroke, hemorrhage, tumor, abscess, or any other condition that results in sustained higher level impairment, which is also known as cognitive deficit. The cognitive disabilities must be addressed because they become barriers to the successful accomplishment of other aspects of the rehabilitation process and achievement of the highest level of independence possible.

ASSESSMENT

How does one identify the patient with cognitive deficits? He is the patient who does not respond appropriately to stimuli. One method of pinpointing the level of dysfunction is through the use of the Rancho Los Amigos Guide to Cognitive Levels. The scale is divided into eight levels that range from no response to purposeful and appropriate response. A description of corresponding behavior and nursing approaches can be correlated to each level. Another possible method of identifying cognitive deficits is by administering a short screening test that takes about half an hour. The test can be given by a specially trained nurse, occupational therapist, or some other designated member of the staff. The examiner assesses memory, attention span, affect and general behavior, sequencing skills, problem solving, insight and judgment, and abstract thinking. The assessment is made by asking the patient questions, giving him directions for specific activity, and noting his responses. General areas of deficit can then be identified. If the patient appears to be having difficulty with these cognitive skills, a complete neuropsychological assessment should be conducted by a qualified neuropsychologist (see Chapter 4 for a description of the test). Based on his findings, the cognitive deficits can be identified and treatment begun. The neuropsychologist is a valuable resource and can offer suggestions on how the team members should approach the patient. He can also begin to see the patient on a regular basis, if that is appropriate.

MANAGEMENT

It is important for the nurse and other team members to discuss the best way of managing the patient so that there is a consistent approach to the patient. Based on the deficits present, realistic goals can be identified for the patient. If the goals are beyond the ability of the patient, he and the staff will feel frustrated.

The patient with severe cognitive deficits will continue to require treatment after his discharge or transfer from the acute care setting. The family should be told what kind of behavior can be expected and how they should interact with the patient. Referrals for follow-up care need to be addressed to provide holistic management of the patient.

PSYCHOSOCIAL CONSIDERATIONS OF NEUROLOGICAL DISABILITY

During the course of recovery from cerebral trauma and other neurological disabilities, several psychological and emotional responses will occur at various points in the rehabilitative process. Common responses include fear, anxiety, depression, denial, anger, emotional lability, frustration, irritability, loss of self-control and inhibitions, reduced tolerance to stress, inability to tolerate the behavior of others, distorted self-image, and loss of sense of personal and gender identity. Many patients experience a sense of loss, grief, and bereavement for any lost body function. (See Chapter 7, Emotional and Behavioral Responses to Neurological Illness.)

The severity of illness, permanency of neurological deficits, age, lifestyle, and roles assumed on the personal, social, and occupational levels are a few factors that influence the patient's response to his illness. The patient responds to the onslaught of illness based on his previous adjustment patterns and personality. The patient who was able to cope effectively in the past will usually be able to cope with his disability and actively participate in his rehabilitation. Those individuals who adjusted poorly in the past will most likely adjust poorly to the threat of serious illness.

In considering the psychosocial aspects of illness and rehabilitation, the family and significant others must be included. The rehabilitative process is directed to returning the patient to his home, family, and previous lifestyle. If this is not possible, adjustments are made within the context of the limitations placed on him. The family will need help in coping with the changes in their lifestyles brought about by illness of a family member. This should be considered as a part of the concerns of rehabilitation.

ASSESSMENT OF PSYCHOLOGICAL ASPECTS OF NEUROLOGICAL DISABILITY

The nurse should listen to and observe the patient in the course of giving care as well as during interactions with the family and other significant people in the patient's life. Both the patient and family can be rich sources of information about the patient's premorbid personality and the type of family and community relationships he had established. The patient and family should also be encouraged to express their perceptions of the impact of the illness and disability on their lifestyles. The empathetic nurse will have a better understanding of the impact of illness on the individual and family unit. By establishing rapport with the patient and family the nurse can collect much information about their values, expectations, and perceptions, which can be helpful in planning nursing management.

LONG-TERM REHABILITATION

Some patients will require long-term rehabilitation, which will necessitate the use of community resources if he is at home, or admission to a rehabilitation center or extended care facility. The nurse should evaluate the patient's level of independence in the activities of daily living to accurately assess how much help the patient will need. This information along with the evaluation of other health-team members will provide a data base for designing a comprehensive rehabilitation plan.

The family members must be assessed to determine their ability to participate in the rehabilitation program. Some families are willing and able to care for the patient at home with the help of various community agencies. Other families do not wish to care for the patient or are unable to do so because of other family responsibilities. The decision of how and where to provide for the long-term rehabilitative needs of the patient must include the physician, nurse, other health-team members, family, and patient, if he is able.

DISCHARGE PLANNING

Regardless of whether the patient is going home to be cared for by family or to an extended care facility, the nurse will need to compile a summary assessment of the patient's needs and his abilities in the activities of daily living. Referral forms must be completed and sent to appropriate resources. (See Chapter 9, Discharge Planning and the Neurological–Neurosurgical Patient).

FAMILY PREPARATION FOR DISCHARGE

If the patient is to return home, modifications in the house may be necessary to provide access for a wheelchair or necessary equipment. As soon as possible the family should be apprised of what the patient can do for himself and what activities will require help. If a family member must learn any special procedures, time should be provided for the nurse to teach the family member. The family should also be told to expect a period of adjustment when the patient returns home. Often there are role changes precipitated by illness and disability. It will take time to work out these changes and deal with them emotionally.

If at all possible, it is advisable for the patient to go home on a weekend pass. This should occur after the family has been pepared and feels ready. After the patient's return to the hospital he should be encouraged to express his feelings about the experience. The family should also be interviewed alone to express their feelings and concerns. Perhaps some things that the family had not even considered in the planning may now be a major concern. The nurse can be helpful in aiding the patient and family to solve problems or direct them to the appropriate person who can provide help.

Patient and family may also be helped through group sessions with other people who have faced similar problems. For example, groups of patients with disabilities can meet with a qualified group facilitator to discuss problems of adjustment. Family members can also benefit from a group experience with family members of other patients with similar problems. The group experience offers the opportunity to discover that others have similar problems and feelings. It also provides the support and friendship to help make the difficult adjustments easier.

PATIENT PREPARATION FOR DISCHARGE

The patient needs help to accept and adjust to his disabilities and the ramifications his illness will have on his life and that of his family. Many patients require counseling to help them make the adjustment.

The weekend visit and group experience with other patients can help to make the transition easier. Many patients experience transfer anxiety as the day approaches when they must leave the hospital setting and return home or go to another health care facility.

In addition, depending on the patient's age, occupation, and disabilities, it may be necessary to include vocational rehabilitation in the plan of care. This may be necessary if the patient's disabilities are such that he cannot return to his former occupation. In the case of a young person who has not yet joined the work force, there may be a need to evaluate and counsel the patient about vocational opportunities so that he may have a productive life as a wage earner.

SUMMARY OF DISCHARGE PLANNING

The goal of discharge planning is to help the patient make the transition from one facility to another or to his home so that the rehabilitative process will continue with few setbacks. A comprehensive approach is necessary to help the patient successfully adjust and realize the greatest rehabilitative potential possible, thereby enabling him to live a worthwhile life of dignity with the greatest level of independence possible.

BIBLIOGRAPHY

Books

Basagian J (ed): Therapeutic Exercise, 3rd ed. Baltimore, Williams & Wilkins, 1978

Benson DF, Blumer D: Psychiatric Aspects of Neurological Disease. New York, Grune & Stratton, 1975

Bitter JA: Introduction to Rehabilitation. St Louis, CV Mosby, 1979

Christopherson V et al: Rehabilitation Nursing: Perspectives and Application. New York, McGraw-Hill, 1974

Ince LP: Behavior Modification in Rehabilitation Medicine. Springfield, IL, Charles C Thomas, 1976

Goldstein G, Ruthven L: Rehabilitation of the Brain-Damaged Adult. New York, Plenum, 1983

Guyton A: Textbook of Medical Physiology, 5th ed, pp 710–728. Philadelphia, WB Saunders, 1976

Lezak MD: Neuropsychological Assessment. New York, Oxford University Press, 1976

Murray R, Kijek JC: Current Perspectives in Rehabilitation Nursing. St Louis, CV Mosby, 1979

Nichols PJ: Rehabilitation Medicine, 2nd ed. London, Butterworth, 1980

O'Sullivan SB, Cullen KE, Schmitz TJ: Physical Rehabilitation: Evaluation and Treatment Procedures. Philadelphia, FA Davis, 1980

Palmer ML, Toms JE: Manual for Functional Training. Philadelphia, FA Davis, 1980

Peszczynski M: Rehabilitation in Hemiplegia. In Licht S (ed): Rehabilitation and Medicine, pp 390–410. Baltimore, Williams & Wilkins, 1975

Pohl M: The Teaching Function of the Nurse Practitioner, 3rd ed. Dubuque, IA, WC Brown, 1978

Redman B: The Process of Patient Teaching, 4th ed. St Louis, CV Mosby, 1980

Rosenthal M et al: Rehabilitation of the Head Injured Adult. Philadelphia, FA Davis, 1983

Rusk H: Rehabilitation Medicine, 4th ed. St Louis, CV Mosby, 1977

Stryker R: Rehabilitative Aspects of Acute and Chronic Care, 2nd ed. Philadelphia, WB Saunders, 1977

Van Meter MJ (ed): Neurologic Care: A Guide for Patient Education. New York, Appleton-Century-Crofts, 1982

Periodicals

Basmajian JV: Biofeedback in rehabilitation: A review of principles and practices. Arch Phys Med Rehabil 62:469, October 1981

Booth K: The neglect syndrome . . . inattention or neglect to one side of their bodies and to one half of space. J Neurosurg Nurs 14:38, February 1982

Burt M: Perceptual deficits in hemiplegia. Am J Nurs 70(5):1026, May 1970

Caplan B: Neuropsychology in rehabilitation: Its role in evaluation and intervention. Arch Phys Med Rehabil 63:362, August 1982

Carlson CE: Psychological aspects of neurological disability. Nurs Clin North Am 15(2):309, June 1980

Demarest CB: Putting biofeedback into perspective . . . to assist treatment and rehabilitation of various disabilities. Patient Care 17(1):37–38, 40–1, January 15, 1983

Egan J: Rehabilitation: The nurse's responsibility in the intensive care unit. Crit Care Q 2(1):105, June 1979

Fozzard E: The psychosexual needs of the neurological disabled. J Neurosurg Nurs 10(3):92, September 1978

Gordon M: Assessing activity tolerance. Am J Nurs 76(1):72, January 1976

Habermann B: Cognitive dysfunction and social rehabilitation in the severely head-injured patient. J Neurosurg Nurs 14(5):220, October 1982

Johnson JH: Rehabilitation aspects of neurologic bladder dysfunction. Nurs Clin North Am 15(2):293, June 1980

Kottke FJ: Philosophic considerations of quality of life for the disabled. Arch Phys Med Rehabil 63:49, February 1982

Kreger SM et al: A procedure for goal setting: A method for formulating goals and treatment plans. Rehabil Nurs 6:23, March/April, 1981

Louis MC, Povse SM: Aphasia and endurance: Considerations in the assessment and care of the stroke patient. Nurs Clin North Am 15(2):265, June 1980

Lynch WJ et al: Brain injury rehabilitation: Standard problem list. Arch Phys Med Rehabil 62:223, May 1981

Mahoney EK: Alterations in cognitive functioning in the brain-damaged patient. Nurs Clin North Am 15(2):283, June 1980

Miller M: Iatrogenic and nurisgenic effects of prolonged immobilization of the ill aged. J Am Geriatr Soc 23(8):360, August 1975

Mills VM et al: Functional differences in patients with left or right cerebrovascular accidents. Phys Ther 63(4):481, April 1983

Moolten SE: Bedsores: An update. Hosp Med 64A, August 1982

Norman, S: Diagnostic categories for the patient with a right hemisphere lesion. Am J Nurs 79(12):2126, December 1979

Pasovac EJ et al: Using a level of function scale (LORS-11) to evaluate the success of inpatient rehabilitation programs. Rehabil Nurs 7(6):17, November/December 1982

Quigley PA: Nursing evaluation in rehabilitation. Rehabil Nurs 6:12, November/December 1981

Rothberg JS: The rehabilitation team: Future direction. Arch Phys Med Rehabil 62:407, August 1981

chapter

9

Discharge Planning

Each person can be located somewhere on the health–illness continuum at any given point in time. Health can be described as a state of physical, psychosocial, and emotional well-being, as defined by the patient and health professionals. When the patient needs help in meeting his health needs, he often becomes a part of the health care system. An integral component of the health care system is discharge planning. It is the patient's right to expect discharge planning as part of his care. It is also the patient's responsibility—or his family's, if he is unable to participate because of the degree of disability—to actively participate in the discharge planning process and identify his specific goals for health. Patients with neurological dysfunction of various types often have extensive and complex health needs that need to be met. Discharge planning is the vehicle through which the patient's health care needs can be met within the continuum of health care delivery services.

CONCEPTUALIZATION OF THE DISCHARGE PLANNING PROCESS

Discharge planning is a logical, coordinated process of decision-making and other activities involving the patient, his family or significant other, and a team of health professionals from various disciplines working together to facilitate a smooth transition of that patient from one environment to another. The transitional environment may be an acute-care facility, a chronic care or rehabilitation hospital, a nursing home of various classifications, or the patient's home. The goal or purpose of discharge planning is to assist the patient to make a smooth transition from one environment or level of care to another without sacrificing the progress that has already been achieved and to provide for other health care needs that are still unmet. The rationale for discharge planning is based on consideration of cost containment and continuity of care.

COST CONTAINMENT

It is now estimated that about 10% of the gross national product (GNP) of the United States is spent on health care. Both public and private sectors are concerned because the cost of health care and the health care industry cannot continue to escalate at the current rate. Since the health care industry had been unsuccessful in regulating itself, the federal and state governments have instituted restrictions on reimbursement that have forced the health care system to comply with regulations directed at cost containment. Four controls on cost and health care should be mentioned: Medicare; Medicaid; professional standards review organizations; and diagnostic related groupings.

Medicare

Because of an increasing number of elderly people with health care needs, Medicare (Title 18 of the Social Security Act) was enacted in 1965 to provide for persons 65 years or older and the disabled. Medicare pays for routine portions of hospitalization such as the cost of the room, and sets limits on other costs to be reimbursed. The legislation affected health care delivery by addressing quality, cost, and access to care. The concept of acute care also began to encompass aftercare, and the terms "levels of care" and "skilled nursing needs" become important considerations in planning for the posthospital needs of the patient. With the enactment of this legislation, discharge planning became an integral part of health care delivery. Currently, Medicare accounts for one third of the nation's hospital revenue. The actual cost of the program has far exceeded any projections, and cost containment is paramount for keeping the program solvent.

Medicaid

Medicaid (Title 19), an amendment to the Social Security Act, was passed in 1968 as the state counterpart to provide for the health care needs of the indigent in the state. The states were given grants to support their medical assistance programs and the latitude to develop the kind of program that best met the needs of their state. The purpose of the legislation is to provide medical benefits to the aged, blind, and disabled, and to families with dependent children who cannot financially provide for necessary medical and rehabilitative care. Medicaid also addresses discharge planning and supports the placement of the patient in an extended care facility deemed necessary for rehabilitative purposes.

Professional Standards Review Organization (PSRO)

A program legislated by the National Health Planning and Resource Development Act of 1972 is the professional standards review organization program. This program developed on a statewide and local level provides a mechanism to review hospital activities according to four basic criteria: need and quality of services, staffing, economic feasibility, and cost containment. A close working relationship is necessary between the PSRO and the discharge planning program. Transfer to intermediate facilities or home is mandated to control cost and to avoid use of inappropriate resources. Discharge planning makes the transition from one facility to another possible.

Diagnostic Related Groupings (DRGs)

Part of the Tax Equity and Fiscal Responsibility Act of 1982 directed drastic changes in Medicare's current system of hospital reimbursement. The act mandates the reduction of the cost of Medicare payments made to hospitals. The Department of Health and Human Services (DHHS) was charged with the responsibility of devising a system of prospective rather than retrospective reimbursement to hospitals for services rendered. Within the system, hospitals would be given clear financial incentives to keep their costs low. Retrospective reimbursement is a system of paying a hospital for costs that have *already* been incurred in treating the patient while prospective reimbursement pays a hospital a fixed fee based on a calculated formula *before* services are rendered. A system was devised that identified 467 diagnostic related groupings (DRGs). In calculating reimbursement, each of the DRGs takes into account the primary diagnosis, the primary procedure, the patient's age, and the presence of a qualifying complication or comorbid condition. The figure calculated is the maximum amount that Medicare will pay for that particular patient. If the hospital's actual cost for treating the patient is less than the Medicare calculated payment schedule, the hospital will be allowed to keep that difference. If the hospital's expenses are greater, it will have to absorb the loss. Thus, the hospital has financial incentive to avoid unnecessary care, treatment, or prolonged hospitalization. Long-term care facilities, psychiatric hospitals, and pediatric hospitals are excluded from this payment system, at least initially.

With the incentive to develop cost containment patient management protocols, the role of discharge planning as a means to control costs is certain to become a major force as hospitals comply with DRGs. It appears that it will be only a matter of time before private health insurers also subscribe to prospective payment schedules.

CONTINUITY OF CARE

Continuity of care is a concept of coordinated delivery of health care on a continuum. The continuum of health services includes various health care facilities such as acute-care hospitals, long-term and rehabilitation hospitals, nursing homes, and day care centers. It also includes various types of services within and outside the hospital setting (e.g., intensive care unit, specialty unit, rehabilitation unit, self-care unit, ambulatory care services) and community resources such as neighborhood health centers, meals on wheels, and specialty organization programs. As the patient moves toward health on the health–illness continuum, his health care needs change and the kind of services necessary to support these needs also change. The appropriate resource or facility that can best support and administer the necessary care by the most economical means should be used. Movement toward health on the health–illness continuum is predicated on selection of the appropriate resources and communication between health care providers. Therefore, continuity of care means quality care by matching the needs of the patient with the appropriate resource. Continuity and quality of care are maintained through the process of discharge planning.

OTHER REQUIREMENTS FOR DISCHARGE PLANNING

The Joint Commission on the Accreditation of Hospitals (JCAH) is a private, nonprofit organization that accredits hospitals who have chosen to voluntarily submit to the process and meet the prescribed standards. Discharge planning is addressed in many different areas of the JCAH Manual of Accreditation as a necessary part of service to the patient and a responsibility of the practitioners.

ORGANIZATIONAL STRUCTURE FOR DISCHARGE PLANNING

Any institution or organization committed to discharge planning must incorporate a mechanism for discharge planning into the organizational or operational structure. In some facilities a separate department for discharge planning will be created. Staff assigned to this department have primary responsibility for discharge planning in that facility. In other situations, the responsibility for discharge planning is vested in the professional nursing staff caring for the patient on the clinical unit. In this instance, the nurse initiates the process with the physician and includes input from other health professionals, depending on the specific needs of the patient.

Discharge planning depends on the conceptualization of discharge planning within the institution, the discharge planning program developed, the resources committed to the program, and the quality control and evaluative mechanisms incorporated in the process. How discharge planning is viewed by the health professionals and administration of the facility will shape the type of discharge planning program developed. The program includes the philosophy, objectives, and specific protocols developed to implement the steps of the discharge planning process. Whatever the program may be, it must be workable and realistic for that facility, and it must have the commitment of the individuals and administration involved to make it a viable and effective process.

THE ROLE OF HEALTH PROFESSIONALS IN DISCHARGE PLANNING

A brief overview of the contributions of each health professional is helpful for understanding the interdisciplinary team approach to discharge planning. With neurological–neurosurgical patients, the services of various health professionals are often necessary because of the complex needs of the patient. Members of the team may include the nurses, primary physician, physiatrist, social worker, physical therapist, occupational therapist, speech therapist, vocational counselor, neuropsychologist, and a member of any other discipline that may be necessary. All disciplines work collaboratively in the discharge planning process.

NURSES

The nursing staff spends more time with the patient and family than members of any other discipline. The responsibility for initiating the discharge planning process often belongs to the nurse, who frequently suggests to the physician that it may be time to proceed in earnest on transferring the patient to a rehabilitation hospital or other agency. Once the formal discharge planning process begins, it is often the nurse who coordinates activities and communications while keeping the patient and family informed of the progress on a day-to-day basis. The nurse completes the nursing portion of the discharge summary form or interagency referral form and communicates with the nursing staff at the transfer facility to coordinate continuity of care. In the summary, the nurse identifies every nursing problem that has not been completely resolved and describes what nursing interventions have been used. Every attempt is made to continue the progress that the patient has made without any setbacks as a result of transfer.

PRIMARY PHYSICIAN

The primary physician coordinates the medical aspects of patient management and requests consultation from specialists as necessary. In discharge planning the primary physician writes a discharge summary, develops a prognosis, and supports continuity of medical management by working collaboratively with the physician at the transfer facility or in the community.

PHYSIATRIST

A physician who specializes in rehabilitative medicine is called a *physiatrist*. He assesses the patient and prescribes a program of physical therapy and occupational therapy to meet the patient's needs. The physiatrist can participate in discharge planning by assessing the patient's functional abilities, formalizing a prognosis, suggesting future needs, and helping to select an appropriate extended care facility that will be most beneficial for the patient who needs extended care.

SOCIAL WORKER

The social worker interviews the patient and/or family to determine family structure, support systems, financial resources and health insurance policies, and any special problems. The social worker periodically meets with the patient or family to advise them on their health care coverage and any special programs that might be available to them. It is often the social worker who is aware of agencies and resources in the area and initiates referrals to particular facilities.

PHYSICAL THERAPIST

The physical therapist assesses the motor function of the patient. Working with the physiatrist, the therapist administers a prescribed exercise, stretching, or gait retraining program. Use of special ambulatory equipment such as walkers and wheelchairs may be necessary for some patients, and the physical therapist will instruct the patient in the proper use of equipment. In discharge planning, the physical therapist will summarize what exercise and motor retraining program has been followed and what progress has been made.

OCCUPATIONAL THERAPIST

The focus for the occupational therapist is helping the patient relearn the activities of daily living. Special equipment may be prescribed for the patient to accomplish activities of daily living and maintain his independence. In discharge planning, the occupational therapist can identify special needs and alterations in environment that could be beneficial to support the patient's independence.

SPEECH THERAPIST

A speech therapist may be needed to evaluate a patient for dysphasia or aphasia. If the patient is receiving therapy for this problem, it will be necessary for the therapist to summarize the treatment in the discharge summary so that necessary therapy can be continued.

VOCATIONAL COUNSELOR

In some instances permanent disability will prevent a person from returning to his previous occupation. A vocational counselor can test a patient and suggest job retraining based on the test results and consideration of the disabilities incurred. If consultation from a vocational counselor has been included in the assessment of the patient, this information and the findings should be recorded in the discharge summary.

NEUROPSYCHOLOGIST

In cases of brain injury, it may be helpful to refer the patient to the neuropsychologist for evaluation of emotional and cognitive abilities. The patient can then begin appropriate retraining and therapy if necessary (see Chapter 4 for a discussion of neuropsychological testing). In discharge planning, if the patient needs cognitive retraining, a facility able to meet these needs must be selected. A summary of the findings of the testing and the prognosis should be included in the discharge summary.

THE STEPS OF DISCHARGE PLANNING

The steps of discharge planning follow the usual flow of steps in any schemata of logical problem solving. The steps include (1) assessment of the patient and his family; (2) analysis of data to identify specific patient and family needs; (3) planning to meet patient and family needs (e.g., exploration for appropriate resources, developing a patient teaching plan); (4) implementation of the plan including actual transfer; and (5) evaluation of the discharge planning process and the results.[1] Even though the steps in the process have been identified as distinct entities, in fact there is much overlap with movement in both directions occurring in the process (Fig. 9–1).

ASSESSMENT OF THE PATIENT AND HIS FAMILY

Discharge planning begins the moment the patient enters the health care system; the initial patient assessment begins the process. Assessment is an ongoing process in which the data base is constantly being refined, clarified, validated, and updated. Data are analyzed frequently to determine their significance. They may point out the need for the collection of other data or they may be of sufficient magnitude to merit immediate planning and implementation of action. The significance of some data may be impossible to determine in some instances, particularly for the unstable or acutely ill patient. It is impossible to predict long-term needs when the impact of illness on the physical, cognitive, emotional, psychosocial, financial, and vocational aspects of a person are uncertain. However, the knowledge and experience of the health care professional will help him to anticipate patient needs and project implications. Although in some instances a "wait and see" attitude is assumed, involving health professionals from other disciplines is helpful when monitoring potential patient and family needs. Once the patient is well stabilized, discharge planning can proceed in a more certain and organized manner.

ANALYSIS OF DATA TO IDENTIFY SPECIFIC PATIENT AND FAMILY NEEDS

Data analysis is an ongoing process because the practitioner must decide the significance and priority of that information. Some information does require immediate action, but most data contribute to a body of information that should be systematically analyzed. Each professional health care discipline collects and analyzes its data and is responsible for sharing its expertise with professionals from other disciplines to work collaboratively in developing a comprehensive discharge plan.

The systematic analysis and sharing of information may be done in several informal and formal ways, such as through informal conversation, interdisciplinary rounds, weekly unit or interdisciplinary conferences, and written records. The written records include progress notes, referral forms (interagency referral forms), consultations, and

FIG. 9–1. Schematic representation of the steps of the discharge planning process.

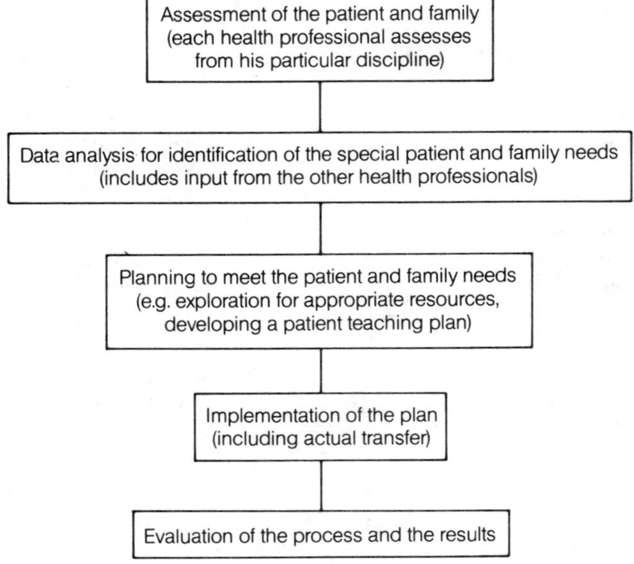

checklist evaluation tools. It is very important to develop an effective mechanism for written documentation of the discharge planning process to keep the various persons involved updated, and also for purposes of reimbursement and quality assurance review.

PLANNING TO MEET PATIENT AND FAMILY NEEDS

Once the specific patient and family needs have been identified, possible alternatives and resources in the community and health care system can be considered. It is most important for the patient and/or family to be an integral part of the process. There are often various alternatives that must be explored to determine what best meets the needs and what is most acceptable to the patient and his family. To be effective, the discharge plan must be individualized, realistic, and acceptable to the patient and/or his family.

If the patient needs to be placed in an extended care facility, nursing home, or rehabilitation center, the social worker or member of the discharge planning department can suggest appropriate facilities in the area that would meet the patient's needs. A site visit can be arranged for the patient or family to assess the facility and talk with staff members at the new facility. Cost, type of programs offered, distance of the facility from home, and other considerations need to be weighed in making a decision on placement. Patients may require referral to community resources for particular needs. Referral forms or telephone contacts are usually necessary to make these arrangements.

For patients and/or families who need patient teaching, a detailed written teaching plan must be developed (see Chapter 8).

IMPLEMENTATION OF THE PLAN INCLUDING ACTUAL TRANSFER

Once a discharge plan has been developed, many activities need to be set in motion and coordinated to ensure a smooth transition to another facility or home. One person must assume the responsibility for the coordination of the plan and keeping all involved persons informed, including the patient and/or his family. Team conferences and conferences that include the patient and family are often very helpful.

The day of discharge finally arrives; it is the culmination of the efforts and cooperation of many people. The patient is prepared emotionally and psychologically for the transition. Most patients will demonstrate some degree of transfer anxiety. By reassuring the patient that he is ready and able to make the transition, the nurse can provide the support for a smooth transition. The day of discharge can be a bittersweet experience for the staff who have worked with the patient, especially if the patient has been hospitalized for a long time. The caregivers must deal with their own feelings about the closure of a relationship.

EVALUATION OF THE DISCHARGE PLANNING PROCESS AND THE RESULTS

The discharge planning process should be evaluated, either in informal conversations or in team conferences. It is important to evaluate what is good about the discharge planning program and process at a facility and what needs to be changed or fine-tuned. Such an evaluation focuses on the opinions of the health professional involved in the process. It is also important to evaluate the process as perceived by the patient, family, and transfer agency. This is accomplished by follow-up telephone calls, conversations, visits from patients, visits by staff to the other facility, and evaluation forms. Evaluation is important for providing quality and continuity of care in the most cost effective means possible. The feedback collected provides the data to make necessary changes in the process and also helps to evaluate the quality of extended care facilities to which the patient has been transferred.

NECESSARY CONDITIONS FOR EFFECTIVE DISCHARGE PLANNING—A SUMMARY

A few basic principles can help to guide the process of discharge planning and include

1. Incorporation of discharge planning as an integral part of delivery of care within the objectives of the institution
2. Incorporation of the responsibility for anticipating a patient's posthospital needs within all professional roles; this responsibility should be written into job descriptions and fulfillment of this responsibility demonstrated
3. Delegation of responsibility to the staff nurse/primary nurse to initiate the formal discharge planning process in enough time to allow for effective discharge planning
4. Utilization of a multi-disciplinary, collaborative approach to discharge planning
5. Development of effective mechanisms and tools for communication among the patient, the family, the health professionals, and others to implement the discharge planning process
6. Written documentation of the steps of the process of discharge planning and the various communications involved in the process must be maintained

APPLICATION OF THE PROCESS TO NEUROLOGICALLY IMPAIRED PATIENTS

The process of discharge planning often becomes very complex when it is applied to neurologically impaired patients because they have many complex and multi-faceted needs. Neurological patients who need discharge planning may include multi-trauma patients who have sustained injury not only to the nervous system but also to other body systems; head injury or spinal cord injury patients; patients with neurological degenerative diseases such as multiple sclerosis and amyotrophic lateral sclerosis; patients with neurological deficits from infectious processes; patients with central nervous system neoplasms; and others. The specific needs of each patient must be individually assessed and the discharge planning process individualized.

The process of discharge planning may need to be organized differently for neurological patients than for patients with other problems although the steps in discharge planning are the same. As with any process the steps involved are not compartmentalized, and there is simultaneous activity in all steps even though the major focus may be on one particular step. The process can also be divided into a *preliminary phase* and an *active collaborative phase*, for it is impossible to proceed with discharge planning until the patient is medically stabilized, and a firm baseline has been established from which deficits and needs can be identified and managed.[2] In the preliminary phase, the practitioners from each discipline work independently from their own perspective to begin assessing the patient even though he is not well stabilized. Care focuses on maintenance of intact function and prevention of complications and new deficits. Once the patient is well stabilized, the team begins to work actively and collaboratively on discharge planning.

ASSESSMENT

On admission to an acute-care setting, it is often necessary for the patient with neurological impairment to be managed by a team of medical specialists. The nursing staff collects an admission history and conducts ongoing assessments. For patients with neurological motor impairment, a physical therapy program is begun to provide passive range of motion exercises to maintain motor function. Until the patient is well stabilized medically, it is impossible to begin formal discharge planning although data are collected and compiled. Therefore, the assessment step of discharge planning can be divided into preliminary and active collaborative phases. The preliminary data gathering phase begins at admission. It is characterized by data gathering (nursing history, complete assessment including a neurological assessment, reassessments) that establishes a baseline by which to evaluate improvement, stabilization, or deterioration. Other members of the health team such as the social worker are also engaged in limited data collection. A pool of information exists for beginning to predict special needs, rehabilitative potential, and expected outcome for the patient.

The second phase commences when the patient has been well stabilized medically. At this point, the extent and degree of deficits and needs can be determined with much more certainty. Consultation and evaluation by various health professionals (e.g., the occupational therapist) can be requested to provide a complete body of data for discharge planning. This phase is called the active and collaborative phase. Input from all disciplines involved with the patient is necessary to plan for the patient's posthospital needs.

DATA ANALYSIS

The pool of information about the patient must be analyzed first by the practitioner from each discipline to consider implications for his discipline. The information then needs to be analyzed by the team members collaboratively to consider interdisciplinary implications and how the information will be used in the overall discharge planning process. Data analysis is considered in conferences within the particular discipline such as weekly nursing conferences or conferences conducted in the physical therapy department for the members of that department. The data are also considered at interdisciplinary team conferences where the persons involved in the care of a particular patient discuss the patient. Written documentation of both individual and interdisciplinary conferences as well as other methods of considering the patient should be available. Although data analysis and planning are two different cognitive activities, they are often addressed at the same time. Once data are analyzed and problems identified, the next logical step is planning to deal with the problem.

PLANNING

Planning, like other steps in the discharge planning process, is ongoing and may be done informally by the individual practitioner and more formally through collaboration with other team members. Planning is based on both short- and long-range realistic goals. The short-term goals become the steps of achieving long-range goals. The plan must be flexible, particularly in the early stages of hospitalization, to accommodate the changes that are apt to occur in the patient. It is impossible to predict with certainty the degree of recovery that can occur when a nervous system is injured. At times, one can be pleasantly surprised by the amount of improvement, while with other patients, hopes for improvement are not realized. Therefore, the health team members must be able to readjust the discharge plan based on changes in the patient's condition and a realistic appraisal of potential outcomes.

Informal and formal conferences with team members or conferences with the patient and/or family are the usual methods for planning. It must be emphasized that inclusion of the patient and/or family is an absolute necessity for effective discharge planning. The plan for discharge should be documented in writing and updated as necessary. A reasonable time frame should be developed so that there is adequate time to complete activities such as patient and family teaching.

IMPLEMENTATION

Implementation of the discharge plan is the collaborative effort of many individuals working together to actualize the plan. A team member, often the social worker, will contact a potential transfer facility if the patient needs to be placed in a long-term or rehabilitative hospital or nursing home. Many times a nursing representative from the transfer facility will visit the patient to assess him for the feasibility of transfer. Rehabilitation beds are usually scarce, and the patient must be able to benefit from the rehabilitation program offered at the facility to make transfer worthwhile. The nurse assessing the patient may decide that (1) the patient is a good candidate for the facility and is ready for transfer; (2) the patient is a good candidate but is not ready for transfer and another assessment of the patient should be scheduled in a few weeks; or (3) the patient is not a good candidate for transfer to the facility. In the case of aggressive rehabilitation hospitals, the patient must be alert, oriented, and able to retain information and follow simple instructions in order to benefit from the rehabilitation program. A patient who is not alert, is not able to comprehend simple instructions, or does not cooperate with the caregiver will not benefit from an aggressive rehabilitation program. Once the patient is accepted for transfer to another facility, it is helpful for the patient or a family member to visit the facility and talk with staff members before transfer plans are formalized.

Once the place of transfer has been selected, information about the patient must be shared by the nursing staffs to promote continuity of care. This may be accomplished through meetings, telephone calls, or written referral forms. Most often, all three methods of communication are used. The physician will communicate with the accepting physician to acquaint him with the medical management of the patient. For the patient who is going home, arrangements should be made for any necessary equipment. If community agencies will provide services to the patient, these arrangements should also be made.

The patient and family must be prepared emotionally and psychologically for the transfer. Transfer can be very frightening to the patient who has been hospitalized for an extended period, so much reassurance must be provided as the day approaches. There may be support groups in the community that would be helpful to the patient or family. One such group is the National Head Injury Foundation, which has chapters throughout the country. If the patient or family could benefit from this group or any other group, information about the purposes of the organization and how to contact it should be provided. Printed materials, visuals, and small group conferences with other patients and families may be helpful. A discharge handbook or any other form of printed material is especially useful because the patient or family member can read it at leisure and then ask questions as necessary.

As caregivers, health professionals often experience mixed emotions about the discharge of a patient with whom they have worked. Many patients with neurological dysfunction have extensive hospitalization, creating strong bonds between patient and caregivers. Health professionals should recognize and deal with their feelings about the transfer of the patient. This may be one topic for discussion at support groups that help the caregivers deal with problems.

EVALUATION

It is important for health team members to evaluate the discharge planning process to identify any areas that need to be changed or improved, either through team conferences or through periodic written reviews of the process. Another focus of evaluation is the patient and his family. How did they view the process? Was it effective? What would have made the transition easier? This information can be collected in a follow-up letter sent to the patient, by return visits, and through other mechanisms designed to provide feedback. It is also important to seek an evaluation from the staff at the transfer facility to gain their perception of the discharge planning process. All of this information can be used to improve the system of discharge planning.

SUMMARY

The discharge planning process is a complex process of problem solving and ongoing independent and collaborative activities and communication directed at helping the patient make a smooth transition from one environment to another without losing the progress that he has already made. The new environment may be home or an extended care facility that will provide continued care based on unmet needs of the patient. Throughout the discharge planning process, the various health professionals work with the patient and/or his family to achieve mutually accepted and specific goals. Unless the health team, patient, and family share mutual and congruent goals, there will be confusion, frustration, discouragement, and fragmentation of effort. If this happens, the patient will not reach his optimum rehabilitation potential.

REFERENCES

1. McKeehan KM (ed): Continuing Care: A Multidisciplinary Approach to Discharge Planning. St Louis, CV Mosby, 1981
2. Hickey JV, McKenna JE: Effective discharge planning and the neurosurgical patient. J Neurosurg Nurs 16(2):101, April 1984

BIBLIOGRAPHY

Books

David J et al: Guidelines for Discharge Planning. Thorofare, NJ, Charles B Slack, 1973

Steffi B, Eide I: Discharge Planning Handbook. Thorofare, NJ, Charles B Slack, 1978

Periodicals

Bristow O, Stickney C, Thompson S: Discharge planning for continuity of care, No 21-1604. New York, National League for Nursing, 1976

Connoly M: Organizing your workday for more effective discharge planning. Nurs '81 11:44, July 1981

DRGs: The new pulse of health policy. Nurs & Health Care, 208, April 1983

Glover J: Reducing discharge planning paperwork with a pocket-size discharge planning record. Nurs '81 11:50, December 1982

Grimaldi PL: Public law 97-248: The implications of prospective payment schedules. Nurs Management 14(2):25, February 1983

Haberman B: Cognitive dysfunction and social rehabilitation in the severely head-injured patient. J Neurosurg Nurs 14(5):220, October 1982

Harvey B: Your patient's discharge plan. Nurs '81 11:48, July 1981

Hicks A, Ashby D: Teaching discharge planning. Nurs Outlook 24:306, 1976

Johnson J, Pachano A: Planning patients' discharge. Supervisor Nurse, 44, February 1981

Korcok M: Payment by diagnosis: US government proposes new fee system. Can Med Assoc J 128:833, April 1, 1983

LaMontague J, McKeehan K: Profile of a continuing care program emphasizing discharge planning. J Nurs Adm 5:22, 1975

National League for Nursing: Patient discharge and referral planning—whose responsibility? No 20-1515. New York, National League for Nursing, 1974

Schreiber H: Discharge-planning: Key to the future of hospital social work. Health Soc Work 6:38, May 1981

Schuman J, Ostfeld A, Willard H: Discharge planning in the acute hospital. Arch Phys Med Rehabil 57:343, July 1976

Spitzer RB: Legislation and new regulations. Nurs Management 14(2):13, February 1983

Stevens M: Post concussion syndrome. J Neurosurg Nurs 14(5):239, October 1982

part four

Special Considerations in Neurological and Neurosurgical Nursing

chapter **10**

Environmental and Occupational Factors in Neurological Nursing

The purposes of this chapter are first, to introduce the nurse to the effects of selected environmental and occupational exposures on the nervous system; second, to identify the nursing implications of environmental and occupational exposures to toxic agents; and third, to identify resources on the local, state, and federal level that can supply information to the nurse and other health professionals about the effects of environmental and occupational exposures on the body.

Every nurse who has worked with neurological patients can usually recall patients with neurological deficits who baffled the physician when he attempted to establish the etiology of the problems. Could it be that some of these patients suffered from neurological deficits that were attributable to environmental or occupational exposures? Sensitizing the nurse to the possibility of environmental and occupational exposures in neurological disease will increase awareness and perhaps prompt the inclusion of questions about environmental exposures and occupational history as data are gathered for the nursing history and overall patient assessment. The nurse who is aware of environmental factors is more apt to be supportive of a patient who develops subjective symptoms of neurological dysfunction that defy diagnosis and cause other health professionals to suspect a psychosomatic basis for symptoms.

SCOPE AND SIGNIFICANCE OF OCCUPATIONAL AND ENVIRONMENTAL EXPOSURES

Many chemicals present in the workplace and home have been identified as causing deleterious effects on the various body systems. Oftentimes, a person is unaware that he is being exposed to material that is harmful to his health. Some exposures cause immediate effects on the body while others require cumulative exposures over the longer term before signs and symptoms are evident. For example, elemental mercury is widely used in thermometers and dental fillings. Exposure to mercury in its various chemical forms has long been associated with serious neurological effects on the central and peripheral nervous systems. The character of the "Mad Hatter" in Lewis Carroll's *Alice in Wonderland* was patterned after persons of the day who used mercuric salts in the manufacture of felt hats, which caused bizarre behavior and poor coordination. The person refinishing a few pieces of furniture in the basement of his home may be similarly exposing himself to toxic substances (the chemicals for stripping the furniture).

Persons working in the hospital environment can be exposed routinely to a variety of chemical agents. For example, ethylene oxide, an agent commonly used for sterilizing equipment, is suspected of causing peripheral neuropathy. Therefore, the nurse should be aware of the hazards of exposure in her own work environment as well as the effects of exposure on the patient.

The risks of exposure to toxins in an industrial, high-technology society are many, and new chemicals, whose effects are unknown, are being introduced at a steady rate. Although this chapter will focus on only the neurological effects of toxic agents, one should keep in mind that many of the chemicals discussed can affect more than one body system.

This chapter was written by Joanne V. Hickey and James E. Hickey, Certified Industrial Hygienist.

SELECTED NEUROTOXIC CHEMICALS

Neurotoxins are substances found in the workplace or environment that are associated with nerve dysfunction. Among the major chemical groups containing neurotoxins are solvents, heavy metals, pesticides, and gases. Solvents are chemicals used in the workplace and the home for cleaning and degreasing and as a vehicle for other materials such as paint and nail polish. The heavy metals that most often affect the nervous system are lead and mercury. The major purpose of pesticides is to affect the nervous system of insects and rodents so it is not surprising that these chemicals can affect the human nervous system. Gases such as carbon monoxide and hydrogen sulfide can have a direct or indirect effect on the nervous system. Carbon monoxide, for instance, exerts its effect by depriving the brain of oxygen. Hydrogen sulfide, on the other hand, acts directly on the respiratory center of the brain.

Table 10–1 has been developed to acquaint the nurse with a variety of neurotoxic chemicals and their effects. The table contains those chemicals that have been the subject of National Institute of Occupational Safety and Health (NIOSH) criteria documents as well as a few other well-documented neurotoxins. The reader should not conclude that this table contains all of the chemicals causing neurological effects and should suspect the possibility of chemical involvement whenever there is a history of significant chemical exposure. Information about the sources of exposure to workers is also included in the table. The table contains those chemicals associated with noncarcinogenic effects on the nervous system. A number of chemicals have been associated with an increased incidence of brain tumors in exposed workers; however, most of these are also associated with an increased incidence of neoplasms throughout the body.

ROUTES OF ENTRY

There are three major routes for entry of foreign chemical substances into the body: inhalation, ingestion, and absorption through the skin. Inhalation of air-borne contaminants is the most common route of industrial exposure. The offending contaminants arise from chemicals introduced or produced during the industrial process or work activity. The respiratory system, with its enormous surface area for the absorption of chemicals into the bloodstream, provides an extremely efficient mechanism for the transport of chemicals to the various organ systems. Solvents such as toluene and trichloroethylene are examples of common industrial air contaminants that are transported by the lungs to the bloodstream and then to the central nervous system.

Ingestion of chemicals because of inadequate personal hygiene is a serious problem in some work situations. Workers' clothes, food, cigarettes, and personal articles are readily contaminated with chemicals such as lead and mercury, which are easily introduced into the mouth during normal activities. Contaminants are then absorbed through the gastrointestinal tract into the bloodstream. Food can also be contaminated from pesticides or other inadvertent exposures during production and processing, or contamination can occur within the home environment. Ingestion of lead paint by small children (pica) is a problem that has led to a national program to identify and treat affected children. Consumption of moonshine whiskey is another cause of lead ingestion.

Many organic chemical liquids are fat soluble and, as such, can be absorbed directly into the bloodstream through the skin and mucous membrane. *n*-Hexane, used as a solvent in industrial processes, is associated with peripheral neuropathy through contamination of the skin.

TOXIC EFFECTS ON THE NERVOUS SYSTEM FROM EXPOSURES

Toxic effects from exposures are generally classified as either acute or chronic. Acute effects are those that are manifest within a short time after exposure and usually require a relatively high exposure level. Exposure to high levels of some toxins such as solvents can lead to unconsciousness. Chronic effects are those that become apparent after a longer course of exposure, which is usually at relatively low levels. Exposure to low levels of solvents over an extended period of time can lead to subtle neurological effects such as sensory and motor deficits (e.g., numbness in the extremities, muscle weakness, generalized deterioration of brain function).

The mechanisms by which chemicals exert toxic effects on the nervous system are not well established. Current toxicological investigations suggest the following mechanisms for various agents:

- Interference with neurotransmitter synthesis
- Interference with release of neurotransmitters
- Promotion of release of neurotransmitters
- Interference with destruction of neurotransmitters
- Mimicking of neurotransmitters either as a postjunctional stimulator or a postjunctional block
- Focal demyelination

The effects of the various mechanisms on the nervous system include swelling of the axon, wallerian-type degeneration, and interference with cell biochemistry. The target site within the central or peripheral nervous system determines the specific function affected. If the central nervous system is involved, cognitive, behavioral, sensory, motor, and cerebellar deficits can result. The sensory and motor deficits that result when a sufficient amount of damage or dysfunction occurs in the peripheral nerves are called peripheral neuropathies. Peripheral neuropathies can be reversible or permanent depending on the degree and length of exposure to toxic agents. For those neuropathies that are reversible, neurological function will slowly return when exposure is eliminated. However, total recovery of function may not occur.

The specific signs and symptoms that are found in a patient will depend on the particular toxic agent to which the

(Text continued on page 221.)

TABLE 10–1. *Neurotoxic Chemicals*

Chemical Agent	*Occupational Groups Potentially Exposed*	*Specific Effect*	*Exposure—Conditions/Comments (ppm = parts per million)*
Acetylene	Used in welding and cutting and as an illuminating agent, a chemical intermediate for products such as acrylonitrile, vinyl chloride, acrylic acid, and ethyl and methyl methacrylate, etc.	Narcosis, anesthesia	Acute exposure required for narcosis. Effects believed to be completely reversible following cessation of exposure.
Acrylamide	Used as a chemical intermediate in the production of vinyl polymers, especially polyacrylamides for water and waste-water treatment	Neurotoxicity as manifested by such symptoms as numbness, tingling, and loss of feeling, especially in the extremities	Both acute and chronic exposure produce peripheral neuropathy as evidenced by reduced nerve conduction velocity.
Arsenic trioxide	Used in agriculture as pesticide and in production of pigments and glass. Exposures occur in smelting and refining of metal ores.	Polyneuritis with numbness and paresthesis of hands and feet. Motor paralyses occur in severe cases. Syndrome characterized by three progressive stages.	Chronic ingestion due to contaminated hands, clothing, etc., may be a problem as well as chronic inhalation.
Carbaryl	Exposures occur in the production, formulation, and use of this organophosphorus pesticide.	Acts as a cholinesterase inhibitor.	Acetylcholinesterase inhibition definitely occurs following acute exposure and probably after chronic exposure. Some prolonged reduction of acetylcholinesterase activity after chronic exposure but little epidemiological data available.
Carbon dioxide	Generated as a byproduct in the production of synthetic ammonia, methanol, and other chemicals. Its main industrial use is in cooling and refrigeration of food and in fire extinguishers.	Muscular twitches, psychomotor excitation	These effects are produced by acute exposure to relatively high concentrations (>100,000 ppm) for a few minutes.
Carbon disulfide	Used in production of regenerated cellulose (viscose rayon and cellulose), manufacture of carbon tetrachloride, vulcanizing rubber, and in neoprene cement.	Neurological, psychological, and behavioral changes occur following both acute and chronic exposure.	These effects are documented mostly through case reports rather than through epidemiological studies.
Carbon monoxide	Major sources of exposure include petroleum refineries, kraft pulp mills, and formaldehyde manufacturing; also in situations where incomplete combustion of fossil fuels occurs.	Neurological effects include changes in reflexes, time discrimination, and visual acuity.	These effects are mainly documented for acute exposures to high levels of carbon monoxide.
Carbon tetrachloride	Used in drycleaning, degreasing, cleaning electric parts, laboratory tests, and as a fire extinguishing agent.	A variety of central nervous system (CNS) effects have been documented.	Acute exposures in excess of 14,000 ppm for 1 minute produce unconsciousness.

(continued)

TABLE 10–1. (continued)

Chemical Agent	Occupational Groups Potentially Exposed	Specific Effect	Exposure—Conditions/Comments (ppm = parts per million)
Cyanide and its salts	Used in extraction and electroplating of gold and silver, heat treating of metals, photography, and chemical manufacture.	Loss of consciousness, vertigo, loss of reflexes, tremor	Acute exposure can produce loss of consciousness whereas tremor and gradual loss of coordination are more characteristic of chronic exposure.
Dichlorophenoxy-acetic acid (2,4-D)	Herbicide used as defoliant in Vietnam as part of mixture known as "Agent Orange." Exposures occurred in manufacture and dispensing. Certain effects may be due to 2,3,7,8-tetrachlorodibenzo-p-dioxin, commonly known as "Dioxin," which is a contaminant in manufacture.	Distal symmetrical polyneuropathy from dermal contact. Mild distal weakness and sensory impairment. Recovery usually occurs when exposure ceases.	Material no longer manufactured or used; however, because of poor biodegradation it continues to be present in environment, e.g., Time's Beach episode.
Dimethylamino-propionitrile (DMAPN)	Used as catalyst in manufacture of polyurethane foams. Use ceased with discovery of widespread effects among workers. May reappear if vigilance slackens.	Unusual features of axonopathy dysfunction. These are followed by polyneuropathy.	Exposures unlikely unless material is reintroduced. Has caused epidemic occurrence of neuropathy in industrial setting.
Dinitro-ortho-cresol	Exposures occur in manufacture and application of this organophosphorus pesticide.	Symptoms of CNS effects include loss of motor function in legs, confusion, tingling, and numbness of extremities.	CNS effects of acute exposures have been documented through case histories or poisoning incidents; little data available on effects of chronic exposure.
Ethylene dichloride	Widely used in the production of vinyl chloride, as a fumigant, an insecticide, and a component of degreasers.	Anesthesia, unconsciousness	Information on these effects comes from acute exposures and poisoning incidents; little epidemiological data available.
Ethylene oxide	A gas widely used in industry and medical care facilities in sterilizing heat-sensitive biomedical materials.	Reported to produce nervous system disease of the distal axonopathy type.	Exposure may occur from leaking sterilizing units or from commercially sterilized packages that have not been properly aged.
Furfuryl alcohol	Exposures are likely to occur in the synthesis of furan resins. It is also used as a solvent and chemical intermediate in many products.	CNS depression	The only real data on human exposures are from cases of persons receiving acute, high-dose exposures.
n-Hexane	The major use is in the formulation of gasolines. Also used as a solvent in glues, varnishes, inks, cements, and as extractants for seed oils.	Polyneuropathy progressing from slight to quadriplegia following chronic exposure	Concentrations of 500 ppm to 2000 ppm of hexane over an extended period (several weeks or more) were associated with severe neurological deterioration.

TABLE 10–1. (continued)

Chemical Agent	*Occupational Groups Potentially Exposed*	*Specific Effect*	*Exposure—Conditions/Comments (ppm = parts per million)*
Hydrogen sulfide	Production of inorganic sulfides, sulfuric acid, and organic sulfur compounds. Exposures may occur in related drilling, mining, smelting, or processing operations or from decomposing organic matter.	CNS depression, loss of consciousness, respiratory arrest	Several fatal accidents have occurred among persons cleaning cesspools. Has disagreeable odor at low concentrations but odor not detected at significant concentrations.
Methyl n-butyl ketone	Widely used as solvent in synthetic resins and coatings, inks, adhesives, and dyes and a variety of other uses.	Chronic exposure has produced peripheral neuropathy with loss of sensory and/or motor functions.	Effects of this material and *n*-hexane thought to be due to common metabolite.
Lead, inorganic	Primary and secondary lead production, manufacture of lead-containing products such as pigments, paints, and automobile batteries.	Peripheral neuropathy as evidenced by numbness, tingling, slowing of nerve conduction velocity	Chronic exposure; extent of neurological impairment related to both concentration and duration of exposure; personal contamination and ingestion are significant problems.
Malathion	An organophosphorus pesticide used on fruit, vegetables, and ornamental plants and to control fleas, lice, and mosquitoes on livestock.	An acetylcholinesterase inhibitor; interferes with neural transmission	Acute exposures produce a variety of CNS symptoms, including unconsciousness, tremor, and other neurological symptoms.
Mercury	Used in production of chlorine and caustic soda; also widely used in plastics, paints, agricultural chemicals, and pharmaceuticals.	CNS effects as manifested by ataxia, tremor, reduction of visual fields; neurobehavioral effects	Chronic exposures produce neurological damage whose onset is insidious and progressive if exposure continues; personal contamination with subsequent inhalation of vapor is significant problem.
Methyl alcohol	Production of formaldehyde, methyl terephthalate, methyl halides, methyl methacrylate, and acetic acid. Also used as a solvent in paints, varnishes, cements, inks, and hair dyes.	Nervous system effects include paresthesias, muscular weakness, unsteady gait, and blindness.	Acute exposures have produced fatalities but there is little specific information on the exact exposure conditions associated with these deaths.
Methyl bromide	Has found use as a fumigant, fire extinguisher, refrigerant, and insecticide.	High exposure can lead to pyramidal tract, cerebellar, and peripheral nerve dysfunction.	
Methylene chloride	Production of paint and varnish removers, insecticides, fumigants, solvents, degreasers, and fire extinguishers.	CNS depression occurs following exposure to several hundred parts per million due to *in vivo* formation of carbon monoxide.	Effects of acute exposure are identical to those from carbon monoxide. Little is known about the effects of chronic exposure.
Methyl parathion	Exposure would occur in the manufacture or application of this pesticide.	Symptoms are related to acetylcholinesterase inhibition, e.g., sweating, bronchoconstriction, muscular weakness, incoordination.	Little is known about the chronic effects of this compound. Available data come from case reports and animal studies.

(continued)

TABLE 10–1. (continued)

Chemical Agent	Occupational Groups Potentially Exposed	Specific Effect	Exposure—Conditions/Comments (ppm = parts per million)
Parathion	Exposure would occur in the manufacture, formulation, and application of this pesticide.	CNS depression characterized by slurred speech, loss of reflexes, convulsions, and respiratory depression.	What little epidemiological data exist concern enzyme changes following acute exposures.
Petroleum solvents	Used in the production of herbicides and insecticides; dry cleaning and degreasing; in paints, inks, and enamels; in laboratories and in adhesive and asphalt coating operations	Narcotic effect at high concentration	Exposure to about 2000 ppm or more for a few minutes makes most people lose consciousness.
Styrene	Used in manufacture of plastic and rubber. Many commercial products are made from styrene-based plastic resins including packaging, insulation, automobile parts, and fiberglass boats.	CNS depression and possible peripheral neuropathy from repeated skin contact	
Tetrachloroethane	Widely used as a solvent for cellulose acetate, fats, waxes, greases, rubber, and sulfur. Its current use is very limited.	Neurological effects induced by chronic exposures include numbness, tingling and paresthesias of the extremities, and loss of reflexes	Little is known about the concentrations required to produce neurological effects. NIOSH noted that neurological effects were mostly associated with acute exposures.
Thallium	Previously widely used as rodenticides and insecticides. Its use is now discouraged in North America.	Peripheral neuropathy resulting from distal axonopathy	Three distinct varieties of peripheral neuropathy follow acute, subacute, or chronic exposure. Intoxication usually stems from homicidal or accidental ingestion (especially in children).
Thiols	These compounds are mainly used in the synthesis of pesticides, defoliants, fungicides, and pharmaceuticals and as stabilizers in plastics.	Neurological effects include skeletal muscle contractions, paralysis of bronchial muscles, loss of consciousness, and amnesia.	Information on neurological effects comes mainly from case reports and appears to be associated chiefly with acute exposures.
Toluene	Exposures are most likely to occur in production or use. Widely used as a solvent for paints, glues, resins, and other coating materials.	CNS depression, including slurred speech, loss of coordination, unconsciousness. Very high exposures can produce permanent encephalopathy.	Exposure to a concentration of 200 ppm for 8 hours produces mild neurological symptoms; 50 to 100 ppm produces drowsiness and mild confusion.
Trichloroethylene	Used mainly in degreasing operations and drycleaning; also limited use in waxes, paint, lacquers, tars, and other similar products.	Acts as a CNS depressant. Large doses depress heart rate, induce defibrillation, and cardiac arrest. Dizziness and loss of senses of smell and touch occur at lower doses.	Chronic exposures produce symptoms such as irritability, sleep disturbances, anxiety, and paresthesias. Concentrations above 100 ppm for several hours are required to produce symptoms.

TABLE 10–1. (continued)

Chemical Agent	Occupational Groups Potentially Exposed	Specific Effect	Exposure—Conditions/Comments (ppm = parts per million)
Triorthocresyl phosphate (TOCP)	Major uses are as an insecticide, a petroleum additive, a high-temperature lubricant, and a modifier in plastic formulations.	Inhibits acetylcholinesterase; also produces unrelated distal axonopathy, which can lead to varying degrees of morbidity including sequelae of both peripheral and nervous system damage.	Because of its oily nature and lipid solubility, skin absorption is significant. Outbreaks have occurred from ingestion of contaminated food products.
Xylene	Used as a solvent for gums and resins, castor and linseed oil, rubber, dibenzl cellulose, paint lacquers, varnishes, cleaning epoxy resins, and as an intermediate in the production of various chemicals.	CNS effects, including narcosis.	Acute exposures to 10,000 ppm for a few minutes produces unconsciousness and death if exposure is continued.

patient was exposed. The signs and symptoms that may be observed from various toxic agents can include the following:

- Motor—weakness; intentional tremors; muscle atrophy; occasionally spastic paraparesis
- Reflexes—selected (Achilles) or diffuse loss of deep tendon reflexes; hyperreflexia and hypertonicity on occasion
- Sensory—numbness and parasthesias especially of the hands and feet; diminished vibration, position, pin, and sometimes temperature sensation in the extremities, often in the hands and feet; pain especially in the hands and feet
- Cerebellar—ataxia; unsteady broad based gait; incoordination
- Cranial nerves—optic atrophy; visual impairment; trigeminal and facial neuropathies with trichloroethylene; cranial involvement is rare
- Autonomic—excessive sweating of feet and hands
- Other—malaise; anorexia; abdominal pain, vomiting, weight loss; irritation of the mucous membranes; hyperkeratosis; urinary hesitancy; partial or complete impotence; coma; Mees' lines (white striae of the nails); alopecia

The signs and symptoms observed in a patient are the same as those observed with neurological disorders of other than toxic origin. This is what makes identification and diagnosis of toxic exposures in neurological patients so difficult.

DIAGNOSIS

Because the neurological signs and symptoms associated with toxic exposures are similar to objective and subjective manifestations of other neurological problems, a differential diagnosis is very difficult unless the patient presents an obvious history of an acute exposure. Other etiologies will usually be investigated through a diagnostic work-up beginning with a complete general physical and neurological examination. Other procedures and tests will be ordered based on the presenting signs and symptoms.

When other etiologies have not been identified, toxic origins should be considered. Criteria for establishing that a condition is related to a toxic exposure include evidence of exposure based on an occupational and/or personal history, bioassay for evidence of the toxic material and/or its metabolites, and, occasionally, specific patterns noted on selected diagnostic tests.

The importance of a complete and detailed exposure history cannot be overemphasized when dealing with conditions of toxic origins. Often a history of exposure is the only clue to the etiology of the health problem. Such information as hobbies, location of residence in relation to industrial sites, and details of work-related procedures should be pursued. An attempt should be made to obtain a list of chemicals with which the patient has had contact. Since the patient does not always know the precise chemical names of his exposures, assistance should be sought from available resources in the hospital and community.

Bioassay procedures may be available for the detection of toxic chemicals and/or their metabolites in blood, urine, cerebrospinal fluid, and other tissue. Normal values and toxic levels for some materials are available in the literature and can be used as a guide for comparison. In some cases, a biopsy of specific tissue may be necessary to establish the presence of a suspected toxic agent. An example of a well-established bioassay procedure that is extensively used is the routine monitoring of the blood and/or urine of workers exposed to lead or mercury. Analysis of exhaled breath with gas chromatography is a procedure being used in some hospital emergency departments to identify the presence and establish the level of toxic gases within exposed patients. This procedure can save the life of an unconscious patient suspected of having an acute toxic exposure to industrial solvents. These are the same chemicals that may be found in products in the home such as glues, paints, aerosols, and cleaning compounds.

Certain signs, symptoms, and diagnostic test results have been consistently associated with exposure to specific toxic agents. Practitioners whose clinical practice has included the observation of workers exposed to specific agents come to recognize the pattern consistent with the exposure. For example, one of the early signs of the effects of mercury exposure on the nervous system is intentional tremors, which are evidenced by examining samples of characteristic handwriting.

Testing of nerve conduction velocities is becoming a standard practice in the examination of patients exposed to agents associated with peripheral neuropathies. Patterns of changes in nerve conduction velocity can be identified and associated with specific exposures and neuropathies. Another test that may be helpful in diagnosis is electromyography. This test may reveal evidence of denervation.

The neurological effects of toxic materials that are probably the most difficult to evaluate are neuropsychological changes. Behavioral toxicology is a developing field of interest that seeks to evaluate these problems. See Chapter 4 for a discussion of neuropsychological testing. For specific information on the application of neurobehavioral testing to monitoring of neurotoxic effects, see the article by Baker and colleagues cited in the bibliography.

Preexisting conditions can be exacerbated by exposure to toxic substances lower than that that would be necessary to affect a normal healthy person. Also, toxic insult is a highly variable phenomenon and the hypersensitivity of a certain number of individuals should be considered.

TREATMENT

The effects of toxic chemicals on the nervous system can result in reversible or irreversible loss of function. Partial recovery of function is also common. Treatment consists of removal of the toxic exposure and institution of supportive and rehabilitative measures while evaluating the extent of recovery as reversible signs and symptoms clear. For those with irreversible disabilities, management is directed toward achieving the highest level of independence possible through a rehabilitation program. In some instances of specific toxic exposure, drug therapy can be used to accelerate the elimination of the toxin from body tissue. For example, chelation therapy, with ethylene diamine tetraacetic acid (EDTA) and penicillamine, can be used to treat severe lead toxicity. Prophylactic use of chelating agents is not accepted protocol because of the possibility of serious side-effects.

NURSES' ROLE AND NURSING IMPLICATIONS

Nurses employed in neurology clinics, neurological units of general hospitals, or in neurologists' offices are more apt to see patients who have had toxic exposures. Nurses should be attuned to the possibility of toxic chemical exposures as a cause of neurological signs and symptoms. It is also helpful for nurses to be aware of the various industries located in their communities that pose potential health hazards to workers.

The nurse's role in managing patients with potential toxic exposures is to be aware of the potential relationship of toxic exposures and neurological signs and symptoms, especially when peripheral neuropathies are present; to include an occupational and environmental exposure history in the patient assessment; to be aware of the resources available for information and assistance when a toxic exposure may have occurred; to teach the patient personal measures that he can use to control any subsequent exposure; and to make appropriate referrals as necessary.

SOURCES OF INFORMATION AND ASSISTANCE

When a practitioner suspects that a case may involve toxic exposure, it is almost always essential to obtain the assistance of health professionals with expertise in environmental and occupational health. Occupational health physicians, occupational health nurses, and industrial hygienists specialize in this field of practice. They are not commonly associated with hospitals but are primarily employed by governmental agencies and private industrial firms. If possible, these resources should be identified before they are needed. However, the hospital laboratory director can usually provide referrals to the appropriate people in the community. Each state health department has personnel knowledgeable in occupational and environmental exposures. The National Institute for Occupational Safety and Health (NIOSH) is the federal governmental agency concerned with research, training, and consultation in occupational health. This agency can provide consultation over the telephone for the medical management of exposed patients and other useful information.

In cases of exposure that are of occupational origin, there is an obligation to report suspected cases to the appropriate governmental jurisdiction so that measures can be instituted to investigate the work environment for possible additional cases and to prevent future toxic exposures.

BIBLIOGRAPHY

Books

Burgess WA: Recognition of Health Hazards in Industry. New York, John Wiley & Sons, 1981

Cralley LV, Cralley LJ (eds): Patty's Industrial Hygiene and Toxicology, Volume I: General Principles; Volume II: Toxicology; Volume III: Theory and Rationale of Industrial Hygiene Practice. New York, John Wiley & Sons, 1979

Cralley LV, Cralley LJ (eds): Industrial Hygiene Aspects of Plant Operations. New York, Macmillan Publishing Co, 1982

Criteria for a Recommended Standard for (Acetophenone to Zinc Oxide). Washington, DC, National Institute for Occupational Safety and Health, 1973–1983

Documentation of the Threshold Limit Values, 3rd ed. Akron, OH, American Conference of Governmental Industrial Hygienists, 1977

Finkel AJ: Hamilton and Hardy's Industrial Toxicology. John Wright, PSG, 1983

Fishbien L: Potential Industrial Carcinogens and Mutagens. Amsterdam, Elsevier Scientific Publishing, 1979

Gosselin RE et al: Clinical Toxicology of Commercial Products, 4th ed. Baltimore, Williams & Wilkins, 1976

Commercial Products, 4th ed. Baltimore, Williams & Wilkins, 1976

Maekison R, Stricoff S, Partiridge LJ (eds): Occupational Health Guidelines for Chemical Hazards. Washington, DC, National Institute for Occupational Safety and Health/Occupational Safety and Health Administration, 1981

Nielson JM (ed): Material Safety Data Sheets, Vol I; Inorganic and Organic Materials, Vol II. Schenectady, NY, General Electric, 1980

Sax NI: Dangerous Properties of Industrial Materials, 4th ed. New York, Van Nostrand Reinhold, 1975

Schaumburg HH, Spencer PS, Thomas PK: Disorders of Peripheral Nerves. Philadelphia, FA Davis, 1983

Xintaras C, Johnson BL, de Groot I (eds): Behavioral Toxicology. Washington, DC, National Institute of Occupational Safety and Health, 1974

Zanetos MA, Warling JC, Marsh GM: Health Effects of Occupational Exposure to Hazardous Chemicals: A Comparative Assessment With Notes on Ionizing Radiation, Vols 1–3. Washington, DC, Nuclear Regulatory Commission, 1983

Periodicals

Baker EL et al: Monitoring neurotoxins in industry: Development of a neurobehavioral test battery. J Occup Med 25(2):125, February 1983

Cavalleri A, Cosi V: Polyneuritis incidence in shoe factory workers: Case reports and etiological considerations. Arch Environ Health 192, July/August 1978

Gross JA, Haas ML, Swift TR: Ethylene oxide neurotoxicity: Report of four cases and review of the literature. Neurology 29:978, July 1979

Polakoff PL: Warning: Nerve poisons at work. Occup Saf Health 15, November 1982

Schaumburg HH, Spencer PS: The neurology and neuropathology of the occupational neuropathies. J Occup Med 18(11):739, November 1976

Sexton DJ et al: A nonoccupational outbreak of inorganic mercury vapor poisoning. Arch Environ Health 186, July/August 1978

chapter 11

Care of the Unconscious Patient

UNCONSCIOUSNESS: IMPLICATIONS FOR NURSING MANAGEMENT

Unconsciousness has been defined as an abnormal state in which the patient is unresponsive to sensory stimuli as a result of trauma, illness, shock, or some other disorder. The episode may take the form of fainting, in which the unconsciousness is very brief and is followed by spontaneous recovery. In most such instances no medical or nursing intervention is required. At the other end of the spectrum is the deep, prolonged unconsciousness of coma, in which continual medical and nursing management is necessary to maintain and support basic physiological functions. Between the two extremes are degrees of unconsciousness varying in length and severity. For coma to occur, there must be damage in both cerebral hemispheres, lesions in the brain stem, or metabolic causes. However, whenever a person is unconscious for more than a few moments, a high standard of care must be provided with the objectives of maintaining and restoring body function and preventing complications that could threaten life itself.

In caring for neurological or neurosurgical patients, the nurse must often provide care for a patient who has been unconscious for a prolonged period. The management of the unconscious patient is an awesome responsibility. Not only is the survival of the patient directly dependent on the quality of care provided, but the occurrence of acute and chronic disabilities that affect the rehabilitative potential of the patient bears a direct relationship to the quality of the care given. See Chart 11–1, Nursing Care Plan for the Unconscious Patient.

SUPPORT OF VITAL FUNCTIONS: RESPIRATORY AND CARDIAC

The support of vital functions is given the highest priority in patient management. A patent airway, necessary for the maintenance of adequate respiratory and cardiac function, is a basic requirement for sustaining life.

RESPIRATORY FUNCTION

Assessment

Respiratory function is assessed by routinely monitoring the depth, rate, and respiratory pattern. The need for oxygen therapy is based on assessment of respiratory function and evidence of inadequate oxygenation (such as cyanosis around the mouth, ear lobes, and fingernails, or dyspnea as evidenced by abnormal breathing, retraction, and restlessness). Adequate oxygen and carbon dioxide blood levels may be determined by the routine assessment of arterial blood gases. Normal values follow:

- Arterial PO_2: 80 mm Hg to 100 mm Hg
- Arterial PCO_2: 35 mm Hg to 45 mm Hg
- Oxygen sat: 94% to 100%
- Arterial pH: 7.35 to 7.45
- Arterial (HCO_3): 22 mEq to 26 mEq/liter

A low level of oxygen saturation in the arterial blood indicates a need for oxygen therapy.

- Routine blood gases should be assessed for any unconscious patient to evaluate adequate oxygen levels. In any patient

(Text continued on page 228.)

CHART 11-1. NURSING CARE PLAN FOR THE UNCONSCIOUS PATIENT

NURSING DIAGNOSIS	EXPECTED OUTCOME	NURSING INTERVENTION
Ineffective airway clearance	Patent airway will be maintained.	• Suction periodically. • Keep the neck in a neutral position. • In the neurological patient, suctioning should be limited to no more than 15 seconds. • If the patient has a tracheostomy tube in place, administer tracheostomy care every 4 hours.
	Drainage of secretions from the oropharynx will be facilitated.	• Position the patient on his side; reposition frequently. • Elevate the head, if possible.
Impaired gas exchange	Oxygen–carbon dioxide gas exchange will be adequately maintained.	• Turn the patient at least every 2 hours. • Provide for periodic chest physiotherapy. • Monitor arterial blood gases. • Hyperinflate the lungs with 100% oxygen for 60 seconds before and after suctioning, with the approval of the physician. • Administer oxygen as ordered.
	Lungs will be completely expanded.	• Ambu the patient every 1 to 2 hours. • Auscultate the chest every 2 hours.
Ineffective breathing pattern	The patient will establish and maintain an effective breathing pattern	• Monitor rate, depth, and pattern of respirations frequently. • Monitor tidal volumes. • Monitor arterial blood gases. • Observe frequently for signs and symptoms of respiratory distress. • Auscultate the chest frequently. • Elevate the head of the bed, if possible. • Position the patient properly. *For ventilator patient* • Adjust ventilator. • Monitor the patient's synchrony or asynchrony on respirator. • Report asynchrony to physician. • If a tracheostomy tube is in place, deflate the cuff periodically. • In weaning the patient from the respirator, assess patient each time for signs of hypoxemia and fatigue.
Alterations in cardiac output	Cardiac output will be maintained within safe limits.	• Monitor vital signs frequently. • Monitor rate, rhythm, and quality of radial and apical pulses. • Document any arrhythmias. • If patient is on a monitor, observe cardiac monitor every ½ to 1 hour. • Note any correlations between pulse and blood pressure and make appropriate observations.
Potential of venous stasis	Venous stasis and associated problems will not develop.	• Apply elastic stockings or Ace bandage to legs. • When using the lateral recumbent position, position upper leg so that it will not cause extreme pressure on lower leg. • Do not use the foot gatch under knees. • Do not apply pillows or constricting objects to back of knees. • Provide range-of-motion exercises to legs four times a day. • Sit the patient in a chair if possible. • Observe patient for a drop in blood pressure and increase in pulse when raising head of bed or sitting patient up.

(continued)

CHART 11–1. (continued)

NURSING DIAGNOSIS	EXPECTED OUTCOME	NURSING INTERVENTION
Increased cardiac workload	Cardiac workload will be maintained at a safe level.	• Synchronize moving of patient with exhalation; prevent Valsalva maneuver. • Elevate the head of the bed, if possible.
Altered level of consciousness: comatose state	The patient will be supported and treated with dignity until he regains consciousness.	• Monitor the neurological signs frequently; compare findings to previous assessments. • Identify signs and symptoms of neurological change.
Potential local edema (dependent edema)	The patient will not develop localized edema.	• Elevate the distal extremities.
Total self care deficit, Level IV	Basic needs will be provided for the patient.	• Provide total care.
Sensory–perceptual alterations: sensory deprivation	Sensory stimuli will be provided for the patient.	• Talk to the patient; tell him what you are doing; present reality. • Open the shades, turn on the radio. • Encourage family members to talk to the patient. • Touch the patient frequently (rub his skin, comb his hair, etc).
Potential of skin breakdown	The skin and mucous membranes will remain intact.	• Give skin care frequently (daily bath; mouth, back, and perineal care every 4 hours). • Lubricate dry skin with cream or lanolin. • Lubricate lips with Vaseline ointment. • Use nonallergenic or burn linen on the bed if the patient develops a rash or irritation from the bed linen. • Observe every square inch of skin at least every shift, some areas more frequently. • Massage reddened areas; do not position patient on reddened areas. • Check the ears, elbows, and heels carefully for signs of skin breakdown. • If the patient has a nasogastric or endotracheal tube taped to his mouth, remove the tape daily, wash the skin, and protect it with tincture of benzoin. Do not apply new tape in the same place. • Keep heels off bed at all times. • Wash the hair at least once a week. • Comb and neatly arrange the hair. • Cut and file fingernails and toenails. • Turn and reposition the patient at least every 2 hours.
Potential of corneal ulceration or eye irritation	The tissue integrity of the eye will be maintained.	• Inspect the eyes every 4 hours for signs of irritation. • Position the patient on his side so that there is no possibility of eye or corneal irritation. • Cleanse the eyes with normal saline and cotton balls frequently. • Instill lubricating eye drops every 3 hours. • Apply eye shield over the eye, as necessary.
Impaired mobility, Level IV	Muscle mass will be maintained.	• Administer passive range-of-motion exercises at least four times a day. • Sit the patient in chair, if possible.
Potential of joint contractures	Joint contractures will not develop.	• Administer passive range-of-motion exercises at least four times a day. • Position in proper body alignment; reposition every 2 hours; use rolls, pillows, etc., as needed; apply splints if ordered. • In decorticate or decerebrate patient, reposition every hour; control noxious stimuli that aggravate abnormal positioning.

CHART 11–1. (continued)

NURSING DIAGNOSIS	EXPECTED OUTCOME	NURSING INTERVENTION
Altered pattern of urinary elimination	Urinary output will be eliminated from the body.	• Maintain an intake and output record. • Maintain a patent drainage system; check tubing for kinks.
Potential of urinary tract infections	Urinary tract infections will not develop.	• Wash the perineal area and catheter–meatus junction every 8 hours. • Secure the catheter to prevent traction on the meatus following prescribed hospital policy. • Pin the tubing to allow for drainage. • Be sure to unpin tubing when turning the patient. • Check tubing for kinks. • Do not allow reflux of urine from the drainage bag back into bladder. • Elevate the head of the bed, if possible. • Maintain a closed drainage system. • Monitor urinalysis and urine for culture and sensitivity. • Monitor patient and urinary output for signs and symptoms of infection.
Potential for urinary tract calculi	Urinary calculi will not develop.	• Turn and reposition every 2 hours. • Maintain patent drainage system.
Alteration in bowel elimination, constipation	The patient will not become constipated.	• Monitor and record frequency of bowel movements. • Monitor characteristics of stool. • Auscultate the abdomen for bowel sounds. • Initiate a bowel program.
Alteration in nutrition: less than body requirements	Adequate nutrition will be provided.	• Monitor weight at least twice a week and record. • Maintain a daily calorie count. • Request a nutritional consultation. • Administer feedings as ordered.
Potential fluid volume deficit	Adequate fluid volume will be maintained.	• Maintain accurate intake and output record. • Evaluate skin turgor and mucous membranes. • Monitor vital signs and specific gravity of urine.
Altered metabolism, potential of electrolyte imbalance	Electrolyte balance will be maintained.	• Monitor blood chemistry reports. • Observe for signs and symptoms of electrolyte imbalance.
Potential of physical injury	The patient will not sustain physical injury.	• Maintain bed in low position with side rails up when not administering direct care. • Pad side rails if patient is agitated. • Restrain, with permission, if patient is trying to dislodge equipment or tubes.
Potential of fear	Fear will be alleviated.	• Talk to patient; tell him what you are doing; reassure him.
Potential of complications	The patient will be observed for early recognition of common complications.	
Gastrointestinal hemorrhage		• Monitor stools for occult blood. • Monitor vital signs for evidence of bleeding.
Diabetes insipidus		• Monitor urinary specific gravity and hourly outputs.
Increased intracranial pressure		• Observe for signs and symptoms of increased intracranial pressure.
Glucose intolerance from steroid therapy		• Monitor urine for sugar and acetone every 6 hours.

receiving oxygen therapy, the testing of routine blood gases can help to determine the best concentration of oxygen to administer. In addition, assessing blood gases can be helpful in diagnosing acidosis or alkalosis of metabolic or respiratory origin. Acidosis or alkalosis must be treated, since both have a direct effect on respiratory and cardiac function.

Maintaining a Patent Airway and Facilitating Adequate Respiration

The Airway. A patent airway is absolutely necessary for adequate oxygen–carbon dioxide gas exchange. Obstruction of the airway may be caused by injury or aspiration of mucus, vomitus, or drainage. It may be necessary to insert an endotracheal tube or tracheostomy tube to maintain the patency of the airway.

Suctioning. Periodic oropharyngeal or tracheal suctioning will probably be necessary to clear the airway of mucus, blood, or drainage (Fig. 11–1). When suctioning, turn the head from side to side so that each bronchus can be suctioned.

- In a patient who is unconscious because of increased intracranial pressure, suctioning must be limited to no more than 15 seconds to prevent the development of hypercapnia, which acts as a potent vasodilator and is a contributory factor to increased intracranial pressure.

In addition, it is recommended that the lungs be hyperinflated with 100% oxygen for 60 seconds before and after suctioning, contingent upon the approval of the physician. Chronic obstructive pulmonary disease is one reason why hyperinflation with pure oxygen would be contraindicated.

Tracheostomy Care. To maintain a patent airway in the patient with a tracheostomy tube in place, tracheostomy care is administered.

- If the patient has a tracheostomy tube and is on a mechanical ventilator, the cuff on the tracheostomy tube should be deflated for 5 minutes every hour to prevent tracheal ischemia or necrosis.
- If the patient has a tracheostomy tube, tracheostomy care should be given at least every 4 hours to remove drainage or secretions that have adhered to the tube; strict aseptic technique should be followed at all times to prevent infection. (The approved procedure for tracheostomy care at the particular hospital should be followed). Observe the stoma for signs of infection.
- If an endotracheal or tracheostomy tube is in place, the physician *may* prescribe the injection of a few milliliters of sterile normal saline into the tube to stimulate coughing, thus raising secretions and increasing lung expansion.

Breathing Patterns

Assessment. The patient's breathing pattern should be considered and adequately supported, if necessary. Respirations must be adequate to provide and maintain a sufficient amount of oxygen to meet the requirements of all body cells, including those of the central nervous system. There are several neurological conditions that can result in ineffective breathing patterns, including the following:

- Any condition that produces secondary pressure on the brain stem because of increased intracranial pressure from cerebral edema, transtentorial herniation, brain tumors, or cerebral aneurysms
- Any condition that results in injury or direct pressure on the brain stem such as brain tumors, aneurysms, or brain stem trauma
- Spinal cord injury in the cervical or thoracic areas that interfere with the function of the diaphragm (phrenic nerve) or intercostal muscles (accessory muscles of breathing)

Clinical evidence of an ineffective breathing pattern includes apnea, dyspnea, shortness of breath, rapid or shallow respirations, prolonged expirations, altered patterns

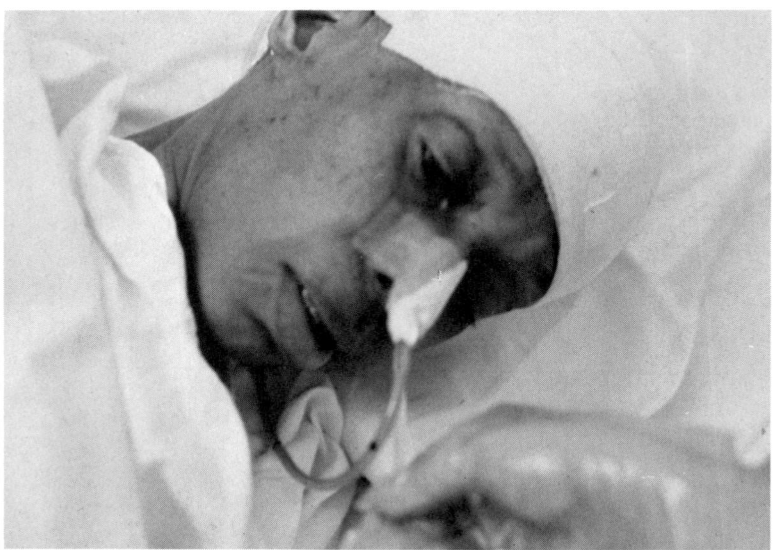

FIG. 11–1. Suctioning of the unconscious patient may be necessary to maintain a patent airway.

associated with neurological impairment (see Chart 5–10), cyanosis, nasal flaring, pursed lips, intercostal or substernal retraction, abdominal breathing, and altered chest expansion. In assessing the patient, the nurse should observe the characteristics of the breathing pattern and the chest movement. Note the facial manifestations of breathing. Next, auscultate the chest for breath sounds. Arterial blood gases and tidal volume should be monitored periodically.

If the breathing pattern is ineffective based on the nurse's assessment of the patient and the laboratory data, the physician should be informed and the patient supported immediately. This may include oxygen therapy by mask or cannula, or ventilation assistance by way of a respirator attached to an endotracheal tube or a tracheostomy tube.

Oxygen Therapy. Based on clinical inspection of the patient and the results of arterial blood gas tests, the patient may need oxygen therapy. There are various methods of administering oxygen to the patient such as by cannula, nasal prongs, or face mask or by attachment of a T-bar to an endotracheal tube or tracheostomy tube. The nurse should know the rate of flow (measured by liters per minute) and the concentration of the oxygen administered. Oxygen is a very dry gas that must be humidified before administration. In some instances, the oxygen is warmed as it bubbles through sterile water. The warming helps to liquify and loosen secretions while oxygen is being provided to the patient.

The patient receiving oxygen therapy should have routine blood gases assessed periodically to be sure that he is being properly oxygenated. Adjustments in the rate of flow and the concentration of oxygen can be made as necessary.

Lung Expansion. Because an unconscious patient cannot respond to instructions to take deep breaths, alternate methods are followed to improve total lung expansion and prevent pooling or stasis of secretions in the lungs. These conditions can lead to pneumonia (hypostatic and bacterial) or atelectasis.

- An Ambu bag can be used for a few minutes every hour to expand the lungs, thus eliminating dead air space that can lead to pneumonia or atelectasis.
- An Ambu bag can be used for a patient with or without a tracheostomy or endotracheal tube.

Positioning and Turning. To prevent pooling of secretions in one area of the lungs, the patient is turned and positioned frequently.

- Turn the patient from side to side every 2 hours to prevent pooling of secretions in one area of the lungs (Fig. 11–2). The unconscious patient is never positioned on his back because his tongue may slip back, obstructing the airway, or he may aspirate.
- Unless contraindicated, the patient's head should be elevated and turned to the side to facilitate drainage of secretions when he is lying in bed (Fig. 11–3).
- If hemiplegia is present, the patient may be positioned on the paralyzed side, but special care and careful observations must be instituted to prevent injury (to soft tissue and nerves), edema, or any compromise of the vascular supply, particularly in the limbs. Because vasomotor tone is decreased in the affected area, adverse effects can develop rapidly from improper positioning. In this case, the patient may need to be turned more frequently than every 2 hours.

Ventilators

Types of Ventilators. *Ventilators* or *respirators* are mechanical devices that maintain breathing when the patient's own breathing pattern is ineffective or absent. Most ventilators used in acute care settings are called positive pressure ventilators, which means that they inflate the lungs by pushing air into them, thus altering the pressure dynamics of normal respirations. A positive pressure ventilator is useful for patients who have a stiff, noncompliant lung or for those who have lost the negative intrapleural pressure within their chest. There are three basic types of positive pressure ventilators used in the adult: the volume-

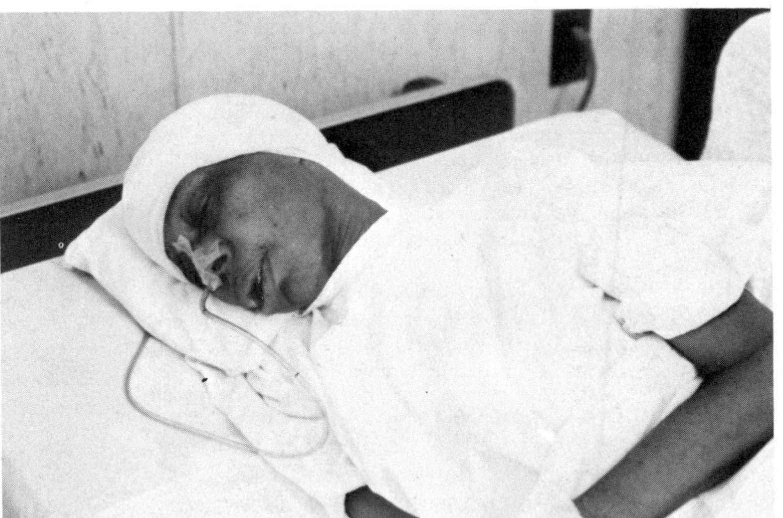

FIG. 11–2. Proper positioning of the unconscious patient.

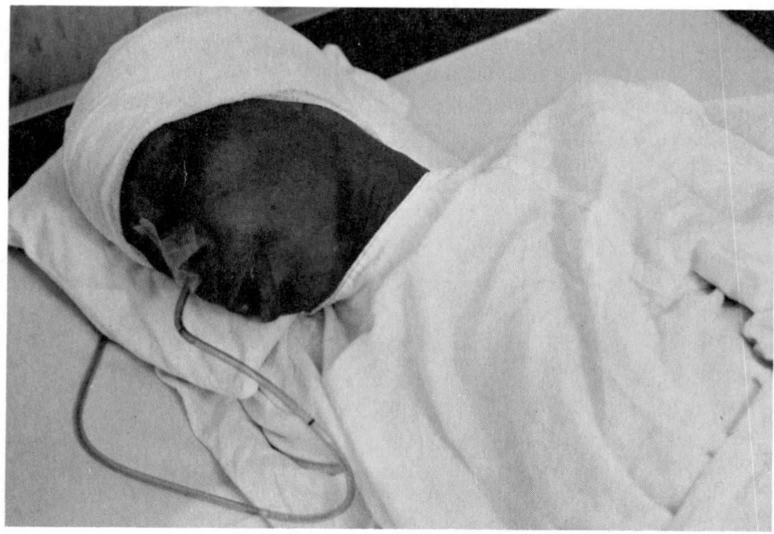

FIG. 11-3. The head of the unconscious patient should be elevated and turned to the side.

cycled ventilator; the pressure-cycled ventilator; and the time-cycled ventilator.

The *volume-cycled ventilator* delivers a certain predetermined tidal volume before terminating an inspiration. Examples of volume-cycled ventilators are the Bennett MA-1 and MA-2 and the Bourns. To prevent injury to the lung, there is a maximum pressure setting that limits the delivery of a high tidal volume to noncompliant or obstructed lungs. This is a versatile ventilator in which sighs and positive end expiratory pressure (PEEP) can be provided. The machine can also be set to provide assisted ventilation, controlled mechanical ventilation, or intermittent mandatory ventilation.

A description and explanation of the purposes of these three settings are as follows:

- With *assisted ventilation*, the ventilator is set to be sensitive to a predetermined level of negative inspiratory effort expended by the patient. If the patient is able to trigger the ventilator, the full preset tidal volume is delivered. If not, the ventilator will still provide a tidal volume. This control is useful for the patient who has some spontaneous breaths although most of his respirations are inadequate. Assisted ventilation supports the spontaneous breathing. A disadvantage of this setting is that an anxious patient can hyperventilate and develop respiratory alkalosis.
- With *controlled mechanical ventilation*, any respiratory attempts by the patient are ignored, and the machine delivers only the number of preset breaths. This control is useful for the patient who is apneic, heavily sedated, or extremely anxious.
- The last type of ventilator control is called *intermittent mandatory ventilation*. The machine is preset to deliver a certain number of breaths, but between those breaths, the patient may take breaths of varying tidal volume on his own.

The *pressure-cycled ventilator* delivers gas to the lungs until a predetermined pressure is reached within the tracheobronchial tree; this stops the inspiration. The tidal volume delivered can vary from breath to breath. Examples of pressure-cycled ventilators are the Bennett PR-1 and PR-2.

The last type of ventilator is called the *time-cycled ventilator*. An inspiration is terminated after a preset time. The tidal volume is regulated by adjusting the length of inspiration and the flow rate of the gas. Examples of time-cycled ventilators are the Engstrom and the Emerson Postoperative Ventilator.

Care of the Patient on a Ventilator. The following outlines the basic points of caring for the patient who is on a ventilator:

- The inspiratory and expiratory cycle of the patient should be synchronized with that of the ventilator. Asynchrony, or being out of phase with the ventilator, is to be avoided because it can result in altered cardiopulmonary hemodynamics and cause arrhythmias, hypotension, and increased tension within the airway. It may be necessary to administer sedation or a muscle relaxant or to paralyze the patient who continues to be asynchronic with the ventilator. A drug frequently administered to produce paralysis and thus ease the patient's resistance to mechanical ventilation is pancuronium bromide.
- Be vigilant to detect airway leakage, which can result from inadequate cuff inflation or fit of the tracheostomy tubes, change in the patient's position, disconnection of the ventilator hoses, or mechanical malfunction. Observe the patient frequently. Search for the source of the leak. Be sure that the safety alarm is on at all times. If necessary, Ambu the patient with oxygen while the leakage is being resolved.
- Airway obstruction can occur because of slippage of the tracheostomy cuff, blockage from a mucus plug, or mechanical obstruction. Try to identify the cause. Suction the patient, deflate the cuff, and then suction again. Ambu the patient as necessary. Adjust the tracheostomy or endotracheal tube.
- Auscultate the chest periodically for breath sounds.
- Monitor tidal volume and arterial blood gases.
- Deflate the tracheostomy or endotracheal cuff periodically to prevent tracheal ischemia. Reinflate the cuff with the same amount of air. Check for air leakage with a stethoscope placed on the side of the trachea on the upper neck. Stop inflating the cuff when the significant air leak has disappeared.
- Maintain strict aseptic technique. Check the dials to be sure that the prescribed settings are maintained.
- Turn the patient every 1 to 2 hours. Coordinate chest physiotherapy with position change. Suction frequently. Be sure to

hyperinflate the lungs with oxygen for 60 seconds before and 60 seconds after suctioning, with the approval of the physician. Limit suctioning to no more than 15 seconds at a time. Allow the patient time to recover between suctioning.
- Record the type, color, and amount of secretions from the oronasopharynx and trachea.

Weaning a Patient From a Ventilator. Weaning the patient from the ventilator is a gradual process and occurs in the following order: he is weaned from the ventilator; the cuff; the tube; and, the oxygen. The patient should be weaned as soon as possible. The decision to wean is based on evidence of adequate baseline measurements of vital capacity, inspiratory force, respiratory rate, resting tidal volume, minute ventilation, fraction of inspired oxygen concentration (FiO_2), and arterial blood gases. Baseline blood gases are drawn. The ventilator is discontinued, and the patient given oxygen and mist by way of a T-adaptor. During this time, the patient should be observed constantly. Blood should be drawn and tested for blood gases after the patient has been off the ventilator for approximately 20 minutes (alveolar arterial equilibration takes 15 to 20 minutes to be established). In addition, the trend of the following values should be closely followed: vital capacity, inspiratory force, respiratory rate, resting tidal volume, fractional inspired oxygen, minute volume, and the blood gases.

In observing the patient the nurse should assess for signs of hypoxemia or increased fatigue (bradycardia, restlessness, a respiratory rate of greater than 35 per minute, and dyspnea). The length of time that it takes to wean a patient from a ventilator will depend on how long he has been on the ventilator and the type of neurological injury sustained. Weaning takes place gradually with several parameters being closely observed to ensure adequate oxygenation of the patient in the process. The amount of time the patient spends off the ventilator is gradually increased on a daily basis. It may take several days to wean a patient who has been on prolonged ventilation therapy.

The process of weaning from the cuff begins after the patient has been weaned from the ventilator. Some patients progress rapidly while others need the cuff for longer periods to prevent aspiration. Each patient must be evaluated individually. Once the patient can manage without the cuff, the next step is to wean him from the tube. This is accomplished by obstructing the external opening of the tracheostomy tube with a special button, sometimes called a "cork," for gradually increasing amounts of time and assessing his tolerance.

Depending on the type of tracheostomy tube used, the means of accomplishing this procedure may vary. In some instances, the inner cannula is removed and the special button or "cork" is inserted and locked. Using such a method, the patient is given the opportunity to breathe completely through his own upper airway. Oxygen therapy is provided by means of a face mask during this phase. Once the patient can tolerate the occlusion of the external opening of his tracheostomy for 8 to 12 hours, breathes adequately, and is able to clear his airway, the tracheostomy tube can be removed. Weaning from oxygen therapy is also a gradual process. The amount of oxygen concentration is gradually reduced and cross-checked with arterial blood gases to ensure adequate oxygenation.

CARDIAC FUNCTION

Assessment

Cardiovascular function is assessed by evaluating blood pressure and the rate, rhythm, and quality of the heartbeat as indicated by the pulse beat and periodic electrocardiogram.

Cardiac Arrhythmias

If there is evidence of cardiac arrhythmias the patient will probably be placed on continuous cardiac monitoring so that any life-threatening arrhythmias can be identified quickly and treatment instituted immediately. Cardiac arrhythmias, depending on the type, are usually treated with drugs.

Abnormalities in blood pressure, either hypotension or hypertension, need immediate attention.

Hypotension and Pulse Changes

Hypotension is rarely due to brain injury. In these rare instances, hypotension is associated with severe cerebral injury and occurs only as a terminal event. The concurrent finding of hypotension and tachycardia should raise suspicion of occult internal hemorrhage (intraabdominal, intrathoracic, pelvic, or long bone injury). Other signs of hypovolemic shock include restlessness, ashen skin color, cold and clammy skin, and a rapid, thready pulse. The combination of hypotension and bradycardia may be secondary to cervical spinal cord injury in which descending sympathetic pathways have been interrupted.

Hypertension and Pulse Changes

Hypertension may reflect a significant increase in intracranial pressure, causing pressure on the brain stem. The combination of elevated blood pressure (hypertension), widening pulse pressure, and bradycardia is called Cushing's response; it signifies decompensation. Hypertension may also be due to preexisting hypertension or pain. Cerebral vascular accident (stroke) caused by hypertension may be the reason for unconsciousness, but there are many other reasons for unconsciousness. The patient must be carefully assessed to determine the underlying cause of hypotension. Regardless of the cause, measures must be taken to control the symptom; drug therapy is often initiated to control hypertension.

Effects on Cardiovascular Function

Because he is unconscious, the patient is immobilized and confined to his bed. The major effects of the immobility on cardiovascular function include thrombus formation, increased work load on the heart, and orthostatic hypotension.[1]

Thrombus Formation. The patient who is immobilized is predisposed to the formation of deep venous thrombus with the potential for pulmonary emboli. Thrombus formation is due to venous stasis, hypercoagulability of the blood, and external pressure against the veins. Muscle contraction in the legs ordinarily promotes venous return to the heart, but in the case of the immobilized unconscious patient, the blood pools and *venous stasis* results.

The second factor contributing to thrombus formation is hypercoagulability of the blood, which is thought to be due to hemoconcentration. Immobility is often associated with dehydration and an increased concentration of the formed elements in the blood. It is also believed that the increased level of calcium found in the blood contributes to hypercoagulation (calcium is liberated from the bones of the patient who is not bearing weight, as is the case of the bedfast patient).

The last factor predisposing to thrombus formation is external pressure on the blood vessels that leads to injury to the intimal layer of the blood vessel. Platelets collect at the intimal injury site, forming a layer that can become the foundation for clot formation. External pressure can be applied by a pillow or Gatch bed supporting the knee, the upper leg resting on the lower leg in the lateral recumbent position, and the heels resting continually on the bed.

Increased Work Load on the Heart. Another effect of immobility on the cardiovascular system is the increased work load on the heart when the patient is in the resting supine position rather than in the resting erect position. The pathophysiological basis for this involves changes in the vascular resistance and hydrostatic pressure associated with the recumbent position because the blood distribution within the body is altered. When the vertical position is abandoned in favor of the horizontal position, part of the blood volume leaves the legs to be distributed to other parts of the body. This increases the total volume of circulating blood that must be handled by the heart. The cardiac output and the stroke volume are also increased when the patient is lying down.

A second factor affecting the work load on the heart is the Valsalva maneuver. The *Valsalva maneuver* is defined as a forced expiration against a closed epiglottis. The physiological alterations at this time include a period of thoracic fixation without expiration, elevating intrathoracic pressure and thus impeding venous blood from entering the large veins. When the patient exhales, there is a dramatic decrease in intrathoracic pressure and a significant surge of blood is injected into heart, thus increasing the work load on the heart. The neurological nurse is also well aware of the effect of spikes in intracranial pressure from the Valsalva maneuver, which can be potentially dangerous in the patient with an already elevated intracranial pressure. Pulling the patient up in bed and improper positioning are some common instances that can initiate the Valsalva maneuver. These are very common occurrences that happen several times a day. The nurse should appreciate this fact and understand the effects on the patient.

Orthostatic Hypotension. The third major effect of immobility on cardiovascular function is *orthostatic hypotension,* which is the inability of the autonomic nervous system to maintain an adequate blood supply in the upper regions of the body. This usually occurs when the body is in the upright position. In the immobilized patient, orthostatic hypotension is due to the loss of general motor tone and the decreased efficiency of the orthostatic neurovascular reflexes (which normally cause contraction of the blood vessel so that blood can flow upward against gravity).

Nursing Management to Support Cardiovascular Function

The nursing management to support cardiovascular function in the unconscious immobilized patient includes the following steps:

- Do not use the foot gatch or place pillows under the knees that will produce pressure and venous stasis.
- When using the lateral recumbent position, position the upper leg so that it will not cause stasis and intimal damage to the lower leg.
- Range-of-motion exercises should be administered at least four times a day to improve blood return to the heart.
- Elastic stockings or Ace bandages are usually applied to the patient's legs to improve the blood return to the heart and minimize venous stasis.
- Turn and position the patient carefully at frequent intervals, usually every 2 hours.
- Elevate the head of the bed, if possible; this will alter the intravascular pressure and stimulate the orthostatic neurovascular reflexes.
- Sit the patient in a chair, if at all possible; this alters intravascular pressure and stimulates the orthostatic neurovascular reflexes.
- Try to synchronize moving the patient with exhalation to prevent initiating the Valsalva maneuver.

Blood Studies

A blood profile should be drawn that includes blood glucose, electrolytes, a possible drug screen, and others, as necessary. A seemingly infinite number of other studies can be done on blood samples. Specific tests ordered in the early stages of diagnosis can be most helpful for establishing or ruling out a possible diagnosis. Because the most common causes of metabolic coma are cerebral ischemia, hypoglycemia, and sedative drug overdose, blood sugar and drug screen tests are routinely ordered for an unconscious patient who has not been diagnosed. An elevated blood glucose level in a newly admitted unconscious patient may be associated with diabetes mellitus and diabetic coma or ingestion of a high-carbohydrate diet shortly before admission. Electrolytes are tested because electrolyte imbalance can result in unconsciousness and cardiac arrhythmias. Normal values are

- Potassium: 3.5 mEq to 5.0 mEq/liter
- Sodium: 135 mEq to 145 mEq/liter
- Chlorides: 96 mEq to 105 mEq/liter

In the unconscious patient who has been hospitalized for

some time, the specific blood studies ordered will be related to the patient's diagnosis. If the patient has been receiving steroid drugs such as dexamethasone, the blood sugar is usually elevated. The blood sugar and fractional urine for sugar and acetone are monitored while the patient is receiving steroid therapy. The blood and urine samples will return to normal levels after drug therapy is discontinued.

ONGOING ASSESSMENT

Once the basic physiological processes have been established and maintained, the patient's condition must be routinely assessed as follows:

1. Assessment of vital signs at prescribed intervals
2. Assessment of neurological signs at prescribed intervals
   - Level of consciousness
   - Pupillary size and reaction to light
   - Eye movement
   - Other cranial nerve check
   - Motor and sensory function
3. Assessment and monitoring of laboratory data
4. Assessment and monitoring of all body systems

Continuous assessment by the observant nurse often uncovers information that helps the physician diagnose the reason for the unconsciousness. The ongoing collection of data also contributes to identifying and refining the nursing diagnoses.

In providing nursing care for the unconscious patient, several nursing protocols must be followed to maintain and restor body function and prevent complication. This information is presented in the following section.

SUPPORT OF OTHER BODY SYSTEMS AND FUNCTIONS

BASIC CARE: THE SKIN AND OTHER STRUCTURES

Skin Care

Care of the skin is a part of basic hygienic care. Giving the patient a sponge bath provides the opportunity to assess, cleanse, refresh, and protect the skin.

- The skin is assessed for color, temperature, and dryness and for the presence of pressure sores. Every square inch of skin should be observed and assessed in an 8-hour period. Many areas are observed more frequently. Bony prominences such as the elbows, iliac crest, or outer aspect of the ankle can become irritated and red. All bony prominences should be checked for redness and massaged to increase the blood supply to the area. The patient should not be positioned on these areas.
- The skin should be washed and thoroughly dried to prevent irritation and possible breakdown. If the skin becomes soiled or wet because of excreta, perspiration, or other agents, the patient should quickly be cleaned and changed to prevent skin breakdown.
- Shaving the male patient is a part of basic daily care. A regular or electric razor may be used. If the patient is receiving anticoagulation therapy, an electric razor should be used.
- Trophic skin changes such as dryness can occur in the neurological patient. Dry skin should be lubricated with lanolin or cream to prevent cracking and breakdown.
- Skin care should be given every 2 to 4 hours when the patient is repositioned.
- The patient is turned every 2 hours to prevent a multitude of problems such as pulmonary stasis, musculoskeletal deformities, and skin breakdown. The position is changed to protect the skin from irritation and to ensure proper circulation. A decreased supply of blood can lead to ischemia and pressure sores. Any reddened areas should be massaged and placed so that no pressure is applied to the area. Other areas that become irritated, such as the ears, should be carefully lubricated and protected from any pressure (Fig. 11–4). The heels should not come in contact with the bed in order to prevent irritation and pressure sores. A decubitus ulcer on the heel will postpone ambulation for months.
- In turning the neurological patient, one must take care not to initiate the Valsalva maneuver, which leads to increased intracranial pressure. The patient should be turned or pulled up in bed with the help of enough staff to prevent isometric contractions. If possible, the patient should exhale when being moved or turned to prevent initiation of the Valsalva maneuver.
- Although the patient is unconscious, it may be possible to synchronize a move with exhalation by observing the patient's respiratory cycle. This may not be possible if the respiratory rate is not too rapid, whether or not he is on a respirator. In a patient at risk of grossly elevated intracranial pressure, any nursing intervention to prevent spikes in intracranial pressure is a worthwhile activity.

In summary, the skin is a protective mechanism and the first line of defense against infection, but it must be intact to be functional. The nurse should assess the patient for potential skin problems and implement nursing protocols to prevent skin breakdown. For example, the folds of skin on an obese patient can easily lead to skin breakdown, while a thin patient is most apt to have bony prominences whose skin is subject to breakdown. Each patient presents special nursing problems for which an individualized nursing care plan must be developed and followed.

Mouth Care

The mouth should be cleansed and lubricated every 3 hours to prevent caries, oral infections, and gum disease. The teeth should be brushed three or four times daily with the aid of a catheter and suction. While the teeth are being brushed with a toothbrush, the suction is used to remove excess fluid from the brush and mouth. In addition, the lips should be lubricated with Vaseline to prevent dryness and cracking, particularly if the patient tends to breathe through his mouth (Fig. 11–5).

Eye Care

The area around the eyes (periocular area) is washed as part of the face. Special attention should be given to the area for signs of edema, ecchymosis, or drainage (from the

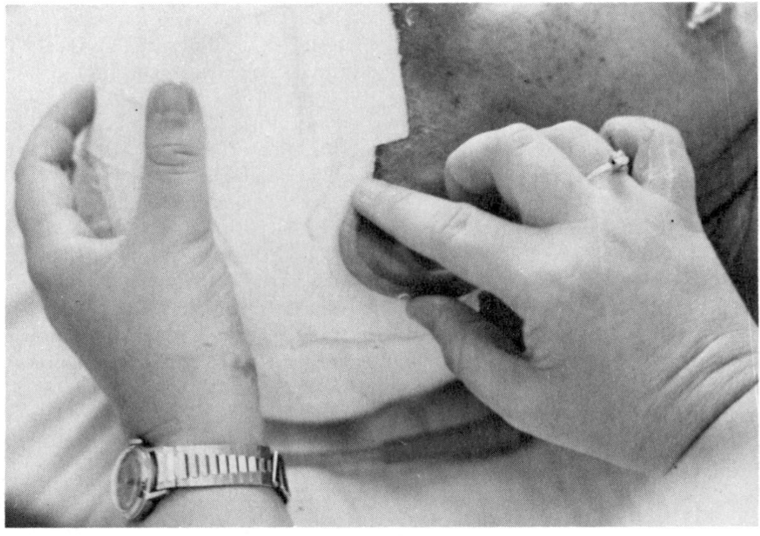

FIG. 11-4. In the unconscious patient, bony prominences and any area subject to pressure, such as the ears, are lubricated and massaged.

eyes). A patient who has sustained either accidental or surgical trauma to the head often develops periocular edema and ecchymosis. Alternate application of warm and cold compresses (½ to 1 hour of cold followed by ½ to 1 hour of warm with continuous alternation) is helpful in reducing edema. Some physicians prefer cold compresses or an ice bag for the first 24 hours, followed by warm compresses. The nurse should check the protocols followed by the particular physician.

- Cotton balls with saline can be used to clean the corners of the eyes, especially if the eyes are swollen shut (Fig. 11-6). The eyes themselves should be irrigated four times a day with normal saline, or a commercially prepared solution (e.g., Tearisol ophthalmic solution) should be instilled because the unconscious patient cannot blink periodically, which moistens the eyes. Drying of the cornea can lead to corneal ulcerations and blindness. Some irrigation preparations contain an antibiotic such as neomycin to control eye infections. Some physicians prefer to order an antibiotic eye ointment, which is applied four times daily, in addition to eye irrigations to prevent eye infections.
- The nurse should also inspect the patient's eyes for signs of irritation or abrasions, since corneal ulcerations can develop from irritation. The eyes can be protected from injury by using an eye shield or by taping the eye closed (Fig. 11-7).
- Other eye deficits commonly seen in the neurological patient are ptosis (cranial nerve III) or inability to close the eye (cranial nerve VII). In these instances special eye care should be provided, such as by protecting the eye with splints or shields or taping the lids closed.

Hair Care

The hair requires regular attention. When a patient with a head injury is first examined, the hair may be matted with blood or soiled with dirt or glass. Such particles may be removed by combing the hair carefully, possibly with ace-

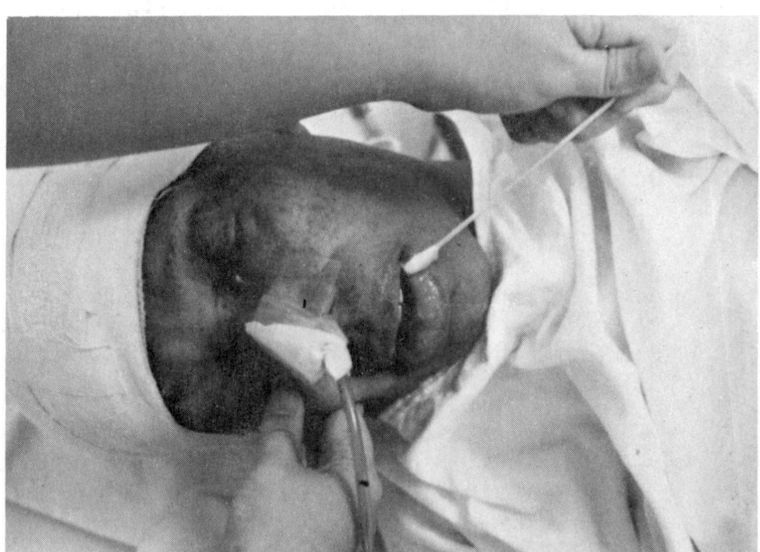

FIG. 11-5. Lubricating the lips is part of regular mouth care in the management of the unconscious patient.

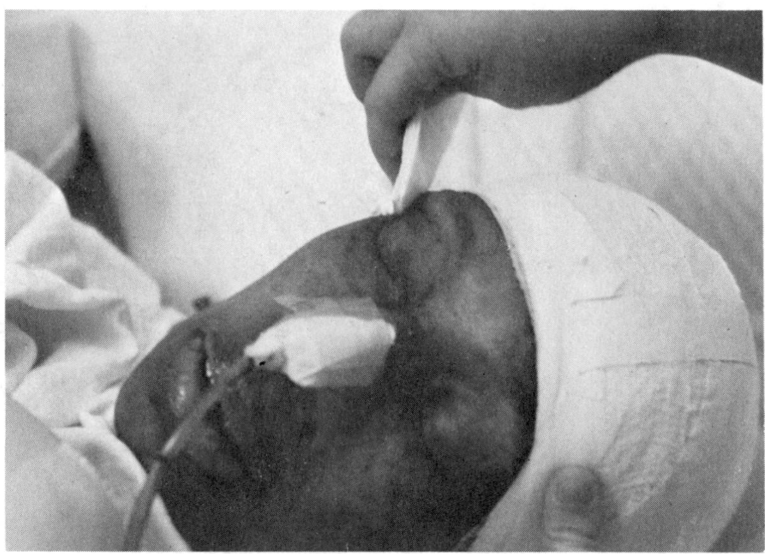

FIG. 11-6. The corners of the eyes should be wiped gently when eye care is given to the unconscious patient.

tone if the hair is bloody and matted. Once the hair is combed, it can be washed at the bedside according to hospital procedure. The hair should be clean and neatly combed as a part of basic care. Part of this routine involves checking the hair for lice.

Fingernails and Toenails

Both fingernails and toenails should be filed and clipped to protect the patient from injury. An unconscious patient often clenches his fists, digging his nails into his hands and causing injury, or he may move his hand near dressings or equipment.

MUSCULOSKELETAL FUNCTION

Maintaining muscle tone and preventing orthopedic disabilities are constant concerns when caring for the unconscious patient. Unless a schedule is rigidly followed, muscle tone and bulk loss, ankylosis, and contractures can develop rapidly. Patients who are on bed rest and not bearing weight loss calcium from their bones, a situation that can lead to osteoporosis and urinary tract calculi

The list below enumerates points of care that should be followed to prevent functional loss.

- Passive range-of-motion exercises should be done for the patient every 4 hours (Fig. 11-8). When a sponge bath is

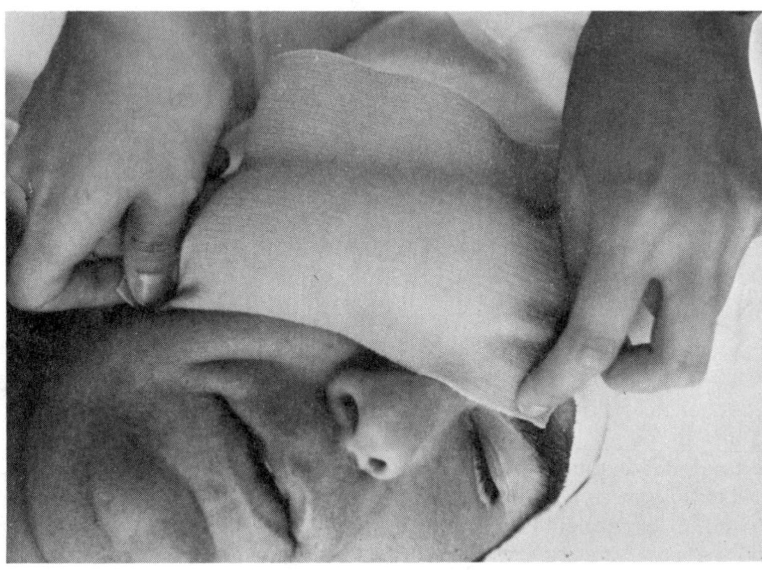

FIG. 11-7. An eye shield may have to be applied to protect the eyes of the unconscious patient.

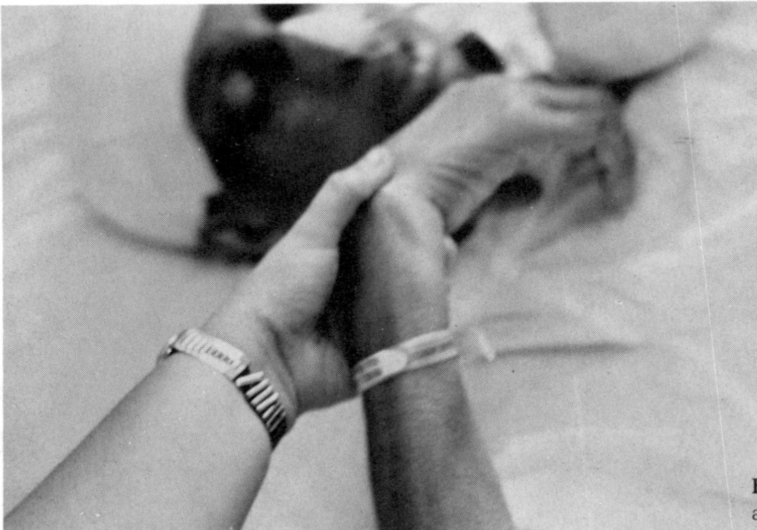

FIG. 11–8. Passive range of motion must be carried out at regular intervals for the unconscious patient.

given, the patient can be put through the normal range-of-motion exercises for all body joints.

- Reposition the patient every 2 hours. Pillows, rolls, and special accessories such as positioner boots, foot boards, or splints can be used. The purpose of repositioning is to maintain good body alignment. An unconscious patient, unlike a conscious patient, is unable to change a malaligned position spontaneously in response to pain or discomfort.
- Reposition weak or paralyzed body parts to prevent deformity. For example, external rotation of the hip can develop if the leg is not properly positioned. The development of an external rotation of the hip substantially prolongs the rehabilitation process. If the patient eventually regained consciousness, gait retraining would be greatly prolonged because of the malalignment of the leg. The external rotation must be corrected before gait retraining can be started.
- Carefully position a limb to prevent dependent edema (for example, a hand should be slightly elevated; Fig. 11–9). Once edema occurs it becomes difficult to guide the wrist and fingers through the normal range-of-motion exercises. Lack of movement contributes to the development of ankylosis and contractures. Therefore, once any deficit impeding normal range of motion develops, the problem is compounded by additional impairments.
- Most patients are placed on a firm mattress with a bedboard to provide optimum support for the musculoskeletal system.

It is difficult to position the decerebrate, decorticate, or restless patient; however, the nurse should routinely reposition the patient to provide the best standard of care to prevent disabilities.

GENITOURINARY FUNCTION

In an unconscious patient an indwelling catheter is usually inserted to manage urinary drainage. The urine can be quantified on a fractional time basis; that is, the urinary output can be measured hourly or at any other time interval to determine adequacy of output. The indwelling catheter that is connected to continuous drainage provides a convenient means for monitoring and measuring urinary output. In addition, for patients receiving diuretic drugs such as mannitol, the therapeutic value of the drug is, in part, assessed by measuring the urinary output. An intake and output record should be maintained.

The indwelling catheter allows for quick and easy access

FIG. 11–9. Proper use of pillows can help prevent dependent edema.

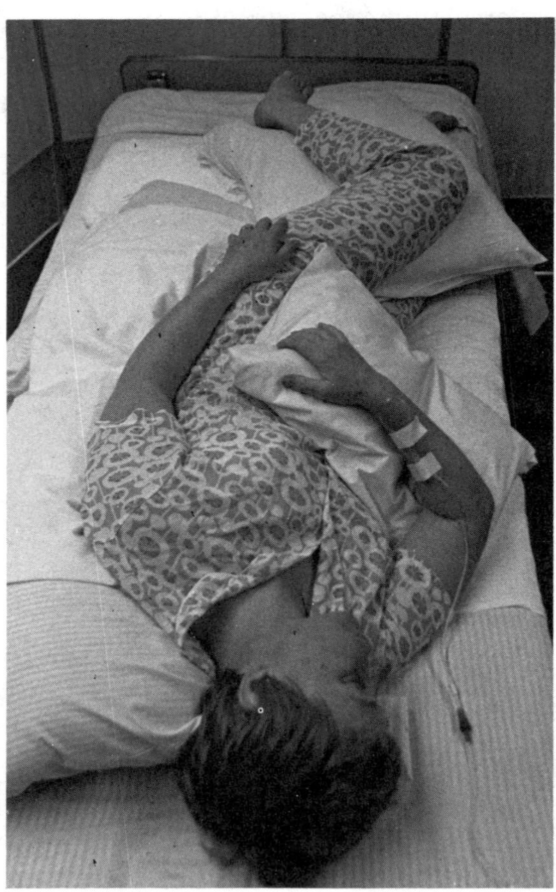

to a urine specimen for urinalysis (specific gravity, color, protein or cell count, and glucose), for a sugar and acetone test, or for a specific gravity test if diabetes insipidus is present. (Diabetes insipidus may be a problem in the neurological patient.) It also enables the nurse to note (at the bedside) the concentration, color, sediment, odor, or other abnormal findings in the urine.

In most instances an indwelling catheter is inserted to keep the patient dry, since urinary incontinence can quickly lead to skin breakdown or infection.

The unconscious patient is subject to two major problems, which develop in every patient who is immobilized for an extended period. These problems are urinary tract infections and kidney and bladder stones. The causes of infection are the catheter and the stasis of urine. The catheter is a source of contamination and causes irritation to the urinary tract. The stasis of urine in the bladder promotes bladder infections and ascending infections, which can involve the kidneys. The stasis of urine in the kidney pelvis and bladder encourages the formation of calculi. The increased levels of calcium being excreted from demineralized bones, another effect of immobilization, also contribute to the formation of urinary tract stones.

The solution to these problems would appear to be removing the catheter, or not inserting one in the first place, and positioning the patient upright. However, this is not always possible or practical. Protocols to prevent urinary tract infections and stone formation must be followed.

Catheter Care

A patient with an indwelling urinary catheter should receive catheter care every 8 hours. The physician's or hospital's catheter care protocol should be followed.

Catheter care is based on strict adherence to meticulous personal cleanliness, control of ascending urinary tract infection, and prevention of trauma to the urethra.

A typical catheter care protocol often includes the following:

- The perineal area and catheter–meatus junction are washed with soap and water, rinsed, and dried.
- The catheter is slightly looped and taped to the lower abdomen or inner aspect of the thigh to prevent traction on the urethra and meatus. (Follow the approved procedure for taping or securing the catheter at your facility.)
- An elastic band is looped around the catheter drainage tubing and pinned to the sheet (*not* into the alternating mattress) so that the tubing is not lying on the floor where someone can trip on it, causing sudden traction and possible injury to the patient. Pinning the tubing also provides proper positioning for urine drainage.

Some physicians prescribe continuous bladder irrigations with a normal saline and antibiotic solution (usually Neosporin) as a means of controlling urinary tract infections.

The catheter in itself is a foreign body and an irritant to the urinary tract. Since the patient with a urinary catheter is at risk for urinary tract infection, the following points of care should be followed:

- Catheters are not routinely irrigated or changed unless obstructed.
- The urinary drainage tubing and catheter are not disconnected for any reason because of the increased risk of ascending infection.
- If the drainage bag does not have a valve to prevent the backward flow of urine into the bladder, the drainage bag should not be lifted; urinary reflux is prevented.
- The tubing is checked routinely for kinks.
- Some physicians prescribe prophylactic Gantrisin, a sulfonamide used for its antimicrobial properties, to control urinary tract infections. Less frequently, urinary tract antiseptics such as Furadantin or Mandelamine are ordered.
- Removal of the catheter as soon as possible is strongly recommended.

Laboratory Data

Periodic urinalysis and urine culture should be scheduled frequently and monitored. If there is any indication of infection, it should be treated vigorously. Urine infections can lead to bacteremia.

Removal of the Catheter

The catheter should be removed as soon as possible. A condom-type catheter that is applied over the penis may be tried. In other instances, a urinal is propped in position. An indwelling catheter is often left in place longer in the female patient because there are no satisfactory atlernatives to the catheter.

GASTROINTESTINAL FUNCTION

Because the unconscious patient is immobilized, physical activity and movement that normally stimulate peristalsis are absent. Constipation and fecal impaction are complications commonly found in the unconscious patient. Other contributing factors are dehydration and the lack of a normal diet that could stimulate peristalsis. The patient may be receiving his nutritional needs from total parenteral nutrition or enteral tube feedings, neither of which stimulate peristalsis. In the patient with increased intracranial pressure, a restricted-fluid diet is commonly used to control cerebral edema; this also contributes to constipation.

Bowel Program

A bowel program must be followed when caring for the unconscious neurological patient. Constipation must be avoided because it increases intraabdominal pressure, which increases intracranial pressure. In a patient with increased intracranial pressure, enemas are contraindicated since they would initiate the Valsalva maneuver which, in turn, would increase the already elevated intracranial pressure.

A drug program of stool softeners and mild laxatives can be given daily to evacuate the bowel and prevent constipation and impaction. Stool softeners can be given to even the unconscious patient if a feeding tube (nasogastric, gastrostomy, or jejunostomy) is in place.

If an enema is not contraindicated, even an unconscious patient can be positioned on a bedpan while lying in bed and given an enema. The nurse will need to wear a glove and hold the rectal tube in position. It is necessary to be certain that the fluid from the enema is expelled. If it has not been expelled, it must be siphoned.

One more point should be made about the gastrointestinal system and the unconscious neurological patient—that is, the need to monitor gastric secretions and stools for occult blood. This is necessary because gastrointestinal bleeding in the neurological patient is not uncommon, especially if a head injury has occurred. A gastric ulcer seen in neurological patients is called Cushing's ulcer. Another factor that increases the possibility of gastrointestinal bleeding is that the drug therapy often prescribed for the neurological patient is irritating to the gastrointestinal tract.

Assessment

In assessing the gastrointestinal tract, the nurse should

- Ascultate the abdomen for bowel sounds
- Note and record the consistency, color, and size of the stools
- Implement a bowel program to promote bowel evacuation
- Test each stool for occult blood and record the results

SPECIAL MANAGEMENT CONSIDERATIONS

MOBILITY AND IMMOBILITY

Kinesis is a word of Greek origin that means motion or to move. The human body, composed to a great extent of muscles and bones, is designed for physical activity and movement. Such activities fine-tune the body and contribute to health while lack of activity leads to physical deterioration. This relationship of exercise and health is relative. But what is the effect on the body of a patient who becomes bedfast or immobilized because of illness, coma, paralysis, or other conditions? The sudden disengagement from physical activity can result in rapid deterioration of several body systems. Bed rest has been said to be the most potentially dangerous treatment prescribed in the hospital today. If the lack of physical activity and movement extends for a prolonged period, which is often the case with comatose, paralyzed, or severely debilitated patients, the effects on the body are extensive and devastating.

Minimal Physiological Mobility Requirement (MPMR)

Mobility has been a topic of extensive study. In examining the body's need for movement, it was noted that the normal healthy adult must change his position during sleep on the average of every 11.6 minutes. This is termed the *minimal physiological mobility requirement*. The immobilized, bedridden patient can no longer effect movement because of his disability, and the multiple complications of immobility may begin to appear. The complications of immobility that affect the skin and pulmonary, cardiovascular, gastrointestinal, musculoskeletal, and genitourinary systems are well known. However, efforts to prevent the ravages of immobility have not been very successful in spite of the best efforts of many nurses and physicians. For example, in 1945 Munro noted that turning the patient every 2 hours is adequate for preventing decubitus ulcers in the acute paraplegic patient. This finding led to the current nursing protocol of turning the patient every 2 hours. Although such a turning schedule is sufficient for preventing decubitus ulcers, it will not prevent the complications of immobility that affect other body systems.

The Kinetic Treatment Table (KTT)

Beginnings of Kinetic Therapy. The advent of kinetic therapy through the development of the Kinetic Treatment Table has demonstrated remarkable results in preventing the complications of immobility. The Kinetic Treatment Table was developed by Dr. F. X. Keane of the Ireland National Rehabilitation Center in the early 1970s and has been widely used throughout Europe as well as in some centers in the United States. Reasoning that if a normal person turned himself or engaged in significant body movement every 11.6 minutes during normal sleep, then a bedridden patient would have to be turned more frequently than every 11.6 minutes by a passive mechanical means to achieve the same degree of protection from the complications of immobility.[2] The Kinetic Treatment Table was designed to turn the patient through an arc of 124 degrees every 3.5 minutes. This time frame has been found to be effective in preventing the complications of immobility. The indications, contraindications, and precautions for the use of the Kinetic Treatment Table are included in Chart 11–2.

Description of the Kinetic Treatment Table. The Kinetic Treatment Table or Roto Bed is a specially designed motor-powered table that provides for continual turning of the patient through a maximum arc of 124 degrees at a minimal rate of 3.5 minutes. This means that the patient can be turned more than 300 times per day. The treatment table has three main hatches, the cervical, thoracic, and lumbosacral (rectal), which allow easy access to all parts of the patient's body including the entire back and rectal area for back care and rectal care (Fig. 11–10). There is easy access to the patient for range-of-motion exercises and other procedures. Other features of this versatile treatment table include

- Ability to stop the table in various lateral positions, such as at an angle of 40 degrees or 70 degrees, so that the nurse can administer care; in most instances, care can be administered without stopping the bed
- Portals for a urinary drainage tube and chest tubes
- A suspension arm to stabilize an endotracheal or tracheotomy tube to oxygen or to a respirator
- Traction of all extremities plus cervical traction
- Built-in fan for control of hyperthermia

CHART 11–2. INDICATIONS, CONTRAINDICATIONS, AND PRECAUTIONS FOR USE OF THE KINETIC TREATMENT TABLE

Indications

- Any immobilized patient
- Patients with spinal cord injury (including cervical or halo vest traction)
- Patients with head injuries (including patients with intracranial pressure monitors)
- Unconscious patients
- Cerebrovascular accident patients
- Craniotomy patients from surgery until ambulatory phase begins
- Patients with Guillain–Barré syndrome
- Multiple sclerosis patients
- Amyotrophic lateral sclerosis patients
- Patients with any chronic debilitating neurological disorder
- Multiple-trauma patients
- Respirator-dependent patients
- Patients with pulmonary complications such as hypostatic pneumonia, atelectasis, adult respiratory distress syndrome (ARDS), chronic obstructive pulmonary disease (COPD), and chronic bronchitis
- Patients with decubitus ulcers
- Burn patients
- Patients with paralytic ileus
- Traumatic hip surgery patients

Contraindications

- Pain while turning the spinal cord injury patient. If patient is properly positioned, turning should be pain free.
- True, severe, uncontrollable claustrophobia
- Unstable cervical fracture with no neurological deficit and no complications of immobility

Precautions

- Patients may have pain when turning onto pathologic or traumatic rib fractures—adjust rotation to avoid weight bearing on the affected side.
- Avoid pressure over a large cranial defect—adjust head pack accordingly.
- Comatose patients in the extreme agitation phase will become more agitated.
- Severe uncontrollable diarrhea—kinetic therapy stimulates peristalsis. Use highly absorbent adult diapers.

- Radiolucent table surface to facilitate diagnostic radiographs
- Accommodation of monitoring lines such as intracranial pressure, Swan–Ganz, and arterial pressure lines
- Ability to weigh the patient on the table
- Trendelenburg and reverse Trendelenburg positions
- A silent motor that does not increase the sensory load or interrupt sleep

There are two models of the treatment table: the Mark I, which is designed for use in the acute-care setting for patients who cannot get out of bed because of traction, coma, multiple injuries, spinal cord injuries, and other immobilizing problems, and the Mark III, which is intended for the patient with reduced mobility who is able to get out of bed during the day. The Mark III model can be used at home. Many health insurance providers will completely cover the cost of renting a Kinetic Treatment Table in the hospital or the home, if it is ordered by the physician.

Effects of the Kinetic Treatment Table on the Body Systems. The effects of the Kinetic Treatment Table on the body systems include

- Skin—prevention of decubitus ulcers and treatment of preexisting decubitus ulcers; easy access to the most common sites of pressure sores
- Pulmonary—continual postural drainage and mobilization of secretions; prevents hypostatic pneumonia and atelectasis or treats these conditions if already present
- Cardiovascular—decreases venous stasis and reduces the occurrence of deep vein thrombosis and emboli as well as postural hypotension
- Gastrointestinal—stimulates peristalsis and reduces constipation and fecal impaction
- Musculoskeletal—reduces muscle wasting, spasticity, and development of contracture; decreases demineralization of long bones; provides immobilization and alignment of the spine and the extremities; minimizes heterotopic bone formation
- Genitourinary—decreases the incidence of kidney and bladder stones and urinary tract infections by the gravitational emptying of the renal pelvis and ureters
- Neurological—decreased anxiety and sleep deprivation, which can decrease the need for sedation

Nursing Considerations. The best reason for using the Kinetic Treatment Table is that it markedly decreases or prevents the major complications of immobility and significantly improves patient outcomes (Table 11–1). It also makes it possible for one nurse to manage a patient easily without back strain and without the help of other busy nurses on the unit. When a patient is placed on the Roto Rest Kinetic Treatment Table, an experienced kinetic therapy nurse will come to your facility to place the patient on the table. This nurse also provides in-service education to the staff caring for the patient around the clock and is available for consultation. This education is very helpful for the staff nurse who is inexperienced in the use of equipment that appears to be complicated, as is the advice from an experienced nurse about the nursing management of the particular patient.

Clinitron Bed

The Clinitron bed is another special bed used for patients who are immobilized for extended periods. The bed is based on the principle of air-fluidization of silicon-coated beads. A flow of warm air passes through a diffuser board at the base of the bed and rises through the beads creating "fluidization" so that an environment is created in which the human body can float. A monofilament polyester filter

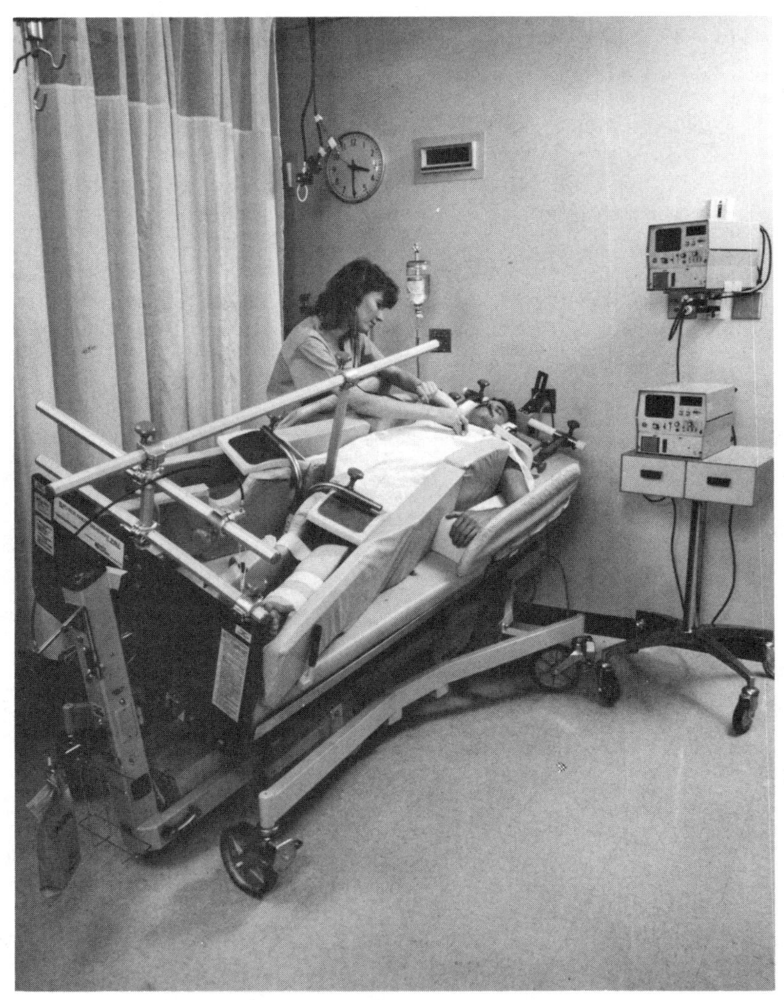

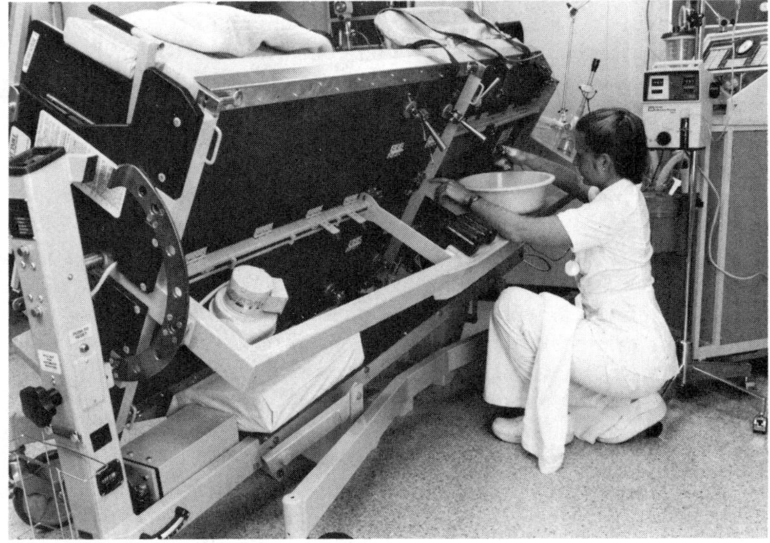

FIG. 11–10. *(Top)* Kinetic bed. *(Bottom)* Hatches in the table surface allow access to all parts of the patient's body. (Kinetic Concepts, San Antonio, TX)

TABLE 11–1. *Incidence of Immobility Complications*

Medical Complication	*Incidence of Complications in Spinal Cord Injury Patients as Reported in Literature*	*Incidence of Complications in Acute Spinal Cord Injury Patients Treated With Kinetic Therapy*
Pulmonary complications	34% severe	1.9%
	100% for complete quadriplegics	
Urinary complications	Calculi—37% in children with spinal cord injury	0%
	infection, virtually 100% at some time after injury	0%
Thrombotic phenomena	100% deep vein thrombosis	Not measured
	15% thrombophlebitis	0%
Pressure sores	49%	6.6%
Heterotopic ossification	16% to 53% in paraplegics	0%
Mortality acutely	30% to 56% for quadriplegics	6.6%
Autonomic dysreflexia	90% of quadriplegics in first 6 months	Rare

(Green B, Green K, Klose K: Kinetic nursing for acute spinal cord injury patients. Paraplegia 18:181–186, 1980. Reproduced with permission)

sheet supports the patient and separates him from the beads. When the air flow is turned off, the consistency of the bed changes from soft and pliable to hard and firm, forming a firm mold in which the body is held.

The purpose of the Clinitron bed is to provide the advantages of floatation without the inherent problems of floatation, which include instability, maceration of the skin, and difficulty in positioning and immobilizing the patient. According to the manufacturer, the features of the Clinitron bed floatation system are

- Significant reduction of constant pressure so that the cutaneous–muscular capillary blood flow cannot be obstructed, nor in most cases, even restricted
- Friction on the body surfaces that come into contact with the filter sheet is eliminated because the filter sheet moves freely.
- Shear force is eliminated because the filter sheet is loose enough to allow the body to sink into the fluid until buoyancy is reached.

In clinical practice, the Clinitron bed is said to (1) prevent the development of decubitus ulcers; (2) prevent further deterioration and infection of existing lesions and aid in their rapid healing; and (3) eliminate the need for frequent turning even in the completely immobilized patient.

Nursing Considerations. The nurse caring for a patient who has been placed on a Clinitron bed must be familiar with the manufacturer's instructions for operating the bed, adaptation of nursing care, and care of the bed. The bed can be instantly defluidized for moving the patient out of bed or performing cardiopulmonary resuscitation or other procedures. Because the bed tends to draw fluid from the body because of the air flow, an adequate fluid intake is needed to compensate. Specific instructions for using the Clinitron bed are outlined in the manufacturer's manual. In addition, a professional nurse employed by the company is available to provide in-service education to the nursing staff and to serve as a consultant.

Other Trauma Beds

There are other special treatment beds and trauma beds available. The various beds differ in design, but the purposes tend to be consistent. Patient comfort, fewer deleterious effects of immobilization, and ease in providing care for the patient are the major advantages cited by the manufacturers.

NUTRITION AND HYDRATION

While unconsciousness may last for weeks, months, or even years, the nutritional needs of the patient must continue to be met to maintain body function, support tissue repair, and combat infections. A nutritional consultation should be ordered as soon as the patient is stabilized (within 24 to 48 hours). At that time the patient's nutritional needs will be assessed and a nutritional program prescribed. The prescribed program should meet the total needs of the individual patient based on consideration of his diagnosis, unusual energy needs (e.g., because of hyperthermia or agitation), requirements for tissue repair, loss of fluid (e.g., from perspiration, diarrhea, or drainage), and basic life functions. The amount of carbohydrates, protein, fats, vitamins, minerals, and water can be determined for the patient.

Methods of administering nutritional support to the unconscious patient include total parenteral nutrition, also known as hyperalimentation, and complete enteral nutritional feedings administered by way of a nasogastric, gastrostomy, or jejunostomy tube. Regardless of the choice of nutritional support or the route of administration, nutritional needs of the patient must be considered early, before the patient is in a catabolic state and losing muscle mass. It is amazing how frequently a basic need for survival such as nutrition is overlooked. Emphasis on diagnosis, monitoring equipment, and technical procedures seems to take top priority while nutrition is neglected. No matter how sophisticated the medical, surgical, nursing, or pharmacological management of the patient may be, the patient will not improve if he is not properly fed! Chapter 6, Nutritional Needs of Neurological and Neurosurgical Patients, should be consulted for a thorough presentation of nutrition.

Although hydration is considered a part of nutrition, a special point should be made about hydration and the neurological–neurosurgical patient. For neurological patients, fluid intake is usually restricted to a specific amount of fluid for a 24-hour period. The purpose of fluid restriction is to control increased intracranial pressure by keeping the patient slightly underhydrated. The intake is correlated with the output; therefore, an accurate intake and output record must be maintained.

When a fluid restriction order is written for a 24-hour period, the amount of fluid allowed is a total figure. It is the nurse's responsibility to divide the intake over the 24-hour period so that the patient will stay within the prescribed allowance. It is often convenient to allow a certain amount per 8-hour shift. The total intake refers to all parenteral, enteral, and oral intake. If the patient has an intravenous infusion, the rate of flow is often slow in order to stay within the limits of the fluid restriction. The intravenous tube may also be established as a "keep open" route so that intravenous medication can be administered.

PREVENTION OF INFECTIONS

The patient who has been unconscious for a prolonged period is usually more prone to infections because his normal body resistance has been compromised for one of several reasons. Frequently, a serious disease process has weakened his overall body defenses, or localized infections (urinary tract or respiratory) have tapped the body's resources that combat pathogens. In some instances the use of antibiotics reduces the number of certain protective bacterial flora so that other organisms can flourish, or an anti-inflammatory steroid medication such as dexamethasone (Decadron), which is used to control cerebral edema, may mask the usual signs of infection. It is possible for the patient to have a serious infection with minimal clinical signs and symptoms of infection. Evidence of infection must be noted and the patient protected from infection by means of aseptic technique when care is provided.

Nosocomial Infections

A *nosocomial infection* is defined as an infection occurring during hospitalization that was not present or incubating at the time of admission. The current nationwide rate of nosocomial infections is about 5%, but the rate is much higher in critical care areas. Although the hospital infectious control department has the overall responsibility for the control of infections, this goal cannot be accomplished without the diligent cooperation of every hospital employee.

Prevention. The single most important method of controlling infection is through strict hand washing technique. The patient at risk should be monitored for evidence of infection. For example, the patient on a mechanical ventilator should have routine sputum cultures at prescribed intervals (e.g., every 3 to 7 days depending on the protocol). A chest x-ray and blood studies are also checked. The patient with an indwelling catheter will have a urinalysis and routine culture and sensitivity tests at frequent intervals. The physicians' and nurses' awareness of the possibility of infections should guide good judgment in monitoring any patient. Table 11–2 lists the most frequent types and causes of infections seen with the comatose neurological patient.

SENSORY DEPRIVATION

Although the unconscious patient appears to be completely unaware of his environment, it is impossible to determine if, in fact, he is aware of any stimulus in the immediate environment. Many patients have recovered from unconsciousness and given accurate details of what happened or what was said to them when they were supposedly unconscious; therefore, it is important to maintain a positive attitude in the presence of the patient and assume that some stimuli will penetrate the complexities of unconsciousness. Stimuli can be provided by playing the radio, touching the patient, and talking to him. Tell the patient what you will be doing; orient him to time, place, and person; and present reality by describing his surroundings (weather and so forth).

Since visual impairment is generally another form of sensory deprivation in the unconscious patient, it is important to be aware that as the patient slowly begins to regain consciousness, there may be some continued visual deficits. (Visual deficits are very common with head injuries because the visual system is a complex network that traverses several areas of the brain.)

RESTRAINING THE PATIENT

The purpose of applying restraints is to protect the patient from injury. If at all possible, restraints should be avoided because the patient may pull against them, causing isometric muscle contractions, which increase intracranial pressure. In addition, the application of restraints seems to make the restless patient even more restless.

There are times, however, when judicious use of restraints is necessary to protect the patient from injury. The vest (Posey) restraint is effective in restraining the patient without restricting movement of the extremities. A hand restraint may be necessary to protect the site of an intravenous infusion if the patient is moving or appears to be picking at the site.

POSITIONING THE PATIENT IN A CHAIR

Positive physiological effects to all body systems, especially the respiratory and cardiovascular systems, are facilitated by getting the unconscious patient out of bed and into a chair (Fig. 11–11). This is not done until the patient is relatively stable and able to tolerate the vertical position without ill effects (lowered blood pressure, raised pulse, pallor, sweating) of orthostatic hypotension.

However, safely positioning and restraining the patient is a challenge to the nurse. Since the patient cannot hold his head up independently, a high-back chair is necessary to support his shoulders, neck, and head. A vest restraint is usually applied to keep the patient in the chair. Other types of restraints may be necessary depending on the size of the patient, other injuries, and neurological deficits.

The patient will need to be observed frequently both to evaluate how well he tolerates being out of bed and also to reposition him as necessary.

TABLE 11-2. *Type, Predisposing Factors, Causes, and Prevention of Infections*

Type of Infection	*Predisposing Factors*	*Common Causative Organisms*	*Prevention*
Urinary tract (most common hospital-acquired infection)	• Indwelling catheters • Straight catheterization • Traction on meatus	*Escherichia coli* (most common cause in nonhospitalized patient); *Proteus, Klebsiella, Enterobacter, Pseudomonas, Serratia* (hospital-acquired infections)	• Maintain sterile closed urinary drainage system • Administer meatal and perineal care • Maintain dependent drainage • Maintain strict aseptic technique • Prevent cross contamination with strict hand washing technique
Respiratory	• Respiratory assistance equipment • Dehydration • Presence of tracheostomy or endotracheal tube	*Staphylococcus aureus* and *Streptococcus;* about half of nosocomial pneumonias are due to *Klebsiella, Enterobacter,* and *Pseudomonas* organisms	• Change ventilation equipment every 24 hours • Change water in respiratory reservoirs every 8 to 12 hours • Maintain aseptic suctioning procedure • Administer tracheostomy care every 4 hours • Adhere to strict hand washing technique • Adhere to principles of aseptic technique
Wound	• Surgical incision • Confused or disoriented patient pulling on his head dressing and contaminating the incision	*Staphylococcus aureus, Escherichia coli*	• Adhere to strict aseptic technique for dressing changes • Change dressing immediately if contamination occurs
Vascular	• Intravenous and arterial catheters • Swan–Ganz catheter • Hyperalimentation	*Staphylococcus aureus, Streptococcus, Klebsiella, Serratia, Enterobacter, Pseudomonas, Escherichia coli*	• Change tubing every 24 hours • Apply iodophor ointment to the site with each dressing change • Change dressing frequently using strict aseptic technique
Cerebrospinal fluid	• Intracranial pressure monitors • Contamination of craniotomy or spinal surgery incisions • Leakage of cerebrospinal fluid as in basal skull fractures	*Streptococcus, Neisseria meningitidis, Hemophilus influenzae, Escherichia coli*	• Maintain a closed system • Use strict aseptic dressing technique • Treat cerebrospinal fluid leakage aggressively with antibiotic therapy

RECOVERY AND AMBULATION

Awaking from unconsciousness is usually a gradual process that tends to vary from patient to patient. Because of prolonged bed rest, the patient must be protected from orthostatic hypotension before being allowed out of bed. Toward this end, the bed is elevated gradually each day and the patient's blood pressure, pulse, and objective signs and symptoms are checked to determine how he is adjusting to the change in position. Once the patient is able to tolerate the vertical position, he will be considered a candidate for sitting in a chair and ambulation unless he is left with neurological deficits that make it unfeasible. A physical therapy program is begun to evaluate his potential for ambulation. Any perceptual deficits or visual impairment that distorts perception can hinder the retraining program because the patient becomes more prone to accidents and injuries and requires special safety precautions. If the patient is a good candidate for ambulatory rehabilitation, any special devices necessary, such as braces, a walker, or crutches, will be provided. The patient must first relearn balance and coordination of body parts in the vertical position. The patient's activity tolerance should be evaluated to provide a schedule of activity and rest. He is most apt to do better with ambulation if he is not too tired.

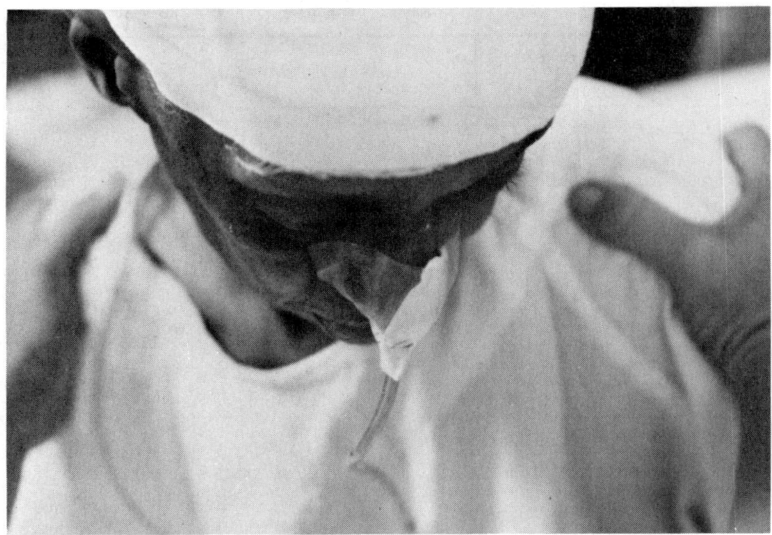

FIG. 11-11. It may be possible to bring the unconscious patient up to a sitting position.

SPECIAL EQUIPMENT

The following pieces of equipment can help the nurse meet the needs of the patient:

- Alternating air pressure mattress—a mattress with chambers that alternately inflate and deflate so that the pressure on skin surfaces of the body is not constant. This aids in preventing pressure areas, skin breakdown, and decubitus ulcers.
- Cooling or hypothermia blanket—a plastic blanket with channels through which a cooled solution of water and alcohol circulates to cool those skin surfaces with which the blanket comes into contact. The cooling blanket is helpful for cooling the patient with an elevated temperature.
- Lapidus or fat pad—a pad upon which a selected area of the body, often the buttocks, is placed to decrease pressure on the skin surface.
- Lifter—a mechanical device to move a helpless patient from the bed to the chair and vice versa.
- Quadriplegia chair—a chair whose back can be lowered so that it resembles a stretcher. When the chair is placed at the level of the bed, the patient can be pulled onto it. The back can then be raised so that the patient assumes the sitting position.
- Mobilizer—a mechanical stretcher that can be raised or lowered to correspond to the level of the bed. It has a movable surface that can be extended under the patient while he is in the bed and then retracted with the patient on it. In essence, this stretcher has the capacity to keep the patient in good body alignment while he is moved from his bed.

REFERENCES

1. Olson E: The hazards of immobility. Am J Nurs 67(4):781, April 1967
2. Keane F: The minimum physiological mobility requirement for a man supported on a soft surface. Paraplegia 16:383, 1978–1979

BIBLIOGRAPHY

Books

Boroch R: Elements of Rehabilitation in Nursing: An Introduction, pp 193–289. St Louis, CV Mosby, 1976

Brunner L, Suddarth D: The Lippincott Manual of Nursing Practice, 3rd ed, pp 706–710. Philadelphia, JB Lippincott, 1982

Brunner L, Suddarth D: Textbook of Medical–Surgical Nursing, 4th ed, pp 1189–1195. Philadelphia, JB Lippincott, 1980

Phipps W et al: Medical–Surgical Nursing Concepts and Clinical Practice, pp 500–511. St Louis, CV Mosby, 1979

Swift–Bandini N: Manual of Neurological Nursing, 2nd ed. Boston, Little, Brown & Co, 1982

Wilson S: Neuronursing, pp 53–77. New York, Springer–Verlag, 1979

Periodicals

Adams N: Prolonged coma. Nurs '77 7:21, August 1977

Allen N: Prognostic indicators in coma. Heart Lung 8(6):1075, November–December 1979

Axnick K: Infection control considerations in the care of the immunosuppressed patient. Crit Care Q 3(3):79, December 1980

Bouvier JR: Measuring tracheal tube cuff pressures: Tool and technique. Heart Lung 10(4):686, July–August 1981

Caronna J: Diagnosis: The comatose patient. Hosp Med 37, July 1980

Collins V: Ethical considerations in therapy for the comatose and dying patient. Heart Lung 8:1084, November–December 1979

Craven D: Antimicrobial therapy of bacterial nosocomial infections. Crit Care Q 3(3):89, December 1980

Darovic G: Ten perils of mechanical ventilation . . . and how to hold them in check. RN 46(5):36, May 1983

Finklestein S, Ropper A: The diagnosis of coma: Its pitfalls and limitations. Heart Lung 8(6):1059, November–December 1979

Flaherty M: Care of the comatose: Complex problems faced alone. Nurs Management 13(10):44, October 1982

Fuller E: Coma—evaluating depth of consciousness. Patient Care 15:127, September 30, 1981

Fuller E: When coma follows drug overdose. Patient Care 15:53, May 15, 1981

Gennis P: Coma. Top Emergency Med 4:47, July 1982

Green B et al: Kinetic nursing for acute spinal cord injury patients. Paraplegia 18:181, 1980

Guzman L, Norton L: Minimizing cuff-related laryngeal–tracheal complications. Focus 23, February/March 1982

Haerer A: Coma: Some differential considerations in the diagnosis and management. Hosp Med 68, April 1976

Henry G: The comatose patient: A case study. J Emergency Nurs 9(2):91, March/April 1983

Hinterbuchner L: Evaluation of the unconscious patient. Hosp Med 83, February 1977

Hoyt N, Caplan E: Identification and prevention of infections in the critically ill trauma population. Crit Care Q 6(1):17, June 1983

Landis K, Smith S: The mechanically ventilated patient: A comprehensive nursing care plan. Crit Care Q 6(2):43, September 1983

Langrehr E et al: Oxygen insufflation during endotracheal suctioning. Heart Lung 10(6):1028, November–December 1981

Loen M, Snyder M: Care of the long-term comatose patient: A pilot study. J Neurosurg Nurs 12(3):134, September 1980

Loen M, Snyder M: Psycho-social aspects of care of the long-term comatose patient. J Neurosurg Nurs 11(4):235, December 1979

Milazzo V, Resh C: Kinetic nursing: A new approach to the problems of immobilization. J Neurosurg Nurs 14(3):120, June 1982

Miller M: Emergency management of the unconscious patient. Nurs Clin North Am 16(1):59, March 1981

Neilsen L: Ventilators and how they work. Am J Nurs 2202, December 1980

Oakes C: Lower respiratory tract infections. Crit Care Q 3(3):57, December 1980

Oermann MH et al: Patient sensations following a tracheostomy: A discussion. Crit Care Q 6(2):53, September 1983

Rainer JK, Hollis J: Evaluation of the comatose patient. J Neurosurg Nurs 15:238, October 1983

Spielman G: Coma: A clinical review. Heart Lung 10(4):700, July–August 1981

Sullivan N: Kinetic nursing: Treating the immobilized patient. Life Support Nurs 4(1):1, 1981

Underwood M: Urinary tract infections. Crit Care Q 3(3):63, December 1980

Vitello–Cicciu JM: Recalled perceptions of patients administered pancuronium bromide. Focus on Crit Care 11(1):72, February 1984

chapter 12

Increased Intracranial Pressure

CONCEPT OF INTRACRANIAL PRESSURE (ICP)

Intracranial pressure is the pressure exerted by the cerebrospinal fluid within the ventricles of the brain (ventricular fluid pressure or VFP). The intracranial pressure is a continually fluctuating phenomenon that responds to such factors as arterial pulsation and the respiratory cycle. Activities such as coughing, sneezing, and straining at stool (the Valsalva maneuver) result in increased intracranial pressure, while activities such as standing up or assuming an erect position will lead to a decrease in intracranial pressure.

Normally, intracranial pressure measures between 80 mm and 180 mm of water (or 0 mm to 15 mm of mercury [Hg]). Intracranial pressure above 15 mm Hg (200 mm water pressure) is considered abnormally elevated.

When one uses the term "intracranial pressure," the implication is that there is only one pressure within the intracranial space. This is a misconception because pressure can vary in different locations or compartments of the brain. For example, the pressure in tissue adjacent to an expanding, space-occupying lesion can be elevated while, at the same time, the intraventricular pressure is within normal range. Elevated intracranial pressure is not consistently conveyed to the lumbar subarachnoid space. It is therefore more accurate to think in terms of intracranial "pressures" rather than a single "pressure."

PHYSIOLOGICAL CONSIDERATIONS

MODIFIED MONRO-KELLIE HYPOTHESIS

Basic to an understanding of the pathophysiology related to intracranial pressure is the *modified Monro-Kellie hypothesis.* This hypothesis can be simply stated as follows: the skull, a rigid compartment, is filled to capacity with essentially noncompressible contents—brain matter—(80%), intravascular blood (10%), and cerebrospinal fluid (10%). The volume of these three components remains nearly constant. If any one component increases in volume, another component must decrease for the overall volume to remain constant; otherwise, intracranial pressure will rise. This hypothesis applies *only* to skulls that are fused. The infant or very young child has a skull with suture lines that have not fused, thus allowing for expansion of the intracranial space in response to increased volume.

THE VOLUME-PRESSURE RELATIONSHIP WITHIN THE INTRACRANIAL CAVITY

Compensatory Mechanism

According to the modified Monro-Kellie hypothesis, reciprocal compensation occurs among the three intracranial components—brain tissue, blood, and cerebrospinal fluid

—to accommodate any alterations of the intracranial contents. The mechanism of compensation, though limited, includes the following buffers that decrease intracranial volume: displacement of some cerebrospinal fluid; compression of the low pressure venous system; and increased absorption of cerebrospinal fluid.

However, the amount of displacement of any of the three components to affect an appreciable change within the intracranial pressure is finite. After a certain level of compensation to maintain homeostasis has occurred, a state of decompensation with increased intracranial pressure results.

Small volume increments can be compensated for much more readily than large volume increments. Increases in volume made over long periods can be accommodated much more easily than a comparable quantity introduced within a much shorter interval. These concepts can be related to the type of space-occupying lesion and to the rate of growth of the lesion. *A patient with an acute subdural hematoma—a rapidly enlarging lesion—will develop clinical evidence of increased intracranial pressure much more rapidly than a patient with a large, slow-growing brain tumor.* The brain tumor can be extremely large before clinically discernible signs and symptoms of cerebral dysfunction and increased intracranial pressure are evident. However, a critical point of decompensation is eventually reached, beyond which a dramatic increase in intracranial pressure is apparent, regardless of how slowly minute volumes are added (Table 12–1).

Limits of Compensation

The limits of compensation can be explained through an understanding of the volume–pressure relationship. Significant animal studies have demonstrated the response of intracranial pressure to the introduction of volume. The volume was provided by an extradural balloon that was rapidly inflated with air. The curve that is plotted demonstrates the relationship (Fig. 12–1). Note that the curve is relatively flat until a certain point is reached (the outer limit of compensation). After this point, the addition of even a small amount of volume will cause a disproportionate elevation in pressure (decompensation). The importance of these studies is their direct application to human subjects.

Two basic concepts are helpful in explaining the volume–pressure relationship: elastance and compliance. *Elastance* is the brain's ability to tolerate and compensate for an increase in volume. It is a measure of the stiffness of the system. High elastance results in a dramatic increase in pressure in response to a small increase in volume.[1] Elastance is represented by the following formula (P = pressure, V = volume):

$$E = \frac{P}{V}$$

Compliance is the reciprocal of elastance and represents an increase or a change in pressure. It is a measure of slackness in the system. Low compliance is seen when a small in-

TABLE 12–1. *Physiological and Clinical Correlation of Progressive, Increased Intracranial Elevation*

Stage	*Intracranial Pressure*	*Effects*
Stage 1	No rise in intracranial pressure is associated with an expanding mass.	*Compensation phase;* no change in vital signs
Stage 2	Slight increase in the mass of the brain results in great elevations of intracranial pressure.	*End stage of compensation;* changes in vital signs are slight to moderate
Stage 3	Intracranial pressure can approach arterial blood pressure.	*Beginning stage of decompensation,* also called the preterminal stage; signs and symptoms that may be observed in the patient include deterioration in the level of consciousness, abnormalities in the respiratory patterns, increase in the systolic blood pressure, a widening of the pulse pressure, bradycardia, and cardiac arrhythmias
Stage 4	The autoregulatory mechanism that normally responds to increased levels of carbon dioxide by dilating cerebral arteries to supply nutrients and oxygen to the brain is nonfunctional. If the condition is not improved, arterial and intracranial pressure will become equal, resulting in cessation of blood flow and death.	*Decompensation phase;* symptoms as noted in stage 3 continue; death results if there is no immediate reversal of the condition

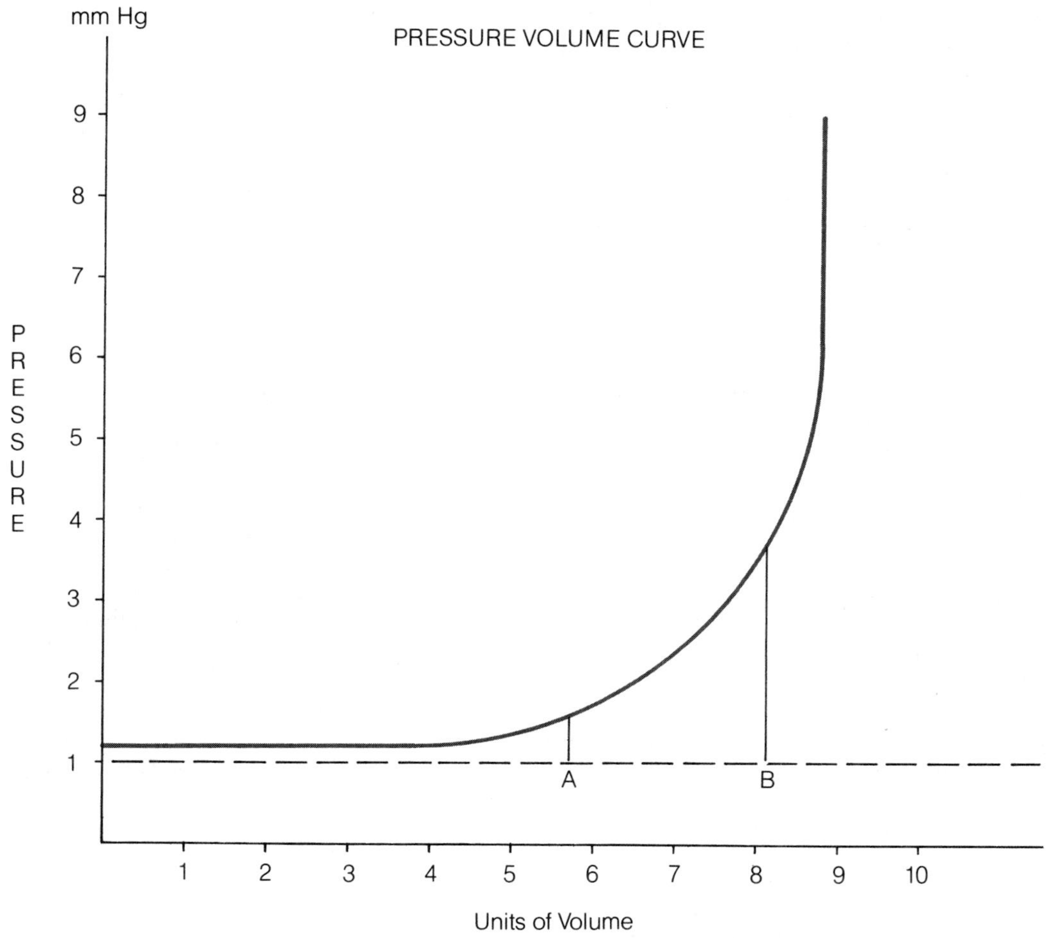

FIG. 12-1. Pressure volume curve. To point "A", addition of volume has little effect on pressure (high compliance); after that point, there is a dramatic increase in response to addition of volume, especially from point "B" onward (low compliance).

crease in volume results in a dramatic increase in pressure. Compliance is represented by this formula:

$$C = \frac{V}{P}$$

Since compliance is the reciprocal or inverse of elastance, low compliance is the same as high elastance.

The Compliance Test

In the clinical setting, compliance can be assessed in a patient who has a ventricular catheter and an intracranial monitor in place. Using sterile technique, a predetermined amount of fluid (usually 1 ml at a time) is rapidly injected into the catheter. The intracranial monitor is immediately observed for a change in pressure. A pressure increase of greater than 5 mm Hg is considered a positive result and suggests that the brain has low compliance. Further administration of fluid would be dangerous to the patient. Before each instillation, a test dose of 0.2 ml should be injected. If there is no change on the intracranial pressure monitor, the remainder of 1 ml can be instilled. If an increase in pressure is noted after injection of the test dose, instilling the remaining amount will cause spikes in intracranial pressure. Therefore, the remaining fluid should not be administered.

Compliance can also be tested by withdrawing a small amount (1 ml) of cerebrospinal fluid and observing the response. If the intracranial pressure drops moderately after the removal, the compliance of the brain is impaired. If the same procedure is followed in an hour with a drastic drop in pressure, the compliance is said to be low. Low compliance is also signified by the presence of plateau or "A" waves. This test was also called the volume–pressure test by Miller and colleagues.

CEREBRAL CIRCULATION

Several terms and abbreviations are used to identify and describe various aspects of cerebral circulation (Table 12–2). An understanding of these terms is necessary to appreciate the dynamics of cerebral circulation.

TABLE 12-2. *Terminology of Cerebral Circulation*

Abbreviation	*Terminology*
CPP	Cerebral perfusion pressure
CBF	Cerebral blood flow
SAP	Systemic arterial pressure
ICP	Intracranial pressure
CVR	Cerebrovascular resistance
CBV	Cerebral blood volume

Cerebral Perfusion Pressure

Cerebral perfusion pressure (CPP) is defined as the blood pressure gradient across the brain and is calculated as the difference between the incoming mean arterial blood pressure and the opposing intracranial pressure on the arteries. It is represented by the following formula (SAP = systemic arterial pressure):

$$CPP = \text{Mean SAP} - ICP$$

CCP is an estimate of the adequacy of cerebral circulation.

To calculate CPP, it is first necessary to compute the mean SAP. This is calculated as

$$SAP = \frac{\text{Systolic} - \text{Diastolic}}{3} + \text{Diastolic}$$

For example, if the patient's blood pressure is 130/82, the difference between the systolic and diastolic blood pressure is 48. The formula states that this figure should be divided by 3, which gives us 16. Now add the difference between the systolic and diastolic, 16, to the diastolic pressure, which is 82 ($16 + 82 = 98$). The mean SAP is 98 mm Hg. (Normally, the SAP is greater than the intracranial pressure.) The second value necessary to substitute in the formula is the intracranial pressure. Let us say that it is 15 mm Hg. The CPP $= 98 - 15$ or 83 mm Hg. The average range of CPP found in the normal adult is approximately 80 mm to 100 mm Hg, with a range of 60 mm to 150 mm Hg. The CPP must be at least 60 mm Hg to provide minimally adequate blood supply to the brain. Below this level, ischemia develops. A CPP of 30 mm Hg or less is incompatible with life and will result in neuronal hypoxia and cell death. When the mean SAP equals the intracranial pressure, the CPP is zero and the cerebral blood flow ceases.

Cerebrovascular Resistance

Cerebrovascular resistance (CVR) is the pressure across the cerebrovascular bed from the arteries to the jugular veins, which is altered by inflow pressure, outflow pressure, the diameter of the vessels, and intracranial pressure. It is the amount of resistance created by the cerebral vessels and is controlled by the autoregulatory mechanism of the brain. The CVR increases with vasoconstriction, decreases with vasodilation, and varies inversely with cerebral blood volume (CBV).

Cerebral Blood Flow

Cerebral blood flow (CBF) is represented by

$$CBF = \frac{CPP}{CVR}$$

Under *normal* circumstances, CBF is maintained at a relatively constant rate regardless of physical activity or changes in blood pressure. The blood supply of the cerebral tissue matches metabolic demands. During times of increased cerebral metabolism in an area, there is vasodilation with subsequent increase in CBF and CBV to the brain (Chart 12-1). When the metabolic demands of cerebral metabolism are low there is decreased CBF and CBV to the brain. If the CBF exceeds the required amount of blood for metabolism, a state of hyperemia is said to exist. *Hyperemia* is an excess of blood to a part of the body. CBF is controlled by an autoregulatory mechanism.

Autoregulatory Mechanism

The autoregulatory mechanism of the brain automatically regulates the diameter of the resistance vessels to maintain constant blood flow. *When systemic arterial pressure increases, there is compensatory vasoconstriction in the resistance vessels, thereby causing the pressure within these vessels to increase.* Although the pressure within the vessel increases, it is still less than the pressure to which the cerebral tissue would be subjected if the full impact of the systemic pressure was allowed to affect the tissue. The converse is also true. Decreased systemic arterial pressure causes vasodilation. The autoregulatory mechanism provides a constant cerebral blood flow, which is maintained within the normal range by adjustment of the diameter of the resistance vessels, which ultimately control the pressure. Cerebral venous pressure rises little, if at all, when systemic arterial pressure increases.

Autoregulation operates within parameters in the healthy adult. The intracranial pressure is below 30 mm to 35 mm Hg and the blood pressure ranges between 60 mm and 160 mm Hg (cerebral perfusion pressure of 50 mm to 150 mm Hg). In patients with chronic hypertension, both the upper and lower limits of autoregulation are elevated.[2]

CHART 12-1. POSSIBLE CAUSES OF INCREASED CEREBRAL BLOOD FLOW

1. Loss of autoregulation
2. Vasodilation of cerebral arteries due to increased $PaCO_2$ or decreased PaO_2 (less than 50 mm Hg)
3. Hypoxemia
4. Cerebral vasodilating drugs
   - Volatile anesthetic agents (halothane and nitrous oxide)
   - Others (histamines, ketamine)
   - Certain antihypertensives

The autoregulatory mechanism can be divided into two types of autoregulation: pressure autoregulatory mechanism and metabolic autoregulatory mechanism.

Pressure Autoregulatory Mechanism. The pressure autoregulatory mechanism within the resistance vessels (arterioles) responds to changes in pressure within the intracranial space and blood pressure. Cerebral blood flow is maintained at a constant level by the vasomotor tone that causes the arterioles to dilate or constrict.

Metabolic Autoregulatory Mechanism. The metabolic autoregulatory mechanism operates in the same manner as the pressure mechanism except that it responds to certain metabolic factors and causes vasodilation of cerebral arteries and, therefore, an increase in cerebral blood flow and cerebral blood volume to the area. Metabolic by-products of cell metabolism cause a localized acidosis to develop because of lactic acid, pyruvic acid, carbonic acid, hypercapnia, and hypoxia.

Carbon dioxide is the most potent vasodilator affecting the brain. The brain is very sensitive to the presence of hydrogen ions.

Carbon dioxide, a by-product of cell metabolism, is found in the blood or locally in the brain as a result of increased cellular activity. The carbon dioxide combines with the water component of body fluid to form carbonic acid which, in turn, dissociates to form hydrogen ions.

$$CO_2 + H_2O = H_2CO_3 \rightarrow H^+ + HCO_3^-$$

The extracellular hydrogen ion is a very potent vasodilator. Lactic acid and pyruvic acid, also by-products of cell metabolism, contribute to the vasodilation because both acids contain hydrogen ions that can be dissociated.

Excessive carbon dioxide in the blood, also called *hypercapnia*, can cause vasodilation just as a localized high level of carbon dioxide can affect the arterioles. (Hypercapnia is most often associated with hypoxia because of respiratory insufficiency.)

In summary, carbon dioxide is a potent chemical autoregulatory mechanism that causes vasodilation and a subsequent increase in blood supply so that metabolic waste will be removed and a renewed oxygen supply be brought to the area to meet the metabolic demands of the cerebral cells.

Loss of Autoregulation. As with most regulatory mechanisms, a critical point is reached when other forces overcome the mechanism, thereby causing it to be impaired or nonfunctional. The autoregulatory mechanisms can be lost locally or globally because (1) the intracranial pressure has exceeded 30 mm to 35 mm Hg (400 mm to 475 mm water pressure); (2) there has been focal or diffuse injury to cerebral tissue; or (3) blood pressure has exceeded the parameters of 60 mm and 160 mm Hg. Without the autoregulatory mechanism, the cerebral blood flow and cerebral blood volume become passively dependent on changes in the blood pressure and the cerebral perfusion pressure.

Cerebral Blood Volume

Cerebral blood volume refers to the amount of blood in the brain at a given time. As mentioned previously, cerebral blood volume occupies about 10% of the intracranial space. The cerebral blood volume is affected by the regulatory mechanisms that control the cerebral blood flow. Another consideration is that the cerebral venous system does not have valves as do other venous vessels in the body. Any condition that obstructs or compromises the venous outflow may also increase cerebral blood volume because more blood is backed up in the intracranial cavity (Chart 12-2).

A limited compensatory mechanism is operational when intracranial pressure begins to rise. It responds by decreasing the cerebral blood volume. However, as the compensatory reserve is exhausted, pressure in the venous system rises, cerebral blood volume increases, and intracranial pressure rises.[3]

Patient Considerations

When increased intracranial pressure exists, certain points need careful consideration. In the patient who already has some compensation by cerebrospinal fluid in response to a space-occupying lesion, even small increases in cerebral blood flow can result in tremendous spikes in intracranial pressure. Increased blood flow can occur as a result of increased local or systemic carbon dioxide. Increased blood flow means increased blood volume. It is said that increased cerebral blood flow and blood volume are responsible for intracranial hypertension. Blood trapped between the arterioles and the sinuses increases cerebral blood volume, thereby resulting in a further increase in intracranial pressure. As the intracranial pressure increases and the autoregulatory mechanism begins to fail, more pressure is communicated to the venous system. As the patient's condition deteriorates, cerebral blood flow begins to fail because of a decreased or lost capacity for vasodilation against the increasing resistance of the veins. Without an intact autoregulatory mechanism, cerebral blood flow passively responds to alterations in cerebral profusion pressures.

In a rapidly expanding space-occupying lesion, vascular collapse begins on the gyri surface of the cerebral cortex and involves both arteries and veins. The collapse continues around the lesion, occurring first on the circumfer-

CHART 12-2. POSSIBLE CAUSES OF DECREASED VENOUS OUTFLOW (CAUSING AN INCREASE IN CBV)

1. Head rotation
2. Lateral flexion of neck
3. Hyperextension of neck
4. Valsalva maneuver
5. Positive end-expiratory pressure (PEEP)

ence and then gradually continuing inward. Cerebral blood flow ceases when intracranial pressure is equal to the cerebral profusion pressure. All remaining arteries, and finally the thick-walled sinuses, collapse.

CONDITIONS ASSOCIATED WITH INCREASED INTRACRANIAL PRESSURE

Three conditions are often associated with increased intracranial pressure: intracranial hypertension, cerebral edema, and hydrocephalus.

INTRACRANIAL HYPERTENSION

Normally, intracranial pressure is less than 10 mm Hg when the measurement is taken at the level of the foramen of Monro in a patient who has assumed the supine position. A sustained intracranial pressure of 15 mm Hg or more is considered abnormal. *Intracranial hypertension* is defined as a sustained elevated intracranial pressure of 15 mm Hg or above. The term "malignant hypertension" has been used by some authors to describe a sustained intracranial pressure of 20 mm Hg or above. The use of this term conveys the idea that this level of intracranial pressure will cause ischemia and neuronal damage.

Conditions that can cause intracranial hypertension can be classified as follows:

1. Conditions that increase brain volume
   - Space-occupying masses (e.g., hematomas, abscesses, tumors, aneurysms)
   - Cerebral edema (e.g., head injuries, Reye's syndrome)
2. Conditions that increase blood volume
   - Obstruction of venous outflow
   - Hyperemia
   - Hypercapnia
3. Conditions that increase cerebrospinal fluid
   - Increased production of cerebrospinal fluid (e.g., choroid plexus papilloma)
   - Decreased absorption of cerebrospinal fluid (e.g., communicating hydrocephalus, subarachnoid hemorrhage)
   - Obstruction to flow of cerebrospinal fluid (e.g., communicating hydrocephalus)

Intracranial hypertension is a symptom of various problems rather than a distinct disease entity. It is often, but not always, associated with cerebral edema. The underlying cause of intracranial hypertension must be identified and treated in order to manage the problem effectively.

CEREBRAL EDEMA

Cerebral edema can be defined as an abnormal accumulation of water or fluid in the intracellular space, extracellular space, or both spaces that is associated with an increase in brain tissue volume.[4] The edema can be a local or generalized problem within the intracranial space. The specific cause of cerebral edema depends on the type of edema present. As mentioned previously, cerebral edema is often, but not always, associated with an increase in intracranial pressure.

Cerebral edema is considered to be a serious and life-threatening occurrence because the increase in brain bulk produces pressure on tissue, resulting in neurological deficit and exacerbation of increased intracranial pressure if present. Severe cerebral edema can produce transtentorial herniation with progressive brain stem compression, herniation, and death. Post mortem examinations have confirmed the finding of severe cerebral edema as the underlying cause of rapid neurological deterioration and death.

Three types of cerebral edema have been recognized: vasogenic, cytotoxic, and interstitial edemas.

Vasogenic Edema

Vasogenic edema, which predominantly affects the *white matter*, is the most common type of cerebral edema seen. The pathophysiological defect is thought to be increased capillary permeability of the arterial walls to large molecules caused by a breakdown of the blood–brain barrier. As a result, there is leakage of a plasmalike filtrate, including large molecules of protein, into the *extracellular space.*

Rate of Development. The rate of development and the extent of involvement of vasogenic edema are influenced by hemodynamic factors; accordingly, systemic arterial hypertension accelerates the process. Lowering an elevated systemic arterial pressure will retard the development of vasogenic edema. Once vasogenic edema becomes established, a sequence of physiological conditions exists that contribute to the development of more edema.

Untreated Vasogenic Edema: Sequence of Events. When vasogenic edema has developed, there is an accumulation of fluid of the extracellular space that increases the brain bulk and raises the intracranial pressure. The sequence of events is as follows (CBF = cerebral blood flow; CPP = cerebral perfusion pressure; ICP = intracranial pressure; SAP = systemic arterial pressure):[5]

$\downarrow$regional CBF $\rightarrow$ $\downarrow$CPP in areas $\rightarrow$ $\uparrow CO_2$ and $\downarrow O_2$ $\rightarrow$ $\uparrow$tissue lactic acid (metabolic by-product) $\rightarrow$ lactoacidosis $\rightarrow$ possible impairment of local autoregulation

Also, the $\downarrow$regional CBF and $\uparrow$ICP activate the vasopressor response $\rightarrow$ $\uparrow$SAP $\rightarrow$ $\uparrow$CBF $\rightarrow$ $\uparrow$vasogenic edema $\rightarrow$ $\uparrow$ICP

This sequence continues until the autoregulatory mechanism is inactivated. The blood flow and cerebral perfusion pressure cannot be maintained in relationship to the dangerously rising intracranial pressure. The cerebral perfusion pressure approaches zero and the blood flow ceases. Cerebral herniation and death follow immediately.

Causes. Vasogenic edema is seen in cerebral trauma such as contusions, lacerations, and epidural and subdural hematomas and in surgical trauma caused by operative procedures. Surgery itself is considered a source of trauma. Vasogenic edema is also seen around brain tumors and abscesses.

Effect of Drugs. The following drugs appear to be beneficial in treating vasogenic edema:

- Furosemide
- Barbiturates
- Corticosteroids: dexamethasone and cortisone preparations (effective with tumors, abscesses, and trauma)
- Osmotic diuretics (helpful in the acute phase)

Cytotoxic Edema

Cytotoxic edema is defined as an increase of fluid within the *intracellular space*, chiefly of the *gray matter*. As the name implies, toxic substances have a negative influence on the cell function. The development of cytotoxic edema is associated with a hypoxic or anoxic episode such as acute hypoventilation or a cardiac arrest. The patient's blood gases will show a significant lowering of oxygen and elevation of carbon dioxide (hypercapnia).

The cerebral cells require oxygen for cell metabolism. In the absence of sufficient oxygen at the cellular level, cell metabolism converts from aerobic to anaerobic metabolism. As a result, there is insufficient energy to maintain the adenosine triphosphate (ATP) dependent sodium pump or active ion transport.[4] Normally, potassium ions are more prevalent within the intracellular space and sodium ions are more prevalent in the extracellular space; this balance is maintained by the sodium pump. If the sodium pump is not functioning properly, more sodium will rush into the intracellular space. Sodium draws water, causing swelling or edema within the intracellular space. Waste products of cell breakdown such as lactic acid accumulate, contributing to the rapid deterioration of cellular function.

Causes. The development of cytotoxic edema is possible in the following conditions:

- Cerebral hypoxia or ischemic episodes associated with acute oxygen deficiency that causes elevation and retention of carbon dioxide (hypercapnia) and other H^+ ion metabolic by-products
- Anoxic episodes, usually associated with cardiac arrest or asphyxiation
- Hypoosmolarity conditions such as water intoxication and syndrome of inappropriate secretion of antidiuretic hormone (SIADH)
- Sodium depletion electrolyte imbalance
- Purulent meningitis

Effects of Drugs. The usual pharmacological therapy of corticosteroids (dexamethasone, cortisone preparations) is not effective in treating cytotoxic edema. It is questionable whether furosemide or barbiturates are helpful. Osmotic diuretics are beneficial in the acute stage when hypoosmolarity is present.

Special Considerations for Vasogenic and Cytotoxic Edema

Vasogenic and cytotoxic edema may be seen concurrently in a patient. For example, a head-injury patient may have vasogenic edema because of the direct trauma to the brain. If his respiratory function is not properly supported, hypoxia and hypercapnia can occur, and cytotoxic edema will develop in addition to the already present vasogenic edema.

Cerebral edema is considered to be proportional to the severity of injury or insult and reaches its maximum level in approximately 24 to 72 hours. It gradually begins to subside in about 2 weeks although it can persist, to some degree, for several months depending on the degree of injury and other circumstances.

Interstitial Edema

Interstitial edema involves movement of cerebrospinal fluid across the ventricular walls so that there is an increase of sodium and water in the periventricular white matter. There is a decrease rather than an increase in the volume of the white matter caused by a rapid disappearance of myelin lipids as the hydrostatic pressure within the white matter increases. The increase of hydrostatic pressure is due to the elevated pressure from the cerebrospinal fluid within the ventricles.

Interstitial edema is associated with obstructive hydrocephalus. Drug therapy is ineffective. Treatment necessitates surgery for the placement of a shunt.

HYDROCEPHALUS

Hydrocephalus refers to a progressive dilation of the cerebral ventricular system because the production of cerebrospinal fluid exceeds the absorption rate. Hydrocephalus is a clinical syndrome rather than a disease entity. Abnormalities in overproduction, circulation, or reabsorption of cerebrospinal fluid can result in hydrocephalus. (See Chap. 1 for a review of cerebrospinal fluid and circulation.)

Hydrocephalus can be subdivided into noncommunicating and communicating hydrocephalus. *Noncommunicating hydrocephalus* is a condition in which the cerebrospinal fluid in the ventricular system does not communicate properly within the subarachnoid space. Obstruction of the ventricular system can be caused by a mass such as a tumor within or adjacent to the ventricular system, or a congenital or inflammatory obliteration. *Communicating hydrocephalus* is described as a condition in which too few or nonfunctional arachnoid villi cannot sufficiently reabsorb the cerebrospinal fluid. Subarachnoid hemorrhage secondary to bleeding from an aneurysm or a head injury can produce transient or lasting communicating hydrocephalus. The arachnoid villi become plugged with the by-products of the breakdown of blood from the bleeding and cannot reabsorb the cerebrospinal fluid. The exudate from meningitis can also obstruct the reabsorption by the arachnoid villi.

The signs and symptoms of hydrocephalus depend on the type of hydrocephalus and the age of the patient. The usual treatment is a surgical shunting procedure, of which there are many variations. Selection of the particular procedure will depend on the age of the patient and any preexisting health problems.

Since the scope of this text addresses itself to adult problems, no discussion of hydrocephalus in the infant or child is included. The reader is directed to a pediatric text for discussion of this topic.

Normal-Pressure Hydrocephalus (NPH)

An important type of hydrocephalus in the adult is called *normal-pressure hydrocephalus;* it is usually reversible. (This syndrome is also called occult hydrocephalus, low-pressure hydrocephalus, normotensive hydrocephalus, and hydrocephalic dementia.)

In normal-pressure hydrocephalus there is ventricular enlargement with compression of the cerebral tissue but with normal cerebrospinal fluid pressure on lumbar puncture. Various circumstances have been associated with the development of normal-pressure hydrocephalus: (1) plugging of the arachnoid villi due to *subarachnoid hemorrhage* from a bleeding aneurysm, arteriovenous malformation, head injury or intracranial surgery, particularly of the posterior fossa; (2) *thrombosis* of the superior sagittal sinus; (3) *head trauma*, either accidental or following surgery, in which scarring of the basal cistern is thought to occur; and, (4) *bacterial meningitis* in which there is plugging and possible fibrotic changes of the arachnoid villi. After careful evaluation of some patients, particularly those in the 60- to 70-year age group, no associated condition has been found which might have precipitated normal-pressure hydrocephalus. This group of patients is said to have *idiopathic normal pressure hydrocephalus.*

Signs and Symptoms. The characteristic onset of normal-pressure hydrocephalus is insidious and slow to develop (over a period of weeks or months). Changes occur so slowly that they can easily be overlooked by the patient and family, or they can be attributed to the aging process when an older patient is involved.

The cardinal symptoms include mental changes and disturbances in gait. Although mental changes usually appear first, it is not uncommon for gait alterations to be noted first.

Early alterations in mental function begin as mild forgetfulness along with a generally diminished level of both mental and physical functions. The patient's ability to actively participate in conversation slowly deteriorates, as does his ability to conduct higher mental functions such as calculating. As the disease process progresses, memory and judgment may be impaired to the degree that he becomes a management problem because of his unreliability. In advanced cases, mutism and hypokinesia may be apparent. The early gait disturbances begin with a slowed pace that includes wide-based, zigzag steps. Ambulation is difficult because of the slow, unsteady pace; subsequently, the patient is prone to falls and injury. Usually no clear cerebellar signs are noted upon neurological examination. Movement of the upper extremities may be unaffected or slowed. As the disease progresses, the patient is unable to ambulate independently or even turn in bed.

Urinary incontinence is not an early sign but usually does appear as the course of the illness progresses. A lack of social inhibition and forgetfulness caused by cerebral atrophy are the probable causes.

No headache or papilledema is noted, although unexplained nystagmus is apparent in many patients. Tendon reflexes, particularly of the lower extremities, are increased. In advanced cases, the Babinski, grasping, and sucking reflexes may be present.

Diagnostic Studies. A history of a slowly developing progression of symptoms is essential in establishing a diagnosis. Various diagnostic procedures can also aid in establishing a diagnosis of normal-pressure hydrocephalus through demonstration of enlarged ventricles in the presence of normal intracranial pressure. The diagnostic studies most commonly used include the computed tomography (CT) scan, pneumoencephalogram, lumbar puncture, cisternogram, and possibly a cerebral arteriogram.

The CT scan can easily demonstrate enlarged ventricles without exposing the patient to the more dangerous invasive procedure of the pneumoencephalogram. If a pneumoencephalogram is done, there would be easy filling of the ventricles but not visible air over the convexities of the cerebral hemisphere in the patient with normal-pressure hydrocephalus. Another valuable diagnostic tool is the cisternogram. A radioactive isotope, usually radioiodinated human serum albumin, is injected into the subarachnoid space by lumbar or cisternal puncture. The patient is kept flat for 2 to 3 hours. Periodic scans are taken within a 72-hour period. In patients with normal-pressure hydrocephalus the isotopes are found in the ventricles, but little or no radioactivity is found over the convexities of the cerebral hemisphere. If the isotope has not cleared in approximately 48 hours, then normal-pressure hydrocephalus is indicated.

If an arteriogram is done, enlarged ventricles will be noted. A lumbar puncture will reveal subarachnoid pressure that is within normal limits unless there is a primary process that includes elevated intracranial pressure as part of its clinical picture.

Treatment. The accepted treatment for normal-pressure hydrocephalus is a ventriculovenous shunt. This surgical procedure is used for treatment of both communicating and noncommunicating hydrocephalus. The shunting device in wide use consists of a primary catheter, reservoir, one-way valve, and terminal catheter. The primary catheter is lodged within the lateral ventricle. Cerebrospinal fluid flows from the catheter in the ventricle to the reservoir, which collects the fluid, and passes by way of the one-way valve through the terminal catheter. The one-way valve prevents fluid from flowing back in the direction of the lateral ventricle. The reservoir is usually accessibly located under the scalp so that cerebrospinal fluid can be withdrawn, if necessary, with a needle and syringe for analysis or rapid reduction of increased intracranial pressure. The terminal end of the catheter empties into the internal jugular vein, the heart, or the peritoneal cavity, depending on the type of shunt selected by the physician.

As with any mechanical system, regardless of how simple the design, shunt malfunctions can occur. The most common causes include (1) plugging of the system with a blood clot or exudate within the ventricular system, (2) malposition of either the primary or terminal catheter, (3) a break in the system by dislodgement of one or more components, and (4) infection of the shunt system. Shunt malfunction usually requires a surgical revision of the shunt.

The most dramatic improvement after a successful shunting procedure is noted in the patient's mental status. He is much more alert, oriented, and manageable. Incontinence is quickly reversed. Gait disturbance takes longer to be rectified, and in some patients a permanent deficit remains. Improvement in mental functions may be evident almost immediately or may develop gradually over several days or weeks.

Pumping a Shunt. Shunts are of various designs. Some shunts have flexible reservoirs positioned on the mastoid bone that allow for pumping. The purpose of pumping a shunt is to flush the system of exudate that might plug the tiny tubing of the shunt apparatus (*i.e.*, to maintain patency). Before a shunt can be pumped, an order must be written by the physician that includes the number of times the shunt should be pumped and the frequency (*e.g.*, every 8 hours).

To pump the shunt, the nurse should lightly palpate the mastoid process on the appropriate side of the head with the index and middle fingers until the reservoir is felt. It will feel bouncy to the touch. Next, with index and middle fingers or the thumb compress and gently release the reservoir the prescribed number of times.

SIGNS AND SYMPTOMS OF INCREASED INTRACRANIAL PRESSURE

A Perspective

The most reliable data for evaluation of increased intracranial pressure is collected from the continuous intracranial pressure monitoring device. However, at present it is not practical or feasible to monitor the intracranial pressure of all patients with an invasive instrument. Clinical inspection and ongoing assessment by the knowledgeable practitioner are the most practical and reliable means of monitoring the patient for neurological change. A baseline assessment and ongoing assessment of neurological and vital signs will provide evidence of neurological change. It is very important to identify *early* signs of neurological deterioration when there is still time for intervention. Waiting until brain stem signs (changes in respiratory pattern, changes in vital signs, decerebration) appear is not advised because these are *late* signs of increased intracranial pressure that become apparent with impending herniation.

There is much confusion in the literature about the signs and symptoms of increased intracranial pressure. The brain stem signs of intracranial pressure are sometimes referred to as the "classical" signs of increased intracranial pressure. The specific "classical" signs and symptoms of the brain stem mentioned are

- A rising systolic blood pressure
- A widening of the pulse pressure
- Bradycardia

These three signs and symptoms are also known as Cushing's response; this is a compensatory mechanism for maintaining blood pressure and cerebral blood flow in the presence of a rising intracranial pressure. Vital signs such as blood pressure and pulse rate are controlled in the vital centers of the brain stem. They are brain stem signs and are seen in the *late* stages of increased intracranial pressure. Other authors refer to the "classical" triad of signs and symptoms associated with increased intracranial pressure. In this instance, the reference is often made to Cushing's triad, which includes

- Hypertension
- Bradycardia
- Respiratory irregularities

These signs and symptoms are also controlled by the vital centers in the brain stem. They are also seen in the *late* stage of increased intracranial pressure. The reader is cautioned to the use of confusing and misleading terminology in the literature.

Before discussing the traditional signs and symptoms associated with increased intracranial pressure, it may be helpful to consider a few points about increased intracranial pressure and how it can be masked or misinterpreted.

CLINICAL VARIATIONS IN INCREASED INTRACRANIAL PRESSURE

Although we rely on clinical examination of the patient for detecting signs and symptoms of increased intracranial pressure, elevations in intracranial pressure that can compromise cerebral perfusion pressure are not necessarily apparent on clinical examination of the patient.[2,6] Elevations in intracranial pressure can *only* be quickly and accurately diagnosed when the patient is being monitored with an intracranial monitoring device. This information is not presented to invalidate the reliability of the neurological clinical assessment. Rather, the point being made is that although a patient does not conform to the usual pattern of signs and symptoms of increased intracranial pressure, he may still have increased intracranial pressure. On clinical inspection, he may be completely asymptomatic or have slight pupillary dysfunction, even with a large slow-growing intracranial mass present. At surgery, a tense brain with a grossly elevated intracranial pressure may be found.

To understand this concept, recall the pressure–volume curve in Figure 12–1. When the compensatory mechanism is at its maximum, brain compliance is decreasing. In other words, you do not know where your patient is in relation to the curve. He may be at the beginning of compensation or close to the end, at which point the slightest increase in intracranial pressure will result in decompensation, elevation in intracranial pressure, and appearance of significant clinical signs and symptoms of increased intracranial pressure.

Many of the signs and symptoms of increased intracranial pressure often cited (decortication, decerebration, respiratory irregularities, loss of corneal reflexes, and blood pressure and pulse changes) relate to brain stem dysfunction. Direct primary injury to the brain stem can produce similar signs and symptoms without the presence of increased intracranial pressure.

Another point is that intracranial pressure is a dynamic rather than a constant pressure. Certain activities such as straining and coughing cause elevation of intracranial pressure. In the patient at risk who already has an elevated intracranial pressure, initiating an activity known to increase intracranial pressure can precipitate *transient* signs and symptoms of increased intracranial pressure (Chart 12-3). The nurse assessing the patient at this time may observe a change in consciousness, a sluggish dilated pupil, or hemiparesis in a patient who had none or less pronounced deficits at the last assessment. If the patient is assessed again in 5 to 20 minutes, the changes noted previously may have disappeared. The transient elevation in intracranial pressure caused *temporary* interference with the cerebral perfusion pressure. Clinical signs and symptoms of neurological deterioration appeared and then disappeared. This may explain why observations of change that you make are not seen by another nurse or the clinical instructor who assesses the patient a little later.

The last consideration is that of *pseudotumor cerebri* or "benign intracranial hypertension." In this condition there is marked elevation in intracranial pressure, often as high as 30 mm to 45 mm Hg, without an intracranial mass or obstruction to the flow of cerebrospinal fluid being present. The condition develops over weeks or months and is seen most often in obese adolescent girls and young women. The patient often complains of headache, or in some instances, of blurred vision, diplopia, slight numbness in the face, or vague dizziness. On physical examination, the patient appears surprisingly alert and aware; the only abnormal finding is papilledema. It is important to rule out any intracranial lesion or problem.

The treatment includes

- Repeated lumbar puncture to remove cerebrospinal fluid until normal pressure is maintained
- If cerebrospinal fluid pressure continues to be elevated and papilledema persists, prednisone or oral hyperosmotic agents (glycerol or acetazolamide) are given to reduce cerebrospinal fluid formation
- If this is ineffective, a lumbar thecoperitoneal shunt may be performed[6]

CHART 12-3. TRANSIENT "PRESSURE SIGNS"

The following signs and symptoms are associated with transient elevations in intracranial pressure and cerebral hypoxia whereby there is temporary interference with cerebral perfusion pressure resulting in transient ischemia. The signs and symptoms last a few minutes, most often occurring at the peak of plateau waves, and then disappear as the pressure decreases and perfusion pressure is once again reestablished. The signs and symptoms of transient "pressure signs" include

- Decreased level of consciousness
- Pupillary abnormalities
- Visual disturbances
- Motor dysfunction (hemiparesis)
- Headache

IDENTIFICATION AND DISCUSSION OF THE SIGNS AND SYMPTOMS OF INCREASED INTRACRANIAL PRESSURE

The signs and symptoms of increased intracranial pressure include

Early findings

- Deterioration in the level of consciousness (confusion, restlessness, lethargy)
- Pupillary dysfunction
- Motor weakness such as monoparesis or hemiparesis
- Possible headache

Later findings

- Continued deterioration in the level of consciousness (coma)
- Possible vomiting
- Hemiplegia, decortication, or decerebration
- Alterations in vital signs
- Respiratory irregularities
- Impaired brain stem reflexes

The presenting signs and symptoms of increased intracranial pressure observed in a patient will depend on

- The compartmental location of the lesion: supratentorial or infratentorial
- The specific location of the mass: cerebral hemispheres, midbrain, cerebellum
- The degree of intracranial compensation

The following signs and symptoms traditionally associated with increased intracranial pressure are worthy of elaboration to clarify their relationship to the cluster of clinical observations. The nurse should implement the guidelines for assessment as discussed in Chapter 5, Assessment of Neurological Signs.

1. Deterioration in the Level of Consciousness

Although deterioration in the level of consciousness can be considered to be a general sign of neurological deficit, it is a reliable and sensitive indicator of neurological deterioration. It may be the first sign of deterioration of the patient's condition for two reasons. First, the most highly specialized cells of the cerebral cortex are the most sensitive to the decreased oxygen supply that occurs with increased intracranial pressure. The patient responds to the oxygen deficit by becoming drowsy or having difficulty with thinking (memory and orientation to time, place, or person). Second, the level of consciousness is altered with increased intracranial pressure because of its impact on terminal arteries, which are more apt to be compromised, thereby decreasing the oxygen supply to the sensitive cells of the cerebral cortex.

The earliest changes in a deteriorating level of consciousness are confusion, restlessness, and lethargy. Disorientation is noted, first to time, then to place, and finally to person. As the intracranial pressure continues to rise, the patient becomes stuporous and finally comatose. In the terminal stages, there is no response to painful stimuli, and the patient is deeply comatose.

2. Pupillary Dysfunction

With increased intracranial pressure caused by supratentorial masses or edema, changes in the pupils' size, shape, and reaction to light are noted. In the early stages, the pupil is small or midposition in size, then it gradually dilates. The pupil may become slightly ovoid, and its response to light sluggish. The hippus response to light may be observed with the beginning of pressure on the oculomotor nerve. Since the source of the rising intracranial pressure (edema, space-occupying lesion) tends to be compartmentalized in the early stages, the pupillary dysfunction is ipsilateral to the edema or lesion. The beginning of compression of the ipsilateral oculomotor nerve from the lesion accounts for the pupillary dysfunction.

In the later stages of increased intracranial pressure, the ipsilateral pupil is dilated and nonreactive (fixed) to light. The pupils become bilaterally dilated and fixed in the terminal stages when a rising intracranial pressure has led to herniation.

3. Visual Abnormalities

Visual deficits that can develop in the early stages of increasing intracranial pressure include decreased visual acuity, blurred vision, and diplopia. The decreased acuity and blurring are probably associated with early hemispheric pressure because the visual pathways transect all of the lobes of the cerebral hemisphere. These findings are quite common. The diplopia is associated with paresis or paralysis of one or more of the extraocular muscles so that eye movement is restricted in certain planes. If the person attempts to focus in that direction, the images from both eyes will not fall on the same area in each retina, resulting in double vision. Therefore, the extraocular muscles that control ocular movement should be evaluated because their function may be inhibited because of pressure from intracranial bulk. As the intracranial pressure continues to rise, the ocular symptoms will usually become more pronounced.

4. Deterioration of Motor Function

In the early stages, monoparesis or hemiparesis develops contralateral to the intracranial bulk because of pressure on the pyramidal tract. In the later stages, hemiplegia, decortication, or decerebration develop because of increasing pressure on the brain stem. Decortication or decerebation may be unilateral or bilateral. In the terminal stages, the patient becomes bilaterally flaccid as death approaches.

5. Headache

In the early stages of rising intracranial pressure, some patients complain of a slight or vague headache. Headaches are not as common as one might expect. The following explanation of headaches and intracranial pathophysiology may be helpful.

Intracranial structures sensitive to pain are the middle meningeal arteries and branches, large arteries at the base of the brain, the venous sinuses and bridging veins, and the dura at the base of the skull.[7] The brain is normally cushioned by cerebrospinal fluid. When the volume of cerebrospinal fluid is reduced, the cushion is decreased or eliminated. When the head is in the erect position, the brain sinks. In the horizontal position the brain shifts to one side. To compensate for the decrease in cerebrospinal fluid and provide an adequate cerebral blood supply, the cerebral vessels dilate, particularly in the venous components. Dilation of the vessels, traction of the bridging veins, and stretching of the arteries at the base of the brain cause a headache.

Headache in the neurological patient with increased intracranial pressure has been described as being worse upon arising in the morning. This can be explained by noting that intracranial pressure is known to rise to very high levels during the rapid eye movement (REM) phase of sleep, which increases metabolism and produces carbon dioxide as a waste product. Hypercapnia can be present because of a variety of reasons. Most likely, there is vasodilation caused by the increased carbon dioxide levels. The traction in connecting venous vessels and the stretching of arteries at the base of the skull are also operational. The net result is headache.[8]

6. Vomiting

Vomiting caused by increasing intracranial pressure is not common in adults. It is a symptom associated with infratentorial lesions or direct pressure on the vomiting center. The reflex is not well understood.

The vomiting center is located in the medulla. The vomiting mechanism can be described as a gastrointestinal reflex with some efferent connections to the muscles of respiration. Vomiting is usually accompanied by nausea and gastrointestinal discomfort that has been precipitated by visceral stimuli. Plum and Posner state that when the vomiting mechanism is directly affected by a neurological lesion, the afferent limb is short-circuited to produce vomiting without nausea. Without the warning of nausea, the vomitus is ejected with unadulterated force because of the suddenness with which the thoracic and abdominal muscles contract, propelling the vomitus forward.[10] The term "projectile vomiting" is used to describe the character of the vomiting.

7. Alteration in Blood Pressure and Pulse

The blood pressure and pulse remain relatively stable in the early stages of rising intracranial pressure. In the later stages of development when there is pressure on the brain stem, changes in blood pressure occur. An ischemic reflex is triggered by ischemia in the vasomotor center in the brain stem and the systemic arterial pressure is increased. The pressure in the cerebral arterial vessels must be greater than the intracranial pressure for the blood to continue to flow. As the intracranial pressure rises, the blood pressure rises reflexively to compensate. Cushing's response or reflex is activated. Cushing's response includes a rising systolic blood pressure, a widening pulse pressure, and bradycardia. The elevation in blood pressure increases cardiac output so that the heart pumps with greater force, thus widening the pulse pressure. Increasing systemic blood pressure with a widening pulse pressure is the compensatory phase of increasing intracranial pressure. As the patient's condition deteriorates and the decompensation phase begins, the blood pressure drops.

In the early stage of increasing intracranial pressure, the pulse is relatively stable. As the pressure continues to rise, the pulse drops to 60 beats per minute or less as it attempts to compensate. The pulse is described as full and bounding. The decreased rate and bounding quality are due to an attempt by the heart to pump blood upward into vessels on which pressure is being exerted from the intracranial bulk. In the decompensatory stage, the pulse becomes irregular, rapid, and thready and then ceases.

8. Alterations in Respirations

Alterations in the characteristics of the respiratory pattern relate to the level of brain dysfunction. The various levels and associated respiratory patterns are discussed in Chapter 5, Assessment of Neurological Signs.

An acute increase in intracranial pressure can trigger the development of acute neurogenic pulmonary edema in the absence of cardiac disease. Other respiratory complications that can develop include adult respiratory distress syndrome (ARDS) and disseminated intravascular coagulopathy (DIC). These three conditions are discussed in Chapter 5.

9. Alterations in Temperature

Temperature elevation is usually associated with hypothalamic dysfunction. In the compensatory phase temperature will probably be within normal limits. In the decompensatory phase, elevations to very high levels are frequently observed. Elevations in either phase can be caused by a superimposed infection in one or more of the body systems but not to the extreme levels that are in evidence with hypothalamic involvement.

10. Loss of Brain Stem Reflexes

In the late stages of rising intracranial pressure, there is pressure on the brain stem that causes loss or dysfunction of reflexes mediated by the brain stem. These reflexes include the corneal, oculocephalic, and oculovestibular reflexes. The prognosis is poor for patients who have lost the brain stem reflexes.

11. Papilledema

Papilledema is a late finding with increased intracranial pressure. It does not occur until the intracranial pressure has reached markedly elevated levels. Papilledema is not a universal observation made in all patients with increased intracranial pressure. In some patients, this may be the first sign observed if an elevated intracranial pressure has developed gradually.

RELATIONSHIP OF INCREASED INTRACRANIAL PRESSURE TO HERNIATION SYNDROMES

Unless increased intracranial pressure, also known as intracranial hypertension, is treated, the outcome will be herniation. *Herniation* is defined as the abnormal protrusion of an organ or other body structure through a defect or natural opening in a covering membrane, muscle, or bone. When one considers herniation in relationship to the brain, the tentorium cerebelli and the foramen magnum come to mind. The tentorium cerebelli is a double fold of dura mater that forms a partition between the cerebrum and cerebellum, and the foramen magnum is the hole at the base of the skull (occipital bone) through which the spinal cord passes. If an elevated intracranial pressure continues to rise unchecked, there will be herniation of a portion of the cerebrum through the tentorium, with pressure being exerted on the brain stem. If this ominous situation is allowed to continue because of continued increased intracranial pressure, the brain stem and cerebellar tonsils will herniate through the foramen magnum, the only opening in the closed cranial vault. Herniation through the foramen magnum is a sure cause of death because of pressure on the vital structures in the medulla of the brain stem.

The most common type of transtentorial herniation is uncal or lateral transtentorial herniation. Central herniation is less common because fewer masses are located on the midline axis.

In summary, there is an important relationship between increasing intracranial pressure (or intracranial hypertension) and herniation syndromes. Increased intracranial pressure will lead to a herniation syndrome with serious consequences or death if not treated aggressively (Chart 12–4).

HERNIATION SYNDROMES OF THE BRAIN

To understand the pathophysiology of mass lesions of the brain, it is most important to understand the principles that govern herniation of the brain caused by cerebral edema or a space-occupying lesion such as a tumor or hematoma. The intracranial cavity is divided into smaller compart-

CHART 12–4. SIGNS AND SYMPTOMS OF IMPENDING HERNIATION

The following lists the signs and symptoms of impending herniation:

- Decreased level of consciousness (coma)
- Pupillary abnormalities
- Motor dysfunction (hemiplegia, decortication, or decerebration)
- Impaired brain stem reflexes (corneal, gag, swallowing)
- Alterations in vital signs including respiratory irregularities

ments by folds of the fibrous, relatively rigid dura mater. The most important dural folds are the (1) falx cerebri, which drops into the longitudinal fissure and partially divides the supratentorial space into a left and right side, and (2) the tentorium cerebelli, which separates the occipital lobes from the cerebellum and much of the brain stem. The tentorium is a tentlike structure higher in the center than on the sides of the skull. To allow the brain stem blood vessels and accompanying nerves to pass through the tentorium, there is an oval opening in the tentorium called the *tentorial notch* or *incisura*.

When cerebral edema or a mass occurs in the semisolid brain within a compartment, the pressure exerted by the lesion is not evenly distributed, resulting in shifting or herniation of the brain from one compartment of high pressure to one of lesser pressure. In the wake of the shifting of cerebral structures, there is pressure or traction on some structures, which is evidenced by malfunction of the particular cerebral tissue.

SUPRATENTORIAL HERNIATION

Three major patterns of herniation, described by Plum and Posner in their classic work, identify syndromes from expanding supratentorial lesions.[9] The descriptive name reflects the end stage noted in the herniation syndrome. The three classifications are (1) cingulate herniation, (2) central or transtentorial herniation, and (3) uncal or lateral transtentorial herniation (Fig. 12–2).

Cingulate Herniation

An expanding lesion in one cerebral hemisphere can cause pressure medially so that the cingulate gyrus is forced under the falx cerebri, displacing it toward the opposite side. The displacement of the falx can create compression of the local blood supply and cerebral tissue, causing edema and ischemia, which further increase the level of increased intracranial pressure. Cingulate herniation is quite common, but little is known about the clinical signs and symptoms that enable one to identify its presence.

Central or Transtentorial Herniation

The usual causes of rostral–caudal downward displacement of central transtentorial herniation are

1. A lesion located around the outer perimeter of the frontal, parietal, or occipital lobe
2. An extracerebral lesion located around the central apex of the cranium
3. Bilaterally positioned lesions in each hemisphere
4. Unilateral cingulate herniation

The lesion produces a downward displacement of the cerebral hemispheres, basal ganglia, diencephalon, and midbrain through the tentorial incisura. The diencephalon can be tightly compressed against the midbrain with such force that edema and hemorrhage result. Often, anterior choroidal artery depression is noted on the cerebral arter-

FIG. 12–2. Cross section of *(left)* normal brain and *(right)* brain with intracranial shifts from supratentorial lesions: herniation of the cingulate gyrus under the falx *(1)*; herniation of the temporal lobe into the tentorial notch *(2)*; downward displacement of the brain stem through notch *(3)*. (Plum F, Posner J: Diagnosis of Stupor and Coma, 2nd ed. Contemporary Neurology Series. Philadelphia, FA Davis, 1972)

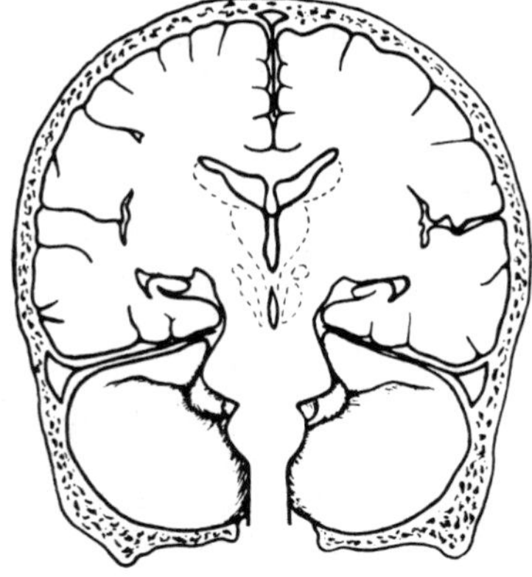

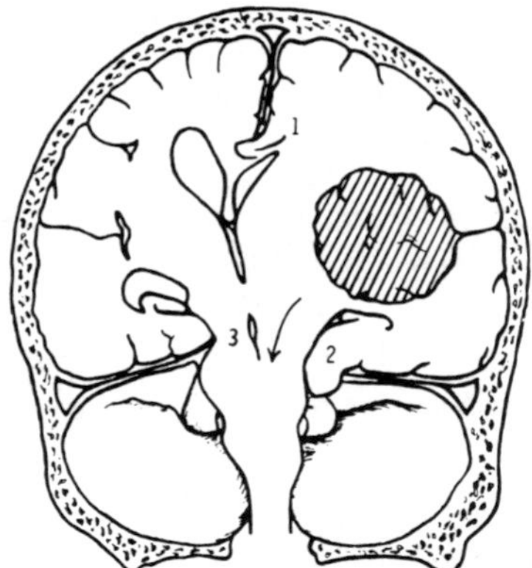

TABLE 12–3. *Progressive Signs and Symptoms of Central and Uncal Herniation**

Uncal Syndrome

	Local Early Signs	*Diencephalon–Midbrain*	*Midbrain–Upper Pons*	*Lower Pons–Upper Medulla*	*Medulla*
Pupils	Unilateral, dilated pupil; sluggish, nonreactive	Unilateral, dilated, and fixed	Bilateral, dilated, fixed	→	→
Extraocular Signs	May have a ptosis Slight weakness → of oculomotor innervated muscles	Slight weakness becomes paralysis	→ →	→ →	→ →
Level of Consciousness	Little effect on consciousness; may notice restlessness *Once deterioration begins, can proceed to deep coma quickly*	Stupor; coma	Deep coma	→	→
Motor		With Kernohan's notch, hemiparesis on side of lesion Contralateral hemiparesis to hemiplegia; decerebration	Bilateral decerebration	Flaccidity with occasional decerebration	→
Sensory	Progressive deterioration	→	→	→	→
Babinski Sign		Bilateral positive	→	No reflexes	→
Respirations		Cheyne–Stokes	Central neurogenic hyperventilation	Shallow	Ataxic, then cease
Other			Bradycardia Elevated systolic blood pressure Widening pulse pressure	Deterioration of vital signs	No vital signs 40.5° C and higher
			Wide variations in temperature; may be grossly elevated	Elevated	40.5° C and higher

Central Syndrome

	Early Diencephalon	*Later Diencephalon*	*Midbrain–Upper Pons*	*Lower Pons–Upper Medulla*	*Medulla*
Pupils	Both small and reactive	→	Not equal in size, but each about midpoint and nonreactive	→	Dilated and fixed
Extraocular Signs	May be normal or slightly roving, then difficulty with upward gaze	Difficulty with → upward gaze	And dysconjugate gaze	→	→

(continued)

TABLE 12–3. (continued)

	Central Syndrome				
	Early Diencephalon	*Later Diencephalon*	*Midbrain–Upper Pons*	*Lower Pons–Upper Medulla*	*Medulla*
Level of Consciousness	Difficulty with concentration and becomes agitated or drowsy; then stuporous	Stuporous; coma	Deep coma	——→	——→
Motor	Contralateral hemiparesis to hemiplegia	Plus paratonic rigidity on ipsilateral side, which becomes decorticate	Bilateral decerebration	Flaccidity with occasional decerebration	——→
Sensory	Progressive deterioration	——→	——→	——→	——→
Babinski Sign	No Babinski sign	Bilateral positive Babinski sign	——→	——→	——→
Respirations	Cheyne–Stokes	——→	And central neurogenic hyperventilation	Shallow	Ataxic, then ceases
Other			Wide variations in temperature (often very high) Many develop diabetes insipidus	Elevated	40.5° C and higher
			Bradycardia	Pulse erratic (fast and then slow)	No vital signs
			Elevated systolic blood pressure Widening of pulse pressure	Blood pressure drops	

* An important point to keep in mind when observing a patient with a possible herniation syndrome is that there is predictable order to the development of signs and symptoms. The neurological deterioration in both central and uncal herniation proceeds in an orderly rostral–caudal scheme; the diencephalon, midbrain, pons, and finally the medulla are affected from the increasing pressure. Signs and symptoms characteristic of each area can be identified. Notice that the last stages of both central and uncal herniation are the same.

iogram. Central transtentorial herniation may or may not be accompanied by uncal herniation.

The early symptoms of central transtentorial herniation include the following:

- Stupor to coma
- Cheyne–Stokes respirations
- Small, reactive pupils (in early diencephalic stage)
- Gradual loss of vertical gaze
- Contralateral hemiplegia
- Ipsilateral rigidity that develops into decorticate and decerebrate posturing

The progression of symptoms with continued pressure can be followed in Table 12–3.

Uncal or Lateral Transtentorial Herniation

The most important herniation syndrome is that of uncal herniation. An expanding lesion of the lateral middle fossa, most often of the temporal lobe, causes shifting of the inner basal medial edge of the temporal lobe. This area contains the uncus and hippocampal gyrus, which is forced through the tentorial incisura. The diencephalon and midbrain are compressed and displaced to the opposite side by the uncal herniation. With this lateral displacement, there *may* be compression of the cerebral peduncle (opposite side to the unilateral uncal herniation) against the firm unyielding edge of the tentorium incisura producing *Kernohan's notch*. This is important because it results in a false localizing sign of hemiparesis on the same side as cranial nerve III deficit rather than on the opposite side as would be expected (Fig. 12–3).

Cranial nerve III and the posterior cerebral artery on the same side of the expanding temporal lobe lesion are frequently caught between the overhanging edematous uncus and the free edge of the tentorium or another resistive structure. The entrapment of the oculomotor nerve results in ipsilateral pupillary dilation, which is usually an early sign of uncal herniation.

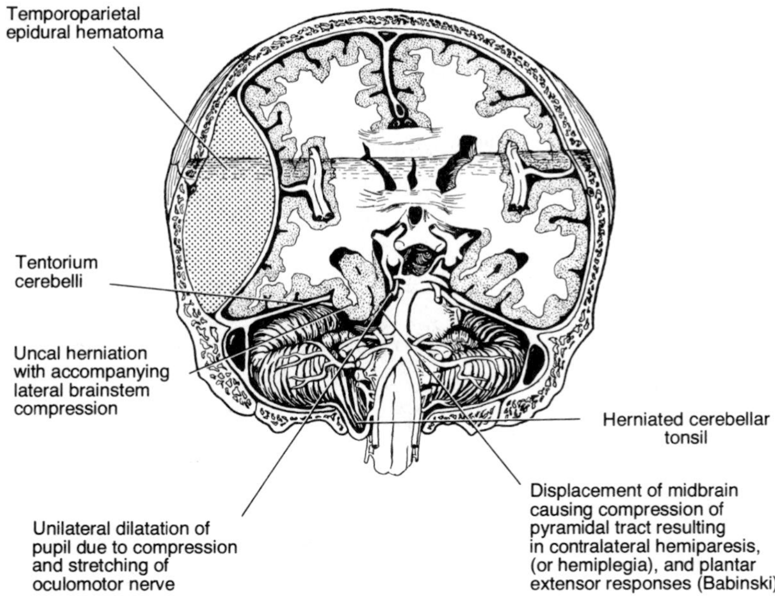

FIG. 12–3. Cross section showing herniation of part of the temporal lobe through the tentorium due to a temporoparietal epidural hematoma. (Kintzel KC: Advanced Concepts in Clinical Nursing, 2nd ed. Philadelphia, JB Lippincott, 1977)

The signs of uncal herniation include

- Ipsilateral pupillary dilation
- Paralysis of the muscles of eye movement (possible ptosis)
- Restlessness, then deteriorating level of consciousness
- Decrease or loss of sensory function
- Contralateral hemiparesis or hemiplegia
- Bilateral Babinski signs
- Respiratory changes (Cheyne–Stokes, central hyperpnea, ataxic)
- Decorticate and decerebrate posturing
- Finally, dilated, fixed pupils, flaccidity, and respiratory arrest.

The progression of symptoms with continued pressure can be followed in Table 12–3.

Any of the supratentorial herniation syndromes can initiate vascular and obstructive complications that can further exaggerate the seriousness of the neurological deterioration. Compression of the aqueducts of the ventricular system can cause cerebrospinal fluid circulation to be interrupted. As a result, hydrocephalus can develop. Cingulate herniation can compress both arterial and venous vessels (portions of the anterior cerebral artery and the great cerebral vein), causing exacerbation of already present ischemia and edema.

When there is uncal or central herniation, the compression through the tentorial incisura compresses the posterior cerebral artery, resulting in occipital lobe infarction and edema. Brain stem edema, ischemia, and hemorrhage can develop from the diencephalon to the pons–medulla area from the rostral–caudal displacement of the precipitating lesion, particularly if it is a rapidly expanding one. Rapid expansion does not allow for compensation by the brain.

The dreaded result of progressive downward displacement from any of the supratentorial herniation syndromes is brain stem herniation in which the medulla herniates into the foramen magnum. Death is immediate and is due to medullary compression. The medulla controls vital functions such as respiration, blood pressure, cardiac function, and vasomotor tone — all absolutely necessary for life.

INFRATENTORIAL HERNIATION

Lesions of the infratentorial compartment contributing to herniation are much less frequent than those of the supratentorial region. The three possible effects of an expanding lesion of the infratentorial compartment are

1. Direct compression of the brain stem, cerebellum, attached cranial nerves, and vascular supply
2. Upward transtentorial herniation of the brain stem and cerebellum through the tentorial incisura, resulting in maximum pressure on the midbrain
3. Downward herniation of both or one cerebellar tonsil through the foramen magnum with compression of the medulla (Fig. 12–4).

An expanding lesion creates increased pressure on selected structures. The increased pressure causes interference with normal function of the involved tissue, edema, ischemia, infarction, and neurosis if the process is not reversed. As the lesion continues to expand, the only sources of egress from the infratentorial compartment are the tentorial incisura or the larger orifice, the foramen magnum.

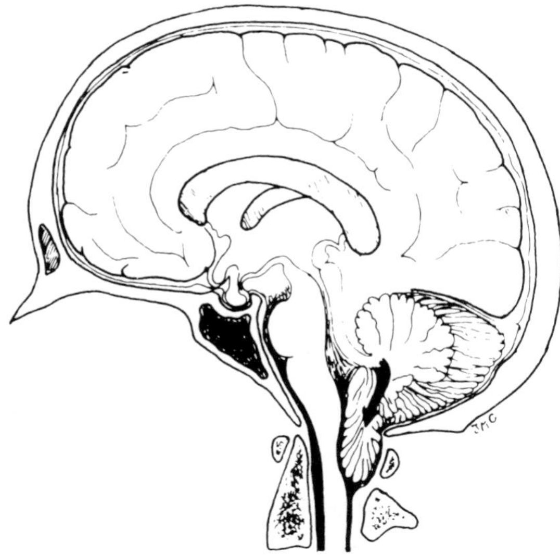

FIG. 12–4. Herniation of the cerebellar tonsils into the foramen magnum is the final outcome of increased intracranial pressure. Respiratory centers within the medulla oblongata are compressed and apnea in sleep frequently leads to cardiac arrest and death. (Smith RR: Essentials of Neurosurgery. Philadelphia, JB Lippincott, 1980)

The brain stem structures, particularly the medulla, contain centers for vital functions such as respiration, vasomotor tone, and cardiac function. If medullary compression develops, the possibility of death from respiratory and cardiac arrests is a dreaded concern. Infratentorial expanding lesions can encroach upon a portion of the ventricular system so that hydrocephalus can develop.

The signs and symptoms noted with the various types of infratentorial herniation syndromes tend to vary depending on the brain stem area most involved.

1. Compression Lesion of the Brain Stem

The most prominent signs include

- Coma
- Abnormal respiratory patterns depending on the area involved (Cheyne–Stokes, central neurogenic hyperventilation, and so forth)
- Pupillary changes; midposition and fixed in midbrain area, small and fixed in pontine area
- Ophthalmoplegias
- Loss of upward gaze
- Hemiparesis and hemiplegia
- Decortication or decerebration, which can progress to flaccidity in medullary injury
- Cranial nerve dysfunction; trigeminal or facial paresis with pontine injury

2. Upward Herniation

There does not appear to be a specific constellation of symptoms characteristic of this phenomenon.

3. Cerebellar–Foramen Magnum Herniation

A wide range of signs and symptoms are common and may include

- Stiff neck
- Arching of the neck
- Paresthesias in the area of the shoulders
- Coma
- Respiratory abnormalities
- Wide range of pulse rates

The reader is cautioned to recognize the wide range of possible signs and symptoms that may be apparent in the patient. Clear-cut syndromes are not present in the infratentorial compartment.

FACTORS THAT INCREASE INTRACRANIAL PRESSURE

Much of the knowledge about the relationship between certain activities and increased intracranial pressure has been gained from the data collected from continuous intracranial monitoring. The nursing research of Mitchell, Mauss, Parsons, and others has been of particular value in defining nursing protocols for managing the patient at risk. The patient at risk is one who already has an elevated intracranial pressure. Any activity that will further increase intracranial pressure is dangerous because plateau waves can occur.

IMPLICATIONS OF PLATEAU WAVES

Clinical symptoms of increased intracranial pressure *do not always* appear, even when the increase in pressure is substantial. If any clinical symptoms of increased intracranial pressure appear, it is most often during the onset and peak of plateau waves. Plateau waves are clinically significant because they peak to levels of 50 mm to 100 mm Hg from an already elevated base of intracranial pressure. The plateau waves correlate physiologically with cerebral hypertension, which leads to cerebral hypoxia, ischemia, and possibly necrosis of selected cerebral tissue. Because cerebral tissue is particularly sensitive to a diminished level of oxygen, symptoms of cerebral dysfunction may be evident. The degree of cerebral dysfunction may be pronounced or subtle. Subtle changes can be difficult to identify and evaluate, but they are indicators of an increasing intracranial pressure. Yet, when the plateau waves subside (in approximately 5 to 20 minutes), the subtle changes may also disappear. If any alterations occur in the vital signs or pupillary reaction, one would expect to observe the changes during peak plateau pressures, if at all.

The signs and symptoms that may occur as a consequence of plateau waves cover a gamut of possibilities. The symptoms most commonly in evidence are those of a change in the level of consciousness (restlessness, confusion) headache and changes in the respiratory pattern (Cheyne–Stokes respirations or forced respirations of central neurogenic hyperventilation). Subtle changes are noted in the alertness of the patient; his orientation to time, place, and person; or possibly recent memory. Other paroxysmal pressure symptoms associated with plateau waves include

- Visual changes (blurred vision, diplopia)
- Pupillary changes (sluggish to fixed pupils that may be dilated)
- Loss of motor function (paresis, paralysis, decerebration)
- Decreased sensory awareness
- Dysphasia
- Nausea and/or vomiting
- Changes in vital signs (elevated blood pressure, decreased pulse, and widening pulse pressure) observed with pressure on the brain stem
- Respiratory changes (central neurogenic respirations, apneustic, cluster, ataxic breathing)

The severity of the symptoms depends on the degree of intracranial decompensation. The plateau waves create cellular hypoxia of the cerebral tissue so that the physiological changes cause deterioration of the patient's condition with possible irreversible damage to the involved cells. The "pressure symptoms" that develop with plateau waves are paroxysmal, transient manifestations, but they may last for a prolonged period after the plateau waves have subsided. Therefore, the nurse's early recognition of any of the subtle changes associated with plateau waves can lead to early intervention, thereby preventing permanent injury or even death.

Since the presence of plateau waves is a dangerous time during which neurological deterioration can occur, identifying and controlling any factors that trigger plateau waves are important nursing considerations.

CONTRIBUTING FACTORS FOR ELEVATION OF INTRACRANIAL PRESSURE

The following is a list of contributing factors that can precipitate sustained spikes in intracranial pressures

- Hypercapnia (PCO_2 greater than 45 mm Hg)
- Hypoxemia (PO_2 less than 50 mm Hg)
- Certain cerebral vasodilating agents such as halothane anesthesia and histamines
- Valsalva maneuver
- Certain body positions (prone, flexion of neck, or extreme hip flexion)
- Isometric muscle contractions
- Coughing or sneezing
- Rapid eye movement sleep
- Emotional upset
- Noxious stimuli
- Arousal from sleep
- Clustering of activities

1. Hypercapnia and Hypoxemia

Hypercapnia (excessive levels of carbon dioxide in the blood) and hypoxemia (decreased levels of oxygen in the blood) are potent vasodilating factors causing cerebral vasodilation, increased blood volume in the brain, and subsequent increased intracranial pressure. Both have been identified as causing substantial pressure peaks and are discussed together because they frequently accompany one another. However, hypercapnia alone will stimulate vasodilation.

Hypercapnia results from underventilation of a patient in such circumstances as

- Sleep
- Sedation by drugs
- Shallow respirations as seen with an anxiety reaction or severe pain or asynchrony with respiration
- Coma
- Improperly calibrated setting for rate or sensitivity on a mechanical ventilator

Hypoxemia can result from

- Insufficient concentration of oxygen used in oxygen therapy
- Inadequate ventilation during surgery
- Inadequate ventilation during intubation
- Insufficient ventilation during and after suctioning

Blood Gas Analysis: Assessing Carbon Dioxide and Oxygen Blood Levels. The most accurate method for determining the oxygenation level of the patient is to draw blood gases. Although maintaining a patent airway is a major objective of patient management, the success of adequate ventilation is best judged by routine blood gas studies. The blood gases are valid criteria for judging patient outcomes and adjusting the plan of care. The following is a list of normal values for arterial blood gases:

- Arterial PO_2: 80 mm to 100 mm Hg
- Oxygen saturation: 94% to 100%
- Arterial PCO_2: 35 mm to 45 mm Hg
- Arterial pH: 7.35 to 7.45
- Arterial (HCO_3^-): 22 mEq to 26 mEq/liter

A level of oxygen below the normal range denotes hypoxemia. Administration of oxygen either by cannula or mechanical ventilation is indicated. A PCO_2 reading above the normal level indicates an abnormally high level of carbon dioxide in the blood. Blood gases have a direct bearing on blood pH, which reflects the acid–base balance of the blood. Normally the blood is slightly alkaline (7.40). An increase in the pH above the normal range is termed *alkalemia*, while a drop in the pH is termed *acidemia*. The pH of the blood is directly affected by the bicarbonate content in the blood. Body fluids contain a number of different acids, but the most important one affecting the acidity of the blood is carbonic acid (H_2CO_3). The production of carbonic acid occurs as follows:

$$CO_2 + H_2O \rightarrow H_2CO_3 \rightarrow H^+ + HCO_3^-$$

The carbonic acid breaks down to bicarbonate and hydrogen ions. The bicarbonate level is associated with the levels of a variety of body ions such as Na^+, K^+, and Cl^- and to the H^+ ion of organic acids.

With any patient, blood gases are helpful in making a diagnosis of metabolic or respiratory acidosis or alkalosis.

Preventing Hypercapnia and Hypoxemia: Principles of Management. To prevent situations that contribute to the development of hypercapnia and hypoxemia, certain principles of patient management can be implemented.

1. In the neurological patient, sedatives should be avoided or given guardedly in reduced doses since even small doses of sedatives can overwhelm the already vulnerable nervous system and lead to respiratory insufficiency. If sedation (or drugs having similar side-effects) must be given, the patient must be observed carefully for signs of respiratory distress.
2. An order for oxygen therapy as needed must be used to provide added oxygenation for the underoxygenated patient.
3. Periodic blood gas analysis is a valid method for determining the need to increase or decrease the amount of oxygen concentration administered to the patient by conventional methods or a mechanical ventilator.
4. Suctioning may be required to remove secretions and aid in the maintenance of a patent airway and adequate ventilation; suction gently and limit the time that the catheter is inserted to no more than 15 seconds.
5. Hyperventilation of the patient with an Ambu bag is a very effective method of reducing carbon dioxide and decreasing intracranial pressure. (Hypocapnia causes vasoconstriction of cerebral vessels.) However, be sure to synchronize the squeezing of the bag with the inspiratory cycle of the patient. If this is not done, intrathoracic pressure is significantly increased obstructing the valveless venous drainage from the brain and increasing blood volume and intracranial pressure in the brain.
6. For the ventilator-dependent patient the following points should be considered:
   - A patient who is out of sync with his ventilator is not being ventilated properly; also, his intrathoracic pressure is raised, impeding venous drainage from the brain. He will develop hypercapnia and hypoxemia. A patient who is at risk and who is fighting the ventilator (asynchrony) may have to be given a curare derivative such as pancuronium bromide to paralyze his respirations. He is then maintained on controlled ventilations.
   - Positive end-expiratory pressure (PEEP) during assisted ventilation is associated with increased intracranial pressure in some patients, particularly at moderate to high levels of PEEP. The effect of PEEP on intrathoracic pressure is the presumed cause. However, the relationship of PEEP to further increases in intracranial pressure is not consistent.[3] The benefit of PEEP to the patient will have to be evaluated.
   - The settings on the ventilator should be checked periodically and recalibrated as necessary. An oxygen analyzer can be used to check the oxygen concentration actually delivered to the patient.

Suctioning. The need to suction the patient is determined by observing the patient's color and any movement of chest and abdomen during breathing, as well as noting the presence of mucus and drainage within the upper respiratory pathways. Color signs to watch for are slight cyanosis or duskiness around the mouth, nail beds, or ear lobes. Natural or artificial light should be sufficient to make this determination.

Chest and abdominal movements during the respiratory cycle should also be noted. If there is excessive abdominal movement, there is a good possibility that respiratory obstruction is creating an added burden on the auxiliary muscles of respiration and the abdominal muscles to move the chest during the respiratory cycle. (Added evidence to support the need to suction will most likely be evident by auscultating the chest.) Contraction of abdominal muscles in abdominal breathing increases abdominal muscle tone during expiration. The increased muscle tone results in increased intracranial pressure.

Noisy respirations caused by mucus and drainage may be noted by auscultating the patient's chest to check clearness of breath sounds. Often, the rasping sound of mucus in the upper respiratory tract is obvious to the naked ear without auscultation. An even more obvious sign is mucus draining from the mouth or tracheostomy tube, if one is present.

It is most important to be alert for the subtle signs of respiratory distress, which can be caused by partial obstruction of the respiratory tract. These subtle symptoms include an increase in pulse rate, perspiration, and restlessness.

Suctioning Protocols. The patient should be evaluated frequently for any obvious or subtle indications of the need for suctioning.

- If suctioning is indicated, it should be limited to *no more than 15 seconds* per catheter insertion.
- Suction gently.
- In the patient at risk, suctioning can cause plateau waves. For the patient who has spikes and maintains the elevation for 20 minutes or more, lidocaine, 50 mg to 100 mg intravenously, has been given before suctioning by some. This is effective in some patients. In patients with endotracheal tubes, instillation of 1 ml to 2 ml of lidocaine elixir into the endotracheal tube may be helpful.
- Hyperinflate the lung with 100% oxygen before and after suctioning, with prior approval of the physician. This protocol helps to maintain levels of oxygen. However, respiratory conditions such as chronic obstructive pulmonary disease would contraindicate use of this therapy. Therefore, oxygen hyperinflation should be incorporated into the nursing care plan only with the prior approval of the physician who has ruled out any contraindications for the therapy.

Positioning to Enhance Respiratory Function. In addition to suctioning, the respiratory system can be aided by changing the patient's position by turning him every 2 hours and asking the conscious, cooperative patient to take a few deep breaths hourly. Both procedures are well-accepted methods for improving aeration of lung tissue and expulsion of drainage.

2. Vasodilating Drugs

Any neurological patient who is receiving drug therapy must be carefully assessed for possible drug side-effects such as cerebral vasodilation, which will aggravate intracranial pressure. Vasodilating drugs increase the blood flow to the brain, which can enhance an already increased level of intracranial pressure. Examples of such drugs include nicotinic acid, cyclandelate, histamine, and nylidrin hydrochloride. When surgery is necessary, the anesthesiologist will select the appropriate anesthetic agent, avoiding drugs such as halothane, enflurane, isoflurane, and nitrous oxide with side-effects detrimental to the neurological patient.

3. Valsalva Maneuver

The *Valsalva maneuver* is defined as exertion against a closed epiglottis. The increased intrathoracic pressure that occurs during the Valsalva maneuver impedes the venous return from the brain, thereby increasing the intracranial pressure. In a patient who is already experiencing compensation from increased intracranial pressure, the increase in intracranial pressure precipitated by the Valsalva maneuver is sufficient to produce plateau waves. The Valsalva maneuver can be initiated by straining at stool or by moving or turning in bed. To prevent the patient from straining at stool, stool softeners should be used in preference to enemas, cathartics, or suppositories. To offset the deleterious effects of turning in bed, the patient should be instructed to exhale while being moved or turned in bed. Exhaling requires an open epiglottis and, therefore, prevents the initiation of the Valsalva maneuver.

4. Body Positions and Turning

Positions that obstruct venous return from the brain cause spikes in intracranial pressure. (The venous cerebral system has no valves. An increase in intraabdominal, intrathoracic, or neck pressure is communicated as increased pressure throughout the open venous system, thus impeding drainage from the brain and increasing intracranial pressure.) The following positions should be avoided because they are known to increase intracranial pressure:

- The Trendelenburg position, which is absolutely contraindicated in the neurological–neurosurgical patient
- The prone position because it increases intraabdominal and intrathoracic pressures along with rotation of the neck
- Extreme flexion of the hips during surgery or in bed
- Angulation of the neck (flexion of the neck, even from a small improperly positioned pillow, and lateral rotation or turning). It has been suggested that turning the head to the right increases the intracranial pressure to higher levels than turning to the left.[10]
- Turning the patient laterally if the head of the bed is up, the knees are flexed on the abdomen, and the neck is angled

It has been demonstrated that positioning the patient so that his head is elevated 30 degrees decreases baseline intracranial pressure (Fig. 12–5). Gravity aids drainage from the brain and head.

The following points of care should be incorporated in the plan of care:

- Avoid positions known to cause spikes in intracranial pressure.
- Elevate the head of the bed 30 to 45 degrees.
- Maintain the head and neck in neutral position at all times. Use a collar or roll, if necessary, to maintain the position.
- Turn the patient laterally in proper body alignment, preventing angulation of the neck.

5. Isometric Muscle Contractions

An isometric muscle contraction results in muscle tension without lengthening the muscle. Such contractions raise systemic blood pressure and further elevate intracranial pressure. Therefore, isometric exercises are contraindicated for patients with increased intracranial pressure. Such exercises include pushing the feet against the footboard or pushing against the bed with one's arms. The patient should be cautioned against these activities.

Passive range-of-motion exercises are not isometric contractions because the length of the muscle *does* change during contraction. As a result, passive range-of-motion exercises do not cause changes in the systemic blood pressure. Therefore, passive range-of-motion exercises should be incorporated into the patient's plan of care to prevent musculoskeletal deformities.

Shivering and decerebration are forms of isometric contractions and should be avoided. Drug therapy has been of some use in controlling these problems: chlorpromazine hydrochloride (Thorazine) has been used for shivering and pancuronium bromide (Pavulon) for severe decerebration.

6. Coughing and Sneezing

Both coughing and sneezing will elevate intraabdominal and intrathoracic pressure. The increased pressure from these areas is transmitted through the spinal subarachnoid space to the intracranial subarachnoid space, as well as through veins that communicate with the dural venous sinuses and intracranial subarachnoid space. The venous

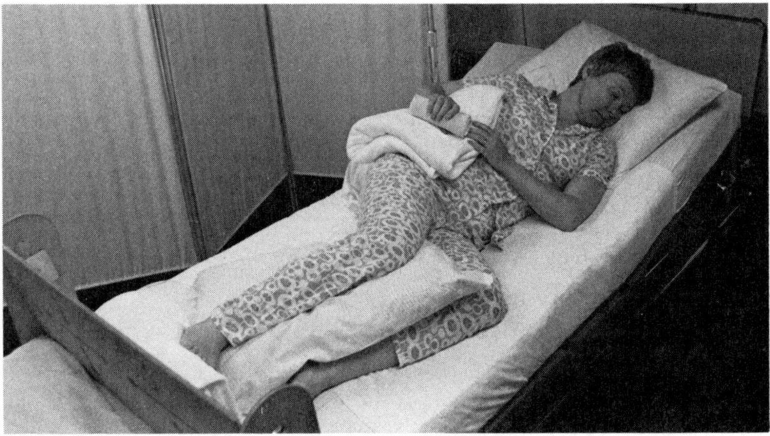

FIG. 12–5. Patient with increased intracranial pressure is positioned with head elevated at 30 degrees.

return from the cranial vault is impeded, resulting in increased intracranial pressure.

Should the patient sneeze frequently, the nurse should attempt to identify the cause of the sneezing (e.g., allergic reaction) and remove the offending agent. Coughing is more difficult to control, should it occur. The normal post-operative routine of having the patient cough is avoided in patients with increased intracranial pressure.

7. REM Sleep and Arousal From Sleep

In REM (rapid eye movement) sleep, which occurs with dreams, there is an increase in blood volume because of a localized increase in cerebral activity. Although the REM stage of sleep cannot be prevented, it can be identified by the obvious fluttering of the eyes under the closed eyelids. Since the intracranial pressure is increased during REM sleep, other activities known to elevate existing intracranial pressure (*i.e.*, turning the patient) should not be initiated during this time. Arousal from sleep will also increase intracranial pressure.

8. Emotional Upset

Conversation that may be emotionally stimulating to the patient such as discussion of his prognosis, condition, deficits, legal proceedings, restraints, or pain should not be conducted within his hearing range. Studies have shown that such conversations overheard by the patient cause elevation in intracranial pressure.[10] Families should also be cautioned about refraining from unpleasant or stimulating conversations.

Soft stimuli such as a soft soothing voice, pleasant conversation, soft music, the voices of loved ones being played on a tape recorder, and gentle therapeutic touching of the skin should surround the patient. The nurse is with the patient most of the time and should guard the patient from emotional upset. Even though a patient is classified as comatose, there is no way to know if his hearing is intact and if he can understand. The most reasonable approach for the nurse and others to take is to assume that the patient can hear and understand at least a few words.

9. Noxious Stimuli

The category of noxious stimuli is perhaps an extension of the previous one, but it broadens the scope of unpleasant stimuli that may affect the patient. Noxious stimuli are unpleasant or painful stimuli. Intracranial pressure will rise as a result of noxious stimuli. Common noxious stimuli that the patient might experience include

- Plugging of a drainage tube (e.g., urinary catheter), which will cause pressure and pain from bladder distention
- Painful nursing or medical procedures (e.g., removing tape from the skin or a lumbar puncture)
- Loud noises or sudden jarring of the bed

Noxious stimuli should be prevented if possible or controlled to a minimal level. Soft stimuli such as that mentioned above under Emotional Upset should be used to decrease the input of noxious stimuli when an uncomfortable procedure must be performed. The value of therapeutic touch cannot be overemphasized.

10. Clustering of Activities

It has been well documented through research that closely spaced activities have a cumulative effect. This means that bathing the patient, turning him to his side for back care (which often includes angulation of the neck), and other common activities of routine care will cause a greater and more prolonged elevation of increased intracranial pressure. Although nursing practice places a high premium on being well organized and doing several care procedures at one time for the seriously ill patient, such a practice in patients with intracranial hypertension may further increase their pressure. Mitchell and colleagues also state that performing closely spaced activities with the patient in the supine position may be the worst possible combination of care activities and most apt to increase pressure. Perhaps procedures such as suctioning should be done after the patient has had a period of rest and with the patient positioned on his side.[10]

Current nursing research may provide a scientific theoretical basis for rethinking the nursing care management of the critically ill neurological–neurosurgical patient who is at risk.

MEASURING AND MONITORING INCREASED INTRACRANIAL PRESSURE

Determining an accurate intracranial pressure at any given time depends on the method of measurement selected and the presence of central nervous system disease, which can influence that measurement.

LUMBAR PUNCTURE

Technically, intracranial pressure can be measured by means of lumbar puncture. An elevated pressure reading (greater than 15 mm Hg or greater than 200 mm water pressure) that is obtained during lumbar puncture can serve as the basis for a diagnosis of increased intracranial pressure. *However, in the presence of a suspected gross increase in intracranial pressure, a lumbar puncture is contraindicated because of the risk of brain stem herniation.*

There are other limits to the use of the lumbar puncture as a means of determining intracranial pressure. For example, a lumbar puncture can give a valid indication of intracranial pressure only if cerebrospinal fluid is flowing freely within the subarachnoid space. Adhesions, constrictions, or a space-occupying lesion can modify the flow of cerebrospinal fluid, thus resulting in a misleading measurement of the intracranial pressure.

CONTINUOUS INTRACRANIAL MONITORING

The continuous intracranial monitoring technique assists in the accurate diagnosis of increased intracranial pressure. It can be used in most patients, regardless of the presence of grossly elevated pressure. Monitoring intracranial pressure requires the use of a sensor, transducer, and recording device. The intracranial sensor, once implanted, transmits changes in intracranial pressure to a transducer that converts the mechanical impulses to electrical impulses. The recording device converts the electrical impulse into visible tracings on an oscilloscope or graph paper; some systems provide a digital readout of pressures.

Three Basic Techniques for Intracranial Monitoring

There are three basic techniques used in continuous intracranial monitoring of ventricular fluid pressure (VFP): intraventricular; subarachnoid; and epidural.

Intraventricular Catheter. The first technique, pioneered by Lundberg and associates, requires implantation through a burr hole of a polyethylene catheter into the anterior horn of the lateral ventricle of the nondominant hemisphere.[11] With the addition of a transducer and recording instrument, recordings of the intracranial pressure are available for interpretation (Fig. 12–6). Insertion of the catheter into the ventricle can be difficult if the ventricle is small. Other problems include leakage of cerebrospinal fluid and the ever-present possibility of infection within the brain.

Subarachnoid Screw or Bolt. The second monitoring technique, developed by Vires and associates, is the subarachnoid screw or bolt.[12] This is the most common intracranial pressure monitoring device used today. A small twist-drill hole is made into the subarachnoid space (see Fig. 12–6). Although cerebrospinal fluid leakage is not a major problem, the possibility of infection is still a major concern, as it is with Lundberg's technique. Another problem is herniation of the brain in the bolt, especially when the pressure is high.

In addition to providing a mechanism for continuous recording of intracranial pressure, both monitoring methods offer other advantages, including (1) the ability to fractionally drain excess cerebrospinal fluid to reduce intracranial pressure; (2) a means of collecting a specimen of cerebrospinal fluid for analysis; (3) a route for inserting medium for radiological examination; and (4) a means of evaluating cerebral compensatory mechanisms (compliance).

Epidural Monitor. Epidural monitoring can be accomplished using various system designs. The first design was introduced by Ladd Research Industries and consisted of a fiberoptic sensor implanted into the epidural space, a transducer, and a recorder. The sensor uses light to ascertain the position of a diaphragm that moves in response to external pressure and air to obtain the measurement by internal balancing. The transducer is not affected by environmental factors and thus there is not a "drift" problem and no need for frequent recalibration as is true of other monitoring devices. A digital readout or a strip-chart recording device can be used to complete the monitoring system.[13]

The disadvantage of this design is the possibility of a "wedge effect," which will result in inaccurate data. In inserting the sensor, care must be taken to free the adjacent dura from the inner table of the skull to avoid a wedge effect. The sensor must be inserted so that it lies completely under the bone. The other disadvantage is that cerebrospinal fluid cannot be removed.

Another epidural monitoring design is the pneumatic flow sensor and monitor produced by Meadox Medicals, Inc. This system includes a sensor, pneumatic system, microprocessor, and display unit. The sensor is placed in the epidural space and acts as a pneumatic flow switch. Air enters the sensor plenum at 40 cc/minute through the inlet tube. The airflow from the plenum at the exhaust port is closed off by the outside pressure exerted against the membrane. The pressure builds within the plenum to overcome the pressure against the membrane and reestablishes the airflow. The pressure required to maintain the airflow represents the intracranial pressure.

The sensor is connected to the pneumatic system in the monitoring device by polyethylene tubing. A bacteriological filter is located within the connector. An air pump circulates the air to a high-pressure chamber and then on to the sensor. Air returns by way of the exhaust tube of the sensor to a low-pressure chamber and then is recycled, thus forming a closed system. A transducer monitors the pressure.[14]

A microprocessor system controls the pneumatic and alarm systems and the data readout. The display unit provides a digital and graphic display of the intracranial pressure. A digital readout of cerebral perfusion pressure, time of day, and time spent on the monitor are also displayed. Data from previous times are stored and may be retrieved, as necessary.

The advantages and disadvantages of a system must be considered. With the pneumatic flow system the advantages are cited as greater accuracy and faster response time to display changes in intracranial dynamics, graphic and digital display of intracranial pressure, digital display of cerebral perfusion pressure, an alarm system, and retreivability of data. The disadvantages include the inability to collect cerebrospinal fluid specimens or to inject material directly into the ventricular system and the possibility of the "wedge effect."

The principal advantage of using epidural monitoring, regardless of the specific design, is that the brain or subarachnoid space is not penetrated and consequently there is less risk of infection. Problems such as uncontrolled loss of cerebrospinal fluid, plugging of the cannula or screw lumens, or surgical difficulties in entering small or collapsed ventricles are also avoided.

PRESSURE WAVES

In monitoring intracranial pressure with a continuous monitoring device, it was found that intracranial pressure is a continuously fluctuating phenomenon as reflected in

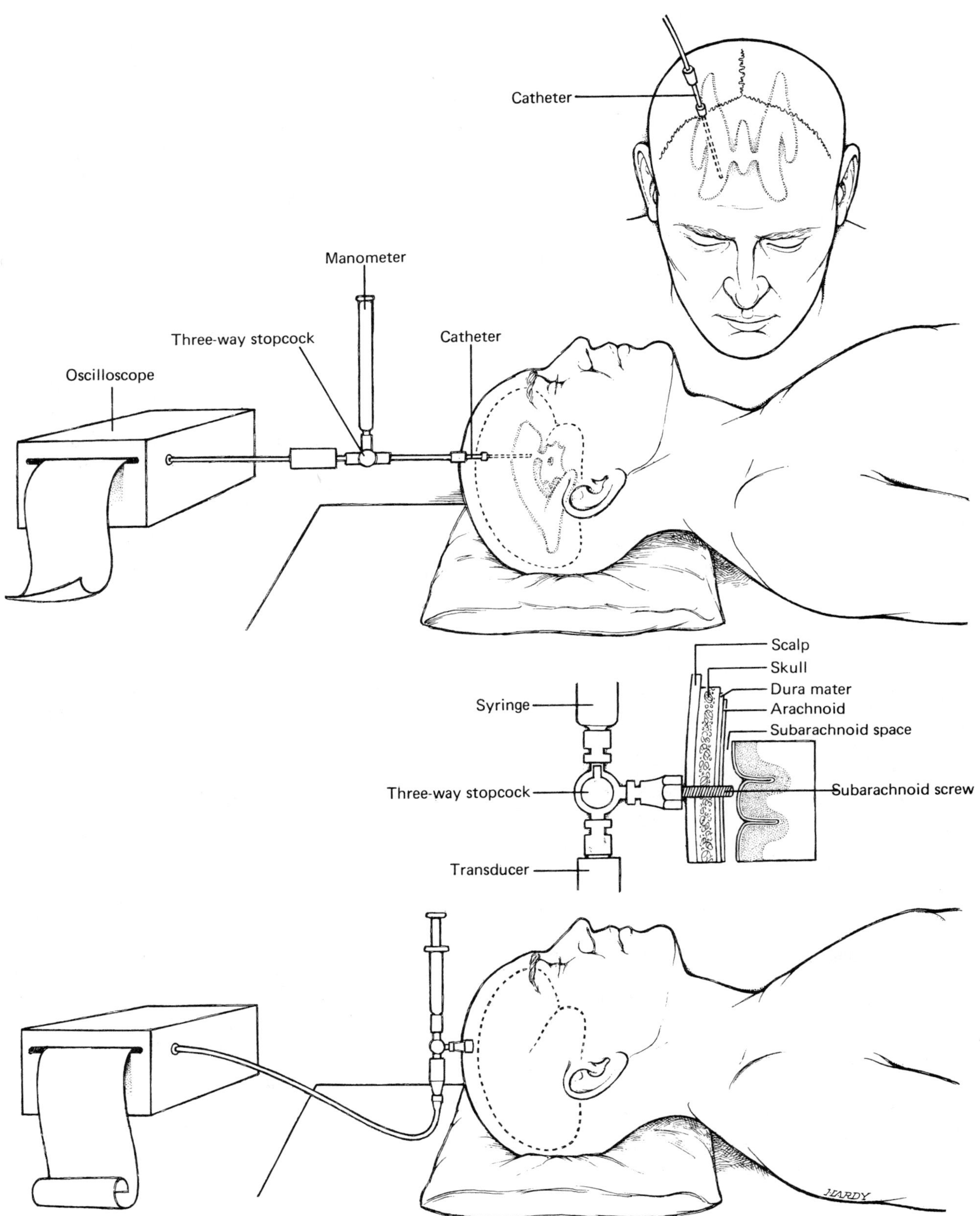

FIG. 12–6. Intracranial pressure monitoring. *(Top)* Ventricular catheter. *(Center)* Subarachnoid or hollow screw. *(Bottom)* Monitoring system connected to pressure transducer and display system. (Brunner LS, Suddarth DS: Textbook of Medical–Surgical Nursing, 5th ed. Philadelphia, JB Lippincott, 1984)

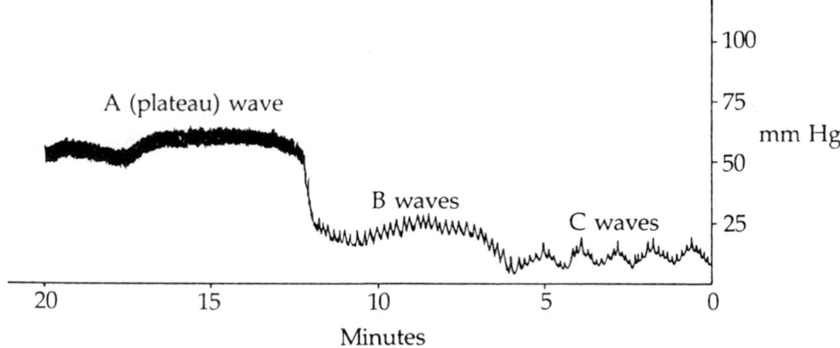

FIG. 12-7. Intracranial pressure waves. Composite diagram of A (plateau) waves, B waves, and C waves. (Holloway N: Nursing the Critically Ill. Menlo Park, CA, Addison-Wesley, 1978)

the pressure waves produced. The pressure waves are defined as spontaneous alterations in the intracranial pressure. Three distinct pressure waves have been identified: A waves, B waves, and C waves (Fig. 12-7). Intracranial pressure measurements are shown in Table 12-4.

A waves are commonly referred to as *plateau waves* and derive their name from the shape of the wave. The clinical significance of A waves is that they increase ventricular fluid pressure and intracranial pressure from 50 mm to 100 mm Hg and are seen in the advanced stages of increased intracranial pressure (>20 mm Hg). The plateau waves are sudden, transient waves lasting 5 to 20 minutes and usually begin from a baseline of already elevated intracranial pressure. The A waves are known to cause cerebral ischemia and brain damage. Transient or paroxysmal symptoms of plateau waves, sometimes called *pressure wave symptoms* or *pressure signs*, are often observed. Symptoms may include deterioration in the level of consciousness, abnormal changes in the respiratory pattern, characteristic changes in vital signs, headache, nausea, vomiting, abnormal pupillary reaction, altered motor function (such as paresis, decerebration, or decortication), dysphasia, and other symptoms related to cerebral dysfunction.

Of all the pressure waves, plateau waves are the most clinically significant because of the cerebral ischemia incurred.

Management of the patient is directed toward implementing measures to prevent the occurrence of plateau waves.

B waves are sharp, rhythmic oscillations occurring every ½ to 2 minutes and peaking the ventricular fluid pressure and intracranial pressure at 20 mm to 50 mm Hg. B waves are seen in relationship to fluctuations in the respiratory pattern, such as Cheyne-Stokes respirations. Decreased wakefulness (due to sleep or an impaired level of consciousness) and B waves tend to occur together.[15]

C waves, also called *Traube-Hering-Mayer waves,* occur every 4 to 8 minutes and increase ventricular fluid pressure and intracranial pressure by as much as 20 mm Hg. C waves relate to the normal changes of the systemic arterial pressure and have no accepted clinical significance.

TABLE 12-4. ***Intracranial Pressure Measurements in mm Hg and mm H_2O (Approximate Figures)***

Description	mm Hg*	mm H_2O
Normal	4-15	50-200
Moderately elevated†	15-40	200-540
Severely elevated	40 or greater	540 or greater
Other approximate figures for comparison		
	10	136
	20	270
	30	410
	40	540
	50	670
	60	800
	70	900
	80	1050
	100	1360

* Also recorded in torr

† Intracranial pressure >20 mm Hg is termed malignant hypertension.

INSERTING THE INTRACRANIAL MONITOR

Regardless of the type of intracranial pressure monitor used, strict aseptic technique must be followed during insertion and whenever the system is used. The procedure for insertion is relatively simple and may be done at the bedside, if necessary, although the sterile environment of the operating room is the usual site of insertion.

Once the sensor is in place a dressing is applied to the insertion site. The connecting tubing can be assembled in many different configurations depending on how the lines will be used. The manufacturer's instruction packet should be consulted. Stopcocks are placed on the lines as necessary. If there is a collection bag for drainage of excessive cerebrospinal fluid, a connection for this purpose is added. Once the system has been assembled, it is connected to the monitor or recording device.

INFECTION CONTROL AND THE ICP MONITOR

Sepsis is the primary concern with any invasive equipment. Care of the dressing at the insertion site depends on the preference of the physician. Some physicians choose to have the dry sterile dressing changed every 24 to 48 hours, with a small amount of gentamicin ointment or other ointment applied around the insertion site. Others prefer to have the dressing changed every 24 to 48 hours without any application of ointment or cleansing. The variations in approach to dressing management are based on the best judgment of the physician concerning the most effective method of preventing infection. Frequent cultures and the advice of the physician from the infection control department are helpful in guiding that judgment.

Many studies suggest that the critical factor in preventing infections in the cerebrospinal fluid is to maintain a closed system. Some systems, by virtue of their design, are not completely closed. Therefore, strict aseptic technique must be followed at all times. Instillation of an antibiotic solution has been suggested by some as an effective means of controlling infections. Instillation of a bacitracin solution or gentamicin followed by flushing with normal saline every 24 to 48 hours are some possible protocols followed. Flushing the line of an intracranial pressure monitor is not a routine procedure. There are serious risks involved, and it is not considered a safe practice by many. The nurse caring for the patient with an intracranial pressure monitor in place should follow the accepted protocol of the physician or hospital.

MANAGEMENT AND TREATMENT OF PATIENTS WITH ACUTE INCREASED INTRACRANIAL PRESSURE

GENERAL MANAGEMENT PRINCIPLES

The medical management of patients with acute increased intracranial pressure (intracranial hypertension) is directed toward (1) identifying and treating the underlying cause; (2) supporting all body systems; and (3) controlling the intracranial hypertension.

Identifying and Treating the Underlying Cause

Common causes of intracranial hypertension include cerebral edema due to direct tissue trauma (severe concussion, contusion, laceration, and surgery); space-occupying lesions such as hematomas, brain tumors, and abscesses; and central nervous system infections such as meningitis. Depending on the cause of the intracranial hypertension, the treatment may be medical, surgical, or both. Specific surgical intervention for treatment of specific neurological problems will be addressed in other chapters.

Supporting All Body Systems

The management of the patient encompasses not only the problem of intracranial pressure but also provision of support to all body systems to prevent complications. This includes respiratory, cardiovascular, gastrointestinal, genitourinary, and musculoskeletal function.

There are a number of complications that can develop as a result of increased intracranial pressure and conditions in other systems such as the respiratory system (adult respiratory distress syndrome, disseminated intravascular coagulopathy, neurogenic pulmonary edema) that will have a negative effect on the intracranial pressure. These complications can lead to permanent neurological deficits and even death. Much of the care included in managing the patient with increased intracranial pressure is directed toward preventing complications.

Controlling Increased Intracranial Pressure

Many of the presenting clinical signs and symptoms relate directly to increased intracranial pressure. This will be discussed in the next section in this chapter.

TREATMENT OF ACUTE INCREASED INTRACRANIAL PRESSURE (INTRACRANIAL HYPERTENSION)

The common protocols used by the physician to treat the patient with increased intracranial pressure include

1. Surgery
2. Drug therapy (osmotic diuretics, steroids, and anticonvulsants)
3. Fluid restriction
4. Hyperventilation
5. Temperature control
6. Cerebrospinal fluid drainage
7. Barbiturate coma

Surgery

If there is a localized hematoma or mass such as a brain tumor or abscess, surgical removal is indicated. A description of surgical intervention and nursing management is included in Chapter 14.

Drug Therapy

Three general classifications of drugs that are commonly administered in the management of increased intracranial pressure are (1) osmotic diuretics such as mannitol (Osmitrol), glucose, and urea, (2) corticosteroids, and (3) anticonvulsants.

Osmotic Diuretics. Osmotic diuretics are also referred to as hyperosmolaric agents. The high osmotic concentration of the drug causes water to be drawn from the edematous tissue. The principle of the diffusion of water depends on the presence of a semipermeable membrane. The direction of flow is from the hypoconcentrated to the hyperconcentrated solution. When a hyperosmolar drug is administered, the flow of fluid is from the edematous brain to the blood. The extracellular fluid of the edematous brain is hypotonic in relationship to the hyperconcentration created in the blood by the drug. The fluid crosses the semipermeable cell membrane, moving into the blood and decreasing the edema in the brain.

Mannitol. Mannitol's (Osmitrol) osmotic effect causes water to be drawn from the cells to the extracellular fluid and from red blood cells to plasma. The result is that extracellular fluid volume, plasma volume, and circulation time are increased so that a dilution of the extracellular sodium ion is achieved.

When mannitol is administered intravenously to the patient with an elevated cerebrospinal fluid pressure, there is a rapid reduction of this pressure within 15 minutes after the intravenous infusion is begun. This effect can last for 3 to 8 hours after the termination of the infusion. Diuresis of fluid will occur within 1 to 3 hours after the drug is begun. Osmitrol does not cross the blood–brain barrier unless very high concentrations are present in the plasma or the patient is acidotic.

The major use of Osmitrol is to greatly reduce increased intracranial pressure prior to and during neurosurgery and to aid in the treatment of cerebral edema. Osmitrol is indicated when there is evidence of developing brain stem compression or herniation. A rebound increase in intracranial pressure may occur 12 hours after osmotic diuretics have been administered, but the occurrence of this phenomenon is less frequent with Osmitrol than with urea.

Osmitrol can produce fluid and electrolyte imbalance. It should not be given to patients with hypovolemic shock, congestive heart failure, dehydration, or kidney disease. There should be monitoring of the following areas when Osmitrol is administered: (1) renal function studies, (2) urinary outputs, (3) electrolytes, (4) serum and urine osmolarities, and (5) central venous pressure. A Foley catheter should be inserted to measure accurate fractional urinary outputs.

The average dose of Osmitrol is 1.5 gm to 2 gm/kg of body weight. It is administered rapidly in a 15%, 20%, or 25% solution (in 500 ml) over a period of 30 to 60 minutes. Another protocol for administering mannitol is to give 100 mg intravenously as a loading dose followed by a maintenance dose of 0.05 gm to 0.15 gm/kg/hour. The goal is to maintain the osmolarity of 305 to 315.

Glycerol. Glycerol is a trivalent alcohol that acts as an osmotic diuretic. Its effect on the brain is similar to that of mannitol. One advantage of glycerol is that it can be taken orally and achieve maximum decrease in intracranial pressure within 30 to 60 minutes. This effect lasts about 4 hours. A rebound effect can develop if the drug is given more often than every 4 hours. Few side-effects have been reported except nausea from the sweet taste. Glycerol appears to be a safe drug for long-term use. It should not be given to patients with liver disease. The patient who needs treatment for cerebral edema usually has neurological deficits such as a decreased level of consciousness that make it impossible for him to take drugs orally. Glycerol is not used widely in clinical settings. The intravenous use of glycerol is associated with many serious side-effects including phlebitis, hemolysis, and acute renal failure. Mannitol is preferable for intravenous use.

Glucose and Urea. Although both glucose and urea are classified as osmotic diuretics, their use in the clinical area is minimal because of side-effects and rebound swelling. Mannitol is usually the drug of choice when osmotic diuretics are indicated.

Loop Diuretics. Furosemide (Lasix) is a potent loop diuretic, its primary site of action being the ascending loop of Henle. Unlike osmotic diuretics, furosemide's dehydration effect appears to have selectivity for injured cerebral tissue. The drug is effective in reducing cerebral edema and lowering intracranial pressure and is especially suited to managing children who respond to cerebral trauma with hyperemia. Furosemide is alleged to have no effect on serum osmolarity, electrolytes, or cerebral volume. The rebound swelling effect is not a problem with furosemide as it is with osmotic diuretics.

Corticosteroids. The use of corticosteroids in the neurological–neurosurgical patient is very controversial. It is generally accepted that the use of steroids in the management of vasogenic edema associated with brain tumors is very effective. The controversy arises in the use of corticosteroids with head injuries. Even those that support the use of corticosteroids differ on recommended dosage of the drug. The drug of choice is usually dexamethasone (Decadron). Although the exact mechanism of action is not clear, it is effective in reducing cerebral edema in selected clinical problems.

For those who support the use of high-dose dexamethasone, the following protocol is typical: after a loading dose of 100 mg given intravenously, give 100 mg every 6 hours intravenously or orally for 8 days, then taper the dose. The drug is usually tapered over the next 7 to 10 days. If a low-dose protocol is selected, a typical drug schedule might be as follows: after giving a 12-mg loading dose intravenously, give 4 mg every 6 hours for 8 days intravenously or orally, then taper the drug as with a high-dose protocol. Dexamethasone is begun intravenously and then switched to the oral route as soon as possible. The intramuscular route is used only if the other two routes are not acceptable.

Dexamethasone cannot be discontinued quickly because the serious side-effect of adrenal insufficiency could develop. As noted above, the dosage is gradually tapered by decreasing the amount and increasing the interval between doses until the drug can be safely discontinued.

There are several side-effects of steroid therapy. One major side-effect that can occur is gastric irritation and gastrointestinal hemorrhage. To control this problem two drugs are frequently ordered: an antacid such as Maalox, 30 ml by mouth or feeding tube every 4 hours, and cimetidine (Tagamet), 300 mg every 6 hours by mouth or parenterally. Cimetidine is a histamine (H2) receptor antagonist administered to reduce gastric secretions. As a result of the use of these two drugs, gastrointestinal hemorrhage is infrequent.

Patients receiving steroid therapy should have their urine tested every 6 hours for sugar and acetone. One of the side-effects seen with dexamethasone is glucose spilling into the urine. If large amounts of glucose are detected in the urine, some physicians order coverage with regular insulin. Stools are monitored daily for occult blood because of the possibility of gastrointestinal bleeding.

Anticonvulsants. The drug of choice for prevention of seizure activity in the patient with increased intracranial pressure is phenytoin (Dilantin). Should the patient display drug reaction or allergy to Dilantin, phenobarbital can be used. The average dosage of Dilantin is 100 mg orally, three or four times daily. It is supplied in capsule or liquid form. Dilantin is strongly alkaline in solution and may produce gastric irritation. Intramuscular injections are very irritating and poorly absorbed. The intravenous route can be used, but the rate of infusion must be slow. It is important to be aware of drug interactions because Dilantin can affect the action of various drugs as well as be potentiated or inhibited by them.

Antihypertensives. Systemic hypertension is frequently seen in patients with acute cerebral injury and increased intracranial pressure. The decision to treat this problem is a difficult one. If the systemic blood pressure is elevated because of the compensatory mechanism, or Cushing's response, it should not be treated. Cushing's response is a compensatory ischemic response that reflexively raises the blood pressure in response to a rising intracranial pressure. If the blood pressure did not rise, the intracranial pressure would be equal to the blood pressure, and the cerebral blood flow would cease. Therefore, blood pressure is not lowered until an elevated intracranial pressure is controlled. It has been suggested by many that the cerebral perfusion pressure is the best guide for the control of systemic hypertension.

If antihypertensive drugs are indicated, the drug chosen should not contribute to increasing cerebral blood flow which will increase intracranial pressure. An antihypertensive drug that is also a vasodilator would increase intracranial pressure if the brain has low compliance. Drugs used to control hypertension include hydrallazine, sodium nitroprusside, and others. Some of these drugs have cerebrovasodilating properties and should be given cautiously.

Fluid Restriction

The physician may choose to limit the patient's fluid intake to a specific amount for the given period (usually written in millimeters [ml] of fluid for a 24-hour period). Fluid intake can range from 900 ml/24 hours to 2500 ml/24 hours. The underlying principle of limiting fluid intake is to cause slight dehydration. By controlling fluid intake, the extracellular fluid will decrease. If the extracellular fluid of body tissue (including the brain) decreases, then the increased intracranial pressure will also decrease. This action will help to stabilize the neurological patient who is at risk.

When fluid restriction is ordered, any fluid intake, regardless of route, is computed as intake. This means that the patient's diet, tube feeding, fluids given to swallow medication, between-meal beverages, and intravenous fluids must all be calculated as part of the total intake. Attention is also given to the restriction of sodium intake because sodium tends to cause fluid retention.

Hyperventilation

Controlled hyperventilation is an important part of the approach for reducing increased intracranial pressure. If the PCO_2 can be reduced from its normal level of 35 mm to 45 mm Hg to a range of 25 mm to 30 mm Hg in the patient with increased intracranial pressure, there will be adequate oxygenation, vasoconstriction of cerebral arteries, reduction of cerebral blood flow, increased venous return, and decreased jugular pressure. The result is a general reduction of intracranial pressure by the reduction of intracranial volume.

Controlled hyperventilation can be achieved for the patient on a ventilator by adjusting the controls on the ventilator. The arterial blood gases and tidal volumes should be monitored frequently and the ventilator adjusted as needed. Controlled ventilation should be maintained as follows: PCO_2, 25 mm to 30 mm Hg; PO_2 greater than 100 mm Hg; and arterial pH between 7.3 and 7.6. If the patient is agitated or bucking the ventilator, he should be sedated with barbiturates or curarelike muscle relaxants (pancuronium, 0.1 mg/kg, or metocurine, 0.3 mg/kg).[16]

For the patient who is not on a ventilator, hyperventilation can be carried out with the use of an Ambu bag. This can be connected to a tracheostomy or endotracheal tube, or a mask attached to the Ambu bag can be placed over the patient's face. (In practice, the hospitalized patient who is ill enough to require aggressive intervention for increased intracranial pressure will probably be comatose and intubated). For the patient who is being monitored for intracranial pressure, spikes in pressure would be reason to Ambu the patient. This is a common practice on most critical care units. The process of Ambuing the patient decreases the carbon dioxide level, causes vasoconstriction, and lowers the pressure to eliminate the spikes on the monitor screen.

Several authors cite two potential problems with hyperventilation. These problems are the potential of hypoxia secondary to the marked reduction of cerebral blood flow and the shift to the left of the hemoglobin dissociation curve. This effect causes an increased oxygen affinity for hemoglobin and may decrease the unloading of oxygen from hemoglobin in cerebral tissue.[17]

The benefits of hyperventilation are well established for the patient with increased intracranial pressure. Precautions should be followed and the patient carefully monitored to attain the optimal effect from reduction of intracranial pressure.

Temperature Control

Hypothermia has been used in varying degrees during intracranial surgery and in the treatment of severe craniocerebral trauma. Hypothermia (<35°C) for the treatment of severe cerebral trauma has become a less common method of treatment because clinical benefit from such treatment has been difficult to demonstrate. The use of hypothermia in neurosurgery is somewhat more accepted, although it is not a standard protocol for all neurosurgical procedures.

The underlying principle for the use of hypothermia is that as the body temperature drops, there is a decrease of all metabolic processes including that of the brain. The systemic blood pressure and the cerebral blood flow decrease. Because the cerebral glucose metabolic curve is directly proportional to oxygen consumption, the production of metabolic by-products such as carbon dioxide and lactic acid will be decreased. The contributing factors for increases in intracranial pressure in the presence of cerebral hypertension have already been discussed.

If any of these factors such as systemic blood pressure, cerebral blood flow, production of the metabolic by-products, and brain bulk can be decreased, the intracranial pressure can be controlled and decreased. Simply stated, by lowering the body temperature, the brain activity diminishes, and the brain can maintain cellular equilibrium for longer periods of time with decreased amounts of oxygen and nutrients than would be required at a higher body temperature.

Of equal importance is the control of an elevated temperature (above 37°C), which causes most body processes to be accelerated. In the patient with existing cerebral hypertension, the increase in systemic blood pressure and cerebral blood flow will contribute to exaggerate the existing increased intracranial pressure. It is therefore important in patient management to control elevated body temperature. This is accomplished with antipyretic drugs such as Tylenol, used alone or in combination with a hypothermia blanket. If shivering occurs, it will increase intracranial pressure; thus, the patient must be closely supervised to prevent this adverse effect. When hypothermia is employed to decrease the body temperature to a subnormal level, shivering (a homeostatic protective mechanism) is controlled by administering the drug chlorpromazine (Thorazine).

The use of hyperbaric oxygen therapy to increased intracranial pressure from head injury, cerebral edema, and cerebral compression is still considered to be controversial. Much more reliable data need to be generated before this treatment method can be incorporated into the routine management of increased intracranial pressure.

Cerebrospinal Fluid Drainage

Some physicians will insert drainage catheters into a cerebral ventricle so that excess cerebrospinal fluid can be easily drained; this controls erratic increases in intracranial pressure. Ventricular drainage is a temporary treatment used in conjunction with the other modalities of care. Ventriculostomy can help sustain the patient through peak periods of cerebral edema by controlling spikes in intracranial pressure. Prophylactic antibiotics are usually given to patients on ventricular drainage because of the ever-present danger of infection.

Because the cerebrospinal fluid provides a favorable environment for an infection to develop rapidly if microorganisms enter the ventricular space, it is imperative that absolutely flawless aseptic technique be maintained. During the procedure an incision is made in the scalp and a burr hole is made in the skull to provide an access route for insertion of the catheter into the ventricle. Regardless of how carefully the suturing has been done to ensure closure around the catheter site, drainage from the incision and around the catheter frequently occurs. This saturates the dry sterile dressing and creates an ideal site for infection; therefore, frequent checking of the dressing and maintenance of absolute sterility is mandatory.

The level of the collection container is adjusted as indicated by the physician. Lowering the collection container increases the amount of cerebrospinal fluid drainage while raising it will diminish the amount of drainage. A too-rapid removal of drainage could lead to brain stem herniation if there is a pronounced level of increased intracranial pressure.

The drainage tubing necessary for ventricular drainage is fine and pliable and prone to kinking, which would interfere with drainage. The tubing must be checked frequently to ensure patency of the tube. If the tubing inadvertently disconnects at the connector site, it should not be reconnected; rather, it should be clamped close to the scalp while sterile equipment is ordered.

Observing and recording the amount of drainage should be conducted at frequent intervals. As mentioned previously, a too-rapid removal of drainage could lead to brain stem herniation and deterioration of the neurological status. The physician may wish to send specimens of cerebrospinal fluid drainage for culture or sensitivity tests or analysis. Specimens must be obtained under sterile conditions.

Barbiturate Coma Therapy

Barbiturate coma therapy is a treatment protocol developed for the management of uncontrolled intracranial hypertension that has not responded to conventional treatment such as surgical decompression, osmotic diuretics, fluid restriction, steroids, hyperventilation, and cerebrospinal fluid drainage. A state of uncontrolled intracranial pressure exists when intracranial pressure remains above 20 mm Hg (20 torr) for 30 or more minutes. When intracranial pressure is within normal range (0 mm to 15 mm Hg), variations in systemic arterial pressure have no effect on cerebral blood flow because the autoregulatory mechanism of the brain maintains the cerebral blood supply at a constant level. But when intracranial pressure is sustained at high levels (20 mm Hg or greater), the autoregulatory mechanism fails and cerebral perfusion pressure is locally or generally reduced, and cerebral blood flow and intracranial pressure become passively dependent on the systemic arterial blood pressure. A self-perpetuating vicious cycle develops in which the primary effects on cerebral cells are hypoxia, ischemia, and finally necrosis caused by cerebral edema, compression, and herniation.

Purposes. Barbiturate therapy, introduced by Shapiro and associates, consists of administering large doses of short-acting barbiturates to induce and maintain coma. The drug most often used is pentobarbital (Nembutal) although some coma protocols use thiopental (Pentothal). The expected outcomes from barbiturate therapy follow.

1. Cerebral vasoconstriction, which will decrease cerebral blood flow and blood volume
2. Decreased cerebral metabolism, promoting stabilization of the cell membrane
3. Preservation of ischemic cerebral cells from irreversible damage by improving and stabilizing the blood supply throughout the entire cerebral arterial system
4. Lowering of the intracranial pressure to an acceptable level
5. Improvement of morbidity and mortality rates for patients who have sustained high levels of increased intracranial pressure

Baseline Data. The following baseline data are collected before barbiturate coma is induced:

Diagnostic Assessment

- CT scan (as necessary)
- Cerebral angiography
- Daily brain stem evoked responses (BSER)

Laboratory Data

- Complete blood count (CBC)
- Coagulation studies (prothrombin time [PT], partial thromboplastin time [PTT], platelets)
- Electrolytes
- Blood urea nitrogen (BUN)
- Creatinine
- Glucose

(Electrolytes, BUN, creatinine, and glucose: maintained within normal limits)

- Serum lactate
- Serum osmolarity (maintained <320 mOsm)
- Arterial blood gases (maintained at PCO_2, 22 to 25 and PO_2, 100 for hyperventilation therapy)

The laboratory studies are monitored on a scheduled basis (usually daily) during therapy.

Once barbiturate coma is induced, the usual parameters of neurological assessment, such as pupillary, oculocephalic, oculovestibular, corneal, gag, swallowing, and other reflexes, are lost. Cortical activity as measured by electroencephalogram (EEG) is depressed, although the brain stem evoked responses, such as the brain stem auditory evoked response (BAER), will remain intact as long as the brain stem is functional.

Monitoring and Support Devices. Before barbiturate coma is induced, the following monitoring and support devices must be in place to maintain the patient:

- Intracranial monitoring device to assess intracranial pressure and calculate cerebral perfusion pressure* continually.
- Assisted ventilation equipment to maintain respiratory function (because of respiratory depression induced by barbiturate therapy)
- Cardiac monitor to monitor sinus rhythm and alert the observer to any arrhythmias or other electrocardiographic changes
- Central venous pressure line or a Swan–Ganz catheter inserted into the pulmonary artery for assessment of intravascular volume
- Blood pressure cuff or continual monitoring device to assess blood pressure (hypotension may occur during coma)
- Endotracheal or tracheostomy tube in place to maintain an airway
- Peripheral and central venous pressure lines for administration of drugs, intravenous fluids, or hyperalimentation
- Other central and peripheral lines, as needed
- Indwelling urinary catheter to facilitate measuring hourly urinary output
- Levin tube and suction to decompress the depressed gastrointestinal tract

Induction. Barbiturate coma is induced by administering a loading dose of pentobarbital, 3 mg to 5 mg/kg of body weight, by slow intravenous push. It is expected that the intracranial pressure will decrease by 10 mm Hg within 10 to 15 minutes. A second loading dose should be administered in 2 hours if the expected drop in intracranial pressure has not occurred. The blood pressure is monitored throughout the protocol but especially during the early phase of induction because there is a tendency toward hypotension, which may require treatment with vasopressor drugs. Once a positive response to the loading dose occurs, the drug is administered hourly at the rate of 1 mg to 3 mg/kg so that a serum blood level of 2.5 mg to 4.0 mg (up to 5.0 mg) can be maintained. Barbiturate coma is continued until intracranial pressure is normal or below 20 mm Hg for 24 to 72 hours when it is gradually tapered. It is reported that coma has been maintained for more than 2 weeks in some patients. The major problems associated with barbiturate coma are hypotension, cardiac depression, and erratic dose response.

Drugs Administered. Steroid drugs (dexamethasone) and osmotic diuretics (mannitol) are given during barbiturate therapy. The following drugs may be administered, depending on the particular needs of the patient:

- Diuretics such as furosemide (Lasix) intravenously as needed to induce diuresis
- Aquamephyton intramuscularly daily or every other day to control bleeding tendency
- Vasopressor drugs such as Dopamine or Levophed intravenously to maintain adequate cerebral and renal perfusion if the systolic arterial pressure falls below 90 mm Hg (a Dopamine drip is often needed to maintain blood pressure).

* Mean systemic arterial pressure minus intracranial pressure equals cerebral perfusion pressure (MSAP − ICP = CPP); ideally, cerebral perfusion pressure should be maintained at 60 mm to 70 mm Hg, although it may be as low as 40 mm to 60 mm Hg during coma therapy.

- Plasma expanders such as salt-poor albumin or Plasmanate to maintain circulating volume
- Multi-vitamin preparations given intravenously and/or hyperalimentation to maintain the nutritional level (hyperalimentation is considered if therapy continues for several days)
- Anticonvulsant drugs, most often phenytoin (Dilantin) intravenously, to prevent seizures upon withdrawal of barbiturate therapy

THE NURSING MANAGEMENT OF THE PATIENT WITH INCREASED INTRACRANIAL PRESSURE

The nursing management of the patient with increased intracranial pressure (intracranial hypertension) is complex. Many neurological patients have some degree of intracranial hypertension that responds well to the basic principles of medical management. Although development of complications such as respiratory distress or intracranial bleeding could lead to neurological deterioration, these patients appear to be well managed. The patient at risk is one who has an elevated intracranial pressure high enough that cerebral perfusion pressure could be compromised. The nursing management of this patient is critical for preventing spikes in intracranial pressure. If the patient with acute intracranial hypertension is not managed properly and the condition controlled, he will go on to develop fulminating intracranial hypertension that will affect the cerebral perfusion pressure, causing hypoxia, ischemia, irreversible neurological damage, and even death. This is the patient who herniates from the extreme pressure (intracranial herniation syndromes).

In the previous sections of this chapter, the dynamics of cerebral circulation, increased intracranial pressure, signs and symptoms of increased intracranial pressure, factors that increase intracranial pressure, and medical management and treatment were discussed. All of this information provides the nurse with a base of knowledge to help identify her unique role in patient management.

The specific responsibilities of the nurse will depend on the condition of the patient. For example, if acute cerebral edema from a closed head injury is the primary cause of an elevated intracranial pressure, the nurse can expect to administer mannitol (Osmitrol) to decrease the pressure. There are several nursing responsibilities associated with the administration of osmotic diuretics. Cerebral edema usually takes approximately 72 hours to reach its maximum development, and then it begins to subside, if all goes well. Other nursing responsibilities in the acute phase will probably include a strict fluid restriction, continual intracranial pressure monitoring, cerebrospinal fluid drainage, and hyperventilation therapy. If the intracranial pressure is out of control, barbiturate coma may be ordered. However, once the intracranial pressure is well controlled, the nursing responsibilities change. The focus of care then tends to be controlling situations that could, once again, raise the intracranial pressure; preventing complications; and providing rehabilitation aspects of patient care.

The following discussion will include the major nursing responsibilities in managing the patient with acute intracranial hypertension. It is suggested that Chapter 5, Assessment of Neurological Signs, and Chapter 11, Care of the Unconscious Patient, also be consulted. See Charts 12–5 and 12–6 for summarization of major nursing points.

The nurse's responsibility for the patient with acute increased intracranial pressure includes

- Neurological assessment
- Maintenance of a patent airway and adequate ventilation
- Hyperventilation
- Prevention of activities that increase intracranial pressure
- Fluid restriction
- Cerebrospinal fluid drainage
- Continuous intracranial pressure monitoring
- General nursing management
- Barbiturate coma

NEUROLOGICAL ASSESSMENT

Frequent assessment of neurological signs (including vital signs) must be made to ascertain any changes in the neurological status of the patient. This means that at frequent intervals (every 15 minutes to every 4 hours), depending on the circumstances, a neurological assessment of the patient is carried out, including

- Level of consciousness
- Pupillary size and direct light reaction
- Eye movement
- Motor function (and sensory function)
- Vital signs

Changes in findings are often subtle. The slight change in points of the assessment can only be detected by periodically evaluating the neurological signs and comparing those findings to results of previous assessments. For example, if the nurse notices that a previously alert and oriented patient is now showing signs of confusion, mental deterioration, and lack of interest, then these findings should be reported to the physician at once. Clinical evidence of this type is often apparent before there are changes in pupillary size or reaction to light, eye movement, motor or sensory function, or vital signs.

Careful observation by the nurse is still the most sensitive indicator of early change. Early recognition allows for definitive action to be taken to reverse the deterioration process. Once the pupillary and other signs mentioned become apparent, the downhill course of events can occur very rapidly, allowing little time or opportunity for intercession.

Noting trends of subtle changes applies not only to the level of consciousness, pupillary size and reaction, eye movement, and motor function, but also to vital signs. It is most important to note trends in vital signs because deterioration in neurological status can herald change from a compensatory neurological state to one of decompensation. Slowing of the pulse, widening of the pulse pressure, and an elevated systolic reading are signs of deterioration, although these are late signs. (Do not wait until these signs are present before acting on other evidence. Cues of change

(Text continued on page 278.)

CHART 12-5. SUMMARY OF NURSING MANAGEMENT OF THE PATIENT WITH INCREASED INTRACRANIAL PRESSURE

Principles of nursing management for the patient with increased intracranial pressure incorporate concepts of physiology and pathophysiology and objectives of medical management. In a patient with cerebral hypertension and increased intracranial pressure, a major objective is to protect the patient at risk from sudden increases in intracranial pressure. The specific points of nursing care outline the nurse's role in providing quality care.

NURSING RESPONSIBILITIES	RATIONALE
Neurological Assessment	
1. Assess baseline neurological signs with periodic reassessment and comparison to previous findings. (Assess level of consciousness, pupillary size and reaction to light, eye movement, and motor/sensory function.)	1. Subtle changes in neurological signs can indicate deterioration or improvement in the neurological status. These changes can only be detected by frequent monitoring and comparison with previous findings.
2. Neurological assessment includes routine monitoring of vital signs. (Compare findings with previous recordings to note trends.)	2. Intracranial decompensation is noted by decreased pulse, increased blood pressure, and widening pulse pressure. Deterioration in neurological status *may* be noted (lowered level of consciousness, pupil inequality and decreased response to light reflex, ophthalmoplegia, paresis, plegia, or abnormal posturing), even though it is generally accepted that vital signs correlate poorly with early neurological deterioration.
3. The temperature should be watched and treatment initiated for elevations. Guard against shivering if a hypothermia blanket is used. Remove patient from blanket when he is 1° or 2° F above normal body temperature because his temperature will drift downward even after the hypothermia blanket has been discontinued.	3. Elevated temperature, increased oxygen consumption, and increased production of by-products of metabolism aggravate increased intracranial pressure
Establishing and Maintaining a Patent Airway and Adequate Ventilation	
1. Assess rate, depth, and pattern of respirations. (Respirations should be regular at a rate of 14 to 16/minute.)	1. Indicates the patency of the airway
2. Assess skin for cyanosis (check around mouth, nail beds, and ear lobes).	2. Indicates adequacy of respirations and the oxygen–carbon dioxide exchange
3. Auscultate chest for normal breath sounds. (Normal breath sounds should be heard in all lobes without rales.)	3. Indicates proper lung expansion
4. Suction, as necessary, for no more than 15 seconds per catheter insertion	4. Time limit prevents the buildup of carbon dioxide, which is a potent cerebral vasodilator able to aggravate increased intracranial pressure
5. Hyperinflate lungs with 100% oxygen for 1 minute prior to suctioning (with previous approval of the physician).	5. Provides adequate oxygenation so that carbon dioxide will not build up and aggravate increased intracranial pressure
6. Check setting on the respirator, if one is in use. Ambu for a few minutes every hour to totally expand all areas of the lungs.	6. Provides for adequacy of oxygenation and prevents development of atelectasis and pneumonia
7. If a tracheostomy is present, give tracheostomy care every 4 hours.	7. Provides for patency of airway
8. Monitor blood gases (PO_2 below 85 mm Hg is considered low).	8. This is a reliable indicator of oxygen and carbon dioxide blood levels. If oxygen concentration is low, oxygen administration may be instituted or increased.
9. Administer oxygen at the ordered percentage.	9. Supplements the need for oxygen
Positioning and Moving Patients	
1. Maintain patient in semi-Fowler's position with head elevated to 30 degrees. Avoid prone position, exaggerated neck flexion, and extreme hip flexion of 90 degrees or greater; Fig. 12-5.	1. Semi-Fowler's position with head elevated provides for drainage from the cranial vault and decreases intracranial pressure. Avoiding the prohibited positions means avoiding occasions of increased intra-abdominal or intrathoracic pressure interference with drainage from the venous vessels from the head and brain.

CHART 12–5. (continued)

NURSING RESPONSIBILITIES	RATIONALE
2. Turn the patient every 2 hours and give skin care.	2. Prevents skin breakdown from pressure and moisture; also aids in respiration by preventing hypostatic pneumonia and atelectasis
3. Patients able to follow simple directions should be instructed to exhale upon turning or moving.	3. Prevents initiation of Valsalva maneuver
4. Assist patient in moving up in bed. Do *not* ask him to push with his heels. Do not allow patient to push or pull with his arms or push against the footboard.	4. Prevents initiation of Valsalva maneuver
5. Do not encourage or suggest isometric exercises for your alert bed patient. Passive range-of-motion exercises *should* be incorporated into the nursing care plan.	5. Isometric exercises initiate the Valsalva maneuver, while passive range-of-motion exercises do not. Muscle tone, atrophy, and contractures are prevented by administering passive range-of-motion exercises.
Fluid Restriction, If Any	
1. Note the total amount of fluid restriction for a 24-hour period and divide by 3. This will give you the amount allowed for your 8-hour shift. If the patient is receiving a tray for meals, you might allow a little more for the day shift because breakfast and lunch are served in that period. Note that fluid intake by the intravenous or oral route is all computed into the restriction. Place a tape conspicuously on the patient's bed to indicate to other personnel the amount of fluid restriction.	1. Fluid restriction aids in decreasing extracellular fluid from the body. Increased intracranial pressure can be controlled or decreased to some degree by control of fluid intake.
Management of the Excretory System	
1. Testing of fractional urinary output and periodic specific gravity of urine will probably be ordered.	1. Indicate the amount of diuresis and urinary dilution. With trauma, diabetes insipidus may be precipitated and would be evidenced by a decrease in specific gravity and an increase in output.
2. Stool softeners should be administered. Avoid enemas or straining at stool.	2. The Valsalva maneuver is initiated by straining at stool or by an enema and must be avoided.
Ventricular Drainage	
1. With ventriculostomy drainage, the elevation of the head of the bed will depend on the physician. The nurse should know how high the drainage bottle should be kept above the level of insertion. Strict aseptic technique must be used to prevent infection.	1. Placing the collection container at too low a level provides for a too-rapid removal of drainage and can lead to brain herniation; placing the collection container at too high a level will prevent drainage from occurring.
2. Maintain sterility at all times.	2. Prevents infection
3. Maintain a closed system.	3. Prevents infection
Continuous Intracranial Monitoring	
1. If this technique is in use, the nurse must be familiar with the specific type of monitoring device in use.	1. The safety of the patient and standards of care must be maintained.
2. The nurse must be aware of her responsibilities of interpreting the readings and what should be done about atypical readings.	2. Same as 1
3. Maintain strict aseptic technique.	3. Prevention of infection is vital.
General Nursing Management	
1. Plan nursing care so that those activities that are apt to produce spikes in intracranial pressure are not clustered together.	1. Contrary to what has been considered good organizational skills in patient management, it is best not to cluster turning and pulling the patient, getting him on and off a bedpan, and suctioning him into the same time period. Individually, these activities may not cause spikes in the patient at risk, but collectively, spikes can be precipitated.

(continued)

CHART 12–5. (continued)

NURSING RESPONSIBILITIES	RATIONALE
2. Review laboratory reports (blood urea nitrogen, electrolytes, blood gases, osmolarities, creatinine, and so forth).	2. Identify abnormal findings and report them to the physician.
3. Check stools for occult blood daily.	3. A side-effect of Decadron administration is gastrointestinal bleeding.
4. Check urine for sugar and acetone every 6 hours; blood sugar should also be monitored.	4. A side-effect of Decadron therapy is hyperglycemia and glucose in the urine.
5. Monitor blood level of anticonvulsive drug.	5. For control of potential seizure activity, a therapeutic drug level must be maintained.
6. Maintain on seizure precautions.	6. Prevents injury to patient should a seizure occur
7. Monitor specific gravity of urine.	7. Gives some indication of osmolarity and development of diabetes insipidus
8. Remove elastic stockings daily to inspect legs for signs and symptoms of thrombophlebitis; then reapply stocking.	8. Thrombophlebitis is a common complication for patients on bed rest. Pulmonary emboli can result from dislodged thrombi.
9. Add all of the other points of good basic nursing care.	9. A high standard of care must be maintained to prevent complications from developing and to reverse the signs and symptoms of increased intracranial pressure.
Drug Therapy	
1. The nurse must be well versed on action, dosage, preparation, route, side-effects, contraindications, and interactions of a drug.	1. Provides for safety of the patient and ensures optimum therapeutic value from drugs
2. Common drugs used include	
• Osmotic diuretics (mannitol, glucose, urea).	• Decreases cerebral edema and increases intracranial pressure
• Dexamethasone (Decadron) 4 mg to 20 mg in divided doses, PO, IM, or IV	• Reduces cerebral edema
• Phenytoin (Dilantin) 100 mg tid, PO	• Prevents seizure activity
• Colace 100 mg tid, PO	• Stool softener to prevent straining at stool (Valsalva maneuver)
• Maalox (or another antacid) 30 ml PO with Decadron	• Prevents gastrointestinal irritation
• Cimetidine (Tagamet) 300 mg qid, PO or IV	• Prevents stimulation of gastric secretions
• Tylenol 650 mg, PO or PR	• Controls elevated temperature
• Prophylactic broad-spectrum antibiotics will probably be ordered if the patient is on ventricular drainage or continuous intracranial monitoring.	• Prevents infection

should be identified from the subtle earlier signs and symptoms.)

The respiratory pattern, although considered to be a vital sign, is more sensitive to change; therefore, it is an earlier indicator of change. The rate and character of the respiratory pattern should be noted. The type of breathing pattern evidenced in Cheyne–Stokes respirations, central neurogenic hyperventilation, or apneustic, cluster, or ataxic breathing can correlate with the site of the neuroanatomical lesion. This information is valuable because it indicates what part of the brain is affected, particularly if a rostral–caudal deterioration is in process. If respirations change from Cheyne–Stokes respirations to central neurogenic hyperventilation, deterioration is occurring (see Fig. 12–3). However, respiratory failure from cardiopulmonary disease, direct muscle paralysis disease (Guillain–Barré syndrome), or injury to the cervical region of the spinal cord must be differentiated from the various abnormal breathing patterns outlined in order to be significant.

MAINTENANCE OF A PATENT AIRWAY AND ADEQUATE VENTILATION

The patency of an airway can be determined by listening to the respirations; examining the patient; noting the rate, depth, and pattern of the patient's respirations; and observing skin color for any signs of cyanosis. Adequate ventilation can best be evaluated by review of the blood gas analysis. The airway is examined for the presence of complete or partial obstruction by foreign materials such as mucus, which interfere with breathing.

CHART 12–6. *NURSING CARE PLAN FOR THE PATIENT WITH ACUTE INCREASED INTRACRANIAL PRESSURE (INTRACRANIAL HYPERTENSION)**

NURSING DIAGNOSIS	EXPECTED OUTCOME	NURSING INTERVENTION
Altered neurological function	The patient will not deteriorate further neurologically.	• Establish a baseline assessment of neurofunction. • To denote change, conduct frequent, ongoing assessments and compare the findings with previous assessments. • Note changes in neurological and vital signs and take appropriate action.
Potential of precipitating activities to increase intracranial pressure	The factors that are known to increase intracranial pressure will be controlled or eliminated.	• Identify each potential factor that can increase intracranial pressure and institute appropriate preventive nursing intervention.
Potential of hypercapnia and hypoxemia	Normal arterial blood gases will be maintained.	• Avoid sedative drugs. • Monitor periodic blood gases. • Provide oxygen therapy as necessary. • Hyperventilate the patient periodically to reduce carbon dioxide. • If hyperventilating with an Ambu bag, maintain rhythm with respiratory pattern of patient. • For patient on ventilator, report asynchrony with ventilator. Administer muscle relaxant (pancuronium bromide) or other similar drug, if ordered. • Maintain a patent airway. • Hyperventilate the lungs with 100% pure oxygen for 60 seconds before and after suctioning, if approved by the physician. • Suction gently. • If suctioning precipitates elevated waves on the intracranial pressure monitor that remain elevated, administer lidocaine, if ordered. • Limit suctioning to no more than 15 seconds per insertion of catheter. • Allow the patient to catch his breath between suctioning. • Pull the patient up in bed so that respirations are facilitated.
Potential of increased cerebral metabolism	Normothermia will be maintained.	• Assess body temperature at least every 4 hours. • Assess for cause of elevated temperature. • Remove excess bed clothes. • Apply cooling (hypothermia) blanket. Do not allow shivering. • Check rectal temperature every 30 minutes while on cooling blanket. • Turn cooling blanket off when temperature drops below 99.8° F (prevents drift).
Potential of impaired venous drainage of the brain	Venous drainage from the brain will be facilitated.	• Prevent initiation of the Valsalva maneuver. *Positioning and turning* • Maintain the neck in a neutral position at all times; use a collar or rolls if necessary. • Use a small pillow placed under the head and shoulders. • Avoid Trendelenburg and prone positions. • Avoid positioning with extreme hip flexion. • Do not turn laterally with the head of the bed up 30 degrees. • When turning laterally, keep the patient's head in a neutral position. • Elevate the head of the bed 30 to 45 degrees. • If patient is conscious, ask him to exhale when he is moved or turned. *Other* • Keep patient from straining at stool. • Implement a bowel program that includes stool softeners. • Keep patient from coughing or sneezing

(continued)

CHART 12–6. (continued)

NURSING DIAGNOSIS	EXPECTED OUTCOME	NURSING INTERVENTION
Potential of isometric contractions	Isometric contractions will be avoided.	• Do not encourage isometric exercises. • Administer passive range-of-motion exercises. • Caution against pushing with the feet against the bed. • Caution against pushing with the feet against the footboard. • Do not ask the patient to grip the siderails when turning him. • Control shivering by adding blankets; lowering the body temperature slowly, if an elevated temperature is present; or using chlorpromazine. • Administer muscle relaxants, if ordered, to control extreme decerebration.
Potential of emotional upset	The patient will not become emotionally upset.	• Maintain a calm, reassuring manner. • Control the environment for noise, odors, temperature, and so forth. • Do not discuss potentially upsetting topics (prognosis, pain) within the patient's hearing range. • Caution the family against discussing upsetting topics in front of patient. • Provide soft, soothing stimuli such as soft music, therapeutic touch, the voice of loved ones on a tape recorder, and so forth.
Sleep–wakefulness disturbance	The patient will not be awakened.	• Avoid arousal from sleep.
Alterations in comfort: noxious stimuli	The patient will be free of noxious stimuli.	• Assess and control for noxious stimuli.
Fluid volume excess	The patient will be maintained in a slightly dehydrated state.	• Institute a fluid restriction diet. • Explain purpose and implementation to patient and family. • Post fluid restriction. • Maintain an intake and output record. • Divide fluid allowance for the 24-hour period. • Calculate intravenous fluids, oral intake, and enteral feeding as part of intake.
Potential of infection	Infection will not develop.	• Maintain a closed system. • Inspect dressing at insertion site for drainage. • Change dressing in approved manner. • Inspect insertion site for signs and symptoms of infection. • Inject antibiotics into line, if ordered. • Monitor complete blood count and culture and sensitivity studies. • Maintain strict aseptic technique.
Potential of alterations in cerebral perfusion	Adequate cerebral perfusion will be maintained.	• Observe for "pressure signs." • Observe the spikes on intracranial pressure monitor. • Control all the factors known to increase intracranial pressure.
Potential of cerebral herniation	Cerebral herniation will not develop.	• Maintain ongoing neurological assessments and compare with previous findings. • Note changes and trends of deterioration in neurological signs. • Observe for signs of herniation. • Institute corrective measures if deterioration is noted (*e.g.*, hyperventilation). • Report findings to physician immediately. • If on continued cerebrospinal fluid drainage, maintain collection bags at prescribed levels. • Do not cluster together activities known to increase intracranial pressure.

* In addition, the Nursing Care Plan for the Unconscious Patient (Chap. 11) should be integrated into this plan of care.

Periodic suctioning can be used to remove mucus and other drainage from the airway. Strict aseptic technique is followed to prevent infection. In the instance of an unconscious patient, or one unable to manage his own secretions, the patient is totally dependent on the nurse to remove secretions.

An endotracheal tube or tracheostomy may be necessary either alone or in conjunction with a mechanical respirator if a patent airway cannot be maintained.

Oxygen can be administered at various concentrations to provide an adequate oxygen supply. The values of PO_2 and PCO_2 obtained from drawing blood gases are accurate and valid indices of oxygenation.

Positioning the patient on his side to allow for drainage of secretions from the mouth can also promote an adequate airway. The patient should be turned from side to side at least every 2 hours so that secretions do not pool in the upper or lower respiratory tract. Turning the patient from side to side is also helpful in preventing atelectasis.

Periodic chest physical therapy should be administered to loosen secretions in all lobes of the lungs.

Routine mouth care should be given to any patient receiving oxygen therapy, patients having copious mucus and other drainage from the mouth, patients requiring frequent suctioning, all unconscious patients, and patients with endotracheal or tracheal tubes (who also require periodic tracheostomy care).

By frequent observation, review of blood gases, suctioning, positioning, and use of oxygen or ventilation therapy as ordered, the patency and adequacy of ventilation can be maintained. For care of the patient on a ventilator, see Chapter 11.

HYPERVENTILATION

The purpose of hyperventilation is to provide for the exchange of larger volumes of air and oxygen so that the carbon dioxide blood level will be reduced. Carbon dioxide is a potent vasodilator when given in excessive amounts, but it will cause vasoconstriction if its level is lower than normal. The goal of hyperventilation therapy is to reduce the $PaCO_2$ level to 25 mm to 30 mm Hg (normal is 35 mm to 45 mm Hg) to cause vasoconstriction and subsequent reduction in intracranial pressure.

The patient on controlled hyperventilation is intubated and attached to a ventilator that has been adjusted for hyperventilation. The nurse should follow these points of care:

- Review the periodic blood gases to be sure that the patient's gases are within the parameters prescribed by the physician.
- If the patient is agitated or bucking the ventilator, try to determine the cause; if he continues, report this to the physician who may wish to order a curarelike muscle relaxant (pancuronium, 0.1 mg/kg, or metocurine, 0.3 mg/kg) or a small dose of morphine sulfate (1 mg to 2 mg every 2 hours) to get the patient synchronized with the ventilator.
- Patients on hyperventilation therapy are usually monitored extensively, including intracranial pressure monitoring; monitor all of the data.
- Do not let the arterial carbon dioxide drop below the prescribed lower level because decreased cardiac output and hypoxia can result.
- If the patient is not on a ventilator, there may be an order to hyperventilate the patient if there are any spikes in intracranial pressure; this can be accomplished by attaching the Ambu bag to the endotracheal tube or tracheostomy tube and Ambuing the patient until the spikes disappear. The nurse should synchronize squeezing the bag with the patient's respirations or else the intrathoracic pressure will be elevated, causing a decrease in the venous drainage from the brain; the intracranial pressure will be raised rather than lowered as a result of the procedure.

PREVENTION OF ACTIVITIES THAT INCREASE INTRACRANIAL PRESSURE

The goal of nursing management is to prevent the development of pressure signs and plateau waves, which compromise the cerebral perfusion pressure. The factors that increase intracranial pressure were discussed previously in this chapter. The nursing management for preventing development of increased intracranial pressure includes

Hypercapnia and hypoxemia

- Keep the patient well oxygenated
- Limit suctioning time to no more than 15 seconds
- Hyperinflate the lungs with 100% oxygen before and after suctioning
- Lidocaine may be administered if the patient has spikes in pressure when suctioned
- See page 264 for respiratory and suctioning procedure

Vasodilating drugs

- Drugs that have a vasodilating effect are not usually given because they increase cerebral blood flow and intracranial pressure.

Valsalva maneuver

- Prevent straining at stool by instituting a bowel program that includes stool softeners
- Keep the neck in neutral position at all times
- Do not administer enemas
- Avoid Trendelenburg and prone positions; turning the patient with the head of the bed up; coughing, sneezing, extreme hip flexion, and isometric contractions
- See page 265 for a more detailed discussion of these areas

Arousal from sleep and REM sleep

- Arousal from sleep and the REM phase of sleep are both known to increase intracranial pressure
- Do not arouse from sleep
- Do not administer other procedures known to increase intracranial pressure when the patient is in REM sleep to prevent the cumulative effect

Emotional upset and noxious stimuli

- Both are known to increase intracranial pressure
- Maintain a quiet and peaceful environment
- Provide soft stimuli
- Assess for presence of pain and take measures to reverse the problem
- See page 266 for a more detailed discussion

Clustering of procedures

- The cumulative effect of scheduling several procedures close together is known to increase intracranial pressure dramatically; avoid clustering procedures in the patient at risk
- See page 266 for a more detailed discussion

FLUID RESTRICTION

The purpose of fluid restriction is to keep the patient slightly underhydrated to help to alleviate cerebral edema and subsequently decrease intracranial pressure. See page 277 for the method of implementing the restriction.

The nursing responsibilities include the following:

- Post a fluid restriction sign on the patient's bed; note on the intake and output record as well as on the parameter and nursing care plan that a fluid restriction is in effect
- Divide the fluid restriction over the 24-hour period by work shifts for the convenience of the nurses (usually there are three shifts)
- Maintain an accurate intake and output record
- Explain the purpose of the fluid restriction to the patient and family and gain their cooperation
- Know that the fluid restriction limit includes all oral and intravenous fluids as well as fluids administered by feeding tube
- Keep the patient within his fluid restriction

CEREBROSPINAL FLUID DRAINAGE

The major nursing responsibilities in caring for a patient with ventricular drainage include (1) maintaining the sterility of the equipment, (2) maintaining the dry sterile dressing at the catheter and incision site for drainage, (3) keeping the collection container at the prescribed level; (4) observing the drainage tubing to ensure that the drainage system is intact without kinks; (5) monitoring the amount of drainage in the collection container, and (6) adhering to the approved procedure for dressing change.

CONTINUOUS INTRACRANIAL MONITORING

As discussed previously, continuous intracranial monitoring is a valid and reliable method for checking the continuous changes in intracranial pressure. At present this technique is most commonly used at larger centers. Continuous intracranial monitoring resembles ventricular drainage with respect to the method of insertion and nursing management. However, the monitoring sensor and transducer are inserted primarily for monitoring the pressure waves of the intracranial pressure, while the ventriculotomy is designed for removing excess drainage. The continuous monitoring is set up in such a way that drainage can be removed, if necessary, but it does not provide a route for continuous drainage.

The nursing management of the patient must be concerned with (1) maintaining sterility, (2) observing the dry, sterile dressing around the insertion site for drainage, (3) positioning the equipment and patient properly, and (4) keeping the system intact and operational. In addition, the nurse must be able to identify the various intracranial pressure waves and know what action, if any, should be taken in response to specific types of pressure waves.

GENERAL NURSING MANAGEMENT

The management of basic needs for the patient with increased intracranial pressure will most likely follow those outlined in Chapter 11. The reader is referred to that chapter.

BARBITURATE COMA THERAPY

Nursing management for the patient undergoing barbiturate therapy is indeed critical. The patient has not responded to conventional treatment methods for increased intracranial pressure and is now being treated with drug induction that will negate all of the usual reflexes (corneal, pupillary, gag, swallowing) and spontaneous respiratory function in an attempt to decrease cerebral metabolism and cause vasoconstriction. The usual focus of a neurological assessment such as the pupillary signs, other reflexes, and consciousness will not be present for the nurse to use as a data base to assess the patient. Several pieces of monitoring and supportive equipment will be in place such as the cardiac monitor, intracranial pressure monitor, ventilator, Swan–Ganz line, central venous pressure line, and others. Using the data from the monitoring devices and the laboratory, decisions will be made for controlling the cerebral perfusion pressure, intracranial pressure, blood pressure, respiratory function, blood level of barbiturates, and body temperature. The reader is directed to the discussion of barbiturate coma earlier in this chapter.

One important point is that the barbiturate, which is usually pentobarbital, is stored in body fat. The decision to discontinue barbiturate coma is not followed by declaring the patient brain dead. The brain death criteria followed by physicians in the United States is based on the absence of spontaneous respirations and brain stem reflexes. These criteria cannot be determined until the drug is cleared out of the body. In an obese person, the clearance time is longer than in a thin person. As a general rule of thumb, one should wait 1 day for every day that the patient was in barbiturate coma. It can be difficult to wait because in some instances the body appears to be deteriorating and organ donation is a consideration. However, there are serious medical–legal implications if the time table is rushed.

REFERENCES

1. Miller J: Volume and pressure in the craniospinal axis. Clin Neurosurg 22:76, 1975
2. Ropper A, Kennedy S, Zervas N: Neurological and Neurosurgical Intensive Care, p 11. Baltimore, University Park Press, 1983
3. Mitchell P: Intracranial hypertension: Implications of research

for nursing care. J Neurosurg Nurs 12(3):145, September 1980
4. Klatzo I: Neuropathological aspects of brain edema. J Neuropathol Exp Neurol 20:1, January 1967
5. Speers I: Cerebral edema. J Neurosurg Nurs 13(2):102, April 1981
6. Adams R, Victor M: Principles of Neurology, 2nd ed, pp 435–436. New York, McGraw–Hill, 1981
7. Howe J: Patient Care in Neurosurgery, 2nd ed, pp 138–139. Boston, Little, Brown & Co, 1983
8. Shillito J Jr, Ojemann R: Hydrocephalus. In Youmans JR (ed): Neurological Surgery, pp 559–587. Philadelphia, FA Davis, 1980
9. Plum F, Posner J: The Diagnosis of Stupor and Coma, 3rd ed. Philadelphia, FA Davis, 1980
10. Mitchell P, Ozuna J, Lipe H: Moving the patient in bed: Effects on intracranial pressure. Nurs Res 30(4):212, July–August, 1981
11. Lundberg N: Continuous recording and control of ventricular fluid pressure in neurological practice. Acta Psychiatr Scand [Suppl] 149(36):1, 1960
12. Vires J et al: A subarachnoid screw for monitoring intracranial pressure. J Neurosurg Nurs 39:416, September 1973
13. Levin A: The use of a fiberoptic intracranial pressure monitor in clinical practice. Neurosurg 1(3):266, November/December, 1977
14. Marcotty SF, Levin AB: A new approach in epidural intracranial pressure monitoring. J Neurosurg Nurs 16(1):54, February 1984
15. Langfitt T: Increased intracranial pressure. Clin Neurosurg 16:436, 1968
16. Jagger J, Bobovsky J: Nonpharmacologic therapeutic modalities. Crit Care Q 5(4):31, March 1983

BIBLIOGRAPHY

Books

Cunitz G, Gaab M: Effect of some analgesics, sedative and IV anesthetics on ICP in man. In Intracranial Pressure IV, pp 619–621. New York, Springer–Verlag, 1980

Davis J, Mason C: Neurological Critical Care. New York, Van Nostrand Reinhold, 1979

Eliasson S et al: Neurological Pathophysiology, 2nd ed, pp 306–312. New York, Oxford University Press, 1978

Fernstermacher JD, Patlak CS: The movements of water and solutes in the brains of mammals. In Pappius HM, Feindel W (eds): Dynamics of Brain Edema. New York, Springer–Verlag, 1976

Fishman RA: Cerebrospinal Fluid in Diseases of the Nervous System, pp 107–128. Philadelphia, WB Saunders, 1980

Guyton A: Textbook of Medical Physiology, 5th ed, pp 373–375. Philadelphia, WB Saunders, 1976

Hossman KA: Development and resolution of ischemic brain swelling. In Pappius HM, Fiendel W (eds): Dynamics of Brain Edema. New York, Springer–Verlag, 1976

Hudak C, Lohr T, Gallo B: Critical Care Nursing, 3rd ed. Philadelphia, JB Lippincott, 1982

Jennett B, Teasdale G: Management of Head Injuries, pp 45–75. Philadelphia, FA Davis, 1981

Klatzo I: Pathophysiology of brain edema: Pathological aspects. In Advances in Neurosurgery I, pp 1–4. New York, Springer–Verlag, 1973

Klatzo I, Sutelburger F (eds): Brain Edema. New York, Springer–Verlag, 1967

Langfitt T: Increased intracranial pressure. In Youmans JR (ed): Neurological Surgery, pp 443–495. Philadelphia, WB Saunders, 1973

Meinig et al: The effects of dexamethasone and diuretics on peritumor brain edema: Comparative study of tissue water content and CT. In Pappius HM, Feindel W (eds): Dynamics of Brain Edema. New York, Springer–Verlag, 1976

Miller JD, Sullivan HG: Severe intracranial hypertension. In International Anesthesiology Clinics: Management of Acute Intracranial Disasters, pp 19–75, 1979

Reulen H, Schurman K (eds): Steroids in Brain Edema. New York, Springer–Verlag, 1972

Smith R: Essentials of Neurosurgery, pp 99–101. Philadelphia, JB Lippincott, 1980

Taylor J, Ballenger S: Neurological Dysfunctions and Nursing Intervention. New York, McGraw–Hill, 1980

Periodicals

Abbey J et al: A pilot study: The control of shivering during hypothermia by a clinical nursing measure. J Neurosurg Nurs 5(2):78, December 1973

Adams R et al: Symptomatic occult hydrocephalus with "normal" cerebrospinal fluid pressure. N Engl J Med 273:117, July 1965

Ambielli M: Drug stop. J Neurosurg Nurs 13(6):344, December 1981

Barson W: Pharmacologic therapeutic modalities: Barbiturates. Crit Care Q 5(4):63, March 1983

Bell M et al: Nursing involvement with monitoring of ICP. J Neurosurg Nurs 7(1):28, July 1975

Bolton M: Hyperbaric oxygen therapy. Am J Nurs, p 1199, June 1981

Bruce D, Gennarelli T, Langfitt T: Resuscitation from coma due to head injury. Crit Care Med 6:254–267, 1978

Calvin R: Continuous ventricular or lumbar subarachnoid drainage of cerebrospinal fluid. J Neurosurg Nurs 9(1):12, March 1977

Clasen R et al: Experimental study of relation of fever to cerebral edema. J Neurosurg Nurs 9(1):12, March 1977

Donegan M, Bedford R: Intravenously administered lidocaine prevents intracranial hypertension during endotracheal suctioning. Anesthesiology 52:96, June 1980

Eilers M: Pharmacologic therapeutic modalities: Osmotic and diuretic agents. Crit Care Q 5(4):44, March 1983

Fishman RA: Brain edema. New Engl J Med 293:706–711, October 2, 1975

Fode N, Laws E, Sundt T: Communicating hydrocephalus after subarachnoid hemorrhage: Results of shunt procedures. J Neurosurg Nurs 11(4):253, December 1979

Foldes F, Arrowood J: Changes in cerebrospinal fluid pressure under the influence of continuous subarachnoid infusion of normal saline. J Clin Invest 27:346–351, 1948

Frank E, Tew J: Normal-pressure hydrocephalus: Clinical symptoms, diagnosis, pathophysiology, and treatment. Heart Lung 11(4):321, July–August, 1982

Gifford R, Plaut M: Abnormal respiratory patterns in the comatose patient caused by intracranial dysfunction. J Neurosurg Nurs 7(1):57, July 1975

Goloskov J et al: A new method for managing extracellular fluid accumulations in central nervous system disorders. J Neurosurg Nurs 8(1):53, July 1976

Graf C, Rossi N: Pulmonary edema and the central nervous system: A clinicopathological study. Surg Neurol 4:319, 1975

Hanlon K: Intracranial compliance interpretation and clinical application. J Neurosurg Nurs 9(1):34, March 1977

Hanlon K: Description and uses of intracranial pressure monitoring. Heart Lung 5(2):277, March–April 1976

Hausman K: Nursing care of the patient with hydrocephalus. J Neurosurg Nurs 13(6):326, December 1981

Hoffman J, Orban D, Podolsky S: Pharmacological therapeutic modalities: Corticosteroids. Crit Care Q 5(4):52, March 1983

Jackson P: Ventriculo-peritoneal shunts. Am J Nurs, p 1104, June 1980

Jimm L: Nursing assessment of patients for increased intracranial pressure. J Neurosurg Nurs 6(1):27, July 1974

Johnson L: If your patient has increased intracranial pressure, your goal should be: No surprises. Nurs '83 13(6):58, June 1983

Johnston I, Paterson A, Besser M: The treatment of benign intracranial hypertension: A review of 134 cases. Surg Neurol 16:218–224, 1981

Jones A: Nursing implications in the administration of urea. J Neurosurg Nurs 7(1):37, July 1975

Jones C, Cayard C: Care of ICP monitoring devices: A nursing responsibility. J Neurosurg Nurs 14(5):255, October 1982

Katzman R et al: Report of the joint committee for stroke resources, brain edema in stroke. Stroke 8(4):512–540, July–August, 1977

Kenning JA, Toutant SM, Saunders RI: Upright patient positioning in the management of intracranial hypertension. Surg Neurol 15:148–152, 1981

Kimball C, Belber C: Protocol for intravenous barbiturate therapy on increased intracranial pressure in a community hospital. J Neurosurg Nurs 11(3):144, September 1979

Klatzo I: Presidential address on the neuropathological aspects of cerebral edema. J Neurosurg 26:1–4, 1967

Lamas E, Lobato R: Intraventricular pressure and CSF dynamics in chronic adult hydrocephalus. Surg Neurol 12:287, 1979

Langfitt T: Cerebral circulation and metabolism. J Neurosurg 40:461, 1974

Lobato R et al: Prognostic value of the intracranial pressure levels during the acute phase of severe head injuries. Acta Neurochir [Suppl] 28:70–73, 1979

Lundberg N et al: Clinical investigations on interrelations between intracranial pressure and intracranial hemodynamics. Prog Brain Res 30:69, 1968

Marsh M et al: Neurological intensive care. Anesthesiology 47:149, 1977

Marshall L et al: The outcome with aggressive treatment in severe head injuries. Part II: Acute and chronic barbiturate administration in the management of head injury. J Neurosurg 50:26, 1979

Marshall L et al: Pentobarbital therapy for intracranial hypertension in metabolic coma (Reye's syndrome). Crit Care Med 6:1, 1978

Martin M: Pharmacologic therapeutic modalities: Phenytoin, dimethyl sulfoxide, and calcium channel blockers. Crit Care Q 5(4):72, March 1983

Mauss N, Mitchell P: Increased intracranial pressure: An update. Heart Lung 5(6):919, November–December, 1976

McNamara M, Quinn C: Epidural intracranial pressure monitoring: Theory and clinical application. J Neurosurg Nurs 13(5):267, October 1981

McQueen J, Jeanes L: Influence of hypothermia on intracranial hypertension. J Neurosurg 19:277, 1962

Michael TA: The esophageal obturator airway. JAMA 246(10):1098–1101, 1981

Miller D, Leech P: Effects on mannitol and steroid therapy. J Neurosurg 42:274, March 1975

Miller J et al: Significance of intracranial hypertension in severe head injury. J Neurosurg 47:503, 1977

Mirr M, Jankowski K, Taylor M: Nursing management for barbiturate therapy in acute head injuries. Heart Lung 12(1):52, January 1983

Mitchell P, Mauss N: Intracranial pressure: Fact and fancy. Nurs '76, 6:53, June 1976

Nikas D, Konkoly R: Nursing responsibilities in arterial and intracranial pressure monitoring. J Neurosurg Nurs 7(2):116, December 1975

Norkool D: Current concepts of hyperbaric oxygenation and its application in critical care. Heart Lung 8(4):728, July–August 1979

Pollack L, Goldstein G: Lowering of intracranial pressure in Reye's syndrome by sensory stimulation. New Engl J Med 304(12):732, 1981

Price M: Significance of intracranial pressure waveform. J Neurosurg Nurs 13(4):202, August 1981

Ramirez B: When you're faced with a neuro patient. RN 42:67, January 1979

Reivich M: Regulation of cerebral circulation. Clin Neurosurg 16:378, 1968

Ricci M: Intracranial hypertension: Barbiturate therapy and the role of the nurse. J Neurosurg Nurs 11(4):247, December 1979

Rudy E: Early omens of cerebral disaster. Nurs '77 7:58, February 1977

Selman WR et al: Management of prolonged therapeutic barbiturate. Surg Neurol 15:9–10, 1981

Shapiro H: Intracranial hypertension. Anesthesiology 43:445, 1975

Stone M: Normal pressure hydrocephalus. Nurs Clin North Am 9(4):667, December 1974

Taylor F, Schutz H: Symptoms caused by intracranial pressure waves. J Neurosurg Nurs 9(4):144, December 1977

Tilbury M: The intracranial screw—A new assessment tool. Nurs Clin North Am 9(4):641, December 1974

Turner M: Intracranial hypertension. Crit Care Q 2:67, June 1979

Weinstein J et al: Experimental study of patterns of brain distortion and ischemia produced by an intracranial mass. J Neurosurg 28:513, 1968

Young MS: Understanding the signs of intracranial pressure: A bedside guide. Nurs '81 11(2):59, February 1981

Zegeer L: Nursing care of the patient with brain edema. J Neurosurg Nurs 14(5):268, October 1982

chapter 13

Water Balance

Water balance is a homeostatic necessity for maintaining health. Fluid and electrolyte balance are controlled by several interrelated mechanisms in the body. When considering fluid and electrolyte balance, the fluid referred to is water and the major electrolytes are sodium, potassium, and chloride. Deviation from the normal limits of fluid and electrolyte balance in the body will cause serious health problems. An understanding of the relationship of fluid and electrolyte balance and neurological–neurosurgical conditions is imperative for the nurse practicing in this specialty area.

The conditions that will be discussed in this chapter include diabetes insipidus (DI), syndrome of inappropriate secretion of antidiuretic hormone (SIADH), hyperosmolar nonketotic hyperglycemia, and various electrolyte imbalances.

DISTRIBUTION OF WATER IN THE BODY

According to Guyton, 57% of the total fat-free body weight is composed of water. It is distributed between two major compartments: the intracellular space, which contains 36% of the body weight, and the extracellular space, which contains 21%.[1] Of the extracellular fluid, plasma accounts for 5% while the other 16% is found in the interstitial spaces. With changes in the overall fluid volume within the body, the water content is redistributed in the body compartments by a process known as osmosis. Electrolytes, mainly potassium and sodium, enter into osmosis. Sodium is the major ion in the extracellular space while potassium is the major intracellular ion.

OSMOLALITY

Osmolality refers to the concentration of solute (ion particles) in a solvent (water) per unit of total volume of solution; it is the ability of fluid to hold water or draw it through a semipermeable cell membrane. Hyperosmolality occurs when there is a depletion of body water or an excess of salt. Hypoosmolality occurs when there is an excess of water or a depletion of salt. Normal values for osmolarity are as follows:

- Serum: 280 mOsm to 295 mOsm/kg water (285 mOsm is considered normal)
- Urine: 50 mOsm to 1400 mOsm/kg water (range)
- The normal ratio of urine to serum osmolality is one to four.

PHYSIOLOGICAL CONTROL OF WATER BALANCE IN THE BODY

Several physiological mechanisms control water balance in the body; these include the neurohypophyseal system, the thirst center, the renin–angiotensin–aldosterone system, and the various receptors and neural stimuli that activate these mechanisms.

THE NEUROHYPOPHYSEAL SYSTEM

The neurohypophyseal system includes the anterior hypothalamus and the posterior hypophysis (neurohypophysis). This system plays a major role in water balance because it produces, stores, and secretes antidiuretic hormone (ADH), which facilitates the reabsorption of water in the body by acting upon the tubules in the kidney. The hypothalamus located slightly above the hypophysis is joined to the neurohypophysis by a ventral projection called the infundibulum or pituitary stalk. (The walls and floor of the third ventricle are created by the hypothalamus.) Within the hypothalamus there are two pairs of nuclear cell groupings called the supraoptic nuclei and paraventricular nuclei, so named for their anatomical location. Nerve tracts located within the nuclear cells, infundibulum, and neurohypophysis control the production of ADH, transportation of ADH through the infundibulum, and storage of ADH in the neurohypophysis. The ADH is stored until needed, when it is secreted into the perivascular space around the neurohypophysis where it enters the blood and the general circulation. The release of ADH is controlled by increased rates of facilitory or inhibitory impulses discharged within the nerve tracts that extend from the supraoptic and paraventricular cells through the infundibulum to the neurohypophysis.[2,3]

Once ADH enters the circulation, it acts on the distal convoluted tubules of the kidney to increase their permeability to water, thus causing water to be reabsorbed. The increased fluid reabsorption results in expansion and dilution of extracellular fluid so that the serum osmolarity is lowered and the volume expanded.

Three types of receptors provide a feedback system to control the secretion of ADH. They include

1. Osmoreceptors located within the hypothalamus that respond to changes in serum osmolarity (associated with the thirst center)
2. Stretch receptors located in the left atrium and large pulmonary veins that respond to changes in volume (hypovolemia/hypervolemia)
3. Baroreceptors located in the carotid sinus and aortic arch that respond to pressure changes (hypotension/hypertension)

Dehydration and hypotension stimulate ADH release while normovolemia or hypervolemia and increased systemic pressure inhibit ADH release.

THE THIRST CENTER

Osmoreceptors in the hypothalamus respond to changes in serum osmolarity. Hyperosmolarity stimulates the hypothalamic thirst center while hypoosmolarity inhibits the center. In the conscious healthy person, stimulation of the center sends a signal that the person is thirsty, thereby encouraging him to drink. However, motor deficits, dysphagia, or a decreased level of consciousness may interfere with the person's ability to respond appropriately to the thirst stimuli. Even a conscious and alert person may not perceive thirst signals when there is direct injury to the hypothalamus or an infectious process (e.g., meningitis), a tumor (e.g., pituitary adenoma), a vascular mass (e.g., aneurysm), or bleeding that involves the hypothalamus or adjacent anatomical structures.

The antidiuretic feedback system and the thirst center in the conscious patient are the major mechanisms for maintaining a normal range of osmolarity in the extracellular fluid. However, aldosterone also contributes to water balance in the body.

The Renin–Angiotensin–Aldosterone System

Aldosterone contributes to the regulation of sodium and water by stimulating the renal tubules to increase reabsorption of sodium ions while increasing excretion of potassium and hydrogen ions. Secretion of aldosterone from the adrenal cortex is activated by stimulation of volume receptors in the juxtaglomerular apparatus in response to a low renal perfusion pressure. Renin, which is released into the blood by the kidney's juxtaglomerular cells, acts on angiotensinogen, which has been produced by the liver, to form angiotensin I. When angiotensin I circulates through the lungs, two amino acids are removed. This reaction results in the formation of angiotensin II, a substance that stimulates the adrenal cortex (adrenal zona glomerulosa) to produce aldosterone. Aldosterone acts on the distal convolutions of the kidney to conserve sodium while excreting potassium and hydrogen ions. Sodium holds water so that water is also conserved.

FACTORS THAT INCREASE ADH RELEASE

Certain conditions or circumstances are known to increase the release of ADH, thereby conserving water in the body. They include the upright position; hyperthermia; hypotension; hyperosmolarity; hypovolemia, especially that caused by severe blood loss; myocardial failure; pain; anxiety; trauma; the stress response; and edematous states associated with hyponatremia.[2,4,5]

Drugs that increase ADH release have also been identified; they include morphine sulfate, chlorpromazine hydrochloride (Thorazine), chlorpropamide (Diabinase), chlorothiazide (Diuril), carbamazepine (Tegretol), barbiturates, angiotensin II, beta-adrenergic agents, cholinergic drugs, clofibrate (Atromid S), cyclophosphamide (Cytoxan), nicotine, vincristine sulfate (Oncovin), acetaminophen (Tylenol), meperidine hydrochloride (Demerol), and nicotine.[3,5]

FACTORS THAT DECREASE ADH RELEASE

There are also conditions and circumstances that decrease the release of ADH. They are the recumbent position, hypothermia, hypertension, hypoosmolarity, and increase in blood volume.

Drugs that decrease the release of ADH include adrenergic agents, anticholinergic agents, ethanol, phenytoin (Dilantin), glucocorticosteroids (e.g., dexamethasone), lithium carbonate, and demeclocycline (Declomycin).[2]

DIABETES INSIPIDUS (DI)

Diabetes insipidus is a condition of abnormal decreased secretion of ADH. The patient voids large amounts of dilute urine daily and is subject to fluid and electrolyte imbalance. The signs and symptoms include

- Polyuria (amounts range from 4 to 10 liters daily; hourly output exceeds 200 ml)
- Low urine specific gravity (1.001 to 1.005)
- Extreme thirst (polydipsia) if the patient is conscious and the thirst center is intact
- Dehydration (if fluids are not replaced)
- High serum osmolarity
- Elevated serum sodium (greater than 145 mEq/liter)
- Low urine osmolarity

PATHOPHYSIOLOGY

The pathophysiology of diabetes insipidus is related to decreased production and/or release of ADH, an increased breakdown of ADH, and, less commonly, a defect in the kidney tubule's response to ADH. The details of these possible defects were discussed in the previous section.

CLASSIFICATION

Diabetes insipidus has been classified by location and etiology (central neurogenic, nephrogenic), pattern of development, and permanency (transient, permanent).

Location or Etiology

Central diabetes insipidus is defined as cessation of the pituitary gland to secrete ADH because of damage from disease or injury to the hypothalamus, the supraopticohypophyseal tract, or the posterior lobe of the pituitary gland (neurohypophysis). Central diabetes insipidus can be subdivided into the following four types:

- Classical severe diabetes insipidus: failure to synthesize or release ADH
- Defective osmoreceptor diabetes insipidus: very high osmolarity fails to trigger secretion of ADH although the hormone is released in response to hypovolemia
- Reset osmoreceptor diabetes insipidus: secretion of ADH is not triggered until the plasma osmolarity is higher than the usual threshold
- Partial diabetes insipidus: although ADH is released at the usual threshold, the amount of hormone secreted is decreased.[6]

The most common cause of central diabetes insipidus is neurosurgery. Less commonly, the disease develops because of familial tendency, or idiopathic causes or because it is secondary to certain infections, neoplasms, vascular lesions, granulomatous disease, or severe head injury such as basal skull fracture. Postsurgical central diabetes insipidus usually occurs any time within 14 days of neurosurgery.[5] Nephrogenic diabetes insipidus is a rare form of the disorder caused by the inability of the kidneys to respond to ADH.

Pattern of Development

Central diabetes insipidus can develop in three distinct patterns following surgery. The patterns include

1. Initial diabetes insipidus: significant polyuria lasts a few days and then gradually subsides over the next 1 to 7 days; it is associated with edema of surgery.
2. Delayed diabetes insipidus, which may be permanent: the hypothalamus is damaged with some destruction of the ADH secretory cells; there is persistent polyuria of varying degree; the polyuria does not begin for about 3 to 4 days after injury because previously synthesized ADH has been released.
3. Triphasic diabetes insipidus: polyuria begins 1 to 2 days after surgery and lasts for 1 to 7 days. This is followed by 1 to 5 days of normal urinary output and then recurrence of polyuria. The period of normal urinary output is probably due to ADH being released until retrograde degeneration of damaged ADH production cells is complete.

Permanency

The classification of diabetes insipidus can also be made according to permanency of the condition. Transient diabetes insipidus can develop after surgery around the supraoptic hypophyseal tract, with skull fractures, or with other disease processes. Edema is thought to be the cause of the problem. The diabetes insipidus tends to be temporary, however, and normal secretion of ADH will usually be reestablished within a few days or a few weeks. The patient may or may not require treatment depending on the severity of the condition and his ability to balance intake and output. A condition of permanent diabetes insipidus will develop only if 80% or more of the ADH-producing nuclei of the hypothalamus and the proximal end of the pituitary stalk are destroyed. In this instance, the patient will require life-long treatment with replacement hormonal therapy.

DIAGNOSIS

The diagnosis of diabetes insipidus is based on the clinical findings of large amounts of urinary output coupled with low urinary specific gravity. However, a dehydration test may be ordered to determine what type of diabetes insipidus is present.

Dehydration Test

The following outlines the steps of the dehydration test:

- Measure serum osmolarity.
- Record patient's weight.
- Withhold fluids for 6 to 18 hours; for the patient with severe diabetes insipidus, begin the fluid restriction at 6 AM so that the patient can be carefully monitored; the test should be terminated if weight loss exceeds 2 kg or untoward clinical signs develop; in this instance, fluids are usually withheld for 4 to 8 hours. In a milder case of diabetes insipidus, begin withholding fluids at 6 PM for 12 to 18 hours.
- Withhold fluids until the osmolarity of at least two consecutive urine specimens collected on an hourly schedule are

stable (*i.e.*, the difference in osmolarity of urine samples is less than 30 mOsm/kg).
- Measure the plasma osmolarity.
- Administer 5 units of aqueous vasopressin subcutaneously.
- Measure the urine osmolarity 1 hour later.

The possible findings on the test include

- Complete central diabetes insipidus: after dehydration, urine osmolality is 50 mOsm to 200 mOsm/kg, urine specific gravity is less than 1.010, and plasma osmolality is 310 mOsm to 320 mOsm/kg; after vasopressin, urine osmolality will increase at least 100%.
- Partial central diabetes insipidus: after dehydration, urine osmolality is 250 mOsm to 500 mOsm/kg, urine specific gravity is 1.010 to 1.015, and plasma osmolality is 295 mOsm to 305 mOsm/kg; after vasopressin, urine osmolality increases 9% to 67%.
- Nephrogenic diabetes insipidus: after dehydration urine and plasma osmolalities are similar to findings in complete central diabetes insipidus; there is no response to vasopressin.[5]

TREATMENT

The treatment of diabetes insipidus initially includes the replacement of fluids and administration of ADH (vasopressin). The various types of drug preparations available and frequently ordered are listed in Table 13–1. For patients with mild diabetes insipidus, other drugs known to stimulate the hypothalamus to produce more ADH or enhance the kidney's response to the hormone may be ordered. These drugs are also included in Table 13–1.

If the diabetes insipidus is a permanent condition, the patient will require a patient teaching program and ongoing medical management.

NURSING MANAGEMENT

Assessment

The nurse caring for the neurological or neurosurgical patient should be aware of the possibility of the development of diabetes insipidus and monitor the patient accordingly. The following parameters are assessed:

- Urinary output every 1 to 2 hours
- Urinary specific gravity every 1 to 2 hours
- Accurate intake and output record
- Periodic serum osmolarity, electrolytes, and blood urea nitrogen
- Periodic urine osmolarity and electrolytes
- Signs and symptoms of dehydration
- Daily weight

In assessing the fractional urinary output for a patient with an altered level of consciousness, an indwelling catheter is usually used to facilitate the measurement of the urinary output on a specific time schedule. The amount of

TABLE 13–1. *Drugs Used in the Treatment of Diabetes Insipidus (DI)*

Name	*Usual Adult Dose*	*Duration*	*Comments*
Aqueous vasopressin	5 to 10 units SC	3 to 6 hours	Short duration; used for patients who have immediate postoperative DI or who cannot be monitored frequently
Vasopressin tannate in oil	5 units IM	24 to 72 hours	Painful injection; must be warmed and shaken to mix properly; need to rotate injection site; used if diabetes insipidus expected to last for a period of time
Lypressin nasal spray	Spray intranasally 3 to 4 times a day	4 to 6 hours	Nasal mucosa must be intact; useful for mild DI; patient may develop nasal congestion which will interfere with absorption
Desmopressin acetate (DDAVP)	0.1 ml to 0.4 ml intranasally	12 to 24 hours	Causes minimal nasoconstriction; administered once or twice a day; used for severe permanent or transient complete central DI
In milder forms of DI (when ADH is secreted in small amounts), the following drugs may be used to enhance the secretion of ADH or to increase the response of the kidney to ADH:			
Chlorpropamide (Diabinese)	250 mg to 500 mg/qd/PO	24 hours	Stimulates release of ADH from the posterior pituitary and enhances its action on renal tubules
Clofibrate (Atromid S)	500 mg/qid/PO	24 hours	Same as above
Carbamazepine (Tegretol)	400 mg to 600 mg/qd	24 hours	Same as above
Hydrochlorothiazide (HydroDiuril)	50 mg/qd or bid/PO	12 to 24 hours	Used for nephrogenic DI

urinary output in just 1 hour can be extraordinary. If the urinary output is 200 ml/hour or more for 2 consecutive hours, this information should be reported to the physician. In most instances, neurosurgical patients and those subject to increased intracranial pressure are kept in a slightly dehydrated state to control intracranial pressure. An output of 200 ml/hour or more for 2 consecutive hours can quickly lead to dehydration in these patients. The nurse will notice that the urine is very pale (straw colored) and dilute. A check of the specific gravity will indicate a reading of 1.005 or less. These two concurrent findings are usual signs of diabetes insipidus. Other findings include a rising serum sodium level and dehydration.

Implementation

The nursing responsibilities for the patient with diabetes insipidus include the hourly monitoring of urine output, specific gravity, and osmolarity. Serum osmolarity, electrolytes, and blood urea nitrogen levels should be carefully observed. The patient should be weighed daily and his oral intake measured and recorded. The patient should also be observed for signs and symptoms of dehydration and electrolyte imbalance.

A major responsibility of the nurse is managing fluid replacement. The oral route may be used if the patient is conscious and able to swallow adequate amounts of fluid. If this is not possible, the intravenous route should be used. The rate of infusion should be monitored frequently and the amount of intake compared with the amount of output. In the patient who has the triphasic pattern of diabetes insipidus, care should be taken to prevent water intoxication during the period of normovolemia of urine. During this period it is thought that patients may secrete an elevated level of ADH, similar to that seen in the syndrome of inappropriate secretion of antidiuretic hormone.

For the patient with permanent diabetes insipidus, a patient teaching plan should be developed and implemented. The following information should be included in the teaching plan:

- Information about diabetes insipidus
- Help in adjusting his daily schedule to living with diabetes insipidus
- Information about the drug protocol (frequency, side-effects, overdose)
- Follow-up care
- Medic Alert bracelet

See Potential of Knowledge Deficit and Potential of Noncompliance in Table 15–1 of the Nursing Care Plan for the Patient With Transsphenoidal Surgery.

SYNDROME OF INAPPROPRIATE SECRETION OF ANTIDIURETIC HORMONE

The condition called *syndrome of inappropriate secretion of antidiuretic hormone* (SIADH) is characterized by an abnormally high level or continuous secretion of ADH so that water is continually reabsorbed from the kidney tubules, resulting in water intoxication. The syndrome can be temporary or permanent with the severity of signs and symptoms depending on the amount of salt depleted and the amount of water retained. The fluid retention involves the total body rather than being restricted to a particular area or compartment of the body such as the lower extremities. The patient is often unaware that he is retaining fluid. The condition of concurrent water retention and hyponatremia is sometimes referred to as "cerebral salt wasting."

PATHOPHYSIOLOGY

The negative feedback mechanisms that normally control the release of ADH fail to function in SIADH. The precipitating factors that are associated with the pathophysiology are

- Bronchogenic carcinoma, especially oat cell carcinoma
- Lung disorders such as pneumonia, lung abscess, or tuberculosis
- Pressure on or injury to the hypothalamic–neurohypophyseal system (e.g., brain tumor, abscess, head trauma, subarachnoid bleeding, hydrocephalus, meningitis, encephalitis, Guillain–Barré syndrome)
- Pain, fear, or temperature change (may cause a temporary SIADH)
- Positive pressure breathing on a respirator (may cause a temporary SIADH)
- Certain drugs increase the secretion of ADH; these drugs were mentioned earlier in this chapter

SIGNS AND SYMPTOMS

The signs and symptoms of SIADH include

- Hyponatremia (serum sodium less than 126 mEq/liter)
- Serum hypoosmolality (less than 280 mOsm/kg of water)
- Increase in urine sodium; also called "salt wasting"
- Urine hyperosmolality
- Decreased urinary output (400 ml to 500 ml/24 hours); the urine appears to be concentrated
- Generalized weight gain
- If serum sodium has fallen below 126 mEq/liter, nausea, vomiting, muscle twitching, seizures, and coma may develop
- In a less dramatic decrease in serum sodium (130 mEq/liter), headache, lethargy, anorexia, muscle cramps, and generalized fatigue are more common

DIAGNOSIS

The possibility of kidney or adrenal disease must first be ruled out before the diagnosis of SIADH is considered. The diagnosis is based on the clinical and laboratory findings associated with the disorder. Associated central nervous system or respiratory system pathophysiology or drug therapy known to increase ADH secretion can usually be identified as the cause.

TREATMENT

The treatment of SIADH depends on its severity and the underlying cause of the problem. If possible, the underlying cause should be managed (e.g., shunting for hydrocephalus, radiation or surgery for oat cell carcinoma). In addition, the principles of treatment include

- Fluid restriction (about 700 ml/24 hours for 3 to 5 days)
- Possible judicious replacement of sodium with a hypertonic solution of sodium chloride given slowly
- Drug therapy

Drug therapy may include the use of furosemide (Lasix) to remove the excess fluid retained in the body. Another drug that may be used for its diuretic effect is mannitol (Osmitrol). The drug of choice for management of SIADH is demeclocycline hydrochloride (Declomycin), 300 mg four times a day. Declomycin is known to suppress the activity of ADH. In rare circumstances, lithium carbonate (Lithonate) may be given, although there is the possibility of serious side-effects from this drug. Two narcotic antagonists have recently been used to treat SIADH with good results. The drugs are butorphanol tartrate (Stadol) and oxilorphan, a drug that is still under investigation. These drugs are thought to decrease ADH secretion by increasing the osmotic threshold at which ADH is released.[7]

It may take several days or a few weeks to correct the condition of SIADH.

NURSING MANAGEMENT

Assessment

The patient whose diagnosis is SIADH should have the following parameters assessed:

- Monitor the intake and output record.
- Check the daily weight for gain.
- Monitor urine and serum electrolytes (particularly the sodium) and osmolalities.
- Monitor the urine specific gravity.
- Monitor the blood urea nitrogen level.
- Observe for signs and symptoms of fluid and electrolyte imbalance (particularly sodium depletion: lethargy, confusion, muscle weakness and cramping, headache, seizures, coma).
- Check the neurological signs.
- Note whether there is any kidney or adrenal disease.

The nurse caring for a neurological patient should be aware that several conditions frequently seen in neurological–neurosurgical nursing practice can precipitate SIADH. Patients should be monitored for the possible development of this condition.

Intervention

The nurse caring for the patient with SIADH must monitor the laboratory parameters of the serum and urine electrolytes (particularly sodium) and the osmolalities. Evidence of kidney or adrenal disease should also be considered so that the blood urea nitrogen level is checked. The intake and output record is carefully monitored. If an intravenous infusion is ordered, it should be administered slowly.

Most patients with SIADH are placed on strict fluid restrictions. The reason for this necessity should be explained to the patient and his family. A strict intake and output record is maintained to keep the patient within his fluid restriction. Frequent mouth care is provided for comfort because the fluid restriction will cause the patient to have a dry mouth.

Since weight gain is common with SIADH, the patient is weighed daily. The accumulation of fluid will also predispose the bedridden patient to skin breakdown. Frequent skin care, turning, and repositioning should be included in the plan of care.

The hyponatremia associated with the disorder can lead to neurological changes in the sensorium, muscle cramping, headache, seizures, and even coma. The nurse must be aware of the signs and symptoms of sodium depletion and be able to identify these changes to the physician so that definitive action can be taken before serious deficits develop.

HYPERGLYCEMIC HYPEROSMOLAR NONKETOTIC COMA

Hyperglycemic hyperosmolar nonketotic coma (HHNC) is a metabolic complication characterized by hyperglycemia, polyuria, dehydration, and hyperosmolality without the presence of ketoacidosis. The reported mortality rate is 40% to 60%. One of the major defining characteristics of HHNC is the accompanying diverse neurological deficits. The condition can develop slowly and is usually seen in the older patient (50 to 70 years old) with a history of non–insulin-dependent diabetes. In some instances, patients with HHNC have had no previous history of diabetes mellitus, and younger patients have developed HHNC. Although hyperglycemic hyperosmolar nonketotic coma was first diagnosed in 1886, the renewal of interest in and attention to the problem are attributed to the report published in 1957 by Sament and Schwartz.[8,9]

Most patients who develop HHNC have concurrent illnesses. The most common associated illnesses are infections (especially those caused by gram-negative organisms such as those seen in certain pneumonias and acute pyelonephritis), severe burns, uremia, myocardial infarction, pancreatitis, intracranial diseases, and acute trauma and physiological stress. About 85% of the patients who develop HHNC have a preexisting renal or cardiovascular disease.[10]

On the neurological–neurosurgical service, many older patients admitted because of multiple trauma have been exposed to extreme physiological stress. These patients are more apt to have chronic diseases such as cardiac, renal, or endocrine diseases (diabetes mellitus). These patients have a high risk for developing HHNC.

The use of certain drugs has been implicated in the development of HHNC. They include some sedatives and diuretics such as furosemide (Lasix); steroids; prolonged use of mannitol (Osmitrol); cimetidine (Tagamet); phenytoin (Dilantin); chlorpromazine (Thorazine); propranolol (Inderal); and diazoxide (Hyperstat). The nurse caring for neurological and neurosurgical patients will be struck by the number of drugs listed that are commonly administered to her patient population.

Other circumstances that have been associated with the development of HHNC are dialysis (both peritoneal and hemodialysis), hyperosmolar tube feedings; and total parenteral nutrition administered by the intravenous route.

PATHOPHYSIOLOGY

HHNC develops from a relative deficiency of insulin in the body and a profound hyperglycemia, often as high as 1000 mg/100 ml, which causes severe osmotic diuresis. Because of the diminished supply of insulin, the glucose is unable to cross the cell membrane into the intracellular fluid; consequently, the extracellular space has an elevated glucose level and is hyperosmolar. The osmotic gradient causes a shift in body fluid from the intracellular compartment to the extracellular compartment, resulting in intracellular dehydration.

Under normal conditions, glucose is filtered by the glomerulus in the kidney (assuming that glomerular filtration rate is normal) and reabsorbed by the proximal tubules. The kidney is only able to function within certain limits—limits that are exceeded by the profound hyperglycemia found in HHNC. The tubules are no longer able to reabsorb the glucose, resulting in glycosuria. The severe hyperglycemia also causes osmotic diuresis, so there is significant dehydration because of the large amounts of fluid lost through the kidneys. The dehydration further elevates the level of glucose and osmolality in the body. The situation is further complicated by the fact that the seriously ill patient is probably not able to replace the fluid loss by the oral route. As the syndrome progresses, the thirst center is impaired. In addition, the extreme dehydration causes electrolyte imbalance, with sodium, potassium, and phosphate being especially affected.

The reason for the absence of ketosis and ketoacidosis in SIADH is not clear although various hypotheses have been proposed. One explanation offered is that there is inhibition of lipolysis from adipose tissue with subsequent lower levels of free fatty acid. Another hypothesis suggests that patients with HHNC have a higher portal venous concentration of insulin that prevents ketone formation.

SIGNS AND SYMPTOMS

The following signs and symptoms are found with HHNC:

- Polyuria that changes to oliguria as dehydration becomes severe
- Glycosuria
- Hyperglycemia (600 mg to 1400 mg/100 ml)
- Negative serum ketone level (normal finding)
- Serum hyperosmolality that elevates to 350 mOsm/liter and then drops to about 304 mOsm/liter
- Dehydration (dry skin; decreased skin turgor; dry mucous membrane; soft, sunken eyeballs; elevated temperature; postural hypotension)
- Rapid respirations
- Decreased level of consciousness, from lethargy, confusion, or drowsiness to coma
- Various neurological deficits (e.g., seizures, usually focal; hemiparesis; hemisensory deficits; nystagmus; hyperreflexia; nuchal rigidity)
- Electrolyte imbalance
  - —Decreased potassium
  - —Sodium may be decreased, normal, or increased
  - —Decreased phosphate
- Other laboratory findings
  - —Increased hematocrit (associated with hemoconcentration from dehydration)
  - —Elevated blood urea nitrogen
  - —Possible elevated creatinine

DIAGNOSIS

Early recognition and diagnosis of HHNC are most important. The high mortality rate is attributed to the delay in proper diagnosis and commencing of aggressive treatment.[10] The diagnosis is based on the clinical findings of profound hyperglycemia, glycosuria, absence of ketonemia, hyperosmolality, dehydration, and central nervous system deficits.

In diagnosing HHNC in the neurological or neurosurgical patient, the cause of central nervous system deficits is difficult to identify. Many patients have been misdiagnosed as having had a cerebral vascular accident because their neurological deficits are misleading. The possible etiologies of the neurological signs and symptoms are numerous although HHNC may not be considered as a possibility. It is important that a thorough clinical and laboratory assessment be conducted. The occurrence of HHNC is not uncommon in the older patient at risk.

TREATMENT

The treatment of HHNC is directed at replacement of fluids; correction of the hyperosmolality, electrolyte imbalance, and hyperglycemia; and treatment of the underlying or prodisposing cause.

The amount of fluid replacement necessary is between 8 and 12 liters.[11] The solution often used for replacement therapy is 0.45 saline to which potassium chloride (20 mEq to 40 mEq/liter) is added to treat the potassium depletion. In some instances normal saline may be given. A common practice is to replace 5 to 6 liters of fluid in the first 12 hours and then to administer another 4 to 6 liters in the next 24 hours. If phosphate replacement is necessary, 20 mmol/liter of potassium phosphate/liter of intravenous fluid is given as necessary. When the blood glucose level reaches approximately 250 mg/100 ml, the intravenous solution may be changed to 5% dextrose in water.[12]

High doses of insulin are not necessary or desirable and can lead to hypoglycemia and vascular collapse. The major problem with HHNC is dehydration, not insulin deficiency. Only regular or crystalline insulin is administered to the patient. The low-dose intravenous infusion of regular insulin at a rate of 4 to 10 units/hour is the preferred method for treating hyperglycemia. This is preceded by a single priming dose of 5 to 15 units of regular insulin by the intravenous route.

Treatment of the underlying cause or predisposing factor will depend on accurate identification. Management of an infection, discontinuation of a suspicious drug, or surgical intervention are examples of interventions used in the overall treatment of HHNC.

NURSING MANAGEMENT

The nurse should assess patients for the development of HHNC if they are older, have a profile of profound hyperglycemia, and have had a recent episode of diuresis. It is often the alert nurse who notifies the physician of a trend of suspicious signs and symptoms. Early diagnosis and treatment is a goal of nursing management.

Assessment

The following parameters are included in the patient assessment by the nurse:

- Clinical inspection of the patient for evidence of dehydration (decreased skin turgor, dry mucous membranes, sunken eyeballs)
- Clinical signs and symptoms of hyperglycemia (headache, blurred vision, nausea and vomiting, abdominal pain)
- Urine for sugar and acetone
- Intake and output record for polyuria and an excessive amount of urinary output
- Weight for evidence of weight lost
- Vital signs for evidence of hypovolemic shock
- Neurological signs for decreased level of consciousness and other deficits
- Fluid and electrolyte imbalance
- Laboratory data including electrolytes, blood glucose, blood ketone level, serum osmolality, blood urea nitrogen, creatinine, blood gases, hematocrit, and white blood count

Intervention

The patient who has been diagnosed as having HHNC is very ill and requires careful supervision and management. The major nursing diagnosis addresses dehydration and can be stated as "fluid volume deficit, actual." Large amounts of intravenous fluids of varying composition will be administered to the patient within a relatively short time. The rate of infusion must be monitored frequently as well as the tolerance of the patient's respiratory, cardiovascular, and renal system. A large number of patients who develop HHNC have preexisting renal or cardiovascular disease as well as other concurrent problems such as infections. Too rapid a correction of dehydration can precipitate circulatory overload, congestive heart failure, and pulmonary edema. These facts further support the need for frequent monitoring of vital signs. Central venous pressure readings are also helpful in monitoring fluid volume. Improvement in the patient's hydration level will be reflected in the serum osmolality values. The patient with a cardiac problem should be monitored by continual electrocardiographic recordings. Electrocardiographic monitoring is also important for the patient with hypokalemia because of the possible development of cardiac arrhythmias.

Insulin is limited to regular or crystalline insulin administered by the intravenous route and to low doses that are correlated with frequent monitoring of blood glucose levels. As hydration improves, the hyperglycemia will also improve. In addition to the correction of fluid depletion, electrolyte depletion will also be corrected. The saline or half saline intravenous solution provides for sodium and chloride loss. Potassium depletion is treated intravenously by the addition of 20 mEq to 40 mEq of potassium chloride per 1000-ml unit of intravenous fluid until balance is achieved. If phosphate must be replaced, potassium phosphate is administered intravenously. The patient with renal disease must be monitored for the development of hyperphosphatemia. The administration of electrolytes is correlated with frequent monitoring of blood electrolyte levels. The nurse should carefully watch these blood chemistries and observe the patient for signs and symptoms of overdose or underdose.

Another major nursing diagnosis is that of "urinary elimination pattern, altered." During the course of HHNC, the patient will experience polyuria and oliguria as dehydration becomes extreme. Many of these patients are known to have preexisting renal disease. Monitoring the blood urea nitrogen and creatinine levels provides an indication of kidney function. Recording urinary output and checking the urine for sugar and acetone are other nursing responsibilities.

Ongoing neurological assessments should be conducted. Several neurological signs and symptoms previously mentioned are characteristic of HHNC. A complication of too much insulin and too rapid an infusion of intravenous fluid is cerebral edema. The underlying cause of the cerebral edema is that the serum osmolality is reduced too rapidly. A typical history of the onset of this complication is that of improvement with treatment, followed by the sudden onset of deepening coma, fever, and circulatory collapse. If this complication occurs, the mortality rate is almost 100%.[10] The nurse should carefully monitor fluid administration and neurological signs for deterioration.

The hemoconcentration associated with dehydration interferes with cardiac output, circulation, and transport of cell nutrients across the cell membrane. Patients are prone to vascular thromboses, pulmonary emboli, and infection. When monitoring the patient for complications, the nurse should be aware of these possibilities and monitor the patient for signs and symptoms of their development.

The patient should be encouraged to take food and liquids as soon as possible. Patient teaching will need to be incorporated in the nursing process. Other principles of management should be included such as weight control, foot and skin care, and an exercise program. These patients should be under medical supervision and have their blood glucose levels tested periodically.

MAJOR ELECTROLYTE IMBALANCES

In considering fluid and electrolyte balance, the nurse should be attuned to the various signs and symptoms of imbalance. The range of normal values for most electrolytes is narrow, and deviation from normal can have significant deleterious effects. It is imperative for the nurse to identify these deviations so that corrective interventions can be instituted. As part of the assessment of patients, a review of the blood chemistry values should be included.

The following information summarizes the major electrolytes and the various states of imbalance.

Potassium (3.5 mEq to 5.0 mEq/liter)

Hyperkalemia (mild symptoms if 5 mEq to 7 mEq/liter; severe if >7.0 mEq/liter)
Signs and Symptoms
- Electrocardiographic changes/cardiac arrhythmias
  - Tall peaked T waves
  - Widening of the QRS complex or shortening of the QT interval
- Ventricular fibrillations leading to cardiac arrest
- Muscle weakness with decreased reflexes
- Bradycardia and hypotension
- Paresthesia
- Respiratory paralysis

Hypokalemia (<3.5 mEq/liter)
Signs and Symptoms
- Electrocardiographic changes/cardiac arrhythmias
  - U waves
  - Prolonged QT interval
  - Depressed ST segment
  - Low, flat T waves

Sodium (135 mEq to 145 mEq/liter)

Hypernatremia (>145 mEq/liter)
Signs and Symptoms
- Dehydration (poor skin turgor; dry skin and mucous membrane; sunken eyeballs)
- Stupor
- Thirst
- Oliguria

Hyponatremia (<135 mEq/liter). Note that signs and symptoms do not become severe until the sodium level is 125 mEq/liter or less)
Signs and Symptoms
- Confusion, lethargy, coma
- Seizure activity
- Hypotension; tachycardia (thready pulse); cold, clammy skin

Chlorides (100 mEq to 108 mEq/liter). Usually seen in combination with depressed sodium levels

Hyperchloremia (>108 mEq/liter)
Signs and Symptoms
- Stupor
- Rapid deep breathing
- Generalized weakness

Hypochloremia (<100 mEq/liter)
Signs and Symptoms
- Hypertonicity of muscles
- Tetany
- Depressed respirations

Calcium (4.5 mEq to 5.5 mEq/liter)

Hypercalcemia (>5.5 mEq/liter)
Signs and Symptoms
- Deep bone pain
- Flank pain from renal calculi
- Muscle hypotonicity
- Nausea and vomiting
- Dehydration
- Stupor to coma

Hypocalcemia (<4.5 mEq/liter)
Signs and Symptoms
- Tingling of fingertips
- Tetany
- Abdominal cramps
- Muscle cramps
- Carpopedal spasms
- Convulsions
- Prolonged QT interval

Phosphorus, in the form of phosphate ions (1.8 mEq to 2.6 mEq/liter)

Hyperphosphatemia (>2.6 mEq/liter)
Signs and Symptoms: usually not present; when high levels are maintained for an extended time, may have phosphate deposits in body; elevated phosphorus often associated with renal failure

Hypophosphatemia (<1.8 mEq/liter)
Signs and Symptoms: not present in acute deficits; in prolonged deficiencies, bone pain, dizziness, anorexia, and muscle weakness; usually associated with hyperparathyroidism

REFERENCES

1. Guyton A: Textbook of Medical Physiology, 5th ed, pp 424–425. Philadelphia, WB Saunders, 1976
2. Coleman P: Antidiuretic hormone: Physiology and pathophysiology—a review. J Neurosurg Nurs 11(4):201, December 1979
3. Guyton A: Textbook of Medical Physiology, 5th ed, pp 1000–1002. Philadelphia, WB Saunders, 1976
4. McLaurin R: Metabolic changes accompanying head injuries. Clin Neurosurg 12:143, 1966
5. Swartz S: Solving antidiuretic hormone puzzles. Patient Care 114, June 30, 1982
6. Streeten DHP, Moses AM, Miller M: Disorders of the neurohypophysis. In Petersdorf RG et al: Harrison's Principles of Internal Medicine, 10th ed, pp 606–607. New York, McGraw-Hill, 1983
7. Miller M: Role of endogenous opioids in neurohypophyseal function of man. J Clin Endocrinol Metab 50:1016, 1980
8. Dreschfeld J: The Bradschawe lecture on diabetic coma. Br Med J 2:356–363, 1886
9. Sament S, Schwartz MB: Severe diabetic stupor without ketosis. S Afr Med J 31:893–894, 1957
10. Sneid DS: Hyperosmolar hyperglycemic nonketotic coma. Crit Care Q 3(3):29–43, September 1983
11. Arieff AI: Nonketotic hyperosmolar coma with hyperglycemia. Medicine 51:73–94, 1972
12. Podolsky S: Hyperosmolar nonketotic coma: Underdiagnosed and undertreated. In Podolsky S: Clinical Diabetes: Modern Management, p 217. New York, Appleton-Century-Crofts, 1980

BIBLIOGRAPHY

Books

Borg N (ed): Core Curriculum for Critical Care Nursing, 2nd ed, pp 326–343. Philadelphia, WB Saunders, 1981

Brunner L, Suddarth D: Textbook of Medical–Surgical Nursing, 4th ed, p 845. Philadelphia, JB Lippincott, 1980

Davis J, Mason C: Neurologic Critical Care, pp 130–134. New York, Van Nostrand Reinhold, 1979

Diagnostics, pp 372–373. Springhouse, PA, Intermed Communications, 1982

Eliasson S, Prensky A, Hardin W (eds): Neurological Pathophysiology, 2nd ed, pp 416–424. New York, Oxford University Press, 1978

Perry M: Metabolic response to trauma. In Shires G: Care of the Trauma Patient, 2nd ed, pp 62–74. New York, McGraw–Hill, 1979

Phipps WJ, Long BC, Woods NF (eds): Medical–Surgical Nursing Concepts and Clinical Practice, pp 665–666. St Louis, CV Mosby, 1983

Podolsky S: Clinical Diabetes: Modern Management. New York, Appleton–Century–Crofts, 1980

Smith R: Essentials of Neurosurgery, pp 35–37. Philadelphia, JB Lippincott, 1980

Tilkian SM, Conover MB, Tilkian AG: Clinical Implications of Laboratory Tests, 3rd ed, pp 25–26. St Louis, CV Mosby, 1983

Periodicals

Anderson B: Antidiuretic hormone: Balance and imbalance. J Neurosurg Nurs 11(2):71, June 1979

Boh D, Van Son A: The water-load test. Am J Nurs 82:112, January 1982

Fairchild R: Diabetes insipidus: A review. Crit Care Q 3(2):111, September 1980

Franco LM: Syndrome of inappropriate secretion of antidiuretic hormone. J Neurosurg Nurs 14(5):276, October 1982

Hamburger S, Rush D: Syndrome of inappropriate secretion of antidiuretic hormone. Crit Care Q 3(2):119, September 1980

Joffle BI et al: Pathogenesis of nonketotic hyperosmolar diabetic coma. Lancet 1:1069, 1975

Khokhar N: Inappropriate secretion of antidiuretic hormone: An overview of the syndrome. Medicine 62:73, October 1977

Kubo G, Grant M: The syndrome of inappropriate secretion of antidiuretic hormone. Heart Lung 7(3):469, May–June 1978

Lancour J: ADH and aldosterone: How to recognize their effects. Nurs '78, 8:36, September 1978

Lane G, Peirce A: When persistence pays off: Resolving the mystery of an unexplained electrolyte imbalance. Nurs '82 12:44, January 1982

Mather HM: Management of hyperosmolar coma. JR Soc Med 73:135, 1980

McLaurin R: Metabolic monitoring of neurosurgical patients. Clin Neurosurg 22:476, 1975

McLaurin R: Recognition and treatment of metabolic disorders after head injuries. Clin Neurosurg 19:281, 1972

O'Dorisio TM: Hypercalcemic crisis. Heart Lung 7(3):425, May–June 1978

Otrakji J: Potassium metabolism disorders. Crit Care Q 3(2):55, September 1980

Ricci M: Water and electrolyte metabolism in patients with intracranial lesions. J Neurosurg Nurs 9(4):165, December 1977

Smith J: Nursing management in diabetes insipidus. J Neurosurg Nurs 13(6):313, December 1981

Winters B: Nursing implications of hyperosmolar coma. Heart Lung 12(4):439, July 1983

chapter 14

General Nursing Care of the Patient Undergoing Cranial Surgery

Surgical intervention is a common means of treatment for some neurological conditions. A craniotomy is the most common of intracranial procedures performed on the neurological patient. The surgical approach to the craniotomy depends on the location of the lesion.

PREOPERATIVE PREPARATION

It is the responsibility of the physician to provide the patient with enough information so that the decision for surgery is based on informed consent. Since the patient's level of consciousness or ability to understand may be altered, it is advisable for a responsible family member to be present for the discussion. Informed consent means that the patient is fully informed about the indications for surgery, possible alternative treatment, potential risks, limitations of the protocol, and temporary or permanent disability following the surgery. Discussing these points honestly and answering questions posed by the patient and family will reduce the possibility of misunderstandings and litigations.

PSYCHOSOCIAL CONSIDERATIONS

For the patient who is conscious and oriented, the prospect of a craniotomy causes overwhelming anxiety. Paramount is the fear of loss of life or possible permanent disability that might affect his ability to speak, ambulate, and take care of basic needs. Of equal concern is the prospect of loss of mental ability, self-control, and those personality characteristics that make an individual unique. Additional stress and worry are stirred up by thoughts of what effect this illness will have on relationships with family and friends. Many patients fear that they will be a burden to their families.

The physician must discuss the purpose of surgery, the possibility of alternate treatment (if any), and the expected outcomes and risk. Questions that the patient or family might have about the surgery must also be answered. Since the nursing staff is with the patient most of the time, the nurse providing care should know what the patient has been told. This knowledge can help her to clarify the patient's misconceptions and enable her to refer special problems to the physician. The patient must be allowed to verbalize his reactions and concerns about surgery. The family will also need the support of the nurse in coping with this crisis.

DIAGNOSTIC PROCEDURES

While special diagnostic or evaluative procedures will be ordered according to the specific problem for which a craniotomy is scheduled, the following procedures will be carried out on all patients:

1. A complete physical examination if one has not already been conducted
2. A complete blood count
3. Fasting blood sugar (FBS) and blood urea nitrogen (BUN)
4. Type and crossmatch
5. Electrocardiogram
6. Chest film

A complete physical examination is necessary to determine the presence and extent of any health problems that might contraindicate the suggested surgery or require that special precautions be instituted before, during, or after surgery. For example, a patient with chronic lung disease would need pulmonary function studies, careful selection of the anesthetic agent and other drugs commonly administered during surgery, and judicious use of oxygen therapy.

A complete blood count may indicate the presence of anemia, infection, low platelet count, and blood dyscrasia. A low hemoglobin would suggest the need for a blood transfusion before surgery to achieve a satisfactory level for the transport of oxygen in the blood. An elevated white blood count (WBC) is indicative of the presence of infection, which is considered a contraindication for surgery. The site and cause of the infection would need to be identified and treated adequately before surgery could be safely rescheduled. A low platelet count or other blood dyscrasia would require evaluation and possible treatment before the plans for surgery would be formalized.

The blood urea nitrogen level would give a general estimate of kidney function, and the fasting blood sugar would determine the presence of diabetes mellitus, which would need to be controlled in the preoperative and postoperative period.

Blood typing and crossmatching are required to make blood available should the patient require blood replacement from surgical loss.

The electrocardiogram is done to identify any cardiac conditions that could be aggravated during the stress of a long surgical procedure and drug therapy.

The chest film is usually taken to rule out lung congestion, pneumonia, atelectasis, or any other pathological condition within the lungs or chest that would compromise respiration.

DAY PRIOR TO SURGERY

On the day before surgery, certain procedures are conducted as a means of establishing baseline data and preparing the patient for surgery. A neurological assessment is carried out; the patient's weight is recorded and the hair washed. (An enema is usually *not* ordered.)

When the hair is washed, a Betadine solution should be used to decrease the count of microorganisms on the hair and scalp. If the patient is a woman with long hair, the hair should be neatly braided. In many hospitals, the hair is cut and the scalp shaved in the operating room. To some patients the thought of having their hair cut can be most distressing. Therefore, the nurse should explain why the hair must be cut, at the same time allowing the patient to express any feelings of dismay.

In general, this entire preoperative period is a time when the patient and family need emotional and psychological support. Since they undoubtedly need an opportunity to express their concerns and fears, this is when the nurse can be most supportive. It may also be helpful to call upon the services of a member of the clergy or other supportive personnel to give reassurance, if necessary.

DAY OF SURGERY

As part of preoperative preparation, the patient is restricted to nothing by mouth after midnight. On the day of surgery, the usual morning care and preoperative preparation routine used for any surgical patient is followed: remove dentures, glasses, and nail polish; complete operative check list; and so forth. Application of Ace bandages to the legs may be ordered. A neurological assessment with vital signs is routinely carried out. Any special orders for preparation are completed and preoperative medication is administered as ordered.

SURGICAL APPROACH TO THE PATIENT

To provide postoperative care, the nurse should have a good idea of the sequence of events that will occur in the operating room. This knowledge serves as the basis for interpreting physiological changes that require specific nursing care or indicate development of complications.

ARRIVAL IN THE OPERATING ROOM SUITE

The period from the arrival of the patient in the operating room suite until surgery begins can be divided into three phases: the preinduction, induction, and postinduction phases.

The Preinduction Phase

After proper identification of the patient has been verified, the patient's chart is reviewed for a signed operative permit and completion of the preoperative orders. Next, the patient is transferred to the operating room table. In some instances, surgery may be performed on a special treatment table such as a Roto Rest bed on which the patient was brought to surgery.

Some monitoring equipment is applied such as a blood pressure cuff, chest leads for an electrocardiogram monitor, precordial stethoscope, and central venous pressure (CVP) line. The patient's vital signs and emotional status are assessed. Emotional support is provided and the patient observed. The anesthesiologist inserts two peripheral lines and an arterial line, and intravenous infusions are started.

The Induction Phase

Induction is oftentimes accomplished with intravenous thiopental sodium (Pentothal). This provides for very rapid induction, usually within 30 to 45 seconds. Other final preparation measures are completed which include

- Ace bandages are applied from the toes to the groin or an antigravity suit is applied to prevent the pooling of blood in the abdomen and lower extremities, which would result in hypotension; without such preparation, hypotension would be severe, particularly in the patient who is placed in the sitting position for surgery.

- A urinary catheter is inserted if one is not already present; this is necessary if hyperosmotic diuretics will be administered or if surgery will be of long duration.
- The eyes are protected from corneal abrasions with the application of a bland eye ointment; they are then taped closed and sterile eye pads applied.
- Other monitoring devices may be added at this time, such as a Swan–Ganz catheter, esophageal temperature probe, indwelling cannula for the continual monitoring of arterial blood pressure, a Doppler ultrasound chest piece (to detect venous air emboli if the sitting position is used), and other equipment, as necessary.
- The patient is intubated after the larynx is sprayed with lidocaine to prevent coughing or retching, which would increase intracranial pressure.
- The head is shaved carefully so that no scalp abrasions occur; these would increase the possibility of postoperative infection; the hair is saved and placed in a labelled envelope.
- The patient is placed in the position (lateral, prone, or sitting) that the surgeon has selected as being most advantageous for the surgical procedure planned; the sitting position is used for posterior fossa surgery because it affords optimal visualization of the operative field.
- The various body supports, such as the head rest, the arm rests, and so forth, are carefully put into place so that no undue pressure is created that will cause ischemia or injury to body tissue.

The Postinduction Phase

The anesthesiologist continues to administer anesthesia while the last-minute preparations are completed. An intravenous 20% mannitol solution is begun to reduce the brain bulk. Dexamethasone to control cerebral edema, phenytoin to control seizures, and antibiotics to control infection are given periodically throughout the procedures.

Throughout the preparation of the patient, the patient has been carefully watched and monitored. The operative written record is begun, and the drugs given and preparation of the patient performed are recorded. The patient is now ready for the neurosurgeon.

Neuroanesthesia

There is no ideal anesthetic agent for neurosurgical procedures. Of the several drugs available, all have actions and side-effects that may cause problems or be unpredictable. Important considerations in choosing drugs are their effects on cerebral metabolism (cerebral metabolic oxygen requirement), cerebral blood flow, intracranial pressure, and vasomotor tone (cerebral vasoconstrictors or vasodilators). Other considerations in selecting anesthetic agents are nonflammability (especially important if cautery instruments will be used); ease of administration; effect on hemostasis and blood pressure; adequate brain relaxation; nonirritability so that coughing and retching are not precipitated; and minimal side-effects and adverse reactions on the various body systems.

For neurosurgical procedures a combination of drugs is given so that one drug offsets the negative side-effects of another. A common combination of drugs is nitrous oxide, oxygen, narcotics (fentanyl), barbiturates (thiopental sodium [Pentothal] or pentobarbital), and muscle relaxants (e.g., pancuronium). Table 14–1 summarizes the major characteristics of the commonly used anesthetic agents.

INTRAOPERATIVE PHASE

During surgery, controlled hypotension, hypothermia, and hyperventilation may be indicated. Increased intracranial pressure, seizure activity, infections, and possible venous air emboli should also be controlled.

Hypotension

In some surgical procedures in which the vascularity is increased, induction of controlled hypotension is advantageous. Hypotension is particularly helpful during the dissection of an aneurysm because the lowered pressure within the blood vessels reduces the pressure on the aneurysmal sac to control bleeding if rupture occurs, and it also increases the plasticity of the aneurysm so that a secure clip or other material can be easily applied. Drug therapy (e.g., trimethaphan [Arfonad] or sodium nitroprusside [Nipride]), the sitting position, and the effects of anesthetic agents such as halothane cause hypotension. The desired level of hypotension is usually 60 mm Hg, although it may be lowered to 40 mm Hg in some instances. The level of arterial pressure is monitored by use of the arterial monitoring cannula.

Hypothermia

The purpose of inducing hypothermia is to provide a bloodless operative site. The less oxygen consumed, the less oxidation and the fewer the metabolic by-products. For every degree lowered from 37°C to 25°C, there is a 6% reduction in oxygen consumption by the brain. The reduction in oxygen consumption and cerebral metabolism results in vasoconstriction. Hypothermia is classified as moderate (37° C to 28° C) and profound (below 28° C). If the temperature is lowered below 28° C, cardiac irritability increases and extracorporeal support of the systemic circulation becomes necessary.[1]

Induction of hypothermia is not a common practice because of its inherent problems. Induction is accomplished through the use of drugs, a cooling (hypothermia) blanket, or an extracorporeal cooling circuit. Each method presents possible side-effects such as shivering and downward drift of the temperature, and asepsis must be monitored and controlled.

Hyperventilation

Controlled hyperventilation can be maintained during surgery with a ventilator. It is an effective means of reducing brain bulk and intracranial pressure. The reduced produc-

TABLE 14–1. *Commonly Used Neurosurgical Anesthetic Agents*

Drug	Side-Effects/Adverse Reactions	Comments
Halothane (volatile liquid)	• Slight cerebral vasodilation and subsequent increase in intracranial pressure (ICP), especially at time of induction • Hypotension • Postoperative shivering • Decreases cerebral metabolic oxygen requirement ($CMRO_2$)	• Begin induction with other drugs using the intravenous route; hyperventilate the patient • Hypotensive effect when given with curare and ganglionic blockers • Useful in inducing hypothermia • Cleared quickly from body when administration is discontinued
Enflurane (volatile liquid)	• Increase in ICP • Decreases $CMRO_2$ • Possible renal failure • Hepatotoxic • Slight hypotension	• Rapid onset • 85% to 90% rapidly excreted from lungs • Used in combination with small amounts of skeletal muscle relaxants
Nitrous oxide (inhalant gas)	• No effect on ICP • Increases cerebral metabolic rate	• Increases possibility of air emboli • Always used in a mixture with oxygen
Ketamine (dissociation agent)	• Elevation in blood pressure (tachycardia) • Increases ICP • Increases $CMRO_2$ • Causes cerebrovasoconstriction • May cause tonic–clonic movements	• Rapid-acting anesthetic agent • Produces analgesia while maintaining normal skeletal muscle tone • Slow recovery from anesthesia state with possible vivid dreams or hallucinations • Barbiturates or narcotics may increase recovery time from ketamine
Innovar (a combination of fentanyl and droperidol; a dissociation agent)	• Decreases $CMRO_2$ and ICP • Hypotension • Bradycardia • Muscle rigidity • Respiratory depression	• Neuroleptanalgesic agent that produces analgesia, reduces motor activity, and alters consciousness • Slow onset and prolonged duration • Used in combination with other drugs
Nondepolarizing muscle relaxants: gallamine (Flaxedil); pancuronium (Pavulon); tubocurarine (Metubine)	• Tachycardia • Muscle weakness • Salivation (an anticholinergic drug is administered to reduce this side-effect) • Dizziness • Hypertension • Respiratory depression • Decreases ICP • Fentanyl decreases $CMRO_2$ while droperidol has no effect on it	• Adjunct to anesthetic during surgery; produces skeletal muscle relaxation • Assists patients on mechanical ventilators • Competitive antagonism of acetylcholine (ACh) at the neuromuscular junction or receptor site • Almost immediate onset that lasts 20 to 60 minutes • Excreted through urine
Depolarizing muscle relaxant: succinylcholine (Anectine)	• Bradycardia or tachycardia • Hypotension or hypertension • Muscle twitching • Respiratory depression • Malignant hyperthermia • Postoperative muscle pain and stiffness • Excessive salivation	• Adjunct to anesthetic during surgery; produces skeletal muscle relaxation • Facilitates intubation procedure • Produces initial muscle fasciculations quickly followed by flaccid paralysis • Almost immediate onset that lasts 2 to 4 minutes • Can be given by intravenous drip for prolonged muscle relaxation • Should not be used with nondepolarizing blocker because prolonged effect results • Excreted through urine • Given with great caution to paraplegics because they tend to become severely hyperkalemic when given this drug
Barbiturates: thiopental and pentobarbital (short acting)	• Decreases $CMRO_2$ • Causes cerebrovasoconstriction • Decreases ICP	• Given intravenously to decrease the effects on intracranial pressure from the halothane and intubation

tion of carbon dioxide results in a reduction in cerebral blood flow and subsequent vasoconstriction. This causes a reduction in brain bulk and intracranial pressure.

Control of Increased Intracranial Pressure

Throughout surgery, intracranial pressure must be controlled by the use of hyperventilation and drugs. The drugs used include hyperosmotic diuretics and dexamethasone.

Control of Seizure Activity and Infections

Phenytoin (Dilantin) is administered to the patient to prevent seizure activity. The drug will also be continued in the postoperative period for prophylaxis of seizures.

The possibility of infection is a concern of everyone involved in patient care. Adherence to strict aseptic technique is imperative. Antibiotics are administered intravenously to prevent infection.

Venous Air Embolus

A potential problem of the sitting operative position is an air embolus. The head is higher than the heart, and a negative pressure is produced in the dural venous sinuses and veins draining the brain and head. If air is introduced into the venous system, it is quickly carried to the right side of the heart. The patient must be monitored with a Doppler sensor. A change in the Doppler signals indicates the presence of air in the heart. When an air embolus is suspected, the surgeon is notified so that he can attempt to identify and occlude the possible site of air entry. Once the problem site has been occluded, the anesthesiologist aspirates air through the central venous catheter using a 20-ml syringe and an air-tight stopcock. Once the air has been aspirated, the entry site closed, and the patient stabilized, surgery can continue. In the event that the entry site cannot be located, the patient is placed in the supine position, and the surgery is terminated. The patient is observed for transient neurological deficits. A mill-wheel murmur heard through an esophageal stethoscope is a late sign of intracardiac air. Air embolus is a serious problem that can lead to death.[2]

COMMON NEUROSURGICAL OPERATIVE PROCEDURES

Definition of Terms

A. Common neurological procedures
   1. Burr hole—a hole made in the cranium with a special drill for evacuation of an extracerebral clot or in preparation for craniotomy. In the case of a craniotomy, a series of burr holes is made. The bone between the holes is cut with a special saw allowing removal of the piece of bone.
   2. Craniotomy—a surgical opening of the skull to provide access to the brain in order to remove a tumor, aneurysm, or so forth. A craniotomy can also be scheduled for surgical repair of a cerebral injury. A bone flap is created by incising the scalp and bone so that the tissue can be turned down (Fig. 14–1). The dura is then incised and the surgery begun. Upon completion of the procedure, the bone flap is replaced and the muscle and scalp are realigned and sutured.
   3. Craniectomy—excision of a portion of the skull without replacement. This procedure may be done for purposes of decompression from cerebral edema.
   4. Cranioplasty—plastic repair of the skull to reestablish the contour and integrity of the skull. This procedure involves the replacement of part of the cranium with a synthetic material.

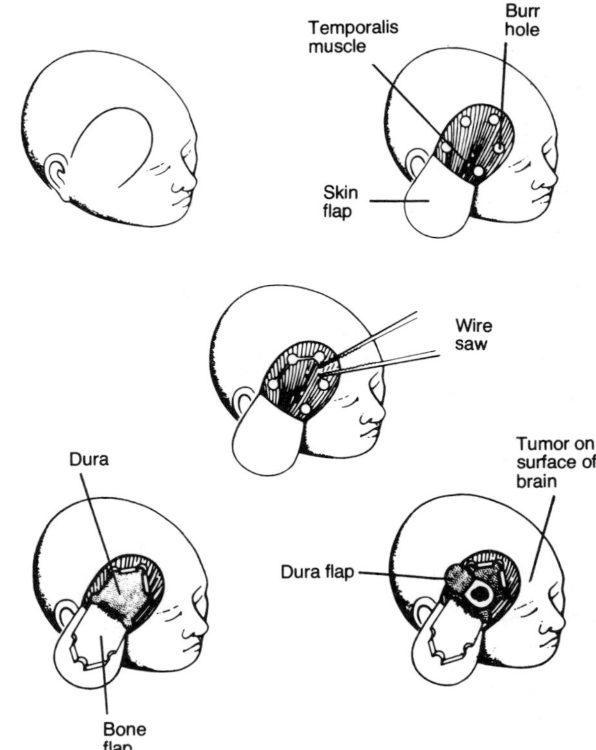

FIG. 14–1. Stages of a craniotomy. (Redrawn from Purchese G: Neuromedical and Neurosurgical Nursing. London, Bailliére Tindall, 1977)

B. General location of surgery. Two terms differentiate areas of the brain upon which surgery is performed (Fig. 14–2):
   1. Supratentorial—area above the tentorium that includes the cerebrum. The tentorium cerebelli is a double fold of the dura mater that forms a partition between the cerebrum and the brain stem and cerebellum. The supratentorial approach is used to gain access to space-occupying lesions (tumors, hematomas, abscesses) in the frontal, parietal, temporal, and occipital lobes of the cerebral hemispheres. Occasionally, temporal or occipital lobe lesions located close to the tentorial margin may be excised through the infratentorial approach.
   2. Infratentorial—area below the tentorium that includes the brain stem (midbrain, pons, medulla) and cerebellum. The infratentorial approach is used to gain access to these areas identified for removal of any type of space-occupying lesion (tumors, hematomas, abscesses).

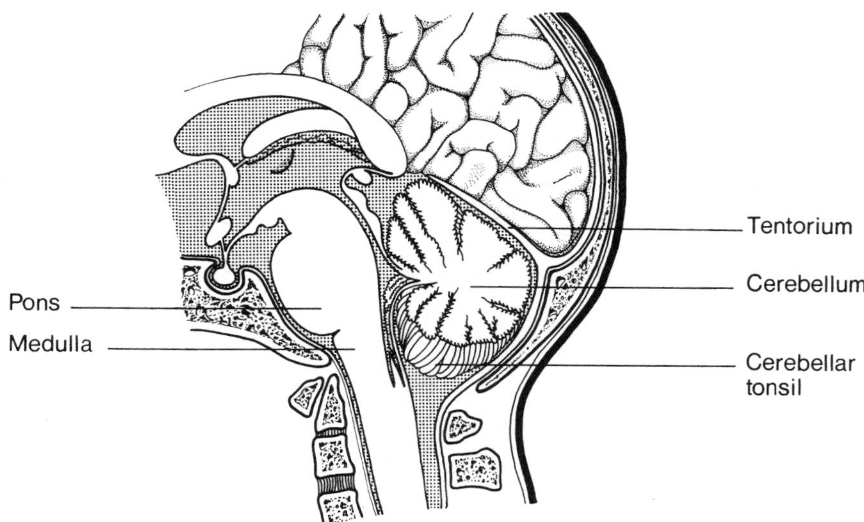

FIG. 14-2. Surgery on area of brain above the tentorium is referred to as *supratentorial;* surgery below the tentorium is referred to as *infratentorial.* (Purchese G: Neuromedical and Neurosurgical Nursing. London, Baillière Tindall, 1977)

SPECIAL NEUROSURGICAL TECHNIQUES AND PROCEDURES

Microsurgery in Neurosurgery

Microsurgery can be defined as any surgery performed with the assistance of an operating microscope that provides magnification of various intensities. The surgical techniques (micro-operative techniques), instruments (microinstrumentation), illumination for visualization, and magnification (operating microscopes), along with a host of other equipment, are specifically designed for this technique. The use of microsurgery has improved several standard neurosurgical procedures such as the removal of brain tumors including acoustic neuromas, aneurysm obliteration, and cervical and lumbar discectomy. It has also provided the means for new neurosurgical procedures such as transsphenoidal removal of pituitary tumors without violating the integrity of the pituitary gland, cerebral anastomosis of intracranial and extracranial arteries previously considered too small to identify or suture with standard surgical procedures, obliteration of previously inaccessible aneurysms, and various brain and spinal cord procedures that require precise structural identification of microscopic neural and vascular areas, delicate dissection of structures, and management of hemostasis.[3]

There are also new demands and considerations that accompanied the advent of microsurgery such as training and education of the surgical team; initial purchase and maintenance of delicate and expensive equipment; and the need for additional space in the surgical suites. Microsurgery requires considerable education and training for the surgeon and other members of the surgical team. It is a new approach to neurosurgery with emphasis on visualization. Use of the special equipment (microscope, illumination devices, instruments, sutures, and so forth) must be mastered in addition to the specific surgical techniques. The nurse who participates in neuromicrosurgery must develop new skills and knowledge to function effectively as a member of the surgical team. The care of all of the equipment involved in microsurgery also becomes a major responsibility of the nurse. The specific care and inspection of equipment requires special protocols that are critical to the success of the surgical procedure.

One of the necessary conditions for microsurgery is a means for accurate and effective coagulation of small cerebral vessels. The bipolar electrocoagulator has been used for this purpose. There are several technical requirements for any piece of electrocoagulation equipment, but the precision required for microsurgery places added demands on the instrumentation design. The microinstrumentation of all equipment—including dissection instruments, retractors, drills, curettes, forceps, needles, and needle holders—requires special designs. In addition to the instrumentation, head fixation devices, operative tables, and suction equipment also must be specifically designed for microsurgery.

The field of neuromicrosurgery is a still-developing area of neurosurgical practice. The extraordinary possibilities for neurosurgery will probably hinge on procedures undertaken through neuromicrosurgery.

Lasers and Neurosurgery

Surgical lasers were first introduced in the early 1960s, but it was not until 1979 that laser neurosurgery slowly began to come into vogue in the United States. The word *laser* is an acronym for *l*ight *a*mplification by *s*timulated *e*mission of *r*adiation. The basic properties of light and electromagnetic radiation govern laser technology. A laser is a device that concentrates light energies into an intense, narrow beam of coherent monochromatic light that can be accurately focused on specific tissue. The selected body tissue absorbs the laser beam. The laser beam is transformed into immense heat energy, and the thermal energy of the laser beam allows simultaneous surgical dissection and coagulation.

There are three types of surgical lasers available to the neurosurgeon: the carbon dioxide, the argon, and the Nd:YAG (neodymium: yttrium aluminum garnet) laser. Each one has its specific advantages and disadvantages. The value of lasers in neurosurgery is that the surgeon, using microscopic visualization, can dissect a precise structure without causing trauma to surrounding tissue, a consequence of traditional surgical techniques. This technique provides an approach for removing tumors from delicate and formerly nonaccessible areas of the brain and spinal cord.

The use of lasers for neurosurgical procedures is still relatively new. Because of limited clinical application, patient selection is important. Patients with tumors located extrinsic to brain tissue but proximal to delicate cerebral tissue are considered good candidates for laser surgery. Acoustic neuromas, craniopharyngiomas, certain brain stem gliomas, pinealomas, ventricular tumors, and meningiomas have been successfully removed with laser surgery.[4,5] The removal of selected intrinsic and extrinsic spinal cord tumors has also been successful. These tumors include intrinsic astrocytomas and ependymomas and extrinsic meningiomas and neuromas.[6]

To summarize, the value of laser surgery is to provide accessibility to neurosurgical sites that were previously prohibited. Lasers can dissect tissue by vaporization while leaving adjacent tissue uninjured, coagulate blood vessels, and, in some instances, shrink tumors. The clinical application of laser is limited, but this so-called "bloodless" surgery is certain to become more refined in the foreseeable future. (See Chap. 21 for additional information.)

Stereotaxis and Neurosurgery

The first practical instruments for stereotactic surgery were developed in 1947. Stereotaxis pertains to precision localization of a specific target point based on the use of three-dimensional coordinates derived with the use of a stereotaxis frame and instrumentation. See Figure 14–3 for examples of representative stereotaxic equipment. Various types of stereotaxic frames and instruments have been developed, which are constantly being updated. Stereotaxis surgery is used in neurosurgery for the precise localization of deep brain lesions for surgical biopsy of dissection. The advantage of the technique is that small lesions can be localized and removed from areas that were previously surgically inaccessible, with minimal trauma to adjacent tissue.

Once the stereotaxic frame is applied to the patient's head, the target site within the brain is located by determining the X, Y, and Z coordinates in relationship to the stereotactic frame. The various coordinates represent the

FIG. 14–3. Some of the components of the BRW CT Stereotaxic System. *(A)* Head ring. *(B)* Localizer ring. *(C)* Arc system. *(D)* Phantom base. (Radiotonics, Inc., Burlington, MA)

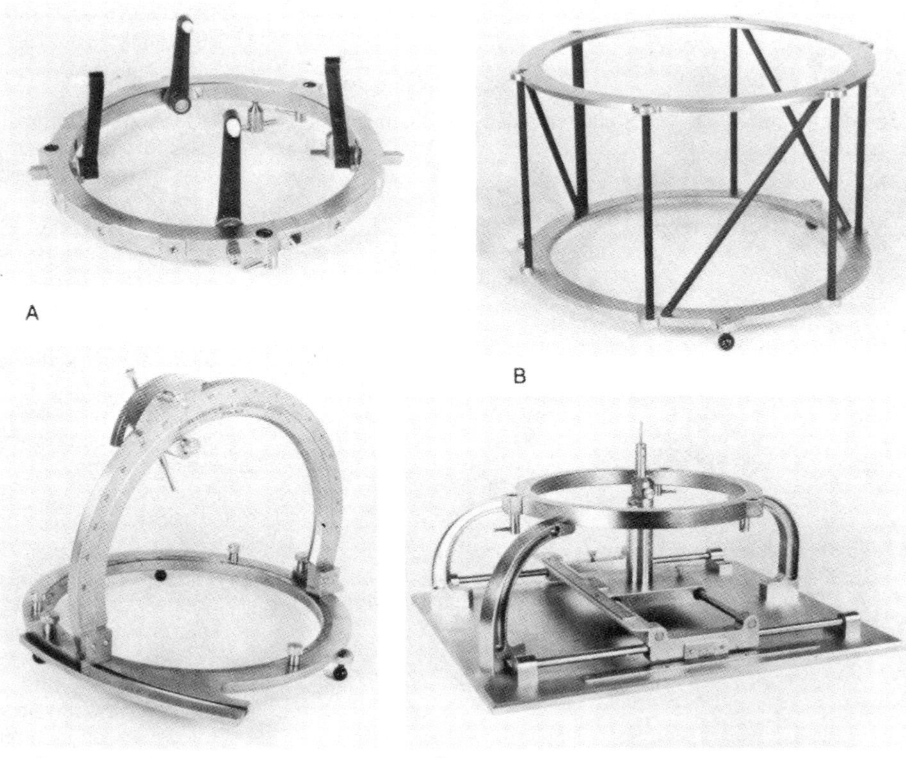

(Text continued on page 304.)

CHART 14–1. NURSING CARE PLAN FOR THE PATIENT SCHEDULED FOR INTRACRANIAL SURGERY

NURSING DIAGNOSIS	EXPECTED OUTCOME	NURSING INTERVENTION
Preoperative Phase		
Potential of fear due to upcoming surgery	• Decrease in observable signs and symptoms of fear • States reason for surgery • Is aware of the preoperative and postoperative care that will be administered • States the anticipated outcome of surgery	• Allow the patient to express his feelings. • Correct any misconceptions. • Provide emotional and psychological support. • Make appropriate referrals to clergy, social worker, or physician, as necessary. • Fill in the gaps in his understanding.
Potential of anticipatory grieving for loss of body function	• Patient will feel that he is not alone and that others are there to support him	• Same as above
Potential of anxiety due to upcoming surgery	• Anxiety will be controlled so that the vital signs will be affected minimally	• Same as above • Use distraction therapy. • Accept the patient's behavior. • Reassure him.
Potential of spiritual distress due to illness and surgery	• Will verbalize some acceptance of his situation	• Allow the patient to express his feelings. • Use reality therapy. • Make referral to clergy or other appropriate person. • Be supportive.
Potential of ineffective coping due to illness and surgery	• Will be able to use adaptive coping skills	• Help the patient to mobilize his coping skills. • Assess how he has dealt with problems in the past. • Help the patient to maintain his dignity and self-respect. • Recognize ineffective use of defense mechanisms; do not reinforce use of these mechanisms. • Help the patient substitute adaptive for maladaptive coping mechanisms. • Set limits.
Immediate Postoperative Phase		
Ineffective airway clearance due to altered consciousness and/or neurological deficits	• Patency of airway will be maintained	• Assess for abnormal breath sounds (rales, rhonchi, wheezing, snoring) • Note increase in respiratory rate and pulse. • Auscultate for chest sounds. • Listen for abnormal repiratory sounds with ear. • Note presence of dyspnea or cyanosis. • Suction as often as necessary. • Encourage expectoration of sputum, if patient is conscious. • Keep neck in neutral position. • Do not position unconscious patient in supine position. • Position on side to facilitate drainage of secretions.
Impaired gas exchange due to hypercapnia	• Adequate oxygen–carbon dioxide gas exchange will be maintained as evidenced by blood gases in normal limits	• Assess blood gases periodically. • Administer oxygen as necessary. • Monitor tidal volumes. • Ambu patient every 1 to 2 hours. • Hyperinflate the lungs with 100% oxygen before and after suctioning, if approved by the physician. • Position to facilitate repirations.

CHART 14–1. (continued)

NURSING DIAGNOSIS	EXPECTED OUTCOME	NURSING INTERVENTION
Altered level of consciousness due to cerebral edema and injury to the brain. As a result of the altered consciousness several nursing diagnoses are made:		
• Cognitive impairment due to cerebral edema and injury to brain	• Extent of cognitive impairment will be identified and patient will be cared for until he is able to assume responsibility for self	• Explain what you are doing. • Maintain his dignity. • Reassure him that cognitive ability will improve. • Do not set unrealistic goals.
• Self-care deficit due to neurological impairment and cerebral edema	• Basic needs will be provided for the patient	• Assess extent of deficits. • Administer basic care. • Provide for basic needs. • Allow patient to do as much as possible for self.
• Health maintenance deficit due to neurological deficits	• Health maintenance will be managed for the patient until he is able to assume responsibility for himself	• Decisions concerning the patient will be made with his best interests in mind. • Family will be consulted. • Although the patient may not understand, he will be told what is being done for him. • Reassure the patient. • Be supportive and maintain his dignity.
• Potential of physical injury	• Physical injury will not occur	• Assess patient's safety needs. • Observe the patient frequently. • Pull up siderails on top and bottom of bed. • Maintain bed in low position when you are not at the bedside. • Restrain when necessary to protect patient from injury (a physician's order will be necessary).
Alteration in comfort; headache due to cranial or intracranial surgery	• Pain will be controlled or absent	• Assess for signs and symptoms of pain (*e.g.,* restlessness, pulling on head dressing, change in vital signs). • Administer analgesic as necessary.
Potential of electrolyte imbalance due to surgery or fluid loss or retention	• Electrolytes will be maintained within normal limits	• Monitor serum electrolytes. • Observe for signs and symptoms of electrolyte imbalance. • Administer replacement therapy as ordered.
Potential of fluid loss or retention due to development of diabetes insipidus (DI) or syndrome of inappropriate secretion of antidiuretic hormone (SIADH)	• Fluid balance will be maintained. Patient will be neither overhydrated nor underhydrated (except as necessary for control of intracranial pressure)	• Maintain an intake and output record. • Monitor blood and urine osmolarity and electrolytes. • Monitor urinary specific gravity. • Weigh patient daily or every other day. • Observe for signs and symptoms of DI and SIADH. • Observe for signs and symptoms of overhydration or underhydration.
Altered nutrition: less than required due to altered consciousness and surgery	• Adequate nutrition will be maintained • Protein will be available for tissue repair	• Request a nutrition consultation. • Monitor dietary intake. • Count daily calorie intake. • Ensure adequate intake.
Altered bowel elimination: constipation due to altered diet, constipating drugs, and dehydration	• Bowel function will be maintained without constipation or straining at stool	• Monitor frequency and characteristics of stool. • Initiate a bowel elimination program. • Administer stool softeners as ordered. • Assess for peristalsis. • Administer mild laxative as necessary. • Include roughage in diet, if possible.

(continued)

CHART 14-1. (continued)

NURSING DIAGNOSIS	EXPECTED OUTCOME	NURSING INTERVENTION
Altered urinary elimination due to decreased level of consciousness, development of DI or SIADH	• Urinary elimination will be maintained	• Maintain intake and output record. • Monitor serum creatinine, serum blood urea nitrogen, urinanalysis, and culture and sensitivity of urine. • Monitor fractional urinary specific gravity. • Report urinary output of 200 ml or more an hour for 2 consecutive hours (DI). • Report diminished urinary output. • Maintain patency of catheter.
Potential of increased intracranial pressure due to cerebral edema	• Intracranial pressure will be controlled and spikes will be prevented	• Maintain aseptic technique. • Monitor neurological signs frequently. • Note signs and symptoms of neurological deterioration. • Prevent activities known to increase intracranial pressure (hypercapnia, Valsalva maneuver, etc.; see Chap. 12). • Observe intracranial pressure monitor, if one is in place. • Maintain on fluid restrictions, if ordered. • Elevate head of bed 30 degrees.

following planes: X, the anterior-posterior; Y, the superior-inferior; and Z, the left-right. The point of intersection of all three coordinates identifies the target tissue. Traditional x-rays of anatomical landmarks have been used to identify the target zone, but newer approaches use the computed tomography (CT) scanner and a computer for target point identification.

Once the target area has been identified, the stereotaxic electrode or probe is passed through the slide carrier, which is attached to the stereotaxic frame, to the target area. It is necessary to verify by x-ray or CT scanner that the target area has been reached. Once placement of instruments is verified, the procedure can continue. Since most procedures are conducted under local anesthesia, the cooperation of the patient must be gained. This is accomplished through a thorough patient teaching program on admission to the hospital.

Stereotaxis neurosurgery is indicated for the removal or biopsy of deep, small subcortical brain tumors. However, this technique has been suggested for or applied to implantation of radioactive seeds into brain tumors; aspiration of intracerebral hematomas, colloid cysts, and abscesses; ablative procedures for extrapyramidal diseases (tremors, rigidity, and others); chronic pain control; and removal of craniopharyngiomas. Additional uses will probably be found as experience with the technique increases.

POSTOPERATIVE NURSING MANAGEMENT

The objectives of nursing care in the postoperative period following a craniotomy are directed toward

- Frequent assessment and evaluation of neurological status to recognize increased intracranial pressure
- Control of contributing factors that can increase intracranial pressure
- Prevention and recognition of complications
- Administration of supportive care
- Rehabilitation

Effective nursing care is based on an understanding of the following points:

- Identification of the reason for surgery, approach, and specific area involved
- Existence of preoperative neurological deficits
- Preexisting medical problems
- Short-term prognosis
- Postoperative regimen as ordered by the physician

All of this information is vital in planning nursing care. The nurse's knowledge and skill as an observer and interpreter are the most critical factors influencing patient outcome. Chart 14-1 provides a summary of nursing consideration in a nursing care plan.

IMMEDIATE POSTOPERATIVE CARE

The site of the immediate postoperative care after craniotomy will depend on the routines followed by the hospital and physician. In many facilities the patient is admitted to the surgical or neurosurgical intensive care unit for about 48 to 72 hours after surgery and then returned to the general neurosurgical unit. In other facilities the patient is returned to the general neurosurgical unit immediately after surgery. Regardless of the postoperative routine followed, the full-support equipment for postoperative neurosurgical emergencies and care must be available:

- Emergency cart (emergency drugs, intravenous solution, and so forth)

CHART 14-2. NURSING CARE FOLLOWING SUPRATENTORIAL OR INFRATENTORIAL SURGERY

SUPRATENTORIAL	INFRATENTORIAL
Incision	
The incision is made within the boundaries of the hairline directly over the area to be explored on the cerebral cortex.	The incision is made slightly above the nape of the neck around the occipital area.
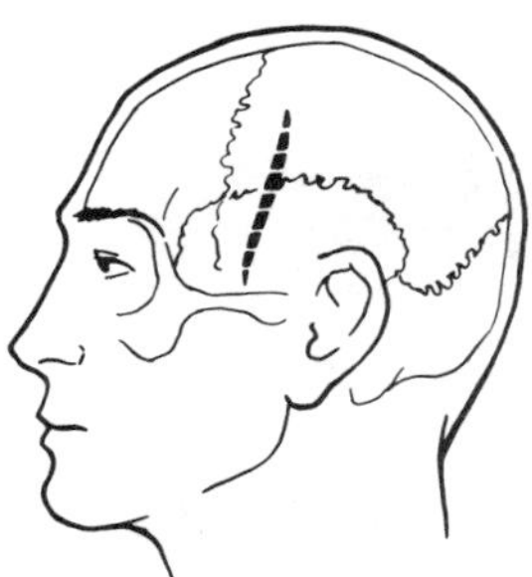	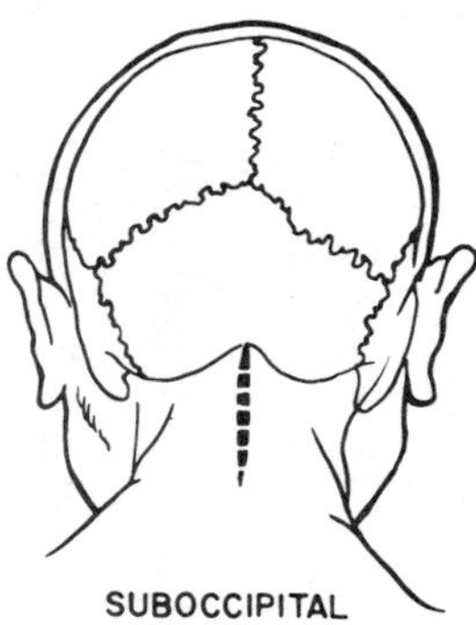
Head Dressing	
A large, turban-style dressing or a dressing covered with stockinette material is worn.	A large, turban-style dressing may be worn with or without added dressings and stiffening in the nape of the neck to prevent flexion of the head.
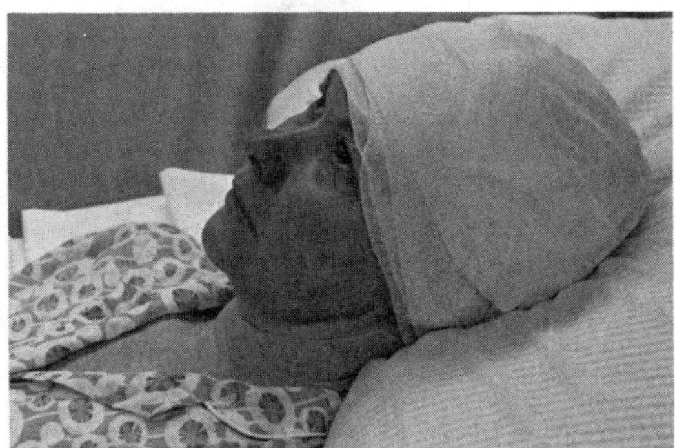	Flexion is contraindicated regardless of infratentorial dressing in order to prevent tearing of the suture line.
Position of the Head of the Bed	
The head is elevated 30 to 45 degrees. A large pillow can be placed under the head and shoulders. This position decreases the chance of hemorrhage, promotes venous drainage from the brain, and improves cerebrospinal fluid circulation.	The patient's head must rest flat with a small pillow under the nape of the neck. This position prevents dizziness and brain stem pressure. The head of the bed is gradually raised in the postoperative period with the physician's approval and based on the tolerance of the patient (no dizziness or light-headedness).
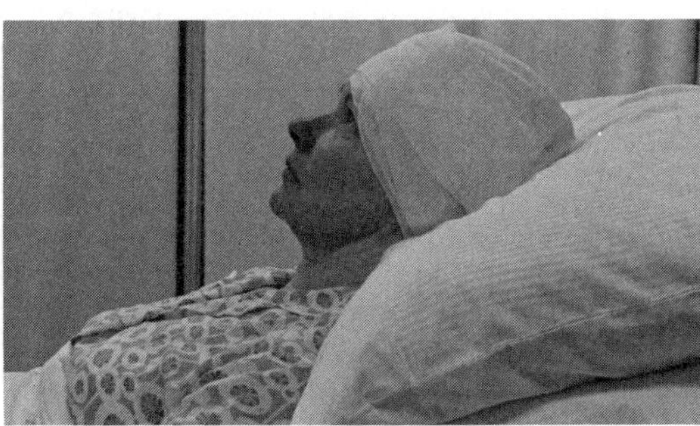	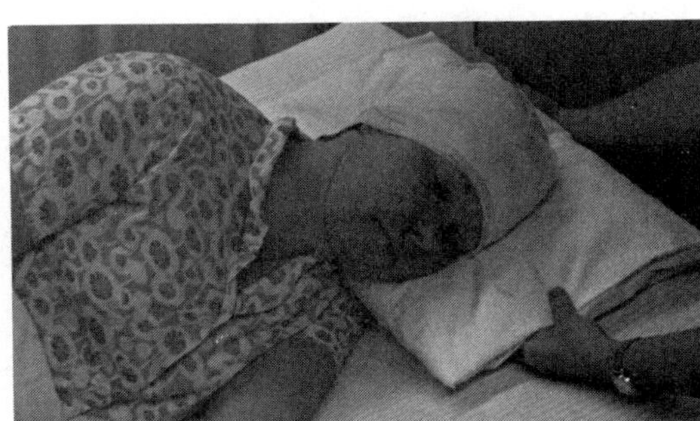

Note: If there is any restriction on the position of the bed, label the head of the bed with a piece of 4-inch tape noting restriction.

(continued)

CHART 14–2. (continued)

SUPRATENTORIAL	INFRATENTORIAL

Turning the Patient

Supratentorial: The patient can be turned to either side or on his back. If a large tumor has been removed, the patient should not be placed on the operative side in order to prevent displacement of cranial contents by gravity.

Infratentorial: The patient can be turned on either side. Some physicians will not permit patients to be on their backs while others do allow this.

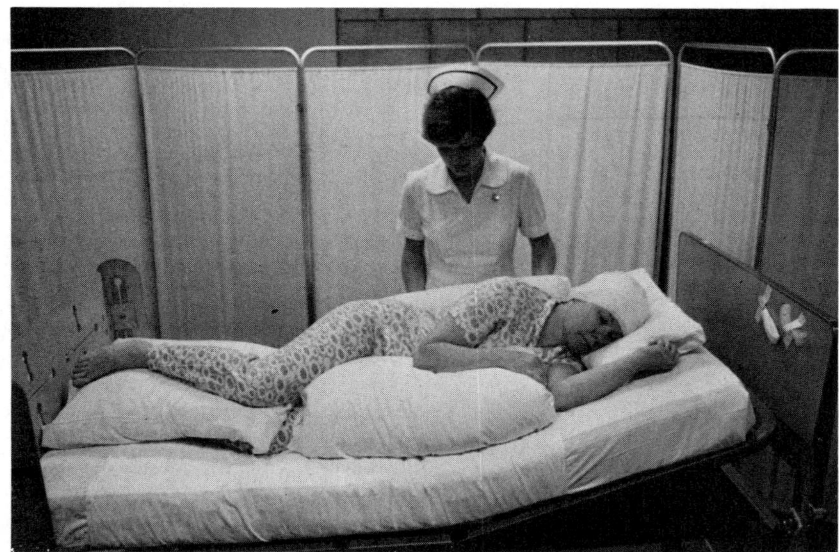

Note: In either case, the patient is placed on his side until he recovers from anesthesia. This position provides for an adequate airway and drainage of secretions.

Ambulation

Supratentorial: The patient is allowed out of bed as soon as tolerated. It will depend on the patient's general condition and the judgment of the physician and nurse.

Infratentorial: The patient is allowed out of bed as soon as the vertical position is tolerated. This patient is often on bed rest longer than the patient with a supratentorial approach. The delay is due to the frequency of dizziness experienced by the patient. This is caused by transient edema in the area of cranial nerve VIII.

Nutrition

Supratentorial:

1. The patient is given nothing by mouth for 24 hours; intravenous fluids are administered slowly.
2. If the patient is not experiencing nausea or vomiting, he is started on clear fluids.

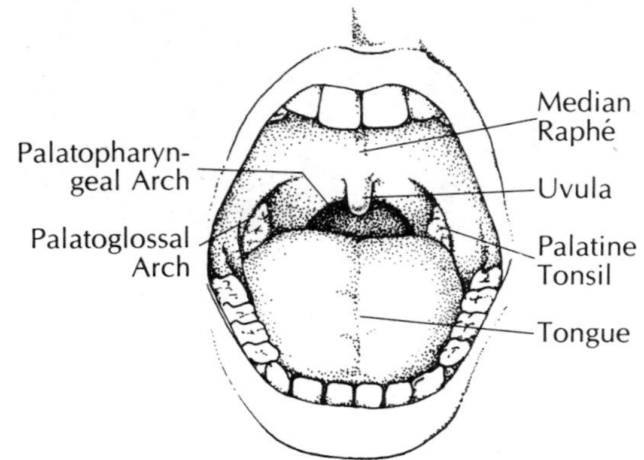

Infratentorial:

1. The patient is given nothing by mouth for *at least* the first 24 hours; intravenous fluids are administered slowly. Nausea tends to be more of a problem with surgery in this region.
2. Edema of cranial nerves IX and X may affect the palatal (swallowing) and pharyngeal (gag) reflexes. The reflexes are tested as indicated in the figure below. If there is no nausea or vomiting noted and the gag and swallowing reflexes are present, the patient is started on water with a straw. Ask the patient to take a small sip and swallow it. (Even though the reflexes are intact, the presence of the palatal reflex is tested by touching the soft palate with a tongue depressor. A normal response is elevation of the palate. The pharyngeal [gag] reflex is checked by touching the posterior wall of the pharynx. The normal response is contraction of the pharynx. Both reflexes should be checked on the left and right sides of the palate and posterior pharynx. There may be slight hesitancy caused by edema). If nausea or vomiting occurs, give the patient nothing by mouth and continue intravenous therapy; after nausea or vomiting has subsided, try again on oral fluids.

CHART 14–2. (continued)

SUPRATENTORIAL	INFRATENTORIAL
3. Progress the diet as tolerated.	**3.** Once the patient is able to tolerate fluids, progress from clear liquids to diet as tolerated.
4. Feed patient for the first few days to prevent fatigue and ensure adequate nutrition.	**4.** Feed patient for the first few days to prevent fatigue and ensure adequate nutrition.
5. If a fluid restriction is ordered, stay within the daily allowance.	**5.** If a fluid restriction is ordered, stay within the daily allowance.

Note: The patient is kept slightly underhydrated to combat cerebral edema.

Elimination

1. In both types of surgery a Foley catheter is usually inserted in the operating room. Catheter care should be provided twice daily to prevent infection.
2. If the area around the sella turcica or the pituitary gland was involved in the surgery, there is the possibility of dysfunction of the posterior pituitary, resulting in diabetes insipidus. A disturbance in secretion of antidiuretic hormone (ADH)—diabetes insipidus—is characterized by large amounts of urine with low specific gravity. Fractional urinary outputs and specific gravity are checked at frequent intervals (every 1 to 4 hours) and recorded.
3. Following both types of surgery, the patient may have difficulty with constipation. A daily stool softener should be given.

Note: Straining at stool initiates the Valsalva manuever, which increases intracranial pressure.

- Emergency tracheostomy tray
- Lumbar puncture tray
- Materials for seizure precautions (padding for siderails, padded tongue depressor, and so forth)
- Siderails
- Suction setup (oropharyngeal and/or tracheal suctioning)
- Oxygen setup (respirator, if necessary)

The patient is placed on an alternating pressure mattress to prevent pressure on an area of the body that could lead to skin breakdown.

Much of the approach to care will depend on whether the patient has undergone supratentorial or infratentorial surgery. (The care is summarized in Chart 14–2.)

ASSESSMENT OF NEUROLOGICAL SIGNS

The neurological signs are assessed routinely to determine the presence and extent of increased intracranial pressure. The knowledge that the patient has recently undergone surgical insult is reason enough to draw the conclusion that increased intracranial pressure is present. However, the nurse, in assessing the neurological signs, should identify changes in condition that may be subtle or rapid. Current findings of the assessment should be compared with baseline findings to determine trends. Neurological assessment includes

- Level of consciousness
- Pupillary signs
- Ocular movement
- Sensory function
- Motor function
- Vital signs (particularly the respiratory pattern)

The frequency with which the assessment is conducted will depend on how stable the patient's condition is and how soon after surgery it is. One would expect neurological signs to be assessed every 15 to 30 minutes for the first 8 to 12 hours postoperatively, then every hour for the next 12 hours. As the patient stabilizes, the frequency of assessment will eventually be every 4 hours.

Blood electrolytes should be checked routinely for electrolyte imbalance. A decreased sodium and chloride level can result in weakness, lethargy, and coma while a decreased potassium level results in confusion. Both can affect the neurological signs and create confusion about the etiology of the change in condition.

BASIC NURSING PROTOCOLS

In addition to the nursing protocols outlined for the patient with a supratentorial or infratentorial surgical procedure, there are basic maintenance and supportive protocols followed for all patients, regardless of the cranial area involved for the surgery. These protocols are summarized in Chart 14–3.

POSTOPERATIVE COMPLICATIONS

Numerous problems and complications may develop after craniotomy, including the following: shock, increased intracranial pressure, cerebral edema, respiratory complications, convulsions, meningitis, wound infection, thrombophlebitis, cardiac arrhythmias, loss of corneal reflex, postoperative hydrocephalus, and diabetes insipidus.

CHART 14-3. BASIC NURSING PROTOCOLS FOLLOWING CRANIAL SURGERY

NURSING RESPONSIBILITY	RATIONALE
1. Give basic hygienic care until the patient is gradually able to participate in self-care (includes bath, oral hygiene, combing hair, cutting nails).	**1.** Conserves patient's energy; maintains cleanliness and dignity
2. Apply elastic stockings and inspect legs daily. Note any signs of thrombophlebitis upon inspection of legs (redness, tenderness, warmth, swelling).	**2.** Improves return of blood to heart and decreases the possibilities of thrombophlebitis
3. Provide skin care every 4 hours.	**3.** Cleanses, lubricates, and provides the opportunity for an inspection of the skin to note irritation or skin breakdown
4. Turn patient every 2 hours, being careful to maintain the patient's body alignment.	**4.** Prevents prolonged pressure on specific areas of the skin; prevents pooling of secretions and development of pneumonia and atelectasis
5. Position the patient in proper body alignment and check every 2 hours. (It will be necessary to use pillows and other similar devices to maintain good body alignment.)	**5.** Prevents the development of musculoskeletal abnormalities
6. Carry out range-of-motion exercises four times daily.	**6.** Maintains muscle tone to prevent atrophy and contractures
7. Provide aseptic urinary catheter care daily. This includes (1) washing the perineal area, (2) applying antiseptic ointment such as Betadine around the meatus, and (3) pinning the catheter to prevent undue traction on the meatus.	**7.** Reduces the incidence of urinary tract infection
8. Apply warm or cold moist compresses to the eye area.	**8.** Relieves signs of periocular edema
9. Inspect eyes every 4 hours for signs of irritation or dryness. Lubricate the eye with normal saline, commercially prepared eye lubricant, or ointment as prescribed by the physician. To protect the eye from injury (corneal ulcerations or abrasions) in the event that the lids do not tightly cover the eye, use an eye shield or tape the eye closed, as prescribed by the physician.	**9.** Prevents injury to or dryness of the cornea and other parts of the eye
10. Pull up siderails and apply protective jacket as necessary.	**10.** Provides for patient's safety.
11. Evaluate periods of restlessness for underlying cause by checking patency of airway, evidence of pain, or a distention of the bladder.	**11.** In the neurological patient, restlessness can be caused by an obstructed airway, pain, or a distended bladder.
12. Administer analgesics as ordered (drug should not mask neurological signs).	**12.** Provides for comfort of patient and control of restlessness
13. Do not cluster together nursing activities that are known to increase intracranial pressure in the patient at risk.	**13.** Prevents dangerous spikes in intracranial pressure
14. Monitor routine vital signs, taking the temperature with a rectal thermometer.	**14.** Provides data that indicate condition of the patient
15. Assess neurological signs at prescribed intervals: • Level of consciousness • Pupillary reaction • Eye movement • Motor function • Sensory function	**15.** Provides data about neurological condition and data for comparison with previous signs to denote change in patient's condition.
16. Review laboratory reports such as electrolytes, BUN, hemoglobin. Normal values for some studies are • Hemoglobin—12.0 gm to 16.0 gm in females 13.5 gm to 18.0 gm in males • Hematocrit—40% to 48% in females 42% to 50% in males • BUN—8 mg to 25 mg • Potassium—3.5 mEq to 5.0 mEq • Calcium—8.5 mg to 10.5 mg • Sodium—135 mEq to 145 mEq • Fasting blood sugar—70 mg to 110 mg • Creatinine—0.6 mg to 0.9 mg/dl in females 0.8 mg to 1.2 mg/dl in males	**16.** Indicates levels of important components of the blood, which indicate physiology of other systems

SHOCK (HEMORRHAGIC, HYPOVOLEMIC, OR INTRACRANIAL BLEEDING)

Hemorrhagic shock is caused by blood loss during surgery or in the postoperative period. Blood may be evident on the dressing, and blood replacement therapy may be required if the loss is significant.

- The nurse should check the dressing frequently to determine the amount of bleeding present and should monitor the patient for signs and symptoms of hemorrhagic shock, including tachycardia; a thready pulse; decreased blood pressure; pallor; cold, clammy skin; and restlessness.
- Tachycardia is perhaps the first sign of shock.

Hypovolemic shock results from general fluid loss (blood, plasma, or water), particularly if osmotic diuretics have been used. The result is a decreased amount of circulating fluid (plasma) in the body.

- The characteristics of hypovolemic shock include a drop in venous pressure and an increase in peripheral resistance. Common signs and symptoms include tachycardia; falling blood pressure; shallow and rapid respirations; cool, pale skin; low urinary output (10 ml to 25 ml/hour), and restlessness to coma.

Treatment is directed toward use of fluid expanders such as dextran, lactated Ringer's solution, or blood. Vasopressor drugs are also commonly given and include such drugs as isoproterenol (Isuprel) and l-norepinephrine (Levophed). The patient should be monitored with a CVP (central venous pressure) line to determine the circulating blood volume. The vital signs should be evaluated frequently.

Intracranial hemorrhage is a serious postoperative complication in the neurological patient, resulting in bleeding into the subdural, epidural, intracerebral, or intraventricular space. Unlike bleeding that is visible externally, bleeding within the cranial vault is characterized by signs or symptoms of a rapidly increased intracranial pressure. A rapid deterioration in the neurological status is often associated with intracranial bleeding; this condition requires immediate intervention to prevent irreversible cerebral damage and death.

INCREASED INTRACRANIAL PRESSURE

Although some increase in intracranial pressure is expected (with the peak occurring about 72 hours after surgery), great spikes in intracranial pressure in the patient are life-threatening events. Great increases in intracranial pressure can result from conditions such as cerebral edema, hemorrhage, meningitis, and surgical trauma. Treatment includes

- Management of the underlying cause
- Initiation of a dehydration regime
- Osmotic diuretics
- Slight underhydration
- Use of corticosteroids
- Possible ventricular drainage

Signs and Symptoms

Frequent assessment of vital signs can be helpful in noting developing trends in the patient's condition. Bradycardia, an elevated systolic pressure, and widening pulse pressure are indicative of increasing intracranial pressure but are not *early* signs and correlate best with posterior fossa hypertension. Massive spikes in body temperature are also associated with extensive increased intracranial pressure although it is not an early sign.

The most sensitive of neurological signs indicating a deterioration of condition appears to be first, the level of consciousness, and second, the respiratory pattern. However, any deterioration in any of the other neurological signs is significant and should be noted and reported.

- For the conscious patient, deep breathing exercises should be included in the nursing care plan to prevent pneumonia and atelectasis.
- In the intubated or comatose patient, the Ambu bag should be used every 1 to 2 hours to expand the lungs completely, preventing sites of dead air that could lead to atelectasis. The development of pneumonia is also decreased by the prevention of stasis of fluid in the lungs.
- Oxygen should be administered as necessary at a concentration sufficient to maintain adequate oxygen blood levels. Routine analysis of blood gases is helpful in determining adequate oxygen concentration within the blood as well as aiding in selection of the best concentration of oxygen for delivery to the patient.
- To prevent aspiration pneumonia, no patient should be given fluids or food unless the pharyngeal (gag) and palatal (swallowing) reflexes are validated. (The gag reflex is tested by touching the posterior wall of the pharynx to determine whether the pharynx contracts; the swallowing reflex is tested by touching the soft palate, which should elevate.)

Preventing Increased Intracranial Pressure

Respiratory Considerations. Certain changes in the respiratory system can contribute to the development of systemic hypercapnia and hypoxia, which increases cerebral edema and intracranial pressure; thus, a patent airway must be maintained at all times. Even partial obstruction of the airway or interference with normal O_2–CO_2 gas exchange because of mucus can contribute to the development of hypercapnia and hypoxia. Therefore, nursing care should include protocols that facilitate adequate respiratory function:

- Maintain the neck in neutral position.
- Place the patient in the side-lying position to promote drainage of secretions. Turn the patient every 2 hours to prevent pooling of secretions, development of pneumonia, and atelectasis.
- Suction as necessary to remove secretion from the oropharyngeal or tracheal areas so that a patent airway can be maintained. To prevent the development of hypercapnia, limit suctioning to no more than 15 seconds for each insertion of the catheter. If not contraindicated, hyperinflate the lungs with 100% oxygen before suctioning to prevent hypoxia and hypercapnia from developing. (Elevating the head of the bed to a 30-degree angle is implemented to facilitate venous drainage from the brain.)

Avoiding the Valsalva Maneuver. The Valsalva maneuver results in an increase in intracranial pressure. Measures must be taken to prevent initiation of the Valsalva maneuver by controlling any precipitating activities such as straining at stool, enemas, coughing, sneezing, pushing against the footboard, and pulling or turning while the glottis is closed. The patient should be instructed to exhale when turning or moving in bed. When one exhales, the glottis is open and the Valsalva maneuver is foiled. To prevent straining at stool, stool softeners are given. Enemas are usually contraindicated for the neurological patient.

Avoiding Isometric Contractions. Since isometric contractions cause an increase in intracranial pressure, exercises of this nature should be omitted from the care plans. In addition, the patient should be prevented from pushing his feet against the footboard.

Cerebral Edema

In the neurosurgical patient the major cause of increased intracranial pressure is cerebral edema. Cerebral edema may have been present before surgery or could develop or increase as a result of the surgical trauma. Postoperative cerebral edema can be controlled by initiation of several nursing protocols:

- Elevation of the head of the bed to 30 degrees to aid in the drainage of blood from the brain. Gravity can be used to enhance drainage because the venous vessels from the brain are valveless. Thirty degrees has been demonstrated to be the best angle of elevation for drainage.
- All intake (oral or by means of a Levin tube, gastrostomy, and intravenous feedings) should be controlled to keep the patient slightly underhydrated. Restricting fluid intake will help control cerebral edema. The amount of fluid for a 24-hour period should be ordered in milliliters and posted conspicuously at the bedside and on the Kardex and care plan to alert all nursing personnel to the restriction. If an intravenous infusion is being administered, it should run slowly.
- To maintain a fluid restriction, an accurate intake and output record should be kept. Fluid restrictions may be as strict as 900 ml/24 hours or as liberal as 2500 ml/24 hours.
- A Foley catheter should be in place if osmotic diuretics are ordered. The urinary output should be measured to quantify the amount of diuresis. Controlled diuresis is helpful in reducing cerebral edema.
- Corticosteroids should be administered as ordered. Dexamethasone (Decadron) is the drug commonly ordered to reduce cerebral edema. The drug is administered with an antacid to prevent gastrointestinal irritation, ulceration, and bleeding.
- The stools should be checked daily for occult blood, which would indicate bleeding somewhere in the gastrointestinal tract. In addition, a gradual drop in hemoglobin on the blood report is suggestive of bleeding somewhere in the body.

Respiratory Complications

Partial or complete obstruction of the airway can occur from improper positioning or accumulation of mucus or other drainage.

- The unconscious patient should never be positioned on his back because the tongue can easily slip backward and obstruct the airway.
- Maintain the neck in neutral position.

If an unconscious patient begins to snore, it is most likely due to obstruction of the airway. This situation must be corrected immediately to prevent not only respiratory failure but cerebral hypoxia as well. The jaw is pulled forward and downward to relieve the obstruction. The patient should be positioned on his side with his head elevated to facilitate drainage.

Elevating the head of the bed 30 degrees is helpful in maintaining a patent airway. If the obstructed airway is not immediately cleared, cerebral hypoxia could develop and lead to a great increase in carbon dioxide. Carbon dioxide, a potent vasodilator, would greatly increase intracranial pressure.

Respiratory difficulty may also result from edema in and around the brain stem, particularly following infratentorial surgery. Aspiration caused by diminished or absent gag and swallowing reflexes can be minimized by properly positioning the patient on his side with his head elevated and withholding oral intake until the presence of the gage and swallowing reflex has been verified.

The nurse should also be aware that adult respiratory distress syndrome (ARDS) and neurogenic pulmonary edema can develop. (See Chap. 5 for discussion of both conditions.) A few words are included here about neurogenic pulmonary edema.

It is thought that a sudden, massive increase in intracranial pressure triggers a pressor response, which results in the development of neurogenic pulmonary edema. The signs and symptoms are the same as those of acute pulmonary edema caused by cardiac decompensation, although in the neurological patient there is no evidence of cardiac disease that could be considered responsible for acute pulmonary edema. Common signs and symptoms of neurogenic pulmonary edema include

- Dyspnea
- Restlessness
- Tachycardia
- Anxiety
- Rapid, moist respirations
- Cold, clammy skin
- Gray or cyanotic skin
- Expectoration of mucus and possible blood

The prognosis is poor even if rapid cranial decompression is possible.

Other pulmonary complications include pneumonia, atelectasis, and pulmonary emboli. Pneumonia and atelectasis have already been discussed. However, pulmonary emboli are a possible complication in any surgical patient especially if surgery is prolonged and hypothermia has been used.

- With any respiratory complication, prophylactic protocols of frequent turning, suctioning, deep breathing techniques, and maintenance of a patent airway should be followed.

Convulsions (Seizure Activity)

Seizures following cranial surgery may take the form of generalized convulsions or focal seizure activity. The most common generalized seizure that might occur is the grand mal seizure. Focal seizures in the form of twitching of selected muscles particularly of the face or hand are also common. Focal seizures in these two areas are common because both occupy large areas on the motor strip of the cerebral cortex; therefore, irritation from surgery or cerebral edema can initiate seizure activity.

Because seizures are common after intracranial surgery, craniotomy patients are usually put on prophylactic phenytoin (Dilantin) to prevent seizure activity.

Seizure precautions should be instituted so that necessary equipment is immediately available should a grand mal seizure occur. Seizure precautions include

- Padded tongue blade
- Oropharyngeal suction
- Padded siderails

For signs and symptoms of seizures see Chapter 27.

Meningitis

Microorganisms responsible for meningitis can be introduced into the meninges or cerebrospinal fluid by spreading from a wound infection, from a head injury in which the dura mater has been punctured, or by contamination at surgery. Evidence of a dural tear, a prime site for entrance of microorganisms, is evident by clear drainage on the head dressing or such drainage from the ear or nose. The drainage on the dressing appears as the *halo sign*—the center of the drainage mark is bloody or serosanguinous, with the outer circle being clear or yellowish. The clear or yellowish drainage suggests cerebrospinal fluid.

Cerebrospinal fluid may also be noticed draining from the ear or nose. To determine if the drainage is cerebrospinal fluid a Dextrostix can be used. Collect some drainage and insert the Dextrostix. If the drainage is cerebrospinal fluid it will be positive in response to the glucose in the cerebrospinal fluid. Mucus does not contain glucose.

- If cerebrospinal fluid is present in drainage from the nose, the patient must not be suctioned nasally or allowed to blow his nose.

Meningitis is treated with large doses of antibiotics and a quiet environment. Most physicians order prophylactic antibiotics routinely after all intracranial surgery for a few days.

Other signs and symptoms associated with meningitis include

- Positive Kernig's and Brudzinski's sign
- Stiff neck
- Photophobia
- Restlessness and hyperirritability
- Elevated temperature

However, prophylactic measures should be taken to prevent the development of meningitis and strict aseptic technique should be followed in the management of the surgical site. Part of the nursing responsibility in this regard is checking for drainage on the dressing and observing its character. A wet head dressing should be reinforced immediately and the physician notified. Because moisture provides organisms with a transport system, a wet head dressing is an ideal medium upon which organisms can grow. The gauze used in most dressings absorbs drainage by capillary attraction. The wicking action helps to remove the drainage from the skin. If a very wet dressing is allowed to remain on the incision, the incision will become contaminated from organisms in the air or on bedclothes by the wicking action of the moist dressing.

When head dressings are changed, strict aseptic technique should be followed. Usually the initial dressing is not touched until the sutures are removed or unless it has become wet. The policy of the hospital and physician should be followed concerning who may change an initial dressing.

Lastly, the nurse should judiciously administer the prophylactic antibiotics ordered by the physician at the prescribed intervals to prevent the development of infection.

Wound Infection

Wound infections can result from poor aseptic technique during surgery or dressing change. The patient may also contaminate his incision by touching it with his hands. To avoid this, the patient must be cautioned against such action and restrained if necessary. The most frequent causative organisms for wound infections are the various staphylococcal organisms. Redness and drainage from the wound are the usual early symptoms. The nurse should observe the incision and dressing for evidence of drainage. A foul odor may also raise suspicion of wound infection. An elevated white blood count would be expected.

Strict aseptic technique should be followed in the management of the wound or dressing. If a wound infection develops, the patient should be placed on "wound precautions" to prevent spreading of the infection. Special moist dressings may be applied to the infected wound to allow for healing from the inside of the incision outward. In addition to wound precautions and application of special dressings, the physician will order antibiotics to treat the infection.

Wound Precautions. When a potentially dangerous organism is identified, special precautions must be followed in handling the contaminated dressing and equipment. Dressings are disposed of in separate double bags that are sealed. Equipment used to dress the wound is sterilized separately, and all linen used by the patient is placed in isolation laundry bags for special handling. In addition, the patient is placed in a private room to safeguard other patients from infection. Most hospitals follow the prescribed "wound precaution" protocol outlined by the hospital infection control (epidemiology) department.

Thrombophlebitis

Any patient on bed rest for even short periods is prone to the development of thrombophlebitis. In addition, techniques used in surgery such as hypothermia and keeping the patient in certain positions for extended periods can be contributory factors in neurosurgical patients. Thrombophlebitis is a serious concern because it can lead to a life-threatening pulmonary embolism.

Treatment of thrombophlebitis follows the usual medical protocol of bed rest, elastic stockings, and elevation of the involved limb. Discretion in the use of anticoagulation therapy, a usual treatment principle, is followed because such drugs may cause bleeding at the surgical site.

The following principles for prevention of thrombophlebitis should be incorporated into the nursing care plan:

- Application of elastic stockings, which are valuable in preventing stasis of blood in the lower legs and improving the venous blood return to the heart
- Range-of-motion exercise to the legs to prevent stasis of blood and improve blood return to the heart
- Observation of the legs for signs and symptoms of thrombophlebitis (redness, swelling, pain)

Cardiac Arrhythmias

Cardiac arrhythmias are not unusual after posterior fossa surgery or if blood has entered the cerebrospinal fluid, a distinct possibility during surgery. A cardiac monitor may be affixed to the patient for the first 24 to 48 hours after surgery. If this is the case, the nurse should periodically observe the rate, rhythm, and pattern on the monitor to determine the presence of an arrhythmia.

If a monitor is not available, the apical pulse should be checked in the postoperative period to identify abnormalities in the heart rate or rhythm. Any abnormalities should be reported to the physician immediately.

Loss of Corneal Reflex

The presence of the corneal reflex is determined by lightly touching the cornea of the eye with a wisp of cotton. The eye should immediately blink. If the corneal reflex is absent, the affected eye must be protected from injury. Corneal abrasion and ulceration can develop from direct injury or from depriving the eye of proper lubrication with moisture. Blindness can be the unfortunate and permanent consequence of corneal ulceration. Applying an eye shield or taping the lids closed can prevent corneal abrasion.

Periodic administration of artificial tears or saline solution can moisten the eye and prevent drying of the cornea. It is usually administered four times daily.

The nurse should determine the presence of the corneal reflex. If it is not present, a special nursing protocol should be developed to prevent eye injury. The eyes should be inspected when administering care to identify any evidence of injury or irritation.

Since the corneal reflex is controlled by the cranial nerve V, other deficits in this nerve may occur such as loss of sensation to touch on the face or weakness of the masseter and temporal muscles used to clench the teeth. In addition, the facial nerve (VII) is closely associated with the trigeminal nerve. It is assessed by asking the patient to wrinkle his brow, show his teeth, open his mouth, close his eyes, smile, and whistle. The anterior two thirds of the tongue is innervated for the sensation of taste. Although these nerves need not be evaluated with every assessment, the nurse should periodically ascertain their functional levels.

Postoperative Hydrocephalus

The postoperative complication of hydrocephalus can develop as a result of edema or bleeding. Bleeding can interfere with the normal production and absorption of cerebrospinal fluid by plugging the arachnoid villi and preventing normal absorption of cerebrospinal fluid. Plugging of the arachnoid villa from bleeding is also associated with primary disease processes such as a ruptured cerebral aneurysm or head trauma. Scarring or obstruction in the ventricular system can also lead to hydrocephalus. The postoperative complication of hydrocephalus occurs more frequently after posterior fossa surgery.

Signs and symptoms of hydrocephalus have been outlined in Chapter 12. The usual treatment requires a surgical shunting procedure to relieve the brain of excessive cerebrospinal fluid and prevent cerebral atrophy.

Diabetes Insipidus

Supratentorial surgery, particularly in and around the pituitary fossa, can lead to temporary diabetes insipidus. Diabetes insipidus is due to a disturbance of the posterior lobe of the pituitary gland, which produces the antidiuretic hormone. If this hormone is not secreted in sufficient quantity, the patient will produce large amounts of urine with low specific gravity. The danger is that the patient will experience a fluid and electrolyte imbalance with dehydration, a serious concern that can affect all body systems.

The development of diabetes insipidus is often a transient problem requiring no specific treatment other than adjusting intravenous therapy based on a correlation with urinary outputs. If the condition does not correct itself, 5 to 10 units of aqueous vasopressin (Pitressin) may be given subcutaneously every 3 to 6 hours. The newest drug used for the treatment of severe permanent or transient complete central diabetes insipidus is desmopressin acetate (DDAVP); 0.1 ml to 0.4 ml are administered intranasally in nasal drops one or two times daily. The duration of the drug is 12 to 24 hours; its side-effects of nasal irritation or vasoconstriction on the nasal mucosa are minimal. Desmopressin acetate is the drug of choice for the treatment of diabetes insipidus.

The nurse should maintain an accurate intake and output record, and fractional urinary outputs should be measured. This is a simple task if a Foley catheter is in place, as is often the case in the early postoperative period when evidence of diabetes insipidus is most apt to occur. The specific gravity of the urine should also be checked about every 1 to 4 hours. A reading of 1.005 or less is considered to be low.

- Large amounts of urine coupled with low specific gravity is indicative of diabetes insipidus.

The patient's hydration level and electrolytes should be monitored regularly to determine the need for replacement therapy. The physician should be made aware of the urinary output and specific gravity. As mentioned above, the condition is often temporary and corrects itself without treatment. See Chapter 13 for a discussion of diabetes insipidus.

Other Postoperative Concerns

Diminished Level of Consciousness. As the cerebral edema subsides, the intracranial pressure will decrease and the level of consciousness will improve. It is often surprising to find a patient fully alert and well oriented after surgery even though there is some cerebral edema present from the surgical procedure.

Deficits in Communications. The patient's ability to express himself verbally and to understand the spoken word will depend on what deficits were present before surgery and what part of the brain was the site of the surgery. If deficits are associated with cerebral edema, they will most likely improve as cerebral edema subsides. If the deficit was prominent before surgery, or if surgical dissection affected the language areas, recovery will be much slower, perhaps requiring a referral to a speech therapist.

The nurse should evaluate the type of communication disability and develop an alternate method of communication. If the patient requires only that the nurse speak more slowly and use simple rather than complex sentences, such an adjustment can easily be made if the nursing diagnosis of the problem has been accurate. A notation on the nursing care plan should be made to describe what alterations are necessary. If this is followed by all personnel, it will greatly reduce the frustration of the patient, as well as that of the staff, in facilitating communication.

Motor and Sensory Deficits. As with consciousness and communication deficits, a decrease in cerebral edema results in functional improvement of the motor and sensory function. The level of improvement is contingent upon the neurological deficit present before surgery and the surgical site.

For patients with motor deficits, a physical therapy program is usually designed to aid in the return of motor function. The nurse must be aware of specific deficits experienced by the patient and participate in the continuity of care that will support the principles of the physiotherapeutic program. Adaptations of nursing care may be necessary to meet the needs of the patient.

The nurse can participate in such ways as encouraging the patient to use a weak limb in the activities of daily living; administering range-of-motion exercises; ensuring proper positioning; applying special braces and splints if these devices are part of the program; and helping the patient in ambulation. Most of all, the nurse is often called upon to provide emotional support as the patient deals with loss of body function and alterations of body image and the "self concept."

Headache. Headache is expected in the first 24 to 48 hours postoperatively and will probably be severe. Much of the pain originates from surgical stretching or irritation of the nerves of the scalp. Pain can also result from traction on the dura, falx, or large blood vessels within the intracranial space. A headache can be intensified by a head dressing that has been applied too tightly. The snugness of the dressing should be assessed for comfort. If a dressing becomes too tight (as evidenced by swelling), the dressing will need to be loosened, cut, or changed.

Codeine sulfate 15 mg to 60 mg or acetaminophen (Tylenol) 650 mg are the drugs most commonly ordered. The particular drug selected will depend on the severity of the headache. A quiet environment with limited direct light or a dimmed room is most soothing. If an ice cap for the head is not contraindicated, it can be used as a comfort measure.

Hyperthermia. Some elevation in temperature is expected in the early postoperative period. A rectal temperature is taken at prescribed intervals to monitor body temperature. Elevation of body temperature above 98.6° F (37° C) can indicate the presence of infection or irritation of the hypothalamus, the area of the brain responsible for regulation of the body temperature. Traction or petechial hemorrhage of the hypothalamus or pons can cause major elevations in body temperature (105° F; 40.6° C). Surgery in or around the third or fourth ventricle can also initiate dramatic spikes in body temperature because of the proximity to the hypothalamus.

As body temperature becomes elevated, there is an increase in arterial and venous blood pressure, an increase in cerebral blood flow, and an increase in the cerebral metabolic rate. The metabolism of glucose, the major nutrient of the brain, is directly proportional to the rate of oxygen consumption. As cerebral metabolism increases, the production of the metabolic by-products (carbon dioxide and lactic acid) increases. Both carbon dioxide and lactic acid are potent vasodilating agents that contribute to the increase in intracranial pressure. Therefore, an elevation of body temperatures contributes to the elevation of increased intracranial pressure.

- It is important to control elevations of body temperature in the neurosurgical patient because hyperthermia may result in increased intracranial pressure.

Hyperthermia is controlled by using antipyretic drugs such as acetaminophen (Tylenol) or sometimes aspirin (650 mg by mouth or rectally). Aspirin is usually not ordered because of its irritating effect on the gastrointestinal tract, which could lead to hemorrhage. Gastrointestinal hemorrhage is possible in a patient who is receiving Decadron to control cerebral edema and another drug that causes gastrointestinal tract irritation as a side-effect.

Drug therapy may be used in conjunction with a hypothermia blanket, control of the environment, removal of excess bedclothes, or sponging of the body with cool water. The lowering of body temperature should be achieved gradually to prevent shivering. If shivering occurs, chlorpromazine (Thorazine) may be ordered by the physician to control this untoward response because shivering causes an increase in intracranial pressure. In addition, it should be mentioned that most physicians order broad-spectrum antibiotics prophylactically after surgery to prevent infections such as meningitis, which causes an elevation in temperature.

Periocular Edema. Swelling around the eyes (periocular edema) is common after cranial surgery because of the manipulation of scalp, skull, and intracranial contents. Periocular edema is usually accompanied by discoloration and ecchymosis.

Alteration of warm and cold saline or water compresses, or cold compresses initially that are followed by warm saline compresses after 24 hours, can be helpful. The eyes should be irrigated about four times daily to prevent crusting and infection. Periocular edema will disappear in 3 to 4 days. Discoloration and ecchymosis will take 10 to 14 days for resolution.

Loss of Pharyngeal or Palatal Reflex. The pharyngeal and palatal reflexes are controlled by cranial nerves IX and X. Both nerves emit from the brain stem at the medulla. Surgery in the posterior fossa (infratentorial area) may cause edema to the brain stem and cranial nerves, resulting in temporary loss of both reflexes. As edema subsides, the reflexes will usually return.

The danger of a temporary loss of either reflex is difficulty in swallowing. There can be regurgitation of food through the nose because the oropharynx is not closed during swallowing, or there is weakness or loss of movement of the throat muscles upon swallowing. Regurgitation or aspiration of food with consequent lung problems and respiratory difficulty are serious possibilities. Therefore, oral intake should not be instituted unless the presence of both reflexes can be validated. Suction equipment should be readily available for use should the need arise.

Visual Disturbances. The vision of the neurosurgical patient should be assessed if he is sufficiently conscious to provide information. The visual field can generally be evaluated by introducing a finger or pencil into the patient's visual field. Temporary visual loss in half or one quarter of the visual field is common after surgery because of the increased intracranial pressure or surgical trauma. Diplopia (double vision) and dimness of vision can also be evaluated by asking the patient to describe changes in vision. If diplopia is evident, an eye patch can be worn.

Even in the noncommunicative patient the nurse can draw a presumptive conclusion about visual loss by observing him. For example, the nurse may observe that the patient does not notice environmental objects on one side of the bed or reacts only when someone approaches him from a specific side. Both situations indicate visual deficits.

Personality Changes. Changes in the normal personality can be temporary or permanent. Permanent changes can occur from cerebral anoxia or surgery in the frontal area. Temporary personality changes can result from cerebral edema, surgery, drugs, or emotional stress.

The reason for any assessed personality change may be difficult to determine, since the cause may be singular or multiple. If personality changes continue after cerebral edema has subsided, a psychological or psychiatric evaluation may be indicated.

Personality changes, although common after cranial surgery, are most disturbing for both the patient and the family. The nurse should be supportive, answering questions as honestly as possible and providing encouragement.

Urinary Bladder Disorders. Cystitis, incontinence, or retention of urine are all possible occurrences after craniotomy. The insertion of a Foley catheter, a usual practice for a craniotomy, can result in cystitis, regardless of how carefully the principles of asepsis are followed. Catheter care should be provided twice daily to reduce infection.

A routine urinalysis and urine culture should be obtained periodically after surgery to indicate the evidence of infection (bacterial). In addition, the urine should be observed for cloudiness, sediment, or foul odor. An accurate intake and output record should be maintained. If bacteria are present in the urine and the colony count is elevated, the drugs most frequently ordered are sulfisoxazole (Gantrisin) or methenamine mandelate (Mandelamine). It is the usual practice to remove the Foley catheter as soon as possible to decrease the possibility of infection to the urethra or bladder.

After the catheter is removed, the amount of urine voided should be measured for the first 24 hours to assess adequate bladder evacuation. Urinary retention with overflow would be evidenced by frequent, small voidings. Retention without overflow would be evidenced by inability to void with distention and lower abdominal discomfort. Incontinence of the bladder is characterized by a constant dribbling of urine.

Continence depends on the patient's awareness of the need to void and his ability to control the urge to void. Both stimuli are mediated in part by the frontal lobes of the cerebral hemispheres. Supratentorial surgery may cause edema, which diminishes the level of consciousness, social control, and judgment. As cerebral edema subsides, the problems of incontinence diminish. With some patients it may be necessary to institute a bladder training program.

Gastric Ulceration. Gastric ulceration (Cushing's ulcer) accompanied by gastrointestinal hemorrhage has frequently been observed in the neurological patient. Neurological procedures as well as acute and chronic central nervous system diseases such as craniocerebral trauma and tumors have been associated with symptoms of active gastric bleeding. The incidence of gastric ulcers is increased with lesions around the anterior hypothalamus. Although the underlying pathophysiology is controversial, it is thought that the stress response is the probable cause.

Some of the drugs used in neurological treatment protocols also contribute to gastric irritation. Examples of such drugs are dexamethasone (Decadron), phenytoin (Dilantin), and certain antibiotics. For this reason, acetaminophen (Tylenol) is often preferred to aspirin for mild discomfort or as an antipyretic drug. When Decadron is administered, Maalox is often given to reduce gastric irritation and cimetidine (Tagamet) to reduce gastric secretions.

Symptoms of gastric ulceration are those of gastric distress. Bleeding may be acute and massive or slow and painless. With slow bleeding, a gradual drop in the hemoglobin and blood pressure along with the presence of occult blood in the stools are the only sublime indications of bleeding. Treatment of active gastric bleeding includes nasogastric suction, fluid and blood replacement, and possible surgical intervention. Steroid drugs are usually discontinued if the evidence of gastric ulceration is apparent.

The nurse should check the stools daily for occult blood. The blood should be routinely drawn to determine the level of hemoglobin and to indicate a drop in the normal level (14 gm to 18 gm in males, 12 gm to 16 gm in females). Complaints of gastric distress should be reported to the physician. The blood pressure should be monitored routinely for a drop, either dramatic or gradual. A drop in hemoglobin and blood pressure should be brought to the attention of the physician.

Drug Therapy in the Postoperative Period

The following is a summary of drugs commonly used in the postoperative period after cranial surgery.

Anticonvulsants. Because cerebral edema and irritation commonly result from surgical trauma, seizure activity is quite probable after surgery. To prevent generalized seizure activity, anticonvulsant drugs are given prophylactically to patients who have undergone intracranial surgery.

The drug of choice is phenytoin (Dilantin), 100 mg administered orally, intramuscularly, or intravenously three or four times daily. The drug is supplied in a liquid suspension for patients who have difficulty swallowing capsules or have a feeding tube in place. For patients who have developed drug idiosyncrasies against phenytoin (Dilantin), phenobarbital may be given orally or parenterally.

The patient may continue on prophylactic anticonvulsant therapy for 6 to 12 months after surgery depending on the management philosophy of the physician. Some physicians no longer use prophylactic anticonvulsant drugs. There are specific nursing responsibilities and side-effects that must be monitored (see Chap. 27.)

Corticosteroids. Corticosteroids are used to combat cerebral edema that results from intracranial surgery. The drug of choice is dexamethasone (Decadron), 10 mg to 40 mg daily, given in divided doses orally, intramuscularly, or intravenously for approximately 10 days. Because of the inherent ability of dexamethasone to cause gastrointestinal irritation, ulceration, and possible bleeding. Maalox, 30 ml, is given orally in conjunction with steroids to prevent gastrointestinal problems. Also, 300 mg of cimetidine (Tagamet) is given four times a day to decrease gastric secretions.

Decadron is a potent drug with many serious side-effects. It cannot be terminated abruptly because acute adrenocortical insufficiency would result. An awareness of the drug's actions and side-effects is necessary to evaluate its effect on the patient.

Osmotic Diuretics. Osmitrol, urea, or glucose may be administered intravenously after surgery to control severe cerebral edema that may be causing serious elevations in increased intracranial pressure. A discussion of the drug's actions, side-effects, and nursing responsibilities can be found in Chapter 12.

Antibiotics. Antibiotics are indicated for most patients who have undergone intracranial surgery as a prophylactic drug to prevent central nervous system infections such as meningitis. A broad-spectrum antibiotic such as Keflin is given by the intravenous route for a period of approximately 5 days or longer, depending upon the specifics of surgery and the potential for infection. The physician may choose to switch to an oral broad-spectrum antibiotic as the patient's condition improves and he is able to tolerate oral intake.

Antipyretics. Antipyretics are given to manage an elevated body temperature. An elevated temperature is a serious concern because cerebral cell activity is increased, thereby requiring more oxygen for cell metabolism. Byproducts of cell metabolism are produced and increased cerebral edema and intracranial pressure result.

To control an elevated temperature acetaminophen (Tylenol) or aspirin 650 mg is given orally or rectally every 3 to 4 hours. The drug may be administered in conjunction with a hypothermia mattress or tepid water sponging.

Antiemetics. Antiemetics are given to control nausea and vomiting. Common drugs given include trimethobenzamid (Tigan), 100 mg to 250 mg or prochlorperazine (Compazine), 10 mg, administered intramuscularly or per rectal suppository every 4 to 6 hours as necessary.

Histamine (H_2) Receptor Antagonist. The drug used in this classification is cimetidine (Tagamet). It acts by blocking the action of histamine at receptors in the acid-secreting parietal cells of the gastric mucosal glands. This drug decreases the possibility of gastric hemorrhage. The usual dose is 300 mg every 6 hours by mouth or parenterally. Antacids interfere with absorption of cimetidine, so cimetidine and antacids should be given at least 1 hour apart.

Analgesics. Analgesics are given to control discomfort and pain from headache, which may be mild or severe. The drug given must be selected carefully so that its action does not mask the neurological signs (level of consciousness and pupillary signs) or depress vital functions (decrease respirations or lower blood pressure). Mild discomfort is controlled by acetaminophen (Tylenol) 650 mg every 3 to 4 hours, while codeine sulfate, 30 mg to 60 mg every 4 hours is reserved for pain that is severe. Morphine sulfate is never given to the neurological or neurosurgical patient because it masks the pupillary signs and decreases respirations.

Hormone Replacement Therapy. Hormone replacement therapy may be necessary if the antidiuretic hormone of the posterior pituitary gland is deficient. Vasopressin (Pitressin), 10 units intramuscularly or inhaled, is the drug of choice to manage diabetes insipidus.

REHABILITATION FOLLOWING CRANIAL SURGERY

Reassessing the postoperative patient is that part of the nursing process related to evaluating the effectiveness of the nursing care plan.

Sufficient time must elapse to allow the patient's status to stabilize and cerebral edema and increased intracranial pressure to subside before neurological deficits can be accurately assessed. Some deficits are temporary and will probably become resolved given additional time. However, it is necessary to identify and plan an approach to maintain the function present and develop a protocol to promote restoration of the functional deficit.

Some deficits may be permanent as a consequence of surgery. However, goals should be realistic because quite often it is not possible to predict with complete certainty what functional loss will be permanent. Both short and long-range goals should be set in measurable terms based on an individual evaluation of the patient's rehabilitative potential and needs. Patient needs must be met by an appropriate plan of nursing action.

The team composed of health professionals from various disciplines can best evaluate and plan a comprehensive rehabilitation program for the patient. Patient needs vary and can be met by specific health professionals. For example, a patient who has personality changes that persist may require a psychological or psychiatric evaluation. Deficits of vision or hearing should be evaluated by an ophthalmological or audiological examination, as the case may be. Physiotherapy is necessary for the patient with paralysis or paresis. An exercise program and assistive device may be ordered to provide for alternate modes of motion. For the patient with speech difficulty, a speech therapist can be most helpful. The important point is that the plan of care must be individualized for the patient.

The patient is involved in his rehabilitation plan by beginning to assume responsibility for personal hygiene and other activities of daily living. The progress possible will depend on his general physical condition, development level, motivation, and neurological deficits.

Any patient who experiences periods of confusion or disorientation needs to be reoriented as often as necessary. Stimulating as many senses as possible and directing the patient's attention to the environment are helpful ways of keeping the patient oriented and aware. This can be done by involving the patient in his surroundings, such as pointing out activity outside his window, referring to greeting cards and family pictures, and posting a calendar with large numbers in the room. The nurse should matter-of-factly correct any misconceptions that the patient may verbalize.

When possible, the patient should be helped to improve his personal appearance. For a female patient, self-image can be greatly enhanced by makeup and an attractive scarf around the head. For the male patient, a daily shave should be part of basic hygiene.

The patient can be encouraged to participate in selected activities of daily living. For example, during meal time, the nurse can pour the beverage in a glass, butter the bread, and cut up the food so that the patient is able to feed himself. He is more apt to eat well if he feeds himself. Such steps will generate positive feelings of independence (Chart 14–4). See Chapter 8 for a discussion of rehabilitation.

PSYCHOSOCIAL CONSIDERATIONS

When the patient is conscious and realizes that he has survived the surgery, he experiences elation at being alive. This period lasts for a few days. Attention then becomes directed to concern about neurological deficits, prognosis, and mutilated physical appearance. Depending on the rea-

CHART 14–4. REHABILITATION NURSING CARE IN THE POSTACUTE PERIOD

NURSING RESPONSIBILITY	RATIONALE
1. Encourage patient to begin taking some responsibility for personal hygiene	1. Encourages independence
2. Prepare meal tray (pour milk, cut up food, and so forth) so that patient can feed himself.	2. Same as above.
3. Encourage progressive ambulation if motor function loss is not prohibitive.	3. Improves general well-being of all body systems as well as motor function
4. Help the patient to set realistic short- and long-range goals.	4. Less apt to be discouraged and depressed if goals are realistic
5. Help patient to improve body image by encouraging use of makeup and wigs for female patients.	5. Improves body and self-image, maintains self worth and dignity
6. Talk to patient, play radio, open shades so that he can see activity around him, show him pictures or cards that might be in his room, and so forth	6. Provides reality orientation
7. For the confused and disoriented patient, present reality through the use of as many senses as possible; correct misconceptions.	7. Provides reality orientation
8. Carry out range-of-motion exercises four times daily; position carefully.	8. Maintains motor function; prevents deformities

son for surgery and the prognosis, the patient or family may need to make major decisions about postacute care facilities and choice of treatment.

Feelings of anxiety, ambivalence, hostility, and depression are common in the postoperative period and continue even after the transition to home has been made. One interesting cause of depression relates to the degree of progress made postoperatively. During the hospital stay and initially after discharge, the patient's recovery and improvement are very rapid. If one were to chart this on a graph, it could be represented by a steeply ascending line; then a plateau would be reached, marking a period of miniscule improvement or no apparent improvement. If the patient is unable to perform activities that he thinks are realistic and feasible, he becomes upset. Discouragement is further augmented by fatigue, which causes the patient to abandon certain activities. This sequence of events reinforces feelings of depression and elicits complaints of constant fatigue or a low energy level. In these circumstances, the patient needs to be helped to set more realistic goals in view of the major insult experienced from surgery. A sympathetic approach and explanation of the postoperative course can prove to be very supportive.

It is impossible to generalize about typical responses to a craniotomy. The experience is unique. For some patients a craniotomy provides a cure from a treatable condition such as a subdural hematoma. For others, intracranial surgery ameliorates symptoms of cerebral compression so that an extension of time can be offered for a terminal prognosis. The implications of the craniotomy on the patient's life can only be assessed individually. Based on a systematic assessment, the nurse can plan a nursing approach best suited to the needs of the patient.

REFERENCES

1. Howe J: Manual of Patient Care in Neurosurgery, p 113–132. Boston, Little, Brown & Co, 1983
2. Potts D: How can I reassure my patient if I've never been in surgery? J Neurosurg Nurs 13(4):211, August 1981
3. Rhoton AL: Micro-operative technique. In Youmans JR (ed): Neurological Surgery, 2nd ed, pp 1160–1193. Philadelphia, WB Saunders, 1982
4. Robertson JH et al: Use of the carbon dioxide laser for acoustic tumor surgery. Neurosurgery 12:286, 1983
5. Strait TA, Robertson JH, Clark WC: Use of the carbon dioxide laser in the operative management of intracranial meningiomas: A report of twenty cases. Neurosurgery 10:464, 1982
6. Walker ML: Using lasers in neurosurgery. AORN 38(2):238, August 1983

BIBLIOGRAPHY

Books

Adams R, Victor M: Principles of Neurology. New York, McGraw-Hill, 1977

Core Curriculum for Neurosurgical Nursing in the Operating Room, 2nd ed. Chicago, The American Association of Neurological Nurses, 1984

Cottrell JE, Turndorf H (eds): Anesthesia for Neurosurgery. St Louis, CV Mosby, 1978

Howe J: Patient Care in Neurosurgery, 2nd ed, pp 11–149. Boston, Little, Brown & Co, 1977

Jennett B: An Introduction to Neurosurgery, 4th ed. Chicago, Year Book Medical Publishers, 1984

Mackety CJ: Perioperative Laser Nursing. Thorofare, NJ, Charles B. Slack, 1984

Malseed R: Pharmacology: Drug Therapy and Nursing Considerations, pp 109–119, 126–136. Philadelphia, JB Lippincott, 1982

Newfield P, Cottrell JE (eds): Handbook of Neuroanesthesia: Clinical and Physiological Essentials. Boston, Little, Brown & Co, 1983

Smith R: Essentials of Neurosurgery. Philadelphia, JB Lippincott, 1980

Van Buren JM, Ratcheson RA: Principles of stereotaxis surgery. In Youmans JR (ed): Neurological Surgery, 2nd ed, pp 3785–3820. Philadelphia, WB Saunders, 1982

Wilson CB, Hoff JT (eds): Current Surgical Management of Neurological Disease. New York, Churchill Livingstone, 1980

Youmans JR (ed): Neurological Surgery, 2nd ed. Philadelphia, WB Saunders, 1982

Periodicals

Apuzzo MLJ, Sabshin JK: Computed tomographic guidance stereotaxis in the management of intracranial mass lesions. Neurosurgery 12(3):277, March 1983

Balestrieri FJ et al: Postcraniotomy diabetes insipidus: Who's at risk? Crit Care Med 10:108–109, 1982

Bertz J: Maxillofacial injuries. Clin Symp 33(4): (entire issue), 1981

Butler VM, Dean LS, Little JR: Positioning the neurosurgical patient in the operating room: "A team effort." J Neurosurg Nurs 16(2):89, April 1984

Calvin R: Continuous ventricular or lumbar subarachnoid drainage of cerebrospinal fluid. J Neurosurg Nurs 9(1):12, March 1977

Camp PE: The newer microsurgical techniques in neurosurgery. Head Neck Surg 4(6):514, July–August 1982

Dickson RA: The scope of microneurosurgery. Radiography 48(576):268, December 1982

Dixon JA: Surgical applications of lasers. AORN 38(2):223, August 1983

Ewy V, Minckley B: The anesthesiologist's view of elective craniotomy. J Neurosurg Nurs 9(2):58, June 1977

Graf, C, Ross N: Pulmonary edema and the central nervous system: A clinicopathological study. Surg Neurol 4:319, 1975

Harris L: The specialized role of the neurosurgical operating room nurse. J Neurosurg Nurs 12(3):128, September 1980

Heilbrun MP et al: Preliminary experience with Brown–Roberts–Wells (BRW) computerized tomography stereotaxic guidance system. J Neurosurg 59:217, August 1983

Huether SE: How lasers work. AORN 38(2):207, August 1983

Jacques S et al: Computerized three-dimensional stereotaxic removal of central nervous system lesions in patients. J Neurosurg 53:816, 1980

Jeffe S: Incidence of postoperative deep vein thrombosis in neurosurgical patients. J Neurosurg 42:201, 1975

Kaminiski D: Air embolism during surgery in the sitting position: Its prevention, detection, and treatment. J Neurosurg Nurs 7(2):65, December 1975

Krieger A, Reed R: Design and optical principles of the surgical binocular microscope. J Neurosurg Nurs 10(1):1, March 1978

Kuhn J, Newfield P: Perioperative anesthetic management of patients operated in sitting postion for posterior fossa tumors. J Neurosurg Nurs 13(4):159, August 1981

Madeja C: Postoperative infections on a neurosurgical service. J Neurosurg Nurs 9(2):84, June 1977

Marinari B: Stereotaxis. J Neurosurg Nurs 16(3):140, June 1984

Martin E, Hummelgard A: Midline transcallosal approach for third ventricle lesions. J Neurosurg Nurs 15(2):50, April 1983

Mattox D: Management of mandibular dislocation. Hosp Med 23, December 1981

Mitchem HL: Experience with a CT guided stereotactic apparatus: A new approach to biopsy and removal of brain tumors. J Neurosurg Nurs 16(5):231, October 1984

Murphy M, Roglitz C: Preoperative teaching, integration of nursing and social work services. J Neurosurg Nurs 9(1):5, March 1977

Potts D: How can I reassure my patient if I've never been in surgery? J Neurosurg Nurs 13(4):211, August 1981

Quest D: Dehydrating agents commonly used in neurosurgery: Advantages and disadvantages. J Neurosurg Nurs 11(3):141, September 1979

Rhodes M: Complications of posterior fossa craniotomy. J Neurosurg Nurs 15(1):9, February 1983

Shelden CH et al: Development of a computerized microstereotaxic method for localization and removal of minute CNS lesions under direct 3-D vision. J Neurosurg 52:21, 1980

Shimko C: The effect of preoperative instruction on state of anxiety. J Neurosurg Nurs 13(6):318, December 1981

Smith J, Geist B: Evaluation and care of the acute craniotomy patient. J Neurosurg Nurs 10(3):102, September 1978

Sutherland M: Informed consent: The informed neurosurgical patient and family. J Neurosurg Nurs 14(3):195, June 1982

Wren L: Nursing care of a craniotomy patient in the operating room. J Neurosurg Nurs 10(2):49, June 1978

Zeidelman C: The patient undergoing craniofacial surgery: Nursing assessment and intervention. J Neurosurg Nurs 13(1):38, February 1981

chapter 15

Transsphenoidal Surgery

DESCRIPTION

The transsphenoidal approach for access to the pituitary gland is a relatively new surgical technique made possible by the development of microsurgical techniques and equipment. Visual and surgical access is provided to areas formerly accessible only by the intracranial approach (Fig. 15–1). Nursing management has addressed the responsibilities for providing safe nursing care in these procedures. The nursing management specific to the problem is outlined.

Pituitary adenomas, craniopharyngiomas, and a hypophysectomy for control of bone pain in metastatic cancer are the usual reasons for which a transsphenoidal surgical approach is used. The transsphenoid hypophysectomy has also been used in patients with diabetic retinopathy to control diabetes mellitus. By achieving better hormonal control of diabetes mellitus, the retinopathy can be arrested so that vision may be preserved.

DESCRIPTION OF PROCEDURE

The transsphenoidal surgical approach is a way of gaining access to the pituitary gland by means of an incision in the upper submucosa gum area, which bilaterally extends to the nasal septum. After the sphenoid sinus floor is resected the sella turcica is visible. The sella floor is removed, and the dura is incised. With the aid of a surgical microscope, the pituitary is partially or completely removed, or the offending tumor excised. A graft of muscle taken from the anterior surface of the thigh is applied to the surgical site as a patch. Nasal Vaseline packings are inserted to control bleeding and to replace the septal mucosa. The upper gum is sutured. A dry, sterile dressing is firmly applied to the donor site on the thigh. The specific tissue surgically excised depends on the reason for surgery. If surgery were scheduled for removal of a pituitary adenoma, the pituitary gland would be left intact, if possible, and the tumor excised. In a patient who has a craniopharyngioma, only the tumor would be excised. Removal of this tumor prevents or alleviates damage to the pituitary, hypothalamus, and optic chiasma.

PALLIATION FROM PAIN OF CANCER

A hypophysectomy for palliation in cancer necessitates total removal of the pituitary. The surgeon attempts to excise the pituitary in one piece, because cells left at the surgical site continue to secrete hormones and decrease the anticipated relief of pain. It is not clear why a hypophysectomy may control further metastasis and bone pain from metastasis. It is thought that the removal of the anterior lobe with cessation of prolactin and the growth-stimulating hormone helps to control breast and prostatic cancer.

PREOPERATIVE PREPARATION

The preoperative preparation begins with patient teaching. The patient should have a realistic expectation of the procedure if it is planned for alleviation of pain from cancer. If the surgery is planned for removal of a pituitary tumor, the patient should know that some of the signs and symptoms associated with the tumor will gradually be alleviated.

Another aspect of the preoperative teaching plan is education about the need for drug replacement. This should be discussed with the physician so that the specifics of the

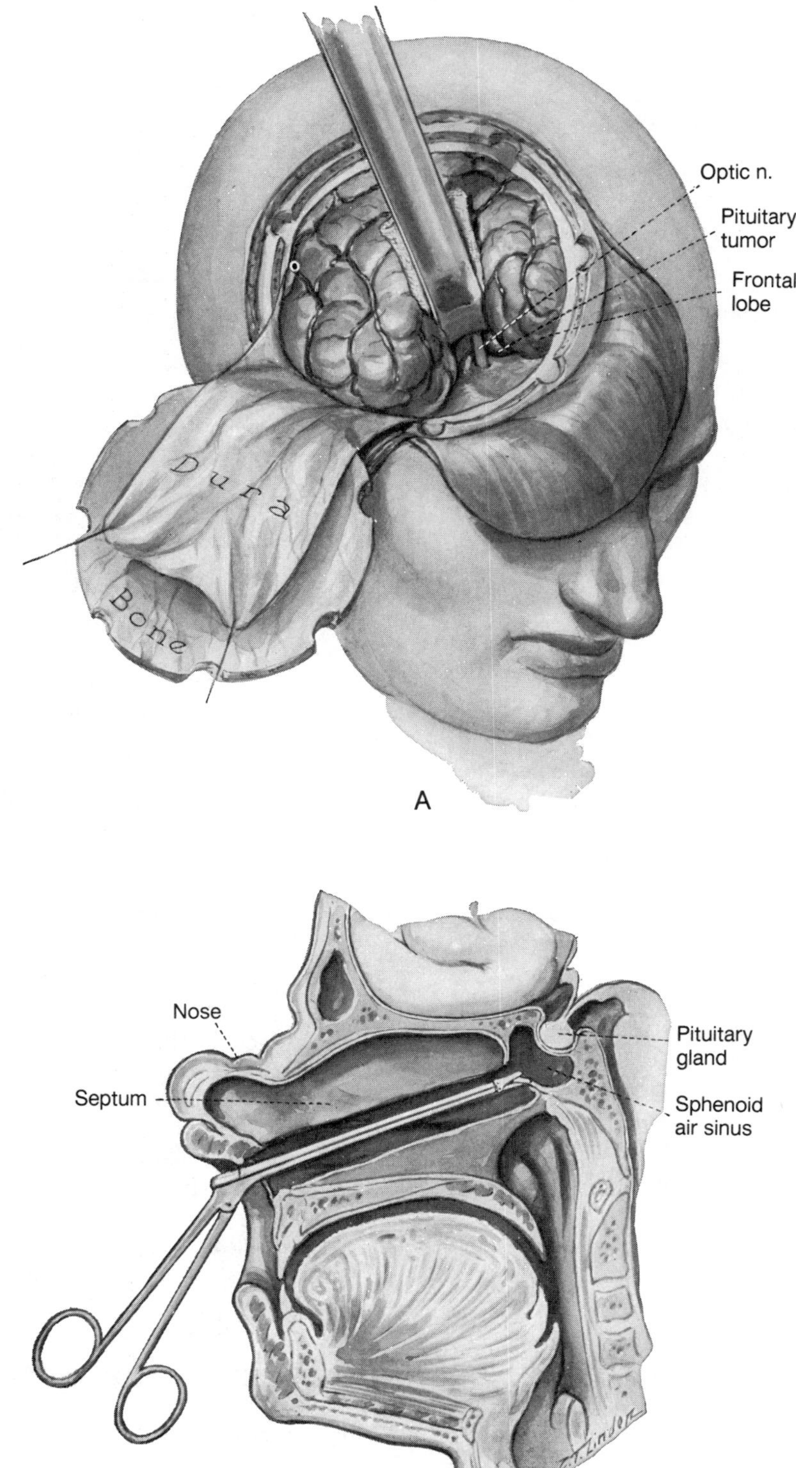

FIG. 15-1. Comparison of the intracranial and transsphenoidal approaches in pituitary surgery. (*A*) Intracranial approach. (*B*) Transsphenoidal approach. (Thorek P: Surgical Diagnosis, 3rd ed. Philadelphia, JB Lippincott, 1977)

drugs that the patient will need to take on a regular basis can be presented to the patient.

Beginning 2 days before surgery, cortisone acetate, 100 mg intramuscularly, is administered daily.

POSTOPERATIVE CONCERNS

HORMONAL REPLACEMENT

In the case of total hypophysectomy, hormonal replacement is necessary. The usual orders are (1) ACTH, 25 mg intramuscularly in the morning and 12.5 mg intramuscularly at night, beginning immediately after surgery, and (2) thyroxin, 0.2 mg to 0.3 mg daily. The thyroid replacement is delayed for 3 to 4 weeks. The patient is also fortified against adrenal insufficiency through the administration of cortisone acetate, 100 mg intramuscularly daily, beginning 2 days before surgery. The drug is continued postoperatively but at a lower dose than that indicated above.

Patient Teaching for Drug Replacement

For the patient who will need replacement drug therapy as a result of a complete surgical excision of the pituitary gland, it is most important that the patient and family understand the purposes of drug therapy. The nurse should begin with a basic overview of the functions of the pituitary gland to help the patient and family understand why drug replacement therapy is necessary. The sophistication with which this information is presented will depend on the learner's level of understanding. It is most important for the nurse to individualize the teaching plan to explain the concepts in terms that are meaningful to the patient and family. To reinforce the verbal explanation, use of visuals is helpful. It is best to develop written material on home care of the hypophysectomy patient because verbal instructions are easily forgotten or misunderstood. Written material also reinforces areas covered during patient teaching.

The teaching plan should include

- Specific information that should be recorded and submitted to the physician, such as daily weight
- Signs and symptoms of undermedication or overmedication of drugs being taken
- Signs of side-effects from drugs
- Any specific alterations in lifestyle necessary as a result of drug therapy

Adrenocorticotropic Hormone. Certain cells of the anterior pituitary gland produce the andrenocorticotropic hormone (ACTH), which is stored until the hypothalamus secretes corticotropin-releasing hormone (CRH), a hormone that signals the pituitary gland to release ACTH. The target organ of ACTH is the cortex of the adrenal glands that affect the sensitive adrenal cortex by way of the bloodstream. The hormones secreted by the adrenal cortex include

- The glucocorticoids such as cortisol (hydrocortisone) and cortisone, its major secretion; these secretions are absolutely necessary for (1) carbohydrate metabolism (promotes glucose production from amino acids), (2) protein metabolism into amino acids for use in tissue repair and cell anabolism, and (3) fat metabolism. At the same time, the glucocorticoids help the body cope with physical and emotional environmental stresses. Cortisone is a hormone that requires daily replacement in order for the patient to survive.
- The mineralocorticoids, particularly aldosterone, which control salt and water metabolism by reabsorbing sodium ions in exchange for potassium in the kidney. This hormone will not require replacement on a daily basis nor is it commercially available.
- Certain male and female hormones that play a minor role in comparison to the secretions of the ovaries and the testes. Replacement therapy is contraindicated if a hypophysectomy was done to control breast or prostatic cancer. In other patients, replacement therapy on a monthly basis may or may not be necessary depending on the patient's age and other considerations. This determination will be made by the physician.

High levels of the corticotropic hormone in the blood inhibit the secretion of CRH so that no more ACTH is secreted by the pituitary gland. The body normally produces larger amounts of ACTH in the early morning hours so that the glucocorticoids necessary for carbohydrate, protein, and fat metabolism are available during the day.

During times of physical and emotional stress the individual will require large amounts of cortisol. ACTH is continually produced to meet this need. Under severe stress, ten times the normal amount of cortisol may be required; approximately 25 mg is the daily requirement under normal circumstances.

In a patient who has had a hypophysectomy the adrenal gland will be deprived of stimulation since the ACTH produced by the pituitary gland is absent. The patient therefore requires ACTH replacement or administration of hydrocortisone (cortisol, Cortef, and so forth), the natural glucocorticoid secreted by the adrenal cortex. This drug also has some of the mineralocorticoid properties secreted by the adrenals.

The patient on cortisone therapy should know the following:

- The drug must be taken daily as ordered; failure to take the drug can be life-threatening.
- The dosage of the cortisone must be increased for periods of emotional stress, illness, excessive exercise, major changes in daily routine, exposure to high altitudes, tooth extraction, fever, or infection.
- Gastric irritation, a side-effect of steroid therapy, can be minimized by taking an antacid (30 ml of Maalox) with each dose of the drug.
- The patient should report the presence of tarry stools to the physician immediately.
- Blood pressure should be checked periodically for hypertension (an elevation in blood pressure is common with cortisone therapy); adjustments in dosage of antihypertensive drugs may be necessary if the patient has been taking such a drug.
- Urine and blood should be checked periodically since there is a tendency toward diabetes mellitus in the predisposed patient.
- Behavioral changes are common with cortisone therapy and should be reported to the physician. Common behavioral mani-

festations may include euphoria, restlessness, sleeplessness, agitation, and depression.

- Signs and symptoms of undermedication (addisonian crisis) include
  - Weakness, dizziness, orthostatic hypotension
  - Nausea and vomiting
  - Sodium and water retention
  - Decreased blood pressure

Management of cortisone insufficiency requires the parenteral administration of hydrocortisone sodium succinate (Solu-Cortef). Failure to treat this condition will lead to circulatory collapse and possible death.

- Signs and symptoms of overmedication include
  - Cushing's signs (moon face, fat pads, buffalo hump, acne, hirsutism, and weight gain)
  - Psychic disturbances
  - Peptic ulcers
  - Headache, vertigo, cataracts, and increased intracranial and intraocular pressure
- A Medi-Alert bracelet should be worn at all times.
- An emergency kit of Solu-Cortef should be carried at all times to be injected in times of stress.

POSTSURGICAL DIABETES INSIPIDUS

Central diabetes insipidus is defined as the cessation of the pituitary gland to secrete antidiuretic hormone (ADH) because of damage from disease or injury of the hypothalamus, the supraopticohypophyseal tract, or the posterior pituitary. The most common cause of central diabetes insipidus is neurosurgery; less common causes are idiopathic, or secondary to certain infections, neoplastic disease, vascular disease or lesions, granulomatous disease, or head trauma associated with basal skull fracture. Postsurgical central diabetes insipidus can occur at any time within 14 days of neurosurgery.[1]

Monitoring the patient for development of diabetes insipidus is a major postoperative concern. Diabetes insipidus is caused by an absence or diminished supply of antidiuretic hormone (ADH) which is secreted by the posterior lobe of the pituitary. The symptoms of diabetes insipidus are copious amounts of pale urine (>200 ml/hour for 2 consecutive hours) and a low urinary specific gravity (<1.005). Monitoring of urinary output is best managed if a Foley catheter has been inserted. In addition, increases in serum osmolarity and serum sodium, concurrent with a decrease in urine osmolarity, are signs of diabetes insipidus. If definitive action is not taken, signs and symptoms of electrolyte imbalance and dehydration will soon be apparent.

Use of osmotic diuretics (such as Mannitol [Osmitrol]) during surgery may give a false indication of the onset of diabetes insipidus because of the copious amounts of urine it may cause to be excreted. However, an excessive amount of urine is an early postoperative occurrence and should reverse itself in about 2 hours after the peak period of drug action has passed.

Other patients may experience a transient period of copious urinary output and low specific gravity. If the patient is able to drink enough fluid to quench his thirst and maintain fluid and electrolyte balance, no medical treatment is indicated. This routine is followed to determine whether the diabetes insipidus is transient or permanent. Some patients may also experience a period of low urinary output 2 or 3 days postoperatively before permanent diabetes insipidus develops.

If a total hypophysectomy has been carried out, one would expect permanent diabetes insipidus to develop. With partial resection or removal of an adenoma from the pituitary, permanent diabetes insipidus is not anticipated. A transient diabetes insipidus may develop, which may or may not require treatment. In the immediate postoperative period, aqueous vasopressin (Pitressin) may be used because of its short duration of action (3 to 6 hours) until the diabetes insipidus can be evaluated to determine if it is transient or permanent. The usual dose is 5 to 10 units subcutaneously. Vasopressin tannate in oil (Pitressin Tannate) is used less frequently because it is painful and dose variation will occur if it is not properly mixed; the dose is 5 mg given intramuscularly. Special precautions of drug administration should be followed, such as (1) give deep intramuscularly, (2) warm before administration, and (3) shake well before giving the preparation. The drug action lasts 24 to 36 hours. With long-term management with Pitressin Tannate, a special nasal spray or snuff called lypressin (Diapid) may be used. This drug is inhaled and absorbed from the nasal mucous membrane. Diapid increases the reabsorption rate of water from the distal renal tubules.

The patient must be instructed in the safe use of Diapid especially if self-administration of the drug is planned. The patient should know that

- The snuff can be irritating to the nasal mucosa, which will interfere with absorption of the drug.
- Overuse of the drug will cause water intoxication (mental confusion, drowsiness). For some patients it may be more convenient and safer to use Pitressin in oil, 2.5 mg to 5.0 mg intramuscularly every 2 to 3 days, to control the diabetes insipidus.
- Record the daily weight.
- Balance the oral intake with the daily output.

The newest addition to the drugs used for treatment of severe permanent or transient complete central diabetes insipidus is desmopressin acetate (DDAVP). It is administered intranasally, 0.1 ml to 0.4 ml in nasal drops one or two times daily. The drug has a duration of 12 to 24 hours and has minimal side-effects—nasal irritation or vasoconstriction of the nasal mucosa. Desmopressin acetate is the drug of choice.

PAIN

After surgery, the patient is relatively free from pain at the oral nasal suture line because the pain receptor fibers have been cut, thereby resulting in loss of pain perception. Regeneration of the fibers will occur, but by that time the

CHART 15-1. NURSING MANAGEMENT AFTER TRANSSPHENOIDAL SURGERY

NURSING RESPONSIBILITY	RATIONALE
Early Postoperative Management	
1. Frequently monitor vital and neurological signs.	1. Provides information for baseline comparisons to indicate trends, deterioration, and complications
2. Maintain in high Fowler's position.	2. Promotes venous drainage from the brain, controls intracranial pressure, and prevents hemorrhage at the operative site
3. Check dressing at donor site on thigh.	3. Observe for bleeding
4. Frequently check nasal drains and packing; mustache dressing should be observed and changed as necessary.	4. Observe for hemorrhage or cerebrospinal fluid drainage from operative site.
Prevention of Complications	
1. Monitor hourly urinary outputs and specific gravity.	1. Indicates signs and symptoms of diabetes insipidus
2. Note patient's complaints of extreme thirst.	2. Same as above
3. Note electrolyte and osmolarity laboratory reports for abnormally high or low readings (serum and urine osmolarity, serum sodium). Normal values are • Serum osmolarity 280 mOsm to 295 mOsm/liter • Urine osmolarity 500 mOsm to 800 mOsm/liter • Serum sodium 135 mOsm to 145 mEq/liter	3. In diabetes insipidus serum sodium is increased, serum osmolarity is increased, urine osmolarity is decreased; also, serum electrolytes can indicate electrolyte imbalance.
4. Give frequent mouth care, but do *not* allow patient to brush his teeth.	4. Prevents injury at the suture line, which allows mouth to be refreshed and cleansed
5. Progress diet from liquid to soft as necessary.	5. Prevents injury to the suture line
6. After packings are removed, caution patient against blowing his nose or sneezing for at least 1 month.	6. Prevents hemorrhage from fragile nasal tissue at operative site
7. Assemble nasal speculum and long forceps.	7. This is stand-by emergency equipment for the physician in case of hemorrhage.
Supportive Care	
1. Give routine hygienic care such as giving bath, combing hair, and cutting fingernails.	1. Maintains well-being
2. Ambulate on second or third postoperative day with assistance.	2. Provides support to prevent falls and injury. If metastasis to bone is present, the patient is very prone to fractures.
3. Assist patient with mouth care.	3. Prevents injury to suture line
4. Offer fluids frequently, as ordered.	4. Maintains hydration and moistening of the oral mucous membrane, which becomes dry from mouth breathing (required when nasal packings are in place)
5. Provide eye care (clean and lubricate).	5. Prevents infection, inflammation, and drying of cornea
6. Supply compresses to the periocular region if periocular edema occurs.	6. Controls and alleviates periocular edema
Patient Teaching	
1. Prepare and implement a patient teaching plan to outline any adjustments in lifestyle, precautions necessary with drug protocol, and discussion of the patient's health problem.	1. Provides for safety as well as including the patient as an involved, informed participant in his health management
2. Provide written material to summarize the major points of home management for the patient.	2. Reinforces the major points of the teaching plan and reduces the possibility of confusion or questions about home protocol
3. Include family in the teaching plan.	3. Includes family in the plan of care so that they can become a knowledgeable support system for the patient

CHART 15–2. NURSING CARE PLAN FOR THE PATIENT WITH TRANSSPHENOIDAL SURGERY

NURSING DIAGNOSIS	EXPECTED OUTCOME	NURSING INTERVENTION
Potential of fluid loss due to development of diabetes insipidus	Fluid balance will be maintained	• Assess for signs and symptoms of diabetes insipidus. • Maintain an intake and output record. • Monitor fractional urinary output every 1 to 2 hours. • Report output of 200 ml/hour or more for 2 consecutive hours. • Monitor urine specific gravity as necessary (every 1 to 4 hours). • Review osmolarity studies of blood and urine. • Observe for signs and symptoms of dehydration. • If patient is able to consume fluids orally, encourage fluid intake.
Potential of electrolyte imbalance	Electrolyte imbalance will not occur	• Monitor blood electrolytes for imbalance. • Observe for signs and symptoms of electrolyte imbalance.
Altered comfort due to nasal packings and oral sutures	The patient will be kept as comfortable as possible	• Offer mouth care frequently. • Assess suture line at least every 4 hours. • Do not allow patient to brush his teeth or place hard objects in his mouth. • Provide a soft diet. • Change mustache dressing as necessary.
Potential of infection due to invasion of incision with microorganisms	Infection will not develop	• Offer mouth care frequently. • Inspect the incision line at least every 8 hours for signs of infection.
Potential of hemorrhage	Hemorrhage will not occur	• Caution the patient against blowing his nose. • Monitor vital signs. • Note the amount and color of drainage on the mustache dressing; note the number of times the dressing has to be changed. • Observe the patient for excess swallowing (may be bloody drainage).
Alterations in body image due to periocular edema and ecchymosis	A positive body image will be supported	• Apply cold or warm compresses under eyes. • Tell the patient that the periocular edema is usual and will disappear. • Encourage female patients to use cosmetics and wear their own clothes.
Potential of knowledge deficit	The patient will learn information about his condition and drug treatment program necessary to manage at home	• Develop a written teaching plan that includes information about drugs, side-effects, and the need to take drugs daily on a permanent basis. • Assess the patient's understanding and knowledge as you teach. • Assess his retention of information. • Provide written material on drugs, side-effects, and so forth.
Potential of noncompliance	The patient will adhere to his prescribed treatment plan	• For patients who will need permanent daily drug replacement, the importance of adhering to the plan must be stressed. • The patient should be able to verbalize the consequences of noncompliance to the drug program.
Potential of depression in patients who have had a transsphenoidal hypophysectomy for control of pain, but for whom the procedure has been unsuccessful	Severe depression will not develop	• Allow the patient to verbalize his feelings. • Accept his behavior. • Point out other methods of pain control. • Recognize signs and symptoms of severe depression and report to physician for possible referral to psychiatrist or other appropriate person. • Assess for evidence of suicidal tendencies, document, and report; observe the patient frequently.

suture line will be healed. Sutures of the mouth will be absorbed in about 7 to 10 days. The nasal mucosa requires at least 1 month to heal satisfactorily. Nasal packings are removed in 3 to 4 days. The sense of smell and taste will return in 2 or 3 weeks. In a patient who has had a hypophysectomy for the control of metastasis and bone pain, relief of pain may be evident within hours after surgery, yet in other patients it will take days to a few weeks to reverse the psychological response to the physical perception of pain. In this instance, a gradual improvement in the response to pain will be noted over several days. Survival rates for these patients may be extended to 2½ years after surgery.

NURSING MANAGEMENT AFTER TRANSSPHENOIDAL SURGERY

Only specific points of nursing care for the management of the patient with the transsphenoidal approach are outlined in Charts 15–1 and 15–2. The areas to be addressed include (1) early postoperative management, (2) prevention of complication, (3) supportive care, and (4) patient teaching.

PSYCHOSOCIAL ASPECTS OF PATIENT MANAGEMENT

A patient with an endocrine disorder precipitated by a pituitary adenoma will be concerned about alterations in body function and appearance. Gigantism and acromegaly greatly alter appearance. Patients with chromophobe adenomas complain of loss of libido, amenorrhea, and low basal metabolism rates. Males develop female characteristics. The threat to the patient's sexuality, body image, and self-esteem is very apparent. Behavior and personality changes caused by hormonal imbalance are common; as a result, disturbances in normal interpersonal relationships develop and the patient may feel that he is losing control of his life as well as his mind.

For the patient with metastatic cancer, the surgery is usually a "last chance" effort to control severe, unbearable pain that has made day-to-day life impossible. The patient may have elected this surgery in hopes of being able to maintain some quality of life for the remaining time. Many patients will express a desire for their families to see them being comfortable without the use of drugs. Patients hope to be given the time and comfort to fulfill certain aspects of their lives before death inevitably occurs.

The nurse's role is a supportive one. Clarifying misinformation and providing necessary information are vital roles. Any activities that improve the body image and self-esteem are worthwhile endeavors.

REFERENCE

1. Swartz SL: CME at "The Brigham": Solving antidiuretic hormone puzzles. Patient Care 114, June 30, 1982

BIBLIOGRAPHY

Books

Bailar J (ed): Modern Concepts in Brain Tumor Therapy: Laboratory and Clinical Investigation. Bethesda, MD, National Cancer Institute, Monograph 46, December 1977

Malseed R: Pharmacology: Drug Therapy and Nursing Considerations, pp 373–376. Philadelphia, JB Lippincott, 1982

Smith R: Essentials of Neurosurgery, p 285. Philadelphia, JB Lippincott, 1980

Periodicals

Anderson B: Antidiuretic hormone: Balance and imbalance. J Neurosurg Nurs 11(2):71, June 1979

Bell M: Preoperative teaching and postoperative care of the hypophysectomy patient. J Neurosurg Nurs 4(2):165–170, 1972

Camunas C: Transsphenoidal hypophysectomy. Am J Nurs, p 1620, October 1980

Clancey J, Abruzzi L: Nursing intervention of patients with pituitary tumors. J Neurosurg Nurs 10(1):24, March 1978

Coleman P: Antidiuretic hormone: Physiology and pathophysiology—a review. J Neurosurg Nurs 11(4):199, 1979

D'Agostino J. Pelczynski L: An overview of cyclotron treatment, Bragg Peak proton hypophysectomy and Bragg Peak radiosurgery for arteriovenous malformation of the brain. J Neurosurg Nurs 11(4), December 1979

Harris L, Park E: Transsphenoidal approach to pituitary ademomas. AORN 23(6):989, May 1976

Hebert P, Breeding P: Self-care after hypophysectomy. J Neurosurg Nurs 11(2):118, June 1979

Kern E et al: A transseptal, transsphenoidal approach to the pituitary. Postgrad Med 63(6):97, June 1978

Nemeroff D: Transsphenoidal hypophysectomy. J Neurosurg Nurs 13(6):305, December 1981

Nevins S: Pre- and postoperative care of patients undergoing transsphenoidal pituitary surgery. J Neurosurg Nurs 8(1):45, July 1976

Newton D et al: Corticosteroids. Nurs' 77 7(6):26, July 1977

Read S: Clinical care in hypophysectomy. Nurs Clin North Am 9(4):647, 1974

Stillman M: Transsphenoidal hypophysectomy for pituitary tumors. J Neurosurg Nurs 13(3):117, June 1981

Tindal G, Mauldin B: Transsphenoidal hypophysectomy. AORN 33(2):246, February 1981

Wachter-Shikora N: ACTH—A review of anatomy, physiology, and structure related to neuroendocrine effects. J Neurosurg Nurs 11(2):105, June 1979

part five

Nursing Care of Patients With Trauma to the Neurological System

chapter 16

The Multi-trauma Patient

The purpose of this chapter is to provide the neurological–neurosurgical nurse with a general approach to the patient who has sustained multiple trauma. A method of assessing the multi-trauma patient based on priorities of care is presented. The information is included because the nurse caring for the neurological–neurosurgical patient must also manage injuries to other body systems that result from the same trauma. An expansion of knowledge and skill are required to safely manage the patient. Details of management for specific conditions or problems are not included in this chapter.

Multi-trauma refers to injuries in more than one body system as a result of vehicular, occupational, household, or sporting accidents or acts of violence. Mortality, morbidity, and the rehabilitative level achieved by the patient depend on the time elapsed from injury to the initiation of health care and the quality of care available to the patient. The development in recent years of critical care medicine, emergency medicine, and traumatology as specialties has been paralleled by the development of critical care nursing and emergency nursing. Critical care nursing has piqued the interest of many nurses, as evidenced by the popularity of seminars and workshops that focus on various issues in critical care, the growth of critical care nursing organizations, and the ever-increasing number of periodicals and textbooks addressing critical care practice. Although this textbook focuses on neurological and neurosurgical nursing, the concept of critical care management of the multi-trauma patient is important because the neurological–neurosurgical nurse cares for many patients with injuries not only to the nervous system but also to several other body systems. No body system is an isolated functional unit. Because the human body is a composite of interrelated physiological and psychosocial systems, every patient must be managed holistically. Yet the nervous system has direct responsibility for controlling functions in all body systems, and many feedback loops control the interaction of the nervous system with each body system. Not only will injury to the nervous system affect the body systems, but dysfunction of a body system will often affect the normal physiology of the nervous system. For example, a patent airway and adequate respirations will support cerebral perfusion and decrease the possibility of the development of secondary injury to the brain such as cerebral ischemia, cerebral hypertension, and increased intracranial pressure. Therefore, the nurse caring for the critically ill neurological–neurosurgical patient must accept the awesome responsibility of caring for the patient holistically while recognizing and appreciating the interrelatedness of body systems. With this approach, the nurse is better able to consider the probability of the development of particular problems and associated nursing diagnoses.

THE TRAUMA VICTIM AND THE HEALTH CARE SYSTEM

How the trauma victim is managed depends on the organizational structure of health care services in the area. Access, resources, and protocols are addressed within the organizational structure. Significant differences exist throughout the country because the United States is both an urban and rural nation with variations in population distribution, topography, and health care resources. It is impossible to generalize except to note that the management of trauma must be organized to meet the needs of the particular area and the people served.

PREHOSPITAL MANAGEMENT

The most critical time for the outcome of a patient who has sustained injury is the time elapsed from injury until admission to an acute care facility. The faster a patient is adequately stabilized and safely transported to the acute care facility, the less chance there is of complications and extension of injuries. It is most important that the medical personnel who attend the patient at the injury site be well trained and knowledgeable in rapid assessment and triage, airway and cardiovascular stabilization, immobilization, and safe transportation of the patient. A mechanism for communication between the medical personnel at the injury site and a physician at a hospital should be available for assessment and instruction concerning patient management. A short-wave radio is often used for this purpose. The hour after injury has been called the "golden hour"; it is the period that makes the critical difference in patient outcomes. Secondary injury and complications rapidly develop without swift and skilled intervention.

ADMISSION TO THE ACUTE-CARE SETTING

The decision concerning the facility to which the patient should be transported is critical because valuable time can be lost if the patient is taken to a facility that is not staffed or equipped to provide the necessary management. The personnel treating the patient at the injury site must triage the patient independently or seek advice from a physician by way of radio contact about the destination of transport. A critically ill patient may be immediately transported by land vehicle or air evacuation to a trauma center, regional head injury center, or spinal cord injury center.

Once the patient arrives at the acute-care setting, he is rapidly triaged and assessed again. He may be admitted immediately to the trauma service, if one exists, stabilized, and managed by a team of specialists. The patient remains on the trauma service until he is well stabilized, and then he is transferred to the service that can best manage his predominant injuries. Management includes any necessary surgery, invasive procedures, ongoing monitoring, and other supportive therapy. The patient is usually admitted to an intensive care unit where he can receive the intensive nursing and medical management that he needs. In hospitals that do not have a trauma service, the patient is stabilized in the emergency department and then admitted to the service that can best manage his predominant injuries. This patient may also be admitted to the intensive care unit for stabilization, management, and ongoing monitoring.

When the patient is well stabilized, he is transferred to the specialty units for continuation of his care. The nursing management required is very challenging because the patient's needs for ongoing monitoring and management to support life are enormously complex, and several complications from the injury that were not immediately evident at the time of injury can begin to develop. The catastrophic event that has critically injured the patient's body has also had tremendous impact on his family system, independence for making critical decisions, and financial resources. Addressing the problems precipitated by injury, the focus of care includes rehabilitation and discharge planning for the multi-disciplinary needs and extended care necessary for achieving the highest level of rehabilitation possible for the patient. All of these processes tend to be very complex and demanding.

THE CONCEPT OF MULTIPLE SYSTEMS FAILURE

In considering the nursing management of the multi-trauma patient, the nurse should be familiar with the concept of multiple systems failure. *Multiple systems failure* is defined as life-threatening failure of two or more physiological systems requiring definitive intervention for the survival of the patient. Physiological complications superimposed on the original problems can produce secondary insult and injury that result in multiple systems failure. For example, a patient with a severe head injury can rapidly develop respiratory complications such as neurogenic pulmonary edema, disseminated intravascular coagulopathy, aspiration pneumonia, and atelectasis; cardiovascular complications such as life-threatening arrhythmias and systemic hypertension; endocrine disorders such as diabetes insipidus or syndrome of inappropriate secretion of antidiuretic hormone; and an unlimited number of other problems.

The development of multiple systems failure depends on several overriding factors such as the following:

- The extent and type of multiple trauma sustained
- Time elapsed before arrival of emergency medical care
- Time elapsed before transport to a hospital
- Immobilization during transport
- Amount of blood and fluid lost
- Patency of the airway and adequacy of respiratory function
- Circumstances of injury (e.g., direction of impact of injury such as head-on collision, wearing of seat belts, speed of impact, drug abuse)
- Pre-existing health problems (e.g., heart disease, chronic lung disease, diabetes mellitus)
- Patient's age

PROBABILITY AND THE EARLY RECOGNITION OF COMPLICATIONS

Probability is defined as the chance of an event occurring or its projected occurrence based on the history of occurrences and the laws of probability. The concept can be applied to the multi-trauma patient to determine the possibility of the development of complications. A baseline assessment and subsequent ongoing assessments are critical sources of data about the possibility of ensuing problems. The data collected in patient assessment; information about contributing factors such as the circumstances of injury and pre-existing health problems; and the nurse's knowledge, skill, and experience help the nurse to predict the development of potential problems. Appreciation of the interrelatedness of various factors helps focus the nurse's assessment of the patient on particular information. At times, it is difficult to identify potential complications and systems failure because so many physiological events occur simultaneously. The usual signs and symptoms that the nurse expects to find may be absent, or they may be masked by other conditions. For example, a patient may develop acute pancreatitis from an injury. The predominant symptom is upper abdominal pain that radiates to the left shoulder and becomes worse when the patient lies flat on his back, but if the patient is unconscious, it will not be possible to localize pain to these specific areas. The nurse may notice that the patient is restless, but the cause of the restlessness may remain a mystery. Laboratory data, and possibly jaundice, may provide the first objective evidence of the problem.

The element of timing is also important in considering the potential development of problems and complications. For example, if an acute subdural hematoma is not present on the initial computed tomography (CT) scan or one taken within 24 to 48 hours of an acute head injury, a subdural hematoma will probably not develop. On the other hand, one would not expect to find evidence of normal-pressure hydrocephalus within the first few days after injury since the probability of its development increases with time after a cerebral hemorrhage.

The goal of management of the multi-trauma patient is early recognition of the development of problems and complications before acute, life-threatening events occur. Even for the expert practitioner, this task is easier said than done.

EARLY ASSESSMENT AND MANAGEMENT OF THE TRAUMA PATIENT

The assessment and management of the multi-trauma patient are concurrent processes because the potentially life-threatening problems involved often require immediate intervention. Appropriate intervention to stabilize and treat the patient are carried out as needed while the assessment process proceeds. Assessment is an ongoing process that is imperative for the unstable patient because his condition is changing so rapidly.

The nurse functions as a team member in the early assessment and management of the patient. In most emergency departments and trauma centers, each member of the team assumes a prescribed role that has been practiced in simulated drills. While each team member assumes a different role and responsibilities, the activities as a whole are designed to complement each other in a coordinated effort to meet the complex needs of the patient.

PRIORITIES IN THE MANAGEMENT OF TRAUMA PATIENTS

The multi-trauma patient has multiple, complex problems and needs that can be overwhelming unless the patient is viewed in perspective. The complex catastrophic situation presented by a multi-trauma patient can be viewed as a series of interrelated, less complex components. Once the various components are recognized, they can be systematically organized based on priorities of management that address the most critical and life-threatening problems first to prevent needless loss of life and rehabilitative potential.

Although the nurse is a team member and a team approach is most effective in managing the patient, the nurse should be able to approach the patient independently with a conceptualization of the assessment and management process. Nurses are familiar with the priority for assessing and maintaining the ABCs of life support in emergency care—ABC stands for Airway, Breathing, and Circulation. A patent airway, adequate respiratory function, and support of circulation are imperative for supporting cardiopulmonary function in order to maintain life. Without maintenance of these conditions, irreversible brain damage and death will occur in a matter of minutes. However, in managing multi-trauma patients a more extensive approach is necessary for assessing the overall needs of the patient. A well-known systematic approach to the assessment of the multi-trauma patient is the ABC approach, which addresses the priorities in which body systems and functions should be assessed. The priorities of care are listed in alphabetical order from A to F so that the higher priorities are managed first and then other priorities are handled in descending order or urgency. See Chart 16–1 for a description of the approach.

DIAGNOSTIC TESTS AND PROCEDURES

Laboratory, radiological, and other diagnostic data are very valuable in assessing, diagnosing, and monitoring the patient with multiple injuries. The nurse includes these parameters in assessing, planning, implementing, and evaluating nursing care. Although the diagnostic protocol will depend on the type of injuries sustained, common tests and procedures include the following:

- SMA 12 (glucose, cholesterol, albumin, total protein, bilirubin, blood urea nitrogen, uric acid, serum glutamic–oxaloacetic transaminase, lactic dehydrogenase, alkaline phosphatase, calcium, and phosphate)
- Electrolytes
- Amylase
- Arterial blood gases
- Complete blood count, hemoglobin, hematocrit, and type and cross match
- Blood coagulation studies
- Drug screen

CHART 16-1. PRIORITIES IN ASSESSMENT OF THE MULTI-TRAUMA PATIENT ACCORDING TO BODY SYSTEMS

In the ABC approach, the letters A through F each stand for a significant function or part of the body system. The body systems are

- A Airway (respiratory system)
- B Bleeding and shock (cardiovascular system)
- C Consciousness (nervous system)
- D Digestive organs (gastrointestinal system)
- E Excretory organs (genitourinary system)
- F Fractures (musculoskeletal system)

The approach for using this system for the trauma patient on initial or early assessment follows:

- In considering each category of the ABCs, assume the presence of every possible injury or problem until it has been ruled out.
- Do not deviate from the prescribed order of assessment; for example, treating a bleeding wound before ensuring a patent airway and adequate respiratory function can result in respiratory arrest while attention is diverted to dressing a wound.
- If possible, a report from the person or persons who brought the patient to the hospital is helpful for learning about the circumstances of injury; a written report may be available; this information is helpful in identifying injuries that may have been incurred.
- Quickly review all written records and reports to learn about how the patient was found, method of transport to the hospital, sequence of activities, specific treatment administered, and other information.
- Collect as much information as possible about the patient's previous medical history; note whether any medication or indication of health problems such as a Medic Alert bracelet was found on the patient.
- Recognize that the information about the patient and injury may be incomplete and fragmented because of the circumstances of injury; try to fill in the gaps in information as soon as possible.
- Each system is assessed and stabilized before going on to the next system.

Initial Assessment Using the ABC Approach

A. Airway (respiratory system)
  1. Patent airway (highest priority of care)
    - If breathing has stopped, resuscitate the patient immediately.

> *Note:* If there is any question of cervical fracture, the neck must be kept in neutral position and immobilized; do not hyperflex, hyperextend, laterally flex, or rotate the head or neck.

    - Check also for cardiac arrest. If an arrest has occurred, immediately institute cardiopulmonary resuscitation.
  2. Assess the breathing pattern
    - Note rate, rhythm, and characteristics of the respirations.
    - Observe chest for symmetry of movement; note any uneven movements or retractions.
    - Auscultate the chest for bilateral breath sounds; note absences of breath sound, rales, or rhonchi.
    - Note presence of cyanosis, air hunger, or dyspnea.
    - Check the chest for open wounds, lacerations, contusions, or fractures of the ribs or sternum.
  3. Possible injuries or problems commonly seen in multi-trauma patients:
    - Obstructed (partial or complete) airway
    - Pneumothorax, hemopneumothorax, lacerated lung
    - Flail chest, fractured ribs, sucking chest wound

B. Bleeding and shock (cardiovascular system)
  1. Assess the vital signs.
  2. Assess for signs and symptoms of hypovolemic shock.
  3. Assess for occult bleeding.
    - The physician checks the abdomen for occult visceral bleeding by peritoneal lavage and palpates the abdomen for evidence of pain or rigidity.
    - Examine the thighs and note any tenderness, pain, and discoloration.
  4. Gunshot wounds
    - Observe for entrance and exit wound.
  5. Impalement injuries
    - Do not remove the penetrating object until surgical hemostasis can be provided; support the object with a dressing to prevent further tissue trauma.
  6. Observe for laceration of tissue or blood vessels.
  7. Possible injuries or problems commonly seen with multi-trauma patients:
    - Hypovolemic shock caused by frank or occult hemorrhage
    - Laceration of viscera or blood vessels; gunshot wounds or impalement objects with subsequent hemorrhage

CHART 16–1. (continued)

C. Consciousness (nervous system)
  1. Assess the neurological signs.
  2. Observe for facial or head lacerations, contusions, or ecchymosis.
  3. Observe for drainage of cerebrospinal fluid or blood from the ear or nose.
  4. Assess for cervical injury (asymmetrical position of the head; loss of motor, sensory, and autonomic function below the level of injury; respiratory difficulty; loss of perspiration; increased space between vertebral spines).
  5. Possible injuries and problems commonly seen in multi-trauma patients:
     - Epidural, subdural, intracerebral, subarachnoid hemorrhage
     - Cerebral concussion, contusion, or laceration
     - Fracture of the facial bones, skull, or vertebral column (including fracture dislocation of the vertebral column and basal skull fracture)
     - Spinal cord injury
     - Dural tears

D. Digestive organs (gastrointestinal system)
  1. Observe for contusions, lacerations, or ecchymosis of the abdomen.
  2. If vomiting occurs, note the presence of blood in vomitus.
  3. Note the presence of distention, rigidity, pain, or local tenderness of abdomen on palpation.
  4. Note the presence of bowel sounds.
  5. Possible injuries and problems commonly seen with multi-trauma patients:
     - Laceration or contusion of the stomach, spleen, liver, small or large intestines, mesenteries, gallbladder, or pancreas

E. Excretory organs (genitourinary system)
  1. Insert indwelling urinary catheter to obtain specimen of urine for urinalysis; note color of urine and presence of blood.
  2. Monitor hourly urinary output.
  3. Observe flank area for signs of contusion or ecchymosis.
  4. Possible injuries or problems commonly seen with multi-trauma patients:
     - Contusion or laceration of the kidneys, ureters, or bladder

F. Fractures (musculoskeletal system)
  1. Observe for bone deformity, contusions, or lacerations.
  2. Assess extremities for pain, pulse, paresthesia, paralysis, and pallor.
  3. Possible injuries or problems common with multi-trauma patients:
     - Fractures, amputations, muscle tears, and soft-tissue injuries

- Central venous pressure line
- Skull, spinal, chest, abdominal, and long bone x-rays
- Other tests as necessary (e.g., C-T scan)

Tests may be repeated periodically as necessary to monitor and treat the patient. The assessment and evaluation of the patient is an ongoing process.

THE STABILIZED PATIENT AND NURSING MANAGEMENT

Once the patient is stabilized he will be transferred to the appropriate nursing unit. The same nursing process is used to provide care whether he is sent to the intensive care unit or a general care unit.

ASSESSMENT

The nurse should review all of the information that has been documented in the patient's record. The nurse begins to compile the nursing history, which is based on available information. Since the patient is often unable to provide information, family members may be interviewed to obtain necessary information. A complete assessment of the patient is the basis for nursing diagnoses and the nursing care plan.

All parameters should be monitored, including neurological signs, vital signs, respiratory function, urinary output, intake (which is usually administered through a peripheral intravenous or central line), central venous pressure readings, pulmonary artery catherization readings (Swan–Ganz catheter), and drainage from various tubes (e.g., chest tubes, sump tube). Careful documentation of the data is essential to note trends in the findings. Laboratory data (e.g., blood gases, electrolytes, cultures, urinalysis) are also monitored. Various equipment (e.g., ventilator, traction, cooling blanket, cardiac monitor, intracranial pressure [ICP] monitor) should be checked periodically to be sure that settings are correct and the equipment is functioning properly.

Information about the drugs that the patient is receiving needs to be correlated to understand their effects on the patient. Patients receiving steroids may have a systemic infection without exhibiting the classical signs and symptoms of infection because steroids are anti-inflammatory drugs that can mask infections. Drug interactions are also possible when patients receive several drugs. In some instances, as with phenytoin, several drug interactions have been well documented. To ensure the therapeutic level of some drugs, blood levels should be drawn periodically and the dosage of the drug adjusted accordingly.

All of the information about the patient must be considered together in order to ascertain a complete and accurate picture of his status. The nurse also assesses each body system for normal function. Skin integrity, nutrition, fluid and electrolyte balance, elimination, and emotional response are but a few of the areas of assessment. Assessment and monitoring are ongoing processes, as are all the steps of the nursing process. The list of nursing diagnoses can become very long as the problems of the critically ill patient are identified.

PLANNING

Planning the nursing management can be very difficult because of the patient's varied needs. For example, turning the patient for back care may be difficult if he has fractured ribs. Patient care goals may need to be met by protocols especially developed for the individual patient. The nurse should also remember that the patient is very prone to infections because he is a compromised host. Attention should be directed to asepsis in planning care.

IMPLEMENTATION

The care that the patient requires is often very complex and time consuming. The nurse should document the implementation of the care plan and the patient's response to that care.

EVALUATION

As with every other step in the nursing process, the nursing management of the patient must be evaluated to determine if it is meeting the patient's needs or if change is indicated.

DISCHARGE PLANNING

The patient with multiple trauma will need extensive discharge planning. As soon as possible after the patient is stabilized, discharge planning should commence, with input from all team members involved in the care of the patient (see Chap. 10).

BIBLIOGRAPHY

Books

Budassi S, Barber J: Mosby's Manual of Emergency Care: Practices and Procedures. St Louis, CV Mosby, 1983

Cowley RA, Dunham CM (eds): Shock Trauma/Critical Care Manual Initial Assessment and Management. Baltimore, University Park Press, 1982

Emergency Department Nurses Association: Standards of Emergency Nursing Practice. St Louis, CV Mosby, 1983

Giving Emergency Care Competently, New Nursing Skillbook. Springhouse, PA, Springhouse Corp, 1983

Harmon AL: Nursing Care of the Adult Trauma Patient. New York, John Wiley & Sons, 1983

Johanson BC et al: Standards of Critical Care. St Louis, CV Mosby, 1981

Mann J, Oakes A: Critical Care Nursing of the Multi-Injured Patient. Philadelphia, WB Saunders, 1980

Moore EE, Eisman B, Van Way C (eds): Critical Decisions in Trauma. St Louis, CV Mosby, 1984

Rosen P (ed): Emergency Medicine: Concepts and Clinical Practice. St Louis, CV Mosby, 1983

Rund DA, Raush TS: Triage. St Louis, CV Mosby, 1981

Shires G: Care of the Trauma Patient, 2nd ed. New York, McGraw-Hill, 1979

Trunkey DD, Lewis FR (eds): Current Therapy of Trauma, 1983-1984. St Louis, CV Mosby, 1984

Warner CG: Emergency Care: Assessment and Intervention. St Louis, CV Mosby, 1983

Zschoche DA (ed): Mosby's Comprehensive Review of Critical Care, 2nd ed. St Louis, CV Mosby, 1981

Periodicals

Boyd DR: Comprehensive regional trauma and emergency medical service delivery systems: A goal of the 1980s. Crit Care Q 1, December 1982

The basics of ballistics. Emerg Med 16(1):26, January 15, 1984

Campbell G: Emergency treatment of chest trauma. Hosp Med 76, April 1980

Cardona V: Trauma post-op: The real nursing challenge. RN 45(3):23, March 1982

Clutter P: Assessment of abdominal trauma. J Emerg Nurs 7(2):47, March/April 1981

Estrada E: Triage systems. Nurs Clin North Am 16(1):13, 1981

Franklin DF, Bargsley L: Comprehensive patient monitoring in a neurosurgical intensive care unit. J Neurosurg Nurs 15(4):205, August 1983

Grover FL: Trauma to the trachea, bronchi, and lungs. Hosp Med 73, January 1983

Heise T: Management of the multiple trauma patient with increased ICP. J Neurosurg Nurs 15(4):201, August 1983

The injured patient's injured neck. Emerg Med 16(7):24, April 15, 1984

Lucas C: Approach to the multiple trauma patient, part 1. Hosp Med 70, January 1982

Lucas C: Approach to the multiple trauma patient, part 2. Hosp Med 86, February 1982

Maher A: A system approach to nursing the patient with multiple system failure. Heart Lung 10(5):866, September/October 1981

Marcum LN, Box CL, Waecherle JF: Priorities in multiple systems injuries. Top Emerg Med 1(1):1, 1979

McSwain N: To manage multiple injury. Emerg Med 16(4):56, February 29, 1984

Molyneux-Luick M: The ABCs of multiple trauma. Nurs77 7:30, October 1977

Parrish N: Evaluation of acute chest pain. Nurs Clin North Am 16(1):25, March 1981

Perry JF: Penetrating abdominal trauma. Hosp Med 33, May 1982

Porgory G, Stanley L: Gunshot victims. RN 47, April 1982

Sigmon HD: Helping your long-term trauma patient travel the road to recovery. Nurs84 14:58, January 1984

Sigmon HD: Trauma: This patient needs your expert help. Nurs83 13:33, January 1983

Siskind J: Handling hemorrhage wisely. Nurs84 14:34, January 1984

Trunkey DD: Trauma: The first hour. Emerg Med 16(5):92, March 15, 1984

Warren JB: Pulmonary complications associated with severe head injury. J Neurosurg Nurs 15(4):194, August 1983

Wells-Mackie J: Clinical assessment and priority-setting. Nurs Clin North Am 16(1):3, March 1981

Worth MH: Managing penetration chest trauma. Hosp Med 53, April 1982

chapter 17

Craniocerebral Trauma

A PERSPECTIVE

This year about 5% of the population will sustain a head injury serious enough to result in loss of time from normal daily activities.[1] This means that about 10 million head injuries are predicted to occur in the United States in any 1 year. Many of the head injuries will result from vehicular accidents, which are often associated with the use of drugs (e.g., alcohol) and noncompliance with the use of seat belts. Other causes of head injury are falls, assaults, and industrial and sporting accidents. Trauma is the leading cause of death for persons under 45 years of age. A large number of these deaths are associated with head injuries. A glance at the statistical breakdown shows that most head injuries occur among 16- to 25-year-olds and that males sustain head injuries about three times more frequently than females. A cursory glance around a trauma, head injury, or neurosurgical unit will confirm this finding.

Head injuries and the disabilities they cause account for billions of dollars a year spent on health care. Because so many of the victims are young, if they survive their needs must be served for many years. The effects of head injury on physical, emotional, psychosocial, vocational, and family relationships are devastating. Although the prehospital and acute management of head injuries have developed rapidly in recent years, rehabilitation facilities, programs, and community resources to meet the long-term needs of these patients and their families have not reached a comparable stage of development. The major challenge for those entrusted with the care of the head-injury patient is to help the patient achieve the highest quality of life with the greatest degree of independence possible.

HEAD INJURY—WHAT DOES THE TERM MEAN?

Head injury can refer to any injury to the scalp, the skull (cranium and facial section), or the brain. When the term *head injury* is used, it usually refers to an injury to the skull, the brain, or both structures that is of sufficient magnitude to require medical attention and to interfere with the person's normal activities. Many times the person is hospitalized for the injury, which may be minor or life threatening.

Another term frequently used is *craniocerebral trauma*. This term refers to injury to the bony cranial vault or to the brain. Craniocerebral trauma covers a variety of conditions including skull fractures, cerebral injuries (concussion, contusion, and laceration), and intracranial hemorrhage.

CLASSIFICATION OF HEAD INJURIES

There are several terms that are used to describe head injuries. The terminology describes the circumstances of injury rather than denoting the type or severity of head injury. Although the value of these old terms is questionable, they are still seen in the literature. Table 17–1 includes these terms and definitions.

Chart 17–1 classifies head injuries according to location and effect on the brain. For purposes of discussion, head injuries are classified into several distinct categories. In fact, most of these injuries do not occur in isolation. A patient may concurrently have several of these problems, which are all related to the same traumatic episode.

TABLE 17-1. ***Descriptive Terms Associated With Classification of Head Injury***

Term	*Description*
Direct (impact) head injury	Direct impact to the head; an object such as a baseball strikes the stationary head or the head in motion strikes an immovable object such as a windshield.
Indirect (impact) head injury	Direct injury to another part of the body that has an indirect rebound effect strong enough to cause injury to the brain; for example, if a person falls from a height and lands on his buttocks, a direct injury to the buttocks will probably occur, but the jarring effect of the fall can cause an injury to the base of the skull and the brain. An indirect impact injury rarely causes a serious head injury unless the height of the fall is extensive.
Open head injury	Penetration or a break in the integrity of the barrier (skull, meninges) between the environment and the intracranial space; for this to occur, there must be a compound or depressed skull fracture, missile injury, or spontaneous tear in the dura. An open head injury also suggests that infection is a major concern; therefore, prophylactic antibiotics and strict aseptic technique are absolute necessities.
Closed head injury	Also called a blunt head injury; this is a nonpenetrating injury to the head in which there is no break in the integrity of the barrier between the outside environment and the intracranial cavity; neither term, closed nor open head injury, gives any indication of the extent of severity of cerebral injury.
Coup injury	Usually cerebral injury; the cerebral injury (contusion, laceration, hematoma) is sustained directly below the site of the impact.
Contrecoup injury	Cerebral injury is sustained in the region or pole opposite the site of impact; the injury (contusion, laceration, hematoma) is caused by the rapid movement of the semisolid brain within the rigid cranial vault.
Missile injury	Penetrating injury to the skull or brain caused by a bullet, knife, scissors, ice pick, or other blunt instrument; usually associated with acts of violence; can cause extensive tissue destruction, contusion, laceration, and herniation; infliction of a "dirty" object is associated with a high incidence of infection.

MECHANISMS OF CRANIOCEREBRAL INJURY

To understand the mechanisms of craniocerebral injury, one must have an appreciation of the anatomical arrangement of the intracranial space that houses the semisolid brain. The intracranial space is divided into compartments by bony buttresses that are often shaped irregularly. The contour of the bony structures that compose the intracranial space is smooth in some areas such as the occipital region and highly irregular in other areas such as the frontal orbital region and the temporal area. The middle meningeal artery is located in a tract etched into the temporal bone in an area where the skull is the thinnest. This artery is frequently torn when the temporal bone is fractured.

The cranial vault is a closed box whose only major opening is the foramen magnum. The brain stem and spinal cord meet at the foramen magnum; the brain stem is attached to the spinal cord. Because the semisolid brain is enclosed by bone, it is subject to bruising and laceration if it is exposed to violent movement. The tips of the brain that lie near irregular bony structures are more often injured than other areas of the brain.

CHART 17-1. CLASSIFICATION OF HEAD INJURIES ACCORDING TO LOCATION AND EFFECT ON THE BRAIN

- I. By location
  - A. Scalp injuries
    1. Contusion
    2. Abrasion
    3. Laceration
  - B. Skull injuries (fractures)
    1. Types of fractures
       - Linear
       - Comminuted
       - Depressed
       - Compound
       - Basal skull
    2. Cranial fractures
    3. Facial fractures
  - C. Meningeal tears (leakage of cerebrospinal fluid)
    1. Otorrhea
    2. Rhinorrhea
    3. Postnasal area (postnasal drip)
  - D. Cerebral injuries
    1. Concussion
    2. Contusion
    3. Laceration
    4. Brain stem injury
  - E. Intracranial hemorrhage
    1. Epidural hematoma
    2. Subdural hematoma
    3. Intracerebral hematoma
    4. Subarachnoid hemorrhage and intraventricular hemorrhage
    5. Injury to blood vessels
- II. By effect on the brain (area of primary injury is localized although secondary effects such as hypercapnia and cerebral edema can lead to a generalized effect on the brain)
  - A. Focal injury
    1. Contusion/laceration
    2. Hematoma
    3. Skull fracture
    4. Gunshot wounds
  - B. Diffuse injury
    1. Concussion
       - Mild
       - Severe
    2. Diffuse axonal injury (DAI)—the old term is *shearing injuries*
       - Mild
       - Moderate
       - Severe

MECHANISM: DEFORMATION, ACCELERATION-DECELERATION, AND ROTATION

Impact injuries of the head are subject to the following forces: (1) skull *deformation*, in which there is a distortion or indentation of the contour or shape of the skull; (2) *acceleration-deceleration*, in which movement of the head in a straight line is affected by increased changes in the velocity vector (acceleration) and decreased speed (deceleration); and (3) *rotation*, in which movement of the head (twisting, lateral flexion, hyperflexion, or hyperextension) results in rotational force experienced by the brain as it twists within the contour of the ovoid, bony skull.

FORCES: COMPRESSION, TENSION, AND SHEARING

Deformation, acceleration-deceleration, and rotation result in intracranial stresses to the brain, which take the following form: (1) *compression* or pushing of tissue together, (2) *tension* or pulling apart of tissue, and (3) *shearing* or sliding of portions of tissue over other portions. In many injuries these three physical stresses operate simultaneously or in rapid succession to produce injury.

Scalp Injuries

In scalp injuries, the velocity and the characteristics of the object creating the impact are important in determining the amount of injury to the scalp. The object may cause compression, tension, and tearing of the scalp.

Skull Injuries

In skull injuries, the amount of deformation will depend on the characteristics of the skull at the point of impact, the weight of the object, and the velocity and force of the impact. When impact occurs, stress waves are set into motion, engulfing both the skull and the assault object.

Impact to the head may or may not result in a skull fracture. If a fracture occurs, it may be linear, comminuted, depressed, compound, or perforated. A high-velocity blow often produces a depressed or perforating skull fracture with dural tearing and laceration or contusion to the underlying brain. A low-velocity blow tends to result in temporary skull indentation or linear fractures.

Brain Injuries

The two major mechanisms responsible for brain injury after impact are (1) acceleration-deceleration with cavitation and (2) skull distortion or head rotation (Fig. 17-1). At the time of impact to the skull, there is *always* a certain amount of acceleration-deceleration of the head, whether the head is fixed or free. The difference in consistency between the skull (a solid substance) and the brain (a semisolid substance) causes the skull to move faster than the intracranial contents. Changes in the intracranial pressure at impact are due to acceleration-deceleration and skull deformation, which creates compression.

The pressure at the point of impact is positive, while at the opposite end of the skull it is negative. The degree of negative pressure created produces cavitation of the tissue. The pressure gradient that develops is due to the positive stress waves produced at the impact site. The negative

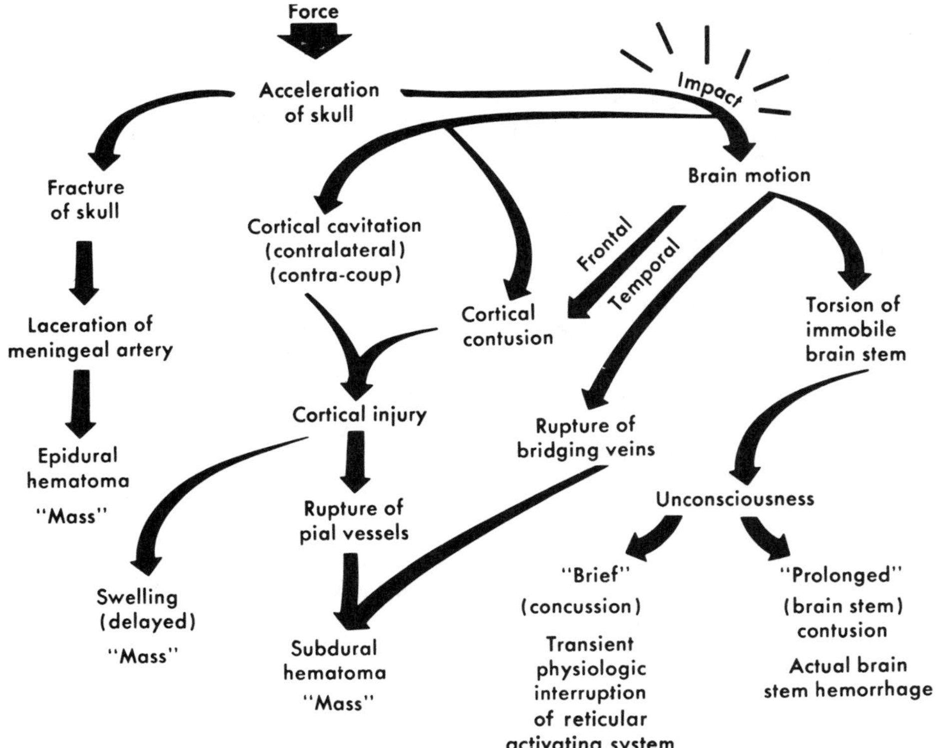

FIG. 17-1. Mechanisms in head injury. (Warner CG: Emergency Care: Assessment and Intervention, 2nd ed. St. Louis, CV Mosby, 1978)

waves continue to the center of the head and then become increasingly negative as they approach the opposite area of the skull. Gas bubbles are released if the pressure is low enough. Maximum stress can be produced at this area of negative pressure in the brain. The cavitation phenomenon partially explains the development of contrecoup injuries. The pressure gradients are particularly strong at the incisura and foramen magnum, and therefore, they can produce movement of the brain stem downward toward the craniospinal junction.[2]

Rotational force on the head is responsible for many severe head injuries. While the brain may "give" a bit on impact, it is not truly compressible. Acceleration–deceleration of the free, mobile head causes much acceleration–deceleration and rotation of the brain tissue. The brain located within the rigid skull (which is compartmentalized by dural sheaths and bony protuberances) responds to force exerted upon the skull by gliding forward and then rotating or turning within the compartment. The rotational force produces distortion of the brain and tension and shearing of involved tissue. The maximum amount of injury is usually found at the tips of the frontal and temporal lobes.

Tension on the brain structures can cause cerebral injury. Certain structures at the upper cervical region, such as ligaments and muscles, may have the built-in ability to stretch and return to normal without injury; however, this is not true of neural tissue, even if the stretching is only momentary. Momentary stretching takes place in many parts of the brain, but especially at the foramen and incisura when the head is hyperflexed as during a head-on collision.

Shearing or sliding of cerebral tissue over other portions implies stresses on two different planes. With rotational acceleration, the stress of shearing is directed toward areas where tough, fibrous tissue and cerebral tissue meet. These areas include the crista galli, the sphenoid wing, the margins of the tentorium or falx, and the foramen magnum. The degree of injury will depend on the extent and direction of the angular acceleration.

PATHOPHYSIOLOGY OF HEAD INJURIES

As part of normal life, people often bump or bang their heads without this impact causing any apparent injury. However, some kinds of craniocerebral impact are capable of causing serious pathophysiological changes as a result of a severe blunt head injury.

In considering head injuries, Bruce and colleagues divided injury into two separate but related sets of events responsible for the pathophysiological changes associated with cerebral injury.[3] The two sets of events were identified as the primary head injury and the second (or secondary) head injury.

PRIMARY HEAD INJURY

The primary head injury is the direct result of the dynamic mechanism (e.g., acceleration–deceleration, rotation) that caused the direct tissue disturbance. The injury can be focal or diffuse, but the effects of injury on the cerebral tissue are a direct result of the initial insult. The primary injury may be a mild concussion or a contusion and laceration that directly injure the nerve cells and nerve fibers. Microscopic examination of a contused or lacerated area demonstrates small hemorrhages around the blood vessels with destruction of adjacent brain tissue. There may be ischemia, infarction, or necrotic areas. Hemorrhage is often found in the overriding meninges as a hematoma or subarachnoid hemorrhage.

At the time of impact, other events have also occurred that affect the normal physiology of the brain and the various mechanisms that maintain the intracranial environment. Loss of autoregulatory control, increased cerebral blood flow, and changes in the efficiency of the blood–brain barrier cause cerebral edema. Cerebral edema is an increase in brain bulk caused by an increase in water in the brain. A rapid increase in intracranial bulk within the limited space of the intracranial cavity causes an increase in intracranial pressure, which is also known as intracranial hypertension. If these initial problems are not quickly controlled and measures taken to restore the normal intracranial physiology, the changes that develop will contribute to the second or secondary head injury.

THE SECOND OR SECONDARY HEAD INJURY

A series of events or complications that contribute to further injury may follow the primary injury. This is called the second (or secondary) head injury and can cause poorer patient outcomes and even death. Events that frequently cause second head injuries are systemic hypotension, hypoxemia, hypercapnia, sustained increased intracranial pressure (malignant hypertension), sustained cerebral edema, respiratory complications, infections, and others.

Second head injuries can continue to occur long after the initial head injury if the patient is not managed properly. The health team has no control over the initial injury, but they can control and prevent the secondary negative events from occurring beginning in the prehospital phase of patient management. The effects of the events that cause the second head injury have been discussed in Chapter 12 and will also be discussed in relationship to nursing responsibilities in this chapter.

MAJOR PATHOPHYSIOLOGICAL CHANGES ASSOCIATED WITH THE PRIMARY HEAD INJURY

Because so many simultaneous, interrelated events occur within the intracranial space with severe injury, it is helpful to focus on separate events to gain a better understanding of the pathophysiology. Cerebral edema, increased intracranial pressure, and hemorrhage will be discussed.

Cerebral Edema

With direct focal injury as well as impact, there is often a simultaneous localized loss of the autoregulatory mechanism of the arterioles. With loss of tone there is a local increase in cerebral blood flow. The combination of increased focal blood flow and dilation of focal blood vessels increases the pressure in the capillaries and venules. There are also alterations in the blood–brain barrier in response to injury. This results in movement of fluid into the cerebral extracellular space resulting in vasogenic edema.

While these vascular changes provide increased profusion to selected areas of the brain, other areas are denied an adequate blood supply, particularly as cerebral edema develops. As portions of the brain are deprived of adequate nutrients necessary for cerebral metabolism, an elevated carbon dioxide level develops. Hypercapnia in inadequately perfused areas contributes to local acidosis and vasodilation, which increase edema. When cerebral tissue is deprived of adequate oxygen and glucose, the sodium pump lacks energy to function properly, so that sodium and water accumulate in the glial cells of the white matter. A vicious cycle develops as the biochemical and vascular alterations perpetuate the cerebral edema.

Cerebral edema is a response to injury just as edema is a common response in other tissue; however, cerebral tissue is particularly sensitive and the corresponding edema is severe.

Cerebral edema can be localized or generalized. Local edema can be extensive and may become a generalized problem. Diffuse cerebral edema of one or both hemispheres may occur even when contusions are mild or are apparently absent. Involvement of one hemisphere is seen most often with an acute subdural hematoma, with edema persisting after evacuation of the clot. One important effect of cerebral edema is that it often exaggerates the amount and severity of the focal neurological deficit present.

Other secondary effects from trauma are associated with cerebral edema. As a rule of thumb, the severity and extent of edema directly correlate with the severity of the head injury. Cerebral edema greatly increases the cerebral mass, although not uniformly in each hemisphere, and taxes the compensatory mechanisms. As decompensation develops, there is a major increase in intracranial pressure so that herniation syndromes can rapidly develop (see Chap. 12).

Effects of Increased Intracranial Pressure. The major sources of increased intracranial pressure in head injuries are cerebral edema and expanding lesions such as hematomas. The effects on cerebral tissue from the cerebral edema, expanding lesion, and increased intracranial pressure will depend on their severity and duration. Compression of any blood vessels can result in ischemia and infarction of particular areas. Several other biochemical changes caused by injury contribute to ischemia. Neuronal necrosis can be due to direct injury or to hypoxia precipitated by the combined forces that cause the cerebral edema.

The normal intracranial pressure is 0 mm to 15 mm Hg, with an average range of 0 mm to 10 mm Hg. The ability of the brain to adjust to volume changes is called *compliance*. As the intracranial bulk increases and the normal compensatory mechanisms are exhausted, intracranial pressure rises.

The clinical importance of increased intracranial pressure (ICP) is its negative effect on cerebral blood flow (CBF) and the viability of neurons. The normal CBF is 50 ml to 55 ml per 100 gm of cerebral tissue per minute. The cerebral perfusion pressure (CPP) is a parameter easily calculated in the clinical setting that can be used to monitor CBF. CPP is calculated by the following formula (MAP = mean arterial pressure):

$$\text{CPP} = \text{MAP} - \text{ICP}$$

A normal CPP is about 80 mm to 100 mm Hg (see Chap. 12 for further discussion). The minimum CPP necessary for maintaining minimal cerebral function is 60 mm Hg. Below 60 mm Hg, cerebral ischemia develops and blood flow begins to be compromised. When CPP is sustained at a low level, irreversible neuronal changes develop and death results.

The two variables controlling CPP are systemic blood pressure and ICP. If the ICP rises, the CPP falls; an episode of systemic hypotension also causes a decrease in CPP. Patient management is directed toward maintaining CBF by supporting CPP and controlling rising ICP. Several methods of preventing a rise in ICP were discussed in Chapter 12, such as elevating the head and preventing the Valsalva maneuver. These points of care are important to incorporate into the plan of care for the patient at risk.

Hemorrhage

Hemorrhage, in the form of epidural, subdural and intracerebral hematomas, and subarachnoid bleeding, can be a secondary result of primary blunt head injury. The cause is laceration of cerebral vessels from the shearing forces of mass movement. A developing hematoma will behave like a rapidly developing space-occupying lesion. The development of cerebral edema around the hematoma, which can rapidly become generalized, is a well-established fact. It is also known that with a hematoma the amount of increased cerebral mass and pressure is not uniform. The hemisphere with the lesion is under great pressure. Both the hematoma and the cerebral edema contribute to an increased intracranial pressure and subsequent herniation syndromes, most often in the supratentorial area.

Subarachnoid hemorrhage is not uncommon with head injuries. This condition contributes to an increase in intracranial pressure. Subarachnoid hemorrhage may be concurrent with other hemorrhage associated with hematomas.

The Effects on Other Structures

Cranial nerves, blood vessels, and cranial structures may be directly contused or torn as a result of the mass movement of the brain. The most commonly affected cranial nerves are the olfactory, optic, facial, and auditory nerves.

Injury to the blood vessels is most common at the cavernous part of the internal carotid artery. A tear in the carotid can give rise to a carotid–cavernous fistula. Tearing of any major blood vessel at the base of the skull, such as the carotid or basilar arteries, will result in major hemorrhage, probably into the subarachnoid space, and death. Contusive injury of any blood vessel can result in cerebral thrombosis.

It is not clear whether damage to the pituitary gland and hypothalamus is due to direct impact or to secondary effects of increased intracranial pressure. Hemorrhagic and ischemic lesions are most characteristic of hypothalamic injury. The heat regulatory mechanism, carbohydrate metabolism, and other important functions are controlled by the hypothalamus. Therefore, injury to this structure can result in grossly elevated temperature, to cite but one consequence of injury.

The pituitary gland is commonly injured in head injuries, with hemorrhage frequently occurring in the pituitary stalk and posterior lobe. (The posterior lobe secretes the antidiuretic hormone for water regulation in the body.) Hemorrhage into the anterior lobe is infrequent, but infarction is a common finding. The many secretions of the anterior lobe regulate several major body functions that are obviously affected by injury.

Summary

In summary, the pathophysiology of head injury is very complex so a simplistic explanation does not accurately reflect the concurrent and interrelated processes that are operational. The degree of severity will depend on several factors directly and indirectly associated with the injury.

SPECIFIC HEAD INJURIES

In this section the major classifications of head injuries will be described and discussed.

SCALP INJURIES

The scalp is composed of three layers: (1) the dermal layer with hair; (2) subcutaneous fascia; and (3) galea. The dermal layer protects the scalp from injury. The subcutaneous fascia is tough fibrotic tissue with a vascular fatty layer that is responsible for profuse bleeding when injury occurs. The galea is a sheetlike tendon layer that connects the frontalis and occipitalis muscles. Below the galea is the subgaleal areolar space, a space in which blood clots can develop. It contains emissary veins that empty into the venous sinus. If infections develop in this area, there is the possibility that they will spread to the brain. The periosteum is located below the subgaleal space. It is a very thin layer of tissue that can be stripped away from the skull.

Injuries to the scalp can be classified as follows:

- *Abrasions*—a scraping away of the top layer of the scalp; minor injury; there may be slight bleeding
- *Contusions*—a bruise to the scalp; an injury to the tissue of the scalp with possible effusion of blood into the subcutaneous layer without a break in the integrity of the skin
- *Laceration*—a wound or tear in the tissue of the scalp; tends to bleed profusely

Diagnosis

The diagnosis of scalp injury is made by physical inspection. The physician may order skull films and other diagnostic procedures if he is concerned about the possibility of skull fracture or associated cerebral injuries.

Treatment

Abrasions require no specific treatment. A scalp contusion may benefit from the application of ice initially to prevent a hematoma from forming. Skull films may be ordered to rule out a skull fracture, but otherwise, no treatment is required.

Scalp lacerations are a common cause of admissions to the emergency room. The bleeding is controlled by direct pressure or the use of instruments such as hemostats or hemostatic clips. Lacerations of the scalp can cause substantial bleeding in any patient, but in infants the blood loss can result in hypovolemic shock. Although there can be severe blood loss in older children and adults, the bleeding does not usually result in hypovolemic shock.

All scalp lacerations are usually explored with a sterile gloved finger to determine if a fracture or foreign body is present. Small fractures are not always seen on x-rays but may be noted by visualization and palpation. Evidence of bone fragments, a depressed skull fracture, or a compound skull fracture will require surgical exploration in the operating room. Digital examination of a scalp laceration is conducted with the help of lidocaine for local anesthesia and epinephrine for vasoconstriction of torn blood vessels.

After bleeding has been controlled, the scalp adjacent to the laceration is shaved. The wound is irrigated with copious amounts of normal saline to ensure that all dirt and foreign materials such as glass are removed. Severely contused tissue may need to be débrided. The subgaleal area is examined for hematomas. If a hematoma is present, some physicians believe that it should be removed before suturing. However, without adequate hemostasis, hematomas tend to recur and be large. A large hematoma may take weeks to reabsorb, but the major concern is that the hematoma site may become infected.[4] The subgaleal area has emissary veins that empty into the venous sinus; therefore, if the subgaleal area is infected, the infection can easily spread to the brain. For this reason, other physicians prefer to leave a subgaleal hematoma alone. Antibiotics are ordered to prevent infection.

Suturing is accomplished in two stages. If possible, the galea is closed separately with interrupted sutures. Next, the dermal layer, subcutaneous fascia, and galea are sutured together tightly (for hemostasis) with through-and-through silk sutures.

When a multi-trauma patient has substained other serious injuries, débridement and definitive suturing of scalp lacerations are often deferred until other emergency treatment and diagnostic measures have been completed. Bleeding is controlled by rapid through-and-through single-layer closure of the scalp. Later, when other priorities of care are completed, the physician can remove these sutures, explore and débride the wound, and suture the laceration properly.

FRACTURES OF THE SKULL

The skull is the bony framework of the head that encloses and protects the brain. The skull consists of two parts, the cranium and the facial sections. The cranium is the domed top, back, and sides of the skull composed mainly of large smooth bones fused together at suture lines. The suture lines make the skull rigid and nonmovable. The facial bones are smaller and more complex than the cranial bones. The mandibular bone is the only movable bone in the facial portion of the skull.

Types of Fractures

The usual classifications of skull fractures are linear, comminuted, depressed, compound, and basal skull fractures. The type of fracture produced depends on the velocity, direction, and momentum of the object causing the impact. Approximately 7% of head injuries result in skull fractures. Accurate statistics are difficult to obtain because so many fractures involving the base of the skull are not visible on radiographic examination; however, clinical evidence, such as leakage of cerebrospinal fluid, indicates the presence of a fracture.

A *linear fracture* of the skull, sometimes called a simple fracture, resembles a line or a single crack in the skull. Seventy percent of all skull fractures are linear.

A *comminuted fracture* refers to fragmentation of the bone into many pieces.

A *depressed fracture* of the skull is characterized by inward depression of the bone fragments to at least the thickness of the skull. In other words, the contour of the skull is indented because of a powerful blow to the skull (Fig. 17–2).

A *compound* or *perforated fracture* implies that a depressed skull fracture and scalp laceration exist, creating a communication pathway to the intracranial cavity. Hair, dirt, pieces of the impact object, and other debris may be found within the wound. The dura may or may not be torn with a compound fracture.

A *basal skull fracture* involves the base of the skull, particularly the anterior and middle fossae. The fracture may be linear, comminuted, or depressed. Most often, a basal skull fracture arises from the extension of a linear fracture into the base of the skull. The frontal and temporal bones are usually affected. It is interesting to note that approximately 75% of basal skull fractures involve the petrous process of the temporal bone. Small basal skull fractures of the posterior fossa may occur when there is upward impact of the cervical vertebrae on the base of the skull.

Basal Skull Fractures: Special Points

When considering fractures of the skull, it is important to distinguish between fractures of the cranial vault and those of the base of the skull. Although the mechanism by which the fractures arise is similar, the secondary lesions and consequences contrast sharply. The consequences of basal skull fractures tend to be much more serious and complex than those of other fractures.

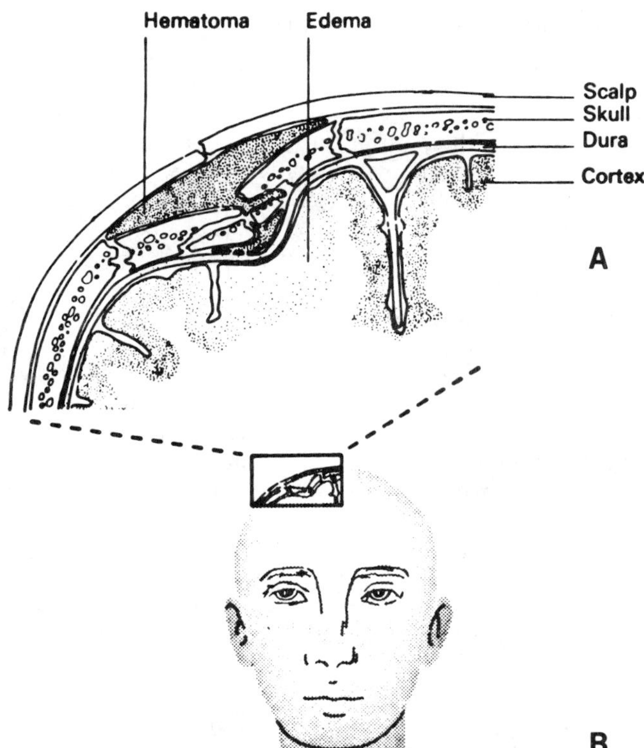

FIG. 17-2. Diagram showing a depressed fracture of the skull. *(A)* The fracture has not punctured the dura, but it has caused compression of the underlying cerebral cortex. *(B)* The relation of the structures after operation and elevation of the depressed fragment. (Brunner LS, Suddarth DS: Textbook of Medical-Surgical Nursing, 3rd ed. Philadelphia, JB Lippincott, 1975)

A unique consequence of basal skull fractures is the frequency in which fractures traverse the paranasal air sinuses (frontal, maxillary, or ethmoid) of the frontal bone or the middle ear, located within the petrous portion of the temporal bone. The fragility of the bones in this area and the intimate adherence of delicate dura account for the frequency of the lesion and the consequent leakage of cerebrospinal fluid through the dural tear. Drainage of cerebrospinal fluid and blood from the nose is called *rhinorrhea*, while drainage of similar components from the ear is called *otorrhea*. When cerebrospinal fluid and blood drain from the paranasal sinuses, they drain into the postnasal area; it is felt as a postnasal drip. Drainage of cerebrospinal fluid is a serious problem regardless of where the fluid drains because an intracranial infection such as meningitis can result from organisms gaining access to the cranium by way of the ear, nose, or paranasal sinuses through the dural tear. A combination of blood encircled by a yellowish stain is called the *halo sign*. This characteristic sign on a dressing or bed linen is highly suggestive of blood encircled by cerebrospinal fluid.

An added complication of basal skull fractures is possible injury to the internal carotid artery at the point where it enters the skull through the foramen in the base of the skull. Fracture in or around the foramen may produce major hemorrhage from laceration or thrombosis or it can result in the development of a traumatic aneurysm or a carotid-cavernous fistula (chemosis, audible bruit, and pulsating exophthalmos of the fistula). Compression of the cavernous sinus may produce ophthalmoplegia of the oculomotor, trochlear, and abducens nerves that pass through this sinus.

Another common complication of basilar fractures is the possible trapping of portions of the frontal arachnoid and dura between the fracture edges, creating a permanent route for leakage of cerebrospinal fluid. There is great difficulty in successful radiological and surgical identification of the exact area of the dural tear. Such identification is necessary to facilitate surgical repair.

Diagnosis. Skull films are the most common radiological procedure used in diagnosing a skull fracture. The ease with which a diagnosis of skull fracture is made depends on the site of the fracture. For example, a linear fracture of the parietal bone may be readily evident on a radiograph. However, determining the presence of a fracture in the basal area may be very difficult because it is not readily visible. Thus, such a diagnosis must be made on the basis of physical findings and the presumptive evidence of leakage of cerebrospinal fluid. Abnormal skull sutures, deep grooves in the inner table of the skull for the middle meningeal artery, or partially healed old fracture lines add to the confusion, particularly in the elderly. If the paranasal sinuses are fractured, air may be evident in the sinuses on x-ray. In the case of fracture of the temporal bone, mastoid sinuses may be opaque.

Basal skull fractures are diagnosed more by physical findings than by x-ray. In addition to leakage of fluid (presumed to include cerebrospinal fluid) from the ear, nose, or postnasal area, other physical findings often found include

- Anterior fossa fracture (fracture of the paranasal sinuses)
  - —Rhinorrhea: cerebrospinal fluid and blood
  - —Subconjunctival hemorrhage
  - —Periorbital ecchymosis (raccoon's eyes)
- Middle fossa (associated with fractures of the temporal petrous bone; involves the middle ear)
  - —Otorrhea: cerebrospinal fluid and blood
  - —Hemotympanum
  - —Conductive hearing loss (may be associated with signs of vestibular dysfunction such as vertigo, nausea, and nystagmus)
  - —Facial nerve palsy (Bell's palsy)
  - —Ecchymosis over mastoid bone called Battle's sign; does not usually develop for 24 to 36 hours; it is seldom seen in the emergency department

Treatment. The treatment protocol for skull fractures depends on the type of fracture. Often a skull fracture is only one of several head and cerebral injuries.

Generally speaking, a simple linear fracture will probably require no special medical management other than bed rest and observation for underlying cerebral injury. Depressed fractures usually require surgery to elevate the bone and débride the underlying structures of bone fragments. With a depressed compound or comminuted fracture a craniectomy of bone fragments may be necessary. A cranioplasty with insertion of a bone or artificial graft may be done immediately or may be postponed for a few months (approximately 3 to 6 months) if cerebral edema is present.

The patient is managed with a course of dexamethasone (Decadron) to reduce cerebral edema.

Any patient who has cranial surgery is managed as a craniotomy patient (see Chap. 14).

The patient who has a basilar skull fracture is managed medically on bed rest (with the bed flat) with frequent observation and assessment of neurological signs. If a dural tear with leakage of cerebrospinal fluid is present, antibiotics are given to prevent infection. The patient is observed to ascertain whether sealing of the dural tear occurs. Most cerebrospinal fluid leaks resolve spontaneously in 7 to 10 days. To aid resolution of the leak, lumbar punctures are made twice daily with large-bore needles and 30 ml or more of cerebrospinal fluid are removed. Another possible method to aid healing is insertion of a lumbar catheter for continual drainage of cerebrospinal fluid.

If leakage of fluid continues, a craniotomy may be necessary to surgically repair the tear. It can be very difficult to identify the actual tear site and manipulate the fragile dura. Injection of radioisotopes (cisternogram) into the cerebrospinal fluid and insertion of sterile cotton pellets into the ear and nose are ways of aiding the physician in identifying the tear site. If there is a tear in the dura of the plugged orifice, the cotton pellets will reveal the presence of the radioisotope.

Since skull fractures are associated with other mild or severe head injury, treatment protocols are designed to manage the various interrelated injuries incurred by the patient.

Facial Fractures

Approximately three out of four people involved in automobile accidents sustain facial injury. The injuries may involve the soft tissue (contusions, lacerations), the facial bones (fractures), or both. The facial bones include most of the paranasal sinuses and the primary receptor organs for the senses of vision, hearing, taste, and smell. Although facial injuries and fractures are usually not fatal, they can result in disfigurement, motor and sensory dysfunction, and deficits in communication. Table 17–2 summarizes the facial fractures most commonly seen.

Skull Fractures: Associated Cranial Nerve Injury

Certain cranial nerves tend to be compressed or injured when fractures of specific bones occur because of the way they transect the brain as they proceed to the base of the skull as well as the way they are attached to vulnerable areas.

Anterior cranial fossa fractures frequently result in injury to the olfactory and optic nerves. Temporal bone injury (middle fossa) most often affects the facial and auditory nerves.

Orbital plate fractures may affect the optic and oculomotor nerves, resulting in loss of vision and impaired eye movement. The orbits are created by many bones that may be fractured in a head injury. Isolated lesions of the trochlear or abducens nerves are rare.

Cribriform plate fractures often produce anosmia owing to injury of the olfactory nerve. The dura at the cribriform plate is very fragile and usually tears with cribriform fracture.

A fracture of the petrous portion of the temporal bone often results in symptoms of paralysis of the facial and/or auditory nerve. Both cochlear and vestibular branches of the auditory nerve are often involved. A tear of the dura is common with otorrhea, a frequent clinical finding.

Major Effects of Skull Fractures: A Summary

The major effects of cranial fractures are (1) tears of the dura with or without leakage of cerebrospinal fluid; (2) contusion and laceration injuries to the underlying brain from displacement of bone parts; (3) contusion or laceration of cranial nerves or blood vessels; and (4) creation of a pathway for intracranial infection from compound, depressed fractures. Simple linear fractures may cause no apparent injury to the brain.

Skull fractures are important because they often cause injury to underlying structures of the intracranial cavity, such as blood vessels, meninges, or the brain.

Nursing Management of Patients With Skull Fractures

The patient who has sustained a skull fracture is usually hospitalized because the injury is serious and most often is associated with cerebral injuries such as concussion, contusion, or laceration.

The objectives of nursing management include

1. Frequent assessment of neurological signs
2. Early recognition of complications
3. Control of cerebral edema
4. Rehabilitation

The patient who requires surgery will be managed with the same nursing protocols as a craniotomy patient (see Chap. 14). Patients with basal skull fractures require special consideration in nursing care, as outlined below. Signs indicative of a basal skull fracture include ecchymosis of the mastoid process of the temporal bone (Battle's sign), conjunctival hemorrhage and ecchymosis of the periorbital areas (raccoon eyes), blood behind the eardrum, (hemotympanum), facial palsy, deafness, or drainage from the ear (otorrhea), nose (rhinorrhea), or postnasal area (postnasal drip).

Basal Skull Fracture. The patient with a basal skull fracture must be kept flat in bed on complete bed rest. The flat position is intended to decrease pressure and the amount of cerebrospinal fluid draining from a dural tear, if one is present. Spontaneous closure of the dural tear may occur while the patient is on bed rest.

- Never suction a patient through the nasal passage if there is any question of a basal skull fracture; since dural tear is common, the catheter and drainage tubes are sources of infection that can lead to the development of meningitis.
- The patient should be cautioned against blowing his nose or

TABLE 17-2. *Most Common Fractures of the Facial Bones of the Skull*

Bone	Fracture	Signs and Symptoms
Mandible • Only movable bone of the face • Composed of lower jaw and ramus portions • Lower jaw or chin portion contains the teeth • Ramus portion is vertical and has condyloid processes that fit into the temporomandibular joint	• Most frequently fractured facial bone • Because of its arch shape, fractures commonly occur in two places	• Malalignment of the teeth • Pain • Bruising and laceration over the fracture site • Ecchymosis in the floor of the mouth • Palpation of a "shelf" defect in the inferior border • Inability to palpate condylar movement when little finger is placed in external ear canal and the jaw is opened
Maxilla • Holds upper teeth • Includes the palate • Forms a portion of the floor of the orbits • Forms part of the floor and outer wall of the nasal fossa • Meets the temporal and zygomatic bones laterally • Contains maxillary sinus	• Involved in midface fractures (involves the maxillae, nasoorbital bones, and the molar [zygoma] bones) • Midface fractures are classified using the system devised by René Le Fort • Le Fort I fracture is a horizontal detachment of the maxilla at the nasal floor; the detached portion normally holds the upper teeth • Le Fort II fracture is a pyramid-shaped fracture of the central part of the face and includes transverse fractures across the medial maxillae and nasal bones, medial half of the infraorbital rim, and the medial part of the orbit and orbital floor • Le Fort III fracture separates the cranial and facial bones; it includes a Le Fort II fracture along with fractures of both molar bones so that the fracture line cuts through both orbits transversely	Midface fractures • Distortion of facial symmetry (elongated face, flattened naso-orbital area) • Possible pushing of the upper and lower molar teeth together • Inability to close jaw • Pain • Edema • Ecchymosis of the buccal mucosa in the lateral portions • Abnormal movement (free-floating maxillary segment)
Molar (also called the zygoma) • Forms the prominence of the cheekbone • Forms part of outer wall and floor of the orbit • Part of temporal and zygomatic fossa	• Often involved in midface fractures • Fractures of the molar are often called tripod fractures because of the shape • Fracture to the molar always involves the orbits	• Flatness of the cheek • Loss of sensation on side of face of fracture • Diplopia • Ophthalmoplegia
Nasal • Forms bridge of nose • Forms part of upper inner orbit	• May occur alone or in conjunction with orbital or Le Fort fractures	• Ecchymosis and edema of the dorsum of the nose • Nosebleed • Laceration
Orbital fractures • Several facial and cranial bones form the orbits	• Fracture may occur with Le Fort fractures or, less frequently, as an orbital blow-out fracture • Blow-out fractures are caused by a spike in intraorbital pressure caused by a blunt object (fist, baseball) directed at the globe; the spike in pressure causes fracture at the weakest point — the orbital floor or medial wall	Blow-out fractures • Sinking of the globe • Diplopia (due to injury of extraocular muscles) • Ophthalmoplegia • Blindness (due to detached retina) • Edema • Ecchymosis • Conjunctival hemorrhage • Paresthesia

(Data from Bertz J: Maxillofacial injuries. Clin Symp 33(4): entire issue, 1981 and Black J, Arnold PG: Facial fractures. Am J Nurs 1086, July 1982)

sniffing in nasal discharge if a basal skull fracture is suspected; the purpose of these precautions is to prevent the introduction of microorganisms that could lead to infection or meningitis.

If there is any drainage, sterile cotton should be loosely placed around the orifice and changed frequently as needed. No attempt should be made to insert anything into the orifice or to irrigate the area. If there is any question of whether the drainage is cerebrospinal fluid, the presence of a halo sign suggests that the drainage is, in fact, cerebrospinal fluid. The halo sign is described as bloody or dark drainage encircled with a lighter halo of drainage. To determine whether the clear drainage is cerebrospinal fluid, some of the drainage should be collected in a test tube and then tested with a Dextrostix reagent strip. If the strip is positive for glucose, the drainage is cerebrospinal fluid. (Glucose is not present in mucus drainage but is present in cerebrospinal fluid.) However, in practice, this is not reliable because blood usually accompanies the cerebrospinal fluid. Blood has glucose in it and will cause a positive reaction on the Dextrostix strip.

A basal skull fracture is considered a serious injury because of the proximity of the fracture line to vital structures of the brain stem. Edema in this area can rapidly lead to respiratory and cardiac arrest. The patient's neurological status must be observed frequently and carefully to identify any dysfunction indicative of cerebral edema or injury.

In addition to the few specific points of care mentioned, nursing management follows the principles of care outlined for head injuries in this chapter.

DURAL TEARS

A tear of the dura mater of the meninges can occur with a basal skull fracture, with a compound fracture involving the temporal or frontal bones, or with some facial fractures. The cerebrospinal fluid may leak from the ear (otorrhea), nose (rhinorrhea), or postnasal area (postnasal drip). There may also be bloody drainage behind the tympanic membrane if the typanic membrane is intact and a temporal fracture has occurred in the middle ear or posterior–superior portion of the external auditory canal. Dural tears are important management concerns because the tear provides a portal of entry for microorganisms that can cause meningitis and cerebritis.

CEREBRAL INJURIES

The major head injuries that are included and discussed in this section are concussions, diffuse axonal injuries, contusions, lacerations, brain stem injuries, missile injuries, and impalement injuries.

Concussions

The word *concussion* is derived from the Latin and means "to shake violently." Concussion is a clinical diagnosis that describes transient, temporary, neurogenic dysfunction caused by head trauma. There is no apparent structural brain damage, and recovery occurs in minutes or hours. Although most patients who sustain a concussion have a period of unconsciousness, loss of consciousness is not necessary for a concussion to have occurred.

Concussions can be divided into mild and severe (classical). The classification is based on the degree of symptoms, particularly those of unconsciousness and memory loss. In a mild concussion there is temporary neurological dysfunction without loss of consciousness, or retrograde or post-traumatic amnesia. The patient may be momentarily dazed. However, a more severe concussion is characterized by temporary neurological dysfunction, a period of unconsciousness, and retrograde and post-traumatic amnesia.

When evaluating memory loss, the time of injury becomes the reference point. Memory loss about events that occurred before the injury is called *retrograde amnesia*, and memory loss about events that occurred immediately after the injury is called *post-traumatic* or *antegrade amnesia*. The term *traumatic amnesia* includes both retrograde and post-traumatic amnesia. The duration of unconsciousness and memory loss are generally accepted as very good indications of the severity of the concussion.

Clinical Signs and Symptoms. The transient signs and symptoms of neurological dysfunction seen with a concussion may include unconsciousness, which is immediate and lasts seconds, minutes, or hours; loss of reflexes; temporary arrest of respirations for a few seconds; a change in vital signs; and retrograde and post-traumatic amnesia, if a memory deficit occurs at all. Other signs and symptoms that are common are headache, visual disturbance, dizziness, giddiness, gait abnormalities, confusion, irritability, drowsiness, and confusion.

Dynamics of Injury. A concussion is a temporary *diffuse* injury of the brain. It is thought that acceleration–deceleration force on the brain and shearing stress on the reticular formation cause the concussion. Several hypotheses have been proposed to explain the neurological dysfunction. Some studies have shown that there is a momentary increase in cerebrospinal fluid, intracranial, and blood pressures; significant changes in the electrocardiogram; and the onset of high-amplitude slow waves in the electroencephalogram on impact. Recovery from concussion usually takes from minutes to hours, but some patients will develop a postconcussional syndrome.

Postconcussional Syndrome. Post-injury sequelae may develop after a mild head injury such as a concussion; these have been termed postconcussional syndrome. The chief complaints are headache and dizziness. Other symptoms include nervousness and irritability, emotional lability, fatigability, insomnia, poor concentration, poor memory, difficulty with abstract thinking, difficulty with judgment, loss of inhibitions, loss of libido, and avoidance of crowds. Symptoms may be experienced for several weeks to 1 year after head injury.

Within the last few years the knowledge and attitude toward minor head injury has changed. The person who sustained a concussion was not considered to have an organic injury of the brain. No abnormalities were evident on computed tomography (CT) scan or other traditional diagnostic tests. Studying minor head-injury patients, Rimel and co-workers found some interesting patterns. The patients in the study group classified as minor head injury met the following criteria: history of unconsciousness of 20 minutes or less; a Glasgow coma scale score of 13 to 15; and hospitalization not exceeding 48 hours.[5]

Follow-up on the patient population at various intervals after discharge revealed that the patient was having difficulty with headache, attention, concentration, memory, and judgment. When employment was considered, one third of the patients gainfully employed before injury were not back at work 3 months after injury. On neuropsychological testing of this population, it was confirmed that they had problems with attention, concentration, memory, and judgment.

The implications of the Rimel study for minor head injuries are important for the nurse to understand. The patient has apparently sustained some organic injury and will have difficulty if he tries to assume his previous lifestyle and responsibilities. The other findings of the study were that emotional stress caused by persistent symptoms seemed to be a significant factor in the long-term disability of these patients and that litigation and compensation have a minimal role in determining outcome after minor head injury. The patient who has sustained a so-called minor head injury needs help and support until he is able to assume his former lifestyle and responsibilities.

Diagnosis of Concussion. The diagnosis of concussion is based on a history, neurological examination, and absence of any focal lesion on CT scan. The patient should be supported and observed to be sure that no other focal lesion such as a subdural hematoma has been overlooked.

Significance of Concussion. Patients who sustain other head injuries such as contusions, lacerations, and hematomas have, in most instances, also sustained a concussion. It is important to bear this in mind when considering the patient's injuries.

Boxer's (Punch-Drunk) Encephalopathy. The cumulative effect of repeated concussions, seen almost exclusively in boxers, leads to the development of a syndrome coined "punch-drunk encephalopathy." The degree of a boxer's neurological impairment appears to be directly related to the number of bouts he has fought. The "slugger" or second-rate boxer sustains more blows to the head and is thus the prime victim. It has been suggested that boxer's encephalopathy begins to develop after an average of 16 years of a boxing career.[6]

The early signs and symptoms include slightly unsteady gait and slight mental confusion. As the condition develops, there is a generalized slowing of muscular movement, shuffling gait, slow cerebration and forgetfulness, speech hesitancy and slurring, mood swings, periods of depression, tremors, and nodding of the head. In severe cases, there is staggering gait, facial characteristics of parkinsonism, and marked mental deterioration that may require commitment to a psychiatric unit. Once the deterioration is established, it is irreversible and progresses steadily. The victim demonstrates little insight into his deteriorating condition.

Autopsies and CT scans have provided evidence of changes in the brain structure of these patients. The findings include cerebral atrophy, dilated ventricles (third and laterals), abnormalities deep in the middle of the brain around the septum pellucidum, cerebellar abnormalities, and cavum septum pellucidum (an abnormal connection between the ventricles). There are those who dispute the development of encephalopathy in boxers and see no reason for concern about the sport of boxing.

Diagnosis. The diagnosis of boxer's encephalopathy is made based on the history, neurological examination, and clinical signs and symptoms. A CT scan and an electroencephalogram are also valuable diagnostic tools.

Diffuse Axonal Injury (DAI)

Diffuse brain injury is characterized by widespread global neurological dysfunction caused by acceleration–deceleration on a 60-degree lateral arc in which the neuronal projections become stretched or torn. This type of injury has been known in the past as a shearing injury. The concept of diffuse axonal injury has been developed by Gennarelli and colleagues.[7] Diffuse axonal injury is characterized by immediate prolonged unconsciousness (more than 6 hours) without any focal lesion noted. There is widespread neurological dysfunction, diffuse white matter degeneration, and diffuse cerebral swelling. This clinical picture has been associated with brain stem injury in the past. However, examination on autopsy failed to confirm this theory.

Diffuse axonal injury can be classified as mild (grade 1), moderate (grade 2), or severe (grade 3). Gennarelli and colleagues described grade 1 as axonal abnormalities mainly restricted to the parasagittal white matter of the cerebral hemispheres; grade 2 as characteristics of grade 1 plus a focal lesion in the corpus callosum (a tear causing hemorrhage); and grade 3 as a much greater degree of axonal hemispheric abnormalities than that incurred in grade 1 or 2 as well as axonal abnormalities of the white matter of the cerebellum and the upper brain stem. The axonal injury in all grades occurred alone and was not associated with infarction, ischemia, contusion, or intracerebral bleeding. The major microscopic finding in diffuse axonal injury is axonal retraction balls or abnormalities of the axons in the white matter of the injured brain. Examination of the brain months after injury reveals degeneration in the long tracts and reduction of the bulk of white matter.[7]

Clinical Course. The clinical picture presented is one of immediate, deep, prolonged coma; initially delayed decerebration; increased intracranial pressure; hypertension; and elevated temperature. The clinical course and outcome depend on the severity of the diffuse axonal injury. With severe diffuse axonal injury, if the patient survives he remains in a comatose state for approximately 3 months. He then remains in a chronic vegetative state, has severe neurological disabilities, and requires complete care and supervision in an extended care facility.

Complications. The clinical course of diffuse axonal injury is riddled with several serious complications that can be life threatening. Examples of complications include respiratory disorders (neurogenic pulmonary edema, disseminated intravascular coagulopathy, pneumonia, atelectasis, aspiration), metabolic disorders (diabetes insipidus, nonketotic hyperosmolar hyperglycemia, syndrome of inappropriate secretion of antidiuretic hormone, electrolyte imbalance), vascular problems (fat emboli, thrombophlebitis), musculoskeletal disorders (decubiti, contractures, spasticity), increased intracranial pressure, vocal cord paralysis, meningitis, gastrointestinal hemorrhage, and seizures.

Diagnosis. The diagnosis of diffuse axonal injury is made on the basis of the clinical picture and lack of treatable focal lesions. On CT scans the following findings are seen early in the clinical course: small midline ventricles, possible small hemorrhagic areas in the corpus callosum, and cerebral edema.

On later scans the hemorrhagic areas become resolved, and there is abnormal focal softening of the brain (encephalomalacia). Other than the findings mentioned, nothing else of significance is noted.

Cerebral Contusions and Cerebral Lacerations

A *cerebral contusion* is a bruising of part of the brain without puncture of the pial covering, although the underlying cortical tissue and white matter may be hemorrhagic. The size and severity of a contusion can vary depending on the area of contact between the striking object and the skull. A *cerebral laceration* refers to a traumatic tearing of the cortical surface of the brain. The distinction between contusion and laceration is one of degree of trauma, although the consequences of a laceration are usually more serious than those of a contusion. However, the circumstances surrounding the infliction of a contusion or laceration are similar, so they are often found together.

Contusions and lacerations can occur any place on the cortical surface. They are commonly found beneath depressed skull fractures and around penetrating injuries inflicted by sharp instruments or missiles. Contusions or lacerations can also occur with closed blunt head injuries.

Dynamics of Injury. A blow to the head, resulting in mass movement of the intracranial contents, may result in a contusion or laceration. An injury directly below the point of impact can produce a coup injury, with or without a skull fracture, caused by the slapping effect of the skull hitting the brain. The contrecoup contusion or laceration can occur at the opposite pole of impact when the brain strikes the irregularities of the skull.

Studies have demonstrated that blows to the front of the head usually produce only coup injuries; on the other hand, a blow to the back of the head results in both coup and contrecoup injuries. A blow to the side of the head produces either coup or contrecoup lesions. A coup injury is most common after a frontal blow because the deformation of the skull slaps the brain with its irregular surface, causing contusion and possible laceration. The mass movement of the brain toward the opposite pole, the occipital region, lags as a result of inertia. The contour of the inner table of the skull is very smooth, and there are few crossing veins or venous sinuses to tear and cause hemorrhage. Therefore, contrecoup injury from frontal impact is rare.

A blow on the back of the head produces both coup and contrecoup injuries because mass movement of the intracranial contents causes the brain to hit the very irregular bones of the frontal area, tearing connecting veins with consequent bruising that results in contrecoup injury. The coup injury at the point of contact arises from the same mechanism as outlined for blows to the frontal area.

Sites of Injury. The major sites of contusions and lacerations are in the frontal and temporal lobes at the frontal poles, the orbital areas, the frontal–temporal junction around the sylvian fissure (brain is close to the lesser wings of the sphenoid bones), and the inferior and lateral surfaces of the temporal lobes (temporal tips) where there is a shelf-like separation between the anterior and middle fossae. The anterior and middle fossae at the base of the skull have irregular, bony structures capable of contusing or lacerating the brain on impact. The distribution of contusions in these particular areas is explained by the movement of the brain within the skull. The frontal–temporal regions are most sensitive to shearing stress injury because of the relatively greater restraint created by the sphenoidal ridges and other irregularities of the base of the skull.[8] These irregular bones not only limit movement by creating buttresses of bone but are also sharp in certain areas. The rotational forces created by movement of the brain cause shearing, tearing, and compression of the brain.

Less common sites of injury are the inferior–lateral angles of the occipital lobes, the medial surfaces of the hemispheres, and the corpus callosum. The presence of the firm, membranous falx cerebri and tentorium cerebelli dural septa creates restrictions of movement of the brain on impact. With lateral blows in the frontal–temporal area the brain may be contused by the falx and tentorium so that surface contusion of the contralateral temporal lobe and deep-seated contusion of the medial surfaces of both hemispheres involving the uncinate gyrus are noted.[9] Contusion of the corpus callosum can also be sustained by this mechanism. Injury to the inferior–lateral angles of the occipital lobe and, less commonly, the inferior surface of the cerebellar and cerebral pendsuncles can occur from impact by the tentorium.[10]

A blow to the vertex of the head may cause cerebellar, cerebellar tonsillar, and brain stem contusions initiated by the downward thrust of the brain toward the foramen magnum.

Brain Stem Injuries

Primary brain stem injury does not occur in isolation but rather is a part of diffuse cerebral injury. However, when symptoms occur in relation to injury in this area, the diagnosis of brain stem injury may be made. Injury can be divided into primary injury as a direct result of impact and secondary injury attributed to distortion and herniation from increased intracranial pressure and cerebral edema. Signs and symptoms of brain stem dysfunction immediately after injury are found in primary injury, while signs and symptoms in secondary injury develop later.

Primary brain stem injury can include cranial nerve injury (III–XII), petechial hemorrhage, and distortion of blood vessels that leads to ischemia, infarction (Fig. 17–3),

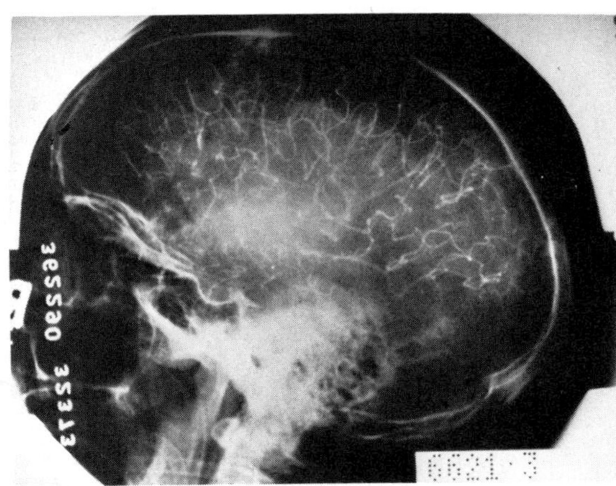

FIG. 17–3. Brain stem infarction.

and necrosis. Associated injury is often found in the superior cerebellar peduncles and the corpus callosum. Major injury to the brain stem, either due to direct or secondary causes, is usually not conducive to life because the brain stem controls vital functions.

Secondary brain stem injury is usually due to supratentorial pressure from cerebral edema, which results in herniation syndromes. In addition to the pathophysiological changes found with primary brain stem injury, patients with secondary injury have been found, at autopsy, to have necrosis of the hippocampal or cingulate gyri, infarction of the medial occipital cortex (due to compression of the posterior cerebral artery), or infarction of the cerebellar tonsils.[10] The severity of the pathology is related to the extent and severity of the cerebral edema and increased intracranial pressure. In clinical practice, most brain stem injuries are secondary, due to the effects of herniation syndromes precipitated by increased intracranial pressure.

Destructive brain stem injury is characterized by immediate loss of consciousness and coma and distinctive patterns of the respiratory, pupillary, oculovestibular, and motor signs that clearly indicate the level of brain stem damage.

The following summary identifies characteristics of injury at specific levels:

- *Midbrain*—deep coma; pupils that are fixed at midpoint or slightly wider; ophthalmoplegia (as noted by oculovestibular testing); decerebration
- *Pons*—coma; small, nonreactive pupils; ophthalmoplegia; decerebration

Missile Injuries

Missile injuries are unlike blunt impact injuries in that the cranium and brain may be penetrated. The cause of this injury is usually the accidental or deliberate discharge of a gun. The wound created by the bullet depends on the size, shape, velocity, direction, and action of the bullet within the intracranial space. As the bullet is propelled and penetrates the skull, it compresses the air in front of it, thereby increasing the destruction of brain tissue not only in the immediate area but also in remote areas.

The wounds from missile injury have been described as (1) tangential injuries in which the missile does not enter the cranial cavity but produces a depressed skull fracture, scalp laceration, and meningeal and cerebral contusion–laceration; (2) penetrating injuries in which the missile enters the cranial cavity but does not pass through it, resulting in the presence of metal, bone fragments, hair, and skin within the brain; and (3) through-and-through injuries in which the missile perforates the cranial contents and leaves through an exit wound.[11] Usually, one tract is created from a missile entering the brain, but two or three tracts are possible if the bullet ricochets.

Extent of Injury. The major effects of missile injuries are focal damage and generalized destruction to the brain in the form of contusions and lacerations, necrosis of some tissue, hemorrhage from tearing of blood vessels, and cerebral edema, both localized and generalized. Hemorrhage and edema may produce increased intracranial pressure and syndromes of distortion and herniation associated with rapidly expanding space-occupying lesions just as in blunt head injury. Other major concerns involving missile injuries are those of infections such as meningitis and brain abscesses, all consequences of the dirty missile.

The amount of injury sustained depends on the structures involved. If brain stem structures associated with vital functions are injured, death may be immediate or may occur shortly thereafter. About 80% of patients with a through-and-through injury die at the time of injury or soon after the injury is inflicted.

Diagnosis. The history and evidence of a gunshot wound are the primary sources of information for diagnosis. Skull x-rays should be taken to visualize any bone fragments. A CT scan is also very helpful in assessing intracranial damage. The patient's entire body should be examined for other gunshot wounds. Both entrance and exit wounds of the head and body should be noted.

Management. If the patient reaches the hospital alive, emergency surgical intervention will be necessary for the following reasons:

1. To control intracranial bleeding by evacuating clots and using drugs such as dexamethasone and mannitol to control the rapidly rising increased intracranial pressure
2. To control infection by débridement of the wound and initiating aggressive antibiotic therapy
3. To provide life support mechanisms (tracheostomy) and repair of any other life-threatening injuries

The management of these patients is a challenge to the staff. Body function must be maintained and the many complications that could occur if the patient survives must be prevented or managed.

Sequelae. Recovery from the injury is frequently a lengthy process with many posttraumatic syndromes often present. Common sequelae include nervous instability (loss of memory, slow cerebration, irritability, and so forth), dementia, psychosis, seizures, and focal symptoms such as aphasia, paresis, paralysis, and cerebellar dysfunction.

Impalement Injuries

To impale means to pierce with something pointed. Impalement injuries of the head refer to piercing of the scalp, skull, or brain. If a patient is found with a foreign body or instrument protruding from his head, it should be left in place to control bleeding until it is removed at surgery. In the meantime, the object is supported to prevent further damage to the tissue.

Diagnosis. The diagnosis is made by clinical inspection. Intracranial trauma is assessed with the aid of a CT scan and skull films to identify bone fragments.

Treatment. Surgery will be necessary to remove the impalement object, control bleeding, and débride the wound. The patient is given antibiotics for 7 to 10 days to control infection, which is a major concern.

INTRACRANIAL HEMORRHAGE

Traumatic intracranial hemorrhage is a common complication of a blunt head injury. Hemorrhage into the extradural, subdural, or subarachnoid spaces, or into the brain or ventricles, may occur. In patients who have sustained contusions and lacerations of the brain, any singular or combined variations of intracranial hemorrhage may develop. Although bleeding may begin soon after the blunt injury, its presence may not be apparent until it is of sufficient dimension to cause the signs and symptoms of a rapidly developing space-occupying lesion. The interval between hemorrhage occurring and clinical symptoms of a space-occupying lesion appearing may be a matter of hours or months, depending on the site and the rate of bleeding.

Intracranial hemorrhage may be a subliminal development in a patient who has sustained a seemingly minor injury in which consciousness has been maintained or quickly restored. This type of clinical finding may be observed with an extradural hematoma. Other patients with hemorrhage may have been rendered unconscious from the moment of impact. It is not necessary for a skull fracture to be present for an intracranial hemorrhage to develop.

Extradural or Epidural Hematoma

An *extradural hematoma*, also known as an epidural hematoma, refers to bleeding into the potential space between the inner table of skull (inner periosteum) and the dura mater (Fig. 17–4). It is a focal lesion. Extradural hematomas account for about 2% of all types of head injury. About 85% of patients who develop an extradural hematoma have sustained a skull fracture.

The most common site of fracture is in the thin, squamous portion of the temporal bone under which is located the middle meningeal artery and vein. A lacerated middle meningeal artery or vein is the source of hemorrhage. Much less commonly, laceration of the superior sagittal sinus from a vertex (frontal–parietal) fracture is implicated. Extradural hematomas are rarely bilateral. As the hematoma develops, it gradually strips the dura from the inner table of the skull and a large ovoid mass develops, creating pressure on the underlying brain, local mass effect, shift and herniation, and brain stem compression. Extradural hematomas are seen most often in children and young people because the dura is less firmly attached to the bone table, as is the case with older people.

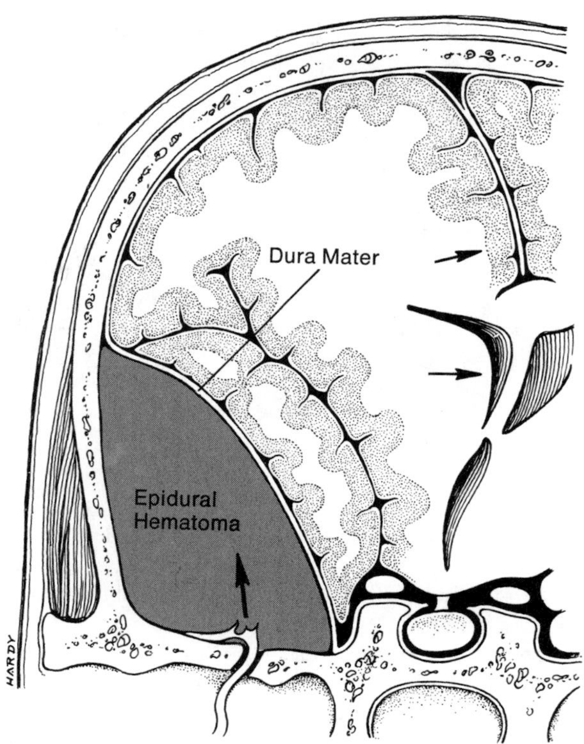

FIG. 17–4. Epidural hematoma. The dark area in the lower left area of the drawing represents the hematoma. Note the broken blood vessel and the shift of midline structures *(small arrows)*. (Cosgriff JH, Anderson DL: The Practice of Emergency Nursing. Philadelphia, JB Lippincott, 1984)

Signs and Symptoms. The classical description of an extradural hematoma is that of momentary unconsciousness followed by a lucid period lasting for a few hours or 1 or 2 days. Occasionally, the interval can last for a few days to 1 week when venous bleeding is involved. The lucid period is followed by deterioration in the level of consciousness (drowsiness, confusion to coma), frequently at a rapid rate. Other symptoms include headache of increasing severity; possible seizure (Jacksonian or generalized); vomiting; hemiparesis, which may be ipsilateral or contralateral; and a dilated ipsilateral pupil, which becomes fixed. As a supratentorial herniation syndrome develops, coma occurs. Hemiparesis may convert to bilateral spasticity of the limbs and there may be positive Babinski signs. Respirations become deeper and more labored, then shallow and irregular, and finally cease altogether. The pulse decreases to 60 or less and is bounding, while the systolic blood pressure and temperature rise, possibly reaching 106° to 107° F (41.1° to

41.6° C). The changes in vital signs are late findings. Death will result if early definitive action is not taken.

The classical clinical picture of an extradural hematoma has been presented. Although the significance of the lucid interval is acknowledged as being characteristic of an extradural hematoma, it should be emphasized that in at least 15% of patients there is no lucid period at all. The lucid period relates to the depth and duration of the initial period of unconsciousness as well as how rapidly the bleeding occurs and what the source of the bleeding is (arterial or venous). The protective mechanism of the brain in which the dura adheres to the skull contributes to the presence of the lucid period. It takes more time for sufficient bleeding to accumulate and apply pressure to the brain before clinical neurological deficits and changes in the level of consciousness are apparent. However, once symptoms develop, the amount of time for definitive action is much shorter than with a subdural hematoma.

Diagnosis. Diagnosis of an extradural hematoma is accomplished by localizing the lesion with a CT scan and sometimes an arteriogram.

Treatment. Treatment is always surgical, with burr holes made into the skull to evacuate the clot and ligate the bleeding vessel. Early diagnosis and treatment are considered synonymous with a good prognosis. If surgery is delayed, the outcome is less optimistic and death may result.

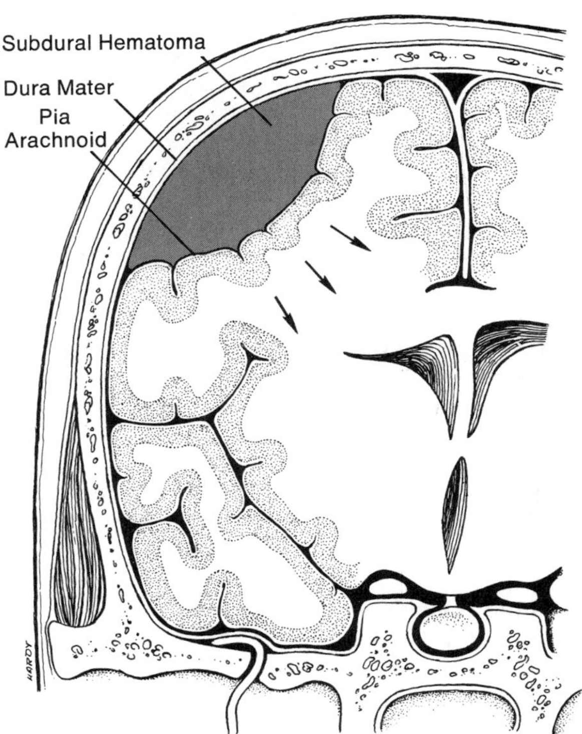

FIG. 17-5. Subdural hematoma. The dark area in the upper left area of the drawing represents the hematoma. Note the shift of midline structures. (Cosgriff JH, Anderson DL: The Practice of Emergency Nursing. Philadelphia, JB Lippincott, 1984)

Subdural Hematoma

A *subdural hematoma* refers to bleeding between the dura mater and arachnoid layer of the meninges (Fig. 17-5). Since the arachnoid-pia layer adheres closely to the brain, bleeding into the subdural space creates immediate, direct pressure on the brain. Bleeding into the subdural space is attributed to

- Rupture of small vessels (bridging veins) that bridge the subdural space
- Rupture of the small branches of cerebral arteries
- Bleeding from contused or lacerated areas of the brain
- Extension from an intracerebral hematoma

Approximately 10% to 15% of head-injury patients develop subdural hematomas. Bilateral subdurals are not uncommon.

Signs and Symptoms. Subdural hematomas are subdivided into three categories based on the interval between injury and the appearance of signs and symptoms of the lesion. The classifications and approximate intervals for the appearance of symptoms are (1) acute—within 48 hours, (2) subacute—from 2 days to 2 weeks, and (3) chronic—over 2 weeks or as long as months.

Acute subdural hematomas are associated with the major cerebral trauma of contusion and laceration. Large hematomas are caused by severe contusion of underlying tissue.

The most common signs of acute subdural hematoma are headache, drowsiness, some agitation, slow cerebration, and confusion, all of which gradually worsen. The ipsilateral pupil is dilated and becomes fixed. Hemiparesis, if present, is a late finding. Bear in mind that acute subdural hematomas are often complications of a contused, lacerated brain, so signs and symptoms of the subdural clot are often not distinguishable within the total clinical picture.

Subacute subdural hematomas are also associated with less severe underlying contusions. Suspicion of the subacute hematoma is raised by the failure of the patient to regain consciousness. The level of consciousness is not improved when a subacute hematoma is present because of unrelenting cerebral pressure. Signs and symptoms correspond more closely to that of the acute subdural hematoma.

Chronic subdural hematomas can develop from seemingly minor head injuries. The lapse of time between injury and development of symptoms may be months, so the initial injury may not be remembered. The chronic subdural hematoma becomes encased within a membrane easily separated from the arachnoid and dura mater. The hematoma slowly increases until it behaves like a space-occupying lesion, probably because of repeated small hemorrhages. The most common symptoms of a chronic subdural hematoma include headache (progressing in severity), giddiness, slow cerebration, confusion, drowsiness, and possibly a seizure. Papilledema may develop, and the ipsilateral pupil will be dilated and sluggish to light. Hemiparesis, a late finding, may be ipsilateral or contralateral depending on whether the temporal lobe has herniated through the tentorial notch and compressed the contralateral cerebral peduncle against the free edge of the tentorium.

It is important to remember that elderly people, because of the cerebral atrophy associated with the normal aging process, are prone to develop subdural hematomas. Cerebral atrophy causes separation of the cortex from the dura so that the fragile bridging veins are more prone to tear and rupture when a blow to the head occurs. The atrophy also provides more free space into which bleeding can occur before symptoms are evident. Symptoms do not develop until the intracranial space is compromised and evidence of a space-occupying lesion slowly becomes apparent. With chronic subdural hematomas the development of symptoms can be subtle because of gradual spatial compensation. The same can be said for chronic alcoholic patients. They, too, undergo a process of cerebral atrophy and are especially prone to subdural hematomas.

Diagnosis. A subdural hematoma can be diagnosed by a CT scan or an arteriogram, but the CT scan is the major tool used today.

Treatment. Small subdural hematomas may be treated medically because they can frequently be absorbed. The neurosurgeon must decide whether surgery is indicated. With large subdural hematomas, surgical evacuation is necessary or death will result from secondary damage caused by increased intracranial pressure and tentorial herniation. Elderly patients and alcoholics who have had an evacuation of a subdural hematoma tend to rebleed.

Burr holes with evacuation of the hematoma is the surgical procedure usually performed for an acute subdural hematoma. However, with some subacute and all chronic subdural hematomas a craniotomy will be necessary because the hematoma has become gelatinous and is not accessible through a burr hole. As previously mentioned, in chronic subdural hematomas a membrane has developed that must be dissected away from the dura and arachnoid layers.

Subdural Hygroma

A *subdural hygroma* is a collection of clear or yellowish fluid (cerebrospinal fluid [CSF] and blood) in the subdural space. If it is of sufficient quantity, the signs and symptoms will mimic those of a subdural hematoma. The accumulation of fluid can be anywhere from a few milliliters to, rarely, as much as 500 ml. The condition follows a head injury, which is usually not severe, and results from a tear in the arachnoid, which allows for escape of the fluid into the subdural space. Concurrent cerebral edema locks the fluid into the space and creates pressure on the brain.

The subdural hygroma is unilateral and may extend over the entire hemisphere or become encapsulated. The fluid has a high protein content, which may be why it occasionally coagulates. Symptoms that correspond to those of a slowly developing subdural hematoma occur beginning with headache, which becomes severe and persistent. Differentiation of a hygroma from a clot is made only at surgery. The only treatment is surgical removal.

Intracerebral Hematoma

An *intracerebral hematoma* refers to bleeding into the cerebral substance, a complication seen in 2% to 3% of head-injury patients (Fig. 17–6). Most intracerebral hematomas are related to contusions and, therefore, tend to occur in the frontal and temporal lobes. They can also occur deep within the hemispheres owing to shearing strain on small vessels. Intracerebral hematomas occur singularly or as multiple lesions. They are uncommon in the cerebellum.

The mode of action is that of a rapidly expanding space-occupying lesion. Occasionally, hemorrhage may be delayed for a few days. It is not certain if slow bleeding or a delay in onset is the underlying cause. Intracerebral hematomas are associated with other serious cerebral injuries such as contusions, lacerations, and other types of hematomas. A large number of intracerebral hematomas are seen at autopsy.

Signs and Symptoms. Unconsciousness, which occurs from the onset of bleeding, is also due to the accompanying serious contusions and lacerations. Signs and symptoms include headache, a deteriorating consciousness to deep coma, hemiplegia on the contralateral side, and a dilated pupil on the side of the clot. As intracranial pressure in-

FIG. 17–6. Intracerebral hemorrhage. The large central dark area represents the hemorrhage. Note the midline shift.

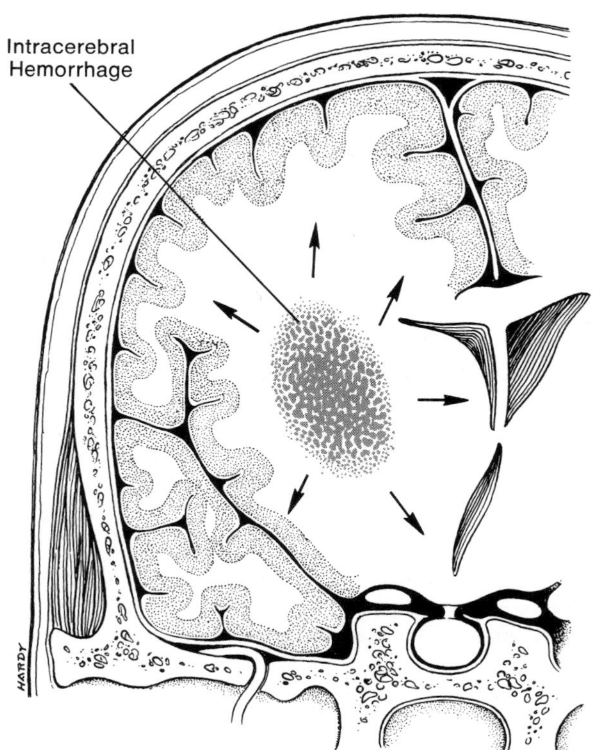

creases, there is evidence of developing tentorial herniation with accompanying changes in pupils, respirations, and other vital signs.

Diagnosis. The most reliable procedures for diagnosing an intracerebral hematoma are the CT scan and the cerebral arteriogram.

Treatment. Craniotomy with evacuation has been beneficial in only a few cases, primarily because widespread cerebral contusion is usually present. Mortality rates are high.

Subarachnoid Hemorrhage and Intraventricular Hemorrhage

A traumatic subarachnoid hematoma is rare; however, subarachnoid hemorrhage is a common finding in severe head injury. Lumbar puncture is often omitted because of the fear of brain stem herniation from increased intracranial pressure. Intraventricular hemorrhage occurs secondary to subarachnoid hemorrhage or as an extension from an intracerebral hematoma.

Nuchal rigidity, headache, deteriorating level of consciousness, hemiparesis, and ipsilateral dilated pupil are the signs and symptoms commonly seen.

The patient is managed on subarachnoid precautions. (See Chap. 24 for specific information.)

Injury to the Blood Vessels

In addition to intracranial hemorrhage (hematomas, subarachnoid hemorrhage), injury to and tears of the cerebral blood vessels can cause vascular spasms, resulting in ischemias to the areas of the brain supplied by the blood vessel. As a result of an intracranial hematoma, cerebral blood vessels can also become deformed or compressed from the traumatic mass or localized cerebral edema. In addition, cerebral blood vessels may become thrombosed or occluded or develop traumatic aneurysms from being stretched or torn at the time of injury.

MANAGEMENT OF THE HEAD-INJURED PATIENT

PREHOSPITAL MANAGEMENT

Prehospital management refers to the immediate resuscitation, stabilization, and immobilization of a patient at the scene of injury and en route to the hospital. Improvements in airway management, fluid replacement, and immobilization of the neck in case of cervical fracture and safe transport by land or air have reduced mortality and secondary cerebral insult, which contributes to poorer patient outcomes.

Depending on the emergency medical system and the facility in which she is employed, the nurse may participate in patient care even before he arrives in the emergency department. This participation may take the form of short-wave radio communications with the emergency vehicle personnel who are managing a patient with neurological trauma. Standing orders are often used to manage the patient at the injury site and during transport. Examples of procedures that may be included in the standing orders are the administration of oxygen and hyperventilation for treatment of hypoxia and hypercapnia. The emergency vehicle personnel will provide the following information about the patient: a brief history (type and circumstances of injury, how the patient was found, including in what position); baseline assessment (vital signs and mini-neurological exam); continual assessment data, and the patient's response to treatment. Personnel assigned to emergency vehicles should be competent in using the Glasgow Coma Scale and in assessing the level of consciousness, pupillary size and response to light, motor function, and vital signs (see Chap. 5). Based on the information supplied to the nurse, she can alert the physician, who will provide additional instruction on immediate patient management. The nurse will also notify necessary personnel of the impending arrival of the patient and the estimated arrival time and prepare the treatment room for the patient. Time is critical, and an organized team approach is imperative in managing the patient.

The professional nurse can also influence the quality of patient care administered in the prehospital period by participation in ongoing teaching of emergency personnel in the safe management of the patient at the injury site and during transport. The importance of treating all head-injury patients for possible cervical fractures by immediately immobilizing the neck and head cannot be overemphasized. All personnel who manage trauma victims must be mindful of the disastrous consequences that will result from manipulation of the neck (cord transection and quadriplegia). The fact that spinal cord injuries may not be noted on physical examination immediately after injury should be emphasized.

Establishing and maintaining a patent airway to prevent hypoxia and hypercapnia is an important concept that has a major influence on patient outcomes. Normal methods of establishing a patent airway must be modified to prevent the extension of possible cervical injuries. Since many trauma patients who have sustained neurological injuries may also have multiple trauma involving other body systems, the patient must be systematically assessed for evidence of multi-systems injuries (see Chap. 16, The Multitrauma Patient, for further discussion).

ARRIVAL IN THE EMERGENCY DEPARTMENT

When the patient arrives in the emergency department of the hospital, a team approach is initiated. In many instances some of the following points of assessment and management are accomplished simultaneously by various members of the team. The approach to the patient includes

Initially

- Quick history of injury
- Baseline assessment of vital signs
- Stabilization and support of vital signs

- Cervical neck assessment
- Triage neurological examination
- Control of seizures, if present
- Intracranial hypertension management
- Laboratory data on blood

Once Stabilized

- Additional information for history
- Ongoing assessment of neurological and vital signs
- Comprehensive physical examination for other injuries
- Radiological data
- Tetanus antitoxin and antibiotics
- Drainage of bladder and stomach
- Other diagnostic tests

Initial Quick History of Injury

Certain information either observed by the emergency vehicle personnel or collected from bystanders is very helpful to the physician in assessing the patient. The information includes

- How did the injury occur? Direct blow to the head, thrown from the car, fell off a bar stool?
- Was the patient wearing a seat belt? What type of seat belt (lap, shoulder)? Was the patient wearing a helmet?
- When did the injury occur?
- Was unconsciousness immediate, or was there a lucid period?
- Was there a documented period of apnea or cyanosis? For how long?
- How was the patient found? Lying face down?
- Was there significant blood loss noted at the scene?

All of this information gives the physician clues about what type of injuries might have been sustained.

Baseline Assessment of Vital Signs

Vital signs are taken and recorded to provide a baseline for future comparison and also to determine what action, if any, should be taken immediately. The parameters assessed include respirations, blood pressure, pulse, and temperature (temperature may be deferred at this time). See Chart 17–2 for assessment of vital signs.

Stabilization and Support of Vital Signs. Airway management is imperative for supporting adequate respirations. The following points of care should be considered:

- Consider any manipulation of the head and neck to be a potential risk to the cervical spine if the status of the cervical spine has not been determined.
- Clear the nose and mouth of blood, mucus, and drainage to ensure patency of the airway.
- Be aware that aspiration prior to admission to the emergency department is very common. This may be true even if chest x-rays are negative.
- Administer an adequate supply of supplementary oxygen.
- If respirations are inadequate, intubation will be necessary. If the status of the cervical spine is unknown, the physician may choose either blind nasotracheal intubation or cricothyroidotomy to prevent manipulation of the neck. Tracheal intubation is contraindicated with midface trauma and sometimes with basal skull fractures. If intubation can be delayed until after the cervical neck has been evaluated by x-rays, it should be. If the x-ray is negative, intubation may be accomplished by whatever method the physician prefers.
- Before intubation, the patient is often given a skeletal muscle relaxant to facilitate intubation; a drug frequently chosen is pancuronium bromide, 0.04 mg to 0.1 mg/kg intravenously; this is also helpful to prevent the patient on a ventilator from bucking the respirator.
- In some facilities, if a patient has a Glasgow Coma Scale of 7 or less the patient is immediately intubated and hyperventilated to ensure a PaO_2 greater than 70 mm Hg and to maintain a $PaCO_2$ within the range of 25 mm to 30 mm Hg.[12] The efficiency of gas exchange is assessed with arterial blood gases.
- If the patient is not breathing adequately, he may be placed on a respirator.
- The airway should be suctioned as necessary, limiting insertion of the catheter to no more than 15 seconds each time. The nasal passage should not be used for suctioning until a basal skull fracture and a dural tear have been ruled out.

Blood pressure must be maintained. If the patient is hypotensive, look for signs and symptoms of occult bleeding. Hypovolemic shock must be treated aggressively. If hypertension is present, it is probably caused by intracranial hypertension. The underlying cause is treated, which will be discussed under Intracranial Hypertension Management. In patients with severely elevated hypertension, the pressure should be lowered gradually to borderline hypertensive levels, usually by nitroprusside infusion.[13]

Pulse is a parameter that indicates cardiac and circulatory function; it is usually considered with blood pressure.

Once vital signs have been stabilized, the cervical neck can be assessed.

Cervical Neck Assessment

Until x-rays of the lateral cervical spine are read as negative, the neck must be immobilized with a hard collar and sand bags. All seven cervical vertebrae must be visualized on the x-ray. To ensure proper visualization, shoulder traction can be used—two people each pull the upper limbs toward the feet. If this approach is unsuccessful, the swimmer's position may be used.

In the conscious patient, be suspicious of cervical injury if the head is tilted to one side and head movement is limited. There may also be local tenderness to palpation over the spinous processes. In the unconscious patient, the examiner may notice an abnormal distance between two adjacent cervical spinous processes.

Signs and symptoms that may be seen if cord injury has occurred follow:

- Response to pain above the shoulders but not below
- Hypotension without evidence of shock
- Flaccid areflexia, especially of the rectal sphincter
- Abdominal or diaphragmatic breathing

If a cervical fracture is discovered, the neurosurgeon will need to decide how it will be managed.

CHART 17–2. ASSESSMENT OF VITAL SIGNS AND THEIR SIGNIFICANCE

Respirations

The rate, pattern (rhythm), and characteristics of respirations should be noted. Head injuries produce a few abnormal respiratory patterns that roughly correlate with the level of neurological injury (see Chap. 5 for abnormal patterns and level of injury). Generally speaking, an initial increase in intracranial pressure results in slowing of respirations. If the rise in intracranial pressure continues, the respiratory pattern becomes rapid and noisy until the end, when respirations cease.

A few points should be mentioned that can affect assessment of respirations:

- Metabolic disorders such as diabetes mellitus can cause changes in the respiratory pattern
- Injury to the cervical spine can cause respiratory difficulty if below C–4 and total arrest if above C–4, the site of phrenic nerve innervation
- Injury to the chest may make assessment of respirations difficult

Blood Pressure

Hypotension is rarely due to cerebral injury. If it occurs, it is a terminal event and is seen with tachycardia. If hypotension and tachycardia are noted in a patient who is not terminal, they usually signify the presence of occult bleeding, most likely in the abdominal, pelvic, or thoracic cavity. An aggressive search for the occult blood should be initiated. Cerebral perfusion pressure depends on systemic arterial pressure and intracranial pressure; it must be adequate for the brain to receive an adequate blood supply. Hypotension will compromise cerebral perfusion and must be treated.

Hypotension, which is usually slight, and bradycardia may also be seen as secondary responses to cervical cord injury if the descending sympathetic pathways have been interrupted.

Hypertension is common and often reflects an increase in intracranial pressure. It may also be a pre-existing condition, or it may be associated with pain, fear, or anxiety.

If hypertension is associated with an increase in intracranial pressure, it is a later sign that correlates with pressure on the brain stem. The presence of hypertension, bradycardia, and a widening pulse pressure is called Cushing's response. This is an ischemic response of the body that maintains cerebral blood flow in the presence of rising intracranial pressure. The triad of hypertension, bradycardia, and irregular respirations is called Cushing's triad. It reflects a rising intracranial pressure in which there is direct pressure on the medullary respiratory center of the brain stem. It is often seen in the terminal stages and is associated with irreversible brain stem damage.

Pulse

Pulse has been discussed in relationship to blood pressure. Bradycardia is associated with a rising intracranial pressure or a cervical injury. Tachycardia is seen with occult hemorrhage and hypovolemic shock. The occult bleeding is not in the nervous system; instead, it is usually found in the abdominal, pelvic, or thoracic cavity. Tachycardia may also be seen as a terminal event in the head-injured patient.

Temperature

Variations in temperature can be caused by variations in weather or temperature at the injury site. Hypothermia may be seen early with cervical cord injury. Since the ability to perspire is lost below the level of the lesion with cord injuries, high cord lesions (cervical) can result in hyperthermia and heat prostration in hot weather if measures are not taken to control body temperature. However, this problem is not usually a concern in the emergency department.

In the head-injured patient, hyperthermia can be associated with direct injury to the hypothalamus or petechial bleeding into the hypothalamus or pons. Hyperthermia must be controlled in the head-injured patient because it increases the need for oxygen and increases the metabolic rate of all body cells including the brain. Oxygen consumption rises 10% for every 1° rise in temperature on the Centigrade scale (an increase from 37° C, which is 98.6° F, to 40.5° C, which is 105° F, causes a 35% increase in oxygen consumption).

Triage Neurological Examination

A mini–neurological examination, also called a triage neurological examination, is done quickly to assess the patient's neurological status. It must be reliable as well as quick. The following areas are assessed in only 2 to 3 minutes:

- Level of consciousness (orientation and cognition)
- Pupillary size, shape, and reaction
- Brain stem reflexes (oculovestibular/cold calorics and corneal reflexes)
- Motor responses (observe for lateralization, which indicates a focal lesion)
- The Glasgow Coma Scale is used in some facilities; it assesses level of consciousness and motor responses; motor response should be tested on both sides to note lateralization.

This first neurological assessment provides a baseline against which subsequent assessments can be compared to denote trends.

Control of Seizures and Temperature

Both seizures and hyperthermia increase cerebral metabolism. It is important to control both of these problems to prevent further demands on the already-challenged brain. Seizures are managed initially by intravenous diazepam (Valium), 10 mg. Later, the patient is begun on phenytoin (Dilantin) by the intravenous route, which is changed to the oral route just as soon as it is feasible.

Hyperthermia is managed by cool sponging and acetaminophen (Tylenol), 650 mg, given rectally every 4 hours. With hypothermia, a temperature of 28° C or below leads to cardiac irritability and the possibility of arrhythmias. The patient should be gradually warmed and monitored for cardiac arrhythmias.

Intracranial Hypertension Management

To control acute ongoing increased intracranial pressure caused by cerebral edema, osmotic diuretics and/or a loop diuretic are usually administered. The drug of choice for osmotic diuretics is mannitol, 0.25 gm to 1.0 gm per kg by the intravenous route. If furosemide (Lasix), a loop diuretic, is used, the dosage is 0.5 mg to 1.0 mg per kg. An indwelling urinary catheter will be necessary to record the diuresis. Unless hypovolemic shock is present, intravenous fluid should be limited. Another drug administered to control cerebral edema is dexamethasone, 20 mg intravenously every 6 hours.

Hyperventilation and drugs are the major means of controlling intracranial hypertension at this time. In some instances, a burr hole will be made and a catheter inserted for continual cerebrospinal fluid drainage. To monitor intracranial pressure, an intracranial pressure monitor may also be inserted.

Laboratory Data

The usual laboratory data ordered initially are included in Chart 17–3. Of this data, the most important are the arterial blood values. Once the patient is stabilized, additional assessment and management are provided.

Additional Information for History

Information about the patient is often collected in a fragmented fashion. The physician may request information about the patient from the family members who have arrived at the hospital. Any information about the past medical history is of value. There may also be clues on the patient's person, such as a Medic Alert bracelet, that provide information about his health status.

Ongoing Assessment of Neurological and Vital Signs

The initial assessment of neurological and vital signs provides a baseline for comparison with future assessments. The subsequent assessments provide evidence of trends of stabilization, improvement, or deterioration. It is most important to continue to conduct these assessments at frequent intervals and record the information.

A more detailed examination of the patient may be possible depending on the injuries present. The patient should be examined for evidence of a basal skull fracture. Drainage from the ear, nose, or postnasal area would raise the suspicion of a basal skull fracture.

If there is a head wound, it should be carefully cleaned under aseptic conditions and dressed with a dry, sterile dressing. Suturing may be necessary to close a scalp wound. For other patients, surgical débridement, burr holes, or a craniotomy may be performed immediately. When a patient has sustained a head injury from a penetrating object that is still within the head, do not remove the object. The physician may choose to remove the object in the operating room where hemorrhage can be adequately controlled. The foreign object can function as a tamponing agent against the injured blood vessels. Once the foreign object is removed, the pressure exerted against the vessels is abruptly withdrawn and serious hemorrhage can result, requiring immediate surgical intervention.

Comprehensive Physical Examination for Other Injuries

The patient with neurological trauma often has sustained trauma to other body systems. Systematic assessment of each body system should be conducted (see Chap. 16).

Radiological Data

In addition to the cervical x-rays, other studies that may be ordered include

- Chest x-rays to assess for the presence of thoracic injury or to validate the position of an endotracheal tube, if one has been inserted
- Skull x-rays to diagnose skull fractures
- A CT scan may be ordered to diagnose the presence of a focal lesion (subdural or epidural hematoma) that may require immediate surgery.

Tetanus Antitoxin and Antibiotics

If an open wound is present, tetanus antitoxin and antibiotics will be given prophylactically. Antibiotics are given for a 7- to 10-day period if the possibility of meningitis or wound infection is high.

Drainage of Bladder and Stomach

An indwelling urinary catheter is usually inserted in a patient who is unconscious or receiving diuretics. If there is spinal cord injury, an atonic bladder may be present. The bladder is also emptied for a urine specimen and, in a multi-trauma patient, to determine whether urinary tract injury has been sustained.

A nasogastric tube is inserted unless there is an anterior fossa basilar skull or midface fracture. With an anterior fossa basilar skull fracture, a nasogastric tube can be inserted through the mouth and guided by a laryngoscope to avoid passing the tube through the fracture area into the brain. The insertion of a nasogastric tube should be delayed

CHART 17-3. LABORATORY DATA FREQUENTLY ORDERED IN THE EMERGENCY DEPARTMENT FOR A NEWLY ADMITTED PATIENT WITH A HEAD INJURY

- Arterial blood gases
- Complete blood count (CBC) including hemoglobin and hematocrit
- Electrolytes
- Blood urea nitrogen (BUN)
- Creatinine
- Calcium
- Glucose
- Serum osmolarity, if mannitol has been given
- Type and cross match for blood replacement for hemorrhage in another body system
- Drug screen (trauma is often associated with drug abuse; it is important to identify the specific drug to determine its effect on the nervous system; also, the patient may need to be treated for the overdose)
- Urinalysis
- Other tests as indicated

until after the endotracheal tube is in position because the insertion of a nasogastric tube may cause vomiting and aspiration.

Other Diagnostic Tests

Depending on the patient, other diagnostic tests may be ordered to establish a diagnosis. These may include blood chemistry, radiological studies, and others.

SUMMARY

The management of the head-injured patient in the emergency department has been directed at resuscitation, stabilization, and diagnosis. Once this has been completed, a decision will be made for further management of the patient based on an overall assessment. The necessary care may include immediate surgery for burr holes or a craniotomy, transfer to another facility better able to provide specialized care, or admission to the intensive care unit or regular neurological-neurosurgical unit.

ACUTE CARE PHASE: THE INTENSIVE CARE NURSING MANAGEMENT FOR THE UNIT

The patient with a severe head injury will usually be admitted to an intensive care unit for neurological intensive management.

TRANSFER AND ADMISSION

Transfer Report

Upon the patient's admission to the unit from the emergency department, operating room, or recovery room, if immediate surgery was necessary, the intensive care nurse should receive a complete report of the patient's diagnosis, circumstances of injury, associated injuries, details of patient management and treatment administered to the present, special observations and concerns, and notification or presence of family.

Admission to the Unit

After a detailed report has been given and the chart reviewed, the patient will be admitted to the unit. The patient may have been transferred to the unit on a traction bed, special trauma bed, or Kinetic Treatment Table or by stretcher. If the patient is to be transferred to another bed from the stretcher, the bed should have a firm mattress and possibly a bedboard and an alternating pressure mattress. All monitoring and support equipment should be connected and checked to be sure that it is operating properly.

GOALS OF INTENSIVE CARE MANAGEMENT

The goals of the intensive care unit are

- Continual assessment and monitoring of neurological function and other body systems for early recognition and treatment of problems and complications
- Prevention of secondary brain injury
- Administration of aggressive forms of therapy

The length of time that the patient remains in the intensive care setting will depend on his condition and response to treatment. In most facilities, if aggressive therapies such as barbiturate coma or continual electroencephalographic (EEG) activity monitoring are instituted, the patient must remain in the intensive care unit for constant surveillance.

OBJECTIVE ONE: CONTINUAL ASSESSMENT AND MONITORING OF NEUROLOGICAL FUNCTION AND OTHER BODY SYSTEMS FOR EARLY RECOGNITION AND TREATMENT OF PROBLEMS AND COMPLICATIONS

To accomplish this goal, several assessment techniques and monitoring devices will be used.

Parameters

Vital Signs. The significance of the vital signs as they relate to neurological function and other body systems was presented in Chart 17–2.

Neurological Parameters. Frequent neurological assessments are conducted by the nurse to assess trends in status (stabilizing, deteriorating, or improving). The importance of ongoing assessment cannot be overstated. (See Chap. 5 for a detailed discussion of assessment.)

The serial neurological assessment is conducted every 15 to 30 minutes, depending on the patient's condition. Once the patient is well stabilized, assessment may be conducted every 2 to 4 hours. The points included in the serial assessment include

- Level of consciousness (orientation and cognition are assessed if the patient is not deeply comatose; they are assessed by the patient's use of language and response to questions)
- Pupillary size, shape, and reaction to light
- Brain stem reflexes (corneal, gag, and oculovestibular; these reflexes may or may not be tested with every assessment depending on the patient's condition)
- Motor function (observe for asymmetry or lateralization, which indicates a focal mass reaction)
- Respiratory pattern

The Glasgow Coma Scale, pupillary responses, brain stem reflexes, and respiratory pattern are the parameters assessed in serial neurological examinations in some institutions.

Neurological Signs and Parameters

Level of Consciousness. The level of consciousness is the most sensitive indicator of neurological change. If the patient is able to respond verbally at all, his orientation to time, place, and person is assessed. Cognition is assessed by the patient's use of language and his responses to questions. If the patient is comatose, painful stimuli are applied and his response is noted. Possible responses are purposeful, nonpurposeful, and unresponsive to painful stimuli.

The level of consciousness will depend on the severity of injury. The patient with a severe head injury is usually in the comatose state for an extended period. The nurse must assume responsibility for providing for the patient's basic needs, including protection from injury.

The Glasgow Coma Scale may also be used to assess the level of consciousness.

Pupillary Size, Shape, and Reaction to Light. Pupils are normally equal in size and midposition, round, and briskly reactive to direct light. Change in the size or reaction of one or both of the pupils should be reported (see Chap. 5 for significance of pupillary size and reaction). With lateral transtentorial herniation (also called uncal herniation syndrome) caused by localized cerebral edema or a focal lesion such as a subdural or epidural hematoma, one pupil will become dilated and unresponsive to light. This is due to compression of the oculomotor nerve by the edematous herniating brain on one side. Immediate intervention will be necessary to prevent continual herniation and irreversible neurological deterioration. An oval or ovoid pupil is also considered to be an early sign of beginning transtentorial herniation. This information should be noted and recorded.

Brain Stem Reflexes. The reflexes assessed are the corneal, gag, and oculovestibular (cold calorics) reflexes. The corneal and gag reflexes can be assessed easily at the bedside. Assessment of the oculovestibular reflex is more involved. Some clinicians assess the oculocephalic reflex (doll's eyes), which also indicates whether the brain stem is functional (see Chap. 5 for assessment technique). The oculovestibular reflex is a stronger reflex that can be elicited when the oculocephalic reflex is absent or provides inconclusive results.

The purpose of testing the brain stem reflexes is to determine whether the brain stem is functional. If the reflexes are absent, it is a poor prognostic sign and the nurse may need to provide special care. The nurse will need to provide special protective eye care and lubricate the cornea periodically if the corneal reflex is absent. Should the gag reflex be absent, the patient is more prone to aspiration.

In assessing the brain stem reflexes, the reflex assessed should be tested individually on each side of the body and recorded. This is necessary because these brain stem reflexes are controlled by pairs of cranial nerves—left and right nerves innervate different sides of the body.

Motor Function. The patient is observed for spontaneous movement as he lies in bed. Techniques for assessing motor function in the comatose patient are found in Chapter 5. Note asymmetry of movement or lateralization, which indicates a focal mass lesion on one side of the brain. Hemiparesis and hemiplegia are signs of lateralization because they involve only one side of the body. The lesion will be located in the hemisphere opposite to the side of motor weakness.

Often, decortication or decerebration posturing is observed in comatose patients who have suffered severe head injury. Bilateral flaccidity may be associated with spinal cord transection or the terminal stage of neurological deterioration.

Motor response can also be evaluated on the Glasgow Coma Scale. The examiner should assess each side of the body to note the presence or absence of lateralizing signs.

Respiratory Pattern. The respiratory rate and pattern are controlled by the brain. Direct pressure on the brain or injury to the brain can cause changes in the pattern and rate of respiratory function that can be roughly correlated with a specific area of the brain (see Chap. 5 for types of abnormal respirations).

Other Observations. The nurse should examine the face and scalp for signs of other injury because abrasions or contusions may have been missed. Note the presence of ecchymosis on the mastoid bone (Battle's sign), periorbital ecchymosis (raccoon eye), or conjunctival hemorrhage. These signs always raise suspicion of basal skull fracture.

Clear or bloody drainage from the ear, nose, or postnasal area should also be reported because these are signs of probable basal skull fracture.

Provided that there is no cervical fracture or dislocation, the neck is assessed for evidence of nuchal rigidity, a sign of meningeal irritation. The rigidity can be caused by meningitis or blood in the cerebrospinal fluid from subarachnoid hemorrhage.

Parameters Used to Monitor Body Systems

Several monitoring devices are used continually to assess the patient such as

- Continual intracranial monitoring
- Swan-Ganz catheter
- Central venous pressure (CVP) line
- Continual cardiac monitor
- Possible continuous recording of the electrical activity of the brain (EEGs)

The patient may also have various support and therapeutic equipment in place such as intravenous lines, an indwelling urinary drainage catheter, a ventilator for respiratory support, continuous cerebrospinal drainage, or a cooling blanket. In some instances, the physician will order the placement of the patient on a Kinetic Treatment Table to prevent the complications of immobility. (See Chap. 11 for a discussion of kinetic therapy.) The equipment and the therapeutic results achieved by its use will also be monitored.

Laboratory Parameters. Laboratory parameters that are closely monitored and the approximate frequency of assessment are included in Table 17-3.

The laboratory data should be recorded on laboratory flow sheets so that trends can be noted easily.

Other Parameters. Other important parameters to monitor will vary from patient to patient. However, common parameters assessed may include tidal volumes, intake and output record, and weight, among others.

Neurological System

Control of Increased Intracranial Pressure. Cerebral edema is the most common cause of increased intracranial pressure in the head-injured patient. The brain responds quickly to injury and becomes edematous with a peak of swelling usually evident in 72 hours. Edema may be generalized or involve only selected areas of the brain. The brain responds to edema by increased intracranial pressure and the development of herniation syndromes. The cerebral edema is aggressively managed to prevent ischemia and necrosis of cerebral tissue and threats to vital functions. The control of elevated intracranial pressure is managed with drug therapy that includes osmotic diuretics, loop diuretics, and corticosteroids.

- Osmotic diuretics such as mannitol (Osmitrol) reduce cerebral edema by excreting excess fluid.
- Loop diuretics act directly on the kidney to excrete fluid.
- Corticosteroids such as dexamethasone (Decadron) are believed to stabilize the cell membrane, thus decreasing cerebral edema.
- Since dexamethasone is irritating to the gastric mucosa and there is also an increased risk of developing Cushing's ulcer with head injuries, Maalox, 30 ml every 3 to 6 hours, is given by feeding tube or orally; some treatment protocols for the critically ill patient require hourly aspirations of gastric contents to assess the pH; the pH is maintained above 3.0 or 4.0 with an hourly administration of an antacid such as Maalox by way of the feeding tube.
- In addition, cimetidine (Tagamet), 300 mg every 4 to 6 hours, is given intravenously or by feeding tube to decrease gastric secretions.

In following this management protocol, it is necessary to maintain the patient on an intake and output record. The blood electrolytes should also be carefully evaluated since diuresis can result in electrolyte imbalance. In any patient receiving steroids such as Decadron, the stools should be checked daily for occult blood. The urine should also be checked for sugar and acetone because steroids tend to cause glycosuria. In addition, to discontinue steroids, the dose must be gradually diminished to prevent adrenal insufficiency.

In addition, other measures helpful for controlling an elevated intracranial pressure follow:

- Elevation of the head of the bed 30 degrees
- Hyperventilation
- Continuous cerebrospinal fluid drainage
- Prevention of the Valsalva maneuver
- Maintenance of the neck and head in neutral position
- Maintenance of normothermia
- Fluid restriction
- Barbiturate coma

These management modalities were discussed in detail in Chapter 12.

Control of Seizures. Seizures are a common occurrence after head injury. Seizures are indications of cerebral irritation caused by direct injury or cerebral edema. Any patient with a head injury should be observed for possible seizures. Seizure precautions should be instituted and anticonvulsant drugs given prophylactically to prevent seizures from occurring. The drug of choice is phenytoin (Dilantin). After a loading dose is administered intravenously, daily doses of 300 mg to 400 mg are given daily in divided doses through the feeding tube or intravenously. Drug levels are checked periodically to maintain the drug level in a therapeutic range of 14 μg to 20 μg/ml.

In administering the drug by the intravenous route, manufacturer's instructions should be followed. Phenytoin should not be given any faster than 50 mg/minute because of the possibility of hypotension and cardiac arrhythmias. It must also be administered in normal saline to prevent precipitation in solution. There are many drug interactions with phenytoin. See Chapter 27 for detailed discussion of this drug.

If seizures occur, they are usually focal or grand mal. Focal seizures frequently involve the face and hands.

TABLE 17-3. *Laboratory Data Commonly Monitored in the Intensive Care Unit for Patients With Acute Head Injuries*

Study and Normal Values	Frequency	Purpose
Arterial blood gases PaO_2: 80 mm to 100 mm Hg $PaCO_2$: 35 mm to 45 mm Hg O_2Sat: 94% to 100% pH: 7.35 to 7.45 HCO_3: 22 mEq to 26 mEq/liter	Every 6 hours	Assesses arterial oxygen, carbon dioxide, and blood pH; indicates respiratory or metabolic acidosis or alkalosis; assesses adequacy of oxygenation and ventilation therapy
Hemoglobin (Hgb) and Hematocrit (Hct) Hgb Male: 13 gm to 16 gm Female: 12 gm to 14 gm Hct Male: 42% to 50% Female: 40% to 48%	Every 6 to 12 hours	In anemic states, there are fewer vehicles (Hgb) to carry oxygen to the brain
White Blood Count (WBC) and Differential WBC: 6000 to 10,000	Daily	Monitors development of sepsis, which can alter neurological function
Fibrinogen Degradation Products (FDP) Screening assay < 10 mcg/ml	Daily for first few days	Aids in the diagnosis of disseminated intravascular coagulation (DIC)
Prothrombin Time (PT) 5 to 10 minutes	Every 12 to 24 hours	Aids in the diagnosis of coagulation deficiencies
Partial Thromboplastin Time (PTT) 20 sec to 45 sec	Every 12 to 24 hours	Aids in the diagnosis of coagulation deficiencies
Serum Electrolytes Sodium: 135 mEq to 145 mEq/liter Potassium: 3.5 mEq to 5.0 mEq/liter Chloride: 100 mEq to 108 mEq/liter	Every 6 hours	Assesses fluid and electrolyte imbalance; serum sodium imbalance states are the most common causes of fluid imbalance in the brain-injured patient
Serum Osmolarity 280 mOsm to 300 mOsm	Every 6 hours	Monitors response to diuretics; assesses hypo-osmolar and hyperosmolar states such as diabetes insipidus and syndrome of inappropriate secretion of antidiuretic hormone (SIADH)
Creatinine 0.8 mg to 1.2 mg in males 0.6 mg to 0.9 mg in females	Every 6 hours	Monitors glomerular filtration rate
Blood Urea Nitrogen (BUN) 8 mg to 20 mg	Every 6 hours	Assesses renal functions
Calcium 4.5 mEq to 5.5 mEq/liter	Every 6 hours	Aids in the diagnosis of arrhythmias, blood-clotting deficiencies, and acid–base imbalance
Glucose 70 mg to 100 mg	Every 6 hours	Monitors for elevation of glucose; may be associated with steroid therapy; screening for diabetes mellitus; screening for hyperosmolar nonketotic hyperglycemia
Urine Osmolarity 300 mOsm to 1090 mOsm	Every 12 to 24 hours	Monitors for development of diabetes insipidus, syndrome of inappropriate secretions of antidiuretic hormone, or water imbalance
Urine Specific Gravity 1.010 to 1.035	Every 1 to 2 hours	Monitors for development of diabetes insipidus (1.001 to 1.005)

TABLE 17–3. (continued)

Study and Normal Values	*Frequency*	*Purpose*
Urine Electrolytes Sodium: 30 mEq to 280 mEq/24 hour Potassium: 40 mEq to 65 mEq/24 hour Chlorides: 70 mEq to 250 mEq/24 hour	Every 12 to 24 hours	Monitors for development of syndrome of inappropriate secretion of antidiuretic hormone; natriuresis (salt wasting)
Urinalysis	Daily to two times a week	Monitors for urinary tract infection and urinary tract disease
Culture and Sensitivity	Twice weekly	Monitors for sepsis, its causative organisms, and drugs sensitive to the organism

Grand mal seizures may occur alone or may follow focal seizures.

Nursing responsibilities center on the following points of care:

- Institute seizure precautions for the patient—have padded siderails, suction, and airway or padded tongue depressor available. If a seizure occurs, necessary equipment will be at hand to prevent injury and aspiration.
- Observe for seizure activity to anticipate this complication and to be ready to institute quick nursing action.
- Administer anticonvulsant drugs as ordered to control or decrease seizure activity.
- If a seizure occurs, the nurse should stay with the patient, guide his movements so that he will not injure himself, maintain a patent airway, and reorient the patient after the episode. In addition, the nurse should observe the sequence of events of the seizure so that the information can be charted and shared with the health team.

Hyperthermia. Hyperthermia can result from local or systemic infections or cerebral injury to the hypothalamus or adjacent area. The danger of hyperthermia is the acceleration of cerebral metabolism, which increases the production of byproducts of cell metabolism, a potent cerebral vasodilator. Therefore, hyperthermia must be controlled to prevent neurological deterioration.

- Monitor rectal temperature frequently (about every 4 hours). The rectal temperature is taken when a patient has altered levels of consciousness because it is the safest method of measurement.
- Administer antihyperthermic measures as ordered (cooling blanket, antipyretic drugs) and monitor temperature to evaluate response to therapy.

Deterioration of Neurological Function. The patient must be observed for the development of herniation from uncontrolled intracranial pressure. Rapid deterioration can occur as a result of intracranial bleeding (subdural or epidural hematoma), subarachnoid hemorrhage, or increasing cerebral edema. The nurse should monitor the neurological signs and watch for transient pressure signs that herald herniation. The transient pressure signs were discussed in Chapter 12.

Respiratory System

Respiratory management of the patient with a severe head injury has developed rapidly over the last few years. The brain, although only 2% of the body's weight, requires 20% of its oxygen supply. The respiratory system supplies oxygen to the brain; therefore, any dysfunction in this system will compromise the delivery of oxygen to the brain. In the injured brain, lack of sufficient oxygen in the blood, or hypoxemia, results in hypoxia at the cellular level. Along with hypoxia, hypercapnia develops, which is a known potent vasodilator. These conditions further increase the already elevated intracranial pressure in the brain-injured patient.

The nurse caring for the acute head-injured patient is concerned about maintaining the patency of the airway and preventing the development of serious respiratory complications.

Patency of Airway. In the patient with a head injury, the patency of the airway relates not only to respiratory function but also to an increase in intracranial pressure. In the acute phase of head injury the patient is neither able to manage his own secretions nor to position himself in the most expeditious way for adequate drainage of secretions. Meeting these needs becomes an objective of nursing care of the highest priority.

- Position the patient on his side to facilitate drainage of secretions.
- Suction as necessary to remove secretions that partially or completely obstruct the airway.
- Follow precautions in suctioning to prevent an increase in carbon dioxide and subsequent hypercapnia, which contribute to cerebral vasodilation, cerebral edema, and increased intracranial pressure.
- To provide increased levels of oxygen to the patient, hyperinflate with 100% oxygen for 1 minute before suctioning (with physician's approval).
- Limit the insertion of the catheter to no more than 15 seconds to prevent an increase in carbon dioxide.
- If the patient has a tracheostomy, give tracheostomy care every 4 hours. This prevents crusting and buildup of mucus and other secretions that can obstruct the airway.

- Monitor blood gases to provide a valid indication of oxygenation.
- Do not hyperextend or hyperflex the patient's neck since such a maneuver creates a partial obstruction of the airway.

Hypoxemia, Hypoxia, and Severe Respiratory Complications. Many patients with head injuries develop hypoxemia, hypoxia, and severe respiratory complications after injury without having any previous history of pulmonary disease. Although the etiology is unclear, it is believed to be related to the stress response of the autonomic system in which there is arteriovenous shunting of blood in the lungs.[14] The respiratory problems related to stress and shunting of blood are neurogenic pulmonary edema, adult respiratory distress syndrome (ARDS), and disseminated intravascular coagulation. Chapter 5 includes a detailed discussion of these conditions.

Pulmonary Fat Emboli. Another potentially lethal respiratory condition seen after trauma is pulmonary fat emboli. This condition, which is associated with long-bone fractures, usually develops 24 to 72 hours after initial injury. It is believed to result from the release of catecholamines, which mobilize fatty acids that develop into pulmonary emboli. Signs and symptoms include petechial rash on the chest and shoulders, apprehension, sweating, fever, tachycardia, pallor, dyspnea, pulmonary effusion, cyanosis, and seizures.

Pulmonary Complications. Pulmonary complications related to immobility are pulmonary emboli, the pneumonias, and atelectasis. Pulmonary emboli can result from deep venous thromboses seen in the immobilized patient. Signs and symptoms include cough, often with hemoptysis; dyspnea; tachypnea; and chest pain. Nursing management is directed at the prevention of thromboses and includes the application of elastic stockings or Ace bandages to the legs to improve the return of blood to the heart and range-of-motion exercises at least four times a day.

Pneumonias. Aspiration pneumonia can result from aspiration at the time of injury, which is a common occurrence. Bacterial invasion and stasis of fluid in the lungs also commonly cause bacterial pneumonia and hypostatic pneumonia, respectively. Patients who have sustained chest trauma in addition to head trauma have an even greater risk of developing respiratory complications. The nurse must assess the patient for signs and symptoms of pneumonia and incorporate nursing measures to prevent its development. To assess the lungs for the development of pneumonia the nurse should

- Auscultate the chest for breath sounds and fluid sounds.
- Listen for rhonchi and rales.
- Monitor the temperature and white blood count for signs of sepsis.
- Monitor the results of chest x-rays.
- Monitor sputum culture and sensitivity.

Nursing management to prevent pneumonia incorporates the following points:

- Turn the patient from side to side every 2 hours to prevent stasis of fluid in the lungs.
- Do not position the patient on his back (this increases the possibility of aspiration).
- Administer chest physiotherapy to loosen and drain pulmonary secretions.
- Maintain a patent airway.
- Remember that the intubated or tracheotomized patient is a compromised host who is very prone to infection; use meticulous aseptic technique.
- Inflate the cuff on the tracheostomy tube to prevent aspiration.
- Be sure that the gag reflex is intact before feeding a patient.

If pneumonia develops, antibiotic treatment is usually prescribed.

Atelectasis. A respiratory problem that can develop very rapidly is atelectasis. *Atelectasis* is defined as a collapsed or airless state of the lung that may involve any part of the lung. It is therefore important to be sure that all areas of the lungs are expanded. To assess the lungs for atelectasis, the nurse should include the following:

- Auscultate the chest for breath sounds; be sure to listen to the entire chest.
- Monitor the chest x-ray.

Nursing management directed at preventing atelectasis includes the following:

- Ambu the patient every 1 to 2 hours to expand all lung tissue for the intubated patient
- If the patient is on a ventilator that can be adjusted for sighs, make this adjustment.
- In the conscious patient encourage deep breathing exercises to expand the lungs and loosen secretions.

For the care of the patient who needs a ventilator to support respiratory function, see Chapter 5.

Cardiovascular System

Cardiovascular function is assessed by monitoring the vital signs and observing the tracings on a continuous cardiac monitor. Patients with acute severe head injuries are prone to life-threatening arrhythmias, especially if there has been bleeding into the subarachnoid space. The patient should be maintained on a continuous cardiac monitor and observed frequently.

Gastrointestinal System

In the early acute phase of serious head injury, the two major concerns for the nurse are gastric hemorrhage and paralytic ileus. As mentioned previously, Cushing's ulcer is common in head-injured patients. Cushing's ulcers occur in the upper gastrointestinal tract, while stress-related ulcerations are usually located closer to the duodenum. The use of cimetidine has decreased the incidence of Cushing's ulcers.

Assessing the gastric pH every hour and maintaining it in the range of 3.0 to 4.0 with antacids has also reduced the incidence of gastric hemorrhage. The patient's stools should be tested for occult blood and the hemoglobin and hematocrit monitored for occult bleeding.

Paralytic ileus may develop, especially if there are abdominal injuries in addition to the head injury. Most severely injured patients will have a nasogastric tube inserted for decompression. The nurse should auscultate the abdomen for peristalsis. Abdominal distention and the absence of peristalsis indicate paralytic ileus. The usual treatment is nasogastric decompression and withholding feedings by the gastrointestinal route.

Fluid and Electrolyte Imbalance

As a result of the stress response, the serum potassium level is decreased after injury. Sodium is retained due to the secretion of aldosterone and water is retained due to increased secretion of antidiuretic hormone. Normally, a few days after injury a diuresis usually occurs. However, there are special problems related to head-injured patients. For the nurse working with patients in the intensive care setting, an awareness of electrolyte and water alteration is essential. The electrolytes should be monitored frequently and replacement therapy may be necessary in some conditions. Osmolarity of the serum and urine should also be monitored to assess water balance.

The special problems to be considered with head-injured patients are diabetes insipidus, syndrome of inappropriate secretion of antidiuretic hormone (SIADH), and nonketotic hyperosmolar hyperglycemia (see Chap. 13 for a detailed discussion).

Nutrition

Just as soon as the patient is stabilized (after about 48 hours), a calorie count should be conducted to keep track of caloric intake and the patient assessed for nutritional needs. A total parenteral nutrition program (hyperalimentation) is begun to prevent a negative nitrogen balance and muscle wasting. The feeding is administered through a large-bore catheter. When the patient is well stabilized and peristalsis has returned, the patient is assessed for extended nutritional needs. Within 7 to 10 days of admission, the patient who will require long-term nutritional management is scheduled for surgical insertion of a gastrostomy tube, if there is no contraindication for using the gastrointestinal tract because of other injuries. At the same time, a tracheostomy is usually performed if the patient with an endotracheal tube will continue to need an artificial airway.

The patient is gradually begun on enteral feedings beginning with water and gradually increasing the feeding to a complete enteral feeding program based on the patient's tolerance and needs. Nutritional needs of the patient are discussed in detail in Chapter 6.

Infections

Infections are a major concern in the compromised host. Sepsis can result from injuries sustained at the time of injury (open head wounds, bullets), from invasive procedures (intracranial pressure monitor, central venous pressure line, Swan–Ganz catheter), and from surgical intervention. The normal body defenses such as the upper respiratory tract, skin, and hematological system are compromised with injury. Drugs such as corticosteroids and antibiotics diminish the body's response to infection and change the flora that keep some microorganisms in check. Bacteremia, osteomyelitis, wound infections, and infections at the catheter insertion sites can cause major sepsis and death in the critically injured patient. Strict aseptic technique and adherence to culture and dressing protocols can control sepsis. The high incidence of nosocomial infections in hospitals is the responsibility of every health worker. A detailed discussion of infections, including causative organisms, is found in Chapter 11.

OBJECTIVE TWO: PREVENTION OF SECONDARY BRAIN INJURY

The accomplishment of this objective is interrelated with the first objective. If there is early recognition and treatment of problems and complications, secondary brain injury will be prevented. Within the discussion of the first objective, the major complications and problems were identified along with nursing actions.

OBJECTIVE THREE: ADMINISTRATION OF AGGRESSIVE FORMS OF THERAPY

The common aggressive therapy used with selected head-injured patients is barbiturate coma. The patient needs the medical and nursing management that can be provided in only an intensive care setting.

Depending on the size and expertise of the medical and nursing staff in a facility, policies may require that a patient undergoing certain forms of therapy must be cared for in the intensive care unit. This internal decision is based on safety and the assurance of quality care.

NURSING MANAGEMENT FOR THE ACUTE CARE PHASE: THE NEUROSURGICAL UNIT

The condition of head-injured patients admitted to the neurological–neurosurgical unit can vary greatly. Some head-injured patients may be admitted directly from the emergency department for observation because the patient had a period of unconsciousness associated with the head injury. The patient may be oriented, slightly confused, and demonstrate no apparent neurological impairment. Because the documented unconsciousness lasted longer than a given time (e.g., 5 minutes) and because of the slight confusion, he is admitted for observation for 24 to 48 hours to be sure that there are no serious developing problems.

Another type of head-injured patient may be transferred from the intensive care unit because he has stabilized. This may be a semicomatose patient who has had an epidural or subdural hematoma evacuated and is now beginning to respond as evidenced by an improved score on the Glasgow Coma Scale or improvement in the overall neurological assessment. In still other instances, the patient may have sustained a severe concussion or diffuse axonal injury and is now stable but deeply comatose. (See Charts 17–4 and 17–5.)

(Text continued on page 369.)

CHART 17–4. SUMMARY OF NURSING MANAGEMENT IN THE ACUTE-CARE PHASE (INTENSIVE CARE AND INTERMEDIATE CARE)

NURSING RESPONSIBILITIES	RATIONALE
1. Collect a concise, complete report about the patient on admission to the unit.	• Provides for continuity of care and safety; establishes a baseline for future assessment; provides a data base for the development of a nursing care plan
2. Establish baseline parameters and note trends and abnormalities in the following: A. Vital signs B. Neurological signs • Level of consciousness including orientation and cognition, if possible • Pupillary size, shape, and reaction to light • Brain stem reflexes (corneal and gag reflexes) Note if oculocephalic or oculovestibular reflexes are present from chart • Motor function • Respiratory function • Glasgow Coma Scale, if used C. Body systems • Intracranial pressure reading • Swan–Ganz readings • Central venous pressure • Cardiac monitor • Continuous EEG monitoring • Others D. Laboratory data • Blood gases • Hemoglobin and hematocrit • Complete blood count and differential • Blood urea nitrogen, creatinine, glucose, calcium, and others as necessary • Serum and urine osmolarities E. Other parameters such as the following: • Tidal volumes • Oxygen concentration	• Provides a baseline against which subsequent assessments can be compared for changes and trends; identifies abnormalities in parameters that may need further assessment, referral, or intervention • Parameters should be recorded on flow sheets, if possible, to graphically identify changes and trends • Multiple parameters recorded on the same flow sheet aids in identifying interrelationships of parameters
3. Monitor for signs and symptoms of increased intracranial pressure • Decreased level of consciousness • Dilated, fixed, or sluggish pupils • Motor dysfunction (weakness, paralysis, abnormal posturing) • Changes in respiratory pattern • Changes in vital signs • Pressure waves on intracranial pressure monitor	
4. Control increased intracranial pressure.	
A. Elevate head of bed 30 degrees.	• Facilitates drainage from brain and decreases intracranial pressure
B. Hyperventilate.	• Decreases carbon dioxide and results in vasoconstriction and decreases intracranial pressure
C. Maintain head and neck in neutral position.	• Prevents obstruction of venous drainage from the brain, which would increase intracranial pressure
D. Prevent initiation of the Valsalva maneuver (straining at stool, coughing, performing isometric exercises, etc.).	• Valsalva maneuver increases intracranial pressure
• Establish a bowel program.	• Prevents constipation and straining at stool
E. Do not position on abdomen or in Trendelenburg position.	• These positions are known to increase intracranial pressure.
F. Do not cluster nursing activities known to increase intracranial pressure.	• Cumulative effect may cause dangerous spikes in intracranial pressure.
G. Maintain normothermia.	• Elevation of temperature increases metabolic rate and need for oxygen; waste products of cell metabolism (carbon dioxide, lactic acid) increase, causing an increase in intracranial pressure.

CHART 17–4. (continued)

NURSING RESPONSIBILITIES	RATIONALE
H. Maintain fluid restriction.	• Patient is kept slightly dehydrated to reduce cerebral edema and intracranial pressure.
I. Maintain continuous cerebrospinal fluid drainage, if a catheter has been inserted. • Maintain bag(s) at specified level. • Maintain strict aseptic technique. • Check tubing periodically for kinking.	• Decrease cerebrospinal fluid, which decreases intraventricular pressure and therefore decreases intracranial pressure.
J. Assist with barbiturate coma, if ordered (special nursing management is necessary; see Chap. 12).	• Causes generalized vasoconstriction (including cerebral vessels) and decreases intracranial pressure
K. Administer drugs as ordered to control intracranial pressure.	• Contributes to lowering of intracranial pressure
• Mannitol (osmotic diuretic)	• Decreases fluid volume
• Furosemide (loop diuretic)	• Decreases fluid volume
• Dexamethasone (anti-inflammatory agent)	• Stabilizes cerebral cell membrane to decrease cerebral edema
5. Monitor specific parameters with drug therapy.	• Assess for development of side-effects and alterations in other systems.
• Mannitol or furosemide—serum and urine osmolarities; electrolytes; intake and output records	• Monitor for dehydration and electrolyte imbalance.
• Dexamethasone—urine for sugar and acetone; stools for occult bleeding	• May cause glycosuria, irritation of gastrointestinal tract; may cause gastrointestinal bleeding.
• Maalox or other antacid—pH of gastric contents	• Decreases gastrointestinal irritation
6. Control seizures.	• Seizures increase metabolic rate and increase carbon dioxide production, leading to an increase in intracranial pressure
• Place on seizure precautions.	• Prevents injury if seizures occur
• Administer anticonvulsants (phenytoin [Dilantin] most frequent choice).	• Prophylaxis against seizures
• Monitor anticonvulsant drug blood levels for maintenance within therapeutic levels.	• Prevents seizure activity
• Observe for seizure activity.	• Assess for reasons seizures not controlled
7. Maintain a patent airway.	• An increase in carbon dioxide causes an increase in intracranial pressure
• Suction as necessary.	• Maintains patency of airway
• Avoid positions known to cause partial or complete airway obstruction.	• Prevents airway obstruction
• Position on side.	• Facilitates drainage from mouth
8. Maintain adequate oxygenation and ventilation.	• Inadequate oxygenation and ventilation cause an increase in carbon dioxide and a subsequent increase in intracranial pressure.
• Monitor blood gases periodically.	• Provides valid data on ventilation and development of respiratory abnormalities
• Do not suction for more than 15 seconds at a time.	• Increases carbon dioxide level, thus increasing intracranial pressure
• Hyperinflate with 100% oxygen before and after suctioning (if approved by the physician).	• Maintains adequate oxygen blood levels during suctioning
• Assess for development of pulmonary complications such as atelectasis, pneumonia, neurogenic pulmonary edema, adult respiratory distress syndrome, disseminated intravascular coagulopathy, pulmonary emboli, and fat emboli. • Monitor blood gases. • Assess other appropriate laboratory data such as differential blood count, coagulation studies.	• Early recognition promotes early, rapid, and effective management of respiratory complications
• Monitor cultures and sensitivity of sputum.	• Identifies presence of pathogens
• Monitor chest films.	• Identifies development of pulmonary problems
• Position properly.	• Facilitates respirations

(continued)

CHART 17–4. (continued)

NURSING RESPONSIBILITIES	RATIONALE
• Turn every 2 hours.	• Prevents pooling of secretions
• Ambu ventilator patient every 1 to 2 hours.	• Expands all areas of lungs
• Prevent aspiration (inflate cuff on tracheostomy tube, check placement of feeding tube before beginning a tube feeding, and so forth).	• Prevents development of aspiration pneumonias
9. Monitor for cardiac arrhythmias.	• Prevents life-threatening arrhythmias
• Assess apical rate and rhythm.	• Identifies abnormalities
• Assess blood pressure and pulse.	
• Assess continuous electrocardiographic (ECG) monitoring.	• Identifies abnormal cardiac patterns
• Report abnormalities.	• Definitive action can be taken before life-threatening arrhythmias result
• Assess for hypokalemia.	• Can cause arrhythmias
10. Control development of thrombophlebitis.	• Prevents development of thrombophlebitis and pulmonary emboli
• Apply elastic stockings or Ace bandages.	• Improves blood return to the heart
• Assess for signs and symptoms of thrombophlebitis.	• Identifies early signs and symptoms to allow early treatment
• Prevent pressure on back or knees.	• Causes circulatory impairment to legs
11. Monitor for gastrointestinal abnormalities (bleeding, paralytic ileus).	
• Check stools for occult blood.	• Indicates bleeding somewhere along gastrointestinal tract
• Monitor hemoglobin.	• A drop indicates internal bleeding
• Auscultate abdomen for peristalsis.	• Lack of peristalsis indicates paralytic ileus
• Assess abdomen for distention.	• Evidence of paralytic ileus
• Assess for other signs and symptoms of paralytic ileus.	
12. Monitor for fluid and electrolyte balance.	• Fluid and electrolyte imbalance can develop rapidly.
• Monitor electrolytes, serum and urine osmolarities, central venous pressure reading, intake and output record, urine specific gravity, and blood acetone.	• Diabetes insipidus can develop because of injury to the hypothalamus or adjacent structures.
• Assess for development of diabetes insipidus (DI), syndrome of inappropriate secretion of antidiuretic hormone (SIADH), hyperosmolar nonketotic hyperglycemia (HNH), and electrolyte imbalance.	• Syndrome of inappropriate secretion of antidiuretic hormone can develop due to administration of inappropriate type or amount of intravenous fluid or in association with the head injury.
• Monitor weight daily or periodically.	• Hyperosmolar nonketotic hyperglycemia can be caused by the stress response to injury in some patients.
• Monitor daily intake and output record.	
• Assess turgor of skin.	
13. Assess nutritional status.	• Catabolic states can rapidly develop from severe injury.
• Assess weight gain or loss since hospitalization.	• Unless the building blocks for tissue repair and anabolism are present, the patient will not recover.
• Assess calorie count on a daily basis.	
• Request nutritional consultation.	
14. Control infection.	• Infection must be rapidly identified and controlled.
• Monitor temperature, white blood count, differential count, wounds, drainage, urinalysis, and cultures for signs of infection.	
• Maintain strict aseptic technique.	
15. Control sequelae of immobility from developing.	• Prevents the major problems of immobility from developing
• Administer passive range-of-motion exercises.	
• Turn and reposition in proper body alignment every 2 hours.	
• Apply special boots to prevent footdrop.	

CHART 17–5. SUMMARY OF COMMON NURSING DIAGNOSES FOR THE PATIENT WITH AN ACUTE HEAD INJURY

NURSING DIAGNOSIS	EXPECTED OUTCOMES	NURSING INTERVENTIONS
Altered overall neurological function due to acute head injury	• Prevention of further deterioration in function • Identification of specific altered function in the neurological parameters	• Assess neurological signs to establish a baseline. • Assess neurological signs at frequent intervals to establish stability, deterioration or improvement in condition. • Note early recognition of deterioration and prompt initiation of intervention to reverse trend.
Potential of increased intracranial pressure and herniation due to increasing brain bulk	• Exacerbation of causative factors responsible for increased intracranial pressure will be controlled. • Cerebral edema will be controlled.	• Institute nursing measures to prevent elevation in intracranial pressure. • Elevate head of bed 30 degrees. • Maintain head and neck in neutral position. • Administer drugs as ordered. • Maintain normothermia. • Do not suction for more than 15 seconds at a time. • Hyperinflate the lungs with 100% oxygen before and after suctioning, if approved by physician. • Avoid positions known to increase intracranial pressure. • Prevent activities known to precipitate the Valsalva maneuver. • Maintain on prescribed fluid restriction.
	• PaCO will be maintained at 25 mm to 30 mm Hg as ordered.	• Hyperventilate as necessary.
	• "Pressure signs," if they occur, will be quickly identified and controlled.	• Assess for "pressure signs" and symptoms. • Hyperventilate the patient and try to identify the cause of "pressure signs." • Observe intracranial pressure monitor, if one is in place.
	• "Herniation signs," if they develop, will be quickly identified and corrective action taken.	• Monitor for "herniation signs"; report at once; try to identify cause; hyperventilate.
Potential of seizures due to head injury	• Seizures will be controlled.	• Administer anticonvulsant medication. • Monitor blood levels of anticonvulsant drug to ensure that it is maintained in therapeutic range. • Maintain on seizure precautions.
Potential of fluid and electrolyte imbalance due to iatrogenic fluid administration problems or head injury	• Fluid and electrolyte balance will be maintained.	• Assess for development of diabetes insipidus, syndrome of inappropriate secretion of antidiuretic hormone, hyperosmolar nonketotic hyperglycemia, and fluid and electrolyte imbalance.
	• If present, diabetes insipidus, syndrome of inappropriate secretion of antidiuretic hormone, or hyperosmolar nonketotic hyperglycemia will be identified and definitive action taken to control the condition.	• Monitor osmolarities, electrolytes, blood acetone, urine specific gravity, weight, and intake and output record; if a Swan–Ganz or central venous pressure catheter is in position, monitor parameters. • For diabetes insipidus—vasopressin (Aqueous Pitressin) will be administered and fluid replacement provided.

(continued)

CHART 17–5. (continued)

NURSING DIAGNOSIS	EXPECTED OUTCOMES	NURSING INTERVENTIONS
		• For syndrome of inappropriate secretion of antidiuretic hormone — fluid restriction and possibly diuretics will be administered • For hyperosmolar nonketotic hyperglycemia — fluid replacement and regular insulin will be administered. • For fluid and electrolyte imbalance — the imbalance will be corrected with replacement or other therapy.
Gas exchange impairment due to inadequate respirator function (associated with head trauma or development of respiratory condition)	• Blood gases will be maintained in normal range; PaCO may be maintained at 25 mm to 30 mm Hg to control intracranial pressure.	• Monitor blood gases. • Auscultate chest for breath sounds. • Monitor results of chest films. • Turn from side to side every 2 hours. • Provide chest physiotherapy periodically. • Expand lungs by hyperventilation and sigh mechanism on ventilator. • Monitor rate, depth, quality, and pattern of respirations. • Provide oxygen therapy as ordered. • Maintain a patent airway. • Suction as necessary. • Position to facilitate respiratory function.
Potential of infection due to decreased resistance, open wounds, and/or poor aseptic technique	• Sepsis will not develop, or if it does occur, it will be identified early.	• Monitor white blood count, differential count, and temperature. • Observe wounds for signs and symptoms of infection. • Monitor routine culture and sensitivity studies on urine, sputum, and wounds. • Maintain strict aseptic technique.
Potential of altered nutrition less than body requires due to injuries and the unconscious state	• Adequate nutrition will be maintained.	• Request a nutrition consultation as soon as feasible (24 to 48 hours). • Maintain a calorie count. • Weigh daily. • Assess for nutritional deficiencies and hydration.
Potential for physical injury due to decreased level of consciousness	• Patient's safety will be preserved.	• Maintain bed in low position when not giving direct care at the bedside. • Siderails on top and bottom of bed should be pulled up at all times. • Restrain the patient's hands if he is pulling at necessary equipment (an order from the physician will be necessary).
Potential of decubitus ulcers due to lack of mobility (unconscious state/head injury)	• Decubitus ulcers will not develop.	• Maintain clean and dry skin. • Maintain wrinkle-free, dry, and clean bed linen. • Assess skin at least every 8 hours for redness or irritation. • Keep off reddened areas. • Massage reddened areas periodically. • Keep heels off bed. • Turn every 2 hours.

CHART 17–5. (continued)

NURSING DIAGNOSIS	EXPECTED OUTCOMES	NURSING INTERVENTIONS
Potential of joint contractures due to unconscious state and head injury	• Contractures will not develop.	• Maintain proper body alignment; reposition frequently. • Provide for range-of-motion exercises at least four times a day. • Patients who are decerebrate or decorticate need repositioning more frequently. • Muscle relaxants may be ordered for the decorticate or decerebrate patient.
Total self-care deficit due to unconscious state and/or cognitive deficits	• Basic care will be provided for the patient.	• Administer basis hygienic care (complete bath daily; back, mouth, and perineal care every 4 hours).
Alterations in bowel elimination: constipation due to immobility and lack of regular diet	• Constipation will be prevented.	• Establish a bowel program using stool softeners and mild cathartics.
Alterations in urinary elimination pattern due to unconscious state	• An adequate urinary elimination pattern will be maintained.	• An indwelling catheter or a condom catheter will drain urine. • Maintain a 24-hour intake and output record.

(See Chap. 11, Care of the Unconscious Patient, for other nursing diagnoses.)

The nurse assigned to this unit must be able to manage a wide gamut of patients, from the critically ill patient who is relatively stable to one who needs assessment and assistance in relearning activities of daily living. The objectives of nursing management include the following:

- Frequent assessment of neurological signs
- Control of increased intracranial pressure
- Prevention, early recognition, and management of complications
- Rehabilitation
- Discharge planning

ADMISSION OF THE PATIENT TO THE UNIT

Admission of the patient to the unit begins with a transfer report from the discharging nurse to the admitting nurse. This is important for continuity of care and safety. The chart should be reviewed and clarification made as necessary.

NURSING PROCESS: NURSING DIAGNOSES AND THE NURSING CARE PLAN

As the first step in the nursing process, the nurse must assess the patient to establish a baseline of information. Necessary data may be collected from a variety of sources including the patient's chart, the nursing history, the nursing care plan (if one exists), the Kardex, and inspection of the patient. Clinical inspection of the patient is most helpful for collecting new information as well as for validating and providing a more thorough perspective of written and verbal data about the patient. Based on all of the information, nursing diagnoses are made and a nursing care plan developed or updated, if one was begun in the intensive care unit. Patients admitted directly from the emergency department rarely have nursing care plans because the focus of care there is rapid resuscitation and stabilization.

FREQUENT ASSESSMENT OF NEUROLOGICAL SIGNS

The neurological signs are assessed frequently and recorded. The assessment may be conducted every hour or at 4-hour intervals. A complete neurological assessment should be conducted initially to establish a baseline against which subsequent assessments can be compared to denote change. The method and areas included on the assessment depend on the condition of the patient and his level of responsiveness. The areas assessed include

- Level of consciousness (orientation, cognition or response to painful stimuli)
- Pupillary size, shape, and response to light
- Brain stem reflexes
- Cranial nerve function
- Motor function
- Sensory function
- Respiratory pattern

Level of Consciousness

Severe head-injury patients are most often in a deep coma. As the patient's condition improves and the coma lightens, he may become restless, confused, and combative and require further measures to protect him from injury. The patient may remain at this plateau for several weeks before his level of consciousness improves.

At the same time, the patient must be evaluated for other possible causes of restlessness, confusion, or combativeness. A patient may be restless as a result of hypoxia, a distended bladder, or pain, or he may display confusion as a result of elevated blood urea nitrogen from inadequate kidney function. A patient may be particularly combative if restraints are applied that allow little opportunity for free movement. Therefore, the nurse must be observant and consider all of the possibilities in evaluating alterations in consciousness.

- Observe the patient frequently to note any subtle changes in the level of consciousness; when necessary, pull up the siderails to protect the patient from injury.
- Consider causes other than neurological ones for alterations in level of consciousness (e.g., diabetic coma, kidney failure, drug abuse).
- Reorient the patient to time, place, and person in the recovery phase from coma. (Use the patient's name: "John, you are in Mercy Hospital in Providence, Rhode Island. It is Thursday morning, May 10, 1979.")
- Provide environmental stimuli for the patient to avoid sensory deprivation for the patient and to help to reorient the patient: turn on the radio, open the shades, place family pictures within the patient's visual field, talk to the patient about what you are doing and interesting things in his environment (room furnishings, weather, unit activity, anticipated activities such as lunch and visiting hours).

It is not enough to assess the patient's orientation to time, place, and person. Cognition should be assessed in the patient able to respond verbally by evaluating the patient's responses to questions and instructions through the use of language skills. A complete discussion of pupillary signs and their significance is included in Chapter 5.

Brain Stem Reflexes

In the unconscious patient the corneal, oculocephalic or oculovestibular, and gag reflexes are assessed. The frequency of the assessment varies based on the condition of the patient. In the conscious patient the corneal and gag reflexes are assessed to determine the need for special eye care and the ability to manage oral intake, respectively. Techniques for assessment are described in Chapter 5.

Cranial Nerve Function

In addition to the pupillary response to light, all other cranial nerves are checked as soon as possible. Conjugate gaze controlled by cranial nerves III, IV, and VI can be collectively checked using the doll's eye maneuver in the unconscious patient or by directing the conscious patient to follow the movement of one's finger through the six cardinal movements. Other cranial nerves, such as the olfactory nerve, cannot be evaluated in the patient; instead, evaluation is deferred until the patient's level of consciousness has improved.

Motor Function

If the patient is able to follow directions, the hand grasps are checked for strength and equality. Hemiplegia and hemiparesis are common motor deficits, which are also lateralizing. Often, decortication or decerebration posture is observed in patients who have suffered severe head injury and are in a coma. The patient is evaluated for motor response to stimuli. Responses may be classified as purposeful, nonpurposeful, or unresponsive. The Babinski sign may also be assessed.

Sensory Function

Sensation from tactile stimulation is evaluated in a patient who is able to indicate awareness to stimuli. Most often the sensory evaluation is deferred in patients with severe head injury until consciousness is regained.

Respirations

In addition to the neurological signs, the vital signs are taken, with special consideration given to the respiratory pattern. The type of respiratory pattern may be indicative of the area of injury. The pulse and blood pressure are important in providing evidence of compensation–decompensation to increased intracranial pressure. The temperature is also monitored to identify high or low readings that require management (see Chart 17–2).

CONTROL OF INCREASED INTRACRANIAL PRESSURE

As discussed in the section on intensive care management in this chapter, cerebral edema is the most common cause of increased intracranial pressure in the head-injured patient. The peak of swelling tends to occur 72 hours after injury. The most common causes of an increase in intracranial pressure in the patient who has been stabilized are rebleeding and hypoxia. If the patient is on an intracranial pressure monitor, the monitor should be observed for increases in pressure. The nurse should also watch for transient pressure signs that indicate ischemic episodes. Changes in neurological signs and changes in pressure seen on the monitor are reliable indicators of deteriorating condition.

The basic management protocols for increased intracranial pressure are discussed in this chapter with intensive care management. They are also discussed in detail in Chapter 11. The usual treatment consists of osmotic and/or loop diuretics, corticosteroids, fluid restriction, hyperventilation, and possibly cerebrospinal fluid drainage. Nursing responsibilities include

- Elevation of the head of the bed 30 degrees
- Prevention of the Valsalva maneuver (prevention of straining at stool, coughing, positioning in prone and Trendelenburg's positions, suctioning more than 15 seconds at a time, and so forth)
- Maintenance of the neck in a neutral position
- Maintenance of a patent airway
- Control of temperature; normothermia
- Adherence to the prescribed fluid restriction
- Planning care to prevent clustering of activities known to cause an increase in intracranial pressure

The nursing management to control increased intracranial pressure is presented in detail in Chapter 12. The nurse caring for the head-injured patient must continually assess for increases in intracranial pressure to protect the patient from the negative effects of this rise on the already-compromised brain.

PREVENTION, EARLY RECOGNITION, AND MANAGEMENT OF COMPLICATIONS

The nurse caring for the head-injured patient provides those basic needs that the patient cannot provide for himself. Nursing management is also directed at maintaining whatever functions are intact and preventing the development of complications. Many of the problems and complications that arise are related to immobility. Chapter 11, Care of the Unconscious Patient, outlines the nursing care associated with prevention of the complications of immobility. A few points will be discussed in this chapter.

Skin Care

The bedridden patient is very prone to skin breakdown because of abrasions and contusions that may have been sustained at the time of injury. In addition, increased perspiration caused by hyperthermia management also causes skin irritation. To guard against these problems, the skin must be inspected daily and kept meticulously clean and dry. In addition, the patient should be turned every 2 hours to relieve pressure and improve circulation. Any evidence of redness or skin breakdown should be aggressively managed to prevent pressure sores.

- Inspect every square inch of the skin at least once daily; areas subject to pressure and possible skin breakdown should be checked every 4 hours.
- Turn the patient every 2 hours, from side to side if unconscious, and if conscious, from side to back to side. This measure will prevent continuous pressure on any particular area of the body.
- Give skin care on a regular basis: wash and dry thoroughly and apply lotion to dry areas. Initiate immediate treatment to any reddened area (rub and apply lotion).

Orthopedic Deformities

Paresis, paralysis, and prolonged confinement to bed frequently predispose the head-injury patient to orthopedic deformities. To prevent these problems, a physiotherapy program should be followed based on an individual assessment of the patient by the physical therapy department. Nursing management is also vital and includes the following points of care as part of the nursing care plan:

- Provide range-of-motion exercises at least four times daily to maintain movement range of the extremities and prevent ankylosis and contractures.
- Reposition the patient every 2 hours in good body alignment to prevent musculoskeletal disabilities; a footboard is used to prevent footdrop.

Eye Problems

Loss of the corneal reflex and periorbital ecchymosis and edema are common problems associated with the eye. Temporary loss of the corneal reflex may be due to dysfunction of the ophthalmic branch of the trigeminal nerve. Special precautions must be taken to protect the eye from injury (corneal abrasions). It may be necessary to tape or suture the eyelids closed. An eye shield should be applied and the eye should be lubricated (normal saline irrigation). Periorbital ecchymosis and edema are managed by warm and cold compresses.

Visual loss or diplopia are also possibilities of head injury. Loss of vision in one or both eyes or hemianopsia can develop. The patient should be evaluated for visual loss as soon as is feasible. Diplopia is managed by applying an eye patch to the eye. This condition tends to disappear spontaneously.

Bladder Dysfunction

The patient may suffer from urinary incontinence or retention, although in all likelihood a Foley catheter will have been inserted. Bladder infections are common; therefore, frequent urinalysis should be monitored. The catheter should be removed as soon as possible and a bladder retraining program begun. The patient needs meticulous perineal care. The female patient should be watched for signs of vaginal yeast infection, which is common with prolonged antibiotic therapy. The drainage of the vaginal infection can be very irritating to the perineal area.

Bowel Dysfunction

Constipation and diarrhea are commonly encountered in the patient. Paralytic ileus can result from abdominal trauma. Bowel distention is avoided to prevent initiation of the Valsalva maneuver. Stool softeners are administered to prevent constipation. Enemas are usually contraindicated, although a Fleet or oil-retention enema may be given if the patient is impacted. Diarrhea can occur as a result of antibiotic therapy or initiation of tube feeding. The multiple trauma patient may not be able to tolerate or digest a particular tube feeding. If diarrhea occurs, the tube feeding should be discontinued. The physician may then prescribe another type of tube feeding or give a combination of fluids such as half water and half skim milk.

Infection

Any patient who has sustained serious trauma requiring long-term management is prone to various types of infections because of a decrease in body defenses and side-effects of drug therapy. The patient must be watched carefully with routine cultures made of urine, sputum, stools, and drainage to indicate the presences of pathogens.

The patient with a head injury is especially prone to meningitis, encephalitis, and abscesses caused by injury. In the patient with an open head injury, prophylactic antibiotics are usually given to prevent infection.

Other Complications

The possibility of complications from head injuries is great in the acute phase of injury. Nursing protocols are initiated as a means of preventing the development of complications. Some problems will develop, regardless of the excellence of management. However, early recognition of signs and symptoms allows rapid control of the problems to minimize disability. (See Charts 17-4 and 17-5.)

REHABILITATION

Rehabilitation is an integral part of nursing management in which the objectives of care are to maintain intact functions, restore lost or deficit body functions, and prevent new complications and disabilities. Throughout the various phases of hospitalization, priorities of care change to meet the most pressing needs of the patient. Although principles of rehabilitation are incorporated into the nursing care plan throughout hospitalization, the specific objectives of nursing care change. For example, in the acute stage of illness, the major goal of care is to stabilize the patient's condition, maintain a patent airway, and provide all of the necessary support systems to maintain life. At this time common rehabilitative activities initiated by the nurse include frequent repositioning, skin care, and range-of-motion exercises. The nursing actions are directed toward preventing skin breakdown as well as musculoskeletal deformities.

During the postacute phase, objectives of nursing care may be directed toward helping the patient to relearn activities of daily living. The focus of management becomes an aggressive rehabilitation program to assist the patient in becoming as independent as possible.

Based on an individual assessment of the patient, the expertise of several health-team specialists may be used to address the particular deficits. The nurse, as the health care provider who spends the most time with the patient, has the responsibility of following through on protocols established for the patient. In this sense, the nurse is the pivotal center for coordinating care. In addition, the nurse initiates referrals if special patient needs become evident in the process.

Since the needs of each patient vary, an individual assessment is an absolute necessity for planning care. Patients respond differently to management and treatment; therefore, ongoing assessment and evaluation of care are needed.

The rehabilitative needs of the head-injury patient are similar to those of other neurologically impaired patients, regardless of specific etiology. Common problems addressed in the rehabilitation of the head-injury patient include

- Motor weakness or paralysis
- Sensory loss or alterations
- Feeding problems
- Visual deficits
- Deficits in communications
- Cognitive impairment
- Personality changes
- Bowel and bladder dysfunction

See Chapter 8 for specific nursing management and rehabilitation of the patient. Cognitive assessment is included in Chapter 4.

Bladder Retraining After Cerebral Injury

With serious cerebral injury, the patient may require bladder retraining. The patient with cerebral injury from trauma, stroke, brain tumor, or other conditions is usually classified as having a mixed neurogenic bladder or incomplete upper motor neuron bladder. This means that the patient has both a diminished perception of bladder fullness and a diminished ability to empty his bladder. Because sensation and control are diminished rather than lost, bladder training is more easily achieved. Patients with a mixed neurogenic bladder often have a feeling of urgency to void and are unable to control this urge until they are in the bathroom or have been given a bedpan or urinal.

Upon admission, an indwelling catheter is usually inserted to manage urinary drainage. As soon as possible, the catheter should be removed and a bladder training program initiated. The chances of retraining the patient are very good. The procedure followed is the same as that outlined for the training of an upper motor neuron bladder.

Bowel Retraining After Cerebral Injury

In the patient with cerebral injury such as severe trauma or stroke, coma and prolonged bedrest contribute to bowel dysfunction. Constipation is the most common dysfunction of the gastrointestinal tract. Diarrhea is commonly associated with intolerance to particular tube feedings or the use of drugs affecting the flora of the gastrointestinal tract. The lack of physical activity, inadequate diet, and frequent limitation of fluids in the patient with cerebral trauma are the major factors contributing to constipation and fecal impaction.

In the patient with cerebral injury there is usually cerebral edema and increased intracranial pressure. Constipation and bowel distention lead to the initiation of the Valsalva maneuver, which is known to increase intracranial pressure; therefore, it is a goal of nursing care to prevent constipation and distention. Stool softeners, mild cathartics, suppositories, and enemas are used to aid in the evacuation of the bowel. In managing the patient in a coma it is necessary to administer a stool softener three times daily by way of a feeding tube. Failure to establish a pattern of bowel evacuation with this program will require the use of a mild cathartic at bedtime. If this is unsuccessful, a medicated, commercially prepared enema may be used. These enemas usually contain approximately 100 ml to 150 ml of fluid so that the bowel is not overly distended. If a soapsuds enema is ordered, the amount of fluid will be limited to approximately 500 ml. Limitation of fluid is necessary to control the initiation of the Valsalva maneuver. An enema may be necessary to evacuate the lower bowel if the stool is hard or impacted before suppositories are given.

Once the patient regains consciousness and is able to eat, a diet high in roughage that includes prune juice should be encouraged to establish a normal evacuation pattern. It is helpful to learn what the normal pattern for the patient prior to injury was because the diversity for "normal" can cover a wide range from individual to individual. Some people evacuate the bowel every day, while for others every 2 to 3 days is normal. Most people tend to have the urge to evacuate the bowel after a meal, particularly breakfast.

The following outlines a bowel evacuation protocol to be followed for the patient with cerebral injury:

- Encourage a diet high in roughage (whole-grain bread and cereal, fresh fruits, and vegetables); in addition, offer prune juice.
- Unless contraindicated by a fluid restriction, increase fluid intake to 2000 ml to 3000 ml/day.
- Administer a stool-softening drug as prescribed by the physician.
- Make sure the lower bowel is clean; an enema may be necessary to begin the training program.
- Establish a time of day for a bowel movement based on the patient's previous pattern; adhere to this designated time of the day rigidly.
- Insert a glycerine suppository on the first day—if it does not work, wait until the next day.
- On the following day, repeat the insertion of the glycerine suppository; if it is effective, continue with the protocol on a daily basis.
- If 2 days have passed with no response to the glycerine suppository, it will be necessary to ask the physician to prescribe a bisacodyl (Dulcolax) suppository.
- Insert the Dulcolax suppository, if this is not effective, an enema will be needed (a mild cathartic should be given as necessary).
- If at all possible the patient should be seated on the commode or taken into the bathroom for defecation.

Hospitals and physicians may have slight variations in the above protocol, but the basic components are found in most bowel-training programs. The nurse should carefully document the steps of the protocol implemented and the results. Once a normal pattern has been established the plan of care should be followed to ensure maintenance of the bowel program.

DISCHARGE PLANNING

Discharge planning begins the moment that a patient is admitted and ends with a discharge from the acute-care setting to the patient's home or appropriate facility if care is still necessary. The process between the entry and exit from the system will depend on the specific needs of the patient and the ability of the professional staff to plan for these needs. As the patient passes through the various stages of hospitalization, it becomes possible to realistically assess his needs and predict outcomes. Some patients, because of multiple serious injuries, have many complex needs that extend beyond the scope of an acute-care setting. Such needs include cognitive retraining, physical therapy, vocational counselling, and speech therapy. Some patients who remain in a chronic vegetative state will need skilled nursing care for the rest of their lives. Other patients will have good rehabilitative potential that can only be realized in an aggressive rehabilitation program. In discharge planning the combined effort of the health team members is directed at matching the patient's needs with community and private resources to achieve the greatest degree of independence possible for the patient.

The nurse is often the person who initiates the active planning process and coordinates the various people and activities involved in the process. Since the nurse is the person who spends the most time with the patient and his family she is in a position to assess both the patient and the family to determine their needs. Head injury is often a catastrophic event for the patient and the family. Learning to cope with the deficits and changes in family structure are major adjustments for all involved. The patient and family need to be educated about their problems and also directed to community resources that offer services and support to them. The process of discharge planning is discussed in some detail in Chapter 9.

One organization that patients and families with head-injured patients should be familiar with is the National Head Injury Foundation (NHIF). The NHIF is concerned with all aspects of head injury from prevention to late rehabilitation. Some of the major objectives of the organization are

- Stimulate public and professional awareness of the problem of head injury
- Provide a central clearinghouse for information and resources for the head-injured and their families
- Develop a support group network for the head-injured and their families
- Establish specialized head-injury rehabilitation programs

The NHIF has chapters throughout the country. Many patients and families have been able to benefit from the "networking" and other services offered by this foundation.

There are other organizations and resources that can be very helpful to the patient and family. The specific resource to which a referral is made depends on the needs of the patient and family and their willingness to participate in the services offered.

POSTACUTE PHASE OF HEAD INJURY

As the patient's level of consciousness improves and plans are made for transfer to an extended care facility or home care, various problems may become apparent, including communication deficits and emotional and cognitive deficits such as emotional lability, memory loss, and decreased mentation.

The communication deficits of dysphasia or aphasia require that alternate methods of communication be developed. A speech therapist may be needed to help the patient or to consult with the nurse to determine appropriate management of the patient.

Emotional deficits are difficult for the patient and family to tolerate. Such deficits influence the patient's ability to learn and make decisions. Maladaptive behavior also has a negative effect on interpersonal relationships and family dynamics. Cognitive deficits such as memory may elicit responses of frustration and alarm as the patient becomes aware of these problems. Assuming a gentle, positive attitude and correcting errors matter-of-factly can be helpful. The patient must be given reassurance that, given time, there will be improvement in these areas.

Other objectives of care in the postacute period are helping the patient relearn any altered activities of daily living such as feeding and eating, walking, and attending to personal grooming. It is often easier and faster for the nurse or family member to do things for the patient, but this approach only deprives the patient of the opportunity to achieve his highest level of independence. Therefore, the patient needs to be encouraged to be as independent as possible by carrying out those self-care activities that are within his range of ability (see Chap. 8).

PREDICTING OUTCOMES FROM HEAD INJURY

There are various definitions of outcome based on criteria such as survival, degree of disability, and return to work. One scale widely accepted and used is the Glasgow Outcome Scale.[15] It has demonstrated reliability in predicting recovery and disability rather than survival in all types of brain injury. The scale developed by Jennett and Bond is used at prescribed time intervals such as 3 months, 6 months, and 1 year (see Chart 17-6 for the Glasgow Outcome Scale). The Glasgow group reported the greatest recovery in the 6-month period after injury. After that period, recovery was rarely sufficient to move the patient to a higher category.

CHART 17-6. GLASGOW OUTCOME SCALE

- *Good outcome*—may have minimal disabling sequelae but returns to independent functioning and a full-time job comparable to preinjury level
- *Moderate disability*—capable of independent functioning but not returned to full-time employment
- *Severe disability*—dependent on others for some aspect of daily living
- *Persistent vegetative state*—no obvious cortical functioning
- *Dead*

(Jennett B, Bond M: Assessment of outcome after severe brain damage: A practical scale. J Neurosurg 4:673, 1975)

In another study, Rimel and co-workers divided head-injured patients into three groups based on the Glasgow Coma Scale (GCS).[5,16] The criteria established were as follows:

- Severe head injury — GCS 3 to 8
- Moderate head injury — GCS 9 to 12
- Minor head injury — GCS 13 to 15

The patients were evaluated 3 months after injury. Their findings were consistent with those of other researchers.

Severe Head Injury

The severely injured patient with head trauma has been studied extensively. This population has post-trauma syndromes and cognitive, emotional, motor, and sensory deficits caused by irreversible brain damage. Their outcome is very poor.

Moderate Head Injury

In the population with moderate head injury there was incidence of mortality and also incidence of focal lesions (most often hematomas) that had to be surgically evacuated. Almost all of the patients complained of persistent headache, memory difficulty, and problems with daily living. Almost 70% of patients who were gainfully employed before injury were not employed 3 months after injury.[16]

Minor Head Injury

In the study, 79% of patients with minor head injury complained of persistent headache and 59% complained of problems with memory.[5] On neuropsychological testing, problems with attention, concentration, memory, and judgment were uncovered. These symptoms were stressful to the patient, and the stress contributed to long-term disability. Another finding related to employment. Of the patients who were gainfully employed before injury, a third were unemployed 3 months later. The findings suggest that the so-called minor head injury is not minor or insignificant at all. The patient appears to have sustained organic brain damage and should be managed more cautiously than has been the practice in the past. It is important for the nurse to understand the implications of minor head injuries so that she can help the patient understand the need to resume activities gradually and to control stress.

Other Predictive Studies

Other predictive studies have dealt with survival, length of post-traumatic amnesia,[17] brain stem reflexes, and others. Bilateral fixed pupils, loss of the oculocephalic or oculovestibular response, and a low score on motor function have been said to indicate a poor prognosis. The other factor that is always cited as critical in outcome is age. Generally speaking, the patient who is 20 years old or older will have a poorer outcome than a younger patient. The prognosis steadily decreases as the age of the patient increases.

Predicting outcome after head injury is still controversial although the Glasgow Outcome Scale is gaining acceptance for the prediction of disability.

SEQUELAE AFTER SEVERE HEAD INJURY

With the passage of time, many of the focal signs and symptoms resulting from craniocerebral trauma gradually abate. A hemiplegia may convert to a mild hemiparesis, aphasis may improve to hesitant speech, and even brain stem dysfunction can improve greatly. Other possible sequelae are discussed below.

POST-TRAUMATIC EPILEPSY

Post-traumatic epilepsy is the most common sequela of craniocerebral trauma; it is seen in about 5% of patients with closed head injuries such as contusion and laceration and in 50% of those with compound depressed skull fractures. The interval between trauma and the development of post-traumatic epilepsy varies greatly. Fifty percent of patients who will develop this sequela show signs of seizure within 1 to 6 months after injury. By the end of 2 years, 80% have experienced the first seizure.

Focal or grand mal seizures are most common. Most seizures are amenable to anticonvulsant drugs, with very few patients requiring excision of the seizure focus if drug therapy proves ineffective. The seizures tend to decrease in frequency with the passage of years. It is estimated that 10% to 30% of patients eventually cease to have seizures.

POST-TRAUMATIC STRESS SYNDROME OR POSTCONCUSSIONAL SYNDROME

The signs and symptoms of post-traumatic stress syndrome include headache, dizziness (giddiness or light-headedness), intolerance of noise, emotional excitement in crowds, tenseness or nervousness, restlessness and apprehension, fatigue, inability to concentrate, and intolerance of usual amounts of alcohol. Headache, either localized or generalized, is the major symptom noted and may be described as pounding, piercing, or aching. The headache is intensified by mental stress and physical exertion. Once this fairly common syndrome is well established, it may persist for months; however, it usually wanes as time passes.

POST-TRAUMATIC HYDROCEPHALUS

The hydrocephalus that occurs is most often the communicating or normal-pressure hydrocephalus (see Chap. 12 for signs and symptoms). A surgical shunting procedure can reverse the symptoms dramatically.

PSYCHIATRIC DISORDERS

Common symptoms of post-traumatic psychiatric disorders include memory disorder, defects of perception and judgment, increased distractibility, perseverance, difficulty in readjusting to work and family life, inability to cope with stress, insomnia, impaired intellectual functions, and manifestations of abnormally abrupt, argumentative, stubborn, and suspicious behavior. As with other post-traumatic sequelae, symptoms gradually subside with time.

PSYCHOSOCIAL ASPECTS OF HEAD INJURY

The impact of head injury on the patient and his family depends on several factors such as (1) the severity of the injury, (2) psychological characteristics of the patient, (3) roles and responsibilities, and (4) family relationships.

SEVERITY OF THE INJURY

An accurate assessment of the injury with reference to temporary and permanent disability will give the patient and family a good idea of what to expect in terms of disabilities and adjustments in lifestyle. If a choice is being made between extended care facilities and home management, consideration must be given to patient needs and available resources. Each patient is evaluated individually by the health team professionals to determine what his needs are and how they can best be met.

PSYCHOLOGICAL CHARACTERISTICS OF THE PATIENT

The patient's age, sex, personality, former adjustment patterns, self-concept, and reaction to illness must be considered. Many studies have been conducted to identify critical factors in positive adjustment to disability. No single factor is predictive of success; therefore, each patient must be evaluated separately. However, the patient who has had successful adjustment patterns in the past is most apt to cope well with disability and a rehabilitation program.

ROLES AND RESPONSIBILITIES

The patient's ability to return to his job or occupation depends on the skills required to do the job, the presence of any residual disability, the attitude of the patient toward work, and the existence of any environmental constraints to mobility. For some patients only minor adjustments are required; for others, the disabilities sustained from the injury make it impossible to return to the same job. Retraining for another career will be necessary. For still others, the disabilities are so severe that gainful employment is not possible.

All roles do not relate to gainful employment. The multiple responsibilities and skills of the homemaker as cook, laundress, child caretaker, and housekeeper are roles that contribute to family well-being, although not necessarily on a payment-for-service basis. Strains can be put on family life if the usual roles assumed by one family member cannot be met or assumed by another.

The occupational therapist can be of great value in helping the injured patient use alternate ways of accomplishing tasks. This may require a change in the usual procedure followed by the patient or special devices so that the task can be accomplished despite certain disabilities.

FAMILY RELATIONSHIPS

Each family must be evaluated separately to determine the degree of participation in the rehabilitative process. If the patient has a spouse, the spouse should be interviewed separately. The prospect of resuming life with a neurologically disabled husband or wife must be considered in terms of the adjustments required.

Role changes in family responsibilities, physical changes to the environment, and psychological alterations occur. The family members may need help to deal with feelings of anger, hostility, and overwhelming responsibilities as the patient recovers. It is not uncommon for a family member to wish that the patient had died of his injuries rather than survive with so many disabilities. The family member usually feels guilty about having such feelings. The family may also go through a feeling of loss, grief, and bereavement.

Each family must be evaluated separately in response to having a family member who has sustained a head injury. Referrals to a mental health helper or agency may be necessary to help them deal with catastrophic injury.

REFERENCES

1. Rimel R: Guest editorial: Head injury: A challenging future for neurosurgical nursing. J Neurosurg Nurs 14(5):207, October 1982
2. Gurdjian E: Impact Head Injury: Mechanistic, Clinical, and Preventive Correlations. Springfield, IL, Charles C Thomas, 1975
3. Bruce D, Gennarelli T, Langfitt T: Resuscitation from coma due to head injury. Crit Care Med 6(4):254, July/August 1978
4. Roberts J: Pathophysiology, diagnosis and treatment of head trauma. Top Emerg Med 1(1):41, May 1979
5. Rimel R et al: Disability caused by minor head injury. Neurosurgery 9(3):221, September 1981
6. Boyle R, Ames W: Too many punches, too little concern. Sports Illustrated 58(15):44, April 11, 1983
7. Gennarelli T et al: Diffuse axonal injury and traumatic coma in the primate. Ann Neurol 12:564, December 1982
8. Ommaya A et al: Coup and contrecoup injury: Observations on the mechanics of visible brain injuries in the rhesus monkey. J Neurosurg 35:503, 1971
9. Gurdjian E et al: Mechanism of head injury. Clin Neurosurg 12:112, 1966
10. Vinken P, Bruyn G (eds): Handbook of Clinical Neurology, Vols 23 and 24, Injuries of the Brain and Skull, Parts I and II. New York, American Elsevier, 1975
11. Purvis J: Craniocerebral Injuries due to Missile and Fragments. In Caveness W, Walker A (eds): Head Injury, pp 133–141. Philadelphia, JB Lippincott, 1966
12. Bowers S, Marshall L: Severe head injury: Current treatment and research. J Neurosurg Nurs 14(5):210, October 1982
13. Epstein F, Hamilton G: Initial approach to the brain-injured patient. Crit Care 5(4):13, March 1983
14. Rossi NP, Graf CJ: Physiological and pathological effects of neurologic disturbances and increased intracranial pressure on the lung: A review. Surg Neurol 5:366, 1976
15. Jennett B, Bond M: Assessment of outcome after severe brain damage: A practical scale. J Neurosurg 4:673, 1975
16. Rimel R et al: Moderate head injury: Completing the clinical spectrum of brain trauma. Neurosurgery 11:344, 1982
17. Lishman WA: Psychiatric sequelae of head injuries: Problems in diagnosis. J Irish Med Assoc 71(9):306, June 30, 1978

BIBLIOGRAPHY

Books

Bakay L, Glassaurer R: Head Injuries. Boston, Little, Brown & Co, 1979

Earnest MP (ed): Neurologic Emergencies. New York, Churchill Livingstone, 1983

Ewing CL et al (eds): Impact Injury of the Head and Spine. Springfield, IL, Charles C Thomas, 1983

Jennett B, Teasdale G: Management of Head Injuries. Philadelphia, FA Davis, 1981

Lindenberg R: Trauma of Meninges and Brain. In Minckler J (ed): Pathology of the Nervous System, Vol 2, pp 1705–1765. New York, McGraw–Hill, 1971

Meirowsky A: Penetrating Craniocerebral Trauma. In Caveness W, Walker A (eds): Head Injury, pp 195–202. Philadelphia, JB Lippincott, 1968

Plum F, Posner J: The Diagnosis of Stupor and Coma, 3rd ed. Philadelphia, FA Davis, 1980

Popp AJ et al (eds): Neural Trauma. New York, Raven Press, 1979

Ropper A, Kennedy S, Zervas N: Neurological and Neurosurgical Intensive Care. Baltimore, University Park Press, 1983

Rosenthal M et al (eds): Rehabilitation of the Head Injured Adult. Philadelphia, FA Davis, 1983

Taylor J, Ballenger S: Neurological Dysfunctions and Nursing Intervention. New York, McGraw–Hill, 1980

Van Meter M (ed): Neurologic Care: Guide for Patient Education. New York, Appleton–Century–Crofts, 1982

Periodicals

Adelstein W: Chronic subdurals. J Neurosurg Nurs 12(1):36, March 1980

Adelstein W: Brain stem injuries. J Neurosurg Nurs 10(3):112, September 1978

Applebury C: Transient loss of consciousness: Assessment and outcome in the emergency room. J Neurosurg Nurs 15(6):321, December 1983

Bracke M, Taylor A, Kinney A: External drainage of cerebrospinal fluid. Am J Nurs 78(8):1355, August 1978

Clum–Mauss N: Bringing the unconscious patient back safely: Nursing makes the critical difference. Nurs82 12(8):34, August 1982

Coleman L, Maudin R: Intracerebral herniation. J Neurosurg Nurs 15(5):287, October 1983

Connolly R, Zewe G: Update: Head injuries. J Neurosurg Nurs 13(4):1981, August 1981

Crockard HA: Early intracranial pressure studies in gunshot wounds of the brain. J Trauma 15:339, 1975

Dagi TF: Penetrating missile injuries of the brain. Crit Care Q 6(1):67, June 1983

DeBard M: Predictors in brain resuscitation. Crit Care Q 5(4):91, March 1983

DeLaurentis D: Resuscitation in the injured patient: Do's and Don'ts. Hosp Med 82, June 1978

Eilers M: Pharmacologic therapeutic modalities: Osmotic and diuretic agents. Crit Care Q 5(4):44, March 1983

Ensin J: Nutritional assessment of a severely head injured, multi-trauma patient. J Neurosurg Nurs 14(5):262, October 1982

Fernandez R et al: Blunt trauma to the neck. Nurs Clin North Am 13(2):191, June 1978

Fleischer A, Barrow D: Axioms on head injury. Hosp Med 66, March 1982

Foster–McGuffin JF: Basic cerebral trauma care. J Neurosurg Nurs 15(4):189, August 1983

Franco LM: Cerebral contusion: A prototype for head injury. J Neurosurg Nurs 16(1):45, February 1984

Franklin DF, Bargsley L: Comprehensive patient monitoring in a neurosurgical intensive care unit. J Neurosurg Nurs 15(4):205, August 1983

Frye B: Brain injury and family education needs. Rehabil Nurs 7(4):27–28, July/August 1982

Gennarelli TA et al: Influence of the type of intracranial lesion on outcome from severe head injury: A multicenter study using a new classification system. J Neurosurg 56:26–32, 1982

Gilmor R: Computerized axial tomography in head trauma. Crit Care Q 2(1):61, June 1979

Gilroy A, Cladwell E: Initial assessment of the multiple injured patient. Nurs Clin North Am 13(2):177, June 1978

Haerer A: Coma: Some differential considerations in the diagnosis and management. Hosp Med 68, April 1976

Haley WE: Behavior management of the brain-damaged patient: A case study. Rehabil Nurs 8(3):26–28, May/June 1983

Hausman K: Head injuries in children. J Neurosurg Nurs 9(3):95, September 1977

Hendler BH: The sites and signs of maxillofacial trauma. Emerg Med 16(6):22, March 30, 1984

Hernesniemi J: Outcome following head injuries in the aged. Acta Neurochir 46:67, 1979

Hinterbuchner L: Elevation of the unconscious patient. Hosp Med 83, February 1977

Hoffman J, Orban D, Podolsky S: Pharmacologic therapeutic modalities. Crit Care Q 5(4):52, March 1983

Hollis J, Kenyan–Rainer J: Evaluation of the comatose patient. J Neurosurg Nurs 15(5):238, October 1983

Hubschmann O et al: Craniocerebral gunshot injuries in civilian practice: Prognostic criteria and surgical management: Experience with 82 cases. J Trauma 19:6, 1979

Jackson F: The pathophysiology of head injuries. Clin Symp 28(3), 1966

Jagger J, Bobovsky J: Nonpharmacologic therapeutic modalities. Crit Care Q 5(4):31, March 1983

Jones C: Monitoring recovery after head injury: Translating research into practice. J Neurosurg Nurs 11(4):192, December 1979

Jordan R: Pathophysiology of brain injury. Crit Care Q 5(4):1, March 1983

Kirkpatrick JB, DiMaio VD: Civilian gunshot wounds of the brain. J Neurosurg 49:185, 1978

Levy D et al: Prognosis in nontraumatic coma. Ann Intern Med 94(3):293, March 1981

Lockwood B: Transport of multisystem trauma patients from rural to urban health care facilities. Crit Care Q 5(3):22, December 1982

Marcotty SF, Levin AB: A new approach in epidural intracranial pressure monitoring. J Neurosurg Nurs 16(1):54, February 1984

Martin M: Pharmacologic therapeutic modalities: Phenytoin, dimethyl sulfoxide, and calcium channel blockers. Crit Care Q 5(4):72, March 1983

Mastrian K: Of course you can manage head trauma patients. RN 45, August 1981

Meyd C: Acute brain trauma. Am J Nurs 78(1):40, January 1978

Minderhoud JM et al: The pattern of recovery after severe head injury. Clin Neurol Neurosurg 84:15–28, 1982

Nelson C, Miner M: Brain injury disseminated intravascular coagulation and fibrinolysis syndrome in children. J Neurosurg Nurs 15(2):72, April 1983

Parkinson J: The ballistics of craniocerebral gunshot wounds. J Neurosurg Nurs 14(5):232, October 1982

Parson LC, Wilson MM: Cerebrovascular status of severe closed head injured patients following passive position changes. Nurs Res 33(2):68, March/April 1984

Perdue P: Life-threatening head and spinal injuries. RN 36, June 1981

Phillips K: Osteomyelitis of the skull. J Neurosurg Nurs 15(1):56, April 1983

Podgorny G, Stanley L: Gunshot victims. RN 47, April 1982

Ranschoff J, Koslow M: Guide to the diagnosis and management of cerebral injury. Hosp Med 127, May 1978

Rimel R: A prospective study of patients with central nervous system trauma. J Neurosurg Nurs 13(3):132, June 1981

Rimel R, Tyson G: The neurological examination in patients with central nervous system trauma. J Neurosurg Nurs 11(3):148, September 1979

Rimel R, Jane J, Edlich R: Assessment of recovery following head trauma. Crit Care Q 2(1):97, June 1979

Rimel R, Jane J, Edlich R: Care of CNS trauma at the site of injury. Crit Care Q 2(1):1, June 1979

Rimel R: Emergency management of the patient with central nervous system trauma. J Neurosurg Nurs 10(4):185, December 1978

Rudy E: Early omens of cerebral disaster. Nurs77, 7:59, February 1977

Samuels M: Meeting neurologic emergencies in primary care. Patient Care 14, May 15, 1981

Saul T: Intensive care of the brain-injured patient. Crit Care Q 5(4):82, March 1983

Seeling JM et al: Traumatic acute subdural hematoma: Major mortality reduction in comatose patients treated within four hours. N Engl J Med 304:1511–1518, 1981

Shpritz DW: Craniocerebral Trauma. Crit Care Nurs 3(2):49, March/April 1983

Snyder M: Cerebral trauma in the chronic alcoholic. J Neurosurg Nurs 10(3):121, September 1978

Stevens M: Postconcussion syndrome. J Neurosurg Nurs 14(5):239, October 1982

Stewart C: Nursing management of gunshot wounds to the head. J Neurosurg Nurs 15(5):277, October 1983

Tyson G et al: Acute care of the head-injured patient. Crit Care Q 2(1):23, June 1979

Voris H: Craniocerebral trauma. Clin Neurol 3:1–45, 1980

Walton J (ed): The treatment of head injuries. Ciba Found Symp 19(1): entire issue, 1967

Ward J: Emergency treatment of major head injury. Hosp Med 58, March 1980

Warren JB: Pulmonary complications associated with severe head injury. J Neurosurg Nurs 15(4):194, August 1983

Warren JB, Goethe KE, Peck EA: Neuropsychological abnormalities associated with severe head injury. J Neurosurg Nurs 16(1):30, February 1984

Williams A: Perceptions of nursing care: Effects of written and verbal instructional methods on families of head injury patients. Heart Lung 7(2):306, March–April 1978

Young JA: Head injuries. Advances in care during the past decade, part 1. Nurs Times 77:766, April 30, 1981

Zettas J et al: Injury patterns in motorcycle accidents. J Trauma 19:833, 1979

chapter 18

Vertebral and Spinal Cord Trauma

A PERSPECTIVE

STATISTICS

The National Institute of Neurological and Communicative Disorders and Stroke (NINCDS) commissioned a study by the National Head and Spinal Cord Injury Survey, which presented its findings in 1980. According to the estimates of the report, there are 200,000 paraplegics in the United States. Approximately 10,000 persons incur permanent spinal cord injuries each year; about half of these become paraplegics and about half become quadriplegics. The incidence of spinal cord injury is 5 per 100,000. By 1980, the estimated cost of caring for one victim for 1 year had exceeded a quarter of a million dollars. The estimated total cost of these injuries to society exceeds $2 billion a year.[1]

The victims of spinal cord injury are the young, as evidenced by the fact that 62% of victims are between the ages of 15 and 30 years. Although the NINCDS findings did not concur, most people believe that there is a higher incidence of spinal cord injuries in males than in females.[2] The causes of spinal cord injury are vehicular accidents, falls, sports-related injuries (e.g., football, lacrosse, diving, skiing), and gunshot or missile injuries.

Advances in medical practice now make it possible for a 15-year-old patient suffering from a serious spinal cord injury to achieve an almost-normal life expectancy. However, he is still expected to develop several injury-related health problems throughout his life that will place a substantial financial burden upon himself or his health insurance underwriters. These ongoing health problems are not only expensive but also detract from the quality of life of the patient. Although the number of patients with spinal cord injury is small in comparison with those suffering from other health problems, the impact on the person's life and the medical expenses incurred are catastrophic.

VERTEBRAL AND SPINAL CORD TRAUMA—WHAT DOES IT MEAN?

In order to appreciate the injuries that can be incurred by the spinal axis and its surrounding structures as a result of trauma, a few points should be made about the relationship of anatomical structures. The anatomical structures among the vertebral column, the spinal cord, the supporting soft tissue, and the intervertebral discs are all interrelated. The vertebrae are the irregularly shaped bones that provide support for the muscles and protection for the spinal cord. There are 33 vertebrae in the vertebral column: 7 cervical, 12 thoracic or dorsal, 5 lumbar, 5 sacral (fused into one), and 4 coccygeal (fused into one). The vertebrae of each area have a rather distinct shape. Stacked one on another to form the vertebral column, the vertebrae are laced into position by a series of supporting structures called ligaments. The ligaments, muscles, and other supporting structures are often called soft tissue.

There are two main parts to a vertebra: the body and the arch. The vertebral bodies are separated by intervertebral discs that serve as shock absorbers for the vertebral column during movement. The arch of the vertebra is created by a series of irregularly shaped projections, that is, the fusion of two pedicles and two laminae along with seven articular processes that create a bony ring. The various projections of the vertebral arch allow for alignment, flexion, and movement of the vertebral column. The soft, vulnerable spinal cord passes through the bony arch of the vertebrae, which offers it protection.

The close anatomical relationship of the vertebrae, ligaments and other soft-tissue structures, intervertebral discs, and spinal cord increases the probability that injury to any one of these structures can cause concurrent injury to any one or all of the other structures. In other instances, injury to one structure, such as a vertebral fracture, can create the potential of injury to another structure, such as the spinal cord, if the primary injury is not treated promptly and effectively. Therefore, in discussing injury to the vertebral column and spinal cord, one must consider the interrelatedness of not only these two structures but also the supporting soft tissue and the intervertebral discs.

Vertebral, spinal cord, and soft-tissue injuries will be discussed in this chapter. Intervertebral disc disease is the focus of Chapter 19.

INJURIES — HOW THEY OCCUR AND HOW THEY ARE CLASSIFIED

To understand the effects of the various mechanisms and forces on the neck, the structural components involved should be reviewed. At the top of the vertebral column is the head, weighing from 8 to 10 pounds and sitting upon seven stacked cervical vertebrae. These vertebrae provide substantial movement of the neck in various directions. The total normal range of flexion and extension possible at the cervical spine is equivalent to an 80-degree arc, 75% of which is extension. Beneath the cervical vertebrae is the thoracic spine, which has little movement due to the restricting ribs. The thoracic region can be considered a fixed point. Because of the interplay of these factors, the neck is extremely vulnerable to injury.

MECHANISMS AND FORCES CAUSING INJURY TO THE SOFT TISSUE, VERTEBRAL COLUMN, AND SPINAL CORD

Mechanisms

A *mechanism* is a process or a technique for achieving a result. The result achieved in this case is injury to the spinal axis and/or associated structures. The four major mechanisms that cause injury are acceleration–deceleration, deformation, axial (vertical) loading, and penetration wounds.[2]

Acceleration–Deceleration. Acceleration and deceleration are discussed together because they often occur in combination. Let us first examine acceleration. At the moment of impact in a rear-end collision (in which external force is applied from the rear), there is sudden acceleration of the portion of the body that is in contact with the seat. The head and upper back that are not in contact with the seat or head rest are bent sharply backward (hyperextension). Once the head strikes the back of the seat or has hyperextended to its limit, it is then thrown forward. The head may strike the steering wheel or dashboard as it slows down or decelerates.

Deceleration is often the major mechanism with head-on collisions. The outside force is exerted from the front, causing the head and body to continue moving forward until contact is made, usually with the dashboard. The person is forcibly hyperflexed as he moves forward, hits the dashboard, and then snaps back into a forced hyperextension position.

Both acceleration and deceleration are the major mechanisms that cause hyperextension and hyperflexion injuries.

Deformation. *Deformation* refers to the various alterations in the spinal cord and supporting cord structures that are necessary to accommodate movement in various positions such as rotation, hyperextension, and hyperflexion. For example, in hyperextension of the cervical neck, the spinal canal shortens, the anterior longitudinal ligaments elongate, and the ligamenta flava are compressed and may bulge into the spinal canal. The result of deformation is injury to the involved tissue or structures.

Axial Loading. Axial loading, which is also known as vertical compression, occurs when a vertical force is exerted on the spinal column. In other words, the force is exerted up or down through the spinal column. Examples of incidents in which axial loading is seen are diving accidents, landing on the feet when falling or jumping from a height, or landing on the derrière when falling from a height.

Penetrating Wounds. Penetrating wounds occur when missiles such as bullets or shrapnel or impalement instruments such as knives, ice picks, or other objects penetrate the spinal column.

Forces

There are four possible vectors or forces that can be applied to the spinal column to cause injury: flexion, extension, rotation, and compression. More than one force can affect the spinal column and cause injury.

Flexion. Excessive flexion tends to produce compression of the vertebral bodies with disruption of the posterior longitudinal ligaments and the intervertebral discs. The extensive flexion causes compression, tension or traction, and shearing (sliding or overriding of one portion onto another) of the involved tissue.

Extension. Excessive extension usually causes fractures of the posterior elements of the spinal column and disruption of the anterior longitudinal ligaments. Excessive extension causes tension (a pulling or traction on the tissue) or shearing (sliding or overriding of one portion onto another) of the involved tissue.

Rotation. Injury from rotation is most apt to produce disruption or rupture of the ligamentous network of structures, fracture and fracture–dislocation of the facets, and possible injury to the midportion of vertebral bodies. Rotational force causes tension or traction, shearing, and compression of the tissue and bony structures.

Compression. Compression can cause explosive fractures of the vertebral body and arch as well as rupture of the supporting ligaments.[3]

Summary of Forces. It is not unusual for various forces to affect the spinal column concurrently. Rotational force is often combined with flexion or extension to produce extensive injuries to the vertebrae, ligamentous support structures, and spinal cord. This is also true for tension or traction, shearing, and compression of structures and tissue. They may occur simultaneously or successively in a specific injury.

Information about forces is included to help the nurse understand the kinds of injuries that can occur that are caused by specific forces exerted on the spinal axis. It also underscores the importance of collecting as much information about the circumstances of injury as possible to help predict the types of injury sustained. This is particularly important for the nurse in the emergency department or at the scene of the accident.

GENERAL CLASSIFICATION OF INJURIES

The velocity, momentum, angle of impact, and type of exaggerated movement produced affect the type of injury sustained. These factors are considered in the classification of injuries.

A patient who has anatomical abnormalities or a disease process in the spinal column is much more vulnerable to injury. Chronic cervical spondylosis, arthritis, and scoliosis are examples of conditions that increase the probability of injury.

A basic classification of causes of injury to the vertebral column, spinal cord, and soft tissue includes the following categories and their characteristics:

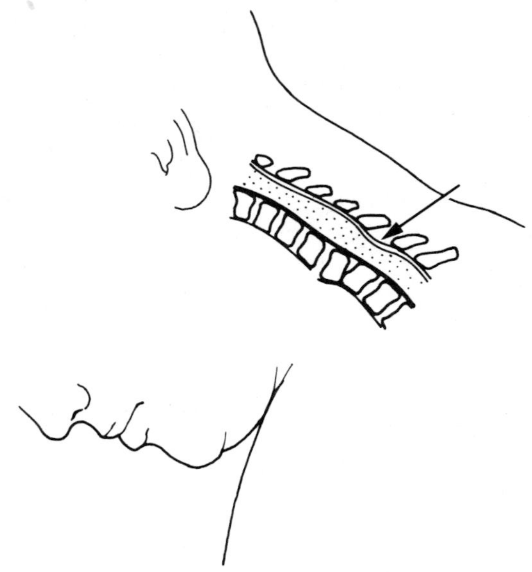

FIG. 18–1. Hyperflexion injury.

Hyperflexion Injuries (Fig. 18–1)

- Caused by hyperflexion of the head and neck as in sudden deceleration. This is seen in head-on collisions and sometimes in diving accidents.
- If the posterior ligamental structures are intact, a wedge or compression fracture of the vertebral body is common; this is considered a relatively stable fracture not usually requiring surgery.
- If the posterior ligamental structures are torn, the facets are usually disengaged and dislocated; this is considered an unstable fracture requiring immediate surgical stabilization.
- The degree of cord damage depends on the amount of compression caused by the dislocated or fractured vertebrae.
- Occur most often in the cervical and lumbar region
- When the cervical area is involved, the greatest areas of stress are at C–5 and C–6.

Lateral Flexion (Rotational Injuries) (Fig. 18–2)

- Caused by extreme lateral flexion or rotation of the head and neck
- There is tearing or rupture of the posterior ligamental struc-

FIG. 18–2. Lateral flexion injury.

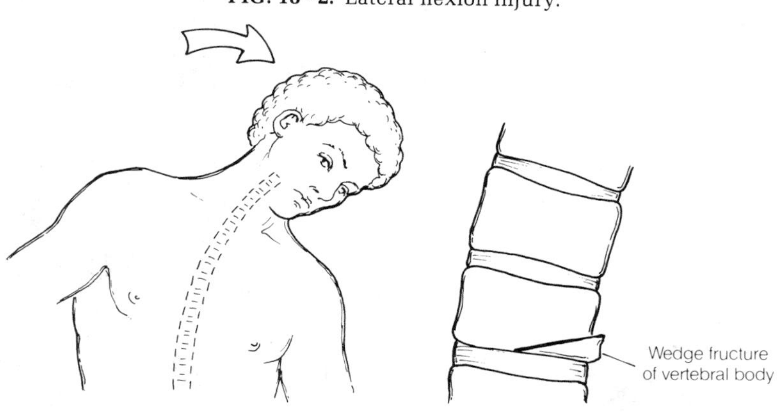

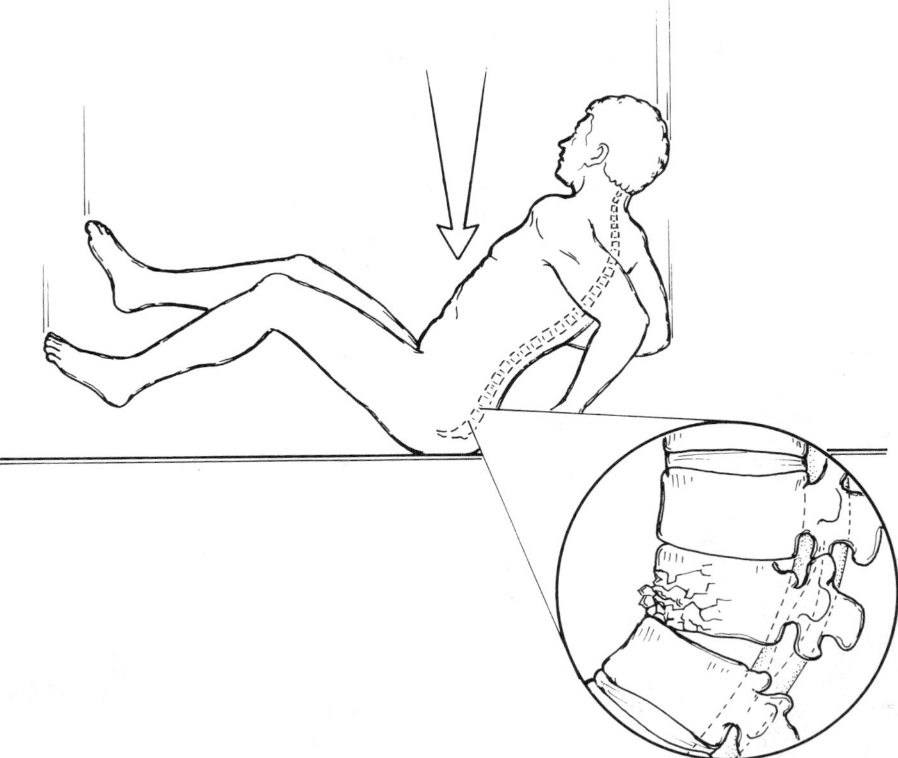

FIG. 18-3. Compression injury.

tures so that the rotational force causes dislocation at the facet joint and fracture at the articular processes.

- There may be one or two facets involved. If one facet is dislocated or locked, there are usually no neurological deficits. More than half of the patients with two facets locked will have neurological deficits. The reduction of the fracture is achieved by traction (cervical traction or halo apparatus with or without a jacket) or surgery to disengage the facets and stabilize the vertebral column.

Compression Injuries (Fig. 18-3)

- Caused by axial loading or vertical pressure such as that which occurs when one falls from a height and lands on one's feet or buttocks
- Burst or explosive fractures occur, which require surgery for the removal of bone fragments and stabilization.

Hyperextension Injuries (Fig. 18-4)

- Caused by hyperextension of the head and neck such as that which occurs in a rear-end vehicular collision
- Hyperextension injuries tend to cause the greatest amount of injury because backward and downward movement includes a larger arc than flexion. If the head flexes forward, the chin strikes the chest and limits the arc. If the head flexes laterally, the head strikes the shoulder.
- The spinal cord is stretched and lies against the ligamenta flava. This type of injury can cause contusion and ischemia to part of the cord resulting in neurological deficits even if the x-ray examination proves negative.
- As a rule, ligamental structures are intact; no fractures or dislocations occur.
- The greatest area of stress for a hyperextension injury is at C-4 and C-5 levels.
- Common injury seen in the elderly if they fall and strike the chin
- A less severe form of a hyperextension injury is called a "whiplash" or an acceleration injury. It is a stress and strain injury to the soft tissue (muscles and ligaments), but there is no vertebral or cord injury.

FIG. 18-4. Hyperextension injury to the cervical spinal cord without fracture or dislocation. (Rockwood CA, Green DP: Fractures. Philadelphia, JB Lippincott, 1977)

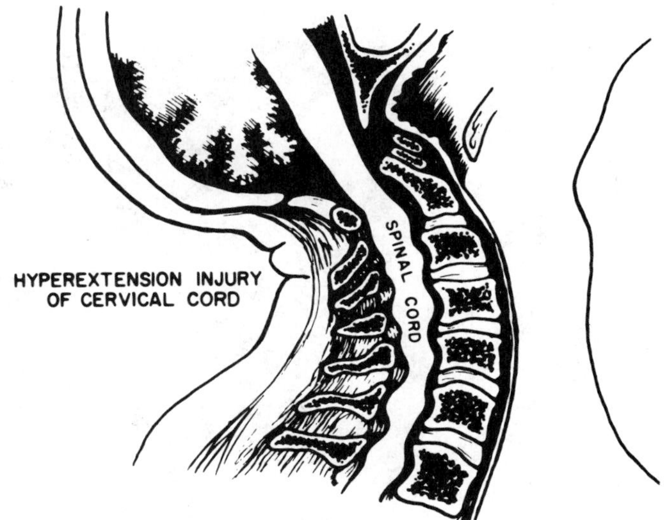

Missile Injuries

- Caused by the penetration of the cord by a blunt object such as a bullet or shrapnel

Stab Injuries

- Caused by a knife that transects a portion or the complete plane of the spinal cord
- There is severe irreversible damage to the spinal cord. Other elements of the spinal column may also be injured.

SPECIFIC CLASSIFICATION OF INJURIES BY SITE: SOFT TISSUE, VERTEBRAL, AND SPINAL CORD TRAUMA

Soft-Tissue Trauma

Whiplash is a lay term used to describe an acceleration injury that causes the head to hyperextend as a result of a rear-end vehicular collision. The ligaments and muscles of the neck sustain stress and strain injury. The usual signs and symptoms—stiff neck, pain in the neck and shoulder, limitation of movement, and muscle spasms—may not begin for 12 to 48 hours after injury. Other signs and symptoms may include headache, paresthesias, dizziness, vertigo, and tinnitus. The findings of the physical examination are normal except for the above-mentioned signs and symptoms. The radiological examination is negative. The diagnosis is based on the history of injury and the presence of the signs and symptoms. This is a very common injury causing much pain and suffering to the patient even though there are no abnormalities noted on radiographic examination.

The pain is thought to be due to the tearing, stretching, microhemorrhage, and edema incurred by the anterior neck muscles (sternocleidomastoid, scalenus, and longus colli muscles). The muscles and possibly the ligaments are strained.[4] Patients with pre-existing cervical spondylosis and some other conditions are at greater risk of developing

FIG. 18-5. Types of rigid cervical collars. (Camp International, Inc., Jackson, MI)

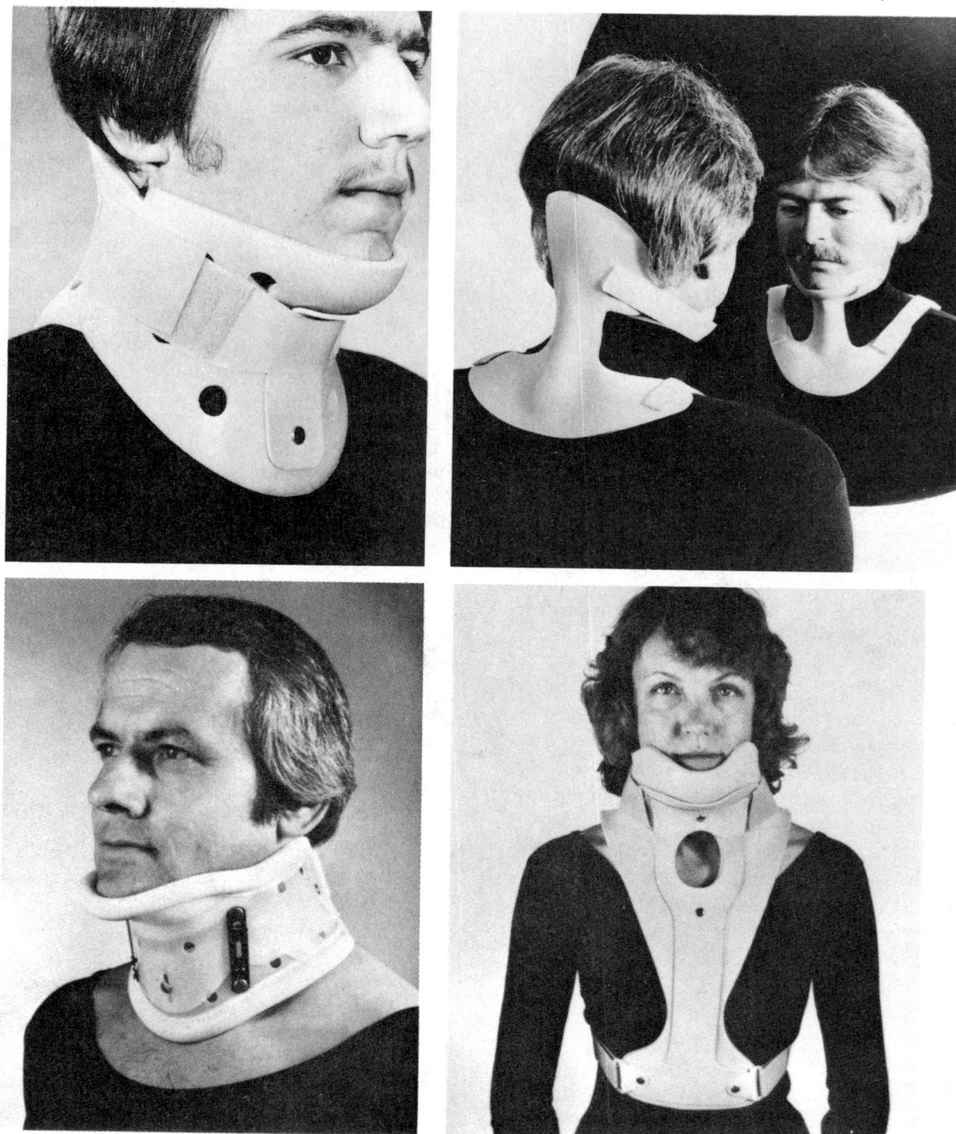

problems if a whiplash injury occurs because of narrowing of the foramina, osteophytes, and increased rigidity of the spinal column.[4]

Treatment. Treatment includes measures directed at comfort. Mild injuries are treated with mild analgesics (aspirin, acetaminophen [Tylenol]), local heat, and rest. More severe injuries are treated with complete bed rest, cervical traction, heat application, pain management, muscle relaxants, and anti-inflammatory agents such as phenylbutazone (Butazolidin), indomethacin (Indocin), and others. Narcotics should be used sparingly. Cervical collars should not be used in mild cases. If they are ordered in more severe cases, they should be worn 24 hours a day for a limited amount of time (Fig. 18–5).

Vertebral Injuries

Classification. Fractures can occur in any part of the vertebra such as the transverse, spinous, lateral, and articular processes. Although fractures can occur singularly in any part of the vertebral arch, most injuries occur in combination with injury to the vertebral body. Anatomically, the vertebrae are highly irregular bony structures that fracture easily. Fractures are caused either by direct or indirect trauma, the latter being the major offender. The "ends" of the vertebral column—the cervical and lumbar portions—have the greatest built-in mobility, thereby predisposing these areas to injury. The thoracic region is less prone to trauma because of the rigidity imparted to it by the rib cage.

Vertebral injuries can be classified into major divisions: simple fractures, compression fractures, comminuted fractures, teardrop fractures, special cervical fractures, dislocations, subluxations, and fracture–dislocations. The concept of stable *versus* unstable fractures is also mentioned.

Simple Fracture. Simple fractures usually occur as fractures to the spinous or transverse process; the facets, pedicles, and vertebral body are rarely involved. The fracture appears as a singular break, with the alignment of the vertebral parts remaining intact. Neural compression is usually not present.

Compression Fracture. A compression fracture, also called a wedged fracture, is one in which the vertebral body is compressed anteriorly due to a hyperflexion injury. Ligaments are usually not ruptured. Neural compression may or may not be present.

Comminuted Fracture. A comminuted fracture, also termed a burst fracture of the vertebral body, results in a shattering of the vertebral body into many pieces, with the possibility that fragments may be driven into the spinal cord, thereby resulting in a serious cord injury. These fractures can occur at the cervical, thoracic, or lumbar regions of the vertebral column.

Teardrop Fracture. As the result of a hyperflexion fracture dislocation, a small fragment of bone from the anterior edge of the vertebra breaks off and is free to lodge within the spinal canal. There is posterior dislocation of the main portion of the vertebral body. Surgical intervention is necessary to remove the fragment. If the fragment has penetrated the cord, neurological deficits will result. The fragment must be removed and a spinal fusion performed to stabilize the area.

Special Cervical Fractures. In the cervical region, the atlas (first cervical vertebra) and the axis (second cervical vertebra) are each different in shape from the other cervical vertebrae (Fig. 18–6). The term *atlantoaxial* refers to the atlas–axis region of the cervical vertebral column. Because a wide range of direction of movement is possible, especially in the upper cervical region, injury can result from excessive rotation of the head.

The following cervical fracture dislocations may result from trauma:

1. A *Jefferson fracture* is a rare fracture of the atlas resulting from a vertically compressing force. At impact the force produces bilateral thrust, which causes fracture at the weakest points, splitting the vertebra into three of four parts (Fig. 18–7, *A*). At the time of fracture the circumference of the circular atlas increases, allowing for a greater space between the circumference of the bone and the spinal canal; therefore, there is usually no immediate damage to the cord. However most patients do not survive a Jefferson fracture because any subsequent movement will cause displacement of bony segments, resulting in severance of the cord and immediate death.
2. *Atlanto–occipital dislocations* are produced by avulsion of the atlas (C–1) body from the occipital bone. Death is immediate with this rare fracture.
3. The *odontoid* or *dens fracture* (C–2) is a common type of traumatic cervical fracture (Fig. 18–7, *B*). The cause of injury is vertical compression alone or in combination with hyperextension, which results from falling on the head, receiving a direct blow, or being thrown through a windshield. The fracture can produce both anterior and posterior displacement, depending on the initial site of trauma. The patient may not have any signs or symptoms of cord deficit. The fracture can be easily missed upon radiographic observation, unless the open-mouth view with flexion–extension aspects are taken. Even though the patient is asymptomatic, odontoid fractures must *always* be treated with immobility and bed rest until the natural healing process stabilizes the fracture.

FIG. 18–6. Specialized articulation between C-1 and C-2 allows for 50% of the rotation in the cervical spine. (Hoppenfeld S: Orthopaedic Neurology. Philadelphia, JB Lippincott, 1977)

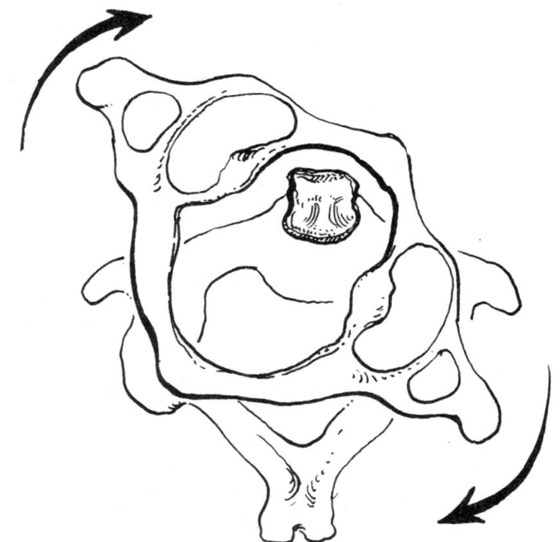

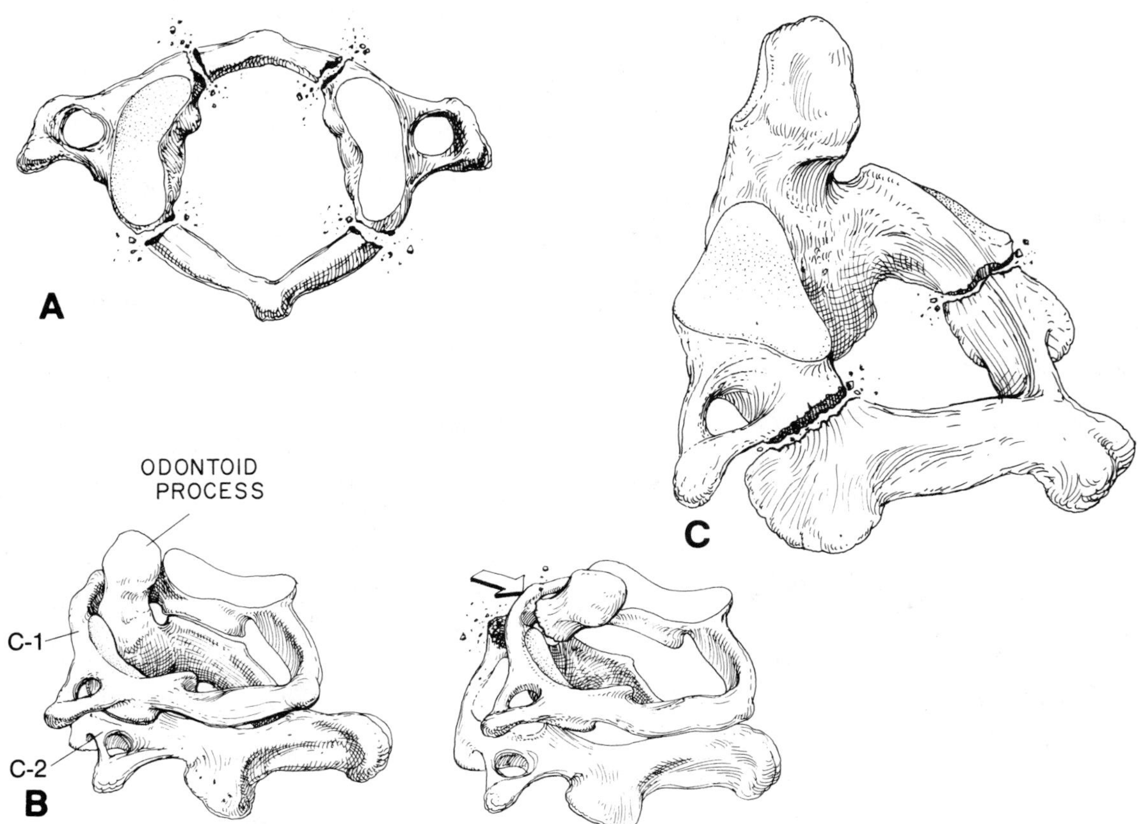

FIG. 18–7. Types of cervical fractures. *(A)* Jefferson fracture—a bursting fracture of the ring of C-1. *(B)* Odontoid fracture. *(C)* Hangman's fracture—a fracture that separates the body of C-2 from its posterior elements. (Hoppenfeld S: Orthopaedic Neurology. Philadelphia, JB Lippincott, 1977)

If rotational force is added to vertical hyperextension, the fractured processes may be driven into the spinal cord, leading to immediate death.

4. The *hangman's fracture* results in a bilateral avulsion fracture through the C–2 arch without odontoid injury (Fig. 18–7, *C*). Fracture–dislocation of C–2 or C–3 may or may not be present. The patient is usually asymptomatic because of the roomy, high, cervical bony canal. Immobilization and bed rest are required and open fusion is not usually necessary.

Dislocation. Dislocation of a vertebra occurs when one vertebra overrides another and there is unilateral or bilateral facet dislocation. Usually the supporting ligaments are injured, and the spinal cord may or may not be injured. There is a disruption in the established alignment of the vertebral column that is noted on the x-ray films.

Subluxation. A subluxation is a partial or incomplete dislocation of one vertebra over another. Cord damage and injury to the supporting ligaments may or may not be present.

Fracture–Dislocation. "Fracture–dislocation" is a descriptive term sometimes used to convey the idea that there is both a fracture and a dislocation. Ligament and cord injury are usually present.

"Stable" Versus "Unstable" Fractures. Vertebral fractures have been traditionally classified as "stable" and "unstable." However, there is increasing concern about the false security of this distinction because many so-called "stable" fractures later result in neurological deficit. Spinal fusion is now recommended as a precaution when managing patients with such fractures. Prudent judgment about using surgical fusion is coupled with the equally important selection of the optimal time after injury.

Vertebral Injuries Below the Cervical Level

Specific cervical injuries have been identified and described. Vertebral injuries at other levels are managed by realignment, stabilization, and decompression based on the type and circumstances of injury. The following information briefly discusses thoracic, lumbar, sacral, and coccygeal injuries.

Thoracic and Lumbar Fractures. Fifty percent of patients with spinal cord injury are paraplegics. Injuries in the thoracic and lumbar regions account for paralysis in the trunk and lower extremities. Normally little movement is possible in the vertebrae of the thoracic region as compared to the lumbar region. The anatomical structures of the thoracic segment provide inherent structural stability.

The spinal cord ends at the upper border of the first lumbar vertebra. The cord gradually tapers beginning at the lower two thoracic vertebrae. As the cord tapers, it forms a cone called the conus medullaris, which continues at the filum terminale. The nerve roots coming off the lower segments of the spinal cord, termed the cauda equina, hang loosely and are susceptible to injury. The contents of the vertebral canal below T-12 or L-1 are similar to peripheral nerves. Injury to these nerves is more likely to result in recovery than injury to the spinal cord, and less likely to require the emergency procedures of decompression, since the roots tolerate trauma far better than the spinal cord itself.

Compression fractures are common in the cervical, thoracic, and upper lumbar regions of the vertebral column (Fig. 18-8). Vertical force or direct force applied to the vertebra itself is responsible for injury. Much direct force must be applied to produce a fracture in the thoracic area. Injury is usually the result of a direct force being applied to one vertebra, with subsequent force and compromise of the underlying cord. When this happens, there is hyperflexion of the vertebra.

A compression fracture in the thoracic or lumbar region may be anteriorly compressed with or without subluxation of the vertebra. The other possibility is total compression of the vertebral body with anteroposterior protrusion (see Fig. 18-8).

Fracture-dislocation injuries of the thoracic and lumbar areas are of three general categories:

1. Either anterior or posterior dislocation of the whole vertebral body with fracture of bony parts
2. Comminuted fractures of the vertebral body with anterior or posterior displacement and rotation, the rotational force usually tearing supporting ligaments
3. Lateral dislocation of the vertebra with fracture

Lesions of the conus medullaris can occur with fractures in the lumbar region. These lesions can be very confusing. Injury to the conus usually results in lower motor neuron symptoms (muscle flaccidity, muscle atrophy, and so forth) because of the disruption of the anterior gray horn cells. A decompression laminectomy may be necessary if there is pressure on the neural elements. Lesions to the cauda equina produce root syndromes of selected roots. A decompression laminectomy may also be necessary.

Sacral and Coccygeal Fractures. Fractures of the sacrum and coccyx usually result from direct trauma. These injuries are most frequently caused by falls. Any fall in the sitting position, such as falling on ice or being thrown from a horse and landing on the buttocks, can result in a fracture. Cord injury in this region can cause bladder, bowel, or sexual dysfunction.

Spinal Cord Injuries

Injury to the spinal cord causes a devastating loss of many bodily functions that make one independent. The loss of function may be permanent or temporary depending on the type of injury. Spinal cord injuries can be classified by type of injury and by syndromes. (Chart 18-1).

Classification by Type of Injury. The spinal cord can be injured by concussion, contusion, laceration, transection, hemorrhage, and damage to the blood vessels that supply the cord.

- Concussion—A concussion of the spinal cord is a rare condition causing temporary loss of function lasting 24 to 48 hours that is due to a severe shaking of the spinal cord. No identifiable neuropathological changes are noted on examination of the cord.
- Contusion—A contusion of the spinal cord refers to a bruising of the cord that includes bleeding into the cord, subsequent edema, and possible necrosis from the compression of

FIG. 18-8. Progressive degrees of compression fracture. *(A)* Severe compression fracture showing the biconcave profile produced by the adjacent discs. *(B)* A more severe degree of fracture. A vertical fracture has joined the deformed, concave end-plates. The anterior body fragment is comminuted and displaced anteriorly. *(C)* A more severe degree of compression fracture. The posterior body fragment is now comminuted and displaced posteriorly into the spinal canal. Neural damage may occur. The neural arch is intact. This spine is stable. (Rockwood CA, Green DP: Fractures. Philadelphia, JB Lippincott, 1977)

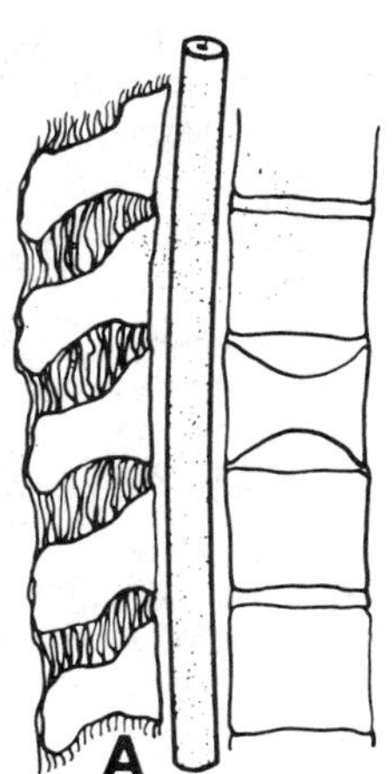

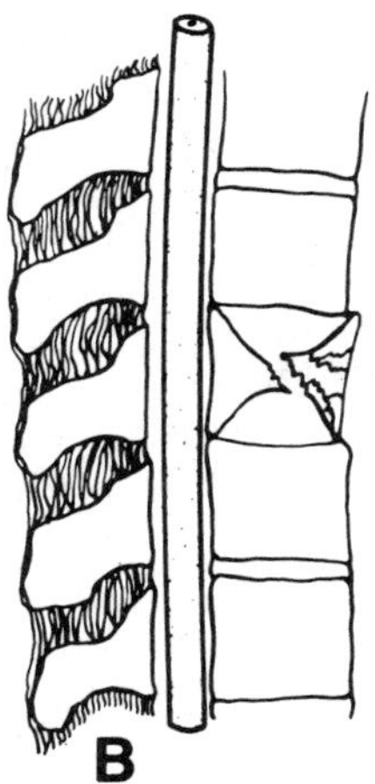

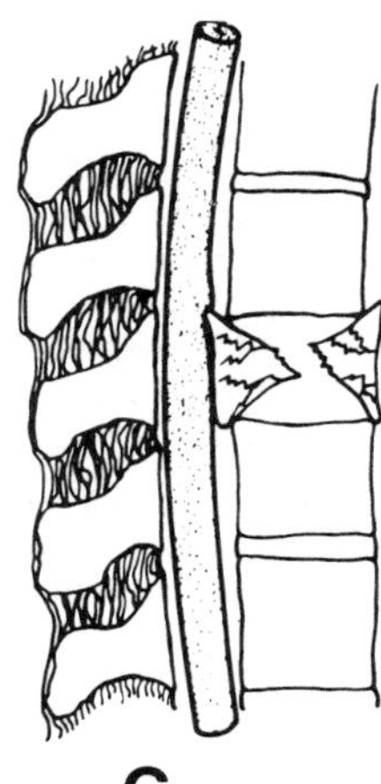

CHART 18-1. DEFINITION OF SELECTED TERMS RELATED TO SPINAL CORD INJURY

Several terms should be defined to clarify the discussion of spinal cord injury and related sequelae (Fig. 18-9).

Paraplegia is defined as paralysis of the lower half of the body with the involvement of both legs.

Quadriplegia (tetraplegia) is defined as paralysis involving all four extremities. The term *complete quadriplegia* is sometimes used to describe the loss of function at the upper cervical region (above C-6), leaving the patient with no potential for independence. An intact C-6 spinal nerve level is the point of demarcation between permanent dependence and the potential for independence. Intact muscle function of the shoulder rotators, deltoid, biceps, brachioradialis, and radial wrist extensors, along with partial strength in the upper pectoral muscle, indicates C-6 function. Although strength in the triceps and hand muscles is lacking, quadriplegics who are described as having mechanical function can generally achieve independence. Therefore, an *incomplete quadriplegic* is one who has loss of cervical spinal function below the C-6 level.

Upper motor neuron lesions are caused by lesions in the corticospinal or corticobulbar tract, producing a characteristic clinical picture. Initially, there is a period of spinal shock with loss of motor, sensory, and autonomic function below the level of injury. There is muscle flaccidity, loss of reflex function, and loss of sensation. After recovery from spinal shock, signs and symptoms of spasticity can develop:

- Muscle hypertonicity (spasticity)
- Postural flexion of arms and extension of legs
- Hyperactive tendon reflexes
- A positive Babinski reflex

Atrophy is not prominent, nor are muscle fasciculations. (Muscle fasciculations are brief contractions of muscle groups that are visible though the skin.)

Lower motor neuron lesions abolish both voluntary and reflex responses of the muscles because of the destruction of the anterior horn cells, ventral nerve roots or motor fibers, or peripheral nerves. The signs and symptoms include the following:

- Paresis or paralysis limited to specific muscle groups
- Gait depends on muscles affected, but flaillike movements are common
- Muscle flaccidity
- Tendon reflexes absent or hypoactive
- Atrophy prominent
- Muscle fasciculations present
- Babinski reflex absent
- Tropic changes of dry and cyanotic skin, which may be ulcerated

Dermatomes and *myotomes* are used to identify the loss of motor and sensory function, which depends on the level of injury. Because of the great overlap of innervation from the spinal nerves, several areas are innervated by more than one spinal nerve. By observing a dermatome and myotome one has a good idea of spinal innervation (Fig. 18-10). A dermatome identifies specific areas of the skin supplied by sensory fibers of a single spinal nerve. A myotome identifies the muscle group or groups innervated by spinal nerves.

the edema or damage to the tissue. The extent of neurological deficits depend on the severity of the contusion and the presence of necrosis. Fractures, dislocations, and direct trauma to the cord can cause a contusion.

- Laceration—A laceration is an actual tear in the cord and results in permanent injury to the cord. Contusion, edema, and cord compression accompany a laceration.
- Transection—A transection is a severing of the cord and can be complete or incomplete. Complete transection is rare, although in a physiological sense, it is frequently seen.
- Hemorrhage—Hemorrhage or bleeding into or around the spinal cord is an irritant to the delicate tissue resulting in changes in the neurochemical components, edema, and neurological deficits.
- Damage to the blood vessels that supply the cord—Interference or damage to the vessels that supply the spinal cord, the anterior spinal artery, or the two posterior spinal arteries results in ischemia and possible necrosis. Episodes of ischemia can cause temporary neurological deficits. Prolonged ischemia and necrosis will cause permanent deficits.

Discussion. With any of these injuries, one can expect cord edema to develop soon after injury, thereby compounding the functional loss, at least on a temporary basis. Edema causes cord compression, which is tolerated poorly by the spinal cord even for short periods.

As is the case with tissues in other parts of the body, edema usually results from trauma. While permanent loss of function may be due to frank damage to the cord itself, cord function may be temporarily inhibited as a result of edema. With resolution of edema, spinal function may return, provided that irreversible damage has not been sustained by the cord. Edema becomes a critical concern, particularly in the upper cervical region, because it can interfere with vital functions, including respiration, because of the proximity of the cervical cord to the brain stem and medulla. As a result, C-1 and C-2 fracture dislocations are fatal. Fractures of C-3, C-4, and C-5 can also result in respiratory paralysis if the phrenic nerve is involved.

It is possible to incur spinal cord injury with clinical symptoms even though there is no detectable damage to the cord or vertebrae upon radiographic examination or surgical inspection. This can occur when a dislocation spontaneously reduces itself at the time of injury; however, by this time serious damage has already been sustained.

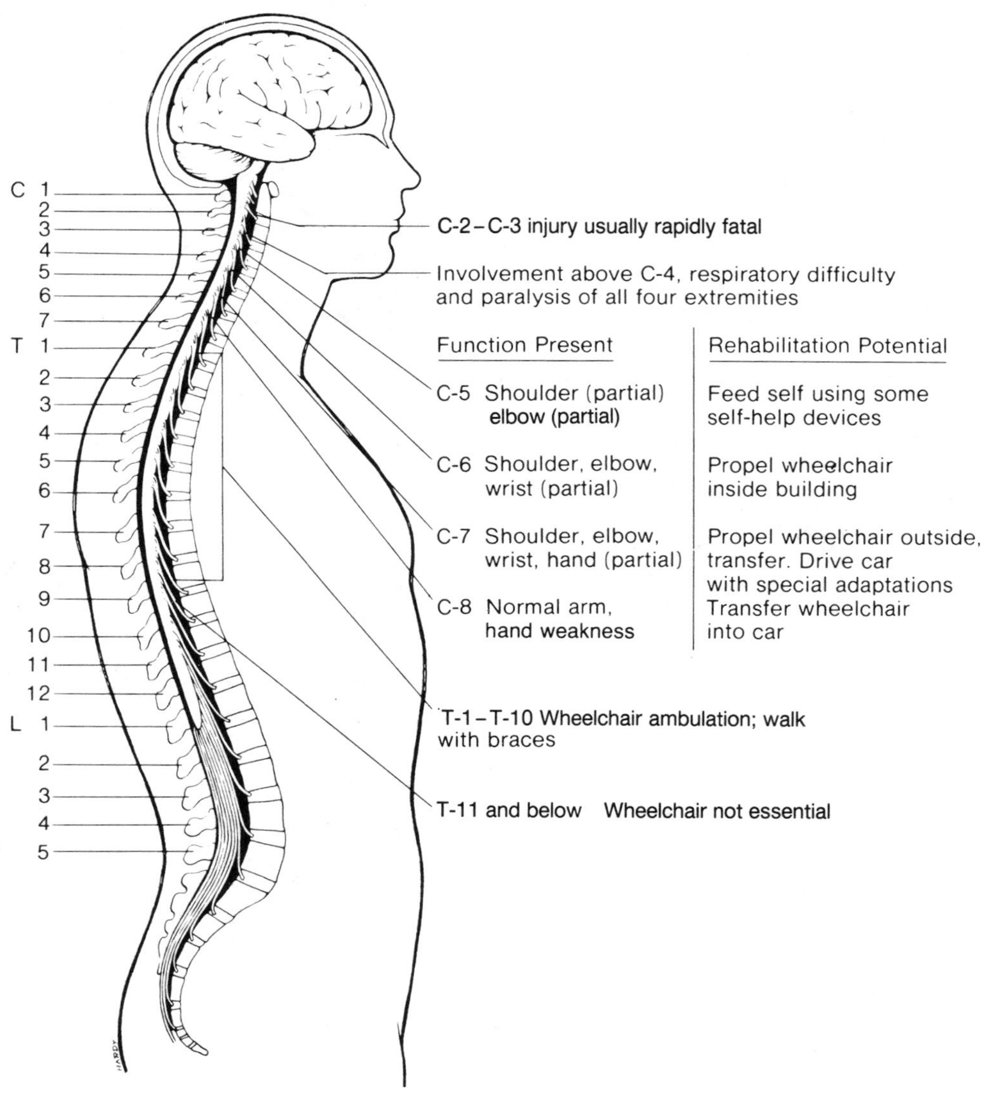

FIG. 18–9. Sequelae of spinal cord injury and rehabilitation challenges. (Brunner LS, Suddarth DS: Textbook of Medical–Surgical Nursing, 5th ed. Philadelphia, JB Lippincott, 1984)

Classification by Syndromes. There are a few syndromes associated with partial spinal cord dysfunction that are seen in clinical practice and cited in the literature. They are the anterior cord syndrome, central cord syndrome, posterior cord syndrome, Brown–Séquard (lateral) syndrome, and sometimes Horner's syndrome. Although root syndromes do not involve the spinal cord *per se,* spinal nerve roots are extensions of the cord and damage to them results in root syndromes. Root syndromes are included because they are possible results of spinal column injury.

Anterior Cord Syndrome. Anterior cord syndrome is due to injury to the anterior part of the spinal cord, which includes the spinothalamic tracts (perception of pain), the corticospinal tracts (perception of temperature), and the anterior gray horn motor neurons. The syndrome can be caused by acute herniation of an intervertebral disc or flexion injuries and fracture–dislocations of the vertebrae. The anterior spinal artery, the singular artery that supplies the anterior two-thirds of the anterior spinal cord, is injured by the compression of the anterior cord from bone fragments or the occlusion of the artery.

Signs and symptoms include loss of pain and temperature sensation as well as motor function below the level of the lesion. The sensations of light touch, position, and vibration remain intact.

Surgical decompression is usually necessary. The prognosis varies with each patient and depends on the degree of structural injury and edema.

Central Cord Syndrome. Central cord syndrome is due to injury and/or edema to the central cord in the cervical region. Hyperextension injuries, particularly if there are hypertrophic spurs from a degenerative process or interruption of the blood supply to the spinal cord, have been cited as frequent causes of the problem. The edema in the central cord exerts pressure on the anterior horn cells. The cervical fibers of the corticospinal tract are located in a

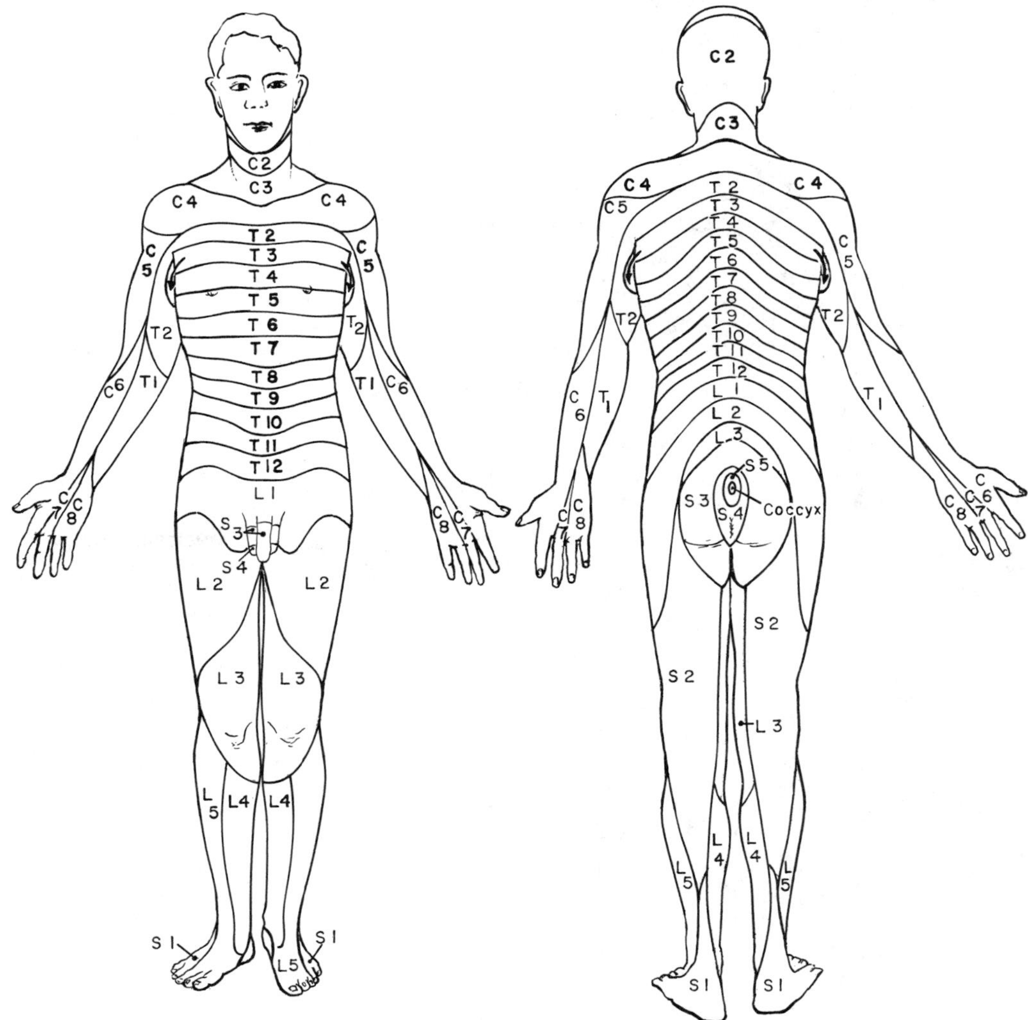

FIG. 18-10. Cutaneous distribution of spinal nerves (dermatomes). (Barr M: The Human Nervous System. New York, Harper & Row, 1979)

more central position in the cord while the sacral fibers are located in the periphery. Accordingly, the motor deficits are less severe in the lower extremities than in the upper extremities in central cord syndrome. On clinical examination of the patient there is a disproportionate motor deficit in the upper extremities as compared with the deficit in the lower extremities. Sensory deficits vary although the loss is more pronounced in the upper extremities. Varying degrees of bladder and bowel dysfunction are common. The sacral area, because it is peripheral, may be spared. On examination of the patient the perineum and genitalia may have escaped motor and sensory deficits. Deficits in these areas are assessed by evaluating sphincter tone, perineal skin sensation, and the reflexes (anal and bulbocavernosus). The sparing of these areas implies a good prognosis because it indicates that the lesion is incomplete.[4]

Treatment of the central cord syndrome includes medical management with steroid therapy to decrease the edema. Complete or partial recovery of function is possible if the edema can be rapidly controlled.

Posterior Cord Syndrome. Posterior cord syndrome is a rare syndrome in which the posterior columns (senses of position and vibration) are involved. The prognosis for recovery is said to be good.[5]

Brown–Séquard Syndrome. Brown–Séquard (lateral cord) syndrome is due to a transverse hemisection of the cord whereby half of the cord is transected from north to south. It results from a knife or missile injury to half of the cord, a fracture–dislocation of a unilateral articular process, or possibly an acute ruptured intervertebral disc. In clinical practice, injury to the cord that is seen has not been so carefully inflicted that precisely half of the cord is transected. The term Brown–Séquard syndrome is generally applied when a relative difference in function is noted from side to side in patients experiencing bilateral cord damage.

The signs and symptoms that result are ipsilateral paralysis or paresis; ipsilateral loss of touch, pressure, vibration, and position sensation; and contralateral loss of pain and temperature. For example, let us suppose that only the left side of the cord has been transected. The following would be present: paralysis of all voluntary muscles below the injury on the left side of the body (lateral corticospinal tract); loss of the perception of touch, vibration, and position on the left side of the body below the injury (fasciculus gracilis and fasciculus cuneatus); and loss of the perception of pain and temperature on the right side of the body below the injury (lateral spinothalamic tracts). This last symptom occurs because the fibers that carry the perception of pain cross to the opposite side of the cord immediately after entering the cord and then ascend. The other tracts that were mentioned do not cross until they reach the brain stem area.

Horner's Syndrome. Horner's syndrome is encountered with partial spinal cord transection at T-1 or above. A lesion of either the preganglionic sympathetic trunk or the postganglionic sympathetic neurons of the superior cervical ganglion will result in Horner's syndrome on the ipsilateral side of the face. The lesion of the sympathetic fibers is due to a partial cord transection in the cervical region.

The signs and symptoms of Horner's syndrome include the following: the ipsilateral pupil is smaller than the opposite pupil; the ipsilateral eyeball sinks; the affected eyelid droops (ptosis); and the ipsilateral side of the face does not sweat.

Root Syndromes. Root syndromes are due to compression of one or more nerve roots that come off the spinal cord rather than compression or injury to the cord itself. Spinal roots and nerves are part of the peripheral nervous system and not the central nervous system as is the case with the spinal cord. Root syndromes can result from compression caused by intervertebral disc herniation or vertebral subluxation. Any area of the cord can be involved (cervical, thoracic, lumbar, or sacral areas).

The signs and symptoms of a root syndrome include tingling, pain, motor weakness of an isolated muscle or muscle group, and absent or diminished reflexes in the involved area. The spinal cord terminates at thoracic level twelve or lumbar level one. The nerve roots that extend from the conus medullaris are collectively called the cauda equina. Lesions of the lumbosacral region may involve multiple roots of the cauda equina with a varying pattern of motor and sensory loss. Deep tendon reflexes are usually diminished or absent. Isolated nerve root involvement is common in the lumbosacral region so that "saddle hypalgesia," diminished or absence of sensation in the saddle region, is possible.[5] Therefore, careful examination of the patient is necessary to identify the erratic sensory or motor loss. When the sacral roots are involved, the patient may experience bladder or bowel dysfunction. If the cervical region is involved, there is usually tingling in the arm, muscle weakness in the arm or shoulder, and pain radiating down the arm and into the shoulder.

Surgery for decompression of nerve roots may be necessary. In some instances, spontaneous motor and sensory recovery is possible even after extended periods. Because the peripheral nervous system is capable of regeneration, the possibility of recovery is greater provided that the nerve roots are intact. The patient may also be treated medically with traction to release the compressed nerve roots and with drug therapy to reduce associated edema, control pain, and reduce muscle spasms.

Pathophysiology. In most instances the spinal cord is not severed at the time of injury; rather, it is bruised or compressed. Yet, in the first few hours after injury, several chemical and vascular changes occur, causing the spinal cord to initiate an intrinsic process of self-destruction and the injury to worsen.

Much of the knowledge about the neuropathological changes associated with spinal cord injury has been generated from experimental studies using a standard low-velocity model of spinal injury in the laboratory. The sequence of events that follows the initial spinal cord injury includes the following[6]:

- Hyperemia and microhemorrhagic areas begin to appear in the central gray matter of the cord within minutes after injury.
- Edema of the spinal cord occurs.
- The blood pressure to the injured areas drops sharply, resulting in ischemia.
- Hemorrhagic areas in the center of the spinal cord (gray matter) are grossly visible within an hour; within 4 hours there may be infarction in the gray matter.
- Edema of the white matter and microhemorrhagic areas develop at this time.
- The highly specialized cells of the central nervous system begin to die due to the ischemia, and hypoxia (noted within 30 minutes), and changes in the normal vasoactive amines are noted (increases in norepinephrine, serotonin, and histamine and a decrease in dopamine in the injured tissue).
- Irreversible nerve damage develops as a result of the replacement of normal neural elements with glial and fibrotic scar tissue; neurological deficits become permanent.

Research. The current research on spinal cord injuries endeavors to discover ways of preventing permanent disability. Several of the studies are supported by the NINCDS. Some of the studies include the use of drugs such as steroids, dimethyl sulfoxide, and endorphin blockers. Other approaches include hyperbaric oxygen therapy and spinal cord cooling. Much interest also centers upon nerve regeneration investigation.

Drugs. One class of drugs under investigation is steroids. Some researchers have advocated the use of large doses of steroids to reduce edema and subsequent neural destruction, while others assert that steroids retard healing and are of no clinical value. A chemical that is used as an industrial solvent, dimethyl sulfoxide (DMSO), is being investigated for its alleged healing and pain-relieving properties. The last category of drugs to be highlighted are endorphin blockers. Endorphins are chemicals produced by the brain that relieve pain in the body. It is now believed that endorphins are also involved in the production of shock because they cause a sharp drop in blood pressure during the acute stage of injury. The resulting hypotension contributes to the cord ischemia. Drugs that would block the hypotensive action of endorphins are under investigation.[1]

Hyperbaric Oxygen Therapy. Hyperbaric oxygen therapy is a medical treatment in which the entire body is under increased atmospheric pressure and the patient breathes pure oxygen. The use of hyperbaric oxygen therapy is not a new medical therapy. What is new is its application as an adjunct treatment for acute spinal cord injury. The proposed benefits of the treatment include reduction of ischemia and the subsequent cord destruction by improving oxygen diffusion into the hypoxia-injured tissue. Some studies of small populations have demonstrated significant reversal of symptoms if the treatment is administered within 12 hours of injury. However, much controversy exists about the efficacy of this treatment.

Spinal Cord Cooling. A small pad through which cool saline solution is circulated is positioned on the epidural layer of the injured spinal cord for 3 to 4 hours. The temperature of the coolant is about 6° C in most protocols. The purpose of the procedure is to reduce the bulk of the edematous cord, thus improving circulation and reducing the intrinsic destructive process. The results of treatment are promising although problems, particularly that of infection from the prolonged exposure of the cord, are cited. Treatment must begin within a few hours after injury, and concurrent high doses of steroids must be administered.

Nerve Regeneration. The basic belief that nerves of the central nervous system are incapable of any regeneration is under scrutiny. Many researchers believe that these nerves may be able to regenerate under special circumstances. This possibility is the focus of investigation at many centers.

Immediate Response to Acute Spinal Cord Injury

Spinal Shock. An immediate response to acute spinal cord injury is called spinal shock. *Spinal shock* is the temporary suppression of reflexes controlled by segments below the level of injury. The normal activity of the spinal cord is dependent on the continual tonic discharge of impulses from the higher centers of the brain. With acute injury, the input of impulses from these higher centers abruptly ceases resulting in spinal shock. After a period that may vary from hours to months, the spinal neurons gradually regain their excitability, thus concluding the period of spinal shock.[7] The earliest indication heralding the end of spinal shock is the return of the perianal reflexes (bulbocavernous and anal reflexes). The bulbocavernous reflex is tested by squeezing the glans penis or pulling the catheter and observing for slight muscle contraction. The anal reflex is present if there is a puckering of the anal sphincter on digital examination of the rectum or scratching of the skin around the anal region. Muscle contraction may also be noted upon the insertion of the rectal thermometer. Perianal reflexes return before deep tendon reflexes. Weeks may elapse between the appearance of the two reflexes. Acute spinal injury does not always produce complete loss of function so varying degrees of spinal shock are possible.

Functional Loss From Spinal Cord Injury. Table 18–1 indicates the different functions and dysfunctions associated with spinal cord injuries at specific levels. In addition to describing motor and sensory losses, the chart contains separate columns delineating respiratory, bowel, and bladder functions. The motor and sensory columns also indicate the functions that are intact. The last column provides information on the rehabilitation potential that might be realistically expected for the patient. By knowing which functions are lost and which remain intact, the nurse can develop a plan of care that will optimize the rehabilitative potential and maintain intact functions that might otherwise be lost.

Assessment. The extent of functional loss with sudden spinal cord injury will depend on the level and degree of injury. By degree of injury, one must consider whether the injury produces a complete or partial cord transection. The patient must be carefully examined to determine if any motor, sensory, or reflex function is intact. If there is absolutely no motor, sensory, or reflex activity seen immediately after cord injury, the possibility of significant recovery is almost nonexistent.[4] Others believe that no determination of prognosis can be made until recovery from spinal shock has occurred.

The Neurological Examination. A complete neurological examination will identify the sensory, motor, and reflex functions that are present or absent. The sensory modality examination for pain, temperature, light touch, deep pressure, position, and vibration provides a reasonable approximation of the level of cord injury. The highest level of sensory appreciation should be noted.

The motor examination should also identify the highest level of voluntary motor function. The examiner also looks for possible sparing of function below the highest level. The examination is conducted systematically and the major muscle groups and movements are evaluated.

The testing of reflexes is also conducted systematically. All deep tendon reflexes are tested. The level of spinal cord injury can be approximated with reflex testing. The significance of sacral sparing is emphasized in the neurological examination. In the discussion of central cord syndrome earlier in this chapter, it was pointed out that the sensory innervation to the sacral area is located in the peripheral area of the spinal cord. Because of its location, it may be spared with certain types of injuries. Therefore, the sphincter tone and the reflexes of the perianal areas should be evaluated, particularly when other reflexes and motor and sensory function are lost. If they are present, the prognosis is hopeful because the patient has not sustained a complete spinal cord injury. A good recovery is possible.

Immediate Signs and Symptoms of Spinal Cord Injury. When the spinal cord is suddenly transected, spinal shock occurs in the portion of the cord severed, with complete loss of motor, sensory, reflex and autonomic function below the level of injury. At time the term *flaccid paralysis* is used to describe the clinical picture seen at this time, because the muscles are flaccid.

Sudden complete transection of the spinal cord results in immediate spinal shock which includes

1. Flaccid, total paralysis of all skeletal muscles below the level of injury
2. Loss of all spinal reflexes below the level of injury
3. Loss of pain, proprioception, and the sensations, of touch, temperature, and pressure below the level of injury. (Pain may be present at the site of the injury due to a zone of heightened sensitivity [hyperesthesia] immediately above the level of the lesion.)
4. Absence of somatic and visceral sensations below the level of injury

(Text continued on page 394.)

TABLE 18–1. *Functional Loss From Spinal Cord Injury*

Level of Spinal Segment Injury	*Motor Function*	*Reflexes, Deep Tendon*	*Sensory Function*	*Respiratory Function*	*Bowel and Bladder Function*	*Rehabilitative Potential*
C–1 to C–4	Quadriplegia (complete) Loss of all motor function from neck down		Loss of all sensory function in the neck and below (C–4 supplies the clavicles)	Spinal nerve C–1 to C–4 forms the phrenic nerve. Innervation to the diaphragm is lost; independent respiratory function is lost. The intercostal muscles are nonfunctional (probably needs a tracheostomy).	No bowel or bladder control	No rehabilitative potential
C–5	Quadriplegia (complete) Loss of all function below upper shoulders Intact: sternomastoids, cervical paraspinal muscles, and the trapezius. (He can control his head.)	C–5, C–6 Biceps	Loss of sensation below clavicle, most of arms and hands, chest, abdomen, and lower extremities. Intact: head, shoulders, clavicle–deltoid areas, part of forearms (C–5 supplies the lateral aspect of the arm)	Phrenic nerve is intact but not intercostal muscles	Same as above	Although there is loss of voluntary use of arms, trunk, and legs, benefit may be derived from training with extremity-powered devices to achieve some useful control of upper limbs. Head control helps in balance in the wheelchair. Adaptive tools held in mouth for typing, writing, and so forth can be helpful.
C–6	Quadriplegia (complete) Loss of all function below shoulders and upper arms; lacks elbow, forearm, and hand control Intact: deltoid, biceps, and external rotators of shoulders (these muscles are usually weak)		Loss of everything listed for C–5 but has more arm and thumb sensation Intact: head, shoulders, arms, palms of hands, and thumbs (C–6 supplies the forearm and thumb)	Same as above	Same as above	Needs assistive devices to use arms. He may be able to feed, groom, and help dress self. He will need a motorized wheelchair. He is completely dependent for transfer from chair, bed, or toilet.

(continued)

TABLE 18–1. (continued)

Level of Spinal Segment Injury	Motor Function	Reflexes, Deep Tendon	Sensory Function	Respiratory Function	Bowel and Bladder Function	Rehabilitative Potential
C–7	Quadriplegia (incomplete) Loss of motor control to parts of the arm and hands Intact: voluntary strength in the shoulder depressors, the scapula stabilizers and shoulder abductors, internal rotators, and radial wrist extensors	C–7, C–8 Triceps	Loss of sensation below clavicle and parts of arms and hands Intact: head, shoulders, most of arms and hands (C–7 supplies the middle finger)	Same as above	Same as above	The intact muscles enhance ability at activities of daily living (ADL). Function of the wrist extensor is important because it can be harnessed with a special splint to induce finger flexion. He can push a wheelchair if it has special handgrasps. Although he still needs some help in dressing and transfer, he is able to participate to a greater degree. May be able to drive.
C–8	Quadriplegia (incomplete) Loss of motor control to parts of arms and hands Intact: some voluntary control of elbow extensors; wrist and finger extension may become stronger; may gain some use of finger flexors		Loss of sensation below chest and part of hands Intact: sensation to face, shoulders, arms, hands, and part of chest (C–8 supplies the little finger)	Same as above	Same as above	Able to do push-ups in wheelchair and can develop improved sitting tolerance. Can grasp and release hands voluntarily. This adds to independence in ADL as well as greatly increasing vocational possibilities. Independent in his wheelchair. With training can harness hand control for catheter irrigation and rectal stimulation for bowel movements
T–1 to T–6	Paraplegia Loss of everything below midchest, including trunk muscles Intact: control of function to shoulders, upper chest, arms, and hands		Loss of sensation from midchest downward, including lower limbs Intact: everything to midchest, including arms and hands (T–1 and T–2 supply inner aspect of arm; T–4 supplies the nipple area)	Phrenic nerve functions independently; some impairment of intercostal muscles; high thoracic injuries	Same as above	Full control of upper extremities and completely independent in wheelchair. Able to be employed full-time and live in a dwelling without major architectural barriers to wheelchair. Independent in managing his urinary drainage, inserting suppositories, and so forth

T-6 to T-12	Paraplegia Loss of motor control below waist Intact: shoulders, arms, hands, and long trunk muscles supporting torso		Loss of everything below waist Intact: shoulders, chest, arms, and hands (T-10 supplies the umbilicus) (T-12 supplies the groin area)	No interference with respiratory function	Same as above	In addition to all of the above, has complete abdominal, upper back, and respiratory control. Very good sitting balance, allowing greater ability for wheelchair operation and athletic activities
L-1 and L-2 L-1 to L-3	Paraplegia Loss of most of the control of legs and pelvis Intact: shoulders, arms, hands, torso, hip rotation and flexion and some flexion of legs	L-2 to L-4—Knee jerk	Loss of sensation to lower abdomen and legs Intact: all of the above, plus some sensation to inner and anterior surfaces of thigh (L-3 supplies the knee)	Same as above	Same as above	Lower lumbar transection Has all of the above abilities
L-3 to L-4	Paraplegia (incomplete) Loss of control of part of lower legs, ankles, and feet Intact: all of above, plus increased control of extension of knee		Loss of sensation to part of lower legs, feet, and ankles Intact: all of the above, plus sensation to upper legs	Same as above	Same as above	Voluntary control of hip extensors and abductors may be lacking to make walking with braces difficult but possible
	Paraplegia (incomplete) L-4, L-5, S-1 control dorsiflexion of the ankle L-5 to S-1 controls eversion of feet L-4 to S-1 controls abductors of hip, internal rotation of hip, and inversion of foot L-4 to S-2 controls knee flexion S-1 to S-2 controls plantar flexion of foot	S-1—Ankle jerk	Lumbar spinal nerves carry impulses generally from upper legs, and part of lower legs and feet. (L-5 supplies the medial aspect of the foot; S-1 supplies the lateral aspect; S-2 supplies posterior aspect of the calf and thigh) Sacral spinal nerves carry impulses from lower legs, feet, and perineum.	Same as above	May or may not be lost S-2 to S-4 controls urinary continence S-3 to S-5 controls bowel continence (perianal muscles)	Can walk with braces or may use wheelchair Can be relatively independent

5. Unstable, lowered blood pressure due to the loss of vasomotor tone
6. Loss of the ability to perspire below the level of injury
7. Bowel and bladder dysfunction
8. Possible priapism (abnormal, painful, and continuous erection of the penis due to disease) in the male

Spinal cord transection can also be partial. Sudden partial transection of the cord will result in immediate spinal shock in those areas transected. The following signs and symptoms of partial cord transection include

1. Flaccid paralysis (asymmetrical) of skeletal muscles below the level of injury
2. Loss of only those reflexes (asymmetric reflex loss) below the portion of the damaged cord
3. Some preservation of pain, temperature, proprioception, and the sensation of touch and pressure below the level of injury. (The paralyzed region is greater than the sensory loss. As with complete transections there may be heightened pain above the level.)
4. Some somatic and visceral sensations below the level of injury may be intact.
5. Less of a problem with vasomotor instability with less subsequent lowering of the blood pressure
6. Ability to perspire probably intact on one side of the body
7. Less bowel and bladder impairment
8. Possible priapism in the male

One should note that the degree of lost function in partial transections is less than that found with complete transections. The symptoms of spinal shock can also occur in portions of the cord that have been injured by causes other than transection, such as concussion, contusion, compression, laceration, hemorrhage, and damage to the blood supply.

Immediate Signs and Symptoms of Cervical Cord Injury. Injury to the cervical spinal cord is characterized by special life-threatening problems that include respiratory insufficiency, neurogenic shock, low body temperature, and possibly Horner's syndrome.

Respiratory Insufficiency. The diaphragm is innervated by C–1 to C–4. If a high cervical injury is sustained, the innervation to the diaphragm is affected and the patient will suffer a respiratory arrest and probably die immediately, If he is attended to immediately after injury, mechanical ventilation will be necessary. If the cord injury is below the innervation to the phrenic nerve and above the innervation to the intercostal muscles, diaphragmatic breathing will be noted. This patient will also need varying degrees of respiratory support.

Neurogenic Shock. Under normal conditions the sympathetic nervous system, which has its origins in the thoracolumbar region of the spinal cord, receives impulses from the brain stem. The input from the brain stem contributes to basic reflex control of vital signs through the cardiac accelerator and vasoconstriction reflexes.[5] With cervical cord injury the modulation of control from the higher centers is lost, and a condition called *neurogenic shock* results. Neurogenic shock is characterized by hypotension due to the vasodilation of the vascular beds below the level of injury, bradycardia due to the suppression of the cardiac accelerator reflex, and loss of the ability to sweat below the level of injury due to lack of innervation of the sweat glands. The patient's temperature tends to be lower than normal (96°F to 98°F) because of the break in the connection between the hypothalamus and the sympathetic nervous system. Body heat is lost by way of the passively dilated vascular bed of the skin.

Horner's Syndrome. If there is a partial cord injury at T–1 or above, Horner's syndrome may be seen. The signs and symptoms include ptosis, miosis, and anhidrosis on the side of the face on which the lesion is located. In addition to the signs and symptoms associated with cervical spinal cord mentioned above, those listed for complete or incomplete cord injury are also applicable. The patient who has sustained injury in the cervical region will be a quadriplegic if he survives. The higher the injury, the greater the functional loss.

Recovery From Spinal Shock. Spinal shock may last from a few days to months, depending on the severity of the injury; however, spinal shock usually lasts for 1 to 6 weeks after injury.

Recovery from spinal shock is a gradual process in which the spinal neurons slowly regain their excitability. Throughout the nervous system neurons that have lost the source of their facilitory impulses seem to compensate by increasing the degree of their own excitability.

Depending on the completeness of the cord transection, one of two possibilities will eventually occur. The first possibility is that the transmission of impulses will resume, resulting in the return of motor, sensory, reflex, and autonomic function below the level of injury. The second possibility is that the isolated cord segment, devoid of any suprasegmental control, will develop its own reflex activity. This autonomous neural activity is divided into a sequence of phases of variable lengths, including the following: (1) minimal reflex activity, (2) flexor spasm activity (superficial reflexes), (3) alteration between flexor and extensor spasm activities, and (4) predominant extensor spasm activity (deep reflexes).

Hyperreflexia. Stretch reflexes return first, followed by the more complex reflexes: the flexor reflexes return next, and lastly the antigravitational or extensor reflexes return. Reflex functions return from the toes to the head. At first, excessive stimulation is necessary to elicit a reflex; later, less intense stimuli, such as passively flexing the toes or merely touching the foot or leg, may be sufficient to evoke a violent flexion of the leg.

Spasticity. Sometimes the functional return is excessive, resulting in hyperactivity of all or most of the cord functions. (Whereas the patient's previous condition was called *flaccid paralysis*, this condition is now termed *spastic paralysis*.) The hyperactivity is particularly remarkable in those patients who have a few intact facilitory pathways between the brain and the cord while the remainder of the spinal cord is transected.

After 1 or 2 years, the patient may be placed in one of the following categories with respect to spastic activity:

1. Extensor spasms predominate over flexor spasms, which is called *paraplegia-in-extension* (accounts for about two thirds of patients)

2. Flexor spasms predominate over extensor spasms, which is called *paraplegia-in-flexion*
3. Flaccid paralysis persists (accounts for less than 20% of patients)

Paraplegia-in-flexion or paraplegia-in-extension occurs in both partial and complete transections. Paraplegia-in-extension often results from cord transections in the cervical region. Midthoracic transections usually result in paraplegia-in-flexion, while upper thoracic injuries can be of either variety.

A few special points should be made concerning cord transections. It is the sudden transection of the cord that results in the initial flaccid paralysis of spinal shock. Transections that occur slowly do not result in flaccid paralysis, instead, spastic paralysis develops slowly. Slow transections can be caused by a spinal cord tumor, syringomyelia, multiple sclerosis, and other slowly developing neurological diseases.

Complications. After recovery from spinal shock, various complications can develop depending on the type and level of injury. Examples of such problems include autonomic hyperreflexia, sexual dysfunction, bladder dysfunction, and autonomic dysfunctions. These topics and others will be discussed later in this chapter in the Postacute and Early Rehabilitation Phases section.

MANAGEMENT OF THE PATIENT WITH SPINAL CORD INJURY

DEVELOPMENT OF REGIONAL SPINAL CORD INJURY CENTERS (RSCIC)

The cost of caring for victims of spinal cord injury is estimated at $2.4 billion annually, a sum much higher than that of other neurological conditions. With ever-mounting costs of hospitalization, it was felt that new treatment methods that would result in better outcomes, be cost-effective, and provide for cost containment were needed. In response to this need Congress provided money through the Rehabilitation Services Administration for demonstration programs of model regional systems designed to improve the delivery of services to those affected by spinal cord injuries. The first project was funded in June of 1970; there are currently fourteen Regional Spinal Cord Injury Centers located throughout the United States. Common objectives shared by all of these programs include

1. Providing a focus of comprehensive rehabilitative services from point of injury through acute care to rehabilitation
2. Developing and evaluating improved equipment for initial care through rehabilitation
3. Improving treatment methods
4. Mobilizing community resources for positive integration of the patient into his community

Of the 10,000 new spinal cord injuries incurred yearly, only about 10% can be managed in the Regional Spinal Cord Injury Centers. Comparing the outcomes of patients managed in the centers with those managed in other facilities reveals some interesting differences. Patients treated at the centers have shorter initial hospitalization and rehabilitation admissions, and their treatment costs less than that of patients treated in other types of facilities. The aggressive, sophisticated treatment available at centers results in better functional recovery, decreasing the need for some types of services and improving the patient's level of independence. Because patients treated at regional centers have better multi-systems management and follow-up, they have fewer complications. Finally, patients managed in centers with a total approach to the management of the patient claim much better vocational, community, and rehabilitative adjustment rates. All of these factors translate into lower cost and better outcome for the patient.

In areas where there is a Regional Spinal Cord Injury Center, there must be a collaborative approach to patient management and triage involving emergency services and the area hospitals. Not all patients with a potential vertebral column injury are candidates for a regional center. A triage system designed to identify appropriate patients, stabilize their injuries, and provide for their rapid and safe transport to the regional center must be operational. Time is of the essence for ensuring optimal patient outcome. Depending on the distance of the victim from the center, transport may be by motor vehicle or helicopter; thus, highly specialized equipment and trained personnel must be available to participate in management of the patient.

For other spinal cord-injured patients who are not admitted to regional centers, the local acute-care community hospital is the usual site of management. After assessment and stabilization in the emergency department, the patient may be admitted to the intensive care unit, a neurological–neurosurgical unit, or a general medical–surgical unit. The setting chosen for management depends on the availability of resources and whether a neurosurgeon is on the staff.

In some instances, particularly when the injuries are numerous and the facility is small or without the services of a neurosurgeon, the patient may be transferred to a larger community hospital. Here acute-care management and early rehabilitation are begun, and community agencies are used to plan for long-term rehabilitation. After the initial hospitalization for acute care, the patient may remain for early rehabilitation or be transferred to a rehabilitation facility where an aggressive rehabilitation program is completed. Another option following acute and postacute care is transfer to a nursing home with a limited rehabilitation program. The plan for each patient must be individualized to his specific needs and matched to the services offered by various facilities.

PREHOSPITAL MANAGEMENT

The prehospital management is critical to the patient's ultimate neurological outcome. The basic objectives of management at the injury site include (1) rapid assessment to determine the extent of vertebral column or spinal cord injury, (2) immobilization and stabilization of the head and neck to prevent extension of injury, (3) extrication of the patient from the vehicle or injury site, (4) stabilization and control of any other life-threatening injuries, (5) triage to the appropriate facility, and (6) rapid and safe transport. The rescue personnel must be well trained because improper handling at the injury site can turn a minor vertebral column injury into a major irreversible spinal cord injury.

Until proven otherwise, each trauma patient should be treated as if he had a spinal cord injury. This rule applies to any patient with a head injury as well as to the inebriated trauma victim whose sensory and cognitive functions are impaired. Although patients may have multiple systems injuries, assessment of the multiple trauma patient is discussed in Chapter 16. The focus of this section is the prehospital management of the vertebral column or spinal cord-injured patient.

The Conscious Injured Patient

Assessment. In the conscious patient the following information can be gathered rapidly without moving him:

- Adequacy of respirations
- Presence of back or neck pain or tenderness
- Presence of neurological deficits as evidenced by absent or diminished sensory or motor function in the arms or legs
- Presence of an associated head injury as evidenced by an altered level of consciousness, content of verbal responses, or other signs and symptoms such as leakage of fluid from the ear or nose or contusions or lacerations of the head

The patient should be instructed not to move. The examiner should make no attempt to flex or rotate the patient's head, neck, or trunk.

Immobilization of the Head and Neck. After the patient has been assessed, his head and neck must be immobilized. Resist the temptation to straighten the head or neck. Immobilize the head and neck in the position in which the patient was found. For example, if the patient was found bent over the steering wheel, he should be kept in this flexed position. A collar is then applied, and towels or other materials may be used to maintain the position. If the patient was found sitting in a vehicle, a short spinal board can be slipped behind the patient while the head and neck are supported. The board will immobilize the upper back and neck. If the injury is lower, a splinting board can be applied to immobilize that portion of the back. The choice of splinting boards and site of application depend on the site of injury and the position in which the patient was found.

Extrication. The patient will finally be moved on a long splinting board and securely immobilized with straps and belts. The process of extrication requires the cooperative assistance of a few people to guide and protect all parts of the body from angulation and injury.

Stabilization and Control of Life-Threatening Injuries. The patient should be rapidly assessed again for the ABC's (airway, breathing, and circulation) of management. If there is any evidence of respiratory insufficiency, supportive therapy should be initiated. This may be the administration of oxygen by mask or the insertion of an endotracheal tube. If intubation is needed, it will have to be done blindly without flexion or hyperextension of the neck. Advice about the need for intubation and the method used should be quick. Hypotension, a rapid pulse, and cool clammy skin are signs of hypovolemic shock, which requires immediate treatment.

Triage. Guidelines based on an initial assessment of the patient should be established to direct the rescue personnel to the appropriate facility. If there is a Regional Spinal Cord Injury Center in the area, the criteria for admission and the transportation protocol should be followed. Transporting the patient to the appropriate facility saves precious time and improves patient outcomes.

Rapid and Safe Transport. The patient should be transported as soon as possible after he has has been well immobilized and stabilized. Transportation may be by land or air depending on the distance to the hospital and the resources available. If transportation is by land vehicle, the operator should drive slowly and avoid bumps, acceleration, and deceleration. These cautions are followed to prevent the extension of injuries. Unless there are life-threatening concurrent injuries, a speedy voyage to the hospital is not essential.

The Unconscious Injured Patient

Assessment. The unconscious patient should be carefully assessed for adequacy of respirations and other vital signs. High cord injuries may have caused injury to the phrenic nerve innervation or intercostal muscles. Respiratory function will need to be supported.

Particular care must be taken for the unconscious patient who cannot call attention to pain or weakness that might lead one to suspect spinal cord injuries. An abnormal position of the head or neck or any angulation of the back or spine is a suspicious sign that warrants careful physical and radiological examination. Subtle cues, such as the "body language" presented by the abnormal positioning or lack of spontaneous movement in one direction, may raise the suspicion of spinal injury. All unconscious head-injury patients should be moved with the utmost care until good lateral spine films can be taken, and spinal column injury can be ruled out.

Other. The other steps of immobilization, extrication, stabilization, triage, and transportion are followed as discussed for the conscious patient. Documentation of how the patient was found, initial assessment, treatment, and method of transportion should be included in the written and oral report submitted to the hospital. This information will be helpful in the evaluation of the patient.

EMERGENCY DEPARTMENT MANAGEMENT

Upon admission to the emergency department a report of the prehospital management and a history of the injury are collected rapidly. The patient is maintained on the splinting board until after x-rays of the spine are taken.

History of Accident

The history of the accident can be obtained from a variety of sources: possibly the patient, a family member, another accident victim, or rescue squad personnel. Information about the mechanism of the injury, neurological status of the patient immediately after injury, treatment at the accident site, and the mode of transport are all vital data. At the same time the following assessment is conducted.

Assessment

1. Adequacy of Respiratory Function. The airway is checked for patency and respirations are evaluated to determine if the diaphragm and intercostal muscles are functional. Skin color, nail beds, and earlobes are also checked as indications of proper oxygenation. If there is cervical injury and respiratory assistance is necessary, special techniques carried out by a specially trained anesthesiologist are necessary to prevent extension of the injury. A tracheostomy or an endotracheal tube may be necessary if an endotracheal tube is not already in place. Any injury compromising ventilation must be treated promptly and effectively.

2. Vital Sign Evaluation. Patients with spinal cord injuries (particularly those in the cervical region) may show signs of hypotension, bradycardia, and lowered body temperature. These are symptoms of spinal shock. The lowered blood pressure is due to vasodilation, which results from the loss of vasomotor tone below the level of injury. In most instances, treatment will not be necessary unless the hypotension is compounded by hemorrhagic shock. Adding blankets will usually control the lowered body temperature.

3. Evaluation of Other Organ Systems. Trauma patients frequently have multiple injuries, including intra-abdominal injury. The presence of tachycardia, in addition to lowered blood pressure and cool and clammy skin, should lead one to suspect visceral hemorrhage. A search for signs of intra-abdominal and/or intrathoracic injury should be conducted. Because of the lack of pain perception in these areas caused by cord injury, pain will not draw attention to the salient, life-threatening, ruptured viscera. Unless the injury is found and treated, the patient may not survive. To summarize, symptoms of two types of shock, spinal and hemorrhagic, can be present in the same patient simultaneously. Assessment must accurately identify the underlying cause, and appropriate treatment must be implemented.

4. Mini-Neurological Examination. A two-fold purpose is accomplished by the examination: first, an estimation of cord involvement is ascertained; and second, a baseline assessment is made so that future neurological examinations can be compared to its findings. The patient is also evaluated for possible head injury.

The physician in the emergency department conducts the neurological examination while the patient is immobilized on the splinting board. The examination focuses on determining the presence, absence, or diminished function of sensory, motor, and reflex systems. The highest level of function and any evidence of sparing should be noted. Obviously, a complete neurological assessment will not be possible at this time. However, a current assessment is collected and compared with prehospital findings to determine the scope of the patient's injuries. Another point of the neurological examination is to rule out head injury.

Other findings that point toward the possibility of spinal cord injury include the following:

- Angulation of the head and neck toward one side
- Local tenderness to palpation of the spinous processes
- Abnormal distance between spinous processes or lack of resistance to digital pressure over the space between them
- Priapism in the male
- Diaphragmatic breathing

5. General Health History. The following information is obtained by observation or inquiry:

1. Preexisting disease (emphysema, asthma, kidney, or liver disease)
2. Use of drugs (e.g., methyldopa [Aldomet], digitalis, alcohol, stimulants, warfarin [Coumadin])
3. Any known allergies
4. Any other injuries or problems missed on the initial assessment, such as long bone fractures, abdominal trauma, and so forth

6. Laboratory Studies. Laboratory studies should include baseline blood studies (such as electrolytes, blood sugar, hemoglobin and hematocrit, blood gases, and so forth), urinalysis, and other studies as indicated. Factors studied and the conditions associated with abnormal values in them follow:

- Electrolytes—electrolyte imbalance
- Glucose—hypoglycemia or hyperglycemia, possibly associated with insulin shock or diabetic coma
- Hemoglobin and hematocrit—blood loss due to hemorrhage
- Blood gases—insufficient oxygen–carbon dioxide exchange indicating a need for oxygen therapy, a tracheostomy, or respirator
- Urinalysis—contused kidneys as indicated by blood in the urine; kidney disease

7. Radiographic Examination. Anteroposterior and particularly lateral films of the spine and any other areas under suspicion should be taken. Every precaution should be used to prevent additional injury caused by moving the patient. This is a dangerous time when spinal cord injury may be extended owing to improper handling by inadequately trained personnel. If at all possible, a physician should accompany the patient in order to supervise the handling of the patient. (The spinal column is difficult to visualize with radiographic examination because of the normal bone irregularity. This is particularly true of the C–7 to T–1 level in obese or heavily muscled patients.) To visualize C–7 and T–1 it may be necessary to pull the patient's shoulders downward toward the foot of the bed while the radiographic examination is conducted. If these x-rays are not satisfactory, the swimmer's position may be necessary. The C–1 to C–2 level, and especially the odontoid process, can be difficult to visualize. In this instance, the x-rays must be taken with the patient's mouth open to visualize the odontoid process.

The physician must decide the specific type of radiographs necessary while considering the risk to the patient.

Summary. Although the discussion of the basic initial assessment in the emergency department has been lengthy, it takes but a few minutes to collect this information as a team in which the nurse participates. If the patient is conscious, he will need to be calmed and reassured in order to gain his cooperation.

Reassessment and Development of a Plan of Care

After the initial data have been collected and the x-rays read, the physician will know what injuries, if any, have been sustained. The patient is reassessed to be sure that nothing has been overlooked. Portions of the neurological examination that may have been deferred because the patient could not be moved may now be tested safely, depending on the x-rays. As mentioned in previous sections, if a cord injury has been sustained, it is important to determine whether the injury is complete or incomplete, and what the highest level of intact function is. Examining the patient for sacral sparing and other sparing is important.

The plan of management that the physician develops may include (1) immediate surgery for life-threatening injuries in other systems (e.g., intra-abdominal bleeding); (2) immediate surgery for decompression, alignment, or stabilization of the vertebral column; or (3) a nonsurgical approach with traction and immobilization. The use of drugs and adjunctive therapy such as spinal cooling may also be initiated.

Measures Initiated in the Emergency Department

In addition to the aforementioned activities, a few other measures may be initiated in the emergency department, including the insertion of a nasogastric tube and an indwelling urinary catheter. If steroid therapy is to be used, an initial dose will be given in the emergency department.

An acute paralytic ileus, which is characterized by the absence of normal peristalsis, abdominal distention, nausea, and vomiting, usually occurs with spinal cord injuries. A nasogastric tube is inserted and connected to suction to decompress the stomach and prevent vomiting, aspiration, and inhibition of free diaphragmatic movement. Paralytic ileus is not only a sign of spinal shock but also can indicate intra-abdominal injury. Normally the patient with an intra-abdominal injury will experience pain, but with a cord injury, the sensation of pain may be lost. Therefore, all parameters must be carefully assessed and reassessed.

The patient with a spinal cord injury and spinal shock will have an atonic bladder that will become overdistended. Urine may be retained and overflow and the bladder may be distended on palpation. An indwelling urinary catheter is inserted to manage the urinary output and prevent injury to the bladder from overdistention.

Steroid therapy is a controversial treatment protocol that may be given to reduce edema in the injured spinal cord. If the physician chooses to use this therapy, an initial dose is administered in the emergency department. An initial dose may be 10 mg of dexamethasone intravenously, followed by 4 mg every 4 hours for 7 to 10 days in tapering doses. Some physicians prefer to use a large loading dose such as 40 mg of dexamethasone followed by 10 mg every 4 to 6 hours in tapering doses for 7 to 10 days. The usual precautions for steroid use should be followed: administering an antacid to prevent gastric irritation or cimetidine to decrease gastric secretions and checking the gastric pH for excessive acidity, stools for occult blood, and urine for glucose.

An intravenous line is routinely inserted if one is not already in place. Depending on the patient's condition, invasive monitoring devices such as a Swan–Ganz tube may be inserted.

DIAGNOSIS

The diagnosis of vertebral column or spinal cord injury can be difficult because the shapes of the vertebrae are so highly irregular.

There may be special problems in visualization that make it necessary to order other diagnostic procedures. The overall diagnostic procedures include

- Physical examination
- Anteroposterior and lateral radiographs (special techniques may be necessary to visualize the C–1 to C–2 and C–7 to T–1 levels (these techniques have been described earlier in this chapter)
- CT scan
- Tomography
- Myelography

EARLY MANAGEMENT OF SPINAL CORD INJURIES

After the initial stabilization and assessment of the patient, he may be admitted to the intensive care unit or another unit for less acute patients.

Selection of Approach: Surgical or Nonsurgical

The basic goals of spinal cord injury management are decompression realignment, and stabilization.[16]

- Decompression of the spinal cord or spinal nerves prevents pain, loss or compromise of neurological function, and ischemia and necrosis to the involved tissue. Decompression can be achieved through the use of skeletal or skin traction or surgery. If surgery is chosen, a decompression laminectomy is done.
- Realignment of the vertebral column and supporting soft tissue is necessary for optimal function of the involved parts, and treatment is often associated with decompression man-

agement. Traction or surgery is possible depending on the type of problem. If the vertebral facets are locked, then surgical intervention will be necessary to align the vertebral column. In other instances, skeletal or skin traction or braces or casts will be effective modes of treatment.

- Stabilization of the spinal column can be accomplished by surgery or by spontaneous fusion during the natural healing process. Skeletal traction, a body cast, or immobilization in a hyperextended position promotes the natural healing process. These treatment methods can be used singularly or they can be combined with surgery to achieve the desired outcome. If surgery is used, a fusion or insertion of Harrington rods is usually planned.

The management of the patient will depend on the type of spinal cord injury and any associated injuries or health problems. Treatment may be surgical, nonsurgical, or a combination. The choice of treatment is based on the professional judgment of the physician after he weighs all data. This data may include the results of consultation with the neurosurgeon, orthopedic surgeon, pulmonary physician, urologist, or physiatrist. The evaluations of these specialists helps the physician who is in charge to maintain intact function and prevent complications and loss of rehabilitative potential.

Surgical Management of Spinal Cord Injuries

If surgery is planned, selecting the best time is critical. Early surgery—that is, within the first 12 to 24 hours—may be undertaken for the following reasons[16]:

1. Evidence of cord compression
2. Progressive neurological deficit
3. Compound fracture of the vertebra (bony fragments may dislodge and penetrate the cord)
4. Penetrating wounds of the spinal cord or surrounding structures
5. A bone fragment in the spinal canal

Early surgery may preserve, improve, or restore spinal cord function, but in order for the patient to tolerate surgery, all body systems must be stabilized, especially the respiratory and cardiovascular systems. Early surgery is contraindicated as outlined in the following circumstances:

1. No patient who has demonstrated rapid and significant improvement in neurological function should have surgery.
2. Surgery should not be performed on a patient if a life-threatening injury or disease exists elsewhere in the body. With severe trauma, the patient may have a head injury, kidney laceration, intestinal rupture, or other problems in addition to cord injury. Death would probably occur as a result of the added insult of general anesthesia and surgery.
3. Skilled personnel and necessary equipment must be available. If either is absent, surgery should not be performed unless the patient is transferred to a facility where both are available.

Types of Procedures. Surgery is the selected mode of stabilization when the physician determines that the nature of the injury requires this form of intervention. The following are among the more common procedures performed[16]:

1. Decompression laminectomies by anterior cervical and thoracic approaches with fusions
2. Posterior laminectomy using acrylic wire mesh and fusion
3. Harrington rods with the correction and stabilization of thoracic deformities

The specific surgical procedures including nursing care will be discussed in Chapter 19.

Nonsurgical Management of Spinal Cord Injuries

Immobilization of the vertebral column to achieve as normal an anatomical alignment as possible is a major concern in the nonsurgical management of the patient with a spinal cord injury. Vertebral subluxation with or without cord involvement is often managed with immobilization and traction.

Cervical Injuries

Immobilization of the cervical region for a cervical fracture is accomplished by means of skeletal traction. Cervical tongs (Vinke, Cone, Crutchfield) and the halo device are types of traction in common use. In either case a regular hospital bed may be used along with a bedboard and a firm mattress, although some physicians prefer using a Stryker or Foster frame or a Kinetic Treatment Table. Circular electric beds are not advocated because of the problems of axial loading and orthostatic hypotension. Shock blocks are usually placed under the head of the bed to provide countertraction.

An alternating pressure mattress may be used on the standard bed as a means of preventing the development of pressure areas. If this device is to be used, it must be checked to see that it is functional *before* the patient is placed upon it! Other pressure-sparing materials include a gel pad or sheepskin.

Although it appears barbaric at first glance, skeletal traction greatly facilitates and enhances patient comfort. Once the traction is operational, pain is greatly decreased. The traction relieves pain by separating and aligning the injured vertebrae and eliminates, or a least reduces, spasms in the distracted muscles. When in traction, the patient can be safely turned with a special technique to allow for skin care and changes in position.

Cervical Tongs (Gardner–Wells, Vinke, Cone, Crutchfield). Gardner–Wells tongs are spring-loaded cervical tongs that are easy to apply. The scalp is prepared with an antiseptic agent such as povidone-iodine (Betadine). It is not necessary to shave or incise the scalp although a local anesthetic is injected at the insertion site. The points of the tongs are applied to the skull immediately in front of the ears. The points are then advanced until the position of the spring-loaded points shows that the proper pressure is being exerted. Once this has been completed, the tongs are tilted back and forth to settle the points. Within 24 hours the tongs are stable so no further tightening should be initiated. Weights are now applied to reduce the fracture–dislocation.

The Vinke tongs are inserted along an imaginary line between the external auditory meatus and the transverse processes of the cervical vertebrae, well above the thin area of the temporal bone. The other types of tongs are inserted in similar fashion (Fig. 18–11). The area of insertion is shaved and prepped, and a local anesthetic is injected. A scalpel is used to make an incision to expose the bone. Since the scalp is very vascular, these minor incisions seem to produce much blood. A special drill is used to penetrate the outer bony table. The tongs are inserted securely. Sutures are used as necessary, and a dry, sterile dressing with polymyxin B (Neosporin) or nitrofurazone (Furacin) ointment is applied. The traction is added at the prescribed weight for reduction. Bedside radiographs are taken at frequent intervals to evaluate the fracture and the effectiveness of the reduction and alignment. Neurological examinations should be performed at prescribed intervals and the results compared with the results of other examinations to determine changes from the established baseline (Fig. 18–12).

The patient in cervical skeletal traction is examined radiologically at least every week to determine alignment and healing of the fracture. When the patient is deemed ready by the physician to shed his traction (after 6 to 8 weeks), he is fitted with a four-poster brace (Florida brace) to provide support and more immobilization. He can be ambulatory with this brace. After wearing this major support device for a few weeks (about 4 to 6 weeks), the patient is weaned to a hard collar and later a soft one. Eventually, he will no longer need the collar. Physical examination and radiographs are needed to guide the progress of this weaning process.

Specific Nursing Management of the Patient in Cervical Skeletal Traction. Chart 18–2 summarizes the major points of care to be followed for the patient in cervical skeletal traction.

The Halo Device. The halo device or apparatus is applied to the skull to provide skeletal fixation to the cervical region for treatment of a fracture–dislocation or subluxation.

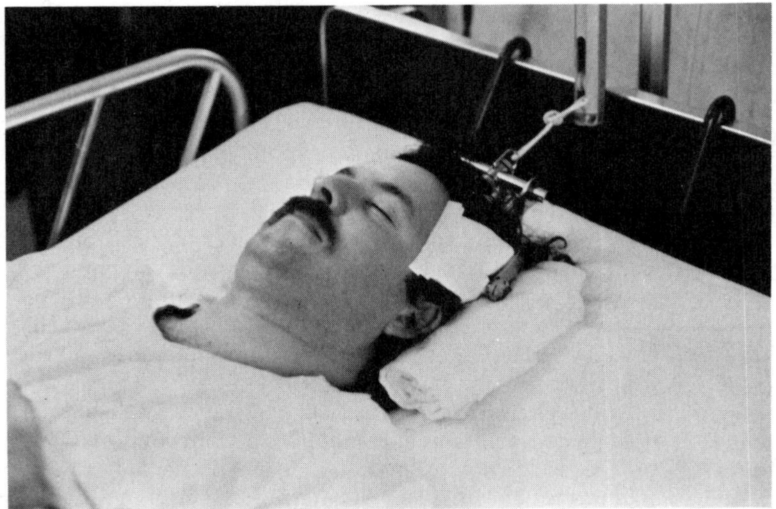

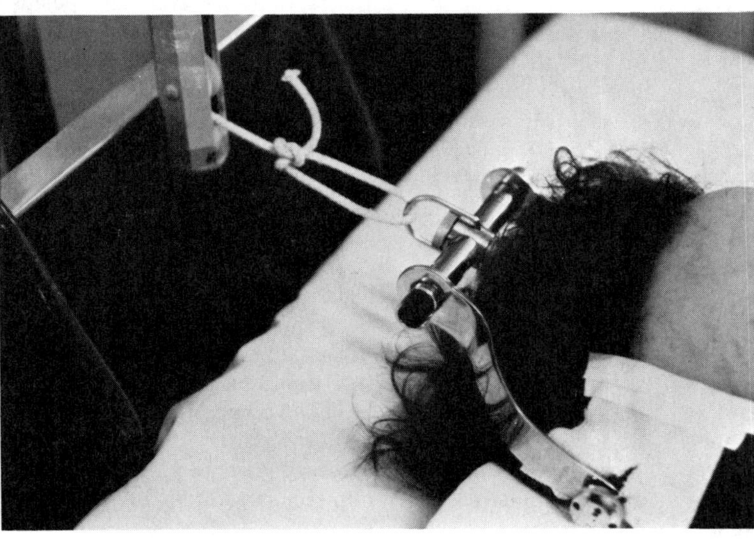

FIG. 18–11. Placement of Crutchfield tongs in the temporal bones. Note placement of dry, sterile dressing around tong site.

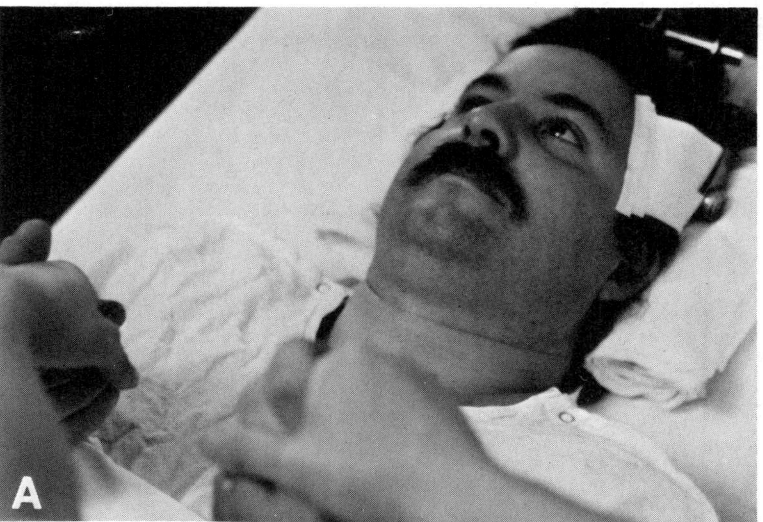

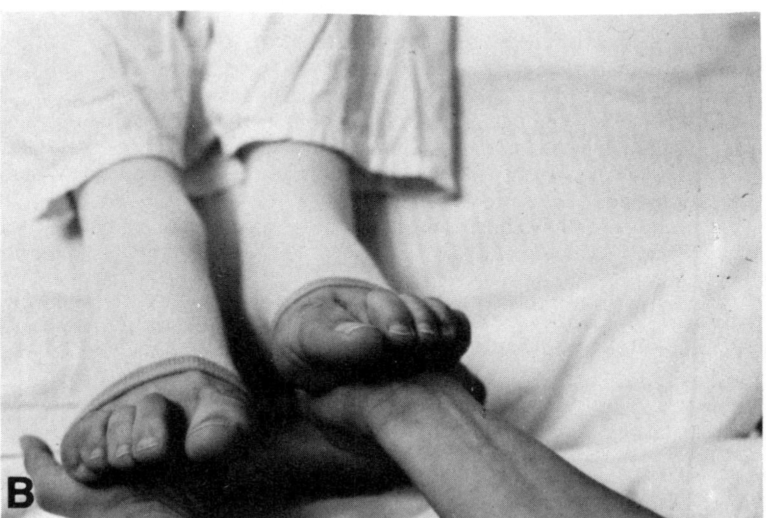

FIG. 18–12. Checking motor function in a patient in Crutchfield tongs by testing hand-grasping ability *(A)* and foot strength *(B)*.

There are two methods of using the halo device:

- It may be used as direct skeletal traction to which hanging weights are applied; the patient is maintained on complete bed rest and managed as a patient with Gardner–Wells, Vinke, or other tongs. See Chart 18–2 for special nursing measures.
- The halo device may also be incorporated with the use of a body vest or jacket to stabilize the spine, thereby allowing the patient to be ambulatory.

The halo device is applied under local anesthesia in what is considered a relatively simple procedure. Preprocedural preparation includes shampooing the hair and shaving the skin in the areas where the pins are to be inserted. The halo (metal ring) is attached to the skull by four pins—two posterior and two anterior—which are inserted into the external bony table of the cranium and connected to the fiberglass or plastic body jacket by adjustable steel rods. As mentioned previously, if direct traction with hanging weights is desired, a jacket would not be applied at this time. Small, dry, sterile dressings are placed around the pins.

One outstanding advantage of using the halo device for immobilization and fixation of the cervical region is that it allows a shorter period of hospitalization. If no paralysis exists, the patient is able to ambulate, thereby counteracting the multitude of potential problems associated with bed rest. The halo device with the jacket is beneficial in cervical and very high thoracic fractures.

It is interesting to note that surgery can be performed while the patient is in halo traction. This is advantageous because it is not necessary to risk malalignment of the injured area with possible infliction or extension of cord injury. This might be sustained if traction were removed. One should remember that the physician often applies skeletal traction prior to surgery to reduce the injury. When the best alignment possible is achieved, then surgery (usually spinal fusion) is scheduled.

The halo apparatus is fairly comfortable despite its bizarre appearance, although some headache is to be ex-

(Text continued on page 406.)

CHART 18–2. SUMMARY OF NURSING MANAGEMENT OF THE PATIENT IN CERVICAL SKELETAL TRACTION

The patient who is in cervical skeletal tongs is on complete bed rest and is totally dependent on the nurse for his every need.

NURSING RESPONSIBILITIES	RATIONALE
The Orthopedic Traction Equipment	
• Check the orthopedic frame and traction daily to make sure that nuts and bolts are secure.	• Ensures safety and integrity of the treatment
• Check the tongs daily to make sure that they are secure.	• Same as above
• Make certain that the traction weights are hanging freely and not resting on any object. Releasing the traction could be very dangerous because cord injury could be extended.	• Same as above
Meticulous Skin Care	
• Inspect the tong site and clean and dress as ordered (pin care). For example, a possible dressing procedure may call for the site to be washed with hydrogen peroxide followed by providone-iodine (Betadine) solution and dressed with a sterile dressing. Another possibility is for the area around the tong site to be washed with hydrogen peroxide and dressed with iodoform gauze.	• Prevents sepsis
• Turn the patient every 2 hours from side to back to other side. Use a triple log rolling technique as described below.	• Helps prevent hypostatic pneumonia and other pulmonary complications as well as preventing pressure sores
• Inspect every square inch of skin for redness, irritation, or breakdown.	• Provides for early identification of skin irritation and breakdown
Turning the Patient at Frequent Intervals	
Steps for Triple Log-Rolling Technique (Fig. 18–13)	
1. One nurse stands behind the head of the bed and places hands firmly on head and neck, being careful not to flex the head and neck.	• Keeps the vertebral column in neutral position to prevent extension of injury to the spinal cord, soft tissue, or vertebra
2. The second nurse is responsible for moving the patient's shoulders.	
3. The third nurse is responsible for moving the patient's hips and legs.	
4. Be sure to explain procedure to the patient *before* you begin.	
5. Be sure to plan ahead, identify the desired position, and place pillows or other equipment in position.	
6. When all three nurses are in position, the patient is turned on the count of three to the desired position. He is turned as a log to maintain proper alignment.	
7. Make sure that the patient is in the middle of the bed. If he is not, he will be uncomfortable. Adjust carefully. Leave patient in good body alignment.	
8. The nurse who moves the head and neck should keep her hands in place until the patient is supported properly with pillows. If the traction slips, she should provide manual traction until help arrives.	

CHART 18–2. (continued)

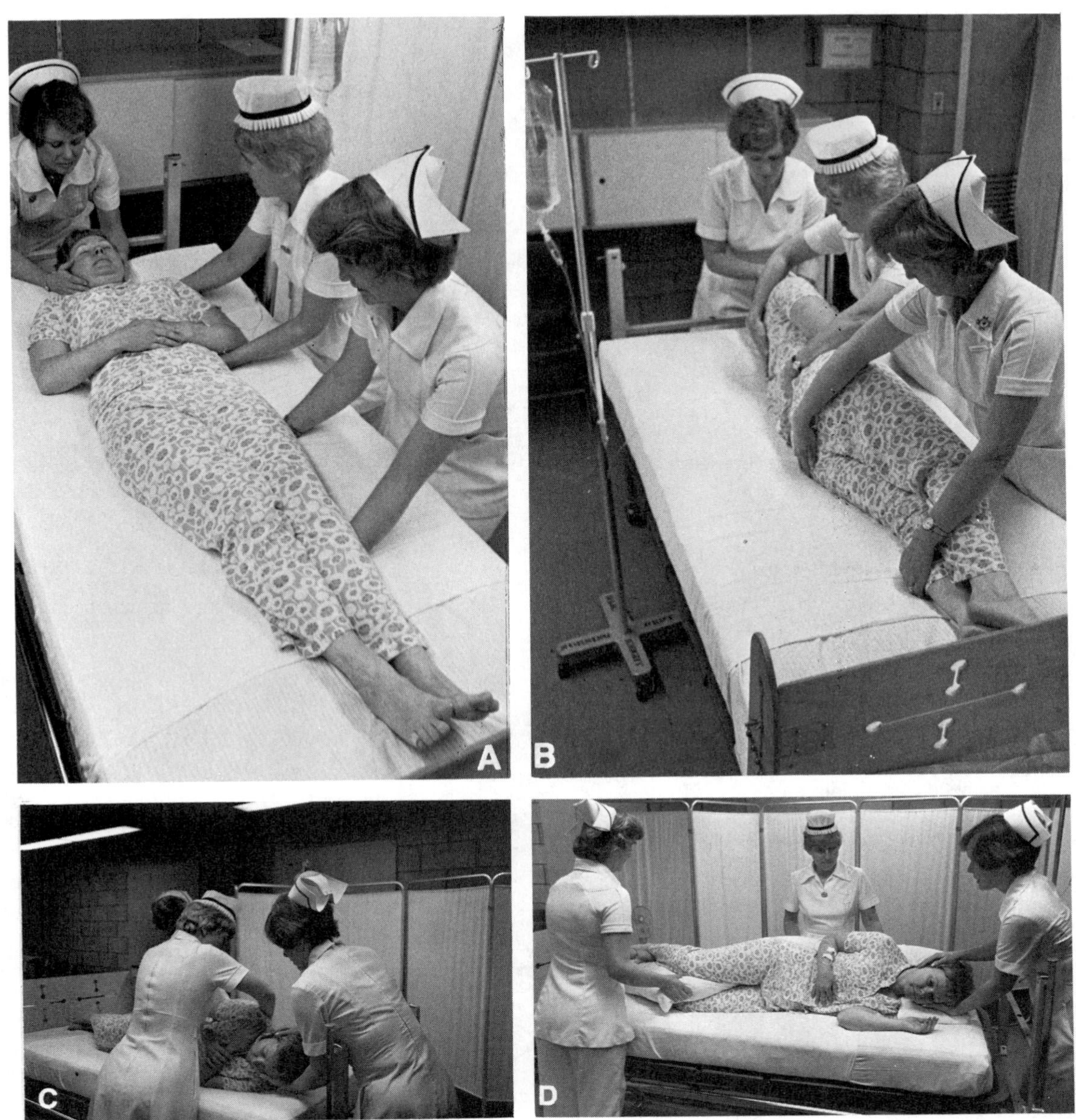

FIG. 18–13. Turning the patient as a triple log roll. *(A)* With patient in the middle of the bed, the three nurses assume their positions. (Note: All pillows and extraneous materials have been removed.) *(B)* At the count of three, the patient is turned to the desired side of the bed. *(C)* With the patient on the side, the two nurses continue to hold the patient in position while the third nurse begins to place pillows to support the patient. (Note: Depending on the weight and height of the patient, as well as the height of the nurses, it may be more comfortable for the nurses responsible for the shoulders and hips to turn from the same side of the bed as seen in *B*. Another possibility is that the nurse responsible for the shoulders moves to the side of the bed where the patient will be turned. At the same time, the nurse responsible for the hips and legs remains on the opposite side of the bed (see *C* and *D*). *(D)* The patient is placed in proper body alignment with the help of pillows. Note that one pillow begins at the top of the patient's head supporting the head, neck, and upper back. Another pillow will be necessary to support the middle and lower back: The nurse responsible for the head continues to hold the head and neck. Another nurse has placed a small pillow or folded bath blanket under the head and neck to prevent angulation of the neck.

(continued)

CHART 18–2. (continued)

NURSING RESPONSIBILITIES	RATIONALE
Assessment Data	
Neurological Signs	
The neurological examination includes the assessment of	
• Level of consciousness • Pupillary signs • Eye movement • Motor function (hand-grasping ability and arm strength; foot strength) (see Fig. 18–11) • Sensory function (reaction to pinprick) • Cranial nerve check • Note the highest level of motor and sensory function	• Establishes a baseline against which subsequent assessments can be compared to denote change
Vital Signs	
Vital signs should be monitored at frequent intervals.	• Establishes a baseline against which subsequent assessments can be compared to denote change and development of complications
Laboratory Data	
Various laboratory studies should be monitored such as • Complete blood count • Electrolytes • Blood gases • Urinalysis • Urine culture and sensitivity • Coagulation studies • Others as necessary or indicated	• Monitors basic parameters for development of complications
Basic Hygienic Care (as Necessary)	
The patient shold be allowed and encouraged to be as independent as possible. The nurse should provide care that the patient is unable to provide for himself.	• Promotes cleanliness and well-being; allows the patient to be independent and in control of some aspects of his life

The following information is directed at prevention of complications in the various body systems. See the section in this chapter entitled "Effects of Cord Injury on the Body Systems: Problems, Complications, and Management."

NURSING RESPONSIBILITIES	RATIONALE
Respiratory Care	
• Maintain a patent airway at all times.	• Provides for adequate oxygenation
• Have suction available at all times.	• Maintains patency of airway
• If patient is able to eat, teach him to take small bites and chew well. Suction should be available and in working order.	• Prevents aspiration
• Provide for deep breathing exercises frequently (may be required hourly).	• Expand lungs and aids in the prevention of complications
• Observe the rate, rhythm, and characteristics of the respiratory pattern for abnormalities; note presence of cyanosis, abdominal breathing, and other indications of inadequate respirations.	• Identifies signs and symptoms of respiratory difficulty
• Auscultate chest at least every shift.	• Allows early identification of the development of atelectasis, pneumonia, and other respiratory complications
• Administer chest physiotherapy at least once every 8 hours (patient may require more frequent therapy depending on his condition).	• Prevents development of respiratory complications and loosens any secretions already present

CHART 18–2. (continued)

NURSING RESPONSIBILITIES	RATIONALE

Cardiovascular Care

NURSING RESPONSIBILITIES	RATIONALE
• Inspect legs and intravenous sites for development of thrombophlebitis and deep vein thrombosis.	• Allows early identification of the development of a potentially life-threatening problem (pulmonary emboli)
• If patient is to receive mini-doses of heparin, administer as ordered and report daily coagulation studies to physician for possible adjustment of dosage.	• Mini-doses of heparin are sometimes ordered prophylactically to prevent development of thrombi. It is necessary to monitor the coagulation studies to maintain a therapeutic blood level.
• If patient is receiving heparin, observe for signs and symptoms of bleeding (occult blood in stools, urine, bleeding from gums, bruising easily).	• Allows early identification of untoward side-effects
• Apply elastic stockings or Ace bandages to the legs and ensure that patient wears them at all times.	• Improves blood return to the heart thus helping to prevent complications (deep vein thrombosis, thrombophlebitis)
• Provide range-of-motion exercises to extremities at least four times a day.	• Improves circulation and maintains muscle tone

Neurological Care

If the patient has cord injury, spinal shock may still be present. Autonomic hyperreflexia will not be a problem while the patient is in traction. As the spinal shock begins to recede, spasticity will become an increasing problem. There may also be pain at or slightly above the site of injury.

NURSING RESPONSIBILITIES	RATIONALE
• Administer analgesics as necessary.	• Provides for comfort
• When spasticity develops, position frequently; see detailed section in this chapter on spasticity.	• Prevents contractures and other complications of spasticity

Musculoskeletal Care

NURSING RESPONSIBILITIES	RATIONALE
• Provide for range-of-motion exercises to all of the extremities at least four times a day.	• Maintains muscle tone and full range of motion of extremities
• Ensure that a physiotherapy consultation and bedside physiotherapy have been ordered.	• Same as above; other exercises may be ordered as necessary such as heel cord stretching
• Position the patient in proper body alignment at least every 2 hours; use pillows, rolls, and other devices to ensure proper position.	• Prevents malalignment problems such as footdrop

Genitourinary Care

NURSING RESPONSIBILITIES	RATIONALE
• Monitor frequency, amount, and character of urinary drainage.	• Early identification of abnormalities
• Monitor frequent urinalysis and urine culture.	• Same as above
• Maintain an intake and output record.	• Same as above
• Provide for adequate fluid intake.	• Provides for flushing of the kidney
• If catheter is in place, prevent traction on the meatus by pinning catheter properly.	• Prevents traction on the meatus
• Assess for bladder retraining as soon as feasible after spinal shock has dissipated.	• Decreases the possibility of infection and other complications
• If patient is receiving steroids, check urine for sugar and acetone.	• Glucosuria is a side-effect of steroid therapy.

Gastrointestinal Care

NURSING RESPONSIBILITIES	RATIONALE
• Auscultate abdomen for bowel sounds.	• Indicates the presence of peristalsis; patient is able to manage feedings if peristalsis is present
• Record frequency and consistency of bowel movements.	• Monitors patient to prevent constipation and impaction
• Provide a bowel program as needed.	• Provides for regular bowel evacuation

(continued)

CHART 18–2. (continued)

NURSING RESPONSIBILITIES	RATIONALE
Nutrition	
• Provide for adequate nutrition just as soon as peristalsis has been reestablished; a nutritional consultation should be suggested.	• Maintains adequate nutrition for maintenance and repair of body tissue
Emotional–Psychological Care	
• Be sensitive to the emotional and psychological response of the patient to his injury; see section in this chapter and Chapter 7.	• Supports patient emotionally and psychologically as he deals with the impact of his injury and the prescribed sensory deficits and immobility resulting from his condition

pected. In addition, any sounds caused by bumping the halo can result in annoying vibrations. Rubber tips added to the pins reduce this problem. Patients in the halo device with femoral pins can be turned.

Specific Nursing Management of the Patient in a Halo Device With a Fiberglass Vest or Jacket. Chart 18–3 summarizes the major points of care to be followed for the patient in a halo device with a fiberglass vest or jacket. If the halo device is connected to direct traction with weights, the points of care to be followed are similar to those for the Gardner–Wells, Vinke, or other traction, with the addition of "pin care," which is found in Chart 18–2.

Thoracic and Lumbar Injuries

When a patient sustains a thoracic or lumbar fracture or fracture–dislocation, various treatment protocols are possible, depending of the specific type of injury. If surgery is indicated, procedures frequently performed include laminectomy with or without a fusion and insertion of Harrington rods or another stabilizing device. To maintain thoracic or lumbar alignment as an adjunct after surgery or as the only management protocol for the injury, the following may be used:

- A fiberglass or plastic body jacket may be applied (the jacket, which is fitted to the patient, provides immobilization and support to the injured area).
- A canvas corset may be applied.
- A Jewett brace extends the spinal column (provides support to the lower thoracic and lumbar region).
- Other specially designed braces may be ordered.

The patient may also be placed on prolonged bed rest in the hyperextended position to allow for healing of an aligned fracture. This treatment is used very infrequently because other more effective methods are now available.

The nursing care of the patient centers on good skin care, frequent inspection of the skin for signs of irritation, proper application and care of the brace or support jacket, assessment of neurological and vital signs, and maintenance of adequate respiratory function.

Sacral and Coccygeal Injuries

The usual treatment of sacral and coccygeal fractures is bed rest. The affected area is supported by a low girdle or special brace. A rubber ring can provide relief from pain and discomfort in the supine position. Pain is increased by sitting on a hard surface, which is therefore avoided. The patient should be evaluated for bowel and bladder dysfunction.

Length of Nonsurgical Management

The nonsurigcal management, in most cases, represents the initial mode of treatment until the patient is able to undergo surgical intervention. This treatment may be all that can be done when severe injuries involving other body systems make the patient a poor surgical risk.

Patients who have sustained cervical fracture or dislocation have traditionally been treated by prolonged immobilization with skeletal traction for approximately 6 to 8 weeks. Some physicians still adhere to this method of treatment. However, this entire area of treatment is changing rapidly to include early spinal fusion that permits mobilization of the patient after a short period of bed rest and traction. The major advantage of this approach is that it reduces the possibility of the many complications of prolonged bed rest, both physical and psychological.

EFFECTS OF CORD INJURY ON THE BODY SYSTEMS AND FUNCTIONS: PROBLEMS, COMPLICATIONS, AND MANAGEMENT

RESPIRATORY SYSTEM

A patient with a spinal cord injury can develop varying degrees of respiratory difficulty depending on the level of the spinal lesion and the groups of respiratory muscles par-

CHART 18-3. SUMMARY OF NURSING MANAGEMENT OF THE PATIENT IN A HALO DEVICE WITH A FIBERGLASS VEST OR JACKET

The patient who is in a halo device with a fiberglass body vest or jacket will remain on bed rest until he has recovered from the procedure. If the patient has had cervical spine surgery, the bed rest may be extended to ensure stability of the spine.

NURSING RESPONSIBILITIES	RATIONALE
Management of the Halo Device and the Body Jacket	
• Check pins on halo traction to be sure they are secure and tight.	• Ensures safety and integrity of the treatment
• Check edges of fiberglass jacket for comfort and fit by inserting small finger or index finger between the jacket and the patient's skin. If the jacket is too tight, skin breakdown, edema, and possible nerve injury can occur.	• Provides for comfort and prevents skin irritation
• The jacket should be supported while the patient is in bed.	• Maintains proper body alignment
• Place rubber cork over the tips of the halo device to diminish magnification of sound if the pin is bumped.	• Provides for comfort
Meticulous Skin Care	
• Pin site is inspected, cleansed, and dressed once or twice daily as prescribed to prevent infection at the pin site.	• Prevents sepsis
• While in bed the patient is turned every 2 hours by means of the triple log rolling technique to prevent the development of hypostatic pneumonia, atelectasis, and skin breakdown.	• Maintains proper body alignment and prevents injury
• Sponge pads should be provided to prevent pressure on prominent body areas such as the forehead and shoulder while the patient is in bed.	• Prevents injury and irritation to the skin
• All exposed areas of skin should be inspected, lubricated, and kept dry.	• Early identification of skin irritation or breakdown
Altered Body Image	
• Help the patient adjust to the distorted body image that the halo device can create.	• Provides emotional support
Control of Pain: Comfort	
• Administer mild analgesics to control headache and discomfort around pin site, which are common.	• Provides for comfort
• Provide a soft diet since many patients have jaw pain if they attempt to chew.	• Provides for comfort
Basic Hygienic Care	
• Allow the patient to do as much of his care for himself as possible.	• Maintains his independence and supports his self-esteem
Support of Body Systems	
• Maintain intake and output record.	• Provides information on urinary tract function and adequacy of fluid intake
• Provide for a bowel program.	• Prevents constipation and maintains a normal pattern of bowel evacuation
• Provide for range-of-motion exercises for all extremities.	• Maintains muscle tone
• Provide for deep breathing exercises at least four times a day.	• Encourages overinflation of the lungs and prevents infections and atelectasis
• Apply elastic stockings or Ace bandages to the legs to improve blood return to the heart.	• Decreases the possibility of thrombus or embolus formation
• Observe the legs for development of thrombophlebitis or deep vein thrombosis.	• Early identification of potential problems so that treatment can be initiated

(continued)

CHART 18–3. (continued)

NURSING RESPONSIBILITIES	RATIONALE
Assessment Data	
• Monitor neurological signs at frequent intervals.	• Establishes a baseline and denotes change
• Monitor vital signs at frequent intervals.	• Same as above
• Monitor laboratory data.	• Denotes deviation from normal and development of complications
Ambulation	
If the patient has intact neurological function, he will be able to ambulate in the halo device and jacket.	
• Start to slowly assess the patient's tolerance in the upright position by having him sit on the edge of the bed ("dangle"). Check vital signs. (Orthostatic hypotension may be an initial problem to overcome in the early stages.)	• Prevents development of untoward side-effects
• Teach the patient to compensate for the lost head and neck movement by making increased use of eye movement to scan the area.	• Provides for safety needs
• Accompany the patient when he ambulates because he is more accident-prone due to his displaced center of gravity, loss of balance, and decreased peripheral vision.	• Same as above
• Consider the patient's use of a walker for ambulation as a means of support and greater safety.	• Same as above
Patient Teaching	
• If the patient is to go home with the halo and jacket in place, begin a patient and family teaching plan.	• Provides for safety and independence

alyzed. A cervical injury in which the function of the diaphragm and intercostal muscles is compromised results in major respiratory disability. Even with the lowest of spinal injuries, one can experience minor deficits in respiratory functions.[8]

After adequate ventilation is established following emergency room care, baseline pulmonary function studies, blood gases, and other laboratory studies are reviewed to define proper management. If mechanical ventilation has been employed, the mode, volumes, flows, and oxygen tension are carefully assessed.[9]

A patient who has a cervical cord injury and must undergo anesthesia and surgery is prone to postoperative pulmonary complications. If surgery is elected, careful consideration should be given to the optimal time for the procedure—when the respiratory system is in the best condition possible.

A patient who cannot cough or manage his own secretions needs a special program to cope with this difficulty. Accumulation of secretions leads to atelectasis, infections, and respiratory failure. Immobilization and injury to the breathing neuromusculature reduces the patient's ability to breathe independently and adequately.

The probability of certain pulmonary complications decreases the lower the injury is on the spinal column because the innervation to the diaphragm and intercostal muscles is spared. The most common respiratory complications that the nurse must consider include respiratory arrest, respiratory insufficiency, bronchial obstruction, pneumonia, atelectasis, pulmonary emboli, and tension pneumothorax, if the patient is on a ventilator.

Assessment Data

In assessing the respiratory system, the following data are considered: chest x-ray, pulmonary function studies, vital capacity, blood gases, complete blood count, other tests as indicated, respiratory pattern (rate, rhythm, depth, character of respirations), chest auscultation, and ventilator settings (mode, volumes, flows, and oxygen tension).

Nursing Management

All patients require an aggressive, comprehensive program of respiratory care to prevent pulmonary complications. This program should include a regimen of intermittent positive pressure breathing, breathing exercises, and assisted coughing and drainage techniques. Points of care include the following:

- Suction equipment to maintain a patent airway should be at hand. Excess secretions must be removed to ensure patency and prevent infection. Another reason for maintaining suction equipment at hand is the tendency of patients in recumbent positions to choke on food and secretions.
- For a patient with a tracheostomy, "trach" care should be given every 4 hours to assure a patent airway. (See specifics of "trach" care in Chap. 11.)
- To avoid choking, the patient should be instructed to take small sips and swallow frequently when taking anything orally. If the patient starts to choke, he must *not* be lifted and tapped on the back.
- Coughing and deep breathing should be encouraged every 1 to 2 hours to prevent atelectasis and pneumonia. Because all the patient's respiratory muscles may not be functioning, it may be necessary to assist the patient in coughing.
- It is necessary to observe the patient for signs of respiratory impairment. Signs of improper ventilation include dyspnea, cyanosis, and lack of chest expansion. These symptoms must be reported immediately and aggressive treatment initiated to treat the underlying etiology.
- Intermittent positive pressure breathing (IPPB) treatments should be carried out, if prescribed, to help liquefy secretions and improve respiratory function.
- Vital capacity may be measured periodically at the bedside since this measurement is an important indication of respiratory function.
- See Chapter 11 for the management of a patient on a ventilator.
- Provide periodic chest physiotherapy.
- Turn the patient at least every 2 hours to prevent pooling of secretions.
- Provide for periodic deep breathing exercises or Ambu technique for ventilator patients to expand all areas of the lungs.
- If a Kinetic Treatment Table is ordered, adapt nursing care to this therapy (it is used to decrease respiratory complications).

Postacute and Long-Term Management

Patients dependent on mechanical respiratory equipment are weaned off these devices as soon as possible. Pulmonary studies are done as necessary to evaluate and plan for the long-term management, which varies depending on the level of the lesion and the specific problems of the patient. Pulmonary studies of cervically injured patients have repeatedly demonstrated the following:

- Lower volumes of air exchange in tidal volumes
- Decreased movement of chest with each respiration
- Decrease of forced expiratory volume (forced expiration after a normal exhalation)
- Reduced responsiveness to chemical stimuli for respiration resulting in chronic alveolar hypoventilation

Use of the Diaphragm Pacer

The diaphragm pacer, also called the phrenic nerve stimulator, has been used for some respirator-dependent patients (patients with a high cord injury). Patients are selected for this newer approach based on their ability to take a few breaths on their own even though the breaths are not sufficient to maintain adequate respirations. Electrodes are surgically implanted bilaterally over the phrenic nerve innervation to the diaphragm. About 2 weeks later, an activator is attached to the electrodes. The patient gradually develops a tolerance to the pacer that allows him to be off the respirator for varying periods. As with a cardiac pacemaker, the implanted electrodes must be replaced periodically.

Patient Teaching

Long-term management requires that the patient and family be instructed to optimize intact function and compensate, as best as possible, for functional loss. Some of the principles of long-term management are carry overs from acute management. The long-term pulmonary teaching plan for patient and family includes

- Respiratory care and suctioning techniques
- Use of the intermittent positive pressure equipment
- Breathing exercises
- Assisted coughing
- Postural drainage techniques

Proper teaching and adherence to the outlined program will prevent major pulmonary complications in most patients. Lifetime management of the respiratory tract, as with all other systems, is necessary for prevention and maintenance of respiratory integrity.

CARDIOVASCULAR SYSTEM

With spinal cord injury, particularly if the cervical cord is involved, the loss of impulses from the higher brain centers deprives sympathetic input to various functions. Bradycardia and vasomotor paralysis with resulting vasodilation of the blood vessels below the level of injury are lost. If blood has been lost because of other injuries, the blood volume decreases and the viscosity of the blood increases. Immobility increases the possibility of vascular stasis while decreasing the blood return to the heart. The major complications that involve the cardiovascular system are cardiac arrhythmias, cardiac arrest, thrombophlebitis, deep vein thrombosis, pulmonary emboli, and orthostatic hypotension.

Assessment Data

The following should be reviewed on an ongoing basis: electrolytes (especially potassium for evidence of hypokalemia), electrocardiograms, blood coagulation studies, vital signs, and response to elevation of the head of the bed (for signs and symptoms of orthostatic hypotension). Continual cardiac monitoring should be employed and the patient should be examined regularly for signs and symptoms of thrombophlebitis.

Special Conditions

Cardiac Arrhythmias and Cardiac Arrest. A low potassium blood level can cause arrhythmias. Initially the electrolytes are monitored at least daily. Deviation from normal limits should be brought to the attention of the physician. If hypokalemia is present, replacement therapy with potassium will be necessary. Since the patient with spinal shock will not have impulses for cardioacceleration, the pulse rate will be low (bradycardia). Excessive vagal stimulation, especially when suctioning, can lead to cardiac arrest; therefore, excessive vagal stimulation that is evidenced by adverse affects should be avoided. The patient with a cervical injury should be monitored on a cardiac monitor for 7 to 10 days after admission to identify any life-threatening arrhythmias.

Nursing Management. Various nursing responsibilities are necessary to preserve adequate cardiac function. In summary, nursing management for controlling cardiac arrhythmias and arrest includes the following:

- Note the electrolytes, especially the potassium, on at least a daily basis; report low or high readings to the physician; administer replacement therapy if ordered; continue to monitor the electrolytes.
- Prevent excessive vagal stimulation especially when suctioning.
- Keep the patient on a continual cardiac monitor for the first 7 to 10 days after admission to determine the presence of life-threatening arrhythmias.
- In most instances the bradycardia will not need to be treated; however, in extenuating circumstances when the heart rate is extremely low the physician may choose to order medication.
- Monitor the vital signs at frequent intervals.

Thrombophlebitis, Deep Vein Thrombosis, and Pulmonary Emboli. Thrombophlebitis with or without embolism is not an uncommon complication in patients with spinal cord injuries. Between 15% and 20% of patients develop deep vein thrombosis. About 5% to 15% of this group develop pulmonary embolism. This problem usually occurs within 3 months of the injury. Immobilization and paralysis contribute to the development of thrombophlebitis.

Anticoagulant drugs (heparin sodium [Heparin] or warfarin [Coumadin]), because of the side-effect of bleeding, must be used cautiously. Some physicians have used low doses of heparin sodium (heparin, 5,000 to 7,500 units every 12 hours subcutaneously) as a prophylactic measure with good results. If pulmonary embolism occurs, it must be treated aggressively. Because prolonged bed rest and vasomotor paralysis (vasodilation of arterioles) below the level of injury increases the possibility of vascular stasis and the development of complications, measures must be taken to increase the return of blood to the heart.

Nursing Management. Various nursing actions and responsibilities are necessary to prevent the development of these potentially life-threatening complications. In summary, nursing management to control for thrombophlebitis, deep vein thrombosis, and pulmonary emboli includes the following:

- Inspect intravenous sites and the legs for the development of thrombophlebitis every 8 hours. Signs of possible thrombophlebitis include
  —Redness
  —Warmth when touched
  —Tenderness to touch
  —Local swelling
  —Red streaking upward on extremity
- Provide for passive range-of-motion exercises as a preventive measure.
- Apply thigh-high elastic stockings or Ace bandages to improve the return of blood to the heart and improve resistance to the veins.
- If ordered, use a Kinetic Treatment Table to help to prevent vascular problems.
- If ordered, administer prophylactic doses (or "mini-doses") of heparin; monitor appropriate blood coagulation studies.
- Give intravenous heparin on a continual basis; run it at the proper rate and check it frequently or administer it at a preset rate using a volume control pump or other machine; notify the physician of the daily PT or PTT blood studies so that the heparin dose can be adjusted.
- Observe for signs and symptoms of bleeding (in stools, urine); note whether the patient bruises easily or has nosebleeds, which are signs of overuse of anticoagulants (heparin) and should be reported to the physician at once.

Orthostatic Hypotension. Immediately after cord injury the blood pressure tends to be unstable and lowered. After 1 or 2 weeks, it gradually rises until it is stabilized at a reading that corresponds to the preinjury norm for the patient. However, problems of orthostatic hypotension can impede the rehabilitative process because the patient cannot be raised in bed or assume the erect position.

Orthostatic hypotension is defined as a rapid drop in blood pressure when the erect position is assumed. Because the blood supply to the brain is inadequate, syncope results. Brain damage and even death can result if the condition is not rectified. This condition is seen in patients who have been bedridden and have not been in the upright position for a prolonged period. It is especially marked in patients who have had a lumbar sympathectomy or those who are paraplegics or quadriplegics.

Physiologically, because of the interruption in the descending central axons controlling vasopressor and cardiac reflexes, there is a profound drop in blood pressure when the patient is placed upright. The systolic pressure drops as low as 40 mm Hg and the diastolic pressure to 0 mm Hg. The drop in the arterial blood pressure is due to the dilation of the blood vessels in the abdomen and the lower extremities under the weight of the volume of blood that accumulates in the lower portions of the body when the patient is upright. Orthostatic hypotension is seen particularly in cord-injured patients with lesions above the T–7 level. Even slightly raising the head of the bed for a quadriplegic patient can result in a drastic lowering of the blood pressure.

Nursing Management. Measures must be employed to counteract orthostatic hypotension so that the patient can proceed with his rehabilitation program.

- Vital signs must be monitored before and after the head of the bed is raised.
- Vasopressor drugs may be ordered to treat the vasodilation.
- Ace bandages, elastic stockings, or an abdominal binder may be ordered to improve the return of blood to the heart.
- When it is permissible to raise the head of the bed or prepare a patient for sitting or ambulation, the process must be car-

ried out gradually and the pulse and blood pressure monitored throughout. Any signs of dizziness or light-headedness should be noted and reported. Frequently a tilt table is used to help the patient gradually assume an upright position.

NERVOUS SYSTEM

In general, any patient who is on prolonged bed rest, regardless of the medical reason, will develop decreased sensory and motor function from lack of stimulation. The patient with a cord injury is subject to this general reaction, in addition to the effects of direct insult to the nervous system.

In the acute stage of cord injury, the devastating effects of the spinal cord injury are apparent. Spinal shock temporarily prevents certain higher level impulses from influencing the cord. However, when spinal shock ceases, a few problems may develop. One problem is autonomic hyperreflexia, which may occur in patients with injuries at T-6 or above; the other problem is pain, which can occur in any patient.

Assessment Data

The data base for diagnosis includes signs and symptoms of autonomic hyperreflexia and subjective symptoms of pain.

Autonomic Hyperreflexia

Autonomic hyperreflexia or autonomic dysreflexia represents a very serious emergency in the rehabilitative phase of the patient with a spinal cord injury. It is characterized by paroxysmal hypertension. Systolic levels can reach as high as 240 mm to 300 mm Hg. Signs and symptoms are pounding headache, vasodilation, flushing, profuse sweating, piloerection above the level of the lesion, nasal congestion, nausea, and possible chest pain. Without reversal of these symptoms, status epilepticus, stroke, and death are possible.

Autonomic hyperreflexia occurs only in patients who have cord injuries above the T-6 level. Not all patients with this type of injury will develop this problem. The problem is not seen until spinal shock has been reversed and reflex activity has returned.

Pathophysiology. The sources of the autonomic nervous system, composed of the sympathetic and parasympathetic systems, are found in the cerebrum, hypothalamus, medulla, brain stem, and spinal cord. Their function is to maintain homeostasis in the body. Large portions of the sympathetic nervous system often become stimulated simultaneously, a phenomenon called *mass discharge.*[7] In contrast, most reflexes of the parasympathetic system are very specific. Signals from the hypothalamus and the cerebrum can affect the activities of almost all of the lower brain stem autonomic control centers. The cord activity is, in turn, controlled by these higher centers. With spinal injury the cord activity below the injury is deprived of the ameliorating effects from the higher regions, and poorly controlled responses result.

Autonomic hyperreflexia results when inhibited sympathetic discharges from below the spinal lesion are elicited by noxious agents stimulating sensory receptors.[10] These discharges, mediated by the spinothalamic tract and the posterior columns, lead to reflex stimulation of the sympathetic nervous system. This causes spasms of the pelvic viscera and the arterioles, causing vasoconstriction *below* the level of injury. Hypertension results, which is sensed by baroreceptors in the aortic arch and carotid sinus. This leads to superficial vasodilation, flushing, profuse sweating, and piloerection (gooseflesh) *above* the level of the lesion. Afferent impulses, generated by high blood pressure, are sent to the vasomotor center of the medulla, and bradycardia develops by way of the vagus nerve. Efferent impulses sent by way of the vagus nerve stimulate the S-A node, directing it to slow down. Ordinarily, the vagus nerve would also send impulses to the constricted blood vessels, forcing them to dilate, but because the cord has been severed, effector organs cannot be reached. The sweating that accompanies autonomic hyperreflexia in patients with upper thoracic and cervical lesions is a prominent feature and represents an outstanding and unique aspect of the autonomic phenomenon.

The mechanism is triggered by a noxious stimuli, most frequently from a distended bladder, caused by a plugged catheter or a spastic sphincter. Other noxious stimuli include constipation or fecal impaction, urinary calculi or severe bladder infection, acute abdominal problems, operative incisions, uterine contractions of labor in the pregnant woman, pressure on the glans penis, and stimulation from skin lesions such as inguinal rash, pressure sores, or ingrown toenails.

Management. Treatment is directed toward the removal of the noxious stimuli. The urinary catheter should be checked for patency and can be irrigated with no more than 30 ml of normal saline, instilled very slowly. If it still will not drain, the catheter should be replaced. Instillation of 30 ml of a 0.25% solution of tetracaine (Pontocaine) into the bladder for 20 minutes has been used in some centers. This is done after the catheter has been drained and the elevated blood pressure has begun to subside.

If the noxious stimulus is from the lower colon, no attempt to disimpact or insert a rectal suppository should be initiated without first applying dibucaine hydrochloride (Nupercaine) ointment to the anus and into the rectum for a distance of 2.54 cm (1 inch). Failure to follow this protocol will result in aggravation of the already-dangerous autonomic response.

If a pressure sore is the triggering mechanism, then it may be sprayed with a topical anesthetic agent.

Nursing Management. The essence of nursing management is directed at preventing the triggering mechanisms by checking the patient for constipation, the possibility of fecal impaction, plugging of the urinary catheter, and any signs of urinary tract infections. Any signs of autonomic hyperreflexia should be reported immediately.

Drug Therapy. Pharmacological intervention may be necessary if the noxious stimuli cannot be removed. The following list includes drugs used for the treatment of autonomic hyperreflexia. Frequent vital signs should be taken to monitor changes in vital signs, regardless of which drug is ordered.

Diazoxide (Hyperstat) may be used for sudden, acute hyperreflexia in the adult. A dose of 300 mg is given by rapid intravenous injection. This dose may be repeated in 3 hours, if necessary. If the blood pressure is not reduced, the administration may have been too slow or the dose too small.

Hydralazine (Apresoline) acts on the smooth muscle of the arterioles and is also classified as a beta adrenergic antagonist. The average dose is 20 mg administered slowly by intravenous push. Blood pressure is monitored to determine if half of the dose has had an effect. If it has not, the remainder of the drug should be given slowly. Since there is the possibility of sudden hypotension, intravenous metaraminol bitartrate (Aramine) intravenous should be available.

Sodium nitroprusside (Nipride) acts directly on the smooth muscle of both arterioles and venous vessels. The blood pressure decreases immediately with no increase in venous return. The drug is given intravenously, 50 mg in 500 ml of 5% dextrose in water. The rate of flow is 0.5 μg to 8 μg/kg/minute.

Ganglionic blocking agents have also been used and include phenoxybenzamine (Dibenzyline), guanethidine sulfate (Ismelin), and mecamylamine (Inversine). Special precautions suggested by the manufacturer should be followed.

Some drugs are suggested for long-term management to prevent autonomic hyperreflexia in the prone patient and include methantheline (Banthine), propantheline (Probanthine), and oxybutynin (Ditropan).

Patient Teaching. It is imperative that patients with cord injury above T-6 be well versed in the causes, symptoms, and treatment of autonomic hyperreflexia. The family also needs specific information, as do those professionals involved in providing health care. A written form should be given to the patient outlining the pertinent information. The nurse should assume the responsibility for patient teaching about this problem.

Pain

Initially, a patient may experience pain at the level of injury although there is anesthesia below the level of injury. As spinal shock resolves, some sensations may become apparent if the lesion is incomplete. These sensations range from mild tingling to severe, intractable pain. Pain may be caused by the scar tissue of surgery or gunshot wounds. It may also be caused by nerve root irritation, in which case the pain tends to diminish or disappear. Pain caused by scar tissue or sympathetic pain, a phenomenon similar to phantom pain, can be much more incapacitating. Methods used to treat severe pain include nerve blocks, nerve stimulators, hypnosis, and biofeedback, although none have been totally successful for long-range management.

Along with pain, paresthesias and hyperesthesias may be a source of discomfort for some patients with spinal cord injury. *Paresthesias* are unusual, annoying sensations (e.g., burning, tingling) along a nerve root. Some patients describe these sensations as pain. These sensations tend to disappear with time although some patients benefit from hypnosis. *Hyperesthesia* is an increased sensitivity of certain areas of the body that may or may not be uncomfortable to the patient. There may be a band of increased sensitivity at or just below the level of the lesion. If the sensation is bothersome to the patient, various treatment methods may be used to relieve the discomfort.

INTEGUMENTARY SYSTEM (SKIN)

Decubitus Ulcers

Decubitus ulcers are among the most common complications that occur with spinal cord injuries. Many factors contribute to the vulnerability of the patient. Patients with cord injuries are usually on bed rest for prolonged periods. Since they cannot position themselves because of paralysis, they are absolutely dependent on the nursing staff to turn and position them. This should be done at least every 2 hours. The patient should be positioned in proper body alignment.

Another contributing factor is the change in the vasomotor tone. Vasodilation tends to allow pooling of fluid in the tissue, thereby inreasing its susceptibility to injury with minimal pressure. Under these circumstances, pressure sores tend to develop rapidly. Once they have developed, they are extremely difficult to heal. Successful treatment is as difficult as with those skin ulcers seen in diabetic patients. With large pressure sores there can be systemic septic absorption from the ulcerative area, resulting in an overall deterioration of the patient's physical condition. Therefore, the key word is prevention. Not only are these ulcers a problem in themselves, but they can also retard the rehabilitative process by months. After all, how can a patient be taught to use a wheelchair when he has a decubitus ulcer on his sacral region? The ulcer must be healed before mobility training can proceed.

Assessment Data. Frequent assessment of the skin for reddened or broken areas is the best source of information about the skin.

Nursing management. Skin care, in general, is a paramount part of nursing management of these patients and should include the following measures:

- Turn the patient every 2 hours around the clock, and then massage any bony prominences or pressure points (back of head, ears, scapula, iliac crest, femur, knees, ankles, and so forth).
- Back care should be given every 2 to 4 hours.
- Every square inch of the patient's skin should be checked every 8 hours to ensure that no pressure areas are developing.
- If a reddened area is noted, it must be massaged well and relieved of pressure. Skin may be painted with tincture of benzoin for added resiliency.
- Lubricate the skin as necessary.

- If the skin is broken anywhere, then the area should be relieved of pressure by keeping the patient off that area.
- The skin must be kept meticulously clean and dry.
- The heels should not be allowed to rest against the bed. Placing a pillow under the lower legs will raise the heels off the bed; however, care must be taken to make sure that the pillow does not cause pressure in the popliteal area of the knee.
- The bed linen must be free of wrinkles and crumbs.
- If a Kinetic Treatment Table is ordered, adapt nursing care as necessary (the table is used to decrease pressure on the skin by continuous movement); use other devices such as an alternating mattress to relieve pressure on the skin.

MUSCULOSKELETAL SYSTEM

Much has been written about the effects of prolonged immobility on the musculoskeletal system. Table 18–2 indicates the initial and advanced changes of bones, joints, and muscles from prolonged immobilization.

As soon as the patient is stabilized after admission, the physiatrist from the rehabilitative medicine department should evaluate the patient to determine his rehabilitative potential and to design an individualized plan of physical therapy.

Assessment Data

The baseline assessment data include a thorough evaluation of the neuromuscular function by the physiatrist or physiotherapist. The nurse will also notice changes as she administers care on a daily basis.

Nursing Management

Nursing measures should be followed to protect the musculoskeletal system as part of routine nursing care:

- Body alignment and repositioning should be checked every 2 hours in conjunction with turning and skin care. This will protect against musculoskeletal deformities such as contractures, ankylosis, and so forth.
- A variety of "props" (pillows, rolls, footboards, and so forth) should be used to maintain good body alignment.
- Range-of-motion exercises should be started as soon as possible and carried out at least four times daily in conjunction with turning and skin care.

TABLE 18–2. *Musculoskeletal Changes Caused by Prolonged Immobilization*

	Initial	*Advanced*
Bone	Skeletal malalignment, loss of calcium	Skeletal deformities and generalized osteoporosis, which can result in an increased amount of cavities and pathological fractures
Joints	Joint stiffness, shortening or stretching of ligaments	Ankylosis
Muscles	Muscle weakness, shortening or stretching of muscles	Muscle atrophy, fibrotic changes, and muscle contractures

Spasticity

After spinal shock has resolved, spasticity develops. Spasticity of the muscles is one of the most incapacitating complications of paraplegia and quadriplegia. These disabling flexor and/or extensor spasms below the level of the lesion interfere with the rehabilitative process.

Spasticity is defined as a state of increased tonus in a weak muscle. Initial increased resistance to passive stretching is followed by sudden relaxation. Associated with spasticity is an exaggeration of deep tendon reflexes and a partial or complete loss of voluntary control. There can be spasms in response to an apparent stimulus or to a stimulus that is not obvious. The latter are called *pseudospontaneous spasms*. Slight touching of the skin can cause an exaggerated response. The following incident illustrates this point: A patient with a cervical cord lesion cautioned those standing at the foot of his bed to step back, because even a slight jarring of the bed provided enough stimulus to precipitate spasticity and a "kick in the face" to the unsuspecting bystander.

The "clasp-knife" analogy has been used in explaining spasticity; the action of the muscles is compared to the "catch" and "give" of a spring-loaded knife blade. Through the initial phase of passive movement on a spastic limb, there is palpable resistance to stretching, as with the opening of the knife blade. Toward the end phase, abrupt loss of muscle resistance occurs, with the muscle completely submitting to the movement, similar to the final phase of the blade action. The term *"clasp-knife" reaction* is derived from this. These characteristics of spasticity are explained to distinguish it from rigidity, with which it is frequently confused.

Spasticity results from hypersensitive protective reflexes, which result from an imbalance of facilitory and inhibitory effects on the gamma efferent neurons. In a cord injury, the distal segment of the cord (below the level of injury) is isolated from the higher inhibitory centers of the brain; thus, the facilitory impulses, entering the spinal cord from the muscles, ligaments, and skin, predominate.

A majority of patients with spinal cord injuries experience spasticity to some degree during the course of their disability. Spasticity can occur from a few weeks (4 to 6) to several months (7 to 8) after cord injury. Muscles are flaccid during spinal shock but develop spasticity with recovery. The height of spasticity in most patients is said to occur approximately 1½ to 2 years after injury. After this period, there is a gradual regression of the spasticity.

Management. Management of spasticity is directed toward prevention of further complications from such effects as contractures, muscle atrophy, urinary tract infections, and pressure sores. It is interesting to note that pressure sores and urinary tract infection, while possibly resulting from spasticity, can also intensify it. This happens because the noxious stimuli from these conditions produce volleys of afferent impulses to the distal cord, and these, in turn increase the degree of spasticity. Cold, fatigue, muscle tightness, and staying in one position for a prolonged period are also precipitating factors that trigger spasms in susceptible individuals. Controlling these factors is helpful in eliminating or moderating spasticity.

The major management approaches used to treat spasticity are pharmacological, medical, and surgical.

Pharmacological Approach. The most widely used drugs for the treatment of spasticity are diazepam, baclofen, and dantrolene sodium. The choice of drug depends on the type of cord injury and the patient's response to the drug. Diazepam (Valium), 2 mg to 10 mg by mouth three or four times a day, is used for its muscle-relaxant effects. Long-term use, however, can cause dependency.

Baclofen (Lioresal), 15 mg to 80 mg in divided doses daily, is a newer antispasmodic drug. The drug appears to be effective in both complete and incomplete spinal injuries but should be used cautiously in impaired renal function, stroke, or epilepsy. It should be administered with a meal to prevent gastric distress. Drowsiness is a common side-effect.

Dantrolene sodium (Dantrium), a skeletal muscle relaxant, is a new drug that has been effective in spasticity control in some patients. The patient should be started on low but gradually increasing doses. The dosage range is from 25 mg three times a day/to 200 mg four times a day. The long-term side-effects have not been established, but there is evidence of liver toxicity; therefore, any patient on this drug should undergo routine liver studies. Drowsiness, vertigo, and general weakness also have been noted.

Medical Approach. Medical management of spasticity includes the application of cold and heat, vibration, biofeedback, relaxation therapy, electrical stimulators, and physiotherapy (passive range-of-motion exercises, heel stretching, and so forth). Another approach to treatment, chemical blocking with alcohol or phenol, administered intrathecally or directly into the peripheral nerve, has been used; however, the relief is temporary and an effect on a specific muscle is difficult to achieve.

Surgical Approach. Surgical procedures to treat spasticity are numerous: tenotomies, myotomies, muscle transplants, peripheral neurectomies, and rhizotomies have all been tried. A surgical intervention such as a rhizotomy should be weighed carefully, since there can be interference with automatic bladder evacuation and reflex erection in males.[11]

Percutaneous radiofrequency thermal selective sensory rhizotomy is a newer method which holds some promise for the treatment of spasticity. This procedure destroys small, unmyelinated sensory fibers that carry noxious stimuli.[12] The larger myelinated motor fibers remain intact. Thermal lesions are created by using a thermal needle at 90° C for 2 minutes. The advantage of this procedure is alleged to be the reduction or complete abolishment of spasms without compromising bladder, bowel, or sexual function. Disadvantages include weakness and anesthesia in the affected area. Anesthesia can contribute to development of injury, since the protective mechanism of pain is absent.

Nursing Management. The major role in managing the day-to-day problems of spasticity belongs to the nurse. The initial appearance of spasticity can be a false ray of hope for the patient. The "movement" noted is often misinterpreted by the patient or family as a return of normal voluntary function rather than a heightened reflex response. Spasticity must be explained clearly and concisely to prevent any misunderstanding of its significance.

Management of spasticity by the nurse includes various nursing actions and procedures directed at preventing, controlling, or reducing spasticity while limiting debilitating effects and complications such as contractures, decubitus ulcers, and bowel and bladder dysfunction. The major nursing problems encountered on a day-to-day basis are the difficulty of positioning the patient and his lack of mobility. Since flexor spasticity develops first, the patient's extremities assume a flexed position. The development of contractures further compounds the problems of positioning.

Several nursing considerations and responsibilities are helpful and include the following:

- Provide passive range-of-motion exercises at least four times a day; stiffness increases spasticity.
- Prevent the development of contractures; flexor spasticity and contractures gravely limit the patient's ability to participate in activities of daily living; he is left lying in bed in the fetal position.
- In touching the patient, limit the amount of tactile stimuli; be gentle, yet firm and steady.
- Avoid circumstances that precipitate noxious stimuli known to increase spasticity (e.g., extremes in temperature, remaining in one position for an extended period, anxiety, pain, bladder or bowel distention, tight clothing or equipment, decubitus ulcers).
- Assume an unhurried manner when working with the patient; allow plenty of time for transfer activities, ambulation, dressing, and so forth.
- Turn and reposition at least every 2 hours; prevent rubbing or irritation of skin.

A sudden increase in spasticity should be viewed as a sign of an underlying cause that is precipitating noxious stimuli. Examples of underlying causes include a kink in the urinary drainage, fecal impaction, a skin abrasion or decubitus ulcer, and stiffness. The nurse and the patient must identify and treat the underlying cause promptly.

Patient Teaching. All of the points listed under nursing management should be taught to the patient. He must understand that these measures will help him improve the quality of his life.

Neurogenic Heterotopic Ossification

Neurogenic heterotopic ossification is seen in the first few months after spinal cord injury. It is defined as osteogenesis in a part of the body that does not normally form bone as soft tissue. The etiology is unknown. About 30% of patients with severe neurological disorders are affected by this anomaly, which is more common in quadriplegics than in paraplegics and occurs more often in spastic disorders than in flaccid ones.

Neurogenic heterotopic ossification is always found below the level of the spinal cord injury in neurologically impaired areas. The most common area of involvement is the hip, followed by the knee and the shoulder.

Signs and symptoms include the following: (1) swelling, either localized or involving the entire extremity; (2) redness and warmth; (3) decreased range of motion; (4) increased alkaline phosphatase; and (5) radiographic evidence of osseous formation. Radiographic evidence is not noted until 3 or 4 weeks after signs (1) through (3) appear.

No definitive treatment exists for neurogenic heterotopic ossification. If ankylosis occurs and limits the patient's joint movement to a sufficient degree, surgery is indicated.

GENITOURINARY SYSTEM

Immediately after spinal cord injury there is a period of spinal shock, during which all reflex activity and motor and sensory functions are lost below the level of injury. Therefore, bladder tone and control from the higher centers of the brain are missing—a condition described as *atonic bladder.* A catheter is inserted to prevent bladder damage. Many physicians start the patient on continuous bladder irrigations to prevent infection; others may select an intermittent catheterization program. After a period of 4 to 6 weeks, there is a gradual return of reflex function as spinal shock diminishes, and the bladder converts to "spastic."

Additional problems include urinary stones and urinary tract infections. The cord-injured patient, as is the case with any patient who does not bear weight, loses calcium from his bones and may develop osteoporosis. Since calcium leaves the body by way of the urinary tract, stone formation is probable, particularly if the urine is alkaline. (An exception is gouty stones, which form in acidic urine.) The use of internal acidifiers (e.g., vitamin C) is therefore indicated for these patients.

Urinary tract infection is a very serious problem because it can lead to renal disease, one of the chief causes of death in long-term management of these patients. Use of prophylactic sulfa drugs such as sulfisoxazole (Gantrisin) is also part of many urinary tract protocols.

Assessment Data

Routine periodic urinalysis and urine tested for culture, sensitivity, and colony count are basic sources of information about the urinary tract. The blood urea nitrogen (BUN) and creatinine levels give some indication of kidney function. If there appears to be abnormal function of the urinary tract, an intravenous pyelogram (IVP) and x-ray films of the kidneys, ureters, and bladder (KUB) will be taken. Based on the findings, other tests can be ordered. The basic diagnostic procedures for assessing bladder function are cystometric studies, which enable the physician to determine the amount of urine that the bladder can hold before a feeling of fullness is perceived and the amount of urine that must be present before the bladder empties. Cystometric studies are ordered after spinal shock has resolved and before a bladder training program is begun.

Other assessment data include color, odor, and character of the urine; intake and output record; and the voiding pattern (amount at each voiding, frequency of voiding).

Nursing Management

General nursing measures related to the urinary system include

- The maintenance of an accurate intake and output record to provide quantitative data on hydration and excretory function
- The forcing of fluids to ensure an intake of 3000 ml/24 hours (necessary to prevent formation of urinary tract calculi)
- The observation of the character of the urine, including concentration, sediment, and so forth with respect to hydration and possible urinary tract infection
- Catheter care twice daily to prevent infection, including
  - —Meticulous perineal washing
  - —Application of a bactericidal or bacteriostatic agent such as povidone-iodine (Betadine) ointment to the urinary meatus
  - —Pinning or taping of the catheter to prevent irritation traction on the meatus

The guidelines for prevention of urinary infection include

- Careful aseptic technique during the catheter phase
- An individualized bladder training program
- Dietary modifications to include copious amounts of fluid
- If intermittent catheterization is used, bladder fullness should be checked periodically to prevent damage to the bladder musculature from overdistention and to protect against hydronephrosis and possible triggering of autonomic hyperreflexia.
- To prevent traction and irritation to the meatus, the catheter should be taped properly: in males, the catheter is taped to the lower abdomen; in females, to the inner thigh. (Traction on the catheter can lead to a fistula.)

General Bladder Training in Spinal Cord Injuries

Although bladder training will not be successful with all patients, each patient should be assessed to determine his potential for success. Regardless of the type of bladder deficit, the goals are similar even though the methods of training are different. See Chapter 8 for a detailed discussion of bladder retraining.

Bladder training is usually initiated in the post-acute phase of the illness. To increase the possibility of successful bladder training, the urinary tract must be maintained in the best possible condition during the acute phase. This is accomplished by careful aseptic attention to the catheter, which represents a potential source of infection and trauma.

A urinary antiseptic such as methenamine mandelate (Mandelamine) is given. A urine pH of 5.5 must be maintained for the drug to be effective; therefore, a urinary acidifier such as vitamin C is also prescribed. The average adult dose is 1 gm to 2 gm, 4 times daily. The patient is instructed about the necessity for large amounts of liquid intake (3000 ml to 5000 ml/24-hour period). Because cranberry juice and apple juice are urine acidifiers, they should be consumed. (Vitamin C must be incorporated into the pharmacological plan for most patients since one would have to drink 2½ quarts of cranberry or apple juice daily to acidify the urine). Milk and dairy products are limited to control the formation of urinary calculi.

As rehabilitation proceeds, the patient's bladder function is evaluated by scheduling cystometric studies. Baseline data are established and plans are outlined based on the individual needs of the patient. The practice of clamping and releasing the catheter with gradually increasing frequency is used by some institutions to improve bladder tone. This must be a gradual procedure, beginning with 1 hour and increasing the time until the bladder will hold 300 ml to 400 ml of urine. By stepwise implementation of the process, bladder spasms are prevented and bladder tone is improved. When the bladder can accommodate 300 ml to 400 ml of urine, the catheter is removed for a trial voiding. Two weeks may be necessary to achieve control. It should be mentioned that other institutions disapprove of the clamping procedure because some believe that it increases the incidence of acute urinary infection.

The optimal time in terms of the patient's physical and emotional readiness is selected for removing the catheter and evaluating voiding.

GASTROINTESTINAL SYSTEM (BOWEL FUNCTION)

Most cord-injured patients are able to regain bowel control with an appropriate bowel training program. The large bowel musculature has its own neural center within the intestinal wall that responds to distention caused by the fecal contents. Dietary intake and digestive activities from the upper intestinal tract also influence bowel evacuation. There can be reflex expulsion as in the infant, or defecation can be postponed by the conscious voluntary inhibition of the reflex. At the appropriate time and place, the bowel can be evacuated by voluntary relaxation of the rectal sphincter and contraction of the abdominal and pelvic muscles.

The neural innervation, located in the lower intestinal wall, is usually not greatly affected by cord injury. The disabilities of neurological injury on bowel evacuation include

1. Loss of the sensation of fullness in the lower bowel
2. Loss of awareness of bowel evacuation
3. Loss of the ability to control the rectal sphincter
4. Loss of the ability to contract the abdominal muscles and to expel the stool

These points are important to note because nursing care will be directed toward helping the patient find alternate ways of creating conditions conducive to bowel evacuation.

Most people have a bowel movement about every 1 to 3 days, frequently after a meal. If the bowel is evacuated routinely, then the possibility of spontaneous defecation is greatly reduced. Defecation should be made as normal as possible. To use the abdominal muscles and diaphragm, the patient should be in a comfortable position with his feet flat on the floor. When the abdominal muscles are impaired, he may be taught to exert pressure on the abdomen with his hands, or an abdominal belt may be suggested for a patient who just cannot strain at stool.

It is important to prevent constipation and fecal impaction for many reasons. Such a problem could trigger autonomic hyperreflexia and aggravate spasticity. A well-balanced diet that is high in roughage and sufficient fluid intake help to forestall the problem by producing a soft stool and stimulating peristalsis. Medications, such as stool softeners, bulk producers, and lubricants are also helpful. Mild cathartics and suppositories may be ordered. Digital dilation may be recommended. If these methods are not successful, then a mild enema of limited fluid content can be administered.

A final important consideration is that selected body rhythms, also known as circadian rhythms, can be effectively utilized to help achieve bowel evacuation at predictable times. For example, the stimulus for defecation commonly occurs after breakfast because food is a stimulus for peristalsis, and peristalsis aids in moving the gastrointestinal contents. The gastrocolic reflex responsible for strong contractions and peristalsis in the gastrointestinal tract can be initiated by feeding the patient warm fluids and food at any time of the day. Therefore, planning for bowel evacuation and retraining immediately after breakfast capitalizes on normal body rhythms.

Bowel training must be a planned activity and must be individually designed. The cooperation of the patient, nurse, and physician is necessary for successful outcomes. Patience and an optimistic attitude on the part of the nurse are necessary to provide a climate for success. See Chapter 8 for a discussion of bowel retraining.

SEXUALITY

While sexuality and sexual adjustment should be an integral part of the patient's overall rehabilitation, this basic need has been a grossly neglected part of patient management. Health personnel have skirted this loaded issue by assuming that somehow the patient has been "neutered" by his injury or is too concerned with other health problems to care about sex. The truth is that sex, as a basic need, is a concern to all human beings. Gratification of one's sexual needs covers a wide range of behaviors and attitudes and is important to that particular individual.

Sexual function is controlled by spinal levels S-2, S-3, and S-4. Several articles have been published about sexual function among patients with cord injury and/or cauda equina lesions. In general, the findings suggest that in

1. *Upper motor neuron lesions in males:* 70% of male patients with complete lesions and 80% with incomplete lesions can consummate coitus; most patients cannot ejaculate or have orgasm and are, therefore, unable to sire children.
2. *Lower motor neuron lesions in males:* 75% of male patients with complete lesions are unable to have erections of any kind, while 25% have psychogenic erections (neither patient can achieve coitus, ejaculation, orgasm, or sire children); 83% of patients with incomplete lesions have psychogenic erections, with 90% able to have coitus (70% of this group are able to ejaculate, and of these, 10% may be able to sire children).
3. *Women regardless of type of lesion:* A woman with a spinal cord injury lacks sensation during intercourse. Women of the childbearing age can become pregnant. Most patients regain menses, with 50% not missing a single period. Vaginal delivery is possible if the pelvic measurements are adequate. Early cesarean section may be selected for patients prone to autonomic hyperreflexia.

Sexually active patients need birth control counseling. Because of the correlation of thrombophlebitis and the "pill," oral contraception is contraindicated for a woman with a spinal cord injury. If she does not wish to become pregnant, another form of contraception or contraception by her partner should be used.

Sex Counseling

To assist the patient in adjusting sexually, two sources of help have been suggested: (1) a primary sex counselor who would take responsibility for providing information, assistance, and support; and (2) informal secondary support by other health-team members.[13]

There should be a coordinated effort between the primary and secondary counselors.

Primary Counselor. It is *not* recommended for any health professional to engage in primary sex counseling without careful personal and academic preparation. Those engaged in dispensing informal secondary support also need preparation. Anyone preparing for the role of primary counselor should explore his or her own attitudes, feelings, values, prejudices, and moral convictions so that these views are not imposed upon the patient. The counselor must be suited to the job by temperament as well as preparation. Educational background should include instruction in human needs and interactions, sexuality, psychological development, and physiological and sociological aspects of sexuality. The primary counselor can be a physician, sex therapist, clinical nurse specialist, psychologist, marriage counselor, or member of the clergy.

Unless the parameters of a professional therapeutic relationship are set for this intimate topic, it is possible for the patient to become emotionally involved with the counselor or vice versa. This situation must be guarded against and carefully handled to prevent serious damage to both the patient and counselor.

The primary sex counselor must have knowledge of the patient's injury, physical status, general background, sexual history, and sexual preference. It is also important to know what the alteration or loss of sexual function means to the patient. The counselor should maintain a positive, realistic, and hopeful attitude toward restoration of sexual functions, since this outcome is difficult to predict. The patient needs to know that sexual experience will probably be different from that before injury, depending on the level of the lesion. Hohmann states that as a general philosophy of patient management, the spinal cord-injured patient should be encouraged to participate in whatever types of sexual activities are "physiologically possible, pleasing, esthetic, gratifying, and acceptable to him and his partner."[14] These few words seem to capture the essence of sound management.

Informal Secondary Support. Although most sexual counseling is provided in the postacute phase where resocialization of the patient is a priority, this topic should be introduced much earlier in the course of the management of the illness. Therefore, those nurses working in areas where patients remain in the acute-care facility need basic knowledge in this critical area.

After the body systems have been stabilized in the acute-care facility, it is appropriate to slowly introduce the whole concept of sexuality by exploring the topic with the patient. As the patient begins to deal with the aspects of this concept, a foundation is created upon which the ramifications of being a sexual being can develop. The nurse who is administering patient care should be able to provide secondary support. However, in-service training must be provided and nursing curricula must be changed so that nurses can fulfill their responsibilities, not only on the cognitive level, but also in the affective domain.

NUTRITION

An assessment of the patient's nutritional status should be made as soon as the patient is stabilized. The method of providing nutritional intake will vary based on the associated injuries that the patient may have, his level of consciousness, and the presence or absence of peristalsis in the gastrointestinal tract. The critical point is to provide adequate nutrition with sufficient fluids, carbohydrates, and protein for energy and tissue repair.

In the postacute and rehabilitative phase, dietary needs should be incorporated into the patient teaching plan. This is important because added protein is needed for muscle maintenance and added fluid is needed to prevent urinary tract infections and calculi. See Chapter 6 for a discussion of nutrition.

PSYCHOSOCIAL–EMOTIONAL RESPONSES TO SPINAL CORD INJURY

A wide range of emotional responses are experienced by the patient with a spinal cord injury as he passes from the period of the initial injury through the rehabilitative process. Although all of the various steps in emotional and psychological rehabilitation will not be evident in acute-care settings, it is important to have an overview of the process.

Sensory deprivation is a major concern for the cord-injured patient. While paralysis negates sensory input from regions of the body, the sensory deprivation encountered is multimodal: visual, auditory, and tactile. Immobilization and confinement to bed by traction or paralysis limits and distorts auditory and visual stimuli. Sound can be distorted if cervical tongs or a halo device is attached to the head. Sight is distorted for a patient on bed rest who may be fully aware of the ceiling, the upper half of the walls, and people from the waist up but who cannot visualize most objects in their totality. Finally, the patient is emotionally, psychologically, and socially deprived because of limited human interaction with loved ones and others.

Immobility from paralysis and the treatment apparatus limits motor function, as is obvious in the extreme example of a paralyzed patient who cannot even scratch his nose. Confinement in the hospital represents limited territoriality with lack of control over access to one's surroundings. Physical immobility can lead to psychological immobility — the inability to cope. Loneliness, powerlessness, hopelessness, and depersonalization further undermine the patient's emotional well-being.

The "self" concept and body image are also threatened. For a man who was conscious of his physique and actively engaged in physical activities such as jogging, weight lifting, and contact sports, paralysis can be a deadly jolt to his body image. For the woman who put great stock in her looks and physical appeal, spinal cord injury not only distorts her body image but also threatens her concept of self as a worthwhile person. For the young person in his or her late teens or early twenties who is not far removed from the dependency–independency struggle of adolescence, a catastrophic injury recasts him into this struggle, negating previous advances in development of self.

The Grieving Process

One way of viewing the adjustment process for these patients is the Kübler–Ross model of denial, anger, bargaining, depression, and final acceptance. While this model was initially structured with respect to a patient's psychological and emotional response to impending death, death can be broadly defined as loss of body function, as well as loss of life. The patient who is permanently paralyzed has sustained such a loss. For reference, the reader is referred to Lindemann, who has described the signs and symptoms of the grief and mourning process for one who has experienced the loss of a "significant other" or a specific body part or body function.[15]

Denial, the first step in the Kübler–Ross model, is really a coping mechanism. With sudden catastrophic disability, the capacity to cope would be nonexistent if the patient knew and accepted the full impact of the disability. With time, the patient begins to comprehend what has happened and what this means in terms of previous lifestyle and future goals. The result is anger, as expressed in such questions as "Why me?" or "What did I do to deserve this?" With this realization, depression sets in. Although depression occupies the fourth position in the model, it occurs in varying degrees throughout the entire grieving process.

The third step is centered around bargaining. The patient thinks that if he would recover, he would act differently, perhaps dedicating his life to charitable acts or that if he could get around on crutches rather than a wheelchair, he would willingly accept the disability. Reality finally indicates that there are no "deals" to be made, and the full impact of the disability begins to define itself in terms of daily living. This, in turn, intensifies the depression felt, to the point where it dominates the situation and becomes the fourth step of the model. However, depression is necessary to gather inner strength in order to regain equilibrium for final acceptance of the disability.

At this junction, health-team members can be supportive and provide information as necessary. The bulk of the depression usually begins in the acute-care facility and lasts in varying degrees throughout the rehabilitative process, from discharge into the community. Even after extensive preparation, about 4 months is required to adjust to the community, at best. This accounts for the fact that psychological rehabilitation takes longer than physical rehabilitation.

Family Consideration

The family experiences many of the same feelings that the patient faces. Along with these emotional responses, there are fear, guilt, and ambivalence. Fear relates to such worries as possible economic disaster, the need for role changes, and an inability to manage with a paralyzed family member. Guilt feelings on the part of the family may stem from feelings of anger directed toward the patient for being injured and from ambivalent feelings about the patient surviving the injury.

Because the family is such an important contributing factor in the patient's ability to adjust to his disability, the family must be helped to adjust also. It should be kept in mind that spinal cord injury happens to a family and not just to an individual.

Assessment Data

Understanding the psychosocial–emotional response to spinal cord injury is based on listening to and observing the patient. The nonverbal cues are just as important as verbal responses in understanding the patient. Sharing and documenting patient responses by all health-team members provides a comprehensive view of the patient. Many patients are evaluated by the psychologist or psychiatrist; their reports should be read carefully.

Nursing Management

Caring for a patient who has sustained a spinal cord injury requires an awareness of the impact that the illness has had on the patient's emotional and psychological equilibrium.

The following general suggestions are offered as an approach to providing patient care:

1. Establish a therapeutic nurse–patient relationship.
2. Cultivate a climate of trust.
3. Allow the patient to verbalize.
4. Accept the patient's behavior without being judgmental.
5. Let the patient know that it will take time to adjust to the disability.
6. Answer questions and refer those that you are unable to answer to the appropriate source.
7. Include written reports of the patient's emotional and psychological reactions.
8. Incorporate steps for meeting the emotional and psychological needs of the patient within the care plan.
9. Maintain good self concept and body image by encouraging the patient to use good grooming habits.
10. Use team conferences to discuss the patient's emotional and psychological status.
11. Involve the patient in the decision-making process about his care. This helps to foster a feeling of some control over himself.

POSTACUTE AND EARLY REHABILITATION PHASES

For purposes of discussion, the course of hospitalization for the patient with a spinal cord injury admitted to an acute-care facility can be divided into four general phases. These phases are the acute phase, the postacute phase, the early rehabilitation phase, and discharge. In most instances, the patient will need long-term rehabilitation. How this need is met will vary from patient to patient. The specific needs of the patient must be matched with the availability of rehabilitation hospitals, extended care facilities, and community resources. Although the aggressive rehabilitation phase of care is a part of the continuum of services necessary for the patient to reach his optimum potential, this type of care is not available in the acute-care hospital. However, planning for a comprehensive, formalized, and aggressive rehabilitation program begins in the postacute and early rehabilitation phases in the acute-care hospital.

There is a transition period that begins after the patient is quite stable physiologically and spinal shock has begun to reverse. A more precise picture of the extent of the patient's overall deficits and how they will affect his former lifestyle begin to emerge. The focus at this time is no longer on surviving the injuries but on coping with the alterations that the injury has imposed upon his daily life. This phase in the acute-care hospital setting may be called the postacute phase. Although the line of demarcation between the acute and postacute phases is identifiable, it is more difficult to separate the postacute phase from what follows. Perhaps the difficulty arises from the differences in degree and purpose of these phases. The postacute and early rehabilitation phases overlap in many instances. In the postacute phase there are ongoing assessments by the nurse, physician, physiotherapist, and others. The purpose of the assessments is to ensure that the patient is still stable and that no complications develop. Although the long-term rehabilitation needs of the patient are considered, there is usually not enough reliable hard data available as a basis for planning except in a very general way. Many pieces of vital information are not available at this time. Care is given to maintain intact body function and prevent the development of complications. An example of such care is range-of-motion exercises. However, much of the care is a general approach to management not based on specific identified needs of the patient.

In the early rehabilitation phase, ongoing assessments are conducted, but now they focus on details and are therefore much more specific. Because the patient's physical condition is much more stable, the information collected is more accurate and reliable. Vital pieces of information previously missing are now available. Because the data base is firmer, specific planning, rather than a generalized approach, can take place. Specific care protocols can also begin based on the specific needs of the patient. In the postacute phase, range-of-motion exercises were administered to maintain musculoskeletal function. Now, specific exercises, based on an identified need, can be administered.

The patient and family, along with the health-team members, contribute to the development of the rehabilitative plans. The nurse must assess the patient to determine his understanding of the goals of rehabilitation. If transfer to a rehabilitation hospital is planned, the patient and family should be oriented to the objectives of this type of facility.

In the early rehabilitation phase of care, the maintenance of existing function and prevention of complications are still primary nursing responsibilities. However, emphasis must also be placed on patient teaching in the activities of daily living (ADL) and on preparation for discharge. The greater the level of independence, the smoother the transition to the community, and the greater the options available to the patient. Therefore, the nurse must be supportive and optimistic to help the patient accept his responsibility for acquiring these skills. The process is slow and can be very discouraging to the patient. Family involvement is always encouraged, because the patient needs to regain his position in this social unit.

Discharge planning is a coordinated effort by all team members. In some instances the group process is used to help with the transition to the community. Groups of patients preparing for discharge meet with a group leader to discuss their concerns about reentry to the community. Family members of patients benefit by similar meetings to discuss their concerns, fears, and adjustments. This is also the time to emphasize vocational rehabilitation. A weekend visit at home should be planned before the actual discharge. When the patient returns to the hospital, he can gain assistance with the problems that he encountered at home.

Contacts with community resource people are made before discharge. The community health (visiting) nurse has a very important function. Arrangements should be made to have the nurse visit the patient in the hospital before discharge. With the establishment of this relationship, a vital transition link is established. The social worker must also make plans for follow-up in the community. To maintain a high level of health in all aspects of the patient's rehabilitation, lifetime follow-up is imperative.

SCOPE OF FORMALIZED REHABILITATION

Rehabilitation, like growth, consists of physical, psychological, and sociological aspects. The complexity and interrelatedness of the elements of the rehabilitative process cannot be overstated. It is important to note that psychological rehabilitation is achieved much later than physical rehabilitation. This point is effectively demonstrated by reemployment patterns of cord-injured patients. Reports indicate that it takes at least 4 to 5 months after discharge for a patient to return to his previous job or employer. Why the delay? The answer is that although physically ready for gainful employment, the patient is still psychologically unprepared. Postponement of employment for 2 years or longer is not uncommon and is generally related to various adjustments, as well as medical and family difficulties. Because of unresolved problems, some patients are never again gainfully employed.

Figure 18–14 depicts the rehabilitative process as analogous to Maslow's hierarchy of needs, the lower levels having to be satisfied before a higher level is relevant. As one ascends the triangle, health personnel exert less and less control of the situations and settings encountered by the patient, indicating less qualitative and quantitative support for the patient from health care personnel.

The quadriplegic and paraplegic represent special categories in rehabilitation. While patients in other rehabilitation programs are helped to achieve an optimal level of function and then remain at that level, quadriplegic and paraplegic disability is such that the patients are at increased risk of medical, social, psychological, and vocational deterioration. Therefore, lifelong follow-up care is an absolute necessity for maintaining rehabilitative status and preventing problems and complications.

THE ROLE OF THE HEALTH-TEAM MEMBERS IN THE REHABILITATION PROCESS

The care of the spinal cord-injured patient requires a well-orchestrated interdisciplinary approach of many health team professionals. Although the focus of this chapter is the acute-care management of the spinal cord-injured patient, much of the care is directed toward achieving the best functional level possible for all body systems in preparation for an aggressive rehabilitation program. This goal, along with the fundamental techniques of early rehabilitation, are part of the purview of the acute-care setting. The contribution of various health-team disciplines is briefly outlined. Not all of the following health professionals are available in all facilities.

The Professional Nurse

The nursing staff becomes the pivotal center for coordinating care because it has the overall responsibility for developing a daily therapeutic schedule of activities. Nurses spend more time with the patient and his family than any other health professional group. A rapport develops between nurse and patient or family that becomes the basis for communications and patient and family teaching. The major responsibilities of the nurse in the postacute–rehabilitative phase in the acute-care setting include the following:

1. Initiate, in collaboration with the physician, the formal phase of planning for discharge and referral for rehabilitation.
2. Assist the patient and family in participating in the planning for discharge from the acute-care facility to a rehabilitation hospital or other extended care facility.
3. Answer questions and clarify information for the patient and family.
4. Assess and document the patient's functional level in activities of daily living.
5. Identify and document those nursing needs and health problems unresolved in the acute-care setting.
6. Work collaboratively with other health-team members to plan for discharge.
7. See Chapter 9 for a discussion of discharge planning.

The Social Worker

With the onslaught of any catastrophic illness or injury, it is imperative that the patient and his "significant others" receive professional help in all of the avenues affected. The

6. Gainful employment

5. Integration into the community

4. Successful adjustment to living at home

3. Accomplishment of ADL, mobility, and self care

2. Early rehabilitative care; PT, OT, social worker's help, use of helping devices, bowel and bladder control

1. Trauma and early posttrauma phase; stabilization of the body system; early psychological support

FIG. 18–14. Hierarchy of rehabilitative process. PT = physical therapy; OT = occupational therapy; ADL = activities of daily living.

social worker contributes to this process by developing a rapport with the patient, getting to know him and his family, and serving as a communication link for other team members. He is the patient's advocate in specific areas. The major areas of concern for the social worker are

1. To help the patient and "significant others" to plan for the rehabilitation program in conjunction with the other team members
2. To help the patient achieve the maximum benefit from his rehabilitation program
3. To explore all avenues for financial help and insurance coverage available to the patient and his family and assist them in using these sources
4. To explore community resources that may be of value to the patient and his family
5. To keep the lines of communication open with the patient, family, and other team members
6. To plan for discharge from the particular facility and/or the health care system (takes place with the patient, family, and other team members)

The Physical Therapist

The physical therapist works closely with the physiatrist in designing a physical therapy program for the patient. Bedside therapy and work in the physiotherapy department provide treatment to maintain the musculoskeletal system.

A physical therapy program for the patient with a spinal cord injury is designed to help him become aware of his capabilities in gross body movement and function. The plan includes the following:

1. Evaluation of the patient in terms of his ability in range of motion, muscle power, and activities of daily living
2. Analysis of all activities of daily living to provide alternate methods of accomplishment where there is functional loss
3. Identification of specific exercises and skills to be accomplished by the patient, including any or all of the following: breathing exercises, muscle strengthening and muscle stretching exercises, mat work, tilt table, wheelchair mobility, crutch walking, and activities of daily living
4. Prescription of appropriate support devices, such as wheelchairs, slings, and braces, that best meet the needs of the patient

The Psychologist

The contribution of the staff psychologist is to aid the patient, family, and also the staff in understanding behavioral and emotional reactions. The major areas of concern for the psychologist are

1. Helping the patient to gain insight into his feelings and reaction about the effects that injury has had on his life
2. Counseling the patient using various techniques, which include traditional psychotherapy methods
3. Establishing a supportive and helping relationship with the family
4. Assisting the staff to understand and cope with their reactions to patients and patients' behavior.

The Occupational Therapist

In the management of patients with spinal cord injuries the objectives of occupational therapy are to achieve independence in self care; eating; dressing; toileting; homemaking; communication; vocational, social, and educational pursuits. The specific areas of concern include

1. Functional motor assessment
2. Teaching the patient the use of selected assistive equipment
3. Training in the use of hand orthosis as a substitute for prehension
4. Homemaking retraining
5. Prevocational assessment
6. Training in communication skills (e.g., special telephone, typewriter, newspaper holder)
7. Introduction to electronic equipment activated by breath or voice for the patient with a cervical injury (C–5 and above)
8. Home planning consultation to deal with the environmental problems of severely disabled individuals that prevent them from functioning as normally as possible in the home setting
9. Driver's training program and introduction to specially equipped vehicles for use by the severely disabled

The Vocational Counselor

The goals of the vocational counselor are to provide individualized service in the following areas:

1. Vocational counseling
2. Educational planning and academic remediation
3. Vocational evaluation
4. Work exposure and experience for exploratory purposes
5. Job placement and follow-up

Although the active vocational rehabilitation phase should coincide with other aspects of the rehabilitative process, vocational rehabilitation should start early in the postacute phase. In this way the patient knows that he is not alone in coping with devastating vocational problems. When the patient's physical condition has stabilized, one can predict, based on a greater data base, what the realistic vocational goals for the patient are. At this point in the rehabilitative process, the services of the vocational counselor are most valuable. There is a great need for follow-up in vocational rehabilitation. Placing a patient in a college program does not ensure successful vocational rehabilitation. Even after successful completion of an academic program, the critical problem is placement for gainful employment. Once the patient is placed in a job, the role of the vocational counselor continues for both the patient and the employer. Help is provided in solving problems, changing jobs, and retraining for a new career. With so many critical steps in achieving gainful employment, it is no wonder that this area is not more successful.

Summary

Finally, it should be said that if the patient is not in a facility that employs all of the above-mentioned personnel, the health specialist, physician, nurse, social worker, and physical therapist are often able to provide some of the services or to make referrals to appropriate governmental and private agencies. The social worker can make referrals for vocational evaluation and help to secure funds for training and equipment. The physical therapist can offer information about prevocational assessment, self-help devices, home consultation, and adaptive methods for various activities.

One of the most satisfying experiences one can have is to play a part in the management and ultimate rehabilitation of a spinal cord-injured patient who is able to assume a useful and satisfying place in society.

REFERENCES

1. Spinal Cord Injury, no. 81-160. Bethesda, U.S. Department of Health and Human Services, Public Health Services, National Institutes of Health, 1981
2. Kalsbeek WD et al: The national head and spinal cord injury survey: Major findings. J. Neurosurg 53:519, November 1980
3. Worth MH (ed): Principles and Practice of Trauma Care, pp 67–68. Baltimore, Williams & Wilkins, 1982
4. Roberts JR: Trauma of the cervical spine. Top Emerg Med 1(1):63, May 1979
5. Tyson GW et al: Acute care of the spinal-cord-injured patient. Crit Care Q 2(1):45, June 1979
6. Heros R: Spinal cord compression. In Ropper AH, Kennedy SK, Zervas NT (eds): Neurological and Neurosurgical Intensive Care, pp 231–232. Baltimore, University Park Press, 1983
7. Guyton A: Textbook of Medical Physiology, 5th ed. Philadelphia, WB Saunders, 1976
8. Haas A et al: Impairment of respiration after spinal cord injury. Arch Phys Med Rehabil 46:399, 1965
9. Larkin J, Moylan J: Priorities in management of trauma victims. Crit Care Med 3:192, 1975
10. Kurtzke JF: Epidemiology of spinal cord injury, part II. Exp Neurol 48:163, September 1975
11. New York University Postgraduate Medical School: Proceedings of comprehensive acute and rehabilitation care of the spinal cord-injured patient. New York, May 14–15, 1977
12. Coleman P: The problem of spasticity in the management of the spinal cord-injured patient and its treatment with special references to percutaneous radiofrequency thermal selective sensory rhizotomy. J Neurosurg Nurs 8(2):97, December 1976
13. Slocombe I: Posterior cervical stabilization with anterior cervical fusion: An alternative approach to cervical fractures. J Neurosurg Nurs 11(1):34, March 1979
14. Hohmann GW: Considerations in the management of psychosexual readjustment in the cord-injured male. Rehabil Psychol 19:50, Summer 1972
15. Lindemann E: Symptomatology and management of acute grief. In Fulton R (ed): Death and Identity. New York, John Wiley & Sons, 1965
16. Youmans JR (ed): Neurological Surgery, 2nd ed. Philadelphia, WB Saunders, 1982

Books

Boroch R: Elements of Rehabilitation in Nursing: An Introduction, pp 64–79. St Louis, CV Mosby, 1976

Brunner L, Suddarth D: Textbook of Medical–Surgical Nursing, 4th ed. Philadelphia, JB Lippincott, 1980

Calenoff L (ed): Radiology of Spinal Cord Injury. St Louis, CV Mosby, 1981

Carlson C, Blackwell B (eds): Behavioral Concepts and Nursing Intervention, 2nd ed. Philadelphia, JB Lippincott, 1978

Clark R: Clinical Neuroanatomy and Neurophysiology, 5th ed. Philadelphia, FA Davis, 1976

Earnest MP: Neurological emergencies. New York, Churchill Livingstone, 1983

Ewing CL (eds): Impact Injury of the Head and Spine. Springfield, IL, Charles C Thomas, 1983

Farrell J: Illustrated Guide to Orthopedic Nursing, 2nd ed. Philadelphia, JB Lippincott Co, 1982

Feldman RC, Young RR, Koella WP (eds): Spasticity: Disordered Motor Control. Chicago, Year Book Medical Publishers, 1980

Guttman Sir L: Spinal Cord Injuries: Comprehensive Management and Research, 2nd ed, pp 107–136. Oxford, Blackwell Scientific Publications, 1976

Jeffrey E: Disorders of the Cervical Spine, p 63. New York, Butterworth, 1980

Kübler–Ross E: Death and Dying. New York, Macmillan, 1969

Maslow A: Motivation and Personality, 2nd ed. New York, Harper & Row, 1970

Pierce DS, Nickel VH (eds): The Total Care of Spinal Cord Injuries. Boston, Little, Brown & Company, 1977

Seeger, W: Microsurgery of the Spinal Cord and Surrounding Structures: Anatomical and Technical Principles. New York, Springer–Verlag, 1982

Seiden MR: Practical Management of Chronic Neurological Problems. New York, Appleton–Century–Crofts, 1981

Tator CH (ed): Early Management of Acute Spinal Cord Injury. New York, Raven Press, 1982

Trieschman RB (ed): Spinal Cord Injuries. New York, Pergamon Press, 1980

Watkins RG: Surgical approaches to the spine. New York, Springer–Verlag, 1983

Worth MH (ed): Principles and Practice of Trauma Care. Baltimore, Williams & Wilkins, 1982

Periodicals

Adelstein W, Watson P: Cervical spine injuries. J Neurosurg Nurs 15(2):65, April 1983

Allmond B: Management of cervical and thoracic spine/cord injured patients. J Neurosurg Nurs 13(2):97, April 1981

Axel SA: Spinal cord injured women's concerns: Menstruation and pregnancy. Rehabil Nurs 7(5):10–15, September–October 1982

Bardack J, Pardone F: Psychological considerations in treatment of the spinal cord injured. In Proceedings of the Spinal Cord Workshop, New York University Institute of Rehabilitative Medicine, New York, May 1977

Barry K: Neurogenic bladder incontinence: The consequence of mismanagement. Rehabil Nurs 6(5):12–13, September–October 1981

Bartol G: Psychological needs of the spinal cord-injured person. J Neurosurg Nurs 10(4):171, December 1978

Bassler S: Achieving continuity of care for the spinal cord injured patient through the problem-oriented approach. J Neurosurg Nurs 13(2):61, April 1981

Bassler S: Development of a resource support system for nurses caring for spinal cord injured patients. J Neurosurg Nurs 12(4):195, December 1980

Beetham W, Hsieh R: Clinical evaluation of neck pain. Hosp Med 60, September 1982

Bolton ME: Hyperbaric oxygen therapy. Am J Nurs 81:1199, June 1981

Buchanan L: Emergency: First aid for spinal cord injury. Nurs82 12:66, August 1982

Buchanan L: Patient preparation and transfer to a regional spinal cord injury center. J Neurosurg Nurs 14(3):137, June 1982

Carol M, Ducker T, Byrnes D: Acute care of spinal cord injury: A challenge to the emergency medicine clinician. Crit Care Q 2(1):7, June 1979

Chui L, Bhatt K: Autonomic dysreflexia. Rehabil Nurs 8(2):16–19, March–April 1983

Cloward R: Acute cervical spine injuries. Clin Symp 32(1):entire issue, January 1980

De Jesus–Greenberg DA: Acute spinal cord injury and hyperbaric oxygen therapy: A new adjunct in management. J Neurosurg Nurs 12(3):155, September 1980

Delaney JF: Medical treatment of spasticity. Curr Probl Surg 17(4):245, 1980

Ducker T et al: Complete sensorimotor paralysis after cord injury: Mortality, recovery, and therapeutic implications. J Trauma 19:837, 1979

Dudas S, Stevens KA: Central cord injury: Implications for nursing. J Neurosurg Nurs 16(2):84, April 1984

Eidelberg E et al: A model of spinal cord injury. Surg Neurol 6 (1):35, July 1976

Errey M: Spasticity: The nursing management. Aust Nurs J 10:43, 1981

Feustel D: Alterations in neuron innervation associated with spinal cord lesions. J Neurosurg Nurs 13(2):48, April 1981

Gamanche FW et al: The clinical application of hyperbaric oxygen therapy in spinal cord injury: A preliminary report. Surg Neurol 15:84–87, 1981

Ginnity S: Assessment of cervical cord trauma by the nurse practitioner. J Neurosurg Nurs 10(4):193, December 1978

Giubilato R: Acute care of the high-level quadriplegic patient. J Neurosurg Nurs 14(3):128, June 1982

Hamric A: A teaching tool for spinal cord injured patients. J Neurosurg Nurs 13(5):234, October 1981

Hart G: Spinal cord injury: Impact on clients' significant others. Rehabil Nurs 6(1):11–15, January–February 1981

Hartman M: Intermittent self-catheterization. Nurs78 8:72, November 1978

Hodges L: Human sexuality and the spinal cord injured: Role of the clinical nurse specialist. J Neurosurg Nurs 10(3):125, September 1978

Hughes J, Percy E: Emergency care of cervical spine injuries. Hosp Med, 53, July 1981

Hummelgard A, Martin E: Management of the patient in a halo brace. J Neurosurg Nurs 14(3):113, June 1982

Isaacs N: The treatment of acute spinal cord injury using local hypothermia. J Neurosurg Nurs 10(3):95, September 1978

James W et al: Cervical accessory respiratory muscle function in a patient with high cervical cord lesion. Chest 71:59, 1977

Kinash R: Experiences and nursing needs of spinal cord-injured patients. J Neurosurg Nurs 10(1):29, March 1978

King R, Dudas S: Rehabilitation of the patient with a spinal cord injury. Nurs Clin North Am 15(2):225, June 1980

Koehler M: Continuity of care for spinal cord injury: A reality. Rehabil Nurs 6(1): 16–18, January–February 1981

Krieger A: Identifying Brown–Séquard syndrome. Hosp Med 60, January 1981

Lagger L: Spinal cord injury: Nutritional management. J Neurosurg Nurs 15(5):310, October 1983

Lamb S: Clinical application of transcutaneous electrical nerve stimulation and high cervical cord stimulation for movement disorders. J Neurosurg Nurs 15(1):1, February 1983

Levitt R: Understanding sexuality and spinal cord injury. J Neurosurg Nurs 12(2):88, June 1980

MacKechnie J: Regional spinal cord injury center nursing care: Prescription for the present and the future. J Neurosurg Nurs 14(3):133, June 1982

Manson R: Autonomic dysreflexia: A nursing challenge. Rehabil Nurs 6(6):18–19, 22–23, November–December 1981

Merritt JL: Management of spasticity in spinal cord injury. Mayo Clin Proc 56:614, 1981

Parkinson J: The spinal cord-injured patient: Autonomic hyperreflexia. J Neurosurg Nurs 9(1):1, March 1977

Roberts J: Trauma of the cervical spine. Top Emerg Med 1(1):6, 1979

Roglitz C: Team approach in the acute phase of spinal cord injury. J Neurosurg Nurs 10(3):117, September 1978

Slocombe I: Posterior cervical stabilization with anterior cervical fusion: An alternative approach to cervical fractures. J Neurosurg Nurs 11(1):34, March 1979

Solomon J: Sex and the spinal cord injured patient. J Neurosurg Nurs 14(3):125, June 1982

Stanton GM: Spinal cord injury: Psychological adaptation. J Neurosurg Nurs 15(5):306, October 1983

Stover J et al: Heterotopic ossification in spinal cord-injured patients. Arch Phys Med Rehabil 56:199, May 1975

Toth L: Spasticity management in spinal cord injury. Rehabil Nurs 8(1):14–17, January–February 1983

Tyson G et al: Acute care of the spinal-cord-injured patient. Crit Care Q 2(1):45, June 1979

Wahlquist G et al: Intermittent catheterization and urinary tract infection. Rehabil Nurs 8(1):18–19, 41, January–February 1983

Wahlquist G: Research news: Regeneration in the central nervous system. Science 209(4454):378, July 18, 1980

Wahlquist G: Regaining urinary continence through intermittent catheterization. J Neurosurg Nurs 12(2):73, June 1980

Wein A: Management of neurogenic bladder dysfunction in the adult. Urology 8:432–453, November 1976

Wing S: Cervical spine injuries: Treatment and related nursing care. J Neurosurg Nurs 9(4):138, December 1977

chapter 19

Back Pain and Intervertebral Disc Trauma

For those health professionals entrusted with the care of the patient with low back pain or intervertebral disc disease, the responsibility can be difficult and frustrating. Back problems, unlike other selected conditions, are usually not "cured" following a treatment protocol. Back problems tend to be chronic conditions characterized by periods of exacerbation and temporary relief. Even after surgical intervention, some patients continue to experience symptoms of varying severity. There are those unfortunate patients for whom second surgical procedures have been suggested, but for whom the results of further surgery have been disappointing in terms of the control of symptoms.

In one respect the problem of back pain can be viewed as one of evolutionary origin. It appears that humans were not designed to ambulate in the erect position. Having assumed the vertical position for many centuries, humans have subjected themselves to the miserable affliction of back problems. For the health professional, caring for these patients continues to be a management dilemma.

FACTORS CAUSING BACK PAIN

CONGENITAL ANOMALIES

Anatomical variations such as scoliosis and kyphosis contribute to anatomical malalignments that produce localized stress problems. Because of the anatomical variations involved, the following result: (1) the vertebrae are maligned in relationship to one another; (2) mechanical movement causes disproportionate stress to selected areas of the spinal column; and (3) the space within the spinal cord is altered. As a result, the person is predisposed to disc and spondylitic changes from the excessive stresses imposed by normal body movement.

Other congenital problems contributing to back pain are spina bifida, which is characterized by an absence of fusion in the laminae of the neural arch, and malformation of vertebrae, particularly of the articular processes, which can interfere with the approximation of bony parts and create areas vulnerable to injury. Specific examples of vertebral malformations in the lumbosacral area include (1) lumbarization of the first sacral vertebra which, in effect, creates a sixth lumbar vertebra, thereby causing increased stress on the lumbosacral joint and (2) sacralization of the fifth lumbar vertebra, which decreases the number of movable lumbar vertebrae to four. Pain is probable if sacralization occurs unilaterally, because of the uneven distribution of stress in the lower back region.

DEVELOPMENTAL CHANGES

As a result of the normal aging process, spinal changes occur. (For example, the fluid content of the nucleus pulposus gradually decreases from 88% in the early 30s to 66% in later years.) As a result, the discs become less efficient shock absorbers for stress from movement and become somewhat smaller so that they can more easily slip from their normal anatomical position. In addition, the aging process causes degeneration of the anulus fibrosus and the posterior longitudinal ligaments that secure the vertebral bodies together. As these ligaments degenerate, they are less able to respond to the various alterations from movement so that stresses, strains, and injuries are much more easily precipitated. The normal anatomical degeneration of aging plus the cumulative effects of everyday activity make the back vulnerable to injury.

NEOPLASMS

Neoplasms of the vertebral column and spinal cord produce pain and cord compression. Such tumors may be classified as benign or malignant and can originate as primary tumors or secondary metastatic lesions (from sites elsewhere in the body; see Chap. 22).

INFECTIONS

Low back pain can be a presenting symptom of both acute pyogenic and chronic infections. Acute pyogenic infections are usually blood-borne from a primary source elsewhere in the body, such as from the respiratory or genitourinary tract. The respiratory tract is often the primary source of infection in the younger population as is the genitourinary tract in the older population. Other sources of infection in any age group are postoperative infections or abscess formations that cause pain. Immobilization and antibiotics are the treatment prescribed.

Chronic infections that can produce low back pain include osteomyelitis, tuberculosis, and those caused by *Brucella* and *Mycobacterium* organisms. The usual treatment consists of bed rest, antibiotics, spinal fusion, and, occasionally, surgical drainage of abscesses.

METABOLIC DISEASE

The metabolic condition most commonly associated with low back pain is osteoporosis. *Osteoporosis* refers to the loss of bone substance due to a failure in the deposition of the bone matrix. The vertebrae are particularly vulnerable because they are composed primarily of cancellous bone, which is an early target of osteoporotic alterations. The patient may be completely asymptomatic or complain of aching pain the thoracic or lumbar region. Slight injury can cause collapse, dislocation, or fracture of the fragile, demineralized vertebrae. Compression of the spinal cord or nerve roots from the collapsed vertebrae can be the result.

Osteoporosis is associated with hormonal changes that occur during the postmenopausal or senile period and with Cushing's syndrome and long-term steroid therapy.

DEGENERATIVE DISEASES

The major degenerative diseases associated with back pain are spondylosis and osteoarthritis.

Spondylosis

Spondylosis is a condition characterized by narrowing of the intervertebral space and changes in the vertebral bodies caused by degenerative changes of the intervertebral discs. Spondylosis of the cervical spine is very common and is often found in middle-aged or older people. The patient may be asymptomatic, with evidence of the degenerative changes noted incidently on radiographic studies of the vertebral column. Signs and symptoms arise when fatigue or injury inflicts additional stress on the spine.

The normal aging process results in loss of fluid from the nucleus pulposus and deformity of the intervertebral disc. The disc also loses its elasticity, becoming more rigid and susceptible to herniation when stress is applied to the spine. The bulging disc creates traction on the longitudinal ligaments and irritates the vertebrae, which can cause osteophyte formation. An *osteophyte*, which is sometimes called a spur, is an irritating outgrowth of bone. Protrusion of the disc can cause collapse of the intervertebral space, narrowing of the intervertebral foramen, and compression of the nerve root or spinal cord. Because the cervical spine has more flexibility than other areas of the vertebral column and degenerative changes and injury are common in this area, cervical spondylosis is a very common problem that causes much pain and suffering to the patient.

Signs and Symptoms

The clinical signs and symptoms of cervical spondylosis include occiput, neck, and shoulder pain; stiff neck; headache; arm pain; muscle weakness; and paresthesia (numbness and tingling along the affected nerve root). If spinal cord compression occurs, there may be motor weakness, spasticity, sensory changes, and a gait disorder. The root syndromes cause signs and symptoms associated with the specific roots compressed.

Diagnosis

The neurological examination will reveal the specific deficits caused by spondylosis. Cervical x-rays are useful, but the most accurate diagnostic procedure is myelography.

Management

More than half of the patients with acute problems associated with cervical spondylosis will improve with nonsurgical management. Bed rest, intermittent cervical traction, drug therapy, and, possibly, a collar to immobilize the neck are used. Drug therapy includes analgesics (nonnarcotic or narcotice as necessary), muscle relaxants such as ibuprofen (Motrin), diazepam (Valium), and others, and anti-inflammatory drugs such as aspirin, phenylbutazone (Butazolidin), and steroids.

If a conservative approach is not effective, then operative procedures such as an anterior or posterior laminectomy will be suggested. The purpose of these procedures is to remove the osteophyte and decompress any neural elements affected by the protrusion of disc material.

Osteoarthritis

Osteoarthritis is a degenerative arthritis that involves the articular cartilages. The cervical region and the lumbar region, in that order, are most often involved, although the entire spine can be affected. Osteoarthritis is an affliction of older age associated with excessive and strenuous stress to the back throughout adolescence and adult life. Symptoms include stiffness, limitation of mobility, and pain in the affected area that is aggravated by movement. Rest usually relieves the pain.

Changes in the vertebrae are described as marked osteophytic overgrowth with spur formations (osteophytes), ridging, and bridging of the vertebrae. Osteoarthritic changes can compress nerve roots or the spinal cord, giving rise to a spondylitic form of myelopathy. Clinical symptoms relate poorly to radiological findings, so that patients with severe pain may demonstrate little pathology upon radiography, while other patients could be completely asymptomatic with blatant radiological changes.

INFLAMMATORY DISEASES

Back pain is a common symptom in rheumatoid arthritis and ankylosing spondylitis (Marie-Strümpell spondylitis). *Rheumatoid arthritis* is a generalized disease process affecting the mesenchymal connective tissue and involving the joints of the spine, hips, and hands. Pain, stiffness, and limited motion are the chief symptoms. The atlantoaxial articulation of the cervical region is commonly affected. When this area is involved, there is limitation of motion in the neck and head. Rheumatoid arthritis is a severely debilitating disease affecting women between the ages of 25 through 45 three times more fequently than men of the same age group.[1] As the disease progresses, pain in the lower back is common due to the degeneration of discs and connective tissue. There may also be anterior displacement of one or more vertebrae, damage to ligaments, particularly in the atlantoaxial area, and possible cord compression or injury.

Marie-Strümpell spondylitis, also known as ankylosing spondylitis, predominantly affects young men. The sacroiliac joints are the primary sites of involvement. The chief symptom is pain in the center of the low back region. The course of the illness is slow, progressing over many years. An early symptom is back stiffness, especially in the morning, due to inactivity. There is also decreased mobility of the hips. Early in the disease, symptoms precede radiological changes.

Continued development of the disease produces destruction and obliteration of the sacroiliac joints with subsequent bridging of the vertebral bodies with bone. These changes create alterations on radiographs that give the visual illusion of a "bamboo spine." The degree of disability is severe. As the disease progresses, there can be complete calcification of the anterior longitudinal ligament, resulting in immobility of the spine.

TRAUMA

This category of causes of back pain includes sprains and strains including whiplash, vertebral fractures, spondylolysis and spondylolisthesis, and protrusion or rupture of an intervertebral disc.

Sprains and Strains

Sprains and strains tend to be vague terms used to describe self-limiting injuries, usually associated with a fall, lifting of a heavy object, or unexpected sudden deceleration, which is common in vehicular mishaps. Since the lifting of patients can place excessive strain on the back, any nurse working with dependent patients must be constantly cognizant of good body mechanics and use appropriate techniques.

Although sprains and strains are self-limiting, they are nonetheless very painful and can predispose a person to chronic back pain. In addition to pain, spasms and local tenderness are experienced in the affected areas. Pain is relieved by rest. If the patient has preexisting disc trouble or muscular, arthritic, or postural problems, a strain or sprain can be the precipitating factor for a chronic or extended period of severe discomfort. Vertebral fractures are capable of producing much pain in the back from injury and spasms. A more detailed discussion of this type of back ailment can be found in Chapter 18.

Spondylolysis and Spondylolisthesis

Most authorities believe that spondylolysis is the precursor of spondylolisthesis. Spondylolysis is caused by a stress fracture of the isthmus of the vertebra. In spondylolisthesis there is a defect in both sides of the vertebra through the isthmus with anterior slipping of the affected vertebral body, pedicle, and superior articular facet, leaving the posterior elements (spinous process and laminae) behind in their normal position (Fig. 19–1). The most frequently af-

FIG. 19–1. Spondylolisthesis, diagrammatic. The defect occupied by fibrous or fibrocartilaginous tissue is represented by cross-hatching. Note its intimate relationship to the fifth lumbar nerve root. (Turek S: Orthopaedics, 3rd ed. Philadelphia, JB Lippincott, 1977)

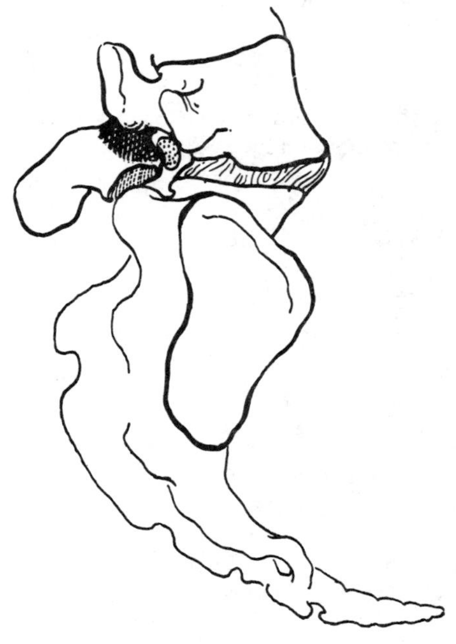

fected vertebra is the fifth lumbar vertebra, with the fourth lumbar vertebra the next most frequent site.

Symptoms are mild early in life but become more pronounced in later life. Symptoms include pain in the lower back radiating to the thighs, limitation of motion, and tenderness over the L-4 and L-5 vertebrae. Nerve root involvement with sensory loss and motor weakness can be present. If there is slippage of the vertebra, narrowing of the spinal canal can occur with possible compression and traction of neural elements. The protrusion or rupture of an intervertebral disc that causes back pain will be discussed later in this chapter.

REFERRED PAIN FROM VISCERA

Pain can be referred to the back from other areas of the body. Common causes of referred pain to the back include aortic aneurysms, fibroids of the uterus, ovarian cysts, pelvic infections, prostatic disease, renal disease, scoliosis, and hip disease.

PSYCHONEUROTIC DISEASE

Psychoneurotic disease applies to the hysterical patient with a conversion reaction experienced as back pain. Also included in this group is the malingerer who feigns back pain for secondary gains, such as relief from normal responsibilities or financial gain in the form of compensation and work-related disability.

For the hysterical patient or malingerer, neurological findings associated with the pain are absent or atypical upon neurological examination. Management of these patients is difficult because the physician must be certain that no pathological changes exist. It is well known that some disabling back conditions cannot be confirmed by radiological changes. The hysterical patient should receive mild sedatives or tranquilizing drugs. In some instances, a psychiatric consultation may be necessary.

SUMMARY

Back pain can be the result of many conditions and disease processes. The initial problem is one of early diagnosis and initiation of appropriate treatment. This is important not only to provide relief from the acute episode but to prevent the development of degenerative changes that lead to chronic conditions. Being aware of the wide range of possibilities that produce back pain can help the nurse focus attention on the importance of observing and recording both objective and subjective symptoms. In planning nursing management, an adequate knowledge base is most helpful in anticipating patient needs as well as helping the patient set realistic goals.

HERNIATED INTERVERTEBRAL DISCS

The herniation of intervertebral discs is the major cause of severe and chronic back pain, particularly in the low back region. The cervical and lumbar regions are the most flexible areas of the spine and are easily susceptible to injury and stress, with the lumbar area most frequently affected by herniated disc disease. Thoracic herniations are uncommon.

Men suffer from intervertebral herniation much more frequently than women. Most patients with disc disease are in the 30- to 50-year age group. About 90% to 95% of lumbar herniations occur at the L-4 to L-5 to S-1 levels. When the cervical region is involved, the most common levels are C-6 to C-7 and then C-5 to C-6. Multiple herniations occur in only 10% of patients.

ETIOLOGY

Trauma accounts for approximately 50% of disc herniations. Examples of traumatic incidents include lifting heavy objects while in the flexed position (most common), slipping, falling on the buttocks or back, and suppressing a sneeze. In a significant number of patients, no history of trauma can be identified. It is alleged that some salient degenerative disc alterations occur prior to a slight trauma that, while too insignificant to recall, nonetheless precipitated the herniation. The herniation syndrome can also occur in other degenerative processes, such as osteoarthritis or ankylosing spondylitis (Marie-Strümpell spondylitis). Patients with congenital anomalies such as scoliosis appear to be predisposed to disc injury because of the malalignment of the vertebral column.

PATHOPHYSIOLOGY

As mentioned earlier, degenerative changes of the posterior longitudinal ligaments and the anulus fibrosus occur in middle and later life. Simultaneously, degenerative changes begin to occur in the intervertebral discs after a peak level of development is reached in the early 30s. Fraying and tears of the anulus fibrosus make the disc vulnerable to posterior displacement in response to a prolapse of the nucleus pulposus. This can occur with slight provocation, such as making an awkward movement, sneezing, or lurching forward. The nucleus pulposus can also protrude through the anulus fibrosus. A fragment may be laterally or centrally thrust into the spinal canal, where it encroaches upon nerve roots (Fig. 19-2). The herniation may be spontaneously reduced or reabsorbed but more often it persists as a source of chronic root irritation. The presence of symptoms, particularly pain, depends on the quantity of disc material that has herniated into the spinal canal, the degree of narrowing of the spinal canal from herniation and edema, and the number of discs involved and the degree of encroachment upon nerve roots.

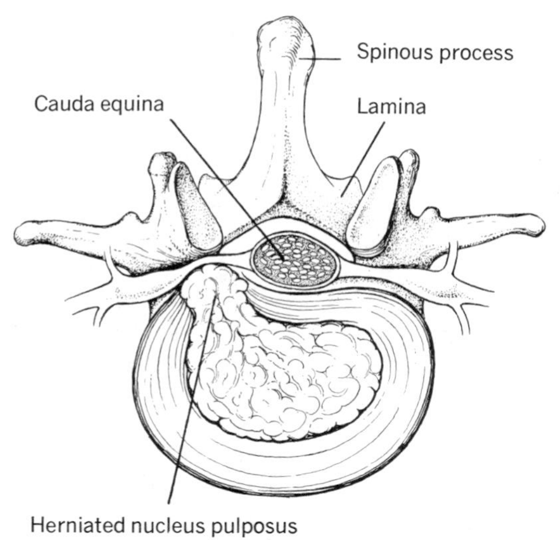

FIG. 19-2. Ruptured vertebral disc. (From Chaffee EE, Lytle IM: Basic Physiology and Anatomy. Philadelphia, JB Lippincott, 1980)

SIGNS AND SYMPTOMS BY LOCATION

Lumbar Area

Herniation of a lumbar disc is usually lateral and only occasionally central. The signs and symptoms of herniated lumbar discs are categorized into the following general areas: pain, postural deformity, motor changes, sensory changes, alterations of reflexes, and specific diagnostic signs.

Pain. Pain is the first and most characteristic symptom of a herniated disc. Initially, after injury, pain is present, varying in the severity of aching and sharpness. The alleged etiology of pain is stimulation of the pain fibers of the posterior anulus and the posterior longitudinal ligament. The low back pain persists for varying periods with radiation across the buttock, thigh, and one entire leg. In some patients, buttock and leg pain develops without back pain. The term *sciatica* is sometimes used to describe a syndrome of lumbar back pain that spreads down one leg to the ankle and is intensified by coughing and sneezing. The nerve roots L-4, L-5, S-1, S-2, and S-3 give rise to the sciatic nerve. The pain in the buttocks is described as deep, aching, or gnawing in character. The intensity of pain is influenced by leg position.

Pain from a herniated disc is aggravated and intensified by coughing, sneezing, straining, stooping, standing, sitting, blowing the nose, spasms of the paravertebral muscles, and any jarring movement while walking or riding. The character of pain can range from mild discomfort to excruciating agony. Sitting is particularly painful. In the acute phase, the patient is most comfortable lying in bed on his back with knees flexed and a small pillow at the head. Other patients prefer the lateral recumbent position, lying on the unaffected side with the knee flexed on the affected side.

Postural Deformity. Upon physical examination, the normal lumbar lordosis is absent in about 60% of herniated disc patients. The sign is also accompanied by lumbar scoliosis and spasms of the paravertebral muscles. Movement of the lumbar spine is limited with lateral flexion restricted.

In the standing position, the patient presents a typical picture of flattened lumbar spine (Fig. 19-3), slight tilting forward of the trunk, and slight flexion on the affected side of the hip and knee. The alterations of normal posture are defense mechanisms to compensate for the pathophysiology. The paravertebral muscles contract to prevent traction on the affected nerve roots, which would intensify pain if the spine were extended. The patient walks cautiously, bearing as little weight as possible on the affected side. His gait may be described as stiff. Movement is very deliberate to prevent jarring. Climbing stairs is particularly painful.

Motor Changes of Involved Nerve Roots. Hypotonia is common with motor root compression. Slight motor weakness may be experienced, although major weakness is rare. Motor weakness is difficult to evaluate because of the defensive reaction precipitated by pain. Weakness may be evident upon plantar flexion or dorsiflexion of the foot and, occasionally, of the hamstring and quadriceps muscles. Atrophy of the affected muscles may develop, although it is not a usual finding and can be minimal. Footdrop has been evident in some patients. Motor weakness is sometimes accompanied by difficulty in micturition and sexual activity.

Sensory Changes of Involved Nerve Roots. The most common sensory impairments from root compression are paresthesias and numbness, particularly of the leg and foot. Tenderness is noted over the L-5 and S-1 vertebral spines and along the tracking of the sciatic nerve (Fig. 19-4).

FIG. 19-3. The spinal signs of lumbar disc herniation. (Smith RR: Essentials of Neurosurgery. Philadelphia, JB Lippincott, 1980)

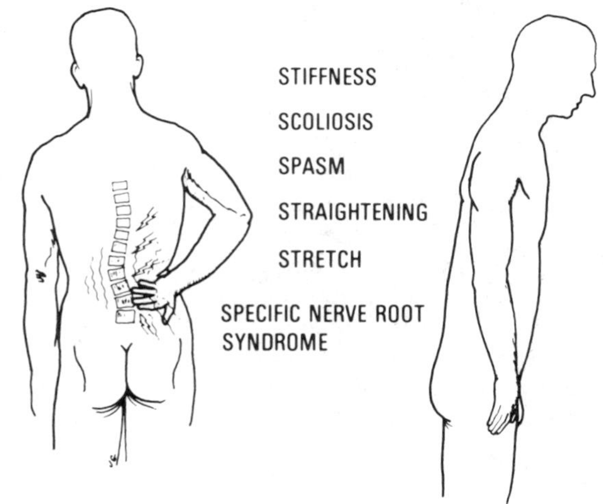

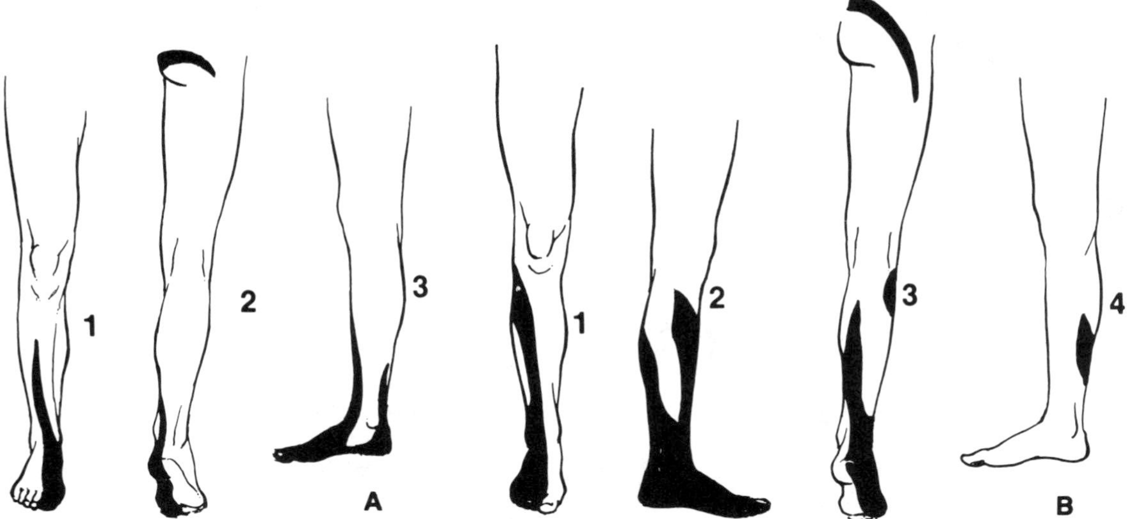

FIG. 19–4. Sensory loss of fifth lumbar nerve root (A) due to compression of the fourth lumbar interspace and (B) from pressure on the first sacral nerve root. (Turek S: Orthopaedics, 3rd ed. Philadelphia, JB Lippincott, 1977)

Alterations of Reflexes. With herniated discs, the knee or ankle reflexes are absent or diminished, depending on the level of the disc herniation.

Other Diagnostic Signs. Other signs that are positive in lumbar herniated disc disease include Lasègue's maneuver, Neri's sign, Naffziger's test, and Kernig's sign.

Lasègue's maneuver refers to straight leg-raising (Fig. 19–5). Normally, it is possible, when lying on the back, to move the straightened leg about 90 degrees with only some slight discomfort in the hamstring muscles. The sciatic nerve becomes stretched upon movement and creates traction on the proximal nerve roots. Traction and movement of the nerve roots begin when the leg is at a 30- to 40-degree angle. In the patient with a herniated low back disc, the stretching of the sciatic nerve during passive, straight leg-raising creates traction on the inflamed or irritated nerve roots, thereby producing severe pain. Patients with severe sciatica will not be able to raise their legs beyond 20 to 30 degrees. Less severe involvement allows straight leg-raising to 50 or 60 degrees.[1] Repeating Lasègue's maneuver on the unaffected leg produces pain of decreased severity on the contralateral side.

FIG. 19–5. Straight leg-raising (Lasègue's sign) in assessment of herniated disc.

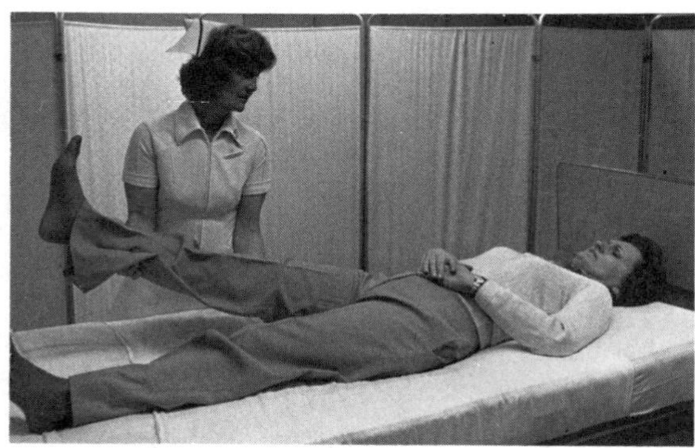

Neri's sign is elicited when the patient bends forward, resulting in knee flexion on the affected side. This is a protective mechanism to prevent stretching of the sciatic nerve.

Naffziger's test is done by compressing both jugular veins while the patient is in a standing position (Fig. 19–6). This

FIG. 19–6. In Naffziger's test, the jugular veins are compressed simultaneously while the patient is standing erect. Radiating components of the pain are usually accentuated by this maneuver. The examiner must avoid bilateral compression of the carotid arteries when performing Naffziger's test. (Smith RR: Essentials of Neurosurgery. Philadelphia, JB Lippincott, 1980)

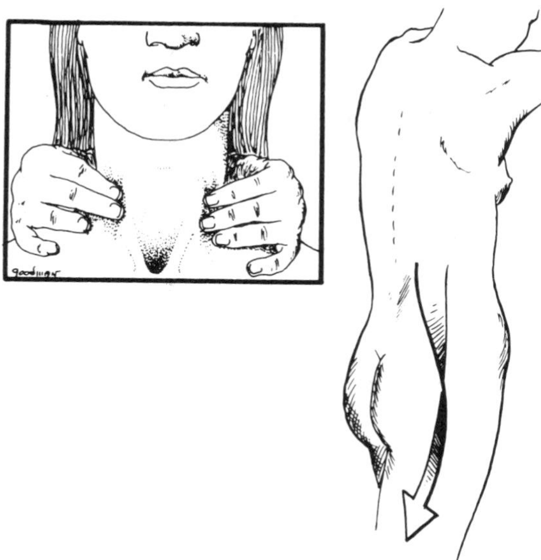

maneuver will produce pain in the patient with a herniated disc. Physiologically, compression of the jugular veins obliterates venous drainage from the brain, thereby increasing intraventricular pressure of the cerebrospinal fluid. The result is an increase in intraspinal pressure, which will produce pain if a herniated disc is present.

Kernig's sign is carried out by attempting to flex the hip and knee while the patient is in the dorsal recumbent position (Fig. 19–7). When the hip is flexed 90 degrees, the knee is slowly extended. In the normal patient, the knee should be able to be extended about 90 degrees. In a patient with a low back herniated disc, severe pain will be precipitated by stretching the nerve roots upon knee extension. It will, therefore, not be possible to extend the knee the normal range in the disc patient. Any manipulation of the leg is painful.

Cerebrospinal Fluid Protein. One last diagnostic test should be mentioned. In many but not all patients with herniated disc disease, the cerebrospinal fluid protein is elevated. The elevation may be 70 mg to 100 mg/100 ml.

Specific Lumbar Levels

The most common sites for lumbar disc herniation are the L–4 to L–5 and the L–5 to S–1 levels, in that order. Lesions at the L–3 to L–4 level are rare.

Each level presents a characteristic syndrome of symptoms distinct from the other levels.

L–4 to L–5 Level. Pain is felt in the hip, groin, posterolateral thigh, lateral calf, dorsal surface of the foot, and the first or second and third toes.[1] Paresthesias may be experienced over the lateral leg and web of the great toe. There is tenderness at the femoral head and lateral gluteal region. There is some weakness upon dorsiflexion of the great toe and foot. Footdrop can occur. The patient has difficulty walking on his heels. Atrophy, if present, is minor. Reflexes are usually not diminished.

FIG. 19–7. Testing for Kernig's sign. Flex one of the patient's legs at hip and knee, then straighten the knee. Note resistance or pain. (Bates B: Guide to Physical Examination. Philadelphia, JB Lippincott, 1974)

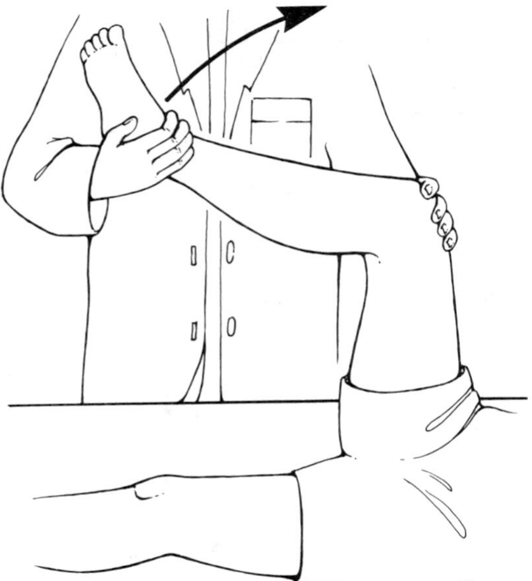

L–5 to S–1 Level. Pain is felt in the mid-gluteal region, posterior thigh, and calf region down to the heel and the outer surface of the foot on the side of the fourth and fifth toes. Paresthesias are found in the posterior calf and lateral heel, foot, and toe. Tenderness is especially apparent in the area of the sacroiliac joint. Weakness in plantar flexion of the foot and great toe is noted. The patient has difficulty walking on his toes. The hamstring muscles may also show signs of weakness. If atrophy is present at all, the gastrocnemius and the soleus are affected. The ankle jerk reflex is diminished or absent.

L–3 to L–4 Level. Pain is located in the lower back, hip, posterolateral thigh, and anterior leg. Paresthesias are experienced in the middle section of the anterior thigh. Weakness is noted in the quadriceps muscles, which may also demonstrate atrophic changes. The knee jerk reflex is diminished.

Remission of Pain. The pain associated with herniated disc disease is recurrent. Patients typically present a history of one or several episodes of low back pain radiating across the buttocks and into one leg to the ankle. Between acute episodes, pain may be completely absent or at least substantially diminished, so that the patient is able to cope with the discomfort. Remissions of acute episodes are probably due to recession of the protruding disc, decreased local edema, relief of root compression, and reabsorption of disc exudate.

Cervical Area

The cervical region of the spine is prone to trauma, degeneration, and spondylitic changes, which predispose the affected person to a wider range of pathological conditions. A serious consequence of nerve root or spinal cord compression is possible interference with vital respiratory functions.

One of the most common causes of neck, shoulder, and arm pain in the middle-aged and older population is disc herniation of the lower cervical region. Symptoms can develop without any apparent injury or may follow trauma such as whiplash or any hyperextension injuries. Upon radiological investigation, salient disc degeneration, arthritis, or spondylitis are frequently identified. The most common sites of cervical herniation are at the C–5 to C–6 and C–6 to C–7 levels, with pain along the affected sensory dermatomes (Fig. 19–8). Herniation may be lateral or central.

Anatomically, there is little free room within the spinal canal to accommodate any extraneous material. The cervical spinal cord is firmly positioned by the ligamenta denticulata. Disc protrusion in the cervical area can result not

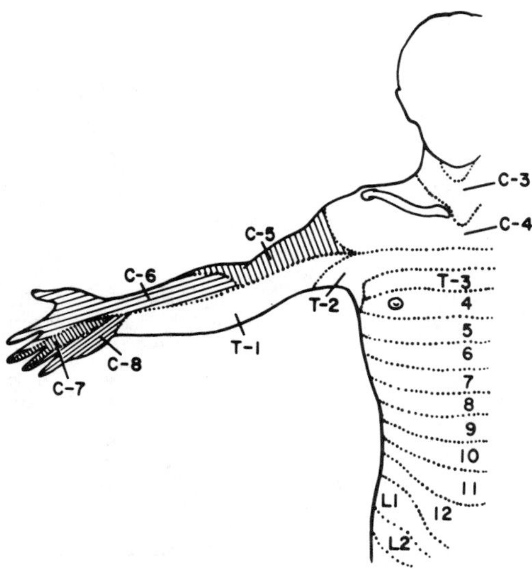

FIG. 19–8. Sensory dermatomes of cervical nerves, including all overlap, document lowest functioning nerve root in traumatic complete quadriplegia. (Rockwood CA, Green DP: Fractures. Philadelphia, JB Lippincott, 1977)

only in root compression but also cord compression due to the lack of free space. The particular presenting symptoms depend on the anatomical point of disc protrusion. The possible locations of disc protrusion include lateral, paracentral, or central herniation.

Lateral Herniation. Symptoms of lateral cervical disc herniation include root pain in the shoulders, neck, and arm (Fig. 19–9) and paresthesias along the dermatome of the compressed nerve root. Paravertebral muscle spasms, which cause a stiff neck, accompany the pain. Reflex loss and possible motor weakness follow. Neck movement is often restricted to some degree in all directions. Tenderness may be experienced when pressure is exerted over the involved cervical spine. Weakness of the hand muscles and forearm may be noted. Atrophy may also be detected upon physical examination. Arm reflexes are absent or diminished.

FIG. 19–9. Pattern of pain radiation with a lateral protrusion of a cervical disc. (Hoppenfeld S: Orthopaedic Neurology. Philadelphia, JB Lippincott, 1977)

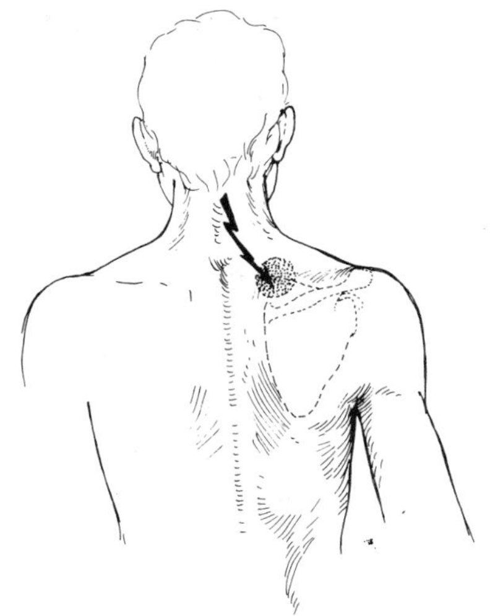

Paracentral or Central Herniations. Symptoms of herniation of this anatomical site can be contrasted with those of lateral herniations. Pain, if present, is usually mild, insidious, and intermittent (Fig. 19–10). An acute or gradual onset of spinal cord compression occurs. Weakness of the lower extremities and an unsteady gait become apparent. As the compression increases, spasticity is noted. There may be difficulty with voiding and sexual function. Reflexes of the lower extremities become hyperactive, while those in the upper extremities vary. Cervical cord compression can simulate degenerative cord disease such as syringomyelia and amyotrophic lateral sclerosis.

Specific Cervical Levels

The most common cervical herniations are at C–5 to C–6 and C–6 to C–7. Each level presents a characteristic syndrome of symptoms distinct from other levels.

FIG. 19–10. Pattern of pain radiation with a midline herniated cervical disc. (Hoppenfeld S: Orthopaedic Neurology. Philadelphia, JB Lippincott, 1977)

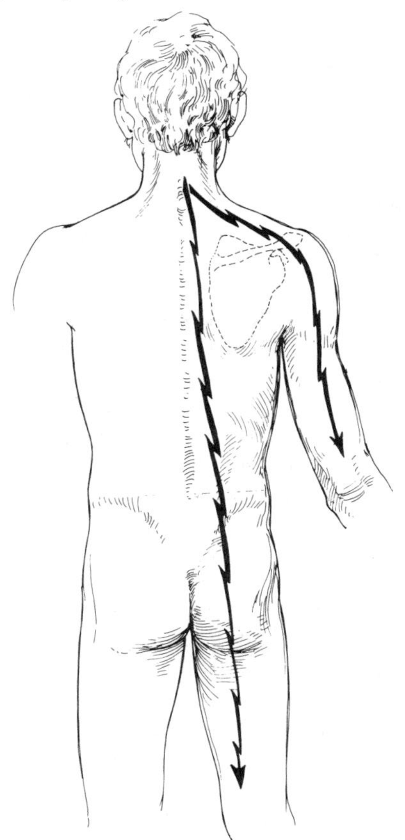

C-5 to C-6 Level (Lateral Herniation). Pain is experienced in the neck, shoulder, anterior portion of the upper part of the arm, radial forearm, and possibly the thumb and forefinger. Less frequently, pain extends to the scapular and clavicular regions. The paresthesias and sensory loss are found in the thumb, forefinger, radial and lateral forearm, and lateral aspects of the upper arm. Weakness is noted upon flexion of the forearm (biceps.). Tenderness is found in both the supraspinal area of the scapula and the biceps region. Reflexes that are diminished or absent include the biceps and supinator reflexes. The triceps reflex is either exaggerated or left intact.[1]

C-6 to C-7 Level (Lateral Herniation). Pain is experienced in the neck, shoulder blade, and the lateral surfaces of upper arm and forearm. The index finger, the little finger, and sometimes the ring finger are plagued by pain, although all of the fingers can be involved. Paresthesias and sensory loss are most prominent in the second and third fingers and lateral forearm. Weakness is found in the triceps and extensor carpi radialis (extensors for forearm and handgrips). Occasional wristdrop may result. Tenderness is most apparent in the area over the medial shoulder blade. Reflexes that are preserved include the biceps and supinator, while the triceps is diminished or absent.

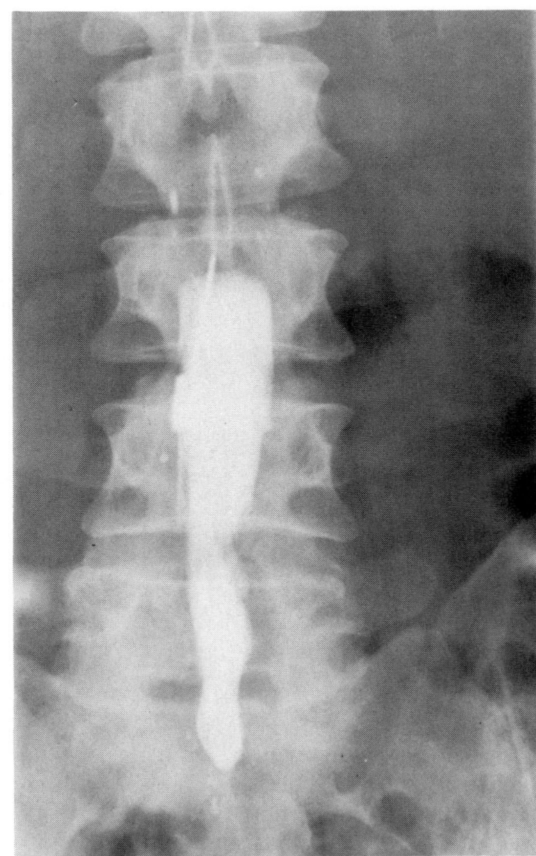

FIG. 19-11. Myelogram showing herniated disc. (Hoppenfeld S: Orthopaedic Neurology. Philadelphia, JB Lippincott, 1977)

DIAGNOSIS

The diagnosis of intervertebral disc herniation must be differentiated from other diseases such as primary tumors, metastatic neoplasms, and all of the other causes of back pain previously mentioned. Making a diagnosis upon clinical examination is difficult, if not impossible. Usual diagnostic procedures ordered to provide additional information include x-ray films of the spine and a contrast myelogram. Other diagnostic tools that may be valuable include spinal fluid studies, spinal dynamics, electromyography, and discograms. X-ray films are not specific but can indicate a narrowing of the intervertebral disc because of disc degeneration. A narrowed disc may or may not be accompanied by a herniated disc. Other findings that may be of value include identification of spurs and hypertrophic osteoarthritis. Contrast myelography is indicated when a disc herniation is suspected. The procedure will usually indicate the presence of a herniated disc and the precise level of herniation, as well as ruling out cord neoplasms. The myelogram is considered the most important diagnostic tool for identifying herniated discs (Fig. 19-11).

The diagnosis of a herniated disc can be accurately concluded from fulfillment of the following criteria: a history of trauma, narrowed intervertebral discs noted on radiographs, and a positive myelogram.

Other diagnostic procedures are ordered for special reasons. Cerebrospinal fluid may be examined for protein elevation; however, elevated protein is possible in both spinal cord tumor and intervertebral disc herniation. Identification of any atypical cell may be ordered if a tumor is suspected. Spinal dynamics or the Queckenstedt test may be conducted to indicate complete or partial blockage to flow of cerebrospinal fluid in the spinal subarachnoid space. More accurate information, however, could be collected from a contrast myelogram. Electromyography may be ordered when the myelogram is not conclusive: it would indicate neural or muscle damage. Discograms, although controversial, sometimes unreliable, and risky, may be done to indicate herniation of a particular disc.

TREATMENT

Treatment of herniated disc disease follows two possible paths: conservative treatment or surgery. The concept that disc disease is caused by repeated trauma with degenerative changes is generally accepted. Most physicians, therefore, propose a course of treatment that will protect the involved area from added trauma and provide an environment that will allow for healing of the injured degenerative discs by fibrosis. These two points plus the control of pain are the goals of conservative treatment.

Conservative Treatment

Conservative treatment may be tried for 2 to 6 weeks. The stringency of rest and avoidance of any stress prescribed depends upon the severity of symptoms. A patient with mild or moderate symptoms is advised to

1. Decrease general activity (bed rest)
2. Avoid any flexion of the spine such as lifting, bending, or twisting
3. Use a support garment such as a corset, brace, or collar (depending on location)
4. Use a firm mattress
5. Possibly participate in physiotherapy—hot or cold packs, diathermy, ultrasound, or dry heat
6. Possible skin traction (pelvic belt or halter traction)
7. Drugs

The patient with severe symptoms is treated with complete bed rest on a firm mattress. Pelvic belt traction for lumbar pain or halter traction for cervical pain may be suggested for home use. Drug therapy and physiotherapy are also included. For the hospitalized disc patient a regime of a few hours in skin traction (Fig. 19–12), followed by 1 or 2 hours out of traction, has been tried. Although it may provide comfort for some patients, there appears to be little therapeutic effect. It does enforce bed rest in the patient who might otherwise resist enforced confinement to bed.

Nursing Management. Nursing management of the hospitalized patient is directed toward maintaining the prescribed bed rest, attending to traction considerations, and preventing complications.

Bed rest for patients with pain in the lumbar region calls for proper positioning on the back with knees flexed. A pillow may be placed under the knees to prevent excess tension on the nerve roots. In addition, pressure must not be allowed to build up on the popliteal nerve. A small pillow may be placed under the head for comfort. For a patient with cervical pain, a small pillow may be placed in the nape of the neck. Since the purpose of bed rest is to reduce strain and pulling on the nerves, the nurse should see that any items the patient may need are within easy reach in order to avoid any undue stretching or moving. While informing the patient about the limitations on activity, the nurse can take the opportunity to discuss the overall purpose and goals of the bed rest regimen and the expected amount of bed rest prescribed by the physician.

FIG. 19–12. Pelvic belt traction. (Farrell J: Illustrated Guide to Orthopedic Nursing, 2nd ed. Philadelphia, JB Lippincott, 1982)

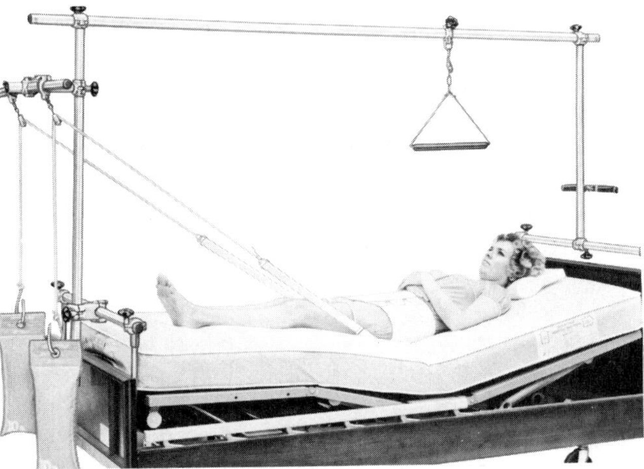

To avoid any complication from the extended period of bed rest, elastic stockings should be applied and the patient encouraged to put his feet through range-of-motion exercises and carry out deep breathing exercises at least four times daily. At the same time, an accurate intake and output record should be maintained to help evaluate bladder function.

If traction is ordered, care must be taken to ensure proper alignment of body and weights. For the patient with lumbar pain, the type of traction ordered is usually pelvic belt traction.

For a patient with pain in the cervical region, a head halter is usually the means of applying intermittent traction to relieve spasms and pressure on the nerve roots. Skin care in this instance would involve checking the chin for irritation from the head gear. Frequently these patients are required to wear a soft or hard collar at all times (when not in traction) to provide added support and comfort. See Chart 19–1 for a summary of conservative management.

Drug Therapy. Analgesics, muscle relaxants, anti-inflammatory agents, and sedative–tranquilizers are types of drugs ordered to control the symptoms and make the patient more comfortable. Muscle relaxants include methocarbamol (Robaxin), carisoprodol (Soma), chlorzoxazone (Paraflex), and metaxalone (Skelaxin), to mention a few.

The use of muscle relaxants is open to discussion because the effectiveness of some of these drugs is questionable, especially since the mode of action of muscle relaxants is unclear. As with any drugs, there are side-effects, such as nausea, vomiting, diarrhea, abdominal distress, drowsiness, vertigo, light-headedness, and headache. There may also be weakness, ataxia, and jaundice. Most drugs are given orally, although in the hospitalized patient, rapid intravenous administration of certain muscle relaxants such as diazepam (Valium) and methocarbamol (Robaxin) is possible. For example, methocarbamol (Robaxin), 500 mg in 5% dextrose in water, can be given intravenously. The dilution in solution decreases the highly irritative quality of the drug. The nurse who is administering any drugs should be familiar with the many side-effects and precautions that should be taken.

Anti-inflammatory drugs are used to diminish the local edema and inflammation from injury. Phenylbutazone (Butazolidin), 100 mg four times a day, may be ordered. Side-effects include gastrointestinal irritation, fluid retention, and blood dyscrasias. The drug should be administered with milk to decrease the gastrointestinal irritation. The patient should be observed for fluid retention. Routine laboratory studies can identify dyscrasias. If ordered, 0.75 mg four times a day of dexamethasone (Decadron), tapered over 1 week, is given. Side-effects are many, including gas-

CHART 19-1. SUMMARY OF THE PROTOCOL FOR THE CONSERVATIVE TREATMENT OF THE PATIENT WITH A HERNIATED INTERVERTEBRAL DISC*

NURSING RESPONSIBILITIES	RATIONALE
1. Maintain a firm mattress with a bedboard.	**1.** Provides support to the vertebral column
2. Maintain on bed rest (bed rest may be complete or bathroom privileges may be allowed).	**2.** Decreases stress and strain on vertebral column and soft supporting structures
3. Assess vital signs at periodic intervals.	**3.** Monitors vital signs for evidence of complications
4. Assess neurological function of involved areas; for cervical disc note motor function, strength, tone, reflex activity and sensation to neck, shoulder, and arms; for lumbar disc note motor function, strength, tone, reflex activity, and sensation to buttocks and legs.	**4.** Identifies motor and sensory function and deficits present
5. Maintain in proper body alignment, which decreases stress of irritated muscles. • For cervical disc provide a small pillow in nape of neck. • For lumbar disc provide a small pillow under the knees to relieve pressure; a small pillow can be placed under the head (avoid pressure on the popliteal area).	**5.** Decreases stress on irritated nerves and muscles; provides comfort
6. Log-roll the patient when turning.	**6.** Maintains proper body alignment
7. Caution the patient against twisting, stretching, straining, pulling, or bending.	**7.** Same as above
8. Apply elastic stockings and ensure that they are worn at all times.	**8.** Improves vascular resistance and venous emptying; prevents thrombus formation in the legs
9. Encourage patient to perform range-of-motion exercises to the extremities at least four times a day.	**9.** Maintains muscle and vascular tone
10. Encourage deep breathing exercises at least four times a day.	**10.** Prevents the respiratory complications of immobility
11. Provide a high roughage diet and stool softener as necessary.	**11.** Prevents constipation, which increases discomfort caused by increased intra-abdominal pressure
12. Administer drugs as ordered: muscle relaxants, analgesics, sedative-tranquilizers, and anti-inflammatory agents.	**12.** Provides for analgesia and resolution of irritation and inflammation
13. Maintain traction schedule as ordered (*e.g.,* 1 to 2 hours in traction followed by 2 to 3 hours out of traction). • For cervical disc, head halter traction is used. • For lumbar disc, a pelvic belt is used.	**13.** Reduces muscle spasms
14. Provide good skin care and inspect skin in contact with traction device.	**14.** Prevents skin breakdown
15. If a soft collar is ordered for a cervical disc, apply with head in slight flexion.	**15.** Maintains normal position
16. For a lumbar disc, exercises may be ordered to be performed when the patient is out of traction; instruct the patient in the conduct of these exercises (*e.g.,* semi-sit-ups, pelvic tilts, and gluteal setting).	**16.** Strengthens the abdominal and back muscles
17. Teach the patient the correct method of applying any support garments for braces.	**17.** Achieves therapeutic goals of treatment
18. Develop and implement a patient teaching plan.	**18.** Promotes good body mechanics and prevents further injury

* Differences in the management of the patient with a cervical or a lumbar disc will be noted where there is variation in management.

trointestinal irritation. Magnesium hydroxide (Maalox), 30 ml orally with dexamethasone (Decadron), is commonly given to prevent gastrointestinal irritation.

Sedative-tranquilizers are given to decrease anxiety, which will subsequently decrease muscle tension and pain. Phenobarbital, 15 mg to 30 mg orally four times a day or diazepam (Valium), 5 mg to 10 mg three or four times a day, are frequent choices. (Note the dual effect of Valium.)

As for analgesics, a few important points should be made. It may be necessary to order narcotics such as codeine, 30 mg orally every 4 hours as needed during the acute phase. The side-effect of constipation should be controlled with a stool softener such as docusate sodium (Colace), 100 mg three times a day, given orally. This is true because constipation increases intra-abdominal pressure and straining at stool, which, in turn, increase pain. Once the acute phase has subsided, it is imperative to change the analgesic order to one that is nonnarcotic; otherwise, one risks the development of drug addiction in the patient. Pain from disc herniation is experienced by the patient in varying degrees for several weeks. Although it is a goal of treatment to control pain, prudent judgment must prevail to prevent added disability to the patient.

Summary. Conservative treatment for herniated disc disease includes

1. Bed rest on a firm mattress
2. Elimination of bending, lifting, and twisting of the spine
3. Intermittent skin traction (head halter, pelvic belt)
4. Use of drugs
5. Physiotherapy

As symptoms subside, activity is gradually increased. Exercises to strengthen back and abdominal muscles are taught to the patient by the physiotherapist, with the nurse being responsible for encouraging and reinforcing the method and purposes of the exercises.

Once the patient has been properly instructed in the exercise program he may do the exercises while in bed during the periods he is out of his traction, if so prescribed. Common exercises ordered include (Fig. 19–13)

1. Semi–sit-ups
2. Pelvic tilts
3. Knee–chest exercises
4. Gluteal setting

In addition, the patient must be instructed in the use of good body mechanics when he is out of bed.

The majority of patients treated conservatively will recover. Unfortunately, there are those who will require surgical intervention.

Chemonucleolysis

Chemonucleolysis is the injection of chymopapain into the nucleus pulposus of an intervertebral disc. Chymopapain is an enzyme extracted from the papaya plant. When injected directly into a herniated intervertebral disc, the enzyme reduces the central disc components by hydrolysis, thus decreasing the size of the protruding disc. With the pressure removed from the spinal nerve roots, pain is significantly diminished.

A few points should be clarified. Recall that the nucleus pulposus is the inner disc material. Chymopapain has little or no effect on the anulus fibrosus, the fibrotic tissue that surrounds the nucleus pulposus. Because of the inherent characteristics of chymopapain, the duration of action is limited to only a few minutes, although it takes from 6 to 12 weeks to determine whether the procedure can be declared successful for the particular patient. In one Canadian study a success rate of 83% was reported for chemonucleolysis with chymopapain.[2] Because the procedure is relatively new in the United States, studies of success rates involving large numbers of patients are just being compiled, yet informal discussions with some physicians indicate success rates of approximately 50%.

Chemonucleolysis with chymopapain has been used since the mid-1960s in Europe, England, and Canada. However, it was not until November 1982 that it was approved for use in the United States. Currently, it is used only for lumbar discs below the L–3 level. The procedure provides an option to selected patients who would otherwise be scheduled for a laminectomy. The advantages of chemonucleolysis over laminectomy are a hospital stay of 1 to 3 days instead of 7 to 10 days; avoidance of a major surgical procedure; and significantly reduced medical costs.

Indications and Contraindications. The careful selection of patients is important for the success of the procedure. The indications for chemonucleolysis include patients with

- Low back pain radiating into the leg
- A positive myelogram that demonstrates a herniated intervertebral disc
- Neurological signs and symptoms consistent with the level of disc protrusion
- Failure to benefit from conservative treatment
- Positive straight leg-raising test (optional with some physicians)[3]

FIG. 19–13. Exercise program for herniated disc includes semi–sit-ups *(left)* and knee–chest exercises *(right)*.

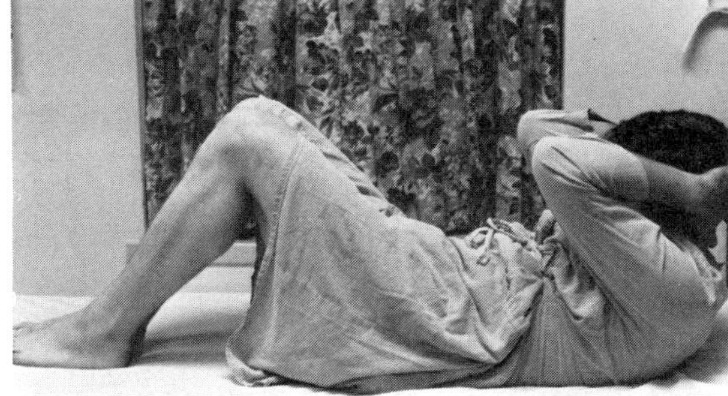

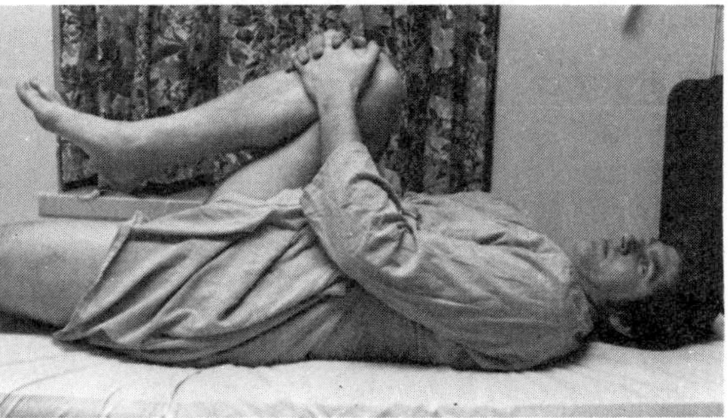

The contraindications for the procedure include

- Rapid progression of neurological deficits
- Bowel or bladder dysfunction
- Discitis
- Previous injection with chymopapain (increased risk of allergic reaction)
- Known allergic response to papaya (e.g., meat tenderizer)
- Pregnancy
- Age less than 18 years or more than 60 years
- More than two levels of disc involvement.
- Presence of lumbar spondylosis or previous surgery in the same area.[2,4]

Procedure. Although chemonucleolysis with chymopapain does not use an open surgical approach, it is considered a surgical procedure. The procedure is performed in the operating room under general anesthesia, although some physicians prefer to use local or epidural anesthesia. An intravenous line and cardiac monitoring should be in place. The patient must be monitored and readied for immediate treatment should an allergic reaction develop. The patient is positioned on his left side and draped after anatomical landmarks have been identified and marked. A fluoroscopic image intensifier is used so that the surgeon can visualize the anatomical structures of the spinal column and the placement of the needle. The suspected discs are injected with a radiopaque dye to verify the herniated disc in a procedure known as a discography. After the herniated disc is identified, a small amount of chymopapain is injected and the patient observed for possible allergic reaction. Barring any untoward response, the therapeutic dose is injected. Upon withdrawal of the needle, a small dressing is applied to the puncture site and the patient is transferred to the recovery room.[2]

Nursing Management. The patient scheduled for chemonucleolysis with chymopapain receives preoperative medication. In some instances, diphenhydramine (Benadryl) may also be given as a precaution against a possible drug reaction. The patient is prepared like any patient who will undergo general anesthesia. Vital signs should be recorded. An assessment of the type, location, and extent of pain and motor or sensory loss or change should be noted as a baseline for comparison.

In the recovery room, nursing observations are directed toward stabilization of vital signs, early recognition of any signs or symptoms of allergic reaction that may lead to anaphylactic shock, and identification of neurological deficits not present before the procedure. Once back in his own room, the patient must continue to be monitored for possible allergic reactions (rash, itching, stuffy nose, hypotension, difficulty in breathing, cardiac arrest). If signs and symptoms of an allergic reaction develop, immediate treatment with epinephrine (Adrenalin), diphenhydramine (Benadryl), hydrocortisone sodium succinate (Solu-Cortef), and other standard drug protocols should be instituted. Some patients will experience transient voiding problems, muscle spasms, pain, and swelling at the injection site. The spasms may continue for several days or even weeks, and pain may continue to be a problem. Both of these conditions are potential sources of altered comfort for the patient.

Bed rest is maintained for 24 hours, and analgesics and muscle relaxants are administered. Ambulation can be resumed after 24 hours and discharge from the hospital scheduled in 1 or 2 days, if the patient progresses well. Upon discharge, it is important to instruct the patient on his activity limitations. Most physicians follow a conservative plan of gradual light exercise followed by gradual resumption of activities in 3 to 6 weeks.

As mentioned previously, it may take from 6 to 12 weeks to judge the success of the procedure. For some patients chemonucleolysis will provide very good results, while others will not be so fortunate and will require an open surgical procedure.

Surgery

Surgery is in order for those patients who do not respond to conservative treatment or for those who, by the very nature of the herniation or symptoms, require immediate surgical intervention. This latter group includes patients with massive central herniations that compress the cauda equina, resulting in motor and sensory paresis along with the loss of sphincter control; compression, resulting in quadriceps weakness or footdrop; severe and unrelenting pain; and prolonged and recurrent sciatica that interferes with normal life, job security, and weekly income.

The possible surgical procedures that may be performed depend on the results of physical examination and myelogram. Possible choices include

- *Hemilaminectomy*—excision of part of the posterior arch of the vertebral lamina
- *Foraminotomy*—surgical removal of part of the intervertebral foramen
- *Anterior cervical discectomy and fusion*—anterior cervical approach to remove a disc fragment and to perform a fusion (can be used in the upper and middle cervical vertebrae)
- *Bone fusion*—immobilization of specific vertebrae by insertion of a wedge-shaped piece of bone usually obtained from the iliac crest, between the vertebrae. (The site from which the bone graft is taken is called the donor site.)

Microsurgical Approaches to Disc Surgery. Microdiscectomy of herniated discs has been made possible with the multiple application of microsurgical techniques to neurosurgery. Both lumbar and cervical microdiscectomies are alternatives to the traditional laminectomy. Although lumbar microdiscectomy appears to be used more widely, cervical microdiscectomy has also achieved very good results. One advantage of microdiscectomy is that it magnifies the operative site for better visualization and identification of anatomical structures, reducing the possibility of dural laceration and cerebrospinal fluid leakage, nerve root trauma, and injury to blood vessels and subsequent development of a hematoma. Because epidural vessels can be identified and coagulated more easily, the possibility of bleeding is decreased. It is also possible to leave the nerve root free, thus decreasing the development of adhesions.[5] The second advantage of the microsurgical technique for disc removal is the improved illumination. Because the illumination and visualization are improved, a smaller incision can be made.

Lumbar Discectomy. The first lumbar microdiscectomy was done in 1978, and modifications to the surgical technique have evolved in the last few years. Patient selection for lumbar microdiscectomy is similar to that of traditional lumbar laminectomy. A patient who has not responded to conservative treatment and has motor or sphincter weakness is a good candidate for disc surgery. The surgical incision is only half an inch to 1 inch long. The value to the patient because of a smaller incision is less pain, less paraspinal muscle disruption (fewer muscle spasms postoperatively), less postoperative spinal instability, a shorter hospitalization, and a faster recovery.

Even though the incision is small, the operating microscope and illumination allow the surgeon to remove sufficient lamina, ligamentum flavum, and disc material. Even very small pieces of disc exudate can be seen and removed. Closure of the small incision is simple, requiring only a few sutures. A small dressing covers the incision.

Postoperatively, the patient is allowed out of bed the same day and is often discharged within 2 days.[5] In addition to the improved comfort of the patient, the cost of hospitalization is substantially decreased. The results of microdiscectomy are considered to be as good or better than the results of traditional lumbar laminectomy. The incidence of recurrence cannot be assessed because of the limited number of patients who have had the procedure. The only complication suggested to result from lumbar discectomy is discitis.

Cervical Microdiscectomy. Various specific surgical techniques are available for the removal of cervical discs under microsurgery. However, the microsurgical approach has many advantages for the patient and surgeon. Some procedures provide for the removal of the entire disc without surgical fusion; within a year of these procedures, immobilization of the involved interspace occurred.[6] Other techniques have also been described in the literature.

NURSING MANAGEMENT OF THE LAMINECTOMY PATIENT

PSYCHOSOCIAL CONSIDERATIONS

By the time that a patient with a herniated disc is seen by the nurse in the clinical setting, the patient has usually experienced pain for varying periods. Some patients may have undergone conservative treatment at home with poor results. Others may have experienced intermittent episodes of pain over a period of months or even years. The decision is finally made by the physician and patient to undergo surgery because the patient's lifestyle has been seriously disturbed by the chronicity of the back problem. There are still other patients who have already undergone one surgical procedure but have experienced continued or renewed pain. Another surgical procedure is perceived as a blatant reminder that surgery does not always produce remission of painful symptoms. The experience shared in common by all patients is disabling pain.

Many patients have taken various analgesics at home for extended periods with unsatisfactory relief of pain. If pain was controlled, the medication might have been a narcotic reluctantly prescribed by the physician. Many patients have developed tolerance to the common analgesics. The patient has probably found that it takes more and more just to take the "edge" off the pain. Sedatives and tranquilizers are often ordered to control anxiety, which enhances the perception of pain. All medications have side-effects that are usually unpleasant. Drowsiness, headache, irritability, and nausea are common distressing symptoms. Side-effects from drugs, compounded by chronic severe pain, deplete the patient of his normal coping mechanisms. The chronicity of pain plus alterations in lifestyle create feelings of anxiety and depression. For some patients, economic security is threatened because of the inability to work due to back pain.

In the clinical setting, these patients are difficult for the nurse to manage. They tend to be irritable, negative, and even hostile. It is difficult, if not impossible, to keep them comfortable because of their severe pain, anxiety, and tolerance to many drugs. It can be frustrating to the nurse not to be able to provide physical comfort for the patient.

The postoperative period can be overwhelmingly disappointing to the patient who experiences muscle spasms and similar or greater pain than he experienced before surgery. Any patient who undergoes surgery, regardless of how explicitly the physician has explained possible outcomes, expects relief. When he finds that he is hurting as much or more than before surgery, he is angry.

There are many things that the nurse can do to help the patient. The first thing is to understand what has preceded hospital admission. The duration of pain, extent of disability, and the effect on the patient's life should be considered. Once the nurse has an understanding of what has happened to the patient, it is easier to understand and accept his behavior. It is most important to listen to the patient so that misconceptions can be corrected and gaps in information can be filled. Ask the patient what the physician has told him about the operation.

It is important that the patient have realistic expectations after surgery. He must understand that he will most likely experience pain because of nerve root irritation and edema, which will gradually subside. The possibility of muscle spasms should also be discussed so that he is not devastated when and if they occur. Tactful handling by the nurse creates a feeling of trust. The patient can be told that many patients experience uncomfortable muscle spasms in the low back, thighs, and abdomen (in lumbar laminectomy) in the early postoperative period. "You may have this experience after surgery. It is a temporary occurrence that passes in a few days. It does not indicate that your surgery was not successful. You will be receiving your pain medication after surgery to keep you comfortable." The patient should be encouraged to discuss his fears.

The basics of good body mechanics and the need to avoid stress to the back should be discussed with the patient long before discharge. Most physicians will approach the subject with the patient, but it is the nurse's responsibility to reinforce this concept. This is one way to alleviate some of the anxiety and fear about the possibility of further back problems.

Summary

A nursing goal is to reduce the patient's anxiety by listening and providing information and a supportive relationship. If anxiety is reduced, the perception of pain is decreased, and the ability to cope is increased.

PREOPERATIVE NURSING CARE

Aside from the regular preoperative preparation, including skin shave, patient teaching, and psychological support, Ace bandages may be required from toe to midthigh (three Ace bandages per leg) to ensure increased blood return to the heart and to guard against vasodilation of the lower extremities from vasomotor changes that could cause a drop in blood pressure.

POSTOPERATIVE NURSING CARE

Postoperative management after cervical or lumbar laminectomy is directed toward the following objective:

- Ongoing assessment and monitoring of parameters for early recognition of complications
- Promotion of comfort
- Promotion of healing at operative site

The specific protocols and nursing responsibilities are summarized in Chart 19–2.

POSSIBLE COMPLICATIONS AFTER SURGERY

Postoperative complications that may develop can be classified into the general problems common to all surgical patients and those seen in laminectomy patients only. The general complications include atelectasis, pneumonia, wound infection, and thrombophlebitis. Prevention and management of these conditions are outlined in a general medical–surgical text. The more common complications specific to the laminectomy patient are outlined below.

Paralytic Ileus

Stimulation of the sympathetic nervous system contributes to the development of the loss of peristalsis in the gastrointestinal tract, resulting in paralytic ileus. The signs and symptoms include

1. Nausea and vomiting (most patients can't even tolerate clear liquids)
2. Major distention of the large bowel and abdomen (the abdomen feels hard)
3. Absence of bowel sounds upon auscultation of the abdominal cavity

In the postoperative period, the nurse will notice that the patient develops an intolerance to fluids and complains of nausea and vomiting whenever fluids are offered. At the same time, an increase in the girth of the abdomen can be noted. Auscultation of the abdominal cavity reveals an absence of peristalsis. All of these symptoms should be reported to the physician.

Patient management for paralytic ileus includes bed rest and the insertion of a nasogastric tube for low, intermittent suction. The patient is given nothing by mouth. A rectal tube can be inserted to relieve flatus. Intravenous therapy is usually ordered to maintain fluid and electrolyte balance. It usually takes a few days of treatment to allow peristalsis to return. Once peristalsis is present, the nasogastric tube and suctioning are discontinued. The patient is gradually started on clear fluids and the diet is progressed gradually based on his tolerance.

Abdominal distention and gastric upset (nausea and vomiting) cause a good deal of discomfort. Comfort measures such as providing frequent mouth care with cold, refreshing solutions and carefully taping and positioning the nasogastric tube are a few of the major points of care to be considered.

Urinary Retention

Painful bladder distention is possible after surgical procedures because of anesthesia and autonomic stimulation. The laminectomy patient, particularly one who has undergone a lumbar laminectomy, is subject to this possible complication.

Signs and symptoms include painful distention of the urinary bladder on palpation and inability to empty the bladder. Because of the concern of preventing urinary tract infections, many physicians do not recommend catheterization unless the patient is painfully distended. It is the nurse's responsibility to assess the patient and implement other nursing interventions to initiate micturition, such as getting the patient up to void and placing spirits of peppermint in the urinal or bedpan. If these measures are unsuccessful, straight catheterization of the patient is necessary. The amount of urine is measured and an intake–output record maintained. The patient should be watched for subsequent inability to void. If this occurs, the physician may order an indwelling catheter for a few days until normal bladder function is reestablished.

Cerebrospinal Fistula

A *cerebrospinal fistula* is an abnormal connection between the subarachnoid space and the incision, causing cerebrospinal fluid drainage on the dressing either alone or in combination with serosanguinous drainage. The dressing is always wet, and the fistula appears to drain larger amounts when the patient is on his back or standing. A major concern is that of infection at the fistula site as well as meningitis, since microorganisms can ascend the fistula and flourish in the ideal environment of the cerebrospinal space.

Formation of a fistula is not an early postoperative complication. It often takes a week for evidence of a fistula to

(Text continued on page 443.)

CHART 19–2. SUMMARY OF NURSING MANAGEMENT OF THE PATIENT AFTER A LAMINECTOMY

NURSING RESPONSIBILITIES	RATIONALE
Bed/Positioning	
1. The patient should be returned to a bed with a firm mattress and bedboard.	1. Provides support for the spine
2. Keep the bed flat or slightly elevated (5 degrees, if permitted). • For a cervical laminectomy, a small pillow may be positioned under the head or nape of neck • For a lumbar laminectomy, a small pillow may be placed under the head and one may be placed under the knees periodically (Fig. 19–14).	2. Reduces strain on the operative site
3. For a cervical laminectomy, a Thomas collar is applied and worn at all times (Fig. 19–15).	3. Prevents flexion of the neck, which could exert stress on the suture line
4. Reposition patient every 2 hours in proper body alignment.	4. Prevents undue stress on the operative site
Neurological and Vital Signs	
1. Assess vital signs frequently.	1. Demonstrates evidence of hemorrhage or other postoperative complications
2. Assess neurological function frequently, especially the patient's ability to move his legs and feel touch on his legs (Fig. 19–16). • For a cervical laminectomy the areas of concern are the arms and shoulders.	2. Indicates alteration of function
Turning	
1. For the first 24 to 48 hours, the log-rolling technique should be used. After 48 hours, a turning sheet may be used with only one nurse doing the turning (Fig. 19–17).	1. Prevents stress and strain on the operative site
2. Do not allow the patient to help to turn himself for the first 48 hours • For the cervical laminectomy patient, do not allow the patient to pull with his arms on the siderail at any time.	2. Same as above
Circulation and Breathing	
1. Ace wraps should be removed on the first postoperative day and replaced with elastic stockings.	1. Improves vascular resistance as a means of preventing thrombus/embolus, or thrombophlebitis

FIG. 19–14. Position of patient following lumbar laminectomy. (Decision Audiovisual Media. Neurological Care Series. Philadelphia, JB Lippincott, 1972)

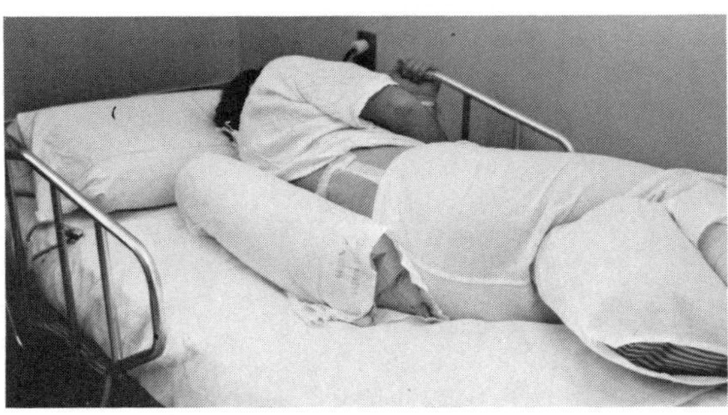

FIG. 19–15. A Thomas collar is used for the patient following a cervical laminectomy. (Decision Audiovisual Media. Neurological Care Series. Philadelphia, JB Lippincott, 1972)

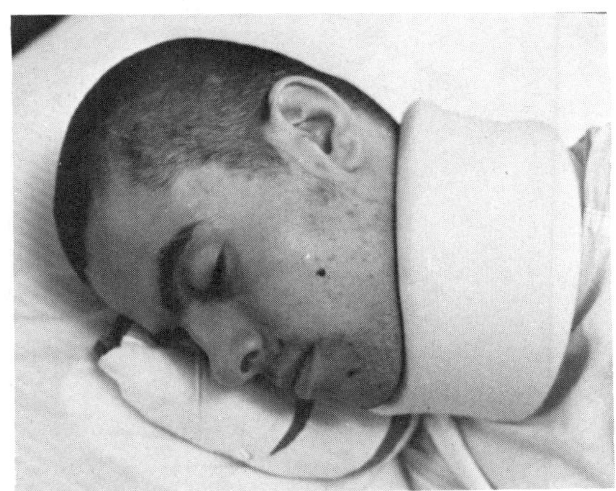

(continued)

CHART 19–2. (continued)

NURSING RESPONSIBILITIES	RATIONALE
2. The patient should be encouraged to move his extremities while in bed (range-of-motion exercises four times a day).	**2.** Improves circulation and motor tone and prevents thrombus/embolus or thrombophlebitis
3. Deep breathing should be encouraged every 2 hours. Because coughing may aggravate the pain, check with physician to see if coughing is to be encouraged. Laminectomy patients (especially those who have had cervical laminectomies) tend to have shallow respirations because of their pain. These patients are therefore more prone to atelectasis and pneumonia.	**3.** Prevents atelectasis and pneumonia
4. Auscultate chest every 4 hours.	**4.** Provides information on development of respiratory complications
5. Assess for atelectasis and pneumonia.	**5.** Same as above
Bowel/Bladder Function	
1. Measure urinary output. • For a lumbar laminectomy, an indwelling catheter will usually be in place; some physicians prefer intermittent catherization every 6 to 8 hours; if no catheter is in place, check frequency and amount of each voiding.	**1.** Ensures an adequate urinary output • Transient voiding problems are common after a lumbar laminectomy; assess for presence of dysfunction.
2. Assess abdomen for distention and bowel sounds.	**2.** Transient paralytic ileus may develop and should be identified early.
3. Administer stool softeners and laxatives as necessary.	**3.** Prevents constipation and pain from straining at stool caused by increased intraspinal pressure
Fluid/Nutrition	
1. Maintain an intake and output record.	**1.** Monitors fluid balance
2. Run intravenous fluids at rate ordered.	**2.** Provides for adequate hydration
3. Once nausea has subsided and bowel sounds are heard, progress from fluid to house diet.	**3.** Provides for adequate nutrition
Dressing	
1. Observe dressing for evidence of drainage (blood or cerebrospinal fluid).	**1.** Indicates hemorrhage or development of a fistula
2. Maintain strict aseptic technique when changing dressing.	**2.** Prevents wound infection or meningitis
3. With a lumbar laminectomy check the dressing to ensure that it has not become wet or contaminated; if this occurs, change immediately.	**3.** Prevents incision contamination

FIG. 19–16. Postoperative assessment of neurological function includes evaluating the patient's ability to move his legs *(A)* and feel sensation on his legs *(B)*. (Decision Audiovisual Media. Neurological Care Series. Philadelphia, JB Lippincott, 1973)

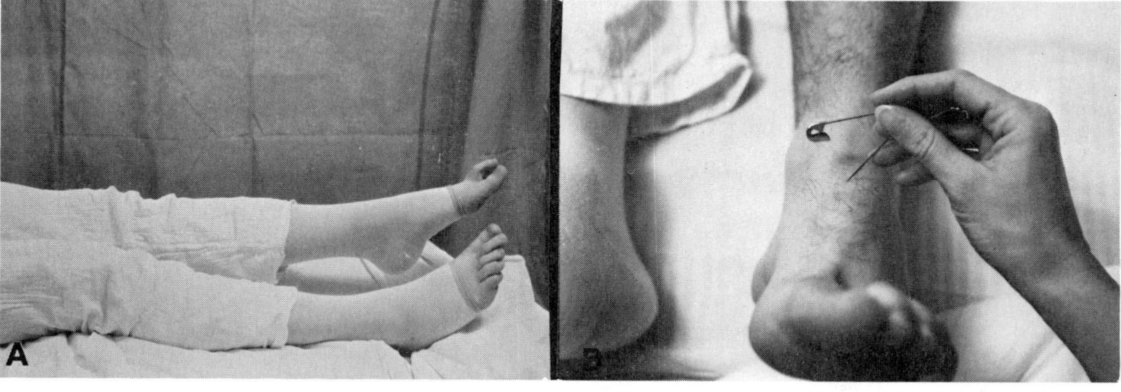

CHART 19–2. *(continued)*

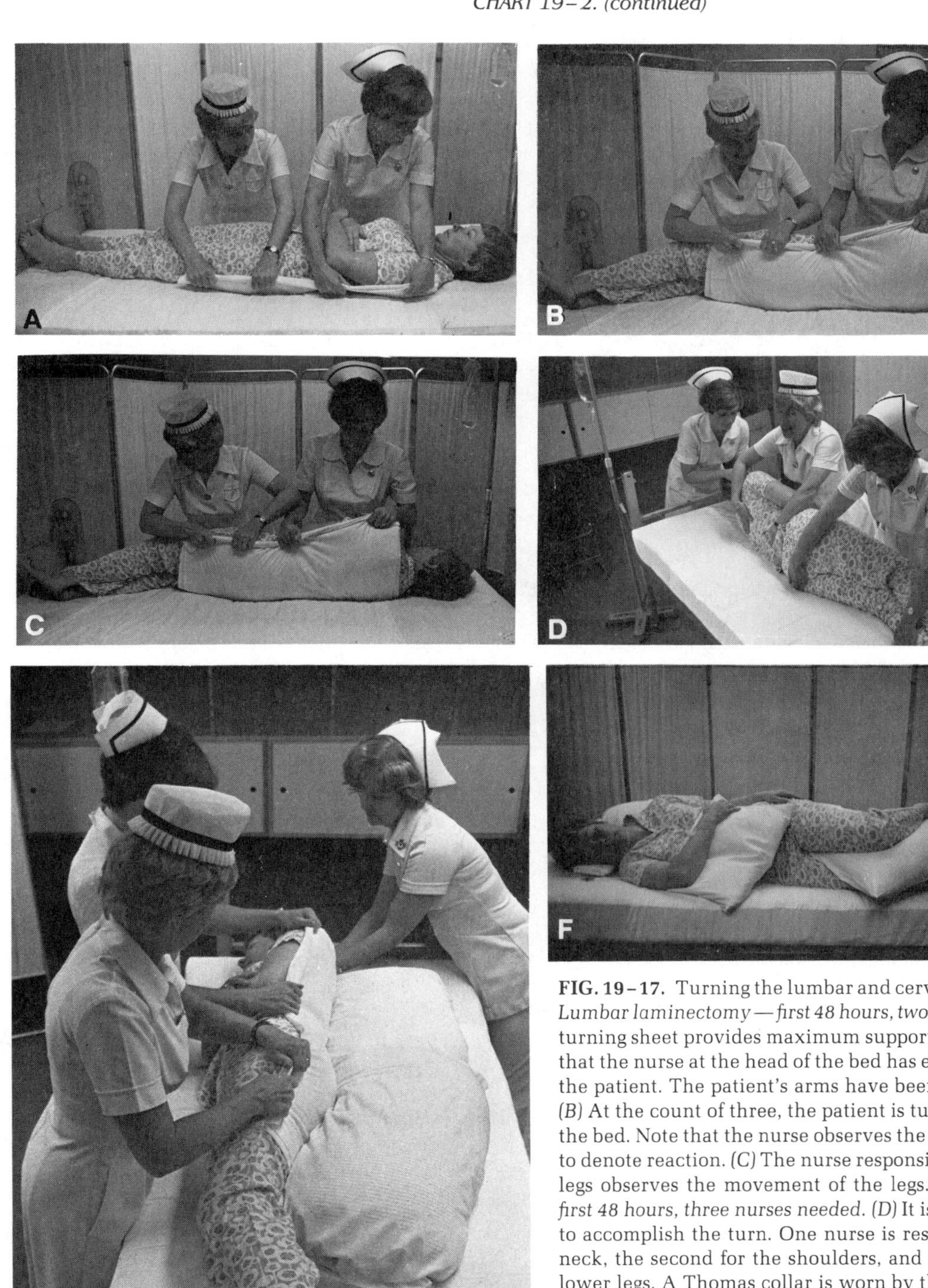

FIG. 19–17. Turning the lumbar and cervical laminectomy patient. *Lumbar laminectomy—first 48 hours, two nurses needed. (A)* Use of a turning sheet provides maximum support and ease of turning. Note that the nurse at the head of the bed has explained the procedure to the patient. The patient's arms have been placed on her abdomen. *(B)* At the count of three, the patient is turned to the desired side of the bed. Note that the nurse observes the patient's facial expression to denote reaction. *(C)* The nurse responsible for the lower back and legs observes the movement of the legs. *Cervical laminectomy—first 48 hours, three nurses needed. (D)* It is best to have three nurses to accomplish the turn. One nurse is responsible for the head and neck, the second for the shoulders, and the third for the hips and lower legs. A Thomas collar is worn by the patient at all times and offers added support to the neck. *(E)* The movement can also be accomplished with a turning sheet and three nurses. *(F)* Regardless of whether patient has had a lumbar or cervical laminectomy, the patient must be positioned with pillows for maximum support of body parts in proper body alignment. *Lumbar and cervical laminectomy turning after 48 hours.* Once the patient has become accustomed to turning, it is possible for the nurse to turn the patient alone with the aid of a turning sheet.

(continued)

CHART 19–2. (continued)

NURSING RESPONSIBILITIES	RATIONALE
Pain/Discomfort	
1. If the patient complains of discomfort or pain because of muscle spasms (lower back, abdomen or thighs with a lumbar laminectomy; upper back, shoulders, neck, or arms with a cervical laminectomy), reassure the patient by explaining that the spasms are probably caused by nerve root and muscle irritation from edema and surgery; the spasms will subside.	1. Relieves the patient's anxiety
2. Medicate the patient for pain and discomfort caused by the incision and muscle spasms.	2. Provides for comfort
3. Following cervical laminectomy, the patient may have a sore throat and find it difficult to expectorate. If permitted, give viscous lidocaine (Xylocaine) to promote comfort.	3. The sore throat is usually caused by the endotracheal tube used for anesthesia; provide comfort measures to reduce discomfort.
Ambulation/Rehabilitation	
The schedule for ambulation will vary according to the type of surgery performed.	
Lumbar Laminectomy	
1. The patient is allowed out of bed to walk only on the second or third postoperative day.	1. Prevents stress and strain on the suture line
2. The patient should not be allowed to sit on the edge of the bed when getting up or out of bed.*	2. Mattress does not provide adequate support to the operative site
3. The patient should be lying flat in bed (or at a 10-degree angle for comfort), standing, or walking. He should not be allowed to assume a sitting position.†	3. Prevents stress and strain on the operative site
4. Toward the end of hospitalization (about the sixth day) the patient is allowed to sit in a hard, straight chair.	4. Provides for adequate support and prepares patient for discharge
5. As part of patient education, the patient should be advised to maintain or achieve his proper weight to reduce stress on back and to use good body mechanics at all times.	5. Educates to prevent further back injury
Cervical Laminectomy	
1. The head of the bed is gradually elevated to accommodate the patient in an upright position. The patient should be evaluated for dizziness and light-headedness during this time.	1. Monitors for possible hypotension caused by transient changes in vasomotor tone
2. The patient is allowed out of bed as soon as possible and must wear a Thomas collar at all times.	2. Provides for early ambulation and support to the operative site
3. Do not allow the patient to pull with his arms when assuming the erect position.	3. Prevents undue stress and strain on the operative site
4. As part of patient teaching instruct the patient in good body mechanics and weight control program, if needed.	4. Educates to prevent further neck injury
Both	
1. Be sure that patient knows and understands limitations of his activity on discharge from the hospital.	1. Prevents further injury

* *Variations in Postoperative Management Protocols After a Laminectomy.* There are variations in the procedure for ambulation of patients from physician to physician. Some surgeons may ask their patient to dangle their feet from the edge of the bed on the evening of the day of surgery or the first or second postoperative day. Other surgeons do *not* allow their patients to dangle their feet at all, since it is believed that excessive stress would be placed on the suture line (see #2). The individual protocols of the surgeon must be followed.

† *Technique for Getting the Laminectomy Patient out of Bed.* If the head of the bed can be raised, the bed is raised with the patient comfortably positioned on the bed close to the edge of the side from which he will get out of the bed. If the bed must remain flat, the patient is positioned on his side with his knees and hips slightly flexed near the side of the bed from which he will rise. In either case, two nurses are necessary. One nurse grasps the patient under his arm and around his upper back and neck. The patient is instructed to place his arm around the nurse's shoulders. The other nurse grasps his hips and legs. At the count of three, the nurses assist the patient to the upright position. If the patient is to walk, the support of two nurses is advisable since weakness, dizziness, and light-headedness are not uncommon. A few steps to the door and back are a sufficient accomplishment for the first venture out of bed. Gradually, the patient will be able to tolerate ambulation for greater distances.

appear. Because drainage on the dressing is the major sign of a fistula, it is important to test the drainage with a Dextrostix strip to determine if glucose, a component of cerebrospinal fluid, is present. Continuous drainage on the dressing should be reported to the physician. If the fistula does not spontaneously seal itself, surgical closure will be necessary. Antibiotics are ordered to control the possibility of infection.

Hematoma at the Operative Site

In some instances, a hematoma will develop postoperatively at the incision because of bleeding. The most prominent symptom is severe, localized incisional pain that may or may not be described as throbbing. The nurse notices that an average dose of an analgesic medication in the postoperative period does not keep the patient comfortable. He complains bitterly about the incisional pain.

If the hematoma is large, surgical evacuation of the clot will be required, thereby necessitating the removal of some of the sutures to allow for evacuation of the clot. Smaller hematomas will often be absorbed spontaneously. The nurse may be required to apply warm sterile saline soaks to the incision to accelerate the process of reabsorption. In other instances, no intervention is necessary.

Nerve Root Injury Resulting in Footdrop or Wristdrop

One aspect of nursing assessment in the postoperative period is the evaluation of sensory and motor function in the extremities. If the operative site was proximal to the cervical region, then assessment would concentrate on arm strength. In lumbar surgery the legs would be the focus of attention. In assessing the motor and sensory function, the nurse compares present motor and sensory function with preoperative function. The patient is asked to move his extremities, wiggle his fingers or toes, and identify the part of the extremity that has been touched or squeezed. If there is apparent motor weakness, paralysis, or lack of awareness of touch or temperature in the postoperative period, nerve root injury is suspected. Such deficits should be reported to the physician, and the motor and sensory function assessed frequently to detect change.

If the patient has sustained nerve root injury, an aggressive program of physiotherapy will be needed, along with slings, braces, or splints, depending on the involved extremity and the extent of injury. Range-of-motion exercises will be incorporated into the nursing care plan, and careful attention will be necessary to prevent contractures, musculoskeletal deformities, and injury to the involved limb. It is possible that even with an aggressive treatment program, the patient will sustain permanent disability.

Arachnoiditis

Inflammation of the arachnoid layer of the spinal meninges can result from infection caused by contamination of the surgical site at surgery or contamination of the dressing. If there is clinical evidence of infection (an increase in temperature and white blood cell count, malaise, headache, redness at the incision, drainage on dry sterile dressings, and so forth), the patient is started on antibiotic therapy. The possibility of arachnoiditis is a particularly worrisome complication because scar tissue and adhesions can form, thereby causing much severe and chronic pain within weeks of surgery. The pain can be so severe that surgical intervention to remove the adhesions may be necessary to control the pain. In this instance a myelogram may or may not demonstrate evidence of adhesions, which may only be evidenced by direct visualization at the time of surgery.

Postural Deformity

A laminectomy at more than one level of the vertebral column can cause spinal column instability and postural deformity. Such abnormality may be noted by observing the patient as he ambulates or by examining his posture in bed. When the surgeon performs a laminectomy on two or more vertebral levels, a spinal fusion may be necessary to ensure stability of the spinal column and prevent disability. If postural deformity develops after a simple laminectomy at a few levels, a spinal fusion may be necessary.

Muscle Spasms

The physiological reason for muscle spasms is not clear, but spasms tend to occur on the third or fourth postoperative day. If a lumbar laminectomy was performed, spasms tend to occur in the lower back and thigh. In a cervical laminectomy, the neck, shoulder, and arm are involved. Overactivity of the patient, irritation of the nerves during surgery, and recovery of nerves from extended compression are proposed reasons for muscle spasms. Management of muscle spasms includes keeping the patient comfortable with analgesic drugs; using muscle-relaxant drugs such as diazepam (Valium) or methocarbamol (Robaxin; an intravenous infusion of 250 ml of 5% dextrose or normal saline with 10 ml of Robaxin, given rapidly over 60 to 90 minutes, can be very effective in relieving muscle spasms); and administering an anti-inflammatory drug such as dexamethasone (Decadron) to control inflammation and edema.

The patient can become very upset and discouraged from the severe pain associated with muscle spasms. It is important to assure the patient that the spasms will abate in a few days. Changing the patient's position frequently, positioning the patient in proper body alignment supported by pillows, and giving frequent back rubs are all nursing measures that can control the onset of spasms as well as provide comfort when they occur.

Elevated Temperature

It is not unusual for the body temperature to be elevated to 102.2° F (39° C) for the first few postoperative days. This is caused by the drainage, which causes aseptic contamination of the cerebrospinal fluid and the normal healing process at the surgical site. Management of the elevated temperature is usually adequately controlled by the use of antipyretic drugs such as aspirin or acetaminophen (Tylenol), 650 mg orally or rectally every 4 hours. In addition, increasing the fluid intake and removing excess bedclothes will aid in controlling an elevated body temperature.

RECURRENT SYMPTOMS AFTER SURGERY

Surgery is not always synonymous with relief of symptoms. For example, a patient who has experienced long-term pain radiating into his leg before surgery will probably continue to have abated pain after surgery. It may persist for several weeks postoperatively. If there has been considerable sensory loss because of nerve root compression preoperatively, pain perception may actually increase because of improvement of the sensory deficit. This patient may experience paresthesias for several months after surgery.[7] There is also the discomfort caused by muscle spasms after surgery, which are troublesome, although expected. Statistics vary greatly on the percentage of patients who continue to have severe to moderate symptoms after surgery. The range is approximately 10% to 40%. Continued long-term pain will require diagnostic evaluation.

Surgery for a herniated disc does not negate the possibility of recurrence of a disc herniation at the same level on the same or opposite side or at other levels. Repeated laminectomies on the same patient are not unusual. This does point out the need for patient teaching in body mechanics, posture, and protection from injury. However, there may be degenerative changes already present that predispose the patient to future problems, even if a teaching program is judiciously followed.

SPECIAL CONSIDERATION: SPINAL FUSION

A spinal fusion is done to stabilize a vertebral column that is weakened or unstable because of degenerative disease or to ensure a stable vertebral column when a multilevel laminectomy is performed. Usually when three vertebrae are involved in a laminectomy, it is necessary to stabilize this area with a spinal fusion to prevent injury to the spinal nerve roots or spinal cord.

A *spinal fusion* consists of the insertion of a wedge-shaped bone graft between the vertebrae to negate movement between these two bones. The bone graft is usually obtained from the iliac crest (the donor site) of the patient. The nurse is responsible for postoperative assessment of the sterile dressing and care of the incision at the donor site.

A spinal fusion results in a firm union. Mobility is lost, and the patient becomes accustomed to a permanent area of stiffness. When a portion of the lumbar spine is fused, the patient usually becomes unaware of stiffness after a short time because motion increases in the joints above the fusion. More limitation of movement is noted when the area of fusion is located in the cervical spine.

When a spinal fusion is done, it is important to immobilize the fused area to allow healing and permanent fusion to occur. In the case of an anterior cervical fusion, a hard collar can be used. Some surgeons prefer application of a Minerva cast, a body cast with a halo apparatus, or a fiberglass body cast. Thoracic or lumbar fusions are also immobilized with the use of various casts. Bed rest following surgery is usually longer than that for simple laminectomy. Dislodgement of the bone graft at the fusion site and infection at the donor site are possible complications.

ANTERIOR CERVICAL FUSION

Anterior cervical fusion is done through an incision in the anterior neck. Postoperative management is similar to that following a posterior cervical laminectomy except that the patient may be out of bed on the first postoperative day with a Thomas collar or brace. He may be relatively pain-free but has difficulty swallowing because of edema or irritation to the pharynx or trachea as a result of endotracheal anesthesia.

ANTERIOR CERVICAL DISCECTOMY WITH FUSION

Complications following anterior cervical discectomy with fusion relate to soft-tissue injuries. Serious injuries can occur, such as perforation of the pharynx, esophagus, or trachea. Vascular injuries to the vertebral, carotid, or jugular vessels are possible but rare.

Because the esophagus and trachea are retracted during surgery, special problems related to these structures should be mentioned. Irritation of the laryngeal nerve and tracheal edema can result in hoarseness and difficulty in coughing. These symptoms are further aggravated when an endotracheal tube is inserted for the administration of anesthesia. The patient complains of a sore throat. Difficulty in managing mucus and secretions can be a problem. The patient is more prone to respiratory complications such as pneumonia.

Viscous lidocaine (Xylocaine), diphenhydramine hydrochloride (Benadryl elixir), and throat lozenges are soothing and help to temporarily alleviate the bothersome symptoms. Ventilation therapy with intermittent positive pressure breathing is helpful. Antibiotics and expectorants are two other types of drugs ordered to manage respiratory symptoms.

REFERENCES

1. Adams R, Victor M: Principles of Neurology, 2nd ed, pp 140–151. New York, McGraw-Hill, 1981
2. Hejna WA, Sinkora G: Chemonucleolysis of the herniated lumbar discs. Am Fam Physician 27(5):97, May 1983
3. Ravichandran G, Mullholland RC: Chymopapain chemonucleolysis: A preliminary report. Spine 5:382, July–August 1980
4. Musolf JA: Chemonucleolysis: A new approach for patients with herniated intervertebral disks. Am J Nurs 83:882, June 1983

5. Hudgins WR: The role of microdiscectomy. Orthop Clin North Am 14(3):589, July 1983
6. Bollati A et al: Microsurgical surgical anterior cervical disk removal without interbody infusion. Surg Neurol 19:329, 1983
7. Hoppenfeld S: Physical Examination of the Spine and Extremities. New York, Appleton-Century-Croft, 1976

BIBLIOGRAPHY

Books

Arbit E, Patterson RH: Extradural spinal cord and nerve root compression from benign lesions in the dorsal area. In Youmans J (ed): Neurological Surgery, 2nd ed, pp 2562-2573. Philadelphia, WB Saunders, 1982

Bates B: Guide to Physical Examination, 3rd ed. Philadelphia, JB Lippincott, 1983

Cauther JC: Lumbar Spine Surgery: Indications, Techniques, Failures, and Alternatives. Baltimore, Williams & Wilkins, 1983

Clark K: Anterior operative approach for benign extradural cervical lesions. In Youmans J (ed): Neurological Surgery, 2nd ed, pp 2613-2628. Philadelphia, WB Saunders, 1982

Davis C: Extradural spinal cord and nerve root compression from benign lesions of the lumbar area. In Youmans J (ed): Neurological Surgery, 2nd ed, pp 2535-2561. Philadelphia, WB Saunders, 1982

Ehni G: Extradural spinal cord and nerve root compression from benign lesions of the cervical area. In Youmans J (ed): Neurological Surgery, 2nd ed, pp 2574-2612. Philadelphia, WB Saunders, 1982

Epstein B: The Spine: A Radiological Text and Atlas. Philadelphia, Lea & Febiger, 1976

Farrell J: Illustrated Guide to Orthopedic Nursing, 2nd ed. Philadelphia, JB Lippincott, 1982

Finneson BM: Low Back Pain, 2nd ed. Philadelphia, JB Lippincott, 1981

Hoppenfeld S: Orthopaedic Neurology. Philadelphia, JB Lippincott, 1977

Howe J: Patient Care in Neurosurgery, 2nd ed. Boston, Little, Brown & Co, 1983

Lin PM (ed): Posterior Lumbar Interbody Fusion. Springfield, IL, Charles C Thomas, 1982

Rothman R, Simeone F: The Spine, 2nd ed. Philadelphia, WB Saunders, 1982

Smith R: Essentials of Neurosurgery. Philadelphia, JB Lippincott, 1980

Spengler DM: Low Back Pain: Assessment and Management. New York, Grune & Stratton, 1982

Stanton-Hicks M, Boas R (eds): Chronic Low Back Pain. New York, Raven Press, 1982

Watkins RG: Surgical Approaches to the Spine. New York, Springer-Verlag, 1983

Wiesel SW, Bernini P, Rothman RH: The Aging Lumbar Spine. Philadelphia, WB Saunders, 1982

Williams PC: Low Back and Neck Pain: Causes and Conservative Treatment. Springfield, IL, Charles C Thomas, 1982

Periodicals

Bartorelli D: Low back pain: A team approach. J Neurosurg Nurs 15(1):41, February 1983

Beetham WP, Hsieh R: Clinical evaluation of neck pain. Hosp Med 60, September 1982

Branson KA: Patient management following amipaque myelography. Orthop Nurs 1(6):38, November-December 1982

Cardea J: Diagnosis: Low back pain of spinal origin. Hosp Med 79, April 1982

Donavan L: Low back pain: Where care is the key to recovery. RN 41(10):71, October 1978

Friedmann L, Cassvan A: Guide to evaluation of low back pain and sciatica. Hosp Med 9, June 1980

Gilbertson B: Low back pain: What to look for . . . What to do. RN 38(10):75, October 1978

Goald H: Microlumbar discectomy: Follow-up of 477 patients. J Microsurg 2:95, 1980

Javid MJ: Treatment of herniated lumbar disc syndrome with chymopapain. JAMA 243:2048, May 23-30, 1980

Lamb S: Neuroaugmentation for the chronic pain patient. J Neurosurg Nurs 11(4):215, December 1979

LaMont R et al: Comparison of disc excision and combined disc excision and spinal fusion for lumbar disc rupture. Clin Orthop 121:212, November-December 1976

Law J et al: Reoperation after lumbar intervertebral disc surgery. J Neurosurg 48(2):259, February 1978

Maida MJ: Chymopapain for herniated lumbar disc disease. J Neurosurg Nurs 15(3):144, June 1983

Maigne R: Low back pain of thoracolumbar origin. Arch Phys Med Rehabil 61:389, September 1980

Mulford EF: Degenerative disease or "slipped" disc? The clues are clear-cut . . . assessment of low back pain. RN 44:44, February 1981

Nwuga VCB: Ultrasound in treatment of back pain resulting from prolapsed intervertebral disc. Arch Phys Med Rehabil 64(2):88, February 1983

O'Brien E: Nursing care following back surgery. Nurs Mirror 144(2):54-56, January 13, 1977

Robb D, Dunsker S: Cervical spondylosis. J Neurosurg Nurs 13(2):72, April 1981

Secor RMC: Rapid triage assessment of low back pain. J Emergency Nurs 9(1):17, January-February 1983

Sharp B: Nursing care of the patient with recurrent back pain after discectomy. J Neurosurg Nurs 13(2):77, April 1981

Stauffer T: Gravity lumbar reduction. J Neurosurg Nurs 13(6):299, December 1981

Terzian M: Neurosurgical interventions for the management of chronic intractable pain. Top Clin Nurs 2(1):75, April 1980

That aching back. Time (cover story) 30, July 14, 1980

Tucker LE: Diagnosis: Back pain of extraspinal origin. Hosp Med 52, April 1981

Williams R: Microlumbar discectomy: A conservative surgical approach to the virgin herniated lumbar disc. Spine 5:366, 1980

Wilson D, Harbaugh R: Microsurgical and standard removal of protruded lumbar disc: A comparative study. Neurosurgery 8:422, 1981

Wilson DH, Campbell DD: Anterior cervical discectomy without bone graft: Report of 71 cases. J Neurosurg 47:551, 1977

Wiltse LL: Chemonucleolysis in the treatment of lumbar disc disease. Orthop Clin North Am 14(3):605, July 1983

chapter 20

Peripheral Nerve Trauma

Peripheral nerve trauma is associated with trauma encountered in active military conflict, mechanized industry, farming, certain sports, and acts of violence. With greater emphasis on energy conservation in a nation dependent on dwindling energy supplies, one can expect to see an increase in peripheral nerve injuries as the weekend woodcutter armed with axe and chainsaw manages to mangle a limb in the process of providing wood for the hearth. The "back-to-nature movement" and the renewed interest in outdoor sports such as skiing also provide activities ripe for injuries that affect the peripheral nerves.

Trauma to peripheral nerves can also develop as a result of exposure to toxic chemicals and substances used in the home workshop and workplace. Occupational exposure to toxins was discussed briefly in Chapter 10.

Although all cranial and spinal nerves constitute the peripheral nervous system, this chapter concentrates on the major peripheral nerves that innervate the extremities.

MECHANISMS OF TRAUMA/INJURY

The specific mechanisms by which peripheral nerves can be traumatized include complete or partial severance; contusion; stretching; compression; ischemia; electrical, thermal, and radiation injuries; and drug injection. It is possible for more than one mechanism of nerve injury to occur simultaneously.

A partially or completely severed nerve usually results from a sharp cutting instrument like a chainsaw or scalpel. Regeneration of the peripheral nerve for some functional return to the involved body part is possible under certain circumstances.

With a contusion, the neuron remains intact structurally, but there is undetermined axonal injury. The injury can occur from a direct blow to a nerve located close to the body surface, as may occur when an elbow is bumped, thereby causing injury to the superficial ulnar nerve; passage of a fast-moving object, such as a bullet or shrapnel, careening close to the nerve; or a compression injury, which may occur to a nerve in a closed fracture or injury to the peroneal nerve caused by pressure on the back of the knee where the nerve crosses the lateral popliteal space and head of the fibula anteriorly.

Stretch trauma injuries result from traction exerted on most of the nerve. Extreme movement and excessive application of weight in orthopedic traction can cause this type of nerve injury. The shoulder joint is a common site for nerve injuries caused by extremes in movement. With traction of the hip or upper leg, the peroneal nerve may be injured by excessive pulling, which is why a major nursing responsibility involves checking the intact motor function of the foot for inversion–eversion and plantar and dorsiflexion.

Compression nerve injuries are caused by extreme or prolonged trauma pressure on a peripheral nerve, such as may be exerted by tumors, herniated intervertebral discs, and osteophytes. Nerve entrapment may also result in compression injury in those areas where peripheral nerves are encased by bone or rigid material. This may be the case with cranial and spinal nerves passing through narrow foramen or with peripheral nerves passing through narrow channels (e.g., the median nerve passing between the carpal ligament and tendon sheath of the flexor arm muscles of the forearm — carpal tunnel syndrome). The narrowness of the foramen and channels, combined with edema from nearby injury caused by fractures or soft-tissue trauma or pressure from a vascular anomaly (hematoma or aneurysm), can easily produce a peripheral nerve entrapment syndrome.

Ischemia as a cause of peripheral nerve injury is closely associated with compression injuries because compression will eventually deprive a nerve of an adequate blood supply. In such circumstances the etiology of nerve injury is more accurately attributed to the compression–ischemia mechanism. Occlusion of a major artery of a limb can lead to nerve injury because of ischemia.

Electrical, thermal, and radiation trauma injuries to peripheral nerves are grouped together. Electrical nerve injury results from current being passed through the peripheral nerve when contact is made with high-tension electrical wires. The resulting injuries produce severe muscle and nerve coagulation in addition to burns of the skin and destruction of bone. Prognosis for muscle reinnervation in these instances is generally poor. Thermal and radiation nerve injury cause similar types of local responses, with major damage resulting from burning and necrosis.

Drug injection into or proximal to a nerve can cause neuropathy, intraneural neuritis, and scarring. The nerves most commonly involved are the sciatic and radial nerves, which are subjected to injury as a result of improper injection technique during the administration of intramuscular drugs; thus, the importance of proper education in drug administration cannot be overstated. Drug injection injuries are preventable problems if proper technique is practiced.

PATHOPHYSIOLOGY

Following transection of a nerve, three degenerative reactions occur: changes in the cell body (chromatolysis), changes in the nerve fiber segment between the cell and body and the point of transection (primary degeneration), and changes in the nerve fiber or amputated stump distal to the injury (secondary or wallerian degeneration). The effect will vary depending on whether the neuron is located entirely within the central nervous system or partly in the peripheral nervous system. (In peripheral nerves the cell body is located in the anterior horn of the spinal cord or in the posterior ganglion.)

A SEVERED NEURON LOCATED ENTIRELY WITHIN THE CENTRAL NERVOUS SYSTEM

A neuron located entirely within the central nervous system undergoes various changes at the time of axonal transection. The effect on the cell body include swelling of the cell body; chromatolysis of the Nissl bodies in the cell body, a process by which the extranuclear ribonucleic acid (RNA) granules appear to dissolve or lose their staining characteristics; and displacement of the nucleus to the side of the cell body. As a result of these events, the cell body usually dies.

At the synaptic junction, swelling of the severed axonal fiber begins to involve the myelin sheath and axis cylinder. (Note that there are no Schwann cells or neurolemma in the central nervous system.) This is a degenerative process, called wallerian degeneration, which destroys the severed axon stump and proceeds backward toward the cell body. Neuroglia cells proliferate in the area, resulting in a phagocytic removal of the breakdown products. Breakdown of the cells and phagocytosis also extends from the point of the transection toward the cell body, a process sometimes referred to as "dying back." Eventually, the entire cell disappears, usually over several months.

It is important to note that this process is replicated in each neuron of the severed nerve. (A nerve is composed of thousands of neurons.) If many nerve fibers are involved, the proliferation of neuroglia cells responsible for phagocytosis can form a dense glial scar. Neurons of the central nervous system do not survive axonal transection.

A SEVERED PERIPHERAL NERVE (AXON LOCATED OUTSIDE THE CENTRAL NERVOUS SYSTEM)

If a peripheral nerve has been completely severed, there is a possibility for self-repair (Fig. 20–1). As with cell injury of the central nervous system, the same changes occur in the cell body of the peripheral nerve; that is, swelling, chromatolysis, and side displacement of the nucleus. Chromatolysis indicates increased protein synthesis, an example of metabolic activity necessary for the regeneration of severed axonal fibers. In the isolated axonal segment, secondary degeneration occurs (wallerian degeneration). The axis cylinder and myelin sheath degenerate and are removed by the phagocytic cells. The only remaining evidence of the severed axonal segment is the Schwann (neurolemma) cells.

The regeneration process begins with the proliferation of Schwann cells in the proximal stump near the transection and in the distal stump. These cells divide mitotically to form continuous cords of Schwann (neurolemma) cells, covering an area that encompasses the proximal stump, the gap across the transected area, the distal stump, and the area up to the sites of the sensory receptors and motor endings. The neurolemmal cords will act as guidelines for the regenerating axon.

Meanwhile, the cell body is directing synthesized protein and metabolites distally to provide the nutritional machinery for axonal regeneration. The axis cylinder of the proximal axon at the transection begins to generate tiny unmyelinated sprouts that grow longitudinally. There may be as many as 50 sprouts. The random growth of sprouts forms an enlargement called a neuroma. Some sprouts will be misdirected and stray, but certain ones will be successful in crossing the transected gap through the guidance of the neurolemma. These sprouts will find their way to the distal stump. The rate of growth of a regenerating sprout is 1 mm to 4 mm/day. If the union is well aligned so that the axon will grow back into its former channel, functional return will be good.

Successful realigned nerves will remyelinate, grow to their former size, and eventually claim a conduction velocity that is 80% of their former capacity. If the realignments are mismatched, functional weakness and unintentional

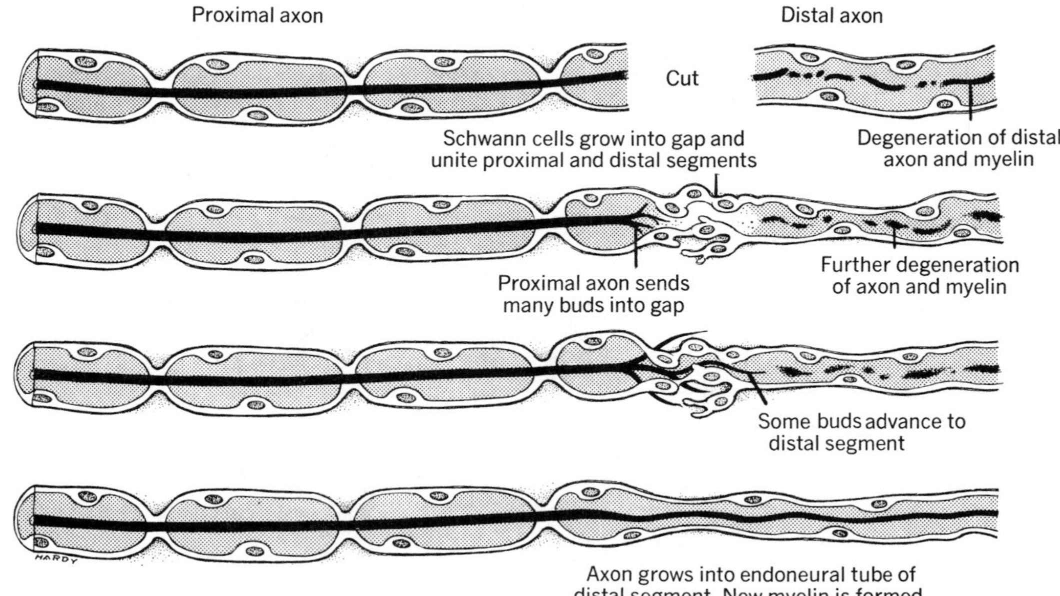

FIG. 20–1. Diagram of changes that occur in a nerve fiber that has been cut and then regenerates.

movements of muscles, as well as poor sensory discrimination and localization of stimuli, may result. Sprouts that are unsuccessful in making connections degenerate.

Collateral Nerve Sprouting

Nerves proximal to the injured neurons are stimulated to produce collateral innervation to denerved areas. This process will provide innervation long before the axon has regenerated to provide innervation. Therefore, some sensory return may occur before regeneration can realistically occur. This process is possible in both the central and peripheral nervous system.

GENERAL SIGNS AND SYMPTOMS OF PERIPHERAL NERVE TRAUMA

Motor, sensory, autonomic, and trophic signs and symptoms are the usual functional changes occurring with peripheral nerve injuries. The degree of deficit in any area depends on the type and extent of injury. Because peripheral nerves arise from spinal nerves, they are lower motor neurons and display signs and symptoms of lower motor neuron (flaccid) paralysis when injured.

Signs and symptoms include

1. Flaccid paralysis of the muscle or muscle groups supplied by the nerve; a paresis results if some, but not all, lower motor neurons innervating the muscle are functional.
2. Absence of deep tendon reflexes of the affected area result if all neurons are affected. If some neurons are functional, deep tendon reflexes are weak.
3. Atonic or hypotonic muscles
4. Progressive muscle atrophy begins early (reaches peak in several weeks).
5. Fibrillations and fasciculations reach a peak 2 to 3 weeks after muscle is denerved. (Fibrillations are transitory muscle contractions caused by spontaneous stimulation of a single muscle fiber. Fasciculations are spontaneous contractions of several muscle fibers innervated by a single motor nerve filament.)
6. Diminished or complete sensory loss
7. Warm or dry skin (anhidrosis) caused by transection of the postganglionic sympathetic fibers
8. Trophic changes

Trophic Changes. Trophic changes can be divided into a warm and then a cold phase. The warm phase lasts about 3 weeks, during which time the skin in the affected areas is dry, warm, and flushed. The cold phase is characterized by cold cyanotic skin, brittle fingernails, loss of hair, dryness and ulceration of skin, and lysis of bones and joints. The digits are affected most. In some incomplete lesions of the median, ulnar, or sciatic nerve with causalgia, the warm phase may persist and be accompanied by sweating.[1]

Causalgia. In 1865 Weir Mitchell coined the name *causalgia* to describe a rare (except in wartime) type of peripheral neuralgia caused by partial injury to the median or ulnar nerve and occasionally the sciatic nerve. True causalgia is associated with penetrating injuries in which some sensory fibers, and usually some muscle fibers, are left intact. The pain, beginning shortly after injury, is described as a constant and intense burning. Symptoms are most pronounced in the digits, palm of the hand, or sole of the foot. Any minor stimulus, such as a draft of air, contact with clothes, noise from a radio, or the immediate environment, can aggravate the pain. The patient is most comfortable when left alone with a cool moist cloth wrapped around the limb.

There are abnormalities of the sweat glands and vasomotor tone in the affected area caused by alteration of autonomic function. The involved hand (or foot, as the case may be) is moist and warmer or colder, and is either pinker or bluer, than the other hand. Trophic changes soon occur in the skin (shiny and smooth, and then scaly and discolored).

The underlying pathophysiology is thought to be caused by short-circuiting of the efferent sympathetic impulses to sensory somatic fibers at the point of injury.

True causalgia may respond to procaine blocks and sympathectomy.

COMMON TRAUMATIC SYNDROMES

Specific traumatic syndromes commonly seen include

1. Brachial plexus injury
2. Upper extremity injuries
   - Median nerve (injury and carpal tunnel syndrome)
   - Ulnar nerve
   - Radial nerve
3. Lower extremity injuries
   - Femoral nerve
   - Sciatic nerve
   - Common peroneal nerve

Brachial Plexus Trauma

The brachial plexus is created from spinal nerves C-5, C-6, C-7, C-8, and T-1 (Fig. 20-2). By a series of division and recombination, three major trunks result: the upper trunk (C-5 and C-6), the middle trunk (C-7), and the lower trunk (C-8 and T-1). Again, these trunks divide and recombine to create three cords that give rise to the following nerves:

1. Lateral cord (chiefly derived from C-5 and C-6)—musculocutaneous and the lateral half of the median nerve
2. Median cord (chiefly derived from C-8 and T-1)—ulnar nerve and the medial half of the median nerve
3. Posterior cord (C-5, C-6, and C-7)—axillary and radial nerve

FIG. 20-2. Brachial plexus showing its various constituents and their relationship to structures in the region of the upper chest, axilla, and shoulder. (DeJong R: The Neurological Examination. New York, Harper & Row, 1979)

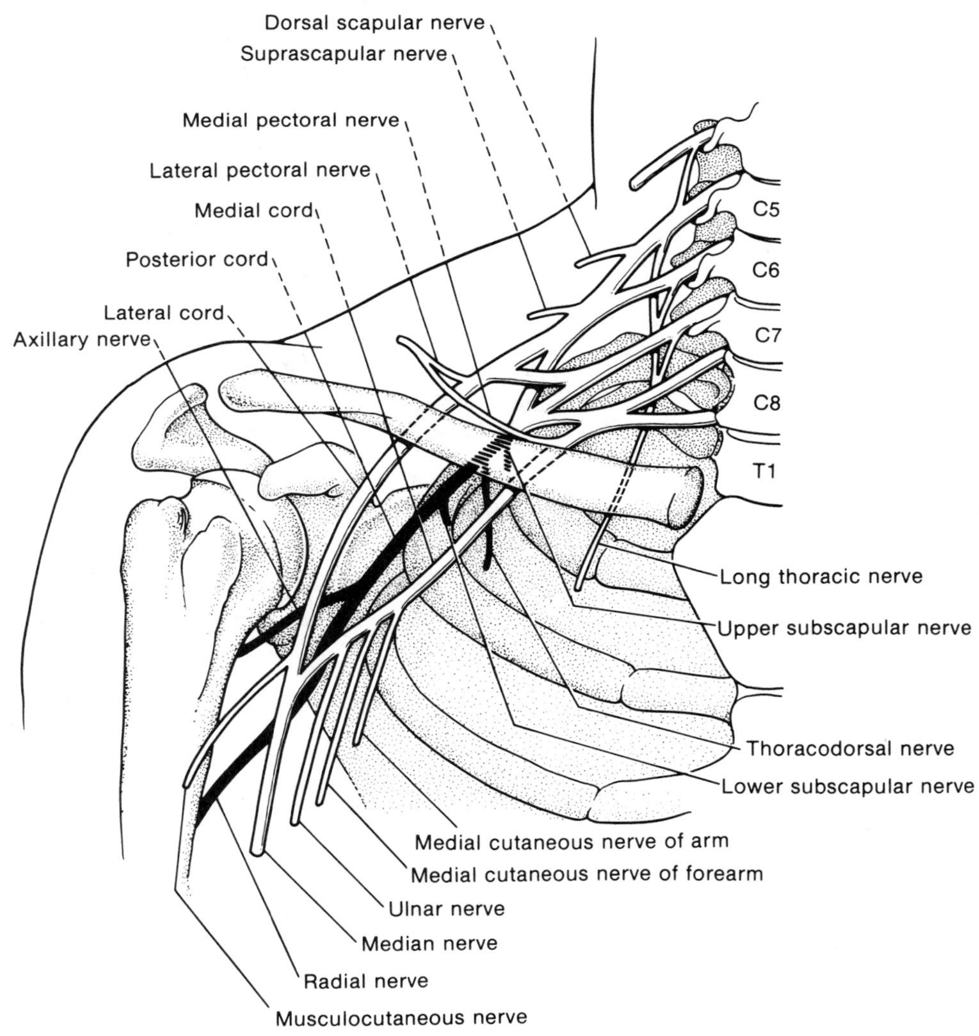

Symptoms. The symptoms seen with particular trunk trauma or injuries follow.

Upper Trunk (C–5 and C–6) Upper Plexus Type (Duchenne–Erb). Most of the shoulder muscles are involved, with the exception of the pectoralis major. There is loss of or difficulty in abduction and external rotation of the arm and weak supination and flexion of the forearm. Sensory deficit is noted in the deltoid region and radial surface of the forearm.

Middle Trunk (C–7). Major, but incomplete, triceps loss, as well as some involvement of the forearm flexors and extensors, are seen. Symptoms include difficulty in extending the forearm and sensory deficit.

Lower Trunk (C–8 and T–1) Lower Plexus Type (Klumpke or Duchenne–Aran). The forearm muscle flexors and the hand muscles are chiefly involved. There is paralysis and atrophy of small hand muscles and wrist flexors, giving the appearance of a "claw hand." Sensory deficit is noted in the medial side of the arm, forearm, and hand.

Causes. The major cause of brachial plexus trauma is traction and stretch injuries. Traction and stretch trauma of the brachial plexus can be caused by birth trauma and vehicular accidents. With traction trauma there may be sensory preservation in spite of total motor loss. A severe traction injury usually involves avulsion of two or more spinal roots from the spinal cord. Simultaneously, other roots have probably experienced severe stretching. The result is total and permanent functional loss to both the avulsed and stretched nerves. The presence of Horner's syndrome is strongly suggestive of C–8 and T–1 avulsion. (Horner's syndrome refers to the sinking of the eyeball, ptosis of the upper eyelid, slight elevation of the lower eyelid, constriction of the pupil, and anhidrosis caused by paralysis of the cervical sympathetic nerve supply.)

Treatment. Each brachial plexus injury is unique. Therefore, it is impossible to generalize about the treatment protocol. Although regeneration is slow, useful recovery is generally not probable in muscles that do not begin to show function by 6 months.

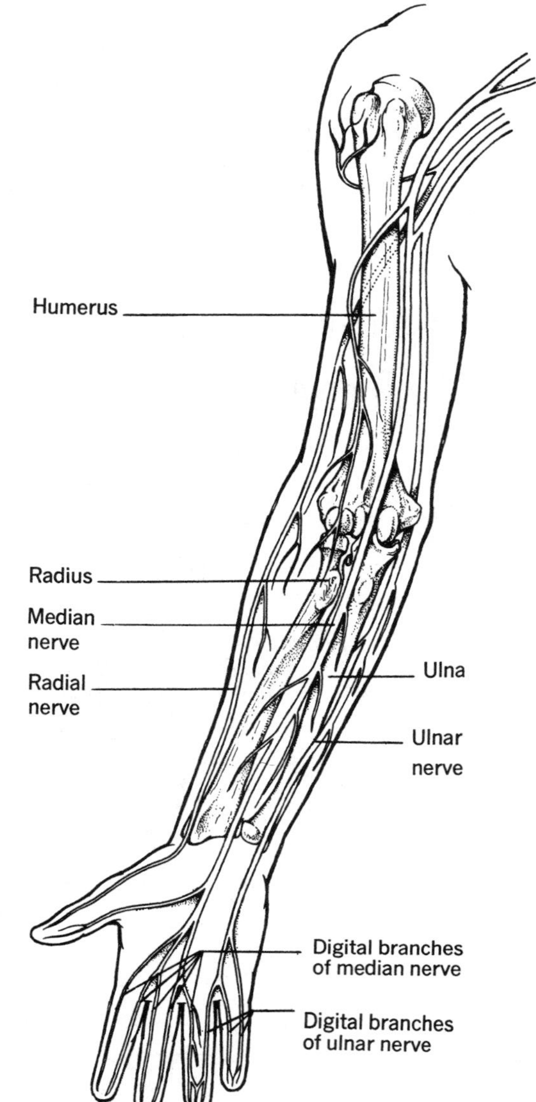

FIG. 20–3. Course of radial, ulnar, and medial nerves in right upper extremity. (Chaffee EE, Lytle IM: Basic Physiology and Anatomy. Philadelphia, JB Lippincott, 1980)

Upper Extremity Trauma

Median Nerve Trauma (Derived from C–5 to T–1, but Mainly From C–6)

Symptoms. The following signs and symptoms are found with median nerve injury (Fig. 20–3):

1. Impairment of pronation of the forearm
2. Weakness of wrist flexion
3. Difficulty in abducting and opposing the thumb
4. Inability to flex the distal phalanges of the index finger and thumb
5. Paralysis of the hand and finer flexors
6. Atrophy of the thenar hand muscles and the flexor–pronator group of the forearm
7. Sensory loss to the radial half of the palm, the palmar surface of the thumb, index and middle fingers, and the radial half of the ring finger
8. Loss of ability to sweat in affected areas

Causes. The median nerve may be injured in the axilla by shoulder dislocation or anywhere along its pathway by laceration, stab wounds, or gunshot wounds. However, the most frequent site of injury is at the wrist, because of its vulnerable anatomical position (Fig. 20–4). The median nerves lie between the tendons of the flexor carpi radialis and palmaris longus. The flexor pollicis longus and the flexor digitorum profundus separate the median nerve from the radius. The nerve crosses the wrist level and enters the carpal tunnel, located beneath the transverse carpal ligament. The carpal tunnel is a narrow tunnel through which the median nerve passes. It is bound superiorly by the transverse carpal ligaments, and laterally and inferiorly by the carpal bones, including fibrous coverings and interosseous ligaments. This syndrome commonly occurs in women between the ages of 40 and 60 years with no obvious etiological factor. If, for any reason, the lumen

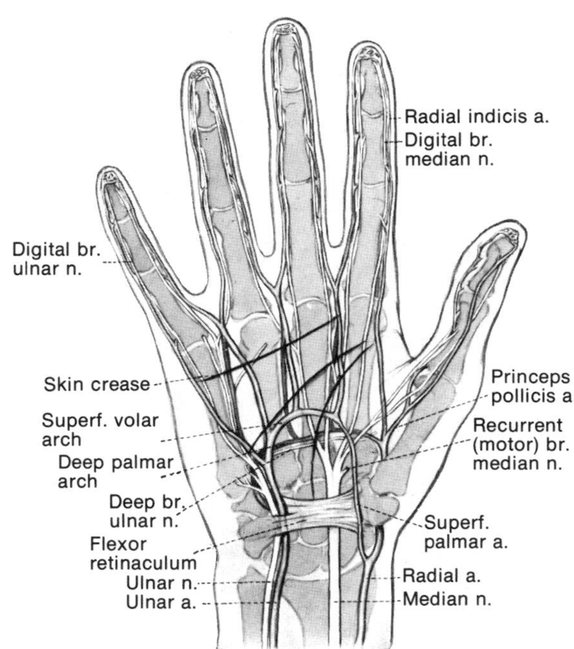

FIG. 20–4. Nerve distribution in the hand. Compression of median nerve in area of the carpal tunnel (flexor retinaculum) produces carpal tunnel syndrome. (Thorek P: Anatomy in Surgery, 2nd ed. Philadelphia, JB Lippincott, 1962)

of this channel is narrowed, the movement of the nerve and muscles is compromised. The result is the development of symptoms.

Carpal Tunnel Syndrome. The carpal tunnel syndrome, an entrapment syndrome, is caused by compression of the median nerve because of edema of tissue in and around the carpal tunnel. Occupation-related activities that require forceful and repetitive movements of the wrists or keeping the wrists in abnormal positions for prolonged periods appear to predispose people to the carpal tunnel syndrome. Such occupational categories include press operators, construction workers who use vibrating equipment, hairdressers, typists, and pianists, to mention a few.

Symptoms. Early symptoms include nocturnal dysesthesias (abnormal sensation) of the involved hand. As the disease progresses, severe dysesthesias accompany the use of the hand during daytime hours. Areas of the hand that are involved are those listed in the general symptoms of median nerve injury. Pain becomes constant, with motor weakness and atrophy. Vasomotor changes are intermittent.

Treatment. Treatment of early carpal tunnel syndrome is directed at immobilization of the wrist so that edema can be resolved. However, if nerve injury is advanced, surgery will be necessary to free the median nerve of compression. Most patients do extremely well with surgical decompression.

Ulnar Nerve (Derived From C–8 and T–1) Trauma. The ulnar nerve is most often injured at the elbow because of a fracture or dislocation of the elbow joint. Injury may also occur from a blow to the elbow that results in a contusion to the ulnar nerve. *Volkmann's contracture* refers to muscle contraction of the arm and hand resulting from ischemic injuries at the elbow (Fig. 20–5).

Symptoms. Symptoms of ulnar nerve trauma include the following:

1. "Claw hand" deformity (results from wasting of the small hand muscles with hyperextension of the fingers at the metacarpophalangeal joints)
2. Weakness of flexion of the wrist
3. Flexion of the fourth and fifth fingers
4. Inability to abduct and adduct the thumb
5. Sensory loss of the fifth finger, the ulnar aspect of the fourth finger, and the ulnar border of the palm
6. In the instance of a contusion to the nerve, the chief symptom may be pain with little, if any, motor deficit. As time passes, motor deficits may evolve (sometimes referred to as a tardy ulnar paralysis).

Radial Nerve (Derived From C–6, C–7, and C–8, but Mainly From C–7 Nerve Root) Trauma. The radial nerve may be injured in the axilla from compression and stretching caused by crutch walking. It is most frequently compressed at the point where the nerve winds around the humerus. Fractures and compression during sleep are the usual causes.

Symptoms. Symptoms of complete radial trauma include

1. Weakness in extension of the elbow, wrist, fingers, and thumb
2. Possible wrist drop
3. Inability to grasp an object or make a fist
4. Sensory impairment over the posterior aspect of the forearm and the radial aspect of the dorsum of the hand

Lower Extremity Trauma (Fig. 20–6)

Femoral Nerve (Derived From the L–2, L–3, and L–4 Nerve Roots) Trauma. The femoral nerve may be injured from compression of a pelvic tumor or during pelvic surgery.

Symptoms. Trauma to the femoral nerve results in

1. Weakness of extension of the knee
2. Wasting of the quadriceps muscles

FIG. 20–5. Volkmann's contracture. (Boyes JH: Bunnell's Surgery of the Hand, 5th ed. Philadelphia, JB Lippincott, 1970)

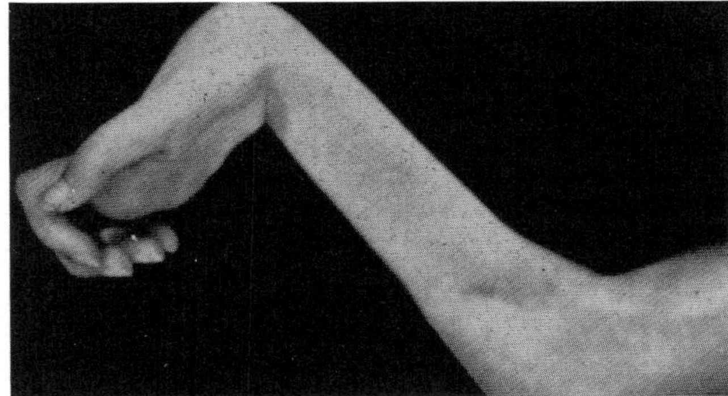

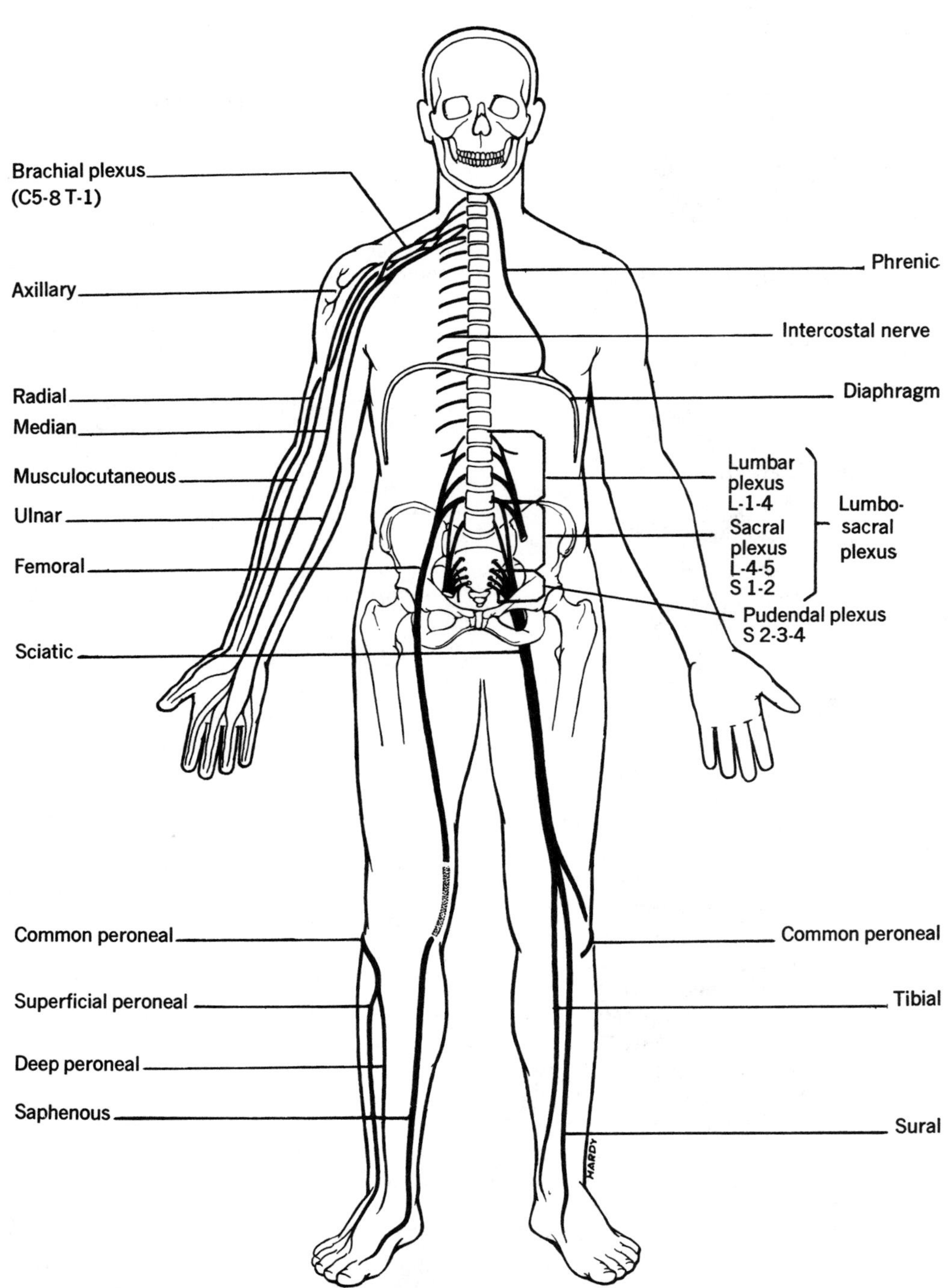

FIG. 20–6. Distribution of certain peripheral nerves, anterior aspect. (Chaffee EE, Lytle IM: Basic Physiology and Anatomy. Philadelphia, JB Lippincott, 1980)

3. Weakness of hip flexion (if injury is near psoas muscle)
4. Absence of the knee jerk
5. Sensory loss of the anterolateral thigh

Sciatic Nerve (Derived From L-4 to S-3 Nerve Roots) Trauma. The sciatic nerve is injured by pelvic or femoral fractures, gunshot wounds, or injection of medication into the nerve. Pelvic tumors and herniated intervertebral discs are other possible causes of sciatic injury.

Symptoms. Symptoms of complete sciatic paralysis include

1. Inability to flex the knee
2. Paralysis of all muscles below the knee
3. Weakened gluteal muscles
4. Pain across buttock and into the thigh
5. Footdrop
6. Sensory loss in the innervated areas

Common Peroneal Nerve (Derived From L-4 to S-3) Trauma. The common peroneal nerve is injured from prolonged traction, prolonged application of a tourniquet, or compression at the lateral aspect of the knees during surgery.

Symptoms. Symptoms of trauma include

1. Paralysis of dorsiflexion of foot and toes (footdrop)
2. Difficulty with eversion of the foot (with involvement of superficial peroneal nerve)
3. Sensory loss of the medial part of the dorsum of the foot and outer side of the leg

DIAGNOSIS

Diagnosis of peripheral nerve trauma is based on a history of injury or presence of an irritative or injurious lesion and a complete neurological examination. A valuable diagnostic aid is Tinel's sign, a tingling sensation experienced at the distal end of a limb when percussion is applied over the site of a divided nerve (Fig. 20-7). A positive Tinel's sign indicates a partial lesion or the beginning of regeneration of the nerve. Some continuity with the nervous system is noted if distal percussion produces some sensory response.

Electromyography and conduction velocity studies are two diagnostic tests that may be ordered to give some indication of an intact nerve.

FIG. 20-7. Tinel's sign is useful in evaluating nerve regeneration. As the sensory fiber proceeds distally from the point of injury, percussion elicits pain response in the distribution of the nerve. (Smith RR: Essentials of Neurosurgery. Philadelphia, JB Lippincott, 1980)

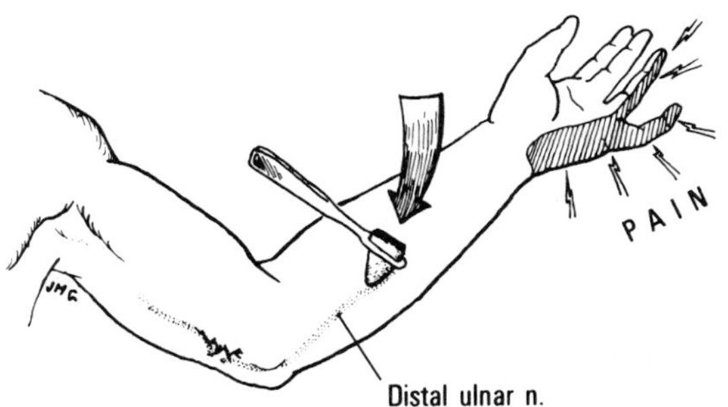

TREATMENT

As indicated earlier, each problem must be evaluated individually. If nerve trauma is secondary to a primary problem such as a tumor, attention is first directed to treatment of the primary problem. Surgery may be indicated for lacerations or transections. Ideally, any associated injuries should be clean and healed. Selecting the optimal time for surgery, however, is most important. To determine the extent of a nerve injury, surgical exploration may be planned immediately after injury. Primary nerve repair is usually scheduled for 3 weeks after injury. Some surgeons may delay surgical anastomosis for up to 2 months, but delays should be no longer. The judgment of the physician in selecting the proper time and surgical procedure is important. Severed nerves may require resection and suturing to reapproximate the ends. Nerve grafts or transplantations are occasionally necessary.

At surgery for anastomosis of the severed nerve, the two nerve segments will have contracted, each having formed scar tissue at the stump. Dissection of the stumps further decreases the lengths of the ends to be joined. To compensate for this situation, the extremity is positioned in exaggerated flexion with a cast or splint applied to maintain the position. However, healing at the suture site takes 3 or 4 weeks. After healing has been ensured, the cast or splint is revised several times, with the degree of extension gradually increased by approximately 10 degrees each time.

Cable grafting with autologous nerve tissue is a newer surgical technique that allows for anastomosis of nerves over large gaps, without exaggerated flexion position being needed.

Because it is known that denerved muscle begins to atrophy almost immediately after injury, it is important to use all available means to retard the process. As previously noted, axonal growth occurs at the rate of 1 mm to 4 mm/day. It is clear that some muscle atrophy will be evident before the slow process of nerve regeneration is completed. Howe endorses the concept of daily use of electrical stimulation to the affected muscles from the time of injury to reduce the inevitable atrophy and facilitate later rehabilitation.[2]

As soon as satisfactory healing has occurred, a physiotherapy program should be implemented to deal with the problems of immobility (stiffness, atrophy, and joint ankylosis). Special spring braces should be used to prevent footdrop or wristdrop. Galvanic stimulation to minimize the atrophic change of muscle to fibrotic tissue is continued daily until the affected muscle demonstrates evidence upon electromyography that it has been reinnervated. Massage, whirlpool treatments, and an exercise program to reeducate the muscles are important contributions that an aggressive physiotherapy program can offer.

The rehabilitation program is a long and arduous one. Depending on the type and location of the injury, the prognosis will vary. It may be necessary to offer a total rehabilitation program at a center that provides vocational rehabilitation, if permanent disability will prevent the patient from assuming his former place in society and the job market. The patient should be kept comfortable with appropriate analgesics, as necessary.

NURSING MANAGEMENT OF THE PATIENT WITH PERIPHERAL NERVE TRAUMA

Specific nursing care depends on the particular problem and the type and degree of injury. The patient with a peripheral injury may be hospitalized for surgery and discharged to recuperate at home. In other instances, a periph-

CHART 20-1. SUMMARY OF NURSING MANAGEMENT OF THE PATIENT WITH PERIPHERAL NERVE TRAUMA

NURSING RESPONSIBILITIES	RATIONALE
Assessment of Function	
1. Assess involved area for motor and sensory function. • Voluntary movement • Abnormal movement or lack of movement • Sensory responsiveness to heat, cold, light touch, and vibration • Reflexes	1. Sets a baseline from which change in function can be determined
2. Assess involved area for texture, warmth, and color.	2. Indicates autonomic changes to the involved area
Maintenance of Function	
1. Maintain immobility of involved area.	1. Provides for rest of an area that has an inflammatory process or allows for healing of area
2. Check skin for trophic changes and provide special skin care to involved area (lanolin, cocoa butter).	2. Prevents breakdown of skin in involved area
3. Avoid exposure of the denerved area to extremes in temperature.	3. Prevents injury to the involved area
4. If a cast has been applied, provide cast care (check if too tight, drainage, and so forth).	4. Prevents injury to involved extremity
Rehabilitation	
1. Help patient set realistic goals by reinforcing what the physician has told him about the time needed for improvement.	1. Decreases anxiety and develops a trusting, honest relationship
2. Be supportive of the patient during rehabilitation process.	2. Provides positive motivation force and support system for the patient
3. Apply splints, slings, and other supportive devices as ordered.	3. Provides support to the affected area
4. Help patient regain his independence in activities of daily living	4. Optimal independence is measured to the degree that activities of daily living skills can be mastered
5. Teach the patient exercises for involved area.	5. Improves muscle strength
6. Provide passive range-of-motion exercises when prescribed by physician.	6. Same as 5
7. Protect involved area from additional injury.	7. Prevents additional disability
8. Be supportive of physiotherapy program by positive attitude, having patient ready on time, and following up on what he has done in physiotherapy.	8. Provides positive motivational force to the patient
9. Prevent development of musculoskeletal deformities (contractures, ankylosis, and so forth).	9. Same as 7
10. Help patient accept altered body image and permanent disabilities.	10. Helps patient to set realistic goals and prevents abnormal emotional response
11. Participate in long-term rehabilitation plans with other team members.	11. Fulfills the nurse's role as the patient's advocate for long-term planning

eral injury may be only one type of injury seen in multiple trauma. The management of the peripheral injury is incorporated into the total nursing management of the patient. However, there are general principles that can be identified and followed when caring for patients with a peripheral nerve injury. These principles can be categorized into the following areas: assessment of function, maintenance of function, and rehabilitation. See Chart 20–1 for summary of nursing management.

ASSESSMENT OF FUNCTION

A neurological assessment of the limb is made to determine which neurological functions are intact. The motor function is assessed by asking the patient to put the limb through the normal range of motion. In an acute traumatic episode, the initial injury should first be evaluated by the physician in the emergency room to determine if movement is contraindicated, as would be the case if there were danger of a broken bone severing a nerve. If movements of the involved extremity are not contraindicated, the movement of the extremity should be assessed. Any evidence of abnormal movements such as tremors, fibrillation, or fasciculations should be reported. Atrophy, contractions, paresis, and paralysis are abnormal findings. The deep tendon reflexes in the limbs should also be checked.

The sensory innervation to the involved limb is tested by using a wisp of cotton for light touch. Pinching the skin or pricking it with a pin can test the patient's reaction to a painful stimulus. Test tubes of both warm and cold water can be individually placed on the skin of the involved limb to test the patient's awareness of differences in temperature. The patient should be questioned about whether he has had any experience of abnormal sensations, such as tingling, a crawling sensation, or pain. All are examples of reportable findings.

The involved limb should also be assessed for color, warmth, and texture. If the skin is cool to the touch or appears cyanotic, circulatory impairment or vasomotor tone may be indicated. Warm, dry, reddish skin indicates possible early trophic changes associated with autonomic alterations. Any evidence of scaling, brittleness of nails, or loss of body hair should be recorded.

The assessment is initially conducted by the nurse to establish a baseline with which subsequent assessments can be compared. After the baseline has been established, subsequent assessments are conducted every 2 to 4 hours or at less frequent intervals, depending on the patient's condition.

MAINTENANCE OF FUNCTION

Following an assessment of the involved area, the nurse plans and implements the nursing care plan with consideration of the goals of medical management.

If the physician has ordered immobilization of the involved area, the immobilization may be accomplished by a splint, cast, or traction. The purpose of immobilization is to provide rest for the involved area if an inflammatory process is present, so that the process can be controlled and resolved. The second reason for immobilization is to allow for the healing of a surgical incision in which there has been a reanastomosis of a severed nerve.

Splint and Cast Care

The splint is usually held secure with an Ace bandage, which can become tight because of edema. The skin around the splint or cast should be checked for tightness, warmth, and color. If the splint or cast is too tight, as evidenced by tingling, discomfort, blanched color, or coolness, it may be necessary to report this information to the physician or physiotherapist so that steps can be taken to provide a better fit. In the case of a tight cast, the physician may choose to bivalve the cast. The two parts of the cast may be held in place with an Ace bandage. Another possibility is removing the cast and replacing it with a new one. A splint can be adjusted in shape or straps fixed to provide a better fit. It is not a nursing prerogative to cut the fastening straps or bend parts of the brace, since irreparable damage can be inflicted when this is done by the inexperienced. It is best to refer the need for adjustments to the department that made the splint or brace originally, since all braces and most splints are custom-made to fit the contour of the wearer. A blanched appearance coupled with coolness to the touch indicates interference with autonomic function and normal blood supply. Any indications of drainage under the cast or splint should be reported immediately.

If the patient has a cast, it should be protected against moisture, injury, and soiling. The cast should be "pedaled" with strips of adhesive tape to prevent crumpling (of the cast) or irritation of the underlying skin.

Positioning the Extremity

If a cast or splint has been applied to the arm, a sling may be necessary to prevent edema because the arm is in a dependent position. In the cast of a leg cast, the physician would probably indicate that the leg was to be supported and elevated on pillows to reduce the occurrence of edema.

Skin Care

Trophic changes of the skin are common signs and symptoms associated with peripheral nerve injury that make the skin susceptible to breakdown and injury. The skin should be examined for evidence of irritation or injury. Washing and careful drying is important, especially between the toes or fingers, as the case may be. If the skin is dry and scaly, lubrication with lanolin or cocoa butter is an effective treatment. The nails should be filed and cut straight across to prevent injury.

Temperature

The involved extremity should be carefully protected from extremes in temperature. Because of the lost or compromised sensory function, the area could be easily injured from extreme heat or cold without the patient being alerted through pain or discomfort.

Ambulation

Depending on the extent of injury of the involved extremity, the physician may limit ambulation and other activities of daily living. The nurse will need to adjust the plan of care based on the limitations imposed by the injury and the medical treatment

REHABILITATION

The length and complexity of the rehabilitative process will vary based on the particular injury and patient. The patient should be allowed to verbalize his concerns about his injury. The nurse should be a good listener, correct misconceptions, and help the patient set realistic goals. Anxiety is decreased and the patient is better able to cope with an altered body image if the nurse can be supportive of the patient. A positive, supportive nurse–patient relationship provides an ideal milieu for the active participation of the patient in the rehabilitative process.

The patient with a peripheral nerve injury requires much teaching to help him regain the greatest level of independence. He may need help in developing alternate methods of fulfilling the activities of daily living. For example, if his dominant arm and hand are encircled by a splint, he will need to be helped to learn to eat with his other hand. If his food is prepared (beverage poured, food cut, and so forth), he will be able to manage with practice.

When an exercise program is initiated for the involved extremity, the patient will have to learn both the active and passive (prescribed) exercises. He should also be taught to protect the involved limb from injury. The process of regaining motor and sensory function can be so slow that the patient becomes discouraged. He needs to be encouraged to follow the outlined physiotherapy program to prevent skeletal deformities and slowly regain as much function as possible. A positive attitude on the part of the nurse conveys the loudest message to the patient about the progress he is making.

The nurse participates in the long-range planning for patient needs with other members of the health team. The rehabilitative process for peripheral nerve injury may be long. Often, the patient with the injury will be treated on an outpatient basis with physiotherapy and supervision by the physician and community health nurse. An assessment of the patient's needs should be conducted to help the patient cope with difficulties related to the limitations imposed by the injury.

PSYCHOSOCIAL CONSIDERATIONS

Peripheral nerve injury is usually synonymous with disability of an extremity. If the arm is involved, the patient is deprived of the normal range of motion, which will usually affect his various roles, whether it be breadwinner, homemaker, handyman, child caretaker, or creative being. Thumb apposition to the index finger is a highly valued skill. Without this skill the patient is unable to pick up objects, feed himself, and perform other acts which would be elements in the activities of daily living. An individual deprived of his ability to perform these activities of daily living will feel limited, especially if the injury is to his dominant side.

Peripheral nerve injury to one of the lower extremities impedes or prevents ambulation and limits the various settings in which the person can function. The inability to ambulate, drive, use public transportation, and move about freely in public settings interferes with normal fulfillment of roles and responsibilities.

The decreased level of independence precipitates various emotional and psychological reactions. The patient experiences changes in body image, self-esteem, and lifestyle. Sensory deprivation, social isolation, and powerlessness result from the limitations imposed by the disability. Common behavioral manifestations from the various physical, emotional, and social disabilities include frustration, hostility, anger, and depression. Many patients go through a process of loss, grief, and bereavement over the lost function. The process of recovery is very slow (approximately 1 year with nerve transections). Physiotherapy is the major approach after surgical intervention has been completed. Anyone who has experience with patient care and physiotherapy is well aware of the painfully slow process involved in rehabilitating a limb. The process is characterized by ups and downs, so the patient can easily become discouraged with the lack of apparent improvement. If disability is permanent, the emotional impact imposes greater demands on the person's coping skills and adjustment patterns; therefore, it is extremely important that the nurse provide the psychosocial support needed at this time.

REFERENCES

1. Haymaker W: Bing's Local Diagnosis in Neurological Diseases. St Louis, CV Mosby, 1969
2. Howe JR: Manual of Patient Care in Neurosurgery, 2nd ed, pp 165–166. Boston, Little, Brown & Co, 1983

BIBLIOGRAPHY

Books

Adams R, Victor M: Principles of Neurology, 2nd ed. New York, McGraw–Hill, 1981

Clark R: Manter and Gatz's Clinical Neuroanatomy and Neurophysiology, 6th ed. Philadelphia, FA Davis, 1982

Eliasson S et al: Neurological Pathophysiology, 2nd ed. New York, Oxford University Press, 1978

Gorgio A, Millesi H, Mingrino S (eds): Posttraumatic Peripheral Nerve Regeneration. New York, Raven Press, 1981

Hudson A, Berry H, Mayfield F: Chronic injuries of peripheral nerves by entrapment. In Youmans J (ed): Neurological Surgery, 2nd ed, pp 2430–2474. Philadelphia, WB Saunders, 1982

Kline DE, Nulsen FE: Acute injuries of peripheral nerves. In Youmans J (ed): Neurological Surgery, 2nd ed, pp 2362–2429. Philadelphia, WB Saunders, 1982

Long DM: Pain of peripheral nerve injury. In Youmans J (ed): Neurological Surgery, 2nd ed, pp 3634–3643. Philadelphia, WB Saunders, 1982

Noback C, Demarest R: The Nervous System: Introduction and Review, 2nd ed, pp 84–85. New York, McGraw–Hill, 1977
Omer GE, Spinner M: Management of Peripheral Nerve Problems. Philadelphia, WB Saunders, 1980
Schaumburg HH, Spencer PC, Thomas PK: Disorders of Peripheral Nerves. Philadelphia, FA Davis, 1983
Sumner AJ: The Physiology of Peripheral Nerve Disease. Philadelphia, WB Saunders, 1980
Sunderland S: The carpal tunnel syndrome. In Nerves and Nerve Injuries, 2nd ed, pp 711–727. New York, Churchill Livingstone, 1979

Periodicals

Bowens B: Carpal tunnel syndrome. J Neurosurg Nurs 13(3):129, June 1981
Bryant W: Wound healing. Clin Symp 29(3):2, 1977
Burg M: Compartment syndrome. Crit Care Q 6(1):27, June 1983
Butterworth G: Interfascicular autologous nerve grafts in the microsurgical repair of peripheral nerves. J Neurosurg Nurs 9(2):63, June 1977
Kline DG: Macroscopic and microscopic concomitants of nerve repair. Clin Neurosurg 26:582, 1979
Lachman T: Some common causes of neuropathy. Hosp Med 19(5):114, May 1983
Lamb C (ed): Investigating the entrapment syndromes. Patient Care 11:64, May 1, 1977
Lamb C (ed): Roundtable: Peripheral neuropathy. Focusing in on peripheral neuropathies. Patient Care 11:20, May 1, 1977
Lupin AE: Head off compartment syndrome before it's too late. RN 43(12):39, December, 1980
Miller BK: How to spot . . . and treat . . . carpal tunnel syndrome . . . early. Nurs 80 10(3):50, 1980
Parry C et al: Rehabilitation of the injured hand. Nurs Times 74:1483, September 7, 1978
Wadsworth T et al: The cubital tunnel external compression syndrome. Nurs Times 73:1357, September 1, 1977
Watson M: Hand injuries: Principles of management of complicated injuries, part III. Nurs Times 74:360, March 2, 1978

part six

Nursing Care of Patients With Tumors of the Neurological System

chapter 21

Brain Tumors

ETIOLOGY AND INCIDENCE

Brain tumors account for about 2% of all cancer deaths each year. Although this is not a large percentage, in terms of human suffering and disability, it is a major concern for nurses caring for these patients.

The American Cancer Society estimates that there are 10,900 cases of primary brain and central nervous system tumors yearly,[1] with a slightly greater number of cases projected for males than females (5900 and 5000 respectively). Other statistics indicate that about 8500 deaths occurred as a result of brain tumors, and 67,000 cases, or 18%, of cancer patients develop metastasis to the brain from other sites.

Intracranial tumors are found in people of all ages, with peaks of incidence occurring in the second half of the first decade, as well as the fourth and fifth decades. The cause of brain tumors is unknown. Certain tumors appear to be congenital (epidermoid, dermoid, and teratoid tumors and craniopharyngiomas). Others may be related to hereditary factors (von Recklinghausen's disease, tuberous sclerosis, and von Hippel–Lindau disease). There is even some suggestion that intracranial tumors can occur secondary to craniocerebral trauma or inflammatory disease; however, no conclusive evidence is currently available to support this hypothesis.

Metastasis of intracranial tumors, both within and outside the central nervous system, is recognized as a more common occurrence than once thought. The spreading within the central nervous system is by transfer of tumor cells by means of the cerebral blood, and by "seeding" through cerebrospinal fluid in the subarachnoid space and ventricles. There are no lymphatics in the brain itself. Metastasis to the spinal cord is not uncommon, and occurs through the leptomeninges.[2] Metastasis outside the central nervous system can occur by "seeding" of the scalp, cerebral blood vessels, and dural sinuses during craniotomy. The lymphatic system also contributes to the spread of tumor cells to other parts of the body.

PATHOPHYSIOLOGY

A brain tumor will usually grow as a spherical mass until it encounters a more rigid structure such as bone or the falx cerebri. The encounter with an aplastic substance necessitates a change in the contour of the neoplasm. Neoplastic cells can also grow diffusely, infiltrating tissue spaces as multiple cells without forming a definite mass. The size of the tumor enlarges because of cell proliferation or as a result of necrosis, fluid accumulation, hemorrhage, or accumulation of by-products of degeneration within the mass.

Tumors affect the brain through compression, invasion, and infiltration. These mechanisms precipitate pathophysiological changes in the brain, resulting in some or all of the following pathophysiological findings:

1. Cerebral edema
2. Increased intracranial pressure
3. Focal neurological deficits
4. Seizure activity
5. Alterations in normal pituitary function
6. Obstruction of flow of cerebrospinal fluid

CEREBRAL EDEMA

In most patients with brain tumors, edema develops in the tissue in the vicinity of the tumor because of compression of the surrounding tissue by the tumor. Physiologically, it is thought that there is increased permeability of the capillary endothelial cells of the cerebral white matter, resulting in the seepage of plasma into the extracellular spaces and the areas between the layers of the myelin sheath. The result is alterations in the cell potential and impairment of cell activity. Some texts refer to this as the vasogenic theory of cerebral edema. Edema of the brain can also rapidly develop from alterations in the blood–brain barrier, which are caused by the neoplastic process.

Cerebral edema, or swelling of the brain, creates signs and symptoms of increased intracranial pressure that include

- Deterioration of the level of consciousness
- Loss of or decreased reactions of the pupils to the direct light reflex
- Unequal pupillary size
- Loss or decreased functional eye movement
- Loss or deterioration of motor function (paresis, paralysis, decortication, decerebration, or flaccidity)
- Deterioration of sensory function
- Changes in respiratory function (Cheyne–Stokes, central neurogenic hyperventilation, apneustic breathing, cluster breathing, or ataxic breathing)
- Changes in vital signs (lowered pulse, elevated blood pressure, and widening of pulse pressure)

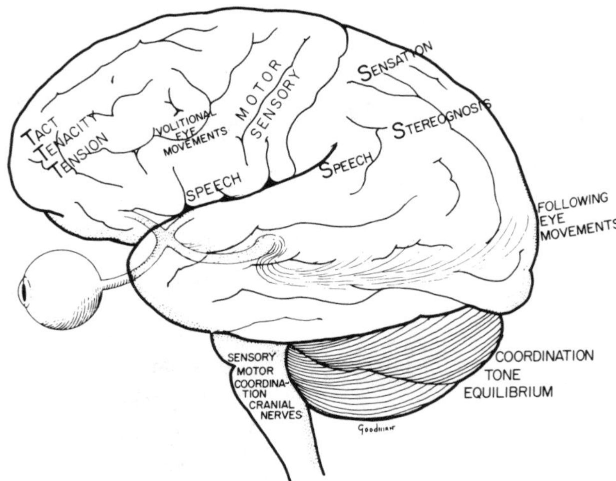

FIG. 21–1. Functional significance of intracranial tumors of the cerebral cortex, cerebellum, and brain stem. (Hardy JD: Rhoads Textbook of Surgery, 5th ed. Philadelphia, JB Lippincott, 1977)

INCREASED INTRACRANIAL PRESSURE

Signs and symptoms of increased intracranial pressure will develop as a tumor expands. Slow-growing tumors allow for greater compensation of intracranial contents than do rapid-growing tumors. However, as the limits of accommodation are reached, intracranial pressure will increase and symptoms will be apparent. This is the period of decompensation.

In the adult most brain tumors are located in the supratentorial region. As the tumor grows, various herniation syndromes, such as those related to cingulate, transtentorial, and uncal herniation, can develop. Characteristic signs and symptoms develop with each syndrome and follow a predictable rostrocaudal deterioration pattern, as explained by Plum.[3] Without definitive treatment of the enlarging neoplasm, intracranial displacement will continue until brain stem–cerebellar herniation occurs through the foramen magnum. The vital centers of the brain stem then become compressed, and death ensues.

FOCAL NEUROLOGICAL DEFICITS

Cerebral tissue is a highly specialized type of tissue. Encroachment upon this tissue caused by compression, infiltration, invasion, or edema will result in functional deficits (Fig. 21–1). Direct pressure on specific neurological tissue, such as the motor strip or visual pathway, will produce related neurological deficits.

Cranial nerves III, IV, and VI are frequently affected by expanding supratentorial tumors. Compression and stretching of cranial nerves and blood vessels can also produce dysfunction. Compression of blood vessels produces a diminished blood supply and possible ischemia to areas supplied by the vessel. Stretching or traction on a blood vessel can cause rupture and subsequent hemorrhage.

Tumors that directly invade cerebral and subcortical substance interrupt neural connections and destroy tissue. Tumor cells can spread to tissue spaces in nearby brain structures without forming a focal lesion. Extensive infiltration of the brain is possible before evidence of neurological deficit is apparent. The particular focal neurological deficits observed will depend on the particular part of the brain compromised.

SEIZURE ACTIVITY

About 30% of adults with brain tumors develop seizure activity. Cerebral edema and alterations in the normal electrical potential of the cell caused by the tumor results in hyperactive cells. This hyperactivity produces abnormal paroxysmal discharge or seizure activity that may be grand mal or focal. Focal seizures can sometimes be of diagnostic value by aiding the physician in the localization of the tumor.

Seizures originate in the gray matter, that is, mainly the mantle of the brain and sometimes the subcortical gray tissue. When seizure activity is the presenting symptom of a brain tumor, one can expect the tumor to be at the surface of the brain, either having arisen on the outer surface or having grown upward into the mantle area.

CHANGES IN PITUITARY FUNCTION

Most pituitary tumors arise from the anterior lobe, although both the anterior and posterior lobes can be severely damaged by tumors in the proximal sella area. Although pituitary adenomas directly affect pituitary function, craniopharyngiomas, some meningiomas, and aneurysms located near the pituitary–hypothalamus can also produce endocrine imbalance.

The implication of the hypothalamus in pituitary dysfunction is well known. It has been established that certain cells in the hypothalamus produce hormones called hypothalamic-releasing and inhibitory factors that control the anterior lobe secretions of the pituitary. These secreting cells release their hormones into the median eminence of the hypothalamus, which, in turn, extends into the pituitary stalk. When hypothalamus-releasing or inhibitory factors are secreted from the hypothalamus, they are immediately absorbed into the hypothalamic–hypophyseal portal capillaries, which then carry the secretions directly to the anterior lobe sinuses.[4]

Each anterior lobe hormone has a corresponding releasing and inhibitory factor. The predominant hormone in most instances is the releasing factor. The exception is prolactin, to which the inhibitory factor is most important.[4] The following is a list of the major secretions and their functions:

1. Thyroid-stimulating–hormone-releasing factor (TRF)—causes release of thyroid-stimulating hormone
2. Corticotropin-releasing factor (CRF)—causes release of adrenocorticotropin
3. Growth-hormone–releasing hormone factor (GRF)—causes release of growth hormone
4. Luteinizing-hormone–releasing factor (LRF)—causes release of luteinizing hormone
5. Follicle-stimulating—hormone-releasing factor (FRF)—causes release of follicle-stimulating hormone
6. Prolactin inhibitory factor (PIF)—causes inhibition of prolactin secretion.

Alterations in any of the pituitary secretions result in major disruptions of body functions, thereby causing conditions such as giantism, acromegaly, Cushing's syndrome, or hypopituitarism.

OBSTRUCTION TO FLOW OF CEREBROSPINAL FLUID

Tumor encroachment from within or outside the ventricles or subarachnoid space interferes with the normal flow of cerebrospinal fluid. This obstruction of cerebrospinal fluid results in hydrocephalus. If the tumor encroachment occurs slowly, the development of an obstruction and/or hydrocephalus will be gradual. However, rapid tumor growth produces acute precipitation of signs and symptoms, such as a massive spike in intracranial pressure with rapid deterioration in neurological status.

CLASSIFICATION OF BRAIN TUMORS

A single, standardized, universally accepted classification system of brain tumors does not presently exist. As the student consults various texts, he is confronted with confusing terminology and assorted criteria used to determine classification of brain tumors. One can find tumors classified according to a histological basis, on a malignant *versus* benign basis, or by intra-axial *versus* extra-axial location.

MALIGNANT *VERSUS* BENIGN BRAIN TUMORS

Using the word "benign" in the classification of brain tumors can be somewhat misleading. When a neoplasm is designated as benign, one concludes that a complete cure is possible; conversely, a malignant tumor would indicate a poor prognosis. This distinction is made on the basis of histological examination. Cells that are well differentiated tend to indicate a much better prognosis than poorly differentiated cells.

However, when a tumor is located within the brain, other factors take precedence. A tumor that is considered to be histologically "benign" may be surgically inaccessible, such as is the case with a deep tumor requiring extensive dissection of tissue or one located in a vital area such as the pons or medulla. A "benign" tumor that is surgically inaccessible with continue to grow, thereby causing an increase in intracranial pressure, neurological deficits, herniation syndromes, and, finally, death. Since the patient has lost neurological function and life, it appears to be grossly inaccurate to suggest that the tumor was "benign." There is also the possibility that tumors can convert to more histologically malignant types as they develop.

INTRA-AXIAL *VERSUS* EXTRA-AXIAL BRAIN TUMORS

Brain tumors may also be classified simply as intra-axial or extra-axial. Tumors originating from glia cells are termed *intra-axial* tumors and affect the brain by invasion and infiltration. *Extra-axial* tumors originate in the skull, meninges, cranial nerves, and pituitary and congenital cells at rest. Compression of the brain is the mode by which extra-axial tumors affect the brain. (For details about specific tumor types, see Table 21–1.)

HISTOLOGICAL CLASSIFICATION OF TUMORS

The following is a histological classification of the major tumors with their relative percentage of incidence. While accurate statistics for the various brain tumors are not available, the figures given provide a general idea of the incidence of specific tumors in the overall patient population.

A. Intrinsic tumors	
1. Gliomas (noncapsulated; tend to infiltrate the cerebral substance)	45%
a. Astrocytoma grades I and II	10%
b. Glioblastoma multiforme (also called astrocytoma III and IV)	20%
c. Oligodendroglioma grades I to IV	4% to 5%
d. Ependymoma grades I to IV	5% to 6%
e. Mixed gliomas	3% to 4%
2. Medulloblastomas	3%

(Text continued on page 471.)

TABLE 21 – 1. *Brain Tumors*

Type of Tumor	Description	Location	Signs and Symptoms	Treatment	Prognosis
Intra-axial					
Astrocytoma Grades I and II*	Grade I: well-defined cells Grade II: cell differentiation less defined	Usually found in frontal, temporal, or parietal lobes of cerebral hemispheres	Neurological deficits depend on specific location of tumor	*Surgical:* complete removal rarely possible; partial removal may prolong life; more than one excision may be done *Radiation:* Grade I: usually not considered; possible radiation necrosis; Grade II: radiation if residual tumor is usual	6 to 7 years average; more years possible
Glioblastoma multiforme (Astrocytoma, grades III and IV)	Grossly undifferentiated cells; necrosis is common with multiple cysts and hemorrhagic areas within the mass; highly malignant and rapid-growing; pinkish gray with soft or granular texture	Frequently involves white matter of anterior or frontal part of the hemispheres; more prevalent in males, 40 to 60 years of age	Depend upon actual location and size	*Surgical:* resection and decompression can alleviate signs of cerebral compression. *Radiation and chemotherapy:* frequently ordered to retard growth of tumor	12 to 18 months (only 10% are alive at 18 months)
Astrocytoma of the cerebellum (Grades I to IV; a childhood tumor)	Cystic tumor; slow-growing; considered benign if completely excised	Cerebellar region; found in children 5 to 9 years of age	Paralysis of cranial (VI) nerve (outward movement of orbit; also nerve VII paralysis – weakness of facial muscles; hemiplegia and sensory loss (long tract signs); gaze disorders; ataxia and incoordination (cerebellar dysfunction)	*Surgery:* removal may be possible with Grade I or II *Radiation:* used if tumor is inaccessible or only partially resected *Shunting procedure:* may be necessary in presence of increased intracranial pressure	Excellent if complete removal is possible (7 to 10 years for partial resection)
Astrocytoma of the Optic Nerves and Chiasma† (also called spongioblastoma in some texts; a childhood tumor)	As tumor grows, it enlarges optic foramen with little distortion of surrounding structures; slow-growing	Found along optic nerves; girls affected twice as often as boys	Early symptoms include dimness of vision and loss of vision in half of visual fields; optic atrophy with or without papilledema; blindness; proptosis (protrusion of eyeball) and hypothalamic imbalance	*Sugery:* removal if possible but often inaccessible *Radiation:* usually responds poorly	10 or more years

Ependymoma Grades I to IV (a tumor of childhood and young adults); more benign form may be called astroblastoma; more malignant may be called ependymoblastoma	A glioma arising from lining of the ventricles; slow-growing tumor	In ventricles, particularly fourth; can attach itself to roof or floor of the ventricle or grow directly into cerebral hemisphere with little or no attachment to ventricles	Rapidly elevated intracranial pressure because of obstruction of cerebrospinal fluid flow; lowered level of consciousness (LOC), pupillary signs, hemiplegia, sensory loss, respiratory changes, vital sign changes, lowered pulse, elevated blood pressure, and widening of pulse pressure; ataxia and incoordination (cerebellar dysfunction)	*Surgery:* removal if surgically accessible, depending upon location *Radiation:* Grades I and II respond poorly; Grades III and IV benefit *Shunting procedure:* may be necessary to reduce increased intracranial pressure from cerebrospinal fluid obstruction	1 month for malignant; 7 to 8 years for benign
Oligodendroglioma Grades I to IV	Calcification noted upon radiological examination in about 50%; deceptively appears encapsulated; slow-growing	Cerebral hemispheres, particularly frontal and temporal lobes; found in 20- to 40-year age group	Depend upon actual location of tumor; seizures first symptom in 50% of patients	*Surgery:* total removal if possible *Radiation:* Should be used if total surgical removal is not possible	5 or more years
Mixed Gliomas (or may be named for the predominant tumor cell present)	Composed histologically of two or more cell types of astrocytoma, glioblastoma, oligodendroglioma, or ependymoma in any combination	Any place where the various glioma types can be found; if glioblastoma cells are present, tumor tends to be malignant	Depend upon actual location of tumor	Depends upon type of tumor; surgery and/or radiation is the usual treatment	If glioblastoma cells are present, 1 to 2 years
Medulloblastoma (a childhood tumor)	Rapidly growing tumor that can obstruct cerebrospinal fluid flow; seeding into the third and lateral ventricles as well as the cisterna magna and along the spinal cord are common	Tumor almost exclusively in the cerebellar vermis; occupies the fourth ventricle and infiltrates its floor; males are affected more frequently; 3- to 5-year age group	Visual disturbances first noted by the child squinting; rapidly elevated intracranial pressure because of obstruction of cerebrospinal fluid flow; ataxia and incoordination (cerebellar dysfunction)	*Surgery:* partial dissection *Radiation:* highly radiosensitive; radiation to entire head and spinal cord because of seeding of malignant cells by way of the cerebrospinal fluid *Shunting procedure:* may be necessary in presence of increased intracranial pressure *Chemotherapy:* with surgery and/or radiation	5 years

(continued)

TABLE 21–1. *(continued)*

Type of Tumor	Description	Location	Signs and Symptoms	Treatment	Prognosis
Extra-axial Tumors: Tumors Arising from the Supporting Structures of the Nervous System					
Meningioma	Firm, encapsulated tumor arising from arachnoid granulations; slow-growing; can become large before symptoms appear, with compression the mode by which the brain is affected	Predilection for areas proximal to venous sinuses. Frequent sites include 1. Superior saggital sinus 2. Over convexities 3. Attached to sphenoid ridge 4. On anterior fossa floor 5. In posterior fossa More common in women; average 50 years	Neurological deficits caused by compression will depend upon area involved	*Surgery:* complete removal, if possible, or partial dissection *Radiation:* with surgery if complete removal is not possible	Excellent if total removal; many years with partial excision and radiation,
Acoustic neuroma (schwannoma, neurofibroma)	Arises from the sheath of Schwann cells; size varies from size of pea to walnut; considered a benign tumor, but located in an area of difficult access; bilateral tumors occasionally found	Vestibular branch of cranial (VIII) nerve; *smaller* tumor confined to internal auditory canal; *larger* tumor displaces cranial (VII) nerve or compresses of cranial (V) nerve; very large tumors will involve cranial (IX and X) nerves; possible cerebellar involvement.	Depend upon size; with a small tumor (confined to internal auditory canal), hearing loss, tinnitus, and dizziness (hearing loss most notable when using telephone or when source of sound close to affected ear); with larger tumor, unilateral weakness of neck muscle (platysma), facial asymmetry, and loss of taste on one side of tongue; larger tumors with cranial (V) nerve symptoms include hyperesthesia including corneal area, facial numbness, paresthesia, and decreased sensitivity to pain; with cranial (IX and X) nerve symptoms, difficulty in speaking or swallowing; ataxia or incoordination if cerebellum is involved; larger tumors may obstruct the flow of cerebrospinal fluid resulting in elevated intracranial pressure	*Surgery:* removal if tumor is not too extensive in area of difficult access (intimate relationship of cranial nerves VII and VIII; about half of patients with incomplete removal have recurrent tumor *Shunting procedure:* if cerebrospinal fluid obstruction is present	Small tumors with complete removal—excellent; 30% mortality in 3 to 4 years with incomplete removal

Von Recklinghausen's disease (neurofibromatosis)	Genetic origin because of autosomal dominant mendelian trait; skin, nervous system, bones, endocrine glands, and other organs sites of congenital anomalies, in addition to the multiple tumors of skin; firm, encapsulated lesions attached to nerve	Benign, multiple, circumscribed dermal and neural tumors with increased skin pigmentation (cosmetically offensive); tumors appear late in childhood or in early adolescence	Spots of hyperpigmentation (café au lait) and cutaneous and subcutaneous tumors	*Surgery:* possible, depending upon location of tumor *Radiation:* radioresistant	Depends upon area involved
Neuromas (cerebellar–pontine angle tumor)	Can be indistinguishable from an acoustic neuroma without visualization; meningiomas, mixed gliomas, or cerebral aneurysms also occur in this region; definitive diagnosis by surgical exposure and histological examination	Cerebellar–pontine angle	Variation of those seen with acoustic neuroma	*Surgery:* If possible; difficult surgical access (near vital centers) *Radiation:* may be selected over surgery	Depends upon type of tumor
Developmental Tumors					
Hemangioblastoma	Vascular tumor; slow-growing	Cerebellum as single or multiple lesion; less common location in medulla and cerebral hemispheres; tumor occurs in adult life	Dizziness, unilateral ataxia, signs and symptoms of elevated intracranial pressure, possible spinal cord involvement	*Surgery:* complete removal, is possible *Radiation:* if recurrent	Usually curable
Craniopharyngioma	Thought to arise from Rathke's pouch; solid or cystic tumors; can compress pituitary gland and may even amputate the pituitary stalk; about three fourths of tumors have calcified areas; growth of tumor directed upward, resulting in invagination of third ventricle and possible blockage of cerebrospinal fluid flow; optic chiasm elevated as a result of tumor, with resulting traction pressure on the optic nerves	In or about sella pituitary area; usually affects children	Signs and symptoms of grossly elevated intracranial pressure because of cerebrospinal fluid blockage; pituitary and/or hypothalamic dysfunction; visual disturbance	*Surgery:* resection by intracranial or transsphenoid approach *Radiation:* after surgery; tumor very sensitive	Excellent if excised, but rarely possible; although a number of total excisions reported, long-term follow-up has shown that because they insinuate themselves around so many structures, there are usually some cells left behind. Almost all tumors recur.

(continued)

TABLE 21–1. (continued)

Type of Tumor	Description	Location	Signs and Symptoms	Treatment	Prognosis
Epidermoid and dermoid cysts	Cysts of congenital origin from ectodermal layer; cysts lined with stratified squamous epithelium; epidermoid cyst contains keratin, cellular debris, and cholesterol; dermoid cyst contains hair and sebaceous glands	On bones of skull or within brain	Depend upon location	Surgery: complete removal usually possible	Very good
Pituitary Tumors					
Pituitary adenomas (in general)	Some texts suggest that all pituitary adenomas are composed of all three cell types: chromophobic, eosinophilic, and basophilic; three cell types originate in anterior lobe; benign, slow-growing, encapsulated tumors	Pituitary gland; most pituitary tumors arising in anterior lobe; both lobes can be damaged from parasellar tumors that crowd the pituitary gland	Pituitary dysfunction; bitemporal hemianopsia; hypothalamic dysfunction; diminished vision; ocular muscle weakness; frontal headache *Serious complications* 1. Pituitary apoplexy syndrome—acute onset of ophthalmoplegia, blindness, drowsiness, and coma; death can result 2. Diabetes insipidus may occur before or after surgery	Depends upon size, type, age of patient, and presenting symptoms; surgery, radiation, or drug therapy (singularly or in any combination) Surgery (indications for) 1. Progessive loss of vision 2. Endocrine dysfunction (some choose radiation first; however, there is concern about producing radiation carcinoma in temporal lobe, hypothalamus, or adjacent areas; if vision continues to deteriorate after radiation or if scotoma increases during radiation, surgery is indicated) If surgery is considered, one must evaluate 1. Fluid and electrolyte imbalance 2. Pituitary–hypothalamic function 3. Visual fields 4. Optic nerves Deficiency in plasma cortical level and addisonian salt loss syndrome can result in	Very good

				cerebral edema, vascular collapse, and death. *Drugs before surgery:* 100 mg cortisone acetate intramuscularly for 2 days prior to surgery (for adrenal insufficiency, which can occur from stress) After surgery, pituitary temporarily nonfunctional—cortisone 37.5 mg daily and thyroid extract 120 mg daily (both in divided doses) *Possible surgical procedures:* 1. Intracranial hypophysectomy 2. Transsphenoid hypophysectomy 3. Stereotactic surgery (cryotherapy) by the transsphenoid approach 4. Yttrium implantation (radiation implant) listed in some texts; this treatment being abandoned since there is often damage to the optic nerve from the radiation *Radiation:* before or after surgery
Chromophobic pituitary adenoma	Accounts for 90% of pituitary tumors; nonsecreting tumor		*Hypopituitarism* 1. Amenorrhea 2. Irregular menses 3. Impotence 4. Decreased libido 5. Decreased body hair 6. Decreased function of glands stimulated by pituitary 7. Diabetes insipidus (in 5% of patients)	

(continued)

TABLE 21–1. (continued)

Type of Tumor	Description	Location	Signs and Symptoms	Treatment	Prognosis
Pituitary Tumors					
Basophilic pituitary adenoma	Secreting tumor producing adrenocorticotropic hormone; evidence of adrenal hyperplasia; can grow rapidly, enlarging sella		*Cushing's syndrome* 1. Moon facies 2. "Buffalo hump" 3. Pendulous abdomen 4. Abdominal stria 5. Thin arms and legs 6. Amenorrhea or impotence 7. Hypertension 8. Muscle weakness 9. Elevated adrenocorticotropin		
Eosinophilic pituitary adenoma	Secreting tumor that produces growth hormone	Affects individuals from childhood to fifth decade	*Giantism* before puberty, or closure of the epiphyses *Acromegaly* after puberty, or closure of epiphyses 1. Thickening of soft tissue of facial features 2. Prominent forehead and lower jaw 3. Enlarged hands and feet 4. Visual loss 5. Joint pain 6. Diabetes mellitus 7. Enlarged heart 8. Possible heart failure		
Metastatic Tumors					
Metastatic brain tumors	10% of all brain tumors metastatic from other parts of body (lungs, breast, stomach, lower gastrointestinal tract, pancreas, and kidney); spread to brain by blood and lymphatic system; usually well differentiated from the rest of the brain	Anywhere; individual tumor or multiple tumors throughout subarachnoid space	Depend upon location	*Surgery*: resection if possible; usually can be shelled out if they are solitary; may treat with steroids first for a period of time and do a CT scan; if no other lesions appear, lesion is removed *Radiation*: in conjunction with surgery	Poor; however, metastatic tumors from the kidney often carry a rather good prognosis
Malignant melanomas		Cerebral hemispheres from a primary lesion in the skin	Depend upon location	*Surgery, radiation, chemotherapy*	Unpredictable; a few months to a few years

* Astrocytomas are graded from I to IV. Some classification systems refer to astrocytomas grades III and IV as glioblastoma multiforme as shown in this table.
† Astrocytoma of the optic nerves and chiasma is called spongioblastoma in some classification systems.

B. Tumors arising from the supporting structures of the nervous system
   1. Meningiomas — 10% to 15%
   2. Neuromas (sometimes called acoustic neuromas or cerebellar–pontine angle tumors) — 5% to 8%
C. Developmental (congenital) tumors — 4% to 5%
   1. Hemangioblastoma
   2. Craniopharyngioma
D. Pituitary tumors — 8% to 12%
   1. Chromophobic
   2. Eosinophilic
   3. Basophilic
E. Metastatic tumors (primary source from another part of the body; carcinomas are much more common than sarcomas) — 10%
   1. Lung, breast, lower gastrointestinal tract, pancreas, kidney
   2. Malignant melanomas

DIFFERENCES IN BRAIN TUMORS IN CHILDREN AND ADULTS

In children (newborns to 16-year-olds), the incidence of brain tumors differs with about two thirds of all childhood brain tumors located in the posterior fossa (infratentorial region).

Type	*Percentage of total primary childhood tumors*
Medulloblastoma	30%
Astrocytoma (grades I and II)	30%
Ependymoma	12%
Craniopharyngioma	10%
Optic pathway glioma (spongioblastoma)	5%
Miscellaneous	13%

SIGNS AND SYMPTOMS OF BRAIN TUMORS

The history of a brain tumor patient usually reflects an evolving progression of symptoms with the rate of progression depending on the location, rate of growth, and type of tumor. Some tumors grow insidiously and are asymptomatic until they become very large. It may be years until symptoms become evident. Other tumors located in vital areas such as the medulla demonstrate clinical presence very early because of encroachment on areas of vital functions (respirations, blood pressure, and so forth). Tumors that grow rapidly (such as glioblastoma multiforme) will cause neurological deficits to develop rapidly.

GENERAL SIGNS AND SYMPTOMS

The general signs and symptoms observed relate to the six areas of pathophysiology, which have been identified as cerebral edema, increased intracranial pressure, focal neurological deficits, seizure activity, endocrine imbalance, and cerebrospinal fluid obstruction. In most cases, symptoms arise from more than one area of pathophysiology.

Most brain tumors in adults are located in the supratentorial compartment. The most frequent initial signs and symptoms of brain tumors are headache, vomiting, and papilledema. Another symptom—alterations in the level of consciousness—is common with intra-axial tumors but not with extra-axial neoplasms.[3] Many tumors initially present symptoms of focal neurological findings before symptoms of increased intracranial pressure, such as headache, vomiting, or papilledema, are evident.

Tumors that arise from the filum terminale may merely result in back pain, which appears to be worse at night. It may take this type of tumor a considerable amount of time to actually compress the spinal nerve roots to the point of creating neurological deficits.

Headache

Headache alone is the presenting symptom in 20% of brain tumor patients. It may also be associated with vomiting or papilledema. The area affected by the headache can be generalized or localized in the frontal or suboccipital region: The headache is often described as intermittent and not severe. It is found in the course of illness in about 70% of patients. Headache, if present, is usually worse in the morning because of irritation, compression, or traction on the dural sinuses or blood vessels.

Vomiting

Vomiting is related to increased intracranial pressure and brain stem compression. Nausea or abdominal discomfort may accompany vomiting, although in most instances the vomiting occurs without symptoms. Vomiting is unrelated to meals and is more common in the morning. It can be caused by direct stimulation of the vomiting center located in the medulla. The vomiting can be projectile. In 10% of patients, vomiting is the initial symptom, although 70% experience vomiting in the course of the illness.

Papilledema

Papilledema is seen in about 70% to 75% of brain tumor patients. Papilledema is associated with visual changes such as decreased visual acuity, diplopia, and deficits in the visual fields. It will be recalled that the visual pathways extend through the lobes of the cerebral hemispheres. It is therefore reasonable to expect a high incidence of visual disturbances in patients with supratentorial lesions. Cranial (VI) nerve palsy is a symptom commonly seen in brain tumor lesions and results in an inability to move the orbit outward.

It is not uncommon for a patient to state that a deterioration in vision was the main reason he was referred to the neurologist. An initial appointment was made with the optometrist or ophthalmologist. If the examiner recognizes the visual deficits, a referral is made to the neurologist, who initiates a diagnostic work-up.

Personality Changes

Another symptom common in adults with brain tumors is personality change. Loss of emotional restraints, impairment of various intellectual functions, and an increase in neurotic traits are general areas of possible deficit.

An increase in intracranial pressure or a focal lesion in the cerebral hemispheres, particularly of the frontal lobe, creates the deficit. Some patients seek out a physician because of behavior and personality changes noted by the patient or family that make it difficult or impossible to continue with the patient's lifestyle and interpersonal relationships.

Local Disturbances

Local disturbances of normal neurological function can be wide and varied depending on the location and size of the neoplasm.

1. Motor, sensory, and cranial nerve dysfunction and alterations in consciousness are possible.
2. In posterior fossa tumors lower cranial nerve dysfunction, ataxia, and incoordination are common symptoms.
3. Seizure activity is a highly suspicious finding in patients who had previously been seizure-free. In 15% of patients seizure activity is the initial symptom of a brain tumor. Thirty percent of patients experience seizures in the course of the illness.

Pituitary Dysfunction

The last major area of general symptoms relates to pituitary dysfunction with all of its ramifications of changes in body function, hypopituitarism, giantism, acromegaly, and Cushing's syndrome, depending on the type of tumor and its location.

SIGNS AND SYMPTOMS RELATED TO TUMOR AREAS

Frontal Lobe

The degree of frontal lobe deficit depends on the extent of involvement caused by the brain tumor. Unilateral involvement results in less functional loss than bilateral, and nondominant involvement produces less of a loss than if the tumor site were in the dominant hemisphere. Collectively, frontal lobe symptoms are referred to as the frontal lobe syndrome. The symptoms include inappropriate behavior, inattentiveness, inability to concentrate, emotional lability, indifference, loss of self-restraint, inappropriate social behavior, impairment of recent memory, difficulty with abstraction, and a quiet but flat affect.

In addition to the frontal lobe syndrome, other possible symptoms include headache (bilateral frontal region), difficulty in expressing oneself in words or in writing (expression aphasia), slowness of movement, incontinence caused by lack of social control, hemiparesis or hemiplegia, seizure activity, particularly jacksonian seizures, and conjugate eye deviation.

Parietal Lobe

The parietal lobe contains the sensory discrimination and association areas for body orientation, vision, and language. The collage of symptoms associated with parietal lobe dysfunction is referred to as the parietal lobe syndrome. Common symptoms include.

1. Hyperesthesia (impaired sensation in which there is decreased response to tactile sensitivity)
2. Paresthesia (abnormal sensation of tingling, crawling, or burning of the skin)
3. Loss of two-point discrimination (unable to determine by feeling if skin is touched by one or two points simultaneously)
4. Astereognosis (inability to recognize an object by feeling its size and shape)
5. Autotopagnosia (inability to locate or recognize parts of the body)
6. Anosognosia (loss of awareness or denial of the motor and sensory defect in the affected parts of the body)
7. Disorientation of external environmental space (a tendency to ignore that part of the environment opposite to the cerebral lesion)
8. Finger agnosia (inability to identify or select specific fingers of the hands)
9. Loss of right–left discrimination (inability to tell the difference between left and right)
10. Agraphia (loss of ability to write)
11. Acalculia (difficulty in calculating numbers)
12. Construction apraxia (if asked to draw an object such as the face of a clock, patient ignores the side opposite to the cerebral lesion)
13. Possible homonymous hemianopsia (loss of half of the visual field in each field so that the inner half is affected in one field and the outer half in the other field)

If the lesion is in the dominant hemisphere and is located in the left angular gyrus of the parietal lobe, Gerstmann's syndrome may be present. Symptoms include finger agnosia, loss of right–left discrimination, acalculia, and agraphia.

Seizure activity is also possible with a parietal lobe lesion.

Temporal Lobe

Neoplasms of the temporal lobe produce salient signs and symptoms. Focal symptoms tend to be few and uncertain, and signs and symptoms of increased intracranial pressure occur late in the illness. Loss in the upper quadrant opposite the lesion is a common finding as are psychomotor seizures. Psychomotor seizures may begin with an aura of peculiar sensations of the abdomen, epigastrium, or thorax. Psychomotor seizures are described as visual, auditory, or olfactory hallucinations; automatism; and amnesia for events of the attack. If the dominant lobe is involved, receptive aphasia caused by encroachment of Wernicke's area is possible. Total destruction of the temporal lobe will result in mental changes such as irritability, depression, poor judgment, and childish behavior.

Occipital Lobe

Tumors of the occipital lobe are infrequent as compared with the other cerebral lobes. When neoplasms do occur, the symptoms tend to be associated with vision. Symptoms include contralateral homonymous hemianopsia (visual loss in half of each visual field on the side opposite the lesion), visual hallucinations, and possible focal or generalized seizures.

Pituitary and Hypothalamus Region

The pituitary and hypothalamus are closely related by location and hormonal production. Common symptoms resulting from tumors in this area are visual deficit caused by optic atrophy and paralysis of one or more of the extraocular muscles, headache, and hormonal dysfunction of the pituitary with the subsequent precipitation of syndromes such as Cushing's, giantism, acromegaly, and hypopituitarism. In addition, tumors ot the hypothalamus can destroy fat and carbohydrate metabolism, water balance, and sleep patterns.

Lateral and Third Ventricle

If the tumor stays small, no apparent signs or symptoms are noted. If the tumor grows into the cerebral hemispheres, deficits will depend on the particular function of the area involved. Tumors that grow within the ventricle may become of sufficient size to obstruct the flow of cerebrospinal fluid. If this occurs, headache, vomiting, and other symptoms of increased intracranial pressure will be obvious. The patient may have relief of symptoms by changing the position of his head. In this case, the position of the obstructing tumor is altered, thereby allowing the normal cerebrospinal fluid flow pattern to be reestablished.

Fourth Ventricle

Tumors of the fourth ventricle obstruct the flow of cerebrospinal fluid and infiltrate and compress the brain stem or cerebellum. Headache, vomiting, and nuchal rigidity are common symptoms. Sudden death caused by compression of the cardiorespiratory center is possible. The lower cranial nerves, which control the gag and swallowing reflexes, become impaired, making aspiration a constant concern.

Midbrain

Neoplasms of the midbrain are rare. If present, they may occlude the cerebral aqueducts, produce cerebellar symptoms if the red nucleus is involved, produce Parinaud's syndrome (conjugate paralysis of upward gaze) if the quadrigeminal plate is involved, possibly cause deafness, and result in ptosis and diminished light reflex as the tumor enlarges.

Brain Stem

Tumors in the brain stem tend to be invasive and spread up and down the neural axis. Symptoms include dysfunction of lower cranial nerves, corticospinal and sensory tract deficits, cerebellar dysfunction, dysphagia, and vomiting throughout the illness. As with fourth ventricle tumors, sudden death can occur from encroachment on vital centers.

Cerebellum

Growth of a tumor in the cerebellar area is accompanied by cerebellar signs (ataxia, incoordination, cerebellar fits, and so forth), obstruction to flow of cerebrospinal fluid, and possible brain stem compression. The usual signs of increased intracranial pressure (headache, vomiting, classical changes in vital signs, and so forth) are common, particularly with cerebrospinal fluid obstruction.

DIAGNOSIS

The first step in diagnosing a brain tumor is taken when the patient visits the family physician or clinic. At that time a history and physical examination are conducted, revealing signs and symptoms suggestive of neurological disease. The next step is usually a referral to a neurologist for further exploration and a definitive diagnosis.

Clinical manifestations of neurological disease can span a wide range of signs and symptoms. In arriving at the diagnosis of an intracranial tumor, the neurologist must rule out other diseases that can demonstrate similar symptoms, such as cerebral arteriosclerosis, chronic subdural hematoma, abscess, and generalized central nervous system degenerative diseases.

In the adult, a history of an unexplained onset of seizure activity is a very suspicious finding. Signs and symptoms of increased intracranial pressure, localizing neurological deficits, and changes in behavior or intellectual ability are highly suggestive of a brain tumor.

To substantiate a suspected diagnosis of brain tumor, the following diagnostic studies are commonly ordered:

1. *Visual field and funduscopic examination*—Careful examination of the visual field provides much information for localizing the lesion. Because the visual pathways encompass portions of the cerebral lobes, visual defects that are specific to particular areas can be detected. A funduscopic examination is included to determine evidence of papilledema, a common sign in brain tumor.
2. *Skull films*—Space-occupying lesions can cause deviation of the calcified pineal body, erosion of bone, and calcification areas within a neoplasm. Such evidence found on radiographic examination indicates the need for further exploration.
3. *Computed tomography (CT) scan*—The procedure can provide definitive data on the presence, size, and location of a tumor (Fig. 21-2).
4. *Electroencephalogram (EEG)*—About three quarters of patients with intracranial tumors have abnormal tracings on electroen-

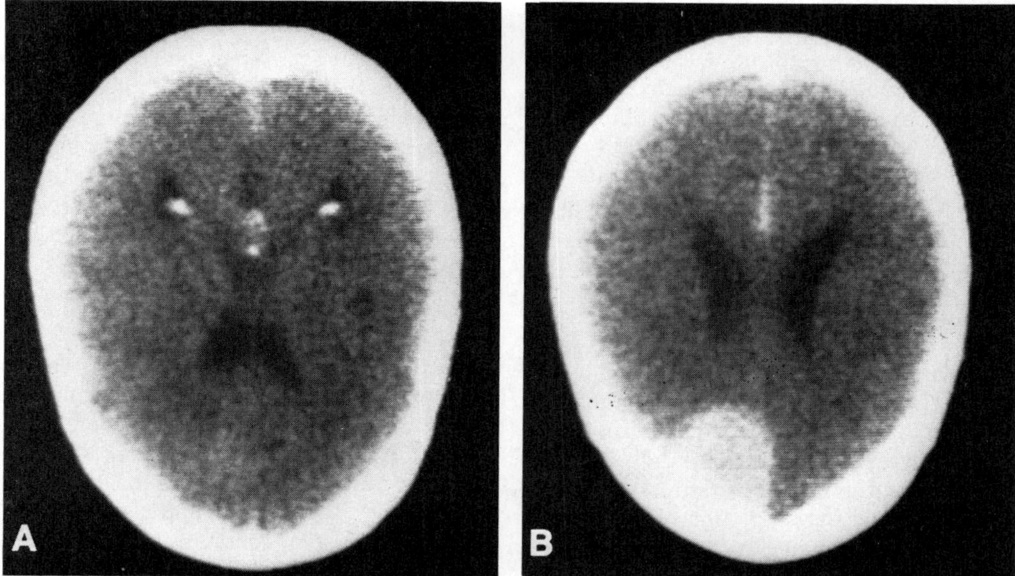

FIG. 21-2. Computed tomography (CT) scan of brain. *(A)* Normal scan. *(B)* Scan showing a large mass in the left frontal lobe.

cephalographic examination. In some cases, abnormal tracings can aid in localizing a tumor.

5. *Brain scan*—Brain tumors tend to disrupt the blood-brain barrier. As a result, the radioactive isotope uptake is increased within the tumor.
6. *Cerebral angiography*—This is a helpful tool for outlining the vascularity within the brain. Deviation of blood vessels by the tumors of high vascularity are apparent by angiography. The vascular pattern of a tumor may give a clue to its pathology. For example, formation of new vessels is frequent with glioblastomas.
7. *Lumbar puncture and cerebrospinal fluid (CSF)*—A lumbar puncture may be contraindicated because of fear of brain stem herniation from greatly increased intracranial pressure caused by the tumor. If a lumbar puncture is done, it should be done cautiously, with careful observation of the patient. The lumbar puncture provides a means by which to measure cerebrospinal fluid pressure and to collect specimens of cerebrospinal fluid for laboratory analysis. Spinal fluid protein is elevated in about one third of patients with brain tumors. Cytological studies may reveal cancerous cells.
8. *Chest films*—Lateral and anteroposterior chest films are taken to rule out carcinoma of the lung. Metastasis to the brain is common, particularly from the lung.
9. *Echoencephalogram*—Brain tumors can displace midline structures. Deviation of midline structure suggests the need for further investigation.

DIAGNOSTIC PROCEDURES USED FOR SPECIFIC TUMORS

Based on the clinical signs and symptoms, the physician may choose to investigate and evaluate certain specific central and peripheral nervous system functions.

- *Audiometric studies*—for tumors that affect hearing such as acoustic neuromas
- *Electromyography*—to record the electrical potentials of muscles for early detection of abnormal function
- *Caloric testing*—evaluates the vestibular branch of cranial VIII nerve
- *Cisternograms*—useful in demonstrating the presence of hydrocephalus when tumors tend to obstruct the flow of cerebrospinal fluid

ENDOCRINOLOGICAL STUDIES

Tumors that influence the endocrine system, such as pituitary tumors, require special endocrinological studies. Pituitary adenomas and craniopharyngiomas are examples of two tumors in which endocrine dysfunction is a prominent feature. The following is a list of the more important endocrine evaluation studies:

1. Growth hormone (plasma)
2. 17-ketosteroids (urine)
3. 17-hydrocorticosteroids (urine)
4. Protein-bound iodine (blood)
5. Thyroid uptake (serum)
6. Thyroid-stimulating hormone (plasma)
7. Glucose tolerance test (blood)

The laboratory finding of each test will depend on the effect of the tumor on the particular endocrine gland. If the tumor causes increased production of the growth hormone, for example, the laboratory report would record an elevation. A tumor that causes a particular gland to become reduced or completely stop secreting a hormone would result in an abnormally low level, likewise recorded upon laboratory analysis.

NURSING MANAGEMENT DURING DIAGNOSIS

While one of the nurse's main responsibilities during this diagnostic period is to provide information to the patient about the tests to be conducted, the possibility of a brain tumor can subject the patient to extreme emotional stress. The impact of such a diagnosis depends on the patient's ability to comprehend what the diagnosis means and how it will affect his life. A patient who has an altered level of consciousness or impaired mental functions will not experience the total impact of his situation but may react merely to the strangeness of the hospital environment, the bed confinement, and the loneliness. However, it is the patient who can comprehend his situation who is most apt to demonstrate profound behavioral responses.

The patient who understands what is happening may initially deny the diagnosis. If such is the case, the patient will refuse to consider treatment, so the informed consent is impossible. If the patient does accept the diagnosis, he may react with anger and hostility. Fear of death, vegetation, and mutilation, as well as loss of independence and mental functions, are terrifying concerns. Mental images of other people with similar diagnoses loom in the patient's mind and threaten body image and the self-concept. A sense of powerlessness can overwhelm the patient.

A positive, supportive approach on the part of the nurse can help the patient cope with the reality of his condition. He should be encouraged to ask questions and express his feelings about his situation. The nurse should provide realistic reassurance for the patient's prospects as an intact total person. At the same time, the patient should be included in the decision-making process as often as possible.

MEDICAL MANAGEMENT

Once the diagnosis of a brain tumor is established, the next major consideration is medical management.

The three general methods for treatment of brain tumors are surgery, radiation, and chemotherapy. These modalities can be used alone or in any combination. The variables that are considered in selecting appropriate treatment are based on the type of tumor, location, size, symptoms, and general condition of the patient. Informed consent for treatment must include the patient in the decision-making process.

DRUG THERAPY

Most patients benefit from administration of dexamethasone (Decadron), which decreases cerebral edema. The reversal of symptoms can be remarkable. Dexamethasone is usually begun when the tumor is diagnosed and the presence of increased intracranial pressure is confirmed. If surgery is recommended, dexamethasone is administered preoperatively, continued postoperatively, and given with chemotherapy, as well as during radiation therapy, to control radiation edema. There is also some evidence that large doses of dexamethasone actually inhibit the growth of tumors.

Regardless of the treatment choice, long-term follow-up is important to assess adverse effects and recurrency of the tumor. Most patients will be sent home with instructions to take phenytoin (Dilantin), 100 mg three times a day, prophylactically to prevent grand mal seizures.

Drugs used during hospitalization to ameliorate symptoms of brain tumors include

1. Dexamethasone (Decadron), 20 mg to 40 mg daily in divided doses—controls cerebral edema
2. Magnesium hydroxide (Maalox), 30 ml orally with dexamethasone—prevents gastrointestinal irritation
3. Cimetidine (Tagamet), 300 mg four times a day—reduces gastric secretions
4. Phenytoin (Dilantin), 100 mg three times a day—prophylactic agent for grand mal seizures
5. Acetaminophen (Tylenol), 650 mg—mild analgesic for headache
6. Codeine, 15 mg to 60 mg as necessary—analgesic for severe headache
7. Docusate sodium (Colace), 100 mg three times a day—stool softener that prevents straining at stool

CONVENTIONAL SURGERY

In most instances, surgery is the last step in positive diagnosis of a brain tumor. Examination of the tissue biopsy by the pathologist will identify the tumor histologically and give a clue to the prognosis. However, malignancy and surgical accessibility are equally important in judging prognosis. Some tumors, although histologically benign, cannot be completely removed; nonetheless, even a partial resection will relieve symptoms temporarily. If the tumor is a slow-growing neoplasm, as is true of meningiomas, the patient may be asymptomatic for years.

Even with malignant tumors (highly undifferentiated cells), a decompression resection is frequently indicated to temporarily relieve symptoms of compression and increased intracranial pressure. Obstruction of the flow of cerebrospinal fluid may require a shunting procedure to relieve cerebrospinal fluid pressure. The nursing care is the same as for the craniotomy patient. See Chapter 14 for general principles of surgical intervention.

LASER SURGERY

Laser surgery is being used more frequently for the treatment of brain tumors. There are three wave lengths in general use, each with its specific uses, advantages, and disadvantages. The three types of lasers are argon, carbon dioxide, and Nd:YAG (neodymium yttrium aluminum garnet).

The argon laser is useful for the coagulation of superficial vessels of less than 1.5 mm in diameter, and at higher energy levels, it causes some vaporization of tissue. The argon laser has been used for the treatment of some vascular tumors although it is less versatile than the carbon dioxide laser.

The carbon dioxide laser is the most popular laser for neurosurgery and is used for the treatment of brain and spinal cord tumors. The carbon dioxide wavelength is instantly absorbed by water in the cells. The brain has a high water content. The laser beam, when directed to a preselected target area with the help of the operating microscope, has a vaporizing effect on the tissue with which it comes in contact. The tissue not touched by the carbon dioxide laser beam remains intact. The ability of this laser wave length to destroy predetermined tissue without the surgeon needing to physically touch the tissue is valuable for destroying cerebral tumors in delicate areas of the brain not accessible to the surgeon, such as the brain stem near the vital centers. It is also valuable for bloodless dissection and extirpation of other tumors. The coagulation value of the carbon dioxide laser is limited to vessels up to 0.5 mm. Larger vessels that need hemostasis must be managed by other means.[5]

The Nd:YAG laser is very powerful and is particularly effective for coagulating large vessels. It heats the tissue with which it comes into contact and denatures the protein but does not vaporize it. This action makes the Nd:YAG laser particularly valuable in shrinking tumors and coagulating vessels.

Tumors that have been treated with lasers include acoustic neuromas, craniopharyngiomas, some brain stem gliomas, pinealomas, ventricular tumors, meningiomas of the brain and spinal cord, and neuromas of the spinal cord. The advantage of using lasers for treatment of brain tumors is that they enable the neurosurgeon to dissect or shrink tumors without inflicting injury on surrounding tissue. Areas of the brain formerly inaccessible to the neurosurgeon are now accessible by this indirect means. Although lasers have limitations, they provide an important treatment modality for brain tumors.[6] (See Chap. 14 for more information on lasers.)

Nursing Management of the Patient Undergoing Laser Surgery

On admission, the patient needs specific preoperative teaching so that he will understand what laser surgery is and what can be expected. The physician discusses the potential complications with the patient. A consent form is signed. In addition, a special consent form may also need to be signed if the procedure or the equipment is considered investigational by the Food and Drug Administration (FDA).

The hospital stay is shorter with laser surgery than with conventional surgery. The specific time that the patient remains in the hospital will depend on the physician. Patient teaching for discharge should be included in the overall teaching plan.

RADIATION THERAPY

The objective of radiation therapy is to destroy tumor cells without injuring normal ones. Tumor cells are more radiosensitive than nontumor cells. A course of radiation treatment can increase survival rates after surgery. The treatment dose for the tumor depends on several variables including histological type, radioresponsiveness, location, and level of tolerance.

The histological identification of a tumor aids in anticipating the treatment needs and prognosis of the patient.

The following types of tumors are general indications for radiation therapy: uncomplicated pituitary adenoma, medulloblastoma, any metastatic lesions, deep and centrally located tumors that would create permanent major neurological deficits from dissection if surgery were attempted, and tumors of vital areas (e.g., pons, medulla) that would cause high mortality rates if surgical resection were attempted.

If tumor excision has been incomplete, a course of postoperative radiation therapy is recommended for the following tumors: astrocytoma, grades II, III, and IV (grades II and IV are also known as glioblastoma multiforme); ependymoma; oligodendroglioma; sarcoma; craniopharyngioma; and chordoma.

Protocols that combine surgery and radiation therapy are of two types: surgery with conventional radiation and surgery with mixed beam radiation. Mixed beam radiation refers to a combination of cobalt and neutron beam. Because the conventional approach is used in most instances, it will be discussed in greater detail.

In a conventional radiation protocol, the amount of radiation varies based on individual differences previously cited. The total tumor dose range is usually from 4000 rad to 7000 rad administered over 4 to 8 weeks.[2] The area to be radiated depends on the anatomical extent of the tumor. Many patients improve remarkably from their symptoms after surgical decompression and radiation. If radiation is not preceded by surgery, radiation accompanied by large doses of corticosteroid can temporarily reverse and control symptoms of increased intracranial pressure.

Unfortunately, not all patients do respond well to radiotherapy. In some, radiation edema exacerbates an already elevated intracranial pressure. The result is an increase in symptoms, which could be falsely interpreted as the progression of tumor growth. In other patients, a recurrence of symptoms is evident in approximately 6 months. Radiation necrosis can be the cause, but it may be difficult to differentiate between tumor progression and radiation necrosis.

Radiation therapy, alone or as adjunctive therapy with surgery, presents special nursing management problems. If the course of radiation therapy is to follow surgery, the incision is allowed to heal well before radiation is begun.

For the patient it is and has been a period of great physiological, emotional, and psychological stress. Radiation is planned for tumors that are surgically inaccessible or for remnants of tumors that could not be completely excised surgically. The patient usually has been advised by his physician of his prognosis and the benefits anticipated from radiation therapy. He is also informed of the possible side-effects that he might experience as a result of the treatment.

Nursing Management During Radiation Therapy

The nurse, as the patient's advocate helps him to receive satisfactory answers to his questions. If the patient's level of consciousness or mental functions have been impaired, the family will be afforded help so that informed consent can be ensured. The nurse's role during radiation therapy is providing emotional support to patient and family, assessing patient needs, managing side-effects, and providing for general comfort and hygienic needs.

The specific nursing responsibilities during radiation therapy include the following:

1. Prior to the start of treatments, inform the patient and family of the various activities that will occur in the radiation therapy department. As with most patient preparation of this kind, informing the patient of what to expect will help allay any fears caused by unfamiliarity with the procedure.
2. Provide proper skin care of the radiation site. Radiation dermatitis can be anticipated (the epidural layer is denuded in a 4- to 6-week period). The skin becomes reddened, tanned, and desquamated. Because the skin is sensitive, do not rub, apply tape, expose to sunlight, or apply alcohol, powder, cream, or cosmetics. The skin markings used to localize radiation exposure should not be washed off.
3. If the patient suffers from nausea, vomiting, or diarrhea, give antiemetics and antidiarrheal agents as necessary.
4. To manage anorexia, offer small portions of food that are both easy to digest and liked by the patient.
5. For general malaise, plan activities to allow for rest periods.
6. Note complete blood count reports, with special attention to white blood cell and platelets count. Bone marrow depression decreases platelets, which, in turn, increases the possibility of hemorrhage (petechiae, purpura, nosebleeds, and so forth).
7. Monitor neurological signs for indications of increased intracranial pressure.
8. Provide emotional support by reassuring the patient that side-effects will pass after the treatment is completed.

See Chart 21-1 for summary of common nursing diagnoses.

CHEMOTHERAPY

The use of chemotherapy for treatment of brain tumors is an accepted approach to the management of malignant brain tumors. Chemotherapy for the treatment of medulloblastomas and glioblastoma multiforme is particularly promising. The drug of choice and its dosage depends on the particular tumor, location, and body tolerance.

The side-effects of the potent chemotherapeutic drugs limit their dosage. Chemotherapeutic drugs currently in use for the treatment of brain tumors are included in Table 21-2. The common side-effects are nausea, vomiting, diarrhea, bone marrow depression, alopecia, stomatitis, and neurological deterioration. The criteria for development of desirable new drugs is high toxicity to cancerous cells that is concurrent with minimal side-effects.

The traditional chemotherapy protocol is to use BCNU or CCNU singularly or in combination with other drugs such as BCNU and procarbazine; BCNU and vincristine; and CCNU, cyclophosphamide (Cytoxan), and vincristine.[2] Nontraditional approaches have also been used. One of these approaches, high-dose BCNU with bone marrow harvest, should be mentioned.

BCNU With Bone Marrow Harvest

Carmustine (BCNU), when given in high doses, is a very effective antineoplastic agent for the central nervous system because of its ability to cross the blood–brain barrier. However, its toxic properties, especially that of bone marrow suppression, create serious drawbacks for its use as a treatment protocol. The active metabolites of BCNU are thought to be excreted into the urine within 96 hours. By removing bone marrow before administering high doses of BCNU, some control of the myelosuppression side-effect is achieved. The protocol, used for patients with grade III and IV astrocytoma, consists of harvesting the bone marrow, administering the BCNU, and infusing the harvested bone marrow.

A clear description of the protocol is found in the literature.[7] Using general anesthesia, the bone marrow is aspirated from the iliac crests by several aspirations with a heparinized needle and syringe. Approximately 1000 ml of bone marrow is removed at the time of the harvest. After appropriate filtering of the marrow, it is stored in blood transfer packs at a temperature of 4°C for future administration to the patient. The patient is made comfortable after the procedure and monitored (vital signs, neurovascular check) for untoward signs and symptoms.

Approximately 4 hours after completion of the marrow harvest, carmustine (BCNU) is administered. Manufacturers' instructions must be followed when preparing the drug. It is administered intravenously in saline over a period of 30 minutes. During this time the patient is monitored for nausea, vomiting, and hypotension. Many protocols include prophylactic administration of an antiemetic. A second dose of BCNU is administered in the same manner approximately 16 hours after the first dose.

The protocol is completed 24 to 36 hours after the second dose of BCNU with the intravenous administration of the bone marrow. The high viscosity of the marrow dictates the need for slow infusion. The patient is monitored for phlebitis at the infusion site and a mild increase in body temperature. Barring any complications, the patient is discharged shortly after completion of the marrow infusion.

Nursing responsibilities during the BCNU–marrow harvest protocol include

- Monitoring for complications and side-effects (e.g., hypotension, phlebitis, increased intracranial pressure, nausea, vomiting)
- Providing for physical comfort (e.g., administering analgesics, antiemetics; positioning)
- Providing emotional support to reduce anxiety

(Text continued on page 481.)

CHART 21–1. SUMMARY OF COMMON NURSING DIAGNOSES MADE FOR PATIENTS UNDERGOING RADIATION AND/OR CHEMOTHERAPY FOR TREATMENT OF A BRAIN TUMOR

NURSING DIAGNOSIS	EXPECTED OUTCOME	NURSING INTERVENTION
Knowledge deficit for purpose, method, and goals of treatment protocol	Patient will be able to verbalize and describe purpose, goals, and method of administering the prescribed protocol.	• Ask the patient to tell you his understanding of his treatment protocol. • Clarify misconceptions. • Expand on areas of partial understanding. • Introduce new information as necessary. • Encourage the patient to ask questions. • Refer questions to resource person, as necessary. • Develop a written teaching plan.
Anxiety due to approaching or current treatment	Anxiety will be reduced or controlled.	• Observe for verbal and nonverbal cues indicating anxiety. • Provide emotional support. • Anticipate needs of the patient.
Nausea due to treatment protocol	Nausea will be controlled or minimized.	• Assess for presence of nausea. • Provide small frequent feedings that are easy to digest. • Administer antiemetics as ordered (prophylactically and as necessary).
Vomiting due to treatment protocol	Vomiting will be absent or controlled.	• Administer antiemetics as ordered. • Give nothing by mouth if vomiting occurs. • Offer mouth care frequently.
Altered bowel elimination: diarrhea	Diarrhea will be absent or controlled.	• Assess for presence, amount, and frequency of diarrhea; document findings. • Administer antidiarrheal drugs as ordered.
Anorexia: nutrition less than required	Patient will maintain adequate nutrition.	• Assess nutritional intake on a 24-hour basis. • Assess patient's likes and dislikes. • Offer small meals frequently (choose easy-to-digest foods).
Stomatitis: altered comfort	Absence or control of discomfort from stomatitis.	• Provide frequent mouth care. • Administer soothing oral rinse or topical solution for oral comfort such as glycerin swabs or Viscous Xylocaine suspension, as directed. • Avoid irritating foods such as citrus fruits. • Provide a soft, bland diet.
Alopecia: altered body image related to hair loss	Patient will accept altered body image.	• Discuss cause of alopecia and regrowth process. • Provide for meticulous personal hygiene. • Encourage female patients to use make-up and wear attractive head cover. • Suggest use of wigs when patient is able to wear one. • Correct any misconceptions. • Allow the patient to verbalize his feelings.

CHART 21–1. (continued)

NURSING DIAGNOSIS	EXPECTED OUTCOME	NURSING INTERVENTION
Generalized malaise: decreased activity tolerance	Feeling of general malaise will be minimized by frequent rest periods.	• Allow patient to express his feelings about general malaise. • Encourage and plan a schedule that allows for frequent rest periods.
Self-care deficits due to general malaise	Personal care needs will be met by patient or nurse.	• Assess patient's ability to perform activities of daily living. • Provide for frequent rest periods. • Adjust schedule as necessary to conserve energy. • Encourage the patient to be as independent as possible. • Reassure the patient.
Neurological deterioration due to intracranial pressure	Neurological changes will be identified early and definitive action taken to control deterioration.	• Assess neurological signs periodically. • Identify neurological deterioration, report changes to physician, and document findings in record. • Elevate head of bed 30 degrees. • Administer drugs and other protocols as ordered. • Continue to monitor the patient.
Increased possibility of infection and bleeding due to bone marrow depression	Bleeding and infection will be absent or identified early. Exposure to infection will be controlled.	• Monitor complete blood count (white blood count, platelet count) and coagulation studies. • Be aware of and discuss with the patient delayed onset of bone marrow suppression (after 3 weeks). • Assess for occult bleeding (stools, urine, gastric). • Assess for easy bruising, petechial bleeding, nosebleeds, and bleeding from gums. • Protect the patient from exposure to infections. • Monitor the patient for signs and symptoms of infection.
Skin integrity, potential impairment of, due to radiation dermatitis (With radiation dermatitis the skin becomes reddened, tanned, desquamatized, and sensitive.)	Skin integrity will be maintained.	• Special precautions will be instituted for the site of radiation. • The skin will be protected from rubbing, application of tape, and exposure to sunlight. • No alcohol, powder, cream, or cosmetics will be used on this area.
	The skin markings for the radiation treatment will not be washed off.	• The skin markings used to localize the radiation exposure site should not be washed off.
Lack of knowledge for follow-up and discharge from the hospital	Patient verbalizes accurate outline of discharge plans and care.	• Develop a written teaching plan for discharge. • Stress the importance of follow-up care. • Provide a written list of signs and symptoms that should be reported to the physician. • Caution against use of any drugs (*e.g.*, aspirin) without prior approval of the physician. • Help the patient understand that some side-effects of the treatment have a delayed onset. • Arrange for follow-up appointment.

TABLE 21–2. *Chemotherapeutic Drugs Commonly Used for Treatment of Various Types of Brain Tumors*

Classification, Drug, Dose	Side-Effects/Toxicity	Laboratory Monitoring and Precautions
Alkylating Agents — Nitrosoureas		
• Carmustine (BCNU) Major drug used in treatment of brain tumors because it crosses the blood–brain barrier 200 mg/m² intravenously every 6 weeks; may be given as a single dose or in a divided dose 100 mg/m² on 2 consecutive days; do not exceed 200-mg dose in less than 6 weeks	• Myelosuppression (bone marrow depression) • Dose related • Most serious/frequent toxic response • Delayed: peaks 4 to 6 weeks after drug therapy; lasts 1 to 2 weeks	• Complete bloodcount weekly • Monitor for infection and bleeding
	• Nausea and vomiting (dose related) begins 2 hours after drug begun and lasts 4 to 6 hours	• Administer antiemetics before giving drug
	• Hepatic toxicity	• Serum transaminase, alkaline phosphatase, bilirubin
	• Nephrotoxicity	• Uric acid
	• Pulmonary infiltrate and/or fibrosis after prolonged BCNU therapy; may be delayed up to 52 weeks	• Chest x-rays
	• Burning at site of intravenous infusion	• Run slowly
	• Skin contact with drug will cause burning and hyperpigmentation	• Wash skin thoroughly, if contact occurs
• Lomustine (CCNU) 130 mg/m² as a single dose orally; do not give more than every 6 weeks Similar to BCNU in action	• Similar to carmustine • Alopecia	• Same as with carmustine
	• Stomatitis	• Provide soothing topical solutions; offer mouth care
Alkylating Agents — Ethyleneamines		
• Thiotepa 0.2 mg/kg intravenously for 5 days every 4 weeks as necessary; used for medulloblastomas	• Myelosuppression is major effect; dose related; delayed 5 to 30 days	• Complete blood count weekly; monitor for infection and bleeding
	• Nausea and vomiting	• Administer antiemetics
	• Anorexia	• Provide small frequent feedings
	• Headache and dizziness • Amenorrhea • Fever	
	• Pain at injection site	• Local anesthetic may be given
	• Nephrotoxicity	• Uric acid, creatine
Antimetabolites		
• Floxuridine (FUDR) 0.1 mg to 0.6 mg/kg daily by intra-arterial infusion *or* 0.4 mg to 0.6 mg/kg daily in hepatic artery	• Most common: nausea, vomiting, diarrhea, enteritis, stomatitis, and localized erythema • Other reactions: anorexia, gastrointestinal tract infections, alopecia, rash, ataxia, hemiplegia, and lethargy	• Complete blood count, alkaline phosphatase, serum transaminase, bilirubin, lactic dehydrogenase
• Fluorouracil (5-FU) 12.5 mg/kg intravenously daily for 3 to 5 days every 4 weeks; administer slowly	• Myelosuppression delayed 7 to 14 days • Nausea and vomiting • Hepatic and nephrotic toxicity • Stomatitis, diarrhea, and alopecia	• Complete blood count • Give antiemetics • Hepatic and renal function
Other		
• Procarbazine hydrochloride (Matulane) 100 mg to 150 mg/m² orally for 10 days	• Myelosuppression • Confusion, depression, and hallucinations • Nystagmus and photophobia	• Complete bloodcount
	• Nausea, vomiting, and anorexia	• Administer antiemetics
	• Stomatitis	• Administer soothing oral solutions
	• Diarrhea	• Administer antidiarrheal drugs
	• Alopecia	

TABLE 21-2. (continued)

Classification, Drug, Dose	Side-Effects/Toxicity	Laboratory Monitoring and Precautions
• Vincristine sulfate (Oncovin) 1 mg to 2 mg/m² intravenously weekly	• Mild anemia and leukopenia • Neuropathies, paresthesias, muscle weakness, and cramps • Depression and insomnia • Diplopia and ptosis	• Complete blood count
	• Nausea, vomiting, stomatitis, anorexia, weight loss, dysphasia	• Give antiemetics; treat stomatitis; monitor weight
	• Constipation	• Give stool softeners and laxatives
	• Alopecia	
	• Phlebitis and cellulitis	• Run intravenous solution slowly

- Supporting an altered body image
- Providing for nutritional needs
- Teaching about the protocol and precautions to be taken on discharge so that the patient will be knowledgeable and compliant
- Arranging for follow-up care (periodic blood work, repeat diagnostic tests)

There are critical points that should be included in the teaching plan. The patient should understand the major side-effects of the drug protocol and the time frame in which they are most apt to develop after completion of the treatment. Bone marrow suppression (myelosuppression) occurs in about 3 weeks, hepatic toxicity in about 4 weeks, and pulmonary infiltration and renal toxicity in 52 weeks. To monitor potential bone marrow suppression, weekly blood studies are ordered for 6 to 8 weeks upon completion of the treatment. Blood studies of liver function are also monitored. Chest films and kidney function studies are evaluated periodically for evidence of the development of complications.

The patient should be followed if he has been exposed to anyone with an infection. Any evidence of infection, respiratory complications, bleeding, or kidney dysfunction should by reported to the physician immediately. A written list of precautions and pertinent information should be supplied to the patient.

Radiation and chemotherapy require management of side-effects and assessment for tolerance. Patients with nausea, vomiting, and diarrhea may require fluid replacement, antiemetics, and antidiarrheal agents. Monitoring of the complete blood count to note hemopoietic depression is necessary so that definitive action can be taken. In this case, whole blood, packed cells, or platelets may be necessary. If a dangerously low white blood count exists, the use of reverse barrier precautions can help to prevent infections in a patient devoid of normal body defense mechanisms.

Nursing Management During Chemotherapy

Much of the same backdrop discussed for radiation therapy applies to the patient who is to receive chemotherapy. The prospect of chemotherapy confronts the patient soon after his brain tumor has been diagnosed. Surgery and perhaps radiation have immediately preceded the plan for chemotherapy. This could accurately be described as a period of crisis. Sufficient information, including the description of possible side-effects, is provided so that informed consent is possible. The side-effects include nausea, vomiting, diarrhea, stomatitis, anorexia, alopecia, and bone marrow depression.

The role of the nurse during chemotherapy generally parallels that followed for radiation therapy. Additional points include measures for management of stomatitis, alopecia, and depressed blood count.

- For stomatitis, give frequent mouth care and apply soothing topical application (such as glycerine swabs or Viscous Xylocaine suspension) to the mucous membrane. Also advise the patient to avoid irritating foods such as fresh fruit and vegetables.
- Alopecia may create problems with body image and self-concept; therefore, advise the patient about the possibility of wearing wigs or attractive scarfs.
- Note the complete blood count to discern indications of white blood cell, red blood cell, and platelet depression. Hemorrhage, increased susceptibility to infection, and gingival bleeding are all possible results. See Table 21-2 for common nursing diagnoses made for the patient receiving treatment.

REFERENCES

1. Walsh J et al: Recent advances in the treatment of primary brain tumors. Arch Surg 110:696, June 1975
2. Rubin P (ed): Clinical Oncology for Medical Students and Physicians, 5th ed, pp 29-50, 181-190. Rochester, NY, American Cancer Society, 1978
3. Plum F, Posner J: Diagnosis of Stupor and Coma, 3rd ed, pp 153-175. Philadelphia, FA Davis, 1980
4. Guyton A: Medical Physiology, 6th ed. Philadelphia, WB Saunders, 1981
5. Dixon JA: Surgical application of lasers. AORN J 38(2):223, August 1983
6. Walker ML: Using lasers in neurosurgery. AORN J 38(2):238, August 1983
7. Gamel-Bentzel C: Nursing management of the patient receiving high-dose BCNU with autologous bone marrow harvest. J Neurosurg Nurs 14(2):98, April 1982

BIBLIOGRAPHY

Books

Adams R, Victor M: Principles of Neurology, 2nd ed, pp 440–474. New York, McGraw–Hill, 1981

Brunner L, Suddarth D: Textbook of Medical–Surgical Nursing, 4th ed. Philadelphia, JB Lippincott, 1980

Butler A, Brooks WH, Netsky MG: Classification and biology of brain tumors. In Youmans J (ed): Neurological Surgery, 2nd ed, pp 2659–2701. Philadelphia, WB Saunders, 1982

Cobb CA, Youmans JR: Brain tumors of disordered embryogenesis in adults. In Youmans J (ed): Neurological Surgery, 2nd ed, pp 2899–2935. Philadelphia, WB Saunders, 1982

Cobb CA, Youmans JR: Glial and neuronal tumors of the brain in adults. In Youmans J (ed): Neurological Surgery, 2nd ed, pp 2759–2835. Philadelphia, WB Saunders, 1982

Cobb CA, Youmans JR: Lymphomas of the brain in adults. In Youmans J (ed): Neurological Surgery, 2nd ed, pp 2836–2844. Philadelphia, WB Saunders, 1982

Eliasson S et al: Neurological Pathophysiology, 2nd ed, pp 305–320. New York, Oxford University Press, 1978

Gamache FW, Posner JB, Patterson RH: Metastatic brain tumors. In Youmans J (ed): Neurological Surgery, 2nd ed, pp 1872–1898. Philadelphia, WB Saunders, 1982

MacCarty CS, Piepgras DG, Ebersold MJ: Meningeal tumors of the brain. In Youmans J (ed): Neurological Surgery, 2nd ed, pp 2936–2966. Philadelphia, WB Saunders, 1982

Matson D: Intracranial tumors. In Cancer: A Manual for Practitioners, 4th ed, pp 100–106. Boston, American Cancer Society (Massachusetts Division), 1968

Merritt H: A Textbook of Neurology, 6th ed. Philadelphia, Lea & Febiger, 1979

Rand RW et al: Acoustic neuromas. In Youmans J (ed): Neurological Surgery, 2nd ed, pp 2967–3003. Philadelphia, WB Saunders, 1982

Shelive GE, Wara WM: Radiation therapy of brain tumors. In Youmans J (ed): Neurological Surgery, 2nd ed, pp 3096–3106. Philadelphia, WB Saunders, 1982

Stein BM: Tumors of the pineal region. In Youmans J (ed): Neurological Surgery, 2nd ed, pp 2863–2871. Philadelphia, WB Saunders, 1982

Wilson CB, Levin V, Hodhino T: Chemotherapy of brain tumors. In Youmans J (ed): Neurological Surgery, 2nd ed, pp 3065–3095. Philadelphia, WB Saunders, 1982

Periodicals

Anchie T: Acoustic neuroma: A benign tumor. J Neurosurg Nurs 12(1):11, March 1980

Blanco K: Acoustic neuroma: Postoperative nursing care and rehabilitation. J Neurosurg Nurs 13(3):153, June 1981

Brain tumors: Hope through research. US Department of Health and Human Services, US Government Printing Office, 1982

Burgess KE: Neurological disturbance in the patient with an intracranial neoplasm: Sources and implications for nursing care. J Neurosurg Nurs 15(4):237, August 1983

Cairncross JG, Joe–Ho K, Posner JB: Radiation therapy for brain metastases. Ann Neurol 7:529, 1980

Cancer statistics, 1976. American Cancer Society, 1977

Clancey J, Abruzzi L: Nursing intervention of patients with pituitary tumors. J Neurosurg Nurs 10(1):8, March 1978

Day A: Axions on brain tumors. Hosp Med 64, April 1980

Epstein B: Guide to cranial and intracranial calcifications, part I. Hosp Med 135, March 1979

Epstein B: Guide to cranial and intracranial calcifications, part II. Hosp Med 64, April 1979

Gehrke M: Identifying brain tumors. J Neurosurg Nurs 12(2):90, June 1980

Hausman K: Brain tumors in children. J Neurosurg Nurs 10(1):8, March 1978

Hill S, Neuwelt E: Intra-arterial chemotherapy following blood–brain barrier disruption in a patient with malignant glioma. J Neurosurg Nurs 14(2):94, April 1982

Krakoff I: Cancer chemotherapeutic agents. CA 23:208–219, 1973

Lamb S: Interstitial radiation for the treatment of brain tumors using the stereotactic method. J Neurosurg Nurs 12(3):138, September 1980

Larson E: The epidemiology of primary brain tumors. J Neurosurg Nurs 12(3):121, September 1980

Magdinec M, Bay J: The brain tumor clinic: Comprehensive, consistent, compassionate care. J Neurosurg Nurs 15(1):36, February 1983

Martin E, Weiss M: Immunological aspects of malignant glial tumors. J Neurosurg Nurs 12(3):161, September 1980

McOuat F: Acoustic nerve tumors: Diagnosis, surgical management, and nursing care. J Neurosurg Nurs 6(1):20, July 1974

Nevins S: Pre- and postoperative care of patients undergoing transsphenoid pituitary surgery. J Neurosurg Nurs 8(1):45, July 1976

Potts D: The preoperative course of brain tumor patients: Better or worse? J Neurosurg Nurs 12(1):18, March 1980

Stewart C: Current concepts of chemotherapy for brain tumors. J Neurosurg Nurs 12(2):97, June 1980

Tedesco MB et al: Total nursing care of vestibular nerve section patient. J Neurosurg Nurs 12(1):2, March 1980

Tortorelli B: Acoustic neuroma: An overview of the disorder and nursing care for these patients. J Neurosurg Nurs 13(4):170, August 1981

Wheeler P: Care of the patient with a cerebellar tumor. Am J Nurs 77(2):263–266, February 1977

chapter 22

Spinal Cord Tumors

Spinal cord tumors constitute approximately 0.5% to 1% of all tumors in the overall population, occurring about one-tenth as frequently as brain tumors. Unlike brain tumors, 85% of intraspinal tumors tend to be benign. Spinal tumors occur about equally in males and females, generally affecting those in the 20- to 60-year age range (median age of 38 years). Rarely are spinal tumors found in children younger than 10 years old or in the elderly.

TYPES OF SPINAL CORD TUMORS

Spinal cord tumors can be described according to location (extradural, intradural, extramedullary, or intramedullary), shape (dumbbell), source (primary or secondary), or consistency (hard or soft).

The definitions of the terms used to describe tumors according to location and shape follow (Fig. 22–1):

- *Extramedullary tumors* arise outside of the spinal cord in the meninges, nerve roots, or vertebrae; they can be further subdivided into extradural and intradural tumors.
- *Extradural tumors* are located outside the dura mater, either in the epidural space or bones of the spinal column or paraspinal tissue.
- *Intradural tumors* are located within or under the dura mater of the meninges.
- *Intramedullary tumors* arise within the substance of the spinal cord.
- *Dumbbell tumors* are shaped like a dumbbell and are located in both the intradural and extradural space as it follows the nerve through tne spinal foramen.

Hospital figures indicate that 55% of spinal tumors are extradural, 40% are intradural–extramedullary, and 5% to 10% are intramedullary.

Spinal tumors may also be described as primary or secondary. Primary tumors constitute 60% to 70% of spinal tumors and arise from the epidural vessels, spinal meninges, or glial elements of the cord. The cause of these spinal cord tumors is unknown.

Secondary spinal tumors arise from intraspinal extension from tumors of the spinal column (periosteal or osteal origin). This category accounts for 5% to 10% of spinal tumors. Secondary spinal tumors also arise from metastatic lesions from primary sources in the lungs, breast, kidney, and gastrointestinal tract. These tumors account for approximately 20% of spinal cord neoplasms.

The regional distribution of spinal tumors by location is cervical, 30%; thoracic, 50%; and lumbosacral, 20%. The most common extramedullary tumors are neurofibromas and meningiomas, which constitute about 55% of spinal tumors. Other extramedullary tumors include sarcomas, chordomas, and dermoid and epidermoid tumors.[1] When metastatic spinal cord tumors occur, they are located epidurally or in the bone of the vertebrae. About 80% of intramedullary tumors are ependymomas and various grades of astrocytomas. Each type of tumor occurs about equally frequently. Other less frequently seen types of intramedullary tumors are lipomas, hemangiomas, and teratomas.

PATHOPHYSIOLOGY

The pathophysiological changes associated with spinal cord tumors result from compression and, much less frequently, invasion of the cord. Common effects on the spinal cord include

1. Compression, irritation, and traction of the spinal nerve roots
2. Compression and displacement of the spinal cord
3. Invasion and destruction of spinal cord tracts
4. Interference with spinal blood supply
5. Obstruction of cerebrospinal fluid circulation

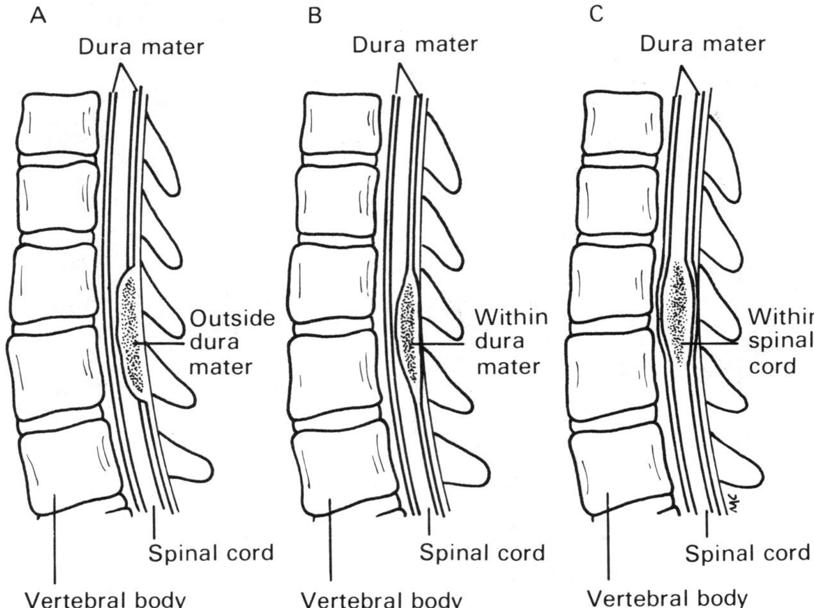

FIG. 22–1. Various possible locations of spinal tumors in a lateral longitudinal section of the vertebrae and spinal cord. Dark shading indicates tumor sites. *(A)* Extradural. *(B)* Intradural or extramedullary. *(C)* Intramedullary tumor sites. (Schott GD: Spinal tumours: I. Classification. Nursing Times 71(52):2055, 1975. Reproduced by permission of Nursing Times, 4 Little Essex Street, London WC2R 3 LF)

Alterations in physiology create the general progressive spinal cord compression, as well as focal signs and symptoms. Focal localizing signs depend on the level, size, and area of the cross section of the cord affected by the tumor.

The time required for the development of neurological signs is directly related to the tumor's rate of growth and its consistency (soft or hard). Slow-growing tumors allow the spinal cord to accommodate itself to the neoplasm. Many cord tumors grow very slowly over a period of years and compress the cord into a thin, ribbonlike substance with minimal neurological deficits. However, with rapid-growing tumors such as malignant or metastatic lesions, the cord fares poorly. The physiological response is substantial edema with major compression of the cord, possibly resulting in rapid paralysis (within a few hours).

A soft tumor can be of a consistency similar to that of the spinal cord. If these tumors grow slowly, they will cause gradual compression of the spinal cord. However, the cord's blood supply is able to respond to this alteration and adequately supply the vascular needs without interruption. The tumor adjusts to the available space for growth, becoming elongated. Neither movement of the spinal column nor normal alterations in blood flow to the cord will produce injury by contusion or ischemia. On the contrary, a hard tumor will respond to movement or vascular changes with spinal contusion, ischemia, and irreversible cord damage. The hard tumor does not conform to the available space, so that encroachment of neurological function is apparent earlier than with soft tumors.

The morphological appearance of spinal cord tumors is described as encapsulated or sharply outlined. The soft tumors are irregularly elongated and can extend for two or more segments. Some tumors are cystic, requiring the draining of fluid.

GENERAL SIGNS AND SYMPTOMS

About 60% to 70% of all spinal cord tumors are located in the posterior or posterolateral part of the spinal cord. The remaining tumors are located in anterior or intermediate positions. The location of the tumor in relationship to the cord segment, spinal tracts, spinal roots, and dura will determine specific signs and symptoms experienced by the patient. Focal signs can aid in determining the level of the lesion; however, they can also be indistinct and misleading and vary intermittently.

The general signs and symptoms of spinal cord tumors can be divided into the following areas: pain, sensory impairment, motor impairment, and sphincter disturbances.

PAIN

Pain, with or without sensory impairment, is the most frequent initial symptom of spinal cord tumors. The symptom is due to compression, invasion of the spinal tracts, tension on the spinal nerve roots, or attachment to the proximal dura.

Cord compression is often accompanied by pain, although in some instances pain is absent. Pain may be the only symptom of a slow-growing tumor for months or years. Severe local pain and tenderness are common in extradural and extramedullary tumors; most intramedullary tumors cause pain, but it is rarely as severe. If radicular pain in present, it can be severe. *Radicular pain* is pain that runs throughout the distribution of the sensory nerve root. It is caused by irritation, tension, or pressure on the nerve roots and can be described as knifelike or as a dull ache with accompanying bouts of sharp, piercing pain. When this type of pain is present, tenderness of the spinous processes over the tumor can be noted in half of patients. Any activity that increases intraspinal pressure, such as the Valsalva maneuver (coughing, sneezing, or straining), will intensify the pain and cause it to radiate to the dermatomes supplied by the nerve root.

Pain can also be exaggerated by lying on a bed because this causes stretching of the spinal nerves. Because of the overlap of dermatomes supplying a particular area, pain can be diffuse and poorly localized. Often, pain is referred so that it mimicks such conditions as angina, acute abdominal, or intercostal neuralgia.

SENSORY IMPAIRMENT

Pain and temperature loss are the most common signs of sensory impairment, with coldness, numbness, and tingling appearing as the early symptoms. Touch, vibration, and finally position sense are areas of later sensory deficit. The slow progression of symptoms commences unilaterally in an arm or leg and continues to spread upward until the level of the lesion is finally reached. Often, the level of sensory impairment is surrounded by a narrow band of hyperesthesia (abnormally increased sensitivity to stimuli) directly above it. This band of hyperesthesia marks the location of the neoplasm.

MOTOR IMPAIRMENT

Motor weakness, a major symptom, develops in conjunction with sensory loss, with functional loss below the level of the lesion. Motor deficits are due to the involvement of the pyramidal or corticospinal tract. The slow progression of early symptoms includes paresis, clumsiness, spasticity, and hyperactive reflexes. One extremity is affected, followed by the gradual involvement of the contralateral or ipsilateral extremities.

Ataxia and hypotonia, common signs of cerebellar impairment, are frequent symptoms of cerebellar dysfunction that are found with spinal cord tumors. Both symptoms are often overlooked in the early stages of spinal tumors and tend to modify the corticospinal tract signs, such as spasticity, that are expected. However, the Babinski sign is found to be positive—a certain sign of corticospinal dysfunction. As the motor tract signs develop, paresis and spasticity are apparent in the areas supplied below the level of the tumor.

The combination of sensory and motor deficits can produce a Brown–Séquard syndrome, characterized by motor loss on the side of the lesion; loss of touch, vibration and position sense on the side of the lesion; and contralateral loss of pain and temperature.

SPHINCTER DISTURBANCES

There may or may not be loss of sphincter control. If it develops, loss of sphincter control of the bladder precedes loss of control of the lower bowel. Early urinary symptoms include urgency and difficulty initiating urination. Symptoms gradually progress so that retention with overflow develops. In the male, impotency can occur. Difficulty in the control of the bowel sphincter is a later occurrence. Lesions producing sphincter disturbance must be bilateral to produce symptoms.

In the instance of a large intramedullary tumor of the cervical cord, "sacral sparing" may occur. Because the perineal sensation is controlled by the spinothalamic tracts that are located on the periphery of the spinal cord, the sensation to the perineum may be spared.[2]

OTHER SIGNS AND SYMPTOMS

Papilledema is not an unusual finding with thoracic and lumbar neoplasms. It is related to the increase in cerebrospinal fluid (CSF), which has an osmotic effect and increases the volume of fluid. Another interesting finding with long-standing tumors is Froin's syndrome. As a tumor grows, it consumes all of the space around the spinal cord, isolating the cerebrospinal fluid below the level of the tumor from the normal cerebrospinal fluid circulation. The cerebrospinal fluid, when aspirated, is characterized by xanthochromia, an increased protein count, few or no cells, and the fact that it clots immediately. This is called Froin's syndrome.

Some types of spinal cord tumor cause a syringomyelic syndrome. A fluid-filled cystic cavity (syrinx) is found in the central intramedullary gray matter of the cord. This syndrome causes a chronic degenerative disorder of the spinal cord with motor weakness, spasticity, and pain.

SIGNS AND SYMPTOMS BY GENERAL LOCATION

CERVICAL REGION

C-4 or Above

A tumor located at the C-4 spinal level or above is particularly dangerous because of the involvement of the diaphragm. If there is bilateral cord involvement, respiratory failure will result. In unilateral cord involvement, signs of respiratory difficulty are observed because of the apparent loss of abdominal and intercostal respirations. Other possible symptoms of high cord tumors include quadriparesis, occipital headache, stiff neck, and downbeat nystagmus, in which the eyes drift upward and then downward when the patient attempts to gaze downward. Physiologically, downward gaze is controlled by pathways that extend from the brain stem to the upper cervical cord. A spinal cord tumor can encroach on this pathway and be evidenced by the nystagmus.

Tumors proximal to the cervical–brain stem junction can trigger symptoms of lower cranial nerve dysfunction such as vertigo, dysphagia, dysarthria, deviation of the tongue, and difficulty in shrugging the shoulders. Atrophy of the sternomastoid muscles, unilateral tongue atrophy, and atrophy and paresis of the shoulder and neck muscles are common. Some high cervical tumors extend upward through the foramen magnum. Occasionally, papilledema is noted.

Below C–4

Lesions below C–4 preserve the integrity of the phrenic nerve. Pain in the shoulders and arms is frequent. If the roots of C–7 and C–8 are involved, pain is felt along the outer side of the forearm and hand. If C–5 and C–6 roots are affected, then pain will be noted along the medial aspect of the arm. Weakness follows pain. Paresthesia may also be present without pain.

The level of a partial lower motor neuron lesion can be generally located by noting what upper extremity functions are intact.

Atrophy of the shoulder, arm, and intrinsic hand muscles is often associated with muscle fasciculations. Unilateral or bilateral Horner's syndrome can result with a lesion of the C–8 spinal nerve roots. It should be recalled that Horner's syndrome includes ptosis of the eyelid, constriction of the pupil, and anhidrosis on the affected side because of the interference of sympathetic innervation.

THORACIC REGION

Localization of a tumor in the thoracic region is more difficult than in the cervical region. One sign that can be helpful in general tumor location is Beevor's sign: when the patient sits up or raises his head from the recumbent position, the umbilicus appears to be displaced toward the head because of paralysis of the interior portion of the rectus abdominal muscle. This is caused by compression at the tenth thoracic segment.

Sensory loss is a more accurate landmark in identifying the level of the lesion. A band of hyperesthesia is frequently found just above this level. Signs of lower motor neuron deficit, spastic paresis of the lower extremities, a positive Babinski sign, and sphincter impairment are all common findings.

LUMBAR–CAUDA EQUINA REGION

The characteristic symptoms of a lumbar tumor are pain, paresis, and atrophy of the muscles of the lower extremities, as well as early loss of sphincter control. Severe low back pain that radiates down one leg and then to the other is common. Occasionally, perineal, bladder, and bowel pain may be experienced. Sensory loss is localized in the legs and saddle area.

Motor weakness usually develops in one leg and involves only certain muscle groups. Atrophy of the affected muscles usually occurs, although it is not necessarily severe. The degree of weakness and atrophy varies greatly within the same patient. The quadriceps, hamstrings, and gastrocnemius, in combination or singularly, can be affected. Footdrop is a common problem. If the nerve roots are affected, the Achilles and patellar reflexes are absent or diminished.

Bladder disturbances such as difficulty in initiating urination and the inability to empty the bladder occur frequently, as do sexual dysfunction in the form of loss of libido and impotency. Bladder and sexual symptoms appear to be more common in tumors of the conus medullaris region.

Because spinal cord problems caused by pressure on the spinal cord from a tumor, disc, or fracture are treatable, it is important that they be diagnosed accurately. None of the intrinsic diseases of the spinal cord are treatable, so making an incorrect diagnosis for these conditions is not nearly as serious as missing a treatable compressing lesion. If there is any doubt about the diagnosis, a myelogram should be done.

TUMORS THAT METASTASIZE TO THE SPINAL COLUMN OR CORD

Tumors that mestastasize to the spinal column account for about 10% to 20% of all spinal tumors. The primary lesions in the body originate in the lungs, breast, prostate, gastrointestinal tract, kidney, and other areas. The cancer tends to spread proximally from the primary organ affected. For example, lung cancer tends to spread to the thoracic spine, while cancer of the uterus or prostate spreads to the lumbar region.

Most metastatic lesions are located in the epidural space and affect the cord by direct compression from the tumor or compression of the cord from a collapsed or eroded vertebra. Infiltration of the cord does not usually occur. The major signs and symptoms include back pain, localized tenderness over the affected vertebra, weakness of the lower extremities, and bladder dysfunction.[3]

Treatment depends on the progression of symptoms and the overall prognosis for the patient. A decompression laminectomy may be performed if neurological function has deteriorated rapidly or if a sudden obstruction to the flow of cerebrospinal fluid has developed. However, if the neurological deficits have existed for some time, or the patient is considered imminently terminal, no surgery will be done. In some instances, radiation therapy will be suggested as a means of shrinking the tumor to control the pain.

DIAGNOSIS

Since several other diseases can mimic the symptoms of spinal cord tumors, it is important but sometimes perplexing for the physician to arrive at a firm diagnosis. Differentiation of a spinal cord tumor is often made by excluding some of the following possibilities: cervical spondylosis, tuberculous granulomas, various granulomatous lesions (syphilic, fungal, and so forth), metastatic lesions, myelomas, lymphomas, protruding intervertebral discs, myelitis, arachnoiditis, syringomyelia, amyotrophic lateral sclerosis, and multiple sclerosis.

The diagnosis of a spinal cord tumor is made on the basis of a careful history, general physical examination, neurological examination, and diagnostic procedures.

HISTORY AND PHYSICAL/NEUROLOGICAL EXAMINATION

The patient will usually provide a history of progressive spinal cord involvement as evidenced by motor and sensory deficits. The progression of symptoms may be gradual or abrupt. Deficits that develop slowly from gradual cord compression are more apt to reverse themselves when the pressure is withdrawn. When compression is acute, recovery is rare. In examining the patient, sensory levels of deficit should be identified even though deficits are often incomplete and erratic. (See Chap. 18, Fig. 18–10, and Tables 2–6 and 2–7.) The sensory modalities that are assessed are pain, temperature, position, vibration, and light touch. When sensory loss is definite and complete, then it usually follows that concurrent motor deficits are permanent.[3]

Motor deficits should be assessed to determine whether the deficits incurred are upper motor neuron or lower motor neuron in origin. It is important to identify the location of the tumor by identifying areas of deficit and the corresponding anatomical location of the spinal cord. Reflexes are also assessed to help in this determination.

The back and spine should be examined to note any localizing signs and symptoms. Localized tenderness, spasms, scoliosis, and stiffness will often signal the location of the tumor site. The importance of the history and physical examination cannot be overstated.

DIAGNOSTIC PROCEDURES

The following diagnostic procedures are the mainstays for the diagnosis of spinal cord tumors:

1. Plain spinal films of the vertebral column are surprisingly helpful in identifying a tumor.
2. Myelography is probably the single most important diagnostic tool for diagnosing a spinal cord tumor. The contrast medium aids in identifying the level, size, and boundaries of the tumor.
3. Lumbar puncture is done cautiously especially if there appears to be a significant elevation in the intraspinal pressure. A Queckenstedt test (spinal dynamics) may be performed. It will indicate if there is partial or complete blockage to the flow of CSF caused by obstruction of the subarachnoid space by a mass such as a tumor.
4. An analysis of CSF reveals an elevation of protein; if the CSF is collected below the level of the spinal tumor, Froin's syndrome may be noted.
5. A computed tomography (CT) scan is helpful in localizing the lesion.
6. Tomograms of suspicious areas of the vertebral column may help in localizing the site of the lesion.
7. Spinal angiography is helpful in delineating a tumor if it is a vascular lesion.
8. Electromyography (EMG) is useful in making a differential diagnosis.

MEDICAL MANAGEMENT

Medical management is directed toward an early differential diagnosis of a spinal cord tumor and control of symptoms. In most cases, surgery is planned. Special supportive care for the maintenance of the normal function controlled by the involved area of the cord must be implemented. For example, even high cervical surgery rarely necessitates a tracheostomy, but equipment for performing a tracheostomy must be ready should the need arise.

To control edema of the cord, dexamethasone (Decadron), 4 mg four times a day, is ordered for 3 or 4 days and then gradually tapered. Maalox, 30 mg orally, is given in conjunction with the dexamethasone to prevent gastric irritation.

The prognosis will vary greatly, depending on the type of tumor and neurological deficits. Recovery of neurological function can occur gradually over a period of approximately 2 years and continue even longer with aggressive physiotherapy. Each patient must be thoroughly evaluated to determine his rehabilitative needs. Based on this assessment, appropriate extended care facilities can be selected, if warranted. Some patients will benefit from an aggressive rehabilitative program at a center.

TREATMENT

The treatment for a specific spinal cord tumor depends on the type of tumor, its location, and the rapidity with which signs and symptoms develop. Surgical excision, decompression, and possibly radiation therapy are the usual methods of management of spinal cord tumors. Chemotherapy and radiation are often used for metastatic lesions of the spinal area.

The following is a list of the general approach to various classifications of spinal cord tumors:

- Intradural–extramedullary tumors should be surgically excised as soon as possible after the diagnostic myelography because there is often neurological deterioration after myelography. A decompression laminectomy with magnification and microsurgical instrumentation will often lead to complete removal of these tumors that are benign (meningiomas and neurofibromas). If a tumor is not clearly delineated, a biopsy followed later by irradiation is the usual approach.
- Extradural–extramedullary tumors are often metastatic cancers or lymphomas. Other types of tumors may also affect

the extradural space. Treatment depends on the type of tumor.

- Metastatic lesions and lymphomas are managed with radiation therapy measures to control pain, and possibly chemotherapy. A decompression laminectomy may be indicated either to preserve neurological function that is threatened by possible collapse of an eroded vertebra or to relieve an obstruction to the flow of cerebrospinal fluid
- Intramedullary tumors are usually ependymomas or astrocytomas, which are not usually amenable to complete surgical removal. Ependymomas can sometimes be removed in a two-stage procedure if the parameters of the tumor are clearly demarcated. In the first stage, the tumor is opened posteriorly in the median raphe so that the central tumor is exposed. The wound is closed without resection of the tumor. In several months, the second stage is initiated. The tumor is examined to see if it has extruded itself.[3] In some instances the tumor can be completely removed because it has extruded itself.
- Tubercular lesions are treated with immobility and drug therapy. In some instances a laminectomy will be necessary.

Variations in the approach to the patient do exist, which depend on the type of tumor and the neurological status of the patient. Noting the rate of progression of symptoms is a key in determining the need to schedule emergency surgery. As a rule, rapid loss of motor and sensory function indicates an immediate need for surgery.

RADIATION THERAPY

When complete excision of a spinal cord tumor is not possible, radiation therapy of the spinal cord should follow surgery. The spinal cord is less tolerant of radiation than other organs. The dosage of radiation therapy varies, but 3500 rad to 5000 rad over a 6- to 8-week period is the usual range. Radiation myelopathy is a possible delayed response to radiation therapy of the spinal column, which should be considered when selecting adjunct irradiation and dosage.

Radiation Myelopathy

If radiation therapy is ordered as part of the treatment protocol, radiation myelopathy must be considered. This is a common complication of radiation, which begins with the development of clinical signs and symptoms at least six months after completion of radiation and, more frequently, 12 to 15 months after therapy. The chronic progressive myelopathy has an insidious onset (sensory impairment to the areas supplied by the affected cord). Pain is not present initially. Symptoms develop slowly over weeks and months. Motor symptoms and changes in pain and temperature develop, so that a Brown–Séquard syndrome is observed. This eventually converts to a transverse myelopathy with spastic paraplegia, loss of sensation to the affected areas, and loss of bowel and bladder control. Death usually occurs within 1 year of the onset of transverse myelopathy.

NURSING MANAGEMENT OF THE PATIENT WITH A SPINAL CORD TUMOR

The nursing management of the patient with a spinal cord tumor is comparable to the management of one with a spinal cord injury (see Chap. 18). Specifics of care depend on the segmental level of the tumor and the presenting symptoms. If the patient is treated surgically, nursing care would follow that for a laminectomy patient (see Chap. 18). The objectives of nursing care for the hospitalized patient are directed toward patient assessment; control of pain, if present; management of sensory and motor deficits; and management of sphincter disturbances. See Chart 22–1 for a summary of assessment data. See Chart 22–2 for a summary of common nursing diagnoses.

PATIENT ASSESSMENT

The nurse should conduct an assessment of the patient to determine baseline data of neurological and vital signs. (Neither the level of consciousness nor pupillary signs are apt to be affected, unless the sympathetic innervation of the cervical spinal nerves are involved. In this instance, a Horner's syndrome with a small pupil would be seen.) Special attention should be given to sensory and motor function. Evidence of deficit in the extremities, bowel, and bladder are the most common deficits encountered.

To evaluate the sensory function, the nurse should do two things. First, pinch the skin on the arms, legs, and trunk to determine the level of feeling, starting with the feet and working upward, and determine the level on the trunk (chest, back, buttocks, abdomen) where the sensory function is lost. (A band of hyperesthesia often exists over the level of sensory loss. Determining this level is helpful in noting progression or regression of the sensory function). Second, the nurse should determine what type of sensory loss, such as temperature, pain, light or deep touch, has occurred.

Motor function is evaluated by asking the patient to move his arms, legs, shoulders, and other body parts. The nurse should then check the hand grasps for strength, comparing the relative strength of each hand. Ask the patient to extend his arms in front of him with his palms up. If any weakness exists, the palm on the affected side will turn downward. This is a more sensitive method of detecting muscle weakness.

Note the movement of the chest when the patient is asked to take a deep breath. The chest should move upward in a symmetrical fashion. If there is paralysis or weakness of any of the muscles innervating the chest, the chest movement will not be symmetrical and the affected side will lag rather than rise (with a deep breath).

Evidence of paralysis or paresis should be recorded as baseline findings to which future assessments should be compared.

Any evidence of abnormal motor tone, such as hypotonia or spasticity, should be noted because they are abnormal

CHART 22–1. ASSESSMENT OF THE PATIENT WITH A SPINAL CORD TUMOR

Sensory Assessment

- With patient's eyes closed, test for sensations of light touch, temperature, pain, and position; depending on the location of the tumor, certain modalities may be spared.
  —The spinothalamic tracts (pain and temperature) are located anteriolaterally in the cross section of the cord; a lesion of the spinothalamic tract will result in loss of the sensations of pain and temperature contralaterally below the level of the tumor because the tract crosses the cord immediately upon entering it.
  —The fasciculus gracilis and fasciculus cuneatus (position and vibration) are located in the posterior columns of the spinal cord; a tumor in this area would affect the sensations of position and vibration.
  —The tracts for the sensation of light touch combine aspects of the two above-mentioned tracts, having some crossed and some uncrossed fibers; light touch is usually spared in unilateral lesions.
- Beginning at the feet and working upward, test each side of the patient individually and compare findings; often sensory loss is asymmetrical.
- Note the highest level of sensation on each side. Helpful sensory dermatome landmarks include C–4, clavicles; T–4, nipple line; T–10, umbilicus; and so forth.
- If pain is present, describe involved area, type of pain, and frequency.

Motor Assessment

- Assess each side of the body separately and compare.
- Note any spontaneous movement.
- Assess muscle strength (see chap. 5).
- Assess gait, if ambulatory.
- Assess reflexes.
- Assess coordination.
- Note presence of spasticity or other abnormal movements.

Sphincter Assessment

- Note patient's voiding pattern.
- Maintain an intake and output record.
- Assess abdomen and suprapubic areas for distention.
- Note bowel evacuation pattern.
- If incontinent, note any associated factors.
- Auscultate abdomen for bowel sounds.

Respiratory Assessment

- Observe chest movement (symmetry, abdominal breathing, apnea).
- Assess rate, depth, and rhythm of respirations.
- Auscultate chest for bilateral chest sounds.
- Monitor arterial blood gases, if appropriate.

Other Signs

- Assess pulse, temperature, and blood pressure.
- Assess for presence of orthostatic hypotension.
- Note any absence of perspiration to areas of the body.

findings. Spasticity is a common occurrence with spinal cord tumors.

Bowel and bladder control are also evaluated. Incontinence in a patient who has been continent is not uncommon. Some patients complain of dribbling of urine, which can excoriate the perineum, therefore having implications for nursing management. Sacral sparing is common with spinal cord tumors. Therefore, bowel and bladder function must be evaluated.

MANAGEMENT OF SENSORY AND MOTOR DEFICITS

Nursing management should be modified to take into consideration the sensory and motor deficits the patient may have. Adaptation of the activities of daily living to meet the specific needs of the patient can allow the patient to maintain his independence. For example, if the patient has paresis of a leg, the use of a cane or walker can provide help in

CHART 22-2. COMMON NURSING DIAGNOSES ASSOCIATED WITH THE PATIENT WITH A SPINAL CORD INJURY

NURSING DIAGNOSES	EXPECTED OUTCOMES	NURSING INTERVENTIONS
Potential of injury due to altered/absent sensory input	• Injury to the patient will be prevented.	• Teach patient to check position of affected limbs with eyes. • Teach patient to check integrity of skin daily, especially on affected parts, for signs of injury. • Teach patient to check temperature with unaffected limb before applying heat to affected area. • Heating devices should be used very cautiously.
Sensory deprivation due to altered sensory function	• Sensory deprivation will not develop.	• Provide for added sensory stimuli to affected area (*e.g.*, touching affected arm while giving care). • Increase output from other intact sensory modalities.
Impaired motor function due to motor weakness/paralysis	• Motor function to involved areas will be supported and maximized.	• Provide range-of-motion exercises to all joints at least four times a day. • Position in good body alignment and reposition every 2 hours. • Use support devices (*e.g.*, splints, footboard) to maintain proper body position. • If spasticity is present, keep involved extremity warm to decrease spasticity. • Encourage use of involved extremities as much as possible.
Potential of skin breakdown	• Skin integrity will be maintained.	• Provide for good skin care. • Keep heels off bed to prevent added irritation and skin breakdown.
Self-care deficits due to neurological deficits	• Self-care needs will be met.	• Help patient develop alternate methods of accomplishing activities of daily living (ADL). • Provide for care that patient is unable to provide for himself.
Impaired urinary elimination: incontinence or retention due to neurological impairment	• An adequate urinary elimination pattern will be maintained.	• Assess bladder function and urinary elimination pattern. • Maintain an intake and output record. • Assess for abdominal distention. • Report urinary outputs to physician. • Encourage adequate fluid intake. • Follow intermittent catheterization or indwelling catheter protocols, if ordered.
	• Urinary tract infection will be prevented.	• Monitor periodic urinalyses and urine cultures. • Begin a bladder retraining program, when feasible.
Altered bowel elimination: constipation or incontinence due to neurological impairment	• An adequate bowel elimination pattern will be maintained.	• Assess bowel elimination pattern. • Assess presence of bowel sounds. • Assess abdomen for distention. • Assess and adjust diet to facilitate a normal bowel elimination pattern for the patient. • Administer drugs as ordered. • Institute a bowel program designed for the patient. • Begin a bowel retraining program, when feasible.

CHART 22–2. (continued)

NURSING DIAGNOSES	EXPECTED OUTCOMES	NURSING INTERVENTIONS
Potential for ineffective breathing pattern	• Effective breathing pattern will be maintained (as evidenced by normal blood gases and lack of respiratory distress).	• Assess adequacy of breathing pattern. • Observe frequently for abnormalities or difficulty in breathing pattern. • Administer oxygen as ordered. • Position to facilitate respirations (with head elevated). • Review arterial blood gases periodically.
Potential for ineffective airway clearance	• Patent airway will be maintained.	• Encourage frequent coughing and deep breathing exercises. • Auscultate chest. • Have suction available; suction as necessary. • Position to facilitate drainage of secretions. • Turn from side to side to prevent pooling of secretions. • Provide for chest physiotherapy as necessary. • Maintain patient's tracheostomy or endotracheal tube, if present, by periodic tracheostomy care and suctioning.
Alteration in comfort: pain due to spinal cord tumor	• Patient will state that pain is controlled and he feels comfortable.	• Assess location and character of pain. • Administer pain medication as ordered. • Provide for comfort measures: — Maintain in proper body alignment. — Reposition every 2 hours. — Apply alternating air mattress. • Provide for measures known to decrease pain: — Provide range-of-motion exercises four times a day. — Prevent chilling. — Decrease anxiety.
Anxiety due to diagnosis of spinal cord tumor	• Anxiety will be reduced to a manageable level.	• Allow the patient to express his feelings. • Correct misinformation and clarify information as necessary. • Refer to appropriate persons, as necessary. • Help patient set realistic goals. • Be supportive of patient. • Help the patient find ways to reduce anxiety (*e.g.*, diversion, relaxation exercises).

ambulation. If spasticity or motor deficits exist, a plan should be initiated to prevent deformities and contractions. Such a plan would include

- Range-of-motion exercises
- Proper positioning
- Use of splints, footboards, and so forth

Additional consideration would aim at teaching the patient to compensate for motor deficits, such as how to transfer from chair to bed, use a cane, walker, or wheelchair, and so forth.

If ambulation is limited, skin care should be given every 4 hours to protect against skin breakdown. If need be, the patient should be turned every 2 hours to facilitate respirations and prevent skin breakdown.

Special attention should also be given to the safety needs

of the patient when sensory or motor deficits exist. For example, if there is a sensory deficit to pain and temperature in the hand, the patient must be cautioned to check the temperature of water, a radiator, and so forth, before putting the affected hand near the material. Serious burns or other injuries can result, especially if the protective mechanism for pain is not intact to warn the person of possible danger.

CONTROL OF PAIN

If medication has been prescribed, the nurse's role is to administer it as directed. However, other measures should be taken into account to provide for comfort. Such measures might include

- Proper positioning and turning every 2 hours
- Range-of-motion exercises
- Use of an alternating pressure mattress

At the same time, activities that might aggravate pain, such as coughing, sneezing, or straining, should be avoided because they tend to increase intraspinal pressure, which, in turn, increases pain.

MANAGEMENT OF SPHINCTER DISTURBANCES

Although not every patient will have sphincter disturbance, the nurse should periodically evaluate the patient for signs and symptoms of this dysfunction. Incontinence or retention are the major symptoms that would occur.

If the patient experiences dysfunction of bowel or bladder, the following points of care would be followed:

- Maintain an accurate intake and output record to provide accurate data on bladder function.
- Force fluids to decrease the possibility of urinary tract infection.
- Note results from urinalysis and culture that would indicate the presence of infection.
- Institute a bowel program to prevent constipation and avoid straining at stool (Valsalva maneuver), which could increase pressure and pain.

PSYCHOSOCIAL CONSIDERATIONS

For the patient with a metastatic cord tumor, death from this lesion is inevitable. Knowledge of the diagnosis may be communicated directly by the physician to the patient. With other patients, the message becomes clear from the evasive, brief conversations with the physician. Unlike the brain tumor patient, the level of consciousness is not usually affected in the cord tumor patient. The patient is perfectly alert, oriented, and perceptive of the verbal and nonverbal communications directed toward him.

Some patients who are suspicious of the prognosis may ask directly for confirmation of the diagnosis; others may completely avoid any but very superficial conversations. It is well established in professional and lay circles that the patient has a right to know that he is dying. However, the actual process of disclosure and support after disclosure is difficult. Disclosure of the diagnosis to the patient is the rightful domain of the physician. In order to function effectively, the nurse must know what information has been conveyed to the patient.

It is extremely difficult for a nurse to care for a patient who is uninformed of the fact that he is terminally ill, although this does not imply that it is easy to manage the informed patient. The best the nurse can do is observe, listen, and record any evidence from the patient's conversation and behavior that indicates that he needs information. In such instances, a team conference aids in planning for individualized patient needs.

Whatever the patient's state of awareness, the nurse assumes a supportive role, ready to listen and talk based on the lead of the patient. The patient needs some time to regain his equilibrium so that he can begin to cope with the crisis. Because behavior manifestations vary from patient to patient, the nurse should accept the patient's behavior and assume an advocacy role.

REFERENCES

1. Adams, RA, Victor M: Principles of Neurology, 2nd ed, pp 638–642. New York, McGraw–Hill, 1981
2. Rosenfield DB: A practical neurological secreening examination. Hosp Med 32A, June 1982
3. Smith RR: Essentials of Neurosurgery, pp 137–146. Philadelphia, JB Lippincott, 1980

BIBLIOGRAPHY

Books

Connolly ES: Radiation therapy of tumors of the spinal cord. In Youmans J (ed): Neurological Surgery, 2nd ed, pp 3222–3226. Philadelphia, WB Saunders, 1982

Connolly ES: Spinal cord tumors in adults. In Youmans J (ed): Neurological Surgery, 2nd ed, pp 3196–3214. Philadelphia, WB Saunders, 1982

Periodicals

Arsenault L: Primary spinal cord tumors: A review and case presentation of a patient with an intramedullary spinal cord neoplasm. J Neurosurg Nurs 13(2):53, April 1981

Livingston KE, Paren RG: The neurosurgical management of spinal metastasis causing cord and cauda equina compression. J Neurosurg 49:839, 1978

Malis LI: Intramedullary spinal cord tumors. Clin Neurosurg 37:512, 1978

McOuat F: The insidious spinal cord tumor. J Neurosurg Nurs 13(1):18, February 1981

Onofrio BM: Intradural extramedullary spinal cord tumors. Clin Neurosurg 38:540, 1978

Schott GD: Spinal tumours: 1. Classification. Nurs Times 2055, December 25, 1975

Schott GD: Spinal tumours. 2. Symptoms and signs. Nurs Times 21, January 1–8, 1976

Schott GD: Spinal tumours. 3. Investigation, treatment and prognosis. Nurs Times 57, January 15, 1976

Stern WE: Localization and diagnosis of spinal cord tumors. Clin Neurosurg 34:480, 1978

part seven

Nursing Care of Patients With Cerebrovascular Problems

chapter

23

Cerebrovascular Accident (Stroke)

Cerebrovascular accident (formerly termed stroke) is ranked as the third cause of death after heart disease and cancer which cause approximately 720,000 and 370,000 deaths per year, respectively. There were 172,500 deaths from stroke in the United States in 1978.

These mortality rates do not reflect the countless individuals disabled by cerebrovascular disease, of whom there are about 2 million in the United States. Although many of these people are in the age range of 25 to 64 years, the older age group is more often affected by stroke, with a sharp increase in frequency noted in people 65 years and older.

Certain families have a tendency to have strokes, with men affected approximately 10% to 15% more frequently than women. There also seems to be a racial component involved, since the black population appears to have a greater incidence of and higher death rate from cerebrovascular disease. It is thought that the higher frequency of hypertension in blacks contributes to the incidence rate.

DEFINITION AND DESCRIPTION

Stroke or *cerebrovascular accident* is a syndrome that is characterized as a sudden, nonconvulsive onset of neurological deficits related directly or indirectly to a deficiency of the cerebral blood supply.

The type and severity of neurological deficits cover a wide range and gradation of symptoms. A patient can experience a mild, transient interruption of neurological function, such as tingling and weakness in one extremity or thick, muddled speech, which passes as quickly as symptoms appear. Symptoms are so mild and nonthreatening that they neither alarm the patient nor require medical attention. These episodes are sometimes called "little strokes" or *transient ischemic attacks* (TIAs).

At the other end of the spectrum are those symptoms characteristic of a *major stroke*, including

- Loss of consciousness
- Hemiplegia
- Aphasia
- Visual field deficits
- Dysarthria

The severity and permanency of symptoms are the factors that differentiate between the so-called "little strokes" and major strokes.

Other terms that refer to the stroke syndrome include apoplexy, cerebrovascular accident, and shock. Distinguishing stroke as a syndrome rather than a disease is important: a syndrome has many etiologies, while a disease has but one. It is clear that the stroke syndrome is caused by abnormalities of the cerebral blood vessels and is generally called cerebrovascular disease.

RISK FACTORS

Much time and research money are being devoted to identifying conditions and primary entities that predispose individuals to the development of the stroke syndrome. Educational programs are planned to inform the general public about stroke and stroke prevention. Programs are also designed for the health professional to increase the awareness of stroke and the methods of identifying high-risk populations that are subject to potential stroke unless appropriate intervention is made available. By drawing high-risk individuals into the health care system, potentially dangerous, preexisting conditions can be managed, thus avoiding needless disability and suffering from stroke.

Generally speaking, strokes that produce symptoms caused by ischemia from occlusion of the blood vessel (thrombus and embolus) or from insufficient cerebral nutrient supply could develop from any of the following conditions: atherosclerosis (atheromas), hypertensive arteriosclerotic changes, subclavian steal syndrome, heart disease, arteritis, diabetes mellitus, and polycythemia vera. Cigarette smoking and use of oral contraceptives in women increase the possibility of stroke. Any condition that leads to the diagnosis of hypertension or heart disease relates closely to the development of cerebrovascular disease. Those conditions that make the patient a high-risk candidate include elevated cholesterol, lipoprotein, and triglyceride blood levels; obesity; and sedentary work with little other exercise.

It should be noted that all of the associated conditions are just that, associations. If these conditions remain silent, there will be no interference with neurological function. The exception is that of cerebrovascular anomalies such as aneurysms or arteriovenous malformations. These conditions can produce neurological deficits by the compression of cerebral tissue.

PHYSIOLOGY AND PATHOPHYSIOLOGY

There are various built-in protective mechanisms of the brain that act to increase blood flow and nutrient supply when the need arises. These mechanisms include arterial tree anastomosis and autoregulatory mechanisms that increase cerebral blood flow and help extract increased amounts of glucose and oxygen from perfusing blood.

ANASTOMOSIS

The brain is able to receive arterial blood from the anastomosing vessels of the extracranial vessels, as well as from the two internal carotids and two vertebral arteries (Fig. 23–1).

Carotid Arteries

Each of the two carotid arteries bifurcates to form an internal and external carotid artery. The internal carotid artery ascends from the point of bifurcation in the neck, penetrating the skull at the petrous portion of the temporal bone. It enters the cranium between the layers of the dura mater at a position just below the gasserian ganglion of the trigeminal nerve. The internal carotid artery does not branch until it penetrates the cranium at the dura. Profuse branching then occurs, giving rise to several arteries including the ophthalmic, posterior communicating, anterior choroidal, anterior cerebral, and middle cerebral arteries. The middle cerebral artery supplies about 80% of the blood received by both cerebral hemispheres. The anterior cerebral artery supplies the frontal pole and medial surface of the frontal and parietal lobes.

FIG. 23–1. Branches of the right external carotid artery. The internal carotid artery ascends to the base of the brain. The right vertebral artery also is shown as it ascends through the transverse foramina of the cervical vertebrae. (Chaffee EE, Lytle IM: Basic Physiology and Anatomy. Philadelphia, JB Lippincott, 1980)

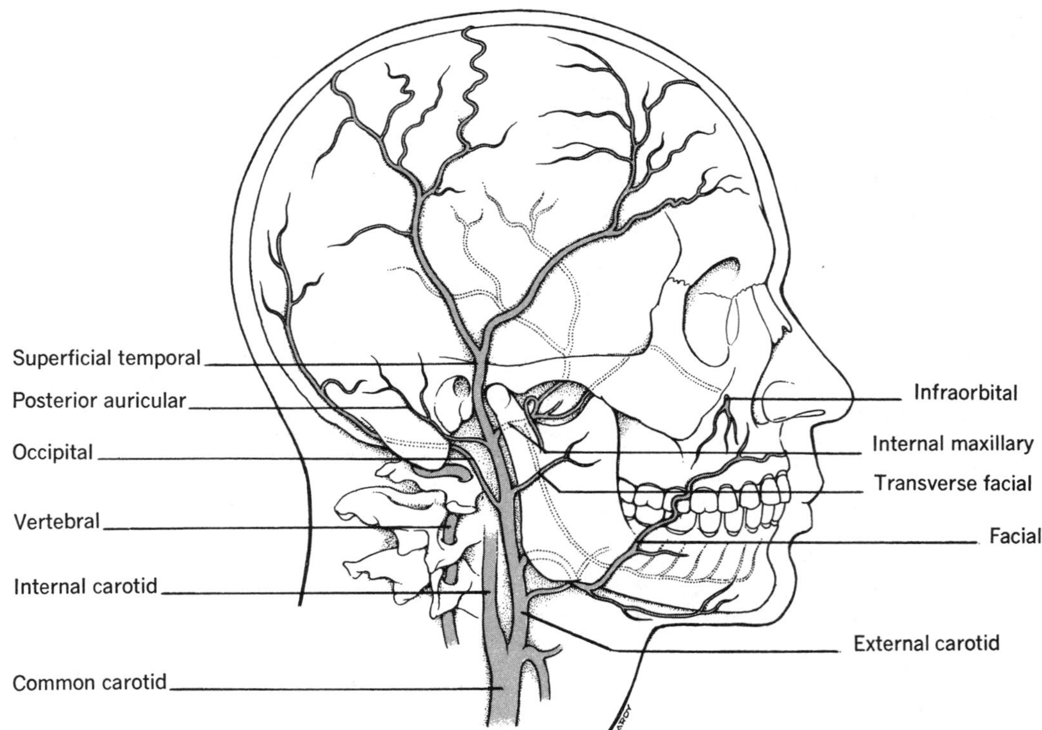

Unlike the internal carotid artery, the external carotid begins to branch profusely immediately after bifurcation and provides a rich blood supply to the face, orbits, and dura mater. In the event of the occlusion of the internal carotid artery, significant amounts of blood can be supplied to the brain from the external carotid artery. The major point at which the anastomosing vessels of the internal and external carotid blood supply meet is the orbit(s) (ophthalmic artery and small external and internal carotid connections).

Vertebral Arteries

The two vertebral arteries arise from the subclavian arteries. The vertebral arteries reach the base of the brain through a bony tunnel formed by the transverse processes of the cervical vertebrae from C-6 to C-1. Entrance to the cranial cavity is gained through the foramen magnum where the vertebrals unite to form the larger basilar artery. The basilar artery divides to form the two posterior cerebral arteries that supply the medial and inferior surfaces as well as the lateral portions of the temporal and occipital lobes (Fig. 23-2).

Circle of Willis

The circle of Willis is an anatomical area where the branches of the basilar and internal carotid arteries unite (see Fig. 23-2). The circle of Willis is composed of the two anterior cerebral, the anterior communicating, the two posterior cerebral, and the two posterior communicating arteries. Small arteries arise directly from the circle of Willis to nourish the diencephalon and basal ganglia. Anomalies of the circle of Willis and vertebral arteries are very common.

Collateral Circulation

With occlusion of a vertebral artery, anastomotic blood flow may be shunted from deep cervical, thyrocervical, or occipital arteries. Blood may also be shunted from the other vertebral artery. Occlusion of the stem portion of a cerebellar artery or a cerebral artery distal to the circle of Willis can be improved by a series of meningeal interarterial anastomoses. The occlusion may be ameliorated but rarely eliminated.

The important point to note is that there are potentially several anastomoses that allow the brain to receive adequate blood supply from any of the four major feeding arteries. The areas from which blood can be connected are the circle of Willis, connections of the internal and external carotid within the orbits, and the pia-arachnoid connection with peripheral branches of the anterior, middle, and posterior cerebral arteries on the hemispheric surface.

Because of the alternate source of the arterial blood supply provided by the anastomotic network, it is possible for one, two, or even three major feeding vessels to become occluded without serious consequences. However, in some individuals cerebral vessels may be anomalous and be of little value as an auxiliary supply of blood. Without angiographic studies, it is difficult to predict which patients can tolerate occlusion of a major feeding vessel(s) and which cannot because of the presence of cerebral anomalies.

AUTOREGULATORY MECHANISM

Oxygen and glucose are the two essential elements for cerebral metabolism and are supplied by means of a continual flow of blood. The cerebral blood flow is maintained at a constant rate of approximately 750 ml/minute. The con-

FIG. 23-2. The circle of Willis as seen at the base of a brain that has been removed from the skull. (Chaffee EE, Lytle IM: Basic Physiology and Anatomy. Philadelphia, JB Lippincott, 1980)

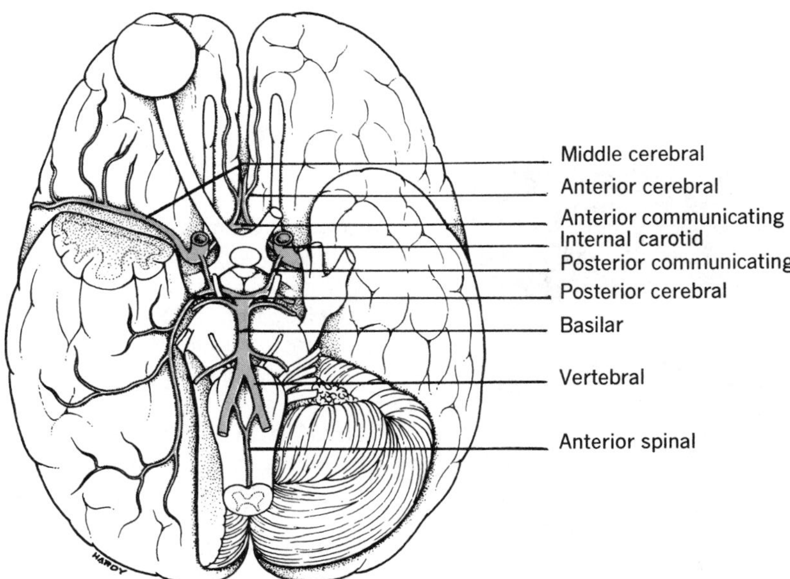

stancy of the rate is maintained by an autoregulatory mechanism within the brain. Various homeostatic mechanisms, both systemic and local, maintain adequate nutrient and blood supplies. However, a homeostatic mechanism can be taxed to the point where it is no longer functional.

These mechanisms can fail under the stress of certain diseases. Interference with oxygen and glucose, the chief cerebral nutrient supply, results in hypoxia or hypoglycemia. If nutrients cannot be delivered to cerebral tissue, ischemia results. Interruption of these elements is related to cerebral infarction, in which the blood supply is cut off as a result of a thrombus or embolus.

INFARCTION

When blood flow to any part of the brain is interrupted as a result of a thrombus or embolus, oxygen deprivation of cerebral tissue precipitates rapid cerebral deterioration, depending on the time involved. Deprivation for 1 minute can produce reversible symptoms such as loss of consciousness. Oxygen deprivation for more than 1 or 2 minutes can produce microscopic necrosis in the deprived area of the brain. If the hypoxia is very severe and prolonged, large areas of both gray and white matter will become necrotic. The necrotic area of the brain is called the *infarction* (Fig. 23–3).

It appears that extension of neuronal ischemia will cause changes in the cell membrane, resulting in cellular edema and compression of the capillaries. The capillary compression interferes with blood supply. The cerebral edema reaches its peak in 72 hours and subsides in approximately 2 weeks. Depending on the extent of the edema, there can be additional neurological deficit and development of herniation syndromes.

ATHEROSCLEROSIS

The cerebral arteries structurally resemble other arteries in that the arterial walls consist of the tunica intima, tunica media, and tunica adventitia. However, the walls of the cerebral arteries are thinner than those of arteries elsewhere in the body. The intima is very thin, with less elastic tissue than in other arteries. The media and adventitia are also thinner and have much less elastic tissue than in noncerebral arteries. Cerebral arteries also lack external elastic lamina. The difference between cerebral and extracranial arteries can be summarized as a difference in the distribution of elastic tissue and the thickness of the layers. Atherosclerosis is a sclerotic disease of the blood vessels that affects the tunica intima or the intimal layer of the artery.

FIG. 23–3. Impairment of cerebral circulation leading to a stroke. Note the area of cerebral infarction.

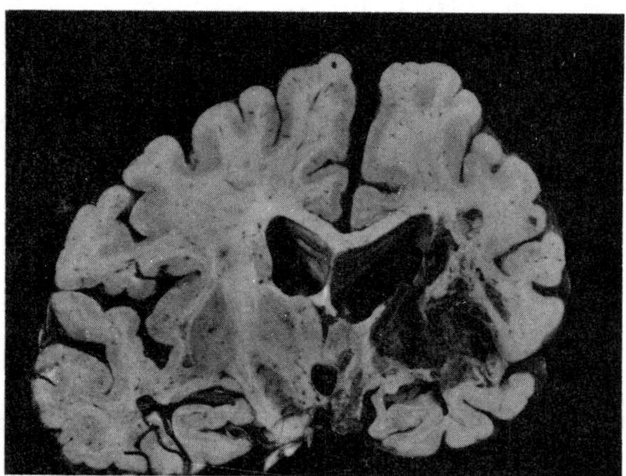

The onset of atherosclerosis can occur as early as the second decade of life. More evidence indicating the relationship between poor nutritional habits and pathological changes of the vascular system continues to mount. Generally, atherosclerosis is considered a problem of older age. Early atherosclerotic changes in the cerebral vessels are evidenced by areas of yellowish or grayish white thickenings called *atheromas*, which may be focal or diffuse. The larger vessels at the base of the brain are affected first, with the points of branching prime areas of involvement. The most frequent sites are (1) the internal carotid artery at the carotid sinus in the neck, (2) vertebral arteries at the subclavian junction, (3) vertebral arteries at the basilar–vertebral junction, (4) the main bifurcation of the middle cerebral artery, (5) the curvature in the posterior cerebral arteries around the midbrain, and (6) the curvature around the corpus callosum in the posterior cerebral arteries.[1]

The initial change that occurs in the artery is the buildup of intimal fibrohyaline plaques. The media layer is usually spared. These plaques develop insidiously over 20 to 30 years. As the disease process continues, there is progressive thickening of the intimal layer due to the addition of lipids and some calcium salts, thereby causing proliferation of the initial fibrohyaline plaques. Changes are apparent in the intimal structures themselves. The intima can become hypertrophied or fragmented or can split longitudinally into thin ribbons. The medial layer undergoes atrophy. The result is an increase in fibrotic tissue. As lipids continue to be deposited into the intima, the atheromas develop further, narrowing the lumen of the artery and eventually interfering with the blood supply to the brain.

CLASSIFICATION OF STROKE SYNDROMES

Stroke syndromes are usually classified according to their etiologic bases and are identified as thrombotic, embolic, or hemorrhagic. Thrombotic strokes may be further classified according to developmental process into transient ischemic attack, stroke in evolution, or completed stroke.

THROMBOTIC STROKE

Thrombotic stroke, the most common type of stroke, is associated with atherosclerosis and causes narrowing of the lumen of the artery. Eventually, there is interference with the blood supply nourishing that portion of the brain. The process is one of stepwise progression. In the initial phase, the thrombus does not always completely occlude the lumen. Complete occlusion may take hours. With complete occlusion, the thrombus may spread distally and proximally to the branching points of the artery and occlude any anastomotic connections. See Chart 23-1.

Transient Ischemic Attacks

When one considers the prolonged evolutionary process of the atherosclerotic-thrombotic phenomenon, it is easy to understand the frequent occurrences of transient ischemic attacks noted in many histories. The transient ischemic attacks last from a few minutes (10 minutes on the average) to hours and tend to replicate the initial symptoms. The symptoms then completely disappear. The transient episodes are observed *only* with cerebral thrombosis and are helpful in establishing the diagnosis. In 75% of patients studied by Adams and colleagues, transient ischemic attacks were foreboding episodes of strokes.[1] The stroke may be preceded by one or two attacks or as many as one hundred. The time between the onset of transient ischemic attacks and the stroke can range from hours to weeks or even years.

The symptoms associated with transient attacks depend on the arteries involved:

Carotid and Cerebral Artery

Blindness in one eye
Hemiplegia
Hemianesthesia
Speech disturbance
Confusion

Vertebrobasilar Artery

Dizziness
Diplopia
Numbness
Visual defects in one or both fields
Dysarthria

Stroke-in-Evolution

The development of the thrombotic stroke has more variables than the embolic or hemorrhagic stroke. It is interesting to note that 60% of thrombotic strokes occur during sleep. The development of a thrombotic stroke occurs in a few possible ways, even if transient ischemic attacks have been experienced prior to the actual stroke. Most often, there is only one attack, with the entire syndrome evolving within a few hours. In other instances, symptoms may evolve stepwise over several hours or days. Sometimes symptoms may develop with temporary improvement for a few hours, followed by a rapid progression of permanent deficits. The process of symptom evolution is referred to as *stroke-in-evolution*. The term *completed stroke* is used to describe the stable, usually permanent, symptoms.

Prognosis

The prognosis in thrombotic stroke is a guarded one. The process of arterial narrowing, thrombus formation, ischemia, and infarction is difficult to predict, particularly soon after the stroke. There is always the possibility that the stroke will extend to other areas of the brain. With a massive thrombotic infarction, there can be extensive cerebral edema with subsequent brain stem herniation and death. In less severe strokes, the cerebral edema with increased intracranial pressure may last for 3 to 5 days and then gradually subside. Recovery depends on the extent of the insult, the area of the brain involved, and the presence of other pathological changes in the brain. Recovery can begin hours or weeks after the stroke. Some patients show no improvement after months. Once having had a thrombotic stroke, the patient is at risk of suffering another.

EMBOLIC STROKE

An embolic stroke is most often the result of heart disease, in which a thrombus within the heart breaks into fragments and is carried to the brain. Patients with atrial flutter are five times more likely to experience embolic stroke than those without flutter. Other less frequent causes of embolic stroke include fat- or tumor-cell emboli, septic emboli, exudate from subacute bacterial endocarditis, or emboli precipitated during cardiac or vascular surgery.

An embolic stroke develops rapidly, evolving within seconds or 1 minute with no warning signs. If the embolus is large, it can plug the internal carotid artery, resulting in severe hemiplegia. Emboli arising from the heart most often enter the cerebral circulation by way of the carotids. Smaller emboli are more common and obstruct a branch of the middle cerebral artery, resulting in monoplegia or aphasia. The left middle cerebral artery is affected more often because it is a straighter vessel and provides the path of least resistance for the embolus. If entry into the brain is by way of the vertebral artery, the posterior cerebral arteries are affected. Homonymous hemianopsia and brain stem edema can result.

As an embolus passes through a vessel, it may produce temporary symptoms. A large embolus may lodge in an area for a few hours, fragment into pieces, and move. When the obstruction breaks down, symptoms will probably be reversed. However, these small fragments will eventually obstruct a smaller vessel, thereby precipitating symptoms of neurological deficit appropriate to that area of the brain.

The prognosis is similar to that for thrombotic stroke. With embolic stroke many patients will have subsequent episodes of stroke, if the underlying cause is not treated aggressively.

HEMORRHAGIC STROKE

The most common causes of hemorrhagic stroke are hypertensive intracerebral hemorrhage, ruptured cerebral aneurysm (see Chap. 24), ruptured arteriovenous malformation

CHART 23-1. SUBCLAVIAN STEAL SYNDROME

Subclavian steal syndrome is a vascular syndrome caused by an occlusion or stenosis proximal to the vertebral artery, most often at the origin of the subclavian artery. Atherosclerosis is the most frequent cause of the obstruction. The blood pressure beyond the occluded-stenotic area of the subclavian artery is decreased and *may* create a gradient of sufficient magnitude to reverse blood flow through the vertebral artery, resulting in siphoning or a "steal" from the basovertebral circulation.

Pathophysiology

A review of the origins of circulation to the brain is helpful for understanding the pathophysiology of the subclavian steal syndrome. (See page 496 of this chapter.) Note that the vertebral arteries arise from the subclavian arteries and that the subclavian arteries also supply the upper limbs and parts of the neck and shoulders. The circulatory insufficiency created in the subclavian steal syndrome is caused by diminished perfusion of areas supplied by the subclavian artery (the brain and the arm). Perfusion is controlled by two hemodynamic parameters—blood pressure and blood flow. In the instance of the steal syndrome, the blood flow to the brain, arm, or both is significantly reduced because of shunting of the blood from one area to the other. The area deprived will also have a decreased blood pressure.[2,3]

With use of the arm, there is related increased demand for blood to the arm. An attempt to meet this need causes a shunting of blood into the brachial circulation at the expense of the basilar-vertebral circulation. This results in the development of cerebrovascular signs and symptoms. If the increased demand for blood in the arm cannot be met, the patient will develop brachial symptoms such as claudication and decreased blood pressure. Retrograde vertebral blood flow is the result of a negative pressure gradient between the vertebral-basilar artery junction and the vertebral-subclavian artery junction. Any hemodynamic changes such as systemic hypertension that will increase the pressure gradient between the basilar and subclavian artery increase the possibility of reversed vertebral blood flow on the affected side.

Signs and Symptoms

The most prominent diagnostic feature of subclavian steal syndrome is the inequality of blood pressure or decreased pulse in one of the upper extremities. Some patients may be completely asymptomatic. When cerebrovascular symptoms are present, they are related to vertebral-basilar insufficiency. These signs and symptoms include vertigo, headache, visual deficits, unconsciousness, dizziness, syncope, ataxia, and motor deficits. A small percentage of patients will present signs and symptoms of brachial ischemia, which include paresthesias, weakness, and feelings of coldness in the arm. Regardless of the signs and symptoms that develop, they are of short duration, lasting a few seconds or minutes or, occasionally, a few days. As the atherosclerosis develops, occluding more and more of the vessel, symptoms develop progressively.

Diagnosis

The diagnosis of subclavian steal syndrome is often difficult to make because the atherosclerosis is usually widespread, mimicking several other vascular disorders such as aortic valve stenosis, anomalous arterial vessel syndrome, arterial stenosis, and labyrinthine disorders.

A simple, noninvasive technique, recording bilateral arm blood pressure, serves as a means for screening patients. A difference of 20 mm Hg between the arms is considered significant. Variations ranging from 10 mm to 180 mm Hg between the arms have been cited in some studies.[4] In some patients the blood pressure in the affected arm is not audible. The major tool for diagnosis of the subclavian steal syndrome is aortic arch and cerebral angiography.

Medical Management

The asymptomatic patient is followed medically. It is generally accepted that generalized atherosclerosis is present. Measures for controlling the risk factors associated with atherosclerosis such as weight reduction, low-sodium diet, control of hypertension, elimination of smoking, institution of a moderate exercise program, and stress control should be included in a patient education program.[2] The patient should also be aware of the signs and symptoms of progressive occlusion. Periodic medical evaluations should be scheduled, and the physician should be notified immediately if any signs and symptoms associated with vascular insufficiency develop.

In the symptomatic patient, surgical intervention is usually necessary although, in some instances, medical management of hypertension will ameliorate the "steal" of blood from the subclavian artery. The goal of surgery is to eliminate the "steal" of blood and restore the antegrade flow of blood in the vertebral artery to relieve transient ischemic attacks and arm symptoms, prevent stroke, and reverse minor neurological deficits.[2] Surgical approaches have included vertebral artery ligation, subclavian endarterectomy, and extrathoracic revascularization procedures (proximal end-to-side vertebral to common carotid artery transposition).[5] The most successful approach is the extrathoracic revascularization procedures because of easy surgical accessibility and the use of local or limited general anesthesia.

CHART 23–1. (continued)

Nursing Management

The nurse may be the first health professional to uncover data suspicious of subclavian steal syndrome. While assessing the patient, differences in bilateral blood pressure may be noted, a finding that is consistent with the steal syndrome. Differences in the quality of the bilateral radial pulses are often noted. Any patient admitted with signs and symptoms of vertebral–basilar insufficiency (*e.g.,* transient ischemic attacks, dizziness, syncope) should be assessed and a careful history taken. Often, the patient is hypertensive. Careful documentation of these findings and frequent ongoing assessment of vital signs (bilateral blood pressure in the arms and bilateral radial pulses), neurological signs, and arm symptoms should be incorporated into the nursing care plan. Along with drug therapy that the physician orders, the nurse will be responsible for developing and implementing a patient teaching plan based on a detailed assessment of the patient's lifestyle and health habits.

If surgery is planned, the patient will need preoperative teaching for the particular procedure. In the postoperative period, the nurse is responsible for continuing to monitor the vital and neurological signs, assessing ischemic responses in the arms, and noting any other vascular deficits. Reinforcement of the patient teaching plan should be included because these patients usually have generalized atherosclerosis, which has implications for their future health.

(see Chap. 25), and hemorrhage precipitated by bleeding disorders.

The hypertensive hemorrhagic stroke is associated with grossly elevated blood pressure. Because of continued pressure on the artery, the vessel ruptures, with bleeding into the brain tissue. Initially, there is no bleeding into the subarachnoid space. However, as the clot enlarges from continued bleeding, there is seepage into the ventricular system in approximately 90% of patients. If the blood pressure were not so grossly elevated, it would be possible for a clot to form at the rupture site and seal off the vessel; however, because the pressure is so high, the force behind the clot is too great to allow the ruptured vessel to be sealed. The intracerebral clot displaces and compresses the adjacent cerebral tissue, resulting in increased intracranial pressure. A major bleeding episode can cause midline displacement, brain stem herniation, and death.

Hemorrhage can be described as massive to petechial in character. Fifty cubic centimeters or more of blood would constitute a major hemorrhage in the cerebrum and would probably result in death. In 50% of hemorrhagic strokes, the site of bleeding is the putamen, with extension into the internal capsule. The other areas most often affected include various areas of the central white matter, the thalamus, the cerebellar hemisphere, and the pons.[1]

Hemorrhagic strokes occur rapidly, with steady development of symptoms over minutes or hours (with an average of 1 to 24 hours). Usually there are no warning signs. Symptoms persist until the clot is absorbed, which takes from weeks to months. With major hemorrhage, many patients lapse into a deep coma and die. About 30% of intracerebral bleeding episodes are less massive, thereby making survival possible.

With hemorrhage some patients may experience some or all of the following symptoms: severe headache, nuchal rigidity, vomiting, focal seizures, hemiplegia, and unconsciousness.

SIGNS AND SYMPTOMS OF STROKE ACCORDING TO THE INVOLVED AREA

Presenting signs and symptoms will depend on the extent and location of the insult. When a cerebral artery is occluded by a thrombus or embolus, classical syndromes are said to develop, although in reality syndromes frequently overlap one another rather than appearing in the "pure" form.

MIDDLE CEREBRAL ARTERY SYNDROME

Middle cerebral artery syndrome is by far the most common of all cerebral occlusions. If the main stem of the middle cerebral artery is occluded, a massive infarction of most of the hemisphere results. Initially, there may be vomiting and a rapid onset of coma, which may last a few weeks. Cerebral edema is extensive.

Symptoms of middle cerebral artery syndrome include

- Hemiplegia (face, arm, and leg flaccidity on contralateral side)
- Sensory impairment (same area as hemiplegia)
- Aphasia (global aphasia if dominant hemisphere is involved)
- Homonymous hemianopsia
- Confusion to coma (deterioration in the level of consciousness)
- Inability to turn the eyes toward the paralyzed side
- Denial of paralysis or lack of recognition of the paralyzed limb
- Possible Gerstmann's syndrome (acalculia, alexia, finger agnosia, and left–right confusion)
- Possible Cheyne–Stokes respirations
- Headache
- Vasomotor paresis

ANTERIOR CEREBRAL ARTERY SYNDROME

The anterior cerebral artery is least often occluded, so that the associated syndrome is not common. If the occlusion occurs proximal to a patent anterior communicating artery, the blood supply will not be compromised. If the occlusion is distal or the communicating artery is inadequate, there will be infarction of the medial aspect of one frontal lobe. Bilateral medial frontal lobe infarction will occur if one anterior cerebral artery is occluded and if the other artery is small and dependent on gross flow.

Symptoms of anterior cerebral artery syndrome (unilateral infarction) include the following (note that aphasia and hemianopsia are not part of the profile):

- Paralysis of the contralateral foot and leg (footdrop a constant finding)
- Impaired gait (contributes to the problem of walking)
- Paresis of the contralateral arm
- Contralateral grasp reflex and sucking reflex may be present
- Sensory loss over the toes, foot, and leg
- Abulia (inability to perform acts voluntarily or make decisions)
- Flat affect, lack of spontaneity, slowness, distractability, and lack of interest in surroundings
- Mental impairment such as perseveration and amnesia
- Cerebral paraplegia (with bilateral involvement), often combined with ataxia and akinetic mutism
- Urinary incontinence (usually lasts for weeks)

POSTERIOR CEREBRAL ARTERY SYNDROME

Approximately 3% of cerebral occlusions occur in the posterior cerebral artery. The usual consequence of the superficial occlusion (peripheral areas) of a posterior cerebral artery is contralateral homonymous hemianopsia. If the penetrating branches (central areas) are occluded, the cerebral peduncle, thalamus, and upper brain stem are involved. There is wide variation in the manifestations of the syndrome.

Symptoms of posterior cerebral artery syndrome include

Peripheral Area

- Homonymous hemianopsia
- Several visual deficits such as color blindness, lack of depth perception, failure to see objects not centrally located, visual hallucinations, and so forth
- Memory deficits
- Perseveration

Central Area

- If the thalamus is involved, there will be sensory loss of all modalities, spontaneous pain, intentional tremors, and mild hemiparesis.
- If the cerebral peduncle is involved, there will be Weber's syndrome (oculomotor nerve palsy with contralateral hemiplegia).
- If the brain stem is involved, there will be deficits of conjugate gaze, nystagmus, and pupillary abnormalities, with the other possible symptoms of ataxia and postural tremors.

INTERNAL CAROTID ARTERY SYNDROME

The patient who has an occlusion of an internal carotid artery may be completely asymptomatic because of efficient anastomotic circulation. Symptoms of the internal carotid artery syndrome sometimes mimic those of main stem middle cerebral artery occlusion.

When there is a difference in carotid and middle cerebral syndromes, it is in the involvement of the anterior and ophthalmic arteries and sometimes the posterior cerebral artery.

Symptoms of the typical internal carotid artery syndrome include the following:

- Repeated attacks of blindness or visual blurring in the ipsilateral eye
- Paresthesia and episodes of weakness the contralateral arm, face, and leg (only parts of the arm may be involved)
- Eventual complete hemiplegia with sensory loss and hemianopsia
- Possible optic nerve atrophy in the ipsilateral eye
- Intermittent dysphasia

POSTERIOR INFERIOR CEREBELLAR ARTERY SYNDROME (WALLENBERG'S SYNDROME)

Posterior inferior cerebellar artery syndrome involves the lateral portion of the medulla because of the occlusion of the posterior inferior cerebellar artery.

Symptoms include

- Dysphagia and dysarthria
- Loss of pain and temperature sensation on ipsilateral side of the face
- Loss of pain and temperature sensation on contralateral side of the trunk and limbs
- Horizontal nystagmus
- Ipsilateral Horner's syndrome
- Cerebellar signs (ataxia and vertigo)

ANTERIOR INFERIOR CEREBELLAR ARTERY SYNDROME

Occlusion of the anterior inferior cerebellar artery is also known as the lateral inferior pontine syndrome.

Symptoms of the anterior inferior cerebellar artery syndrome include

Ipsilateral Side

- Deafness and tinnitus
- Facial paralysis
- Loss of facial tactile sensation
- Horner's syndrome
- Cerebellar signs (ataxia, nystagmus)

Contralateral Side

- Impaired pain and temperature sensation of trunk and limbs (may also involve face)
- Horizontal nystagmus

SUMMARY OF DEFICITS INCURRED WITH STROKE SYNDROME

A stroke syndrome is a form of cerebral injury. The injury to the brain results from a ruptured blood vessel in the case of hemorrhagic stroke or from ischemia that develops either over time or suddenly, as may be the case in thrombotic or embolic strokes. In all cases of stroke syndrome, areas of the brain are deprived of an adequate oxygen supply. If the blood supply is cut off for an extended period, the involved cerebral tissue may become necrotic, resulting in permanent neurological deficits. In instances of ischemia, temporary neurological impairment may result. Similar hemodynamic changes occur with other forms of cerebral injury such as head injuries, cerebral aneurysms, or cerebral edema.

The particular type and degree of neurological deficits depend on the particular area of the brain involved. Because the brain is composed of the most highly specialized tissue in the body, the deficits incurred will depend on the area compromised. (The common deficits seen in the stroke patient are summarized in Chart 23-2. The rehabilitation and management of the deficits are discussed in Chap. 8.)

GENERAL DISABILITIES WITH LEFT- AND RIGHT-SIDED HEMIPLEGIA

In predicting the type of disabilities incurred from stroke, knowledge of "handedness" and the side of the brain in which the stroke occurred is helpful. "Handedness" refers to the preference for use of one hand over the other. Ninety-three percent of the population is right-handed. This means that their dominant cerebral hemisphere is on the left. Of the 7% of the population who are left-handed, about 60% have their dominant speech center located in the left hemisphere, just as right-handed people do.

Based on this information, certain generalizations can be made about the deficits experienced by left- and right-sided hemiplegics. This information is listed in Table 23-1.

DIAGNOSIS

The diagnosis of stroke syndrome is made on the basis of history and physical inspection. It is important to identify the underlying cause because treatment protocols differ. Diagnostic procedures that may be ordered include computed tomography (CT) scan, brain scan, cerebral arteriography, digital subtraction angiography, lumbar puncture, and blood studies. Before using any diagnostic procedures, one must weigh the risks against the possible benefits of collecting valuable diagnostic data.

Thrombotic Stroke

With thrombotic stroke the CT scan will show necrotic areas in a few days, but lacunar infarctions* are usually too small to be identified. A brain scan will show major infarct areas but not as early as with the CT scan. The cerebral arteriogram is a definitive method of identifying arterial thrombosis or vascular narrowing. However, it should not be used indiscriminately because of the danger that a stroke could be extended by the use of this procedure.

Cerebrospinal fluid is clear, but protein may be elevated. Cerebrospinal fluid pressure can be elevated (> 200 mm of water pressure). Serum cholesterol or triglycerides are also elevated in thrombotic stroke.

EMBOLIC STROKE

Embolic stroke will be evident by CT scan, brain scan, or arteriogram. If the occlusion produces a hemorrhagic infarction, there may be blood in the cerebrospinal fluid. This would be important to know if anticoagulation therapy were contemplated. If the embolus were septic, an elevation in the white blood cell count of the cerebrospinal fluid would be present.

HEMORRHAGIC STROKE

With a hemorrhagic stroke the patient will most often have a grossly elevated blood pressure. The CT scan is effective in noting intracerebral bleeding, except for small areas such as a small pontine hemorrhage. Blood is usually found upon lumbar puncture, and the pressure is somewhat elevated (> 200 mm of water pressure). A shift on an echoencephalogram indicates a clot of sufficient size to shift midline structures.

MEDICAL MANAGEMENT OF THE PATIENT WITH A STROKE SYNDROME

When a stroke syndrome occurs, the medical management is directed toward (1) acute care management; (2) diagnosis of the type and cause of the stroke syndrome; (3) measures to restore cerebral circulation and control or reverse patho-

* A *lacunar infarction* is defined as softening areas of cerebral tissue ranging in diameter from 0.5 mm to 1.5 cm and caused by the occlusion of penetrating arteries, chiefly from middle cerebral, posterior cerebral, and basilar arteries supplying the basal ganglia or pons. As the softened tissue sloughs away, a small cavity or lacuna remains. There may be from four to six lacunae noted in a specimen, and as many as ten to fifteen may be found on occasion. The location of the lacunae will determine whether any signs or symptoms of neurological deficit will be experienced by the patient.

CHART 23-2. COMMON DEFICITS AND EMOTIONAL REACTION TO STROKE WITH GENERAL NURSING INTERVENTION

COMMON MOTOR DEFICITS	NURSING INTERVENTION
1. { Hemiplegia (side of the body opposite the cerebral episode) Hemiparesis (side of the body opposite the cerebral episode)	1. Position in proper body alignment, use a hand roll to keep the hand in functional position. • Provide frequent passive range-of-motion exercises. • Reposition every 2 hours.
2. Dysarthria (muscles of speech impaired)	2. Provide for an alternate method of communication.
3. Dysphagia (muscles of swallowing impaired)	3. Test the patient's palatal and pharyngeal reflexes before offering nourishment. • Elevate and turn the patient's head to the unaffected side. • If able to manage oral intake, place food on patient's unaffected side of mouth.

COMMON SENSORY DEFICITS	NURSING INTERVENTION
1. Visual deficits (common deficit because the visual pathways cut through much of the cerebral hemispheres)	1. Be aware that variations of visual deficits may exist.
a. Homonymous hemianopsia (loss of vision in half of the visual field on the same side) 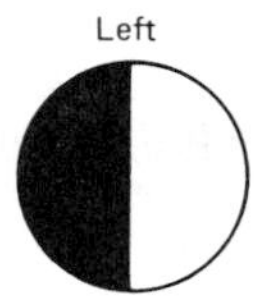 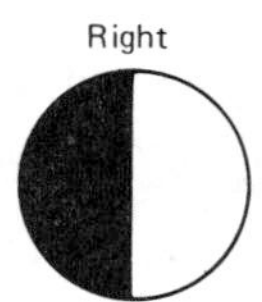	a. Approach patient from the unaffected side; remind patient to turn his head to compensate for visual deficits.
b. Double vision (diplopia)	b. Apply eye patch to affected eye.
c. Decreased visual acuity	c. Provide assistance as necessary.
2. Absent or diminished response to superficial sensation (touch, pain, pressure, heat, cold)	2. Increase the amount of touch in administering patient care. • Protect the involved areas from injury. • Protect the involved areas from burns. • Examine the involved areas for signs of skin irritation and injury. • Provide the patient with the opportunity to handle various objects of different weight, texture, and size. • If pain is present, assess location, type, and duration of pain.
3. Absent or diminished response to proprioception (knowledge of position of body parts)	3. Teach the patient to check the position of his body parts with his eyes.
4. Perceptual deficits (disturbance in correctly perceiving and interpreting himself and/or his environment)	
a. Body scheme disturbance (amnesia or denial for paralyzed extremities)	a. Protect the involved area. • Accept patient's perception of himself. • Position patient to face the involved area.
b. Disorientation (to time, place, and person)	b. Control the amount of change in patient's schedule. • Reorient the patient as necessary • Talk to patient; tell him about his environment. • Provide a calendar, clock, pictures of family, and so forth.
c. Apraxias (loss of ability to use objects correctly)	c. Correct misuse of objects and demonstrate proper use.
d. Agnosias (inability to identify the environment by means of the senses)	d. Correct misinformation.
e. Defects in localizing objects in space, estimating their size, and judging distance	e. Reduce any stimuli that will distract the patient.
f. Impaired memory for recall of spatial location of objects or places	f. Place necessary equipment where patient will see it, rather than telling the patient "It is in the closet" and so forth.
g. Right-left disorientation	g. Use terms like "Lift this leg." (Point to the leg.)

CHART 23–2. (continued)

LANGUAGE DEFICITS	NURSING INTERVENTION
1. Expressive aphasia (difficulty in transforming sound into patterns of understandable speech) Can speak in single-word responses	**1.** Ask patient to repeat individual sounds of alphabet as a start at retraining.
2. Receptive aphasia (impairment of comprehension of the spoken word) Able to speak, but uses words incorrectly and is unaware of these errors	**2.** Speak clearly and in simple sentences; use gestures as necessary.
3. Global aphasia (combination of expressive and receptive aphasia) Unable to communicate at any level	**3.** Evaluate what language skills are intact, speak in very simple sentences, ask patient to repeat individual sounds, and use gestures or any other means to communicate.
4. Alexia (inability to understand the written word)	**4.** Point to written names of objects and have the patient repeat the name of the object.
5. Agraphia (inability to express ideas in writing)	**5.** Have the patient write words and simple sentences.

INTELLECTUAL DEFICITS	NURSING INTERVENTION
1. Loss of memory	**1.** Provide necessary information as necessary.
2. Short attention span	**2.** Divide activities into short steps.
3. Easily distractible	**3.** Control any excessive environmental distractions.
4. Poor judgment	**4.** Protect patient from injury.
5. Inability to transfer learning from one situation to another	**5.** Repeat instructions as necessary.
6. Inability to calculate, reason, abstract	**6.** Do not set unrealistic expectations for patient.

EMOTIONAL DEFICITS	NURSING INTERVENTION
1. Emotional lability (exhibits reactions easily or inappropriately)	**1.** Disregard bursts of emotions; explain to the patient that emotional lability is part of the illness.
2. Loss of self-control and social inhibitions	**2.** Protect the patient as necessary so that his dignity is preserved.
3. Reduced tolerance to stress	**3.** Control the amount of stress experienced by the patient.
4. Fear, hostility, frustration, anger	**4.** Be accepting of the patient; be supportive.
5. Confusion and despair	**5.** Clarify any misconceptions; allow the patient to verbalize.
6. Withdrawal, isolation	**6.** Provide stimulation and a safe, comfortable environment.
7. Depression	**7.** Provide a supportive environment.

BOWEL AND BLADDER DYSFUNCTION	NURSING INTERVENTION
Bladder: Incomplete Upper Motor Neuron Lesion	Do not suggest insertion of an indwelling catheter immediately after the stroke.
1. Unilateral lesion from the stroke results in partial sensation and control of bladder so that the patient experiences frequency, urgency, and incontinence	**1.** Observe patient to identify characteristics of voiding pattern (frequency, amount, forceful, or constant dribbling).
2. If stroke lesion is in the brain stem, there will be bilateral damage, resulting in an upper motor neuron bladder with loss of all control of micturition.	**2.** Maintain accurate intake and output record.
	Nursing note: Incontinence after consciousness is usually due to urinary tract infection caused by a urinary catheter that has been in place.

(continued)

CHART 23–2. (continued)

BOWEL AND BLADDER DYSFUNCTION	NURSING INTERVENTION
3. Possibility of establishing normal bladder function is excellent	3. Try to allow patient to stay catheter-free: Offer the bedpan or urinal frequently. Take patient to the commode frequently. Assess patient's ability to make his need for help with voiding known. If a catheter is necessary, remove it as soon as possible and follow a bladder training program (see Chap. 8).
Bowel	
1. Impairment in stroke patient due to Deterioration in the level of consciousness Dehydration Immobility	1. Develop a bowel training program: Give foods known to stimulate defecation (prune juice, roughage) Initiate suppository and laxative regimen
2. Constipation most common problem with potential impaction	2. Institute a bowel program. Enemas are avoided in the presence of increased intracranial pressure.

logical processes; (4) a rehabilitation program; and (5) patient management and education to prevent future stroke syndromes.

ACUTE CARE MANAGEMENT

Basic support measures such as maintenance of vital signs (with oxygen therapy, intravenous fluids, drug therapy) and control of cerebral edema and subsequent increased intracranial pressure, if present, are instituted upon admission or as problems develop early in the hospitalization. The usual management of cerebral edema and increased intracranial pressure includes drug therapy (dexamethasone) and other measures outlined in Chapter 12. The patient is stabilized as quickly as possible so that a definitive diagnosis can be established.

TABLE 23–1. *Comparison of Signs and Symptoms Associated With Right-Sided and Left-Sided Hemiplegia*

Stroke Syndrome on Left Side of Brain—Right-Sided Hemiplegia	*Stroke Syndrome on Right Side of Brain—Left-Sided Hemiplegia*
• Expressive aphasia or	• Spatial–perceptual deficits
• Receptive aphasia or • Global asphasia	• Denial and deficits of affected side require special safety consideration • Tends to be distractible
• Intellectual impairment	• Impulsive behavior; appears to be unaware of deficits
• Slow and cautious behavior	• Poor judgment
• Defects in right visual fields	• Defects in left visual fields

DIAGNOSIS

It is important to establish the type of stroke syndrome present before instituting definitive treatment because certain treatment protocols, such as anticoagulation therapy used in thrombotic stroke, are contraindicated in hemorrhagic stroke. Although some diagnostic procedures such as cerebral angiography may be postponed until the patient's condition has improved, a differential diagnosis can usually be established based on criteria discussed in the section on diagnosis in this chapter.

MEASURES TO RESTORE CEREBRAL CIRCULATION AND CONTROL OR REVERSE PATHOLOGICAL PROCESSES

The medical management of the patient will depend on the type of process present. Therefore, transient ischemic attack and thrombotic stroke, embolic stroke, and hemorrhagic stroke will be discussed separately.

Transient Ischemic Attacks and Thrombotic Stroke

Once a thrombotic stroke has occurred, it may be too late to prevent irreversible neurological damage. Therefore, the emphasis is on preventing the process from developing by aggressively managing transient ischemic attacks. A transient ischemic attack is regarded as a warning sign of impending stroke caused by the occlusion of an intracranial or extracranial artery. This process is most often associated with atherosclerosis (atheromas). The most common sites of atherosclerosis in the extracranial arteries are at the bifurcation of the common carotid artery and also at the origins of the vertebral arteries. The middle cerebral artery is the most common site of atherosclerosis in the intracranial arterial system.

Drug Therapy. Drug therapy is used to improve and restore circulation to the brain. Anticoagulation drug therapy using heparin sodium followed by warfarin (Coumadin) or warfarin therapy alone is usually administered. The dosage of the drug is calculated based on the prothrombin activity time or the coagulation time. According to Adams and Victor, anticoagulant drugs are of no value in the fully developed stroke. Another drug category that prevents clotting by reducing platelet adhesiveness is antiplatelet drugs. Aspirin, 600 mg twice a day, dipyridamole (Persantin), 50 mg every 8 hours, and sulfinpyrazone (Anturane), 200 mg every 8 hours, are possible choices of drugs in this drug group.[1] Some physicians have also prescribed vasodilating drugs as a means of improving cerebral circulation, but this therapy is controversial because it tends to lower blood pressure.

In the hypertensive patient, the elevated blood pressure must be gradually reduced so that infarction does not develop from too rapid a lowering of pressure. In the patient who has sustained a thrombotic stroke, this is particularly important to observe because more areas of the brain could become infarcted with too rapid and aggressive a reduction of hypertension.

Surgical Procedures. Selected patients with extracranial or intracranial atherosclerotic disease that is located in accessible sites (areas previously mentioned) may be good candidates for surgery. The goal of the surgical procedure is to correct the condition directly predisposing the patient to transient ischemic attacks or stroke. Carotid endarterectomy or extracranial graft may benefit the patient with narrowing of the extracranial artery. A bypass grafting procedure may be of value for the patient with an intracranial occlusion such as internal carotid or middle cerebral artery occlusion. The procedure most often used for intracranial involvement is the superior temporal artery anastomosis to the middle cerebral artery (STA–MCA).

Not all patients with cerebral occlusive disease are good surgical candidates. The criteria for selection of patients is based on the neurological examination, history, and several diagnostic procedures, which include cerebral angiography, skull films, cerebral blood studies (especially noting the effectiveness of the autoregulatory mechanism), and the CT scan of the head and neck. In addition to these procedures, patients being evaluated for the STA–MCA anastomosis also need electroencephelogram, chest films, pulmonary and cardiac consultations, electrocardiogram, blood gases, coagulation time, and a serum lipoprotein profile. The presence of any major uncontrolled systemic disease is reason to reject a candidate for STA–MCA anastomosis.

Carotid Endarterectomy. A carotid endarterectomy of the internal carotid artery at the bifurcation of the internal and external carotid arteries consists of removal of the atheroma from the innermost lining of the artery after a temporary bypass shunt has been created to provide an adequate blood supply to the brain. The atheroma is removed after the artery is temporarily occluded both above and below the atheroma. Upon removal of the plaque, circulation is reestablished.

Nursing management after carotid endarterectomy includes frequent monitoring of neurological signs for evidence of neurological deficit as well as the usual postoperative nursing care. Many patients receive a continuous intravenous infusion with a mini-dose of heparin sodium, an anticoagulant, to prevent clot formation at the surgical site.

STA–MCA Anastomosis. A microneurosurgical bypass procedure that is used to provide collateral circulation to the areas of the brain supplied by the middle cerebral artery consists of the anastomosis of the superior temporal artery, a branch of the external carotid artery, to the middle cerebral artery. The desired result of an STA–MCA anastomosis is improved collateral circulation to the brain, thereby correcting the preoperative problem of transient ischemic attacks.

Postoperatively, the patient is admitted first to the surgical intensive care unit for 1 or 2 days, and then to the neurosurgical unit for another 5 to 10 days. The postoperative nursing management includes frequent assessment of vital and neurological signs. The neurological assessment provides for the detection of any developing deficits, which, in turn, suggest compromised cerebral blood flow or increased intracranial pressure. Another important parameter that is assessed each time the vital and neurological signs are assessed is the superior temporal artery pulse. This assessment checks the patency of the graft. The major complications of surgery are interruption of the blood flow through the graft, stroke, or subdural hematoma caused by bleeding at the surgical site. Therefore, the nurse must be alert for any neurological changes that are indicative of these complications.

The head of the bed is elevated to 30 degrees and the patient is kept from lying on the operative site. Initially, the patient will probably have in place a central venous line, intravenous infusion line, urinary catheter, cardiac monitor, and oxygen therapy equipment. In addition to the usual nursing management of the craniotomy patient, a continuous intravenous infusion with a minimal dose of heparin sodium to prevent clot formation at the surgical site may be instituted. In the postoperative period, the patient will be gradually changed to an oral anticoagulant, warfarin sodium (Coumadin). Some physicians prefer to administer antiplatelet drugs such as dipyridamole (Persantin) or aspirin rather than anticoagulants. There appears to be a trend toward the use of antiplatelet drugs.

Regardless of the drug chosen, the medication is usually continued for approximately 3 to 6 months after surgery. The patient will need periodic blood studies to monitor platelets or coagulation times.

Embolic Stroke

The onset of an embolic stroke is an acute and rapid event created by the movement of a thrombus to the cerebral circulation, thus obstructing the flow of blood to a selected area of the brain. The source of the thrombus is usually the heart. Because of the rapidity of onset, collateral circulation, such as that seen with thrombotic stroke, does not have time to develop. The key to management is prevention by the aggressive management of conditions known to precipitate emboli such as heart disease, recent cardiovascular surgery, vegetative exudate of acute bacterial endocarditis, and thrombophlebitis. Patients at risk should be on anticoagulation therapy and monitored frequently.

The stroke develops rapidly, becoming fully developed in a few minutes. Once an embolic stroke has developed and been diagnosed, anticoagulation therapy is instituted. In some instances when the site of the emboli can be confirmed and it is surgically accessible, an embolectomy may be performed. The surgery is scheduled as soon after the stroke episode as possible in the hope of reversing neurological deficits already present and preventing the extension of further cerebral injury.

Cerebral edema and increased intracranial pressure are managed by the protocols outlined in Chapter 12.

Hemorrhagic Stroke

A hemorrhagic stroke syndrome has many possible causes such as hypertensive intracranial hemorrhage, ruptured cerebral aneurysm, and arteriovenous malformations. The features of the stroke syndrome are similar regardless of etiology. The physician must correctly diagnose the type and cause of the stroke syndrome. Cerebral aneurysms and arteriovenous malformations will be discussed in Chapter 24. The hemorrhagic stroke syndrome to be considered in this chapter is one caused by hypertensive intracranial hemorrhage.

Hypertensive intracranial hemorrhage is caused by essential hypertension that has not been controlled. It has an abrupt onset with signs and symptoms gradually developing over minutes to hours. Severe headache and increased intracranial pressure develop and must be managed. A bloody lumbar puncture tap indicates a hemorrhagic episode. The presenting neurological signs and symptoms vary with the size and location of the hemorrhage. The control of the hypertension with drugs and the management of the increased intracranial pressure are the chief medical approaches to this patient.

As noted with the other types of stroke syndromes, prevention is the best approach. Control of essential hypertension with drug therapy and control of risk factors associated with stroke are the most effective deterrents to an actual stroke syndrome.

REHABILITATION PROGRAM

Once the patient is stabilized and the specific type of neurological deficit present has been determined, the focus of management is restoration of function. Although this may not be possible in all patients, a complete assessment and therapy program should be developed by the various health-team professionals. Depending on the deficits of the patient, he may need physical therapy, occupational therapy, speech therapy, and nutrition counselling. The role and focus of the rehabilitation process are outlined in Chapter 8. The quality of life for the patient and his family rests on the quality of the rehabilitation program offered to him.

PATIENT MANAGEMENT AND EDUCATION

Once the patient is discharged from the acute-care facility and is involved in a rehabilitation program, it is important for him to be followed by a physician in a private office or clinic. As the patient is managed for his current health problems, prevention of future stroke episodes can be stressed by control of risk factors and precipitating health problems. The physician may choose to provide the health counselling himself, or he may choose to refer the patient to the nurse for a formalized education program. Community resources such as the American Heart Association should be used to provide the patient's needs.

GENERAL NURSING MANAGEMENT

When the nursing management of cerebrovascular disease and stroke is planned, five areas should be considered:

1. Initial management during the acute phase
2. Maintenance of body functions and prevention of complications
3. Psychological needs
4. Rehabilitation within the hospital
5. Discharge planning

MANAGEMENT DURING THE ACUTE PHASE

The acute phase of a cerebrovascular accident generally applies to the period from admission until the patient is stabilized, which is usually the first 24 to 48 hours of hospitalization. However, the period may be longer in certain situations.

During this period, nursing activity is directed toward maintaining the patient's vital functions and helping him survive the cerebral assault. While initial diagnostic procedures may be carried out, some studies may be postponed until the patient is more stable.

Because the patient has undoubtedly suffered a change in the level of consciousness and is frequently unconscious, special management is necessary to stabilize and maintain him. Any patient with subarachnoid hemorrhage should be maintained on subarachnoid precautions, as described in Chapter 24. Nursing management of the unconscious patient is outlined in Chapter 11.

The quality of the initial nursing management will have a major influence on the outcome for the patient in terms of complications and permanent disabilities. Even relatively minor complications can lead to major ones that can, in turn, threaten the patient's life. It is therefore important to manage the patient aggressively to prevent the development of any and all potential threats. The main points of

CHART 23-3. NURSING CARE OF THE PATIENT WITH A STROKE

NURSING RESPONSIBILITIES	RATIONALE
Acute Phase	
1. Maintain a patent airway, administer oxygen as ordered, and position the patient on his side.	1. Provides for adequate oxygenation. An airway, endotracheal or tracheostomy, may have been inserted. Position on side to prevent aspiration.
2. Remove secretions from airway. Precautions should be taken to avoid prolonged suctioning (> 15 seconds), which would increase intracranial pressure.	2. If the patient cannot manage his own secretions, suction as necessary.
3. Monitor respiratory function by auscultating, measuring arterial gases, and observing chest movement.	3. Pneumonia, atelectasis, and other respiratory problems can easily develop.
4. Carry out frequent assessment of vital signs.	4. Provides a baseline assessment and can indicate development of increased intracranial pressure, respiratory or cardiac decompensation (elevated intracranial pressure, elevated blood pressure, lowered pulse), widening pulse pressure, tachycardia, thready pulse, and elevated respirations
5. Carry out frequent assessment of neurological signs • Level of consciousness • Pupillary signs • Motor and sensory function • Eye movement • Cranial nerves • Reflexes	5. Indicates baseline and subsequent changes in patient's condition; deficits can be identified and monitored and special nursing management can be planned and implemented
6. Monitor urinary function. (A Foley catheter is usually inserted.)	6. Measure output routinely and maintain an intake and output record.
7. Evaluate fluid and electrolyte balance by maintaining intake and output record and reviewing blood chemistry for electrolytes.	7. Provides quantitative data to assess function • Potassium: 3.5 mEq to 5.0 mEq/liter • Sodium: 135 mEq to 145 mEq/liter • Chlorides: 96 mEq to 105 mEq/liter
8. Review other diagnostic studies such as electrocardiogram report, urinalysis, and so forth.	8. Provides both quantitative and qualitative data of function
9. Establish seizure precautions as necessary (see Chap. 27).	9. Provides for safe management if seizure activity occurs
10. If the patient is unconscious, incorporate points of care outlined in Chapter 11.	10. Provides a standard of care necessary for the unconscious patient
Postacute Phase	
1. Provide routine hygienic care as necessary.	1. Maintains cleanliness and, therefore, supports self-esteem
2. Carry out routine monitoring of vital and neurological signs.	2. Provides baseline assessment and comparative data to denote change
Neurological Signs • Level of consciousness • Pupillary signs • Motor and sensory function • Eye movement • Cranial nerves • Reflexes	
Vital Signs • Blood pressure • Pulse • Respiratory function	
3. Carry out passive range-of-motion exercises four times daily to all joints.	3. Maintains muscle tone and prevents musculoskeletal deformities

(continued)

CHART 23–3. (continued)

NURSING RESPONSIBILITIES	RATIONALE
4. Give skin care every 4 hours.	4. Inspect skin for redness, irritation, and breakdown. (A broken area on the heel can postpone gait retraining for months, thus greatly compromising the rehabilitative potential of the patient.)
5. Position every 2 hours with the hand higher than the elbow and the elbow elevated.	5. Prevents development of contractures and dependent edema in extremities. Use support devices (splints, as necessary).
6. Turn every 2 hours.	6. Prevents pressure on the same skin area and improves respiratory function
7. Elevate the head of the bed 30 degrees.	7. Aids in venous drainage from the brain, thus controlling the increased intracranial pressure
8. Maintain patent airway and remove secretions. If patient is able to cough and deep breathe, encourage this every hour; if patient is unable, use suction, intermittent positive pressure breathing (IPPB), and chest physical therapy to control secretions.	8. Provides for adequate oxygenation; prevents a buildup of carbon dioxide, a potent cerebral dilator that would increase intracranial pressure; and prevents the development of respiratory complications.
9. Apply elastic stockings.	9. Prevents thrombus and embolus formation in the legs
10. Initiate a bowel program (stool softeners and so forth).	10. Prevents straining at stool and initiation of the Valsalva maneuver
11. Maintain an intake and output record to assess kidney function and hydration level.	11. Provides a good indication of fluid and electrolyte balance
12. Attend to catheter care twice a day (if present) • Wash perineal area • Apply bacteriostatic ointment to urinary meatus • Pin catheter to prevent traction on catheter	12. Prevents bladder infection, which would postpone bladder retraining
13. Institute a bladder retraining program at the proper time (see Chap. 8).	13. Decreases possibility of bladder infection and increases independence
14. When the patient is conscious, evaluate ability to swallow by checking the palatal and swallowing reflexes.	14. Prevents aspiration of oral intake
15. Evaluate communication system for both expressive and receptive aphasia by talking to the patient and evaluating his responses and questions.	15. Aids in planning alternate method of communication and identifies deficits
16. Adjust communications to those appropriate for the patient's deficits (*e.g.,* speak slowly in a normal voice, listen carefully, explain procedures, and so forth).	16. Provides for environmental stimulation; decreases frustration and confusion
17. Provide for reality orientation with calendar, radio, and family picture, noting activity in patient's environment.	17. Aids in reorientation of confused patient
18. Evaluate vision and visual field deficits such as diplopia and homonymous hemianopia.	18. Nursing care can be planned to compensate for visual deficiencies by approaching patient from the unaffected side, placing all necessary equipment in visual field, and telling patient to turn his head to compensate for limited visual field.
19. Provide eye care as necessary; protect from injury; lubricate.	19. Prevents infections and corneal abrasions
20. Institute seizure precautions as necessary (see Chap. 27).	20. Depending on the type of stroke, seizure activity may be a part of the stroke syndrome.
21. Enhance intact body image by positioning patient *facing paralyzed extremity* if there is denial of paralyzed side of the body. Maintain attractive personal appearance of patient.	21. Improves self-concept and body image, thus decreasing possibility of depression
22. Provide for nutritional needs (low-salt diet may be ordered if fluid retention or hypertension are present). Provide for adequate nutrition.	22. Therapeutic diet may be ordered to control hypertension and edema. Prevents dehydration, constipation, and so forth

CHART 23–3. (continued)

NURSING RESPONSIBILITIES	RATIONALE
23. Observe patient for any complications such as paralytic ileus, infection, pulmonary embolus, myocardial infarction (hydrocephalus in hemorrhagic stroke), and so forth.	**23.** Definitive action can be promptly instituted.
24. Monitor other identified diseases and conditions such as diabetes mellitus, obesity, hypertension, subacute endocarditis, arterial fibrillation, and so forth.	**24.** Such conditions increase the risk of complications and another stroke.
25. Review laboratory data to note abnormalities (blood urea nitrogen, hemoglobin, sodium, potassium, chloride).	**25.** Definitive action can be instituted if abnormality is noted.

care are directed at maintaining a patent airway and monitoring both vital and neurological signs until the patient's condition stabilizes. The details of nursing care during this acute phase are outlined in Chart 23–3.

Chart 23–4 summarizes the common nursing diagnoses made for a patient with a cerebral vascular accident.

MAINTENANCE OF BODY FUNCTIONS AND PREVENTION OF COMPLICATIONS

Once the patient's condition has stabilized, nursing management shifts to the postacute phase of care, which is aimed at maintaining body function and avoiding complications so that the patient will be in the best possible condition for a rehabilitative program (see Chart 23–3). It should be recalled that the patient has an increase in intracranial pressure because of cerebral edema and possibly a hematoma if there has been intracerebral bleeding. The nursing protocols for managing increased intracranial pressure must be incorporated into the nursing care plan. Such measures include limiting suctioning to 15 seconds, elevating the head of the bed 30 degrees, and limiting fluid intake to a specific amount in a 24-hour period (see Chapter 12). Subarachnoid precautions are continued during the subacute phase for any patient who has sustained a subarachnoid hemorrhage (see Chapter 24).

PSYCHOLOGICAL NEEDS

Although the psychosocial aspects of care are an integral part of the nursing care plan, an overview of the wide range of behavioral and emotional deficits experienced with a stroke will be helpful. Stroke patients will behave differently depending on the area of the brain affected. There may also be a pattern of inconsistency in the degree and frequency of deficits; that is, the patient may have good days and bad days, or even good hours and bad hours. Although there is a wide range of possibilities in behavioral and intellectual abilities, a few general classifications of deficits can be identified.

Deficits can be categorized as emotional lability (reacts quickly and inappropriately to stimuli), loss of self-control, and reduced tolerance for any type of stress. The deficits that a particular patient will experience depend on the area and extent of cerebral injury and the prestroke personality. These deficits can be augmented or minimized depending on how the nurse and others approach the patient.

Emotional lability refers to emotional instability, resulting in inappropriate responses. For example, the patient may weep profusely after a nurse hands him a glass of water, stating that the nurses are so good to him but that he has no money to pay for it. Although the patient may comment that he doesn't know why he is crying, he has no control over his emotions.

Loss of self-control can be described as the loss of social restraint and cultural norms of behavior. The patient may swear, expose himself, or make advances toward the nursing staff. He may make fun of other patients in the room.

When a person's tolerance to stress is reduced, any stimuli, no matter how light or benevolent, can be perceived inappropriately. For example, a patient who cannot reach the box of tissues on his bedside stand may scream and throw things. If his family arrives 5 minutes after visiting hours start, he sulks and won't speak to them.

Initially after a stroke, there is some change in the level of consciousness. The patient may have periods of confusion. Confusion, in addition to sensory, perceptual, and intellectual disabilities, creates distorted stimuli. The responses generated by the patient reflect all of these deficits as well as emotional deficits. The patient also experiences sensory and social deprivation and may be deprived of speech. The body image and self-concept are greatly altered.

The patient reacts to these assaults by demonstrating behavior identified as fearful, hostile, frustrated, withdrawn, negative, and depressed.

The Nurse's Role in Providing Emotional and Psychological Support

The following points serve as general principles to guide the nurse in supporting the patient.

1. Reassure the patient and family that the behavior is caused by the brain injury and that it is not intentional. The behavioral deficits will improve with time.
2. Ignore behavior such as swearing or exposure. If the patient has exposed himself, simply cover him.

CHART 23-4. SUMMARY OF COMMON NURSING DIAGNOSES FOR THE PATIENT WITH A CEREBROVASCULAR ACCIDENT*

NURSING DIAGNOSES (Potential or Actual)	EXPECTED OUTCOMES	NURSING INTERVENTIONS
Ineffective airway clearance due to unconsciousness or cough reflex dysfunction	• Airway will be patent, allowing for increased air exchange. • Decreased risk of aspiration • Decreased risk of elevated CO_2, which contributes to cerebral hypoxia and cerebral edema	• Position to facilitate drainage of oropharyngeal secretions; turn from side to side every 2 hours. • Elevate the head of the bed to 30 degrees. • Clear secretions from airway with suction, as necessary. • Provide for chest physical therapy. • Provide for coughing and deep breathing exercises. • If patient is receiving oxygen therapy, be sure that it is adequately humidified.
Alteration in respiratory function related to cerebral edema, ischemia of vital centers, or primary injury to vital centers	• Adequate respiratory function • Adequate oxygen supply to the brain	• Assess respiratory function by —Auscultating the chest for breath sounds —Noting characteristics of respiratory pattern —Observing chest movement —Checking vital capacity and blood gases —Monitoring vital signs • Note contributing factors that alter respiratory function (*e.g.,* a cold, smoking). • Note signs and symptoms of respiratory distress. • Administer oxygen therapy and ventilator support as ordered.
Ineffective breathing pattern due to increased intracranial pressure or injury to respiratory center	• Decrease the work of breathing and support an effective respiratory rate and gas exchange.	• Note anxiety in the use of auxiliary muscles of breathing. • Administer oxygen therapy and ventilator support as ordered.
Impaired gas exchange due to partial airway obstruction	• Preserve pulmonary function.	• Provide for periodic pulmonary hygiene. • Adjust activity level to enhance gas exchange. • Administer supplemental oxygen therapy as ordered. • Control increased intracranial pressure to support oxygen to the brain.
Increased intracranial pressure due to cerebral insult	• Early identification and management of intracranial pressure	• Establish a baseline and continue to monitor neurological signs to identify increased intracranial pressure. • Institute nursing measures to control development of increased intracranial pressure (see Chap. 12).
Potential of seizure activity due to cerebral irritation	• If seizures occur, patient will not sustain injury.	• Maintain on seizure precautions. • Assess for possible seizure activity (*e.g.,* prodromal signs).

CHART 23–4. (continued)

NURSING DIAGNOSES (Potential or Actual)	EXPECTED OUTCOMES	NURSING INTERVENTIONS
Altered urinary elimination pattern (incontinence) due to cerebral injury/altered level of consciousness/motor impairment	• An adequate urinary elimination pattern will be established. • Incontinence will be eliminated or reduced.	• Assess for contributing factors. • Measure urinary output routinely and maintain on an intake and output record. • Monitor urinalyses and urine cultures to identify urinary tract infections. • Provide a bladder retraining program as soon as possible. • Provide perineal care four times daily.
Altered bowel elimination pattern (constipation) due to cerebral injury/altered level of consciousness/motor impairment	• An adequate bowel elimination pattern will be established. • Constipation will be eliminated; straining at stool or constipation increase intracranial pressure; this will be avoided.	• Assess premorbid bowel elimination pattern. • Assess bowel sounds. • Assess fluid intake and presence of dehydration. • Begin a bowel program. • Prevent straining at stool.
Alterations in fluid and electrolyte balance related to altered level of consciousness/motor deficits	• Fluid and electrolyte balance will be maintained.	• Assess for dehydration, fluid overload, and electrolyte imbalance by —Clinical inspection —Laboratory data. • Maintain on fluid restriction, if ordered, to control intracranial pressure. • Monitor intake and output record.
Altered nutrition due to inability to consume an adequate amount of food	• Adequate nutrition will be maintained.	• Assess caloric intake. • Monitor weight periodically (*e.g.*, twice a week).
Potential of injury due to poor judgment and/or neurological deficits	• Use safety measures to prevent injury. • Reduce or eliminate factors causing or contributing to injury.	• Orient patient to his surroundings. • Provide patient with his glasses and/or hearing aid. • Provide proper lighting. • Assist with ambulation, as necessary. • Remove hazards from the area.
Impaired physical mobility due to neurological deficits	• Alternate methods of mobility will be provided. • Passive movement will be provided to prevent the negative effects that immobility has on the nervous system.	• Assess the type and degree of impairment. • Provide slings, braces, support shoes, and so forth, as necessary. • Teach patient alternate methods of mobility. • Provide for range-of-motion exercises four times per day.
Impaired skin integrity due to immobility/altered blood supply to the area	• Skin integrity will be maintained.	• Assess skin for redness or signs of breakdown. • Massage reddened areas. • Turn and reposition every 2 hours. • Provide skin care every 4 hours.
Altered venous return/possibility of pulmonary emboli due to immobility	• Venous return to the heart will be supported.	• Apply Ace bandages or elastic stockings to the legs. • Assess for signs and symptoms of thrombophlebitis/venous stasis.
Sleep-pattern disturbance due to cerebral injury	• An adequate sleep–wakefulness pattern will be established that meets the patient's requirement for sleep.	• Assess sleep–wakefulness pattern. • Assess sleep requirement. • Provide for an environment conducive to sleep. • Provide for comfort measures to induce sleep.

(continued)

CHART 23–4. (continued)

NURSING DIAGNOSES (Potential or Actual)	EXPECTED OUTCOMES	NURSING INTERVENTIONS
Self-care deficits due to altered level of consciousness	• Self-care needs will be provided or an alternate method of achieving these activities will be established.	• Assess patient's ability to provide for his own self-care needs. • Develop alternate methods to perform activities of daily living. • Provide for needs that the patient cannot accomplish for himself (hygiene, eating, toileting).
Communications impairment due to cerebral injury/altered level of consciousness	• An alternate method of communications will be established. • Support the patient's attempts to communicate.	• Assess type of communication deficit present. • Develop appropriate methods for communications.
Sexual dysfunction due to altered libido or neurological deficits	• The patient's sexuality will be supported.	• Assess sexuality needs. • Discuss sexuality changes with the patient. • Support the patient's sexuality.
Alterations in thought processes due to cerebral injury/altered level of consciousness	• The patient will be able to: —Differentiate between reality and fantasy —Understand and explain the rationale for treatment	• Assess type and degree of alterations. • Protect the patient from injury, humiliation, and embarrassment. • Control the environment as necessary.
Sensory–perceptual alterations due to cerebral injury (particularly if lesion is on the right side of the brain)	• Optimal contact and sensory input will be experienced.	• Assess type(s) and degree of sensory–perceptual deficit(s). • Provide added sensory stimulation. • Prevent injury to involved body parts. • Assist patient as necessary.
Knowledge deficit due to cerebral injury/altered level of consciousness	• Necessary information will be provided in a manner that is understandable to the patient.	• Assess degree and type of knowledge deficit. • Provide information as necessary. • Correct misinformation. • Anticipate the need for more information.
Emotional–psychological responses to stroke include fear; ineffective coping; anxiety; grieving; social isolation; altered self-concept; or powerlessness due to presence of neurological deficits	• The specific emotional–psychological response(s) will be identified and managed appropriately.	• Assess for presence of these responses. • Identify the underlying cause. • Develop nursing strategies to manage the problem.

* For nursing diagnoses related to unconsciousness, see Chapter 11.

3. Control the environment by reducing or removing stimuli that are upsetting to the patient.
4. Anticipate the patient's needs to decrease his frustration.
5. Provide positive feedback for the patient's accomplishments.
6. Encourage the patient to relearn skills by encouraging him and breaking the task down into small steps.
7. Provide for reality orientation (orient to time, place, and person) and reorient as necessary.
8. Explain emotional deficits to the family. Be supportive.
9. Because most patients are easily distractible, unacceptable behavior can sometimes be controlled by distracting the patient to a more productive activity.
10. Repetition is necessary because many patients have difficulty in transferring learning to similar situations.

Because the behavior manifestations demonstrated by a patient depend on the particular part of the brain injured, the scope of possible behavior is varied. It is therefore impossible to generalize about expected behaviors. Based on an individual assessment, the nurse can plan an approach to the patient.

REHABILITATION WITHIN THE HOSPITAL

Rehabilitation within the hospital requires a systematic assessment and evaluation of the patient's deficits and intact functions. Based on this data, a team conference should be convened so that a comprehensive rehabilitative program can be formulated. The core members of the team include the physician, nurse, physical therapist, and social worker. Assistance from other specialists, such as the dietitian, psychologist, psychiatrist, and vocational counselor, may be necessary depending on the needs of the particular patient. Nursing responsibilities in the rehabilitation process are outlined in Chart 23–5.

The focus of care is directed at helping the patient relearn lost skills so that he can regain as much independence as possible. In some hospitals the patient may be sent to the stroke unit for rehabilitation. In other hospitals, he will remain on the same unit to which he was originally admitted. Although the focus in this phase is on rehabilitation, the patient is monitored carefully for the development of any complications.

Before gait retraining can begin, muscle strength must be regained. Simple quadriceps and gluteal setting exercises are valuable for this purpose and will help augment the exercise program that is initiated by the physical therapist.

Sitting balance must be established before one can regain standing balance. To achieve this aim, the head of the bed is gradually raised to determine the presence of any vasomotor deficits that could cause a change in vital signs (elevated pulse, lowered blood pressure) or dizziness.

Standing balance will probably require the use of support devices such as a walker, four-point cane, or a brace. Braces, splints, or slings should be applied first to help the patient maintain his center of gravity. See Chapter 8 for a discussion of rehabilitation.

The patient and family must be well aware of the plan and goals of the rehabilitative phase. Their active participation is encouraged and is absolutely necessary for optimum success. The nurse must provide much support and positive feedback so that the patient will not be too discouraged. Unlike recovery from some illnesses, recovery from a stroke is a slow process. There are many excellent publications available through the American Heart Association that are written for both lay and health professionals about stroke and rehabilitation. This literature can be a valuable aid for the patient and family.

DISCHARGE PLANNING

Discharge planning, although listed last, is taken into account early in the rehabilitative program. It begins upon admission, when information is being gathered about family, living situation, and patient needs. The process is formalized and intensified as the patient's condition stabilizes and his rehabilitative potential and needs are determined. The family situation must be realistically evaluated by the health team. The social worker, in conjunction with the nurse and physician, is able to gather information from the family. Because each patient and family are unique, the degree to which the family can participate in the program will vary from family to family.

Once the patient's needs are determined, it must be decided where and how the needed care can best be provided. For some, the needs are so great that a nursing home or rehabilitation hospital is the best choice. For others, the family can manage well with the help of community ser-

CHART 23–5. REHABILITATION MEASURES FOLLOWING STROKE

NURSING RESPONSIBILITIES	RATIONALE
1. Encourage the patient to do as much of his own personal hygiene as possible.	1. Increases independence
2. Teach the activities of daily living (ADL) with respect to ways to compensate for the patient's disability. (ADL includes dressing, toileting, bathing, eating, gait training, and so forth.)	2. Provides for alternate methods to overcome disability and increases the patient's level of independence
3. Instruct the patient in bed exercises such as quadriceps and gluteal setting.	3. Improves muscle tone
4. Teach the patient transfer techniques (*e.g.,* bed to chair, chair to bed).	4. Increases independence and provides for a greater number of environmental settings available to the patient
5. Give special skin care, such as lubrication and protection from extremes in temperature, for tropic skin areas.	5. Trophic skin changes are possible when flaccidity occurs.
6. Have the patient dress in his own clothes rather than a hospital gown.	6. Improves self-image and dispels image of the "sick role"
7. Provide for patient's privacy by screening when he is learning new skills such as relearning to feed self.	7. Preserves self-esteem and decreases patient's embarrassment if "accidents" happen
8. Provide emotional support and encouragement.	8. Aids in motivation of patient
9. Encourage the patient to express feelings.	9. Decreases anxiety and allows for correction of misinformation
10. Be emphathetic with patient's feelings.	10. Able to be more sensitive to patient's needs
11. Know what the physiotherapist is doing with the patient.	11. Activities can be reinforced by the nurse.
12. Encourage family to participate (*e.g.,* demonstrate range-of-motion exercises to family).	12. Allows family member to feel that he is "doing something to help"

vices such as the public health nurse, senior citizens' transportation, and home physiotherapist, to mention but a few.

If the patient is to return to his home, a home assessment visit should be made by a health professional to evaluate feasibility. After the necessary equipment has been assembled and adjustments have been made, the patient ideally should have a weekend (home) pass so that difficulties can be identified and corrected with the help of the health team. A conference should be scheduled with the family to discuss the experience after the weekend. A similar interview should be conducted with the patient.

Once the patient is discharged home, he and the family should have someone whom they can contact for help and reassurance. This should be the professional nurse who was part of the hospital setting and has had good rapport with the patient and family.

RECOVERY

Patients who survive a stroke will usually have some potential for recovery of function. The extent of the stroke and the preexisting disease exert great influence on recovery. In small strokes, recovery can begin within hours after the stroke. For others, no recovery at all may be evident after months of a rehabilitation program. If motor and speech functions do not show some improvement after 1 or 2 months, the outlook is guarded. Deficits of apraxia, the various agnosias, and emotional lability usually improve within a few weeks. Visual deficits of hemianopsia tend to become permanent if they are still present after a few weeks.

Although walking, dysarthria, and aphasia can improve for up to 1 year, the rule of thumb states that deficits present after 6 months will most likely be permanent.

REFERENCES

1. Adams RD, Victor M: Principles of Neurology, 2nd ed, pp 529–593. New York, McGraw–Hill, 1981
2. Greenfield NN: Subclavian steal: A review. Heart Lung 11(4):327, July–August, 1982
3. Herring M: The subclavian steal syndrome: A review. Am Surg 43:220, 1977
4. Lawson JD et al: Subclavian steal: Review of the clinical manifestations. South Med J 72:1369, 1979
5. Booth K: Subclavian steal syndrome: Treatment with proximal vertebral to common carotid artery transposition. J Neurosurg Nurs 12(1):28, March 1980

BIBLIOGRAPHY

Books

Adams R, Victor M: Principles of Neurology, 2nd ed. New York, McGraw–Hill, 1981

Clifford RF (ed): Advances in Stroke Therapy. New York, Raven Press, 1984

Crickmay M: Helping the Stroke Patient to Talk. Springfield, IL, Charles C Thomas, 1977

Downey JA: A Guide for Patient and Family. New York, Raven Press, 1984

Eliasson S et al: Neurological Pathophysiology, 2nd ed. New York, Oxford University Press, 1978

Fisher CM: Management of occlusive cerebrovascular disease. In Ropper AH, Kennedy SK, Zervas NT (eds): Neurological and Neurosurgical Intensive Care, pp 189–206. Baltimore, University Press, 1983

Johnstone M: The Stroke Patient: Principles of Rehabilitation, 2nd ed. New York, Churchill Livingstone, 1982

O'Brien M, Pallett P: Total Care of the Patient With Stroke. Boston, Little, Brown & Co, 1978

Sharpless JW: Mossman's Problem Oriented Approach to Stroke Rehabilitation, 2nd ed. Springfield, IL, Charles C Thomas, 1982

Smith G: Care of the Patient With a Stroke: A Handbook for the Patient's Family and Nurse. New York, Springer, 1976

Periodicals

Allwood A, Lundy C: Cerebral artery bypass surgery. Am J Nurs 80(7):1284, July 1980

Ball PM: Preventing stroke through non-invasive carotid artery assessment. J Neurosurg Nurs 14(4):182, August 1982

Bashor P: A communication assessment guide. Rehabil Nurs 8(1):20–21, 30, January–February 1983

Behrends E: Intraoperative monitoring of cortical oxidative metabolism. J Neurosurg Nurs 12(1):22, March 1980

Behrends E: Superficial temporal artery anastomosis to middle cerebral artery. J Neurosurg Nurs 8(2):113, December 1976

Bell BA, Ambrose J: Smoking and the risk of stroke. Acta Neurochir 64:1, 1982

Blanco KM: The aphasic patient. J Neurosurg Nurs 14(1):34, February 1982

Booth K: The neglect syndrome. J Neurosurg Nurs 14(1):38, February 1982

de Weerd A et al: Effect of the extra-intracranial (STA–MCA) arterial anastomosis on EEG and cerebral blood flow: A controlled study of patients with unilateral cerebral ischemia. Stroke 13:674, 1982

Fedum P: Preoperative evaluation of patients undergoing microanastomosis for brain ischemia. J Neurosurg Nurs 12(1):46, March 1980

Graham L: Stroke rehabilitation: A creative process. Can Nurse 72(2):22, February 1976

Groteboer J: Stroke, carotid endarterectomy, and the neurosurgeon. J Neurosurg Nurs 10(2):52, June 1978

Hargrove R: Feeding the severely dysphagic patient. J Neurosurg Nurs 12(2):102, June 1980

Hirsh LF: Subclavian steal syndrome. Hosp Med 50, April 1980

Kirkman K: Functional differences in patients with left and right cerebrovascular accident. Phys Ther 63(4):481, April 1983

Louis MC, Povse SM: Aphasia and endurance: Considerations in the assessment and care of the stroke patient. Nurs Clinics N Am 15(2):265, June 1980

Mills VM et al: Functional differences in patients with left and right cerebrovascular accident. Phys Ther 63(4):486, April 1983

Nicholson C: Cranial bypass: A case study. J Neurosurg Nurs 15(3):136, June 1983

Paulshock BZ (moderator): A primary care focus on stroke. Patient Care 16(7):15, April 15, 1982

Polhopek M: Stroke: An update on vascular disease. J Neurosurg Nurs 12(2):81, June 1980

Schoonmaker FW, Vijay NK: Identifying aortic arch syndrome. Hosp Med 62, June 1982

Stoker R: Impact of disability on families of stroke clients. J Neurosurg Nurs 15(6):360, December 1983

Tilton CN, Maloof M: Diagnosing the problems in stroke. Am J Nurs 82(4):596, April 1982

Tyler HR: Answers to questions on stroke. Hosp Med 26, June 1977

Tyler KL, Tyler HR: Answers to questions on stroke (Part 2). Hosp Med 89–104, August 1983

chapter 24

Cerebral Aneurysms

Subarachnoid hemorrhage (SAH) is defined as bleeding into the subarachnoid space within the intracranial vault. The causes of subarachnoid hemorrhage include primary hypertensive hemorrhage, ruptured cerebral aneurysm, ruptured arteriovenous malformation, head injury, and others. This chapter focuses on a major cause of subarachnoid hemorrhage, cerebral aneurysms.

DEFINITION AND DESCRIPTION

A *cerebral aneurysm* is a round, saccular dilation of the arterial wall that develops as a result of weakness of the wall. Most aneurysms are called berry aneurysms because they look like a berry and have a stem and neck. Others appear as a puckering or ballooning of the blood vessel, without a neck (Fig. 24–1). The anatomical structure of the aneurysm is an important consideration when surgery is considered for the patient.

Aneurysms are usually small, most being 1 cm in diameter; however, in some instances, an aneurysm can dilate to as much as 5 cm. Not all aneurysms cause problems for the patient or manifest any clinical signs. Many remain silent throughout life and are uncovered by chance during postmortem examination.

POSSIBLE CAUSES

The cause of aneurysms is uncertain, although many theories have been proposed. Other diseases, such as hypertension and polycystic disease, have been correlated with aneurysms, but no direct cause-and-effect relationship has been proven. One explanation suggests that aneurysms are caused by congenital defects in the media of the cerebral arteries. The wall of the aneurysm is thin and usually composed of intimal and subintimal connective tissue, without any muscle or elastic tissue in the sac itself.

Other theories propose that aneurysms represent vestigial remains of the embryonic circulatory system or result from arteriosclerotic changes in the blood vessels. The present status of these theories is still speculative. Research continues in an attempt to uncover an accurate explanation for this problem.

More recently, trauma has been added to the list of possible causes of cerebral aneurysms. A traumatic cerebral aneurysm can be correlated to the shearing force responsible for many head injuries. Basal skull fractures and penetrating head wounds, especially those caused by missiles such as bullets, can be potential offenders. The wall of any artery may be weakened at the fracture line or by a careening missile. With each pulsation, the damaged arterial wall expands until clinical symptoms or bleeding occurs. The diagnosis of traumatic cerebral aneurysm can be missed if the physician does not consider the possibility of its existence. Some head-injury patients who have been treated for subdural hematomas may, in fact, have had traumatic cerebral aneurysms.

CLASSIFICATION

The following is a general classification system for aneurysms.[1]

- *Berry aneurysms*—thought to be due to a defect in the anatomical development of the muscle wall; possible association with polycystic disease
- *Giant (fusiform) aneurysm*—3 cm or more in diameter; behaves like a space-occupying lesion and produces neurological deficits of compression of cerebral tissue and/or cranial nerves; associated with hypertension

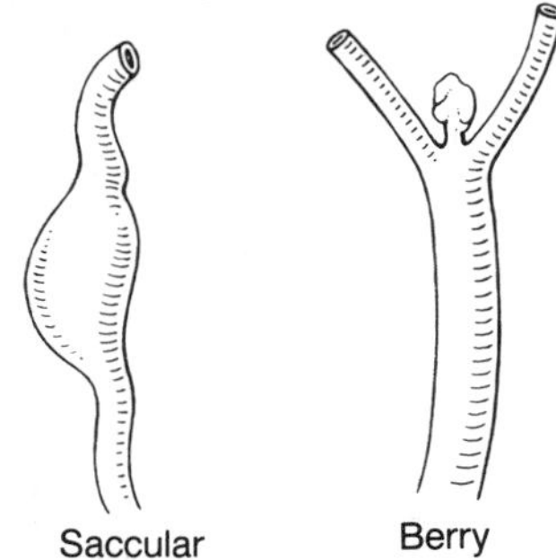

FIG. 24-1. Saccular and berry aneurysms.

- *Mycotic aneurysms*—rare; septic emboli from infections may lead to aneurysmal formation
- *Charcot-Bouchard aneurysms*—microscopic aneurysmal formation associated with hypertension and involving the basal ganglia or brain stem
- *Traumatic aneurysms*—associated with head injuries

LOCATION

Most aneurysms (85%) develop in the anterior portion of the circle of Willis, primarily in the internal carotid artery, the posterior and anterior communicating arteries, the middle cerebral artery, or the anterior cerebral artery (Fig. 24-2). The most frequent site of occurrence is the juncture of the posterior communicating artery and the internal carotid artery. A small percentage (15%) arise within the vertebral-basilar system. It should be noted that aneurysms, with rare exception, occur at the point of bifurcation of arterial vessels. It appears that a site of potential weakness exists when two arteries form a junction.

FIG. 24-2. Major locations for cerebral aneurysms. (Beeson PB, McDermott W: Textbook of Medicine. Philadelphia, WB Saunders, 1970)

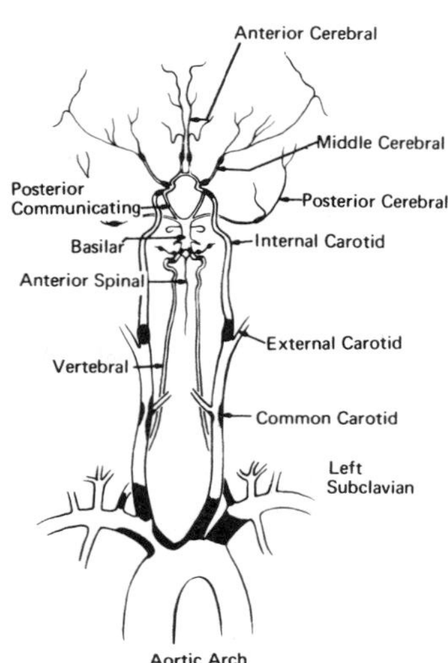

PATHOPHYSIOLOGY

Rupture of a cerebral aneurysm results in bleeding into the subarachnoid, subdural, or intracerebral areas. A stroke syndrome develops, with associated increased intracranial pressure. The specific signs and symptoms associated with the event depend on the location of the hemorrhage and degree of increased intracranial pressure.

SIGNS AND SYMPTOMS

Cerebral aneurysms are most prevalent in the 35- to 60-year age group. Symptoms arising from an aneurysm may be divided into two categories: before rupture or bleeding and after rupture or bleeding. *Rupture* means that there is a forcible tearing apart or a major break in the aneurysmal sac. The term *bleeding* is used to mean a weeping or "sweating" of blood from a very thin aneurysmal sac without actual rupture. These terms are frequently interchanged, but they both convey the idea that blood is lost through the aneurysmal sac into the cerebral tissue and subarachnoid space.

BEFORE RUPTURE OR BLEEDING

Most patients are completely asymptomatic until the time of bleeding. Other patients may complain of generalized headache with subsequent lethargy, neck pain, and localization of headache. Warning signs are noted in about 49% of patients. Localized signs and symptoms depend on the size and the location of the aneurysm. Dysfunction of the optic, oculomotor, or trigeminal cranial nerve may also be present. Some patients may describe a "strange noise" in their heads, which is clinically referred to as a *bruit*. A bruit is a murmur that is related to circulation and can be heard upon auscultation.

If the patient experiences any of the previously mentioned symptoms to a sufficient degree, it is possible that he may seek medical evaluation. However, because many of these symptoms are vague and unspecific, they are often disregarded by the patient. Even if the patient does seek advice from his family physician, he most likely will be referred to a specialist. While arrangements for referral are being made, precious time can be lost before the diagnosis is reached.

AFTER RUPTURE OR BLEEDING

The bleeding aneurysm may hemorrhage into the subarachnoid space, into the cerebral substance, or into both areas. Bleeding into the subarachnoid space is called a subarachnoid hemorrhage. Bleeding into the cerebral substance results in an intracerebral hematoma.

At the time of rupture or bleeding, the patient experiences a violent headache commonly described as "explosive." Other signs and symptoms include a decreased level of consciousness, deficit of the cranial nerves (especially the oculomotor nerve), visual disturbances, deficit of voluntary muscles resulting in hemiparesis or hemiplegia, and possible vomiting. *All of these signs and symptoms are related to increased intracranial pressure.* If the blood from the bleeding aneurysm has come into contact with the meninges as in subarachnoid hemorrhage, symptoms of meningeal irritation will be present. These symptoms include stiff neck, positive Kernig's and Brudzinski's sign, pain in the neck, photophobia and blurred vision, irritability and restlessness, and possible elevation of temperature. The presence and severity of symptoms depend on the amount, location, and extent of the bleeding. Regardless of what symptoms are present, the patient's condition is extremely serious and the prognosis is guarded.

PHYSIOLOGICAL BASIS OF SYMPTOMS

The proximity of the circle of Willis, the internal carotid artery, the cranial (III, IV, VI) nerves, the hypophysis, and the optic nerves plays a role in the development of symptoms. Symptoms of oculomotor nerve dysfunction are noted with many aneurysms because the cranial (III) nerve lies directly beside the internal carotid artery, the most common vessel associated with aneurysms. The oculomotor nerve is also the only neural pathway that cuts through the cerebrum directly and horizontally. The normally functioning oculomotor nerve elevates the upper eyelid, constricts the pupil, and innervates four of the six muscles responsible for moving the eyeball. With cranial (III) nerve dysfunction, the patient has difficulty looking upward, downward, and medially; there is ptosis and a dilated pupil on the affected side, and diplopia may also be present. Thus, pupillary reaction and the movement of the eye provide valid data in assessing the patient's condition.

Lastly, the proximity of the hypophysis to the area of the aneurysm explains why some patients develop diabetes insipidus after surgery. This gland is so close to the surgical site that if surgery is performed, it is reasonable to predict a possible, temporary malfunction in the form of clinical symptoms of diabetes insipidus.

DIAGNOSIS AND CLASSIFICATION

The diagnosis of a cerebral aneurysm is made by an accumulation of data, which include

1. History and physical examination—including a neurological examination
2. Lumbar puncture—to ascertain the presence of blood in the cerebrospinal fluid caused by hemolyzed red blood cells (*xanthochromia*). In addition, the cerebrospinal fluid pressure may be elevated 250 mm (water pressure) in about 50% of the patients. Upon analysis of the cerebrospinal fluid, the protein content is usually elevated (80 mg to 130 mg/100 ml or higher). The white blood cell count is elevated after hemorrhage as meningeal irritation develops. Lastly, the glucose content may be decreased in some patients.
3. CT scan—demonstrates the presence of a subdural hematoma, an intracerebral hematoma, or hydrocephalus, as well as an aneurysm. This information is valuable in planning the management of the patient.
4. Cerebral arteriogram—outlines the cerebral vascularity and is most valuable in identifying abnormalities such as aneurysms (Fig. 24–3). If vasospasms occur, the aneurysm may not be detected initially, so another arteriogram may be scheduled in a few days or 1 week.
5. Serial regional blood flow studies—multiple regional cerebral blood flow studies can provide guidelines for the proper timing of aneurysmal surgery; a means for detecting vasospasms and providing a physiological correlation to neurological deficits; and guidelines for postoperative patient management. In the intraoperative phase of aneurysmal surgery, cerebral blood flow studies help detect impaired autoregulation during induced hypotension thereby identifying those patients at risk for postoperative complications.
6. Other diagnostic tests—including electroencephalogram and brain scan, although these procedures provide less exacting information than other tests

A preliminary diagnosis is made based on the history, physical examination, and lumbar puncture. Other diagnostic tests are then scheduled as soon as possible. The serial regional cerebral blood flow studies are scheduled periodically to guide the neurosurgeon in scheduling surgery and monitoring the patient. A computed tomography (CT) scan and follow-up CT scan are other important diagnostic tests.

Classification of the patient by grade (Table 24–1) has proven to be a most worthwhile step in reducing mortality and morbidity, since it provides an accurate baseline assessment. From this reference point, changes in the patient's condition can be noted and evaluated. This tool guides the physician in making decisions about the timing of surgery, if indicated. The patient is assigned to one of the categories shown in Table 24–1 on admission. It is then revised as his condition changes.

PROGNOSIS AND COMPLICATIONS

Death rates statistics vary for the initial bleed of cerebral aneurysms, but between 20% and 40% of patients succumb at this time.

At the time of rupture about 10 ml to 20 ml of blood escapes, and a clot forms. Loss of 30 to 50 ml of blood would institute a massive hemorrhage and would probably result in death. The clot must withstand a pressure that is the difference between the surrounding pressure of the clot and cerebral tissue and the intra-aneurysmal pressure. The aneurysmal pressure is determined by the central blood pressure. Thus, the patient's arterial blood pressure must be controlled to decrease the possibility of rebleeding.

REBLEEDING

Rebleeding is shown to be the greatest cause of mortality in patients with ruptured aneurysms. Of those surviving the initial bleed, 35% to 40% bleed again in the early weeks, with an approximate mortality rate of 42%.

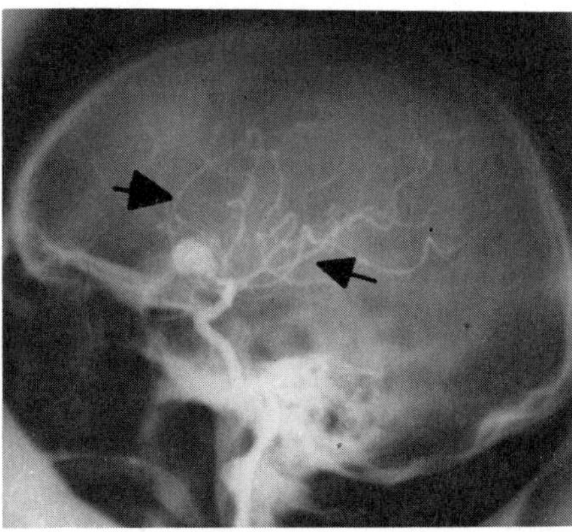

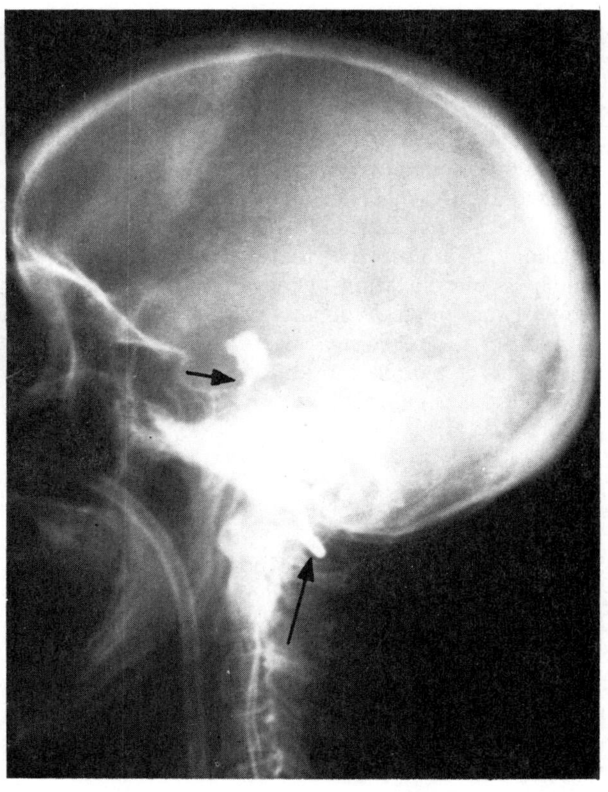

FIG. 24-3. Carotid angiography indicates a large aneurysm of the anterior communicating artery. *(Left)* The anterior cerebral artery *(large arrow)* and the middle cerebral group *(small arrow)* are also illustrated. *(Right)* Catheter angiography demonstrates the vertebral artery *(long arrow)*, the basilar artery *(short arrow)*, and a large, lobulated basilar artery aneurysm. (Hardy J: Rhoads Textbook of Surgery. Philadelphia, JB Lippincott, 1977)

Rebleeding is not immediate but occurs most frequently from the third to the eleventh day, with a peak incidence around the seventh day after the original bleed. There is a sharp drop in rebleeding 4 weeks after the postinitial bleed. The solution to this problem would seem to be early surgery, but it has been documented that patients subjected to early surgery do poorly. Improvement in the patient's clinical condition and time elapsed from the date of bleed seem to be very influential factors in a favorable outcome for the patient. Some authorities state that 5 to 10 days after the initial bleed is an appropriate time for surgery because it corresponds to the peak time of rebleeding. Others suggest a delay of 2 to 3 weeks. The initial category grade assigned to a patient and his level of improvement are important variables to consider in scheduling surgery. Any evidence of a subdural hematoma, an intracerebral hematoma, or development of acute hydrocephalus might suggest an earlier surgical date. A CT scan would demonstrate evidence of any of these conditions.

CEREBRAL VASOSPASMS

Cerebral vasospasms are well-documented events that occur in some patients following subarachnoid hemorrhage. It has been reported that 30% to 50% of all patients

TABLE 24-1. *Classification of Cerebral Aneurysms*

Category	*Criteria*
Grade I (minimal bleed)	Asymptomatic; alert with minimal headache, slight nuchal rigidity, and no neurological deficit
Grade II (mild bleed)	Alert, mild to severe headache, nuchal rigidity, minimal neurological deficit (as third nerve palsy)
Grade III (moderate bleed)	Drowsy or confused, nuchal rigidity; may have mild focal deficits
Grade IV (moderate to severe bleed)	Stupor, mild to severe hemiparesis, nuchal rigidity, possible early decerebration
Grade V (severe bleed)	Deep coma, decerebrate rigidity, moribund appearance

with subarachnoid hemorrhage develop cerebral vasospasms preoperatively. An even larger number (about 65%), develop vasospasms in the postoperative period.[2] Since rupture of cerebral aneurysms is the major cause of subarachnoid hemorrhage, cerebral vasospasms are a significant consideration in patient management.

Cerebral vasospasm is defined as a constriction or narrowing of an artery or branch of an artery compared to the corresponding vessel on the other side of the brain, as noted on angiography. The diagnosis of cerebral vasospasms is made by cerebral angiography although clinical evidence of neurological deterioration may be highly suggestive of spasms. Vasospasms may be localized or diffuse. They frequently occur in the vessel adjacent to the ruptured aneurysm, causing a localized constriction. Depending on the magnitude of the spasm, the vasospasm may then spread to other major vessels, creating a state of diffuse vasospasms. The significance of cerebral vasospasms is that they result in ischemia of the cerebral tissue supplied by the affected blood vessel and can lead to infarction or even death, if they persist.

It has been suggested that after subarachnoid hemorrhage, all patients demonstrate a certain amount of cerebral vasospasms.[3] However, not all patients develop serious neurological deterioration as a consequence of vasospasms. The sequence of vasospasm development, as outlined in the literature, helps to clarify the biphasic nature of the phenomenom.[4] The initial hemorrhage is followed by an initial or acute phase of vasospasms, which decrease blood pressure and control bleeding. It is a protective mechanism that lasts several hours. The second phase of vasospasms, the chronic phase, follows the acute phase and may persist for several days to 4 weeks. Angiographic or clinical evidence of vasospasms is usually not evident until 4 to 10 days after the initial hemorrhage. The peak incidence for vasospasms and rebleeding are the same, 7 to 10 days after the initial bleed.

Clinical signs and symptoms vary depending on the specific function of the brain undergoing the ischemic episode. In general, the patient may experience deterioration in consciousness, motor weakness or paralysis, visual deficits, and changes in vital signs, particularly the respirator pattern. There may also be focal or generalized seizure activity.

Vasospasms are not only a concern after the initial hemorrhage but also after surgery. A patient can die after very successful surgery if vasospasms of sufficient magnitude have developed.

Etiology

The etiology of cerebral vasospasms is not clear, although it is a topic of intense investigation. Various theories have been proposed to explain cerebral vasospasms. Researchers have found that cerebral vasospasms can be precipitated by many naturally occurring substances, such as the by-products of blood breakdown (5-hydroxytryptamine, lysed erythrocytes, prostaglandins, serotonin, and catecholamines). Currently the most popular explanation of vasospasms is that all of these substances can increase the influx of calcium into the vascular smooth muscle, which precipitates vasospasms. Calcium initiates muscle contraction and also regulates the degree of that contraction.

Pathophysiology

The pathophysiological changes caused by vasospasms are reflected in the altered cerebral perfusion pressure. The subsequent effect of decreased cerebral blood flow, especially to a brain that is already experiencing some degree of edema and increased intracranial pressure from the initial bleed, can be disastrous when the collateral circulation is insufficient. The autoregulatory mechanism that normally controls constant blood flow during changes in perfusion pressure is often lost. This additional consequence also compromises adequate cerebral blood supply.

Treatment With Drugs

A review of the literature indicates that there is no widely accepted method of treatment for vasospasms. Some of the drug protocals that have been tried include papaverine hydrochloride, a smooth-muscle relaxant; aminophylline–isoproterenol, which acts on enzymes active in vasomotor contraction[5]; and serotonin antagonists, which control serotonin, a substance thought to precipitate vasospasms. The latest drug group used to manage cerebral vasospasms is calcium-blocking agents. For those who believe that vasospasms are caused by an increased influx of calcium into the cell, pharmacological agents designed to block or antagonize this action may prevent or reverse the action of cerebral vasospasms already present. Cerebral artery smooth muscle is dependent on calcium for contraction and is unable to contract properly without it. Therefore, a certain amount of calcium is necessary.

Two calcium blockers are currently approved and available for treating cerebral vasospasms: verapamil (Isoptin) and nifedipine (Procardia). Verapamil appears to be of value as an antiarrhythmic drug. Nifedipine appears to be of value in controlling cerebral vasospasms by two mechanisms: inhibition of calcium influx into the cerebral artery muscle and interference with the lysis of erythrocytes and platelet aggregation.[6,7] Nifedipine is administered by mouth in divided daily doses of 30 mg to 120 mg. The reported side-effects are hypotension, headache, nausea, and flushing. Several other calcium-blocking agents are under investigation, so new drugs appropriate for the control of cerebral vasospasms can be expected.

Treatment of Cerebral Ischemia Associated With Vasospasms

The newest treatment for the cerebral ischemia associated with vasospasms is intravascular volume expansion and induced arterial hypertension, normotension, or hemodilution. The development of vasospasms after subarachnoid hemorrhage results in narrowing of the the arterial lumen, increased cerebral vascular resistance, and lowered focal perfusion pressure. Cerebral ischemia with neurological deficits then develops. The goal of therapy is to restore adequate blood flow to the ischemic cerebral tissue before infarction develops.

The protocol for hypervolemic–hypertensive therapy discussed by Kassell and colleagues achieved intravascular volume expansion with transfusions of whole blood or packed cells that maintained the hematocrit at approximately 40.[8] Plasma fractionate or albumin is also administered along with the blood. Fluids are administered to raise the central venous pressure to 10 mm Hg or the pulmonary wedge pressure to 18 mm to 20 mm Hg. To manage the vagal depressor response (reflex bradycardia and hypotension), 1 mg of atropine sulfate is administered by the intramuscular route every 3 to 4 hours. Vasopressin (Aqueous Pitressin), 5 units intramuscularly, is injected to maintain the uninary output at less than 200 ml/hour. To maintain the hypertensive state, levarterenol, metaraminol, isoproterenol, dopamine, or dobutamine is used. The maximum level of systolic blood pressure for patients with obliterated aneurysms was 240 mm Hg and for those with untreated aneurysms, 160 mm Hg. The patients are monitored for systemic arterial pressure, central venous pressure or pulmonary artery wedge pressure, electrocardiographic abnormalities, and, for those patients with intracranial hypertension, intracranial pressure. The hemoglobin, hematocrit, creatinine, blood urea nitrogen, glucose, blood gases, and electrolytes and osmolarities of urine and serum are monitored extensively.

The results of maintaining a patient on a hypervolemic–hypertensive protocol for a week or longer have been encouraging. Many patients demonstrated reversal of ischemic neurological deficits. Complications experienced during therapy included pulmonary edema, dilutional hyponatremia, aneurysmal rebleeding, coagulopathy, hemothorax, and myocardial infarction. In the discussion of the protocol, Kassell states that fluid restriction had been used in the past as an adjunct to control arterial pressure preoperatively but that this approach has been abandoned in favor of a normal to high fluid intake because it appears that hypovolemia contributes to the development of vasospasms and cerebral ischemia.[8] This is an important addition to the body of knowledge of neuroscience because the practice, in the past, has been to restrict fluids.

In another study, patients with subarachnoid hemorrhage had their volume expanded while blood pressure was maintained at normotensive levels with centrally acting vasodilator drugs and only small amounts of diuretics. Parameters monitored were similar to those followed in the Kassell report. Although the study group was small, a decreased incidence of vasospasms was reported.[9]

Still another report advocated hypervolemic hemodilution for the treatment of focal cerebral ischemia.[10] There appears to be a relationship between blood viscosity and hematocrit levels and the amount of cerebral ischemia in this report. By using an intravenous infusion of 5% albumin to expand intravascular volume and to thin the blood, the flow of blood to the ischemic area is increased. The increased blood supply relieves cerebral ischemia, prevents infarction, and provides time for collateral blood vessels to dilate and improve blood supply to the area. The hematocrit level was reduced to about 33%. Improvement was noted within 24 hours in some patients. The protocol is maintained for 3 to 4 days before being tapered. The value of this approach is that it does not raise blood pressure, which can contribute to rebleeding and cerebral edema. The protocol does, however, augment cerebral blood flow and perfusion. In addition to vasospasm and ischemia management, some institutions use this protocol during cerebral arterial bypass surgery and for 2 to 3 days immediately after surgery.[10]

In summary, the most direct treatment of vasospasms is prevention or management of the problem. However, because there is no therapy currently meeting this goal, other methods such as hypervolemic hypertension, hypervolemic normotension, and hypervolemic hemodilution have been proposed and used in various institutions. The reversal of ischemia-induced neurological deficits and the prevention of cerebral infarction has been very encouraging. The practice of fluid restriction for patients with cerebrovascular conditions has come under question and has been abandoned in some institutions.

GENERAL APPROACH TO MEDICAL TREATMENT

The patient who survives the initial rupture of an intracranial aneurysm and the subsequent subarachnoid hemorrhage is beset by both short- and long-term problems that require joint medical and surgical management.

The generally accepted treatment for a cerebral aneurysm is surgery. However, surgery is postponed for some time, usually 2 or 3 weeks, so that the patient's neurological status can improve and cerebral edema and spasms can be controlled. The brain has been described as "soft and mushy" because of the edema and local response to the presence of free blood in the area. The postponement of surgery has greatly reduced the high mortality rates that were seen when surgical intervention was immediate. During the preoperative period, the patient is maintained on complete bed rest, subarachnoid precautions, and drug therapy.

Some patients are poor candidates for surgery because of age, preexisting health problems, or location of the aneurysm. For these patients a conservative regime of complete bed rest and drug therapy, similar to the preoperative approach used in managing the patient for whom surgery is planned, is used.

CONSERVATIVE MEDICAL TREATMENT

If the patient is comatose, ventilation assistance and/or oxygen therapy might be indicated. Blood gases should be checked at prescribed intervals for any comatose patient. Excessive carbon dioxide is a potent vasodilator and could increase the intracranial pressure. An electrocardiogram should be taken, because possible injury to the central nervous system could result in electrocardiographic changes. In some instances, cardiac monitoring may be instituted.

Changes frequently seen with bleeding aneurysms include complete heart block and pronounced abnormalities of the S–T segment and T wave. The goal of management is to maintain the patient until his neurological status improves enough to allow surgery to be performed and also to prevent the development of any other problems that would make him a poor surgical risk.

To control the patient's arterial blood pressure and increased intracranial pressure, the plan of care usually includes

- Complete bed rest with the head of the bed elevated 30 to 40 degrees
- Subarachnoid precautions (Chart 24–1)
- Routine monitoring of vital and neurological signs
- Limited fluid intake (1500 ml to 1800 ml) in a 24-hour period
- Possible control of cerebrospinal fluid by means of ventricular drainage system
- Drug therapy (steroids, antihypertensives, antipyretics, stool softeners, antifibrinolytics, anticoagulants, analgesics, sedatives, and drugs to control cerebral vasospasms.

All of these medical management protocols will be addressed in relationship to the specific points of care.

DRUG THERAPY

The following drug groups are usually administered to the patient with a ruptured cerebral aneurysm.

Steroids

Anti-inflammatory corticosteroids are used to treat cerebral edema. The drug of choice is dexamethasone (Decadron), a very potent drug requiring careful supervision and observation for side-effects and toxicity. Dexamethasone does not retain sodium ions, thereby eliminating the subsequent problem of fluid retention that is characteristic of other steroids. However, the usual precautions of gradually tapering the doses of the drug must be observed. Because dexamethasone is alleged to be very irritating to the gastrointestinal tract, the drug is frequently administered with Maalox or Mylanta. In addition, cimetidine (Tagamet) may be given to decrease gastric secretions.

Antihypertensives

Hydralazine hydrochloride (Apresoline) is an effective antihypertensive agent, particularly when used in combination with other drugs for treatment of the patient with moderately severe hypertension. Apresoline is the drug frequently selected to control the arterial blood pressure of the patient with an aneurysm. The drug's effect is primarily by direct action on the smooth muscles of arteries. This action reduces vascular resistance by producing arteriolar vasodilation but has little effect on the venous system. In combination with rauwolfia or thiazides, it often lowers diastolic blood pressure in both the recumbent and upright positions. Toxicity decreases when Apresoline is given in combination with other drugs. Dosage and frequency of administration are correlated with frequent assessment of arterial blood pressure. Other drugs used to manage hypertension are methyldopa (Aldomet) and reserpine.

Antipyretics

Because an increase in temperature causes increased metabolism in cerebral tissue, treatment to control temperature is important. Acetaminophen (Tylenol) or aspirin given orally or rectally are choices commonly ordered when the temperature reaches a certain level. A hypothermia blanket may be prescribed in conjunction with antipyretic drugs. The patient should be observed for shivering, since shivering is known to increase intracranial pressure. The use of chlorpromazine (Thorazine) has been effective in controlling this problem.

Stool Softeners

Straining on defecation must be avoided since it initiates the Valsalva maneuver and causes an increase in intra-abdominal pressure. The mechanism of the Valsalva maneuver involves forcible exhalation against the closed glottis, increasing intrathoracic pressure and impeding venous return to the heart. The result is an increase in intracranial pressure. To avoid this phenomenon and to prevent constipation, which could result from decreased physical activity and use of a drug like codeine, a stool softener should be prescribed. A common choice is docusate sodium (Colace) or a similar drug given orally.

Antifibrinolytics

The use of antifibrinolytics is rapidly decreasing because of new risks and problems being reported. If the drug group is used, the drug administered is aminocaproic acid (Amicar). Antifibrinolytic agents delay the lysis of the clot by preventing the dissolution of the fibrin that forms the foundation of the clot. Fibrin is normally broken down by plasmin, a proteolytic enzyme that resembles trypsin. Plasmin is converted from naturally occurring plasminogen by various enzyme activators. It is thought that such activators are present in thrombin, cerebrospinal fluid, and the meninges, which contribute to the lysis of the blood within the meningeal space. Aminocaproic acid (Amicar) inhibits these activators, thereby preventing plasminogen from being converted to plasmin.

The usual dosage of aminocaproic acid (Amicar) is 24 gm to 36 gm daily. It is supplied in 500 mg tablets, 25% syrup, and 5 gm vials for intravenous use. Dosage must be planned to maintain a constant level in the blood. Reports vary as to the effectiveness of this drug; some are very encouraging, while others are more cautious.

Serious cautions must be considered; use of this drug is contraindicated in patients with uremia, cardiac problems, or hepatorenal disease; intravenous administration must not be rapid since it may induce hypotension, bradycardia, or arrhythmias; pulmonary emboli have also been reported after the use of aminocaproic acid (Amicar). Symptoms of pulmonary emboli may not occur until 1 or 2 weeks after administration of the drug.

CHART 24-1. SUBARACHNOID PRECAUTIONS

Purpose of subarachnoid precautions: to provide a nonstimulating environment

NURSING RESPONSIBILITY	RATIONALE
1. Single room with control of both natural and artificial light; blinds are kept drawn or turned to prevent direct light from shining into the room; artificial light is also controlled so that the room is dim.	**1.** Assigning the patient to a single room makes it possible to control the environment. Closing the blinds decreases light, which would be an irritant to photophobia. A quiet environment will help to keep the patient calm and the blood pressure low.
2. Dimmed light over sink or an indirect light may be used for care.	**2.** A dim light gives the nurse the opportunity to assess the skin color and general appearance of the patient. It also prevents the nurse from tripping or bumping into objects, which might startle the patient and raise his blood pressure.
3. Head of the bed is elevated to 30 to 45 degrees.	**3.** The head of the bed is elevated to promote drainage from the venous system. There are no valves in the cerebral veins so drainage is responsive to gravity, particularly in the patient with cerebral edema.
4. Patient is turned from side to side every 2 hours.	**4.** The patient is turned to prevent skin breakdown and respiratory problems. An alternating pressure mattress may be placed on the patient's bed. The patient should not be asked to help turn himself or pull himself up in bed since the Valsalva maneuver could be activated.
5. Back care is given very gently.	**5.** Back care is given gently to prevent stimulation of the circulatory system, with subsequent increased blood pressure and intracranial pressure.
6. Blood pressure, pulse, respirations, and neurological signs are taken every 30 minutes initially but may be altered by the physician.	**6.** The nurse is responsible for frequent checks of vital signs. The vital signs are monitored as frequently as every 15 to 30 minutes during the acute stage, with the interval increasing as the patient's condition stabilizes.
• The blood pressure is also monitored to regulate the antihypertensive medication. • With an intracranial hemorrhage, the pulse slows to 40 to 50/minute and is bounding. The pulse pressure widens with an increase in the systolic and a drop in the diastolic pressure.	• These are cardinal signs of increased intracranial pressure.
• Rectal temperature may be taken.*	• Although early elevated temperature is indicative of hypothalamic irritation, its significance is not considered critical. However, a febrile state increases the cerebral metabolic rate. This is why hypothermia is often employed to minimize unnecessary cerebral activity.
7. *All* nursing care must be administered. The patient must be fed and bathed.	**7.** All care is administered to prevent any exertion that would raise the blood pressure.
8. Patient must be cautioned against coughing, sneezing, and straining of any kind.	**8.** Coughing, sneezing, and straining cause an increase in intracranial pressure.
9. All of the patient's physical and mental activities must be kept to an absolute minimum. The patient is maintained on complete bed rest	**9.** Minimal activity and control of stress will keep the blood pressure and intracranial pressure low.
10. No external stimuli, that is, no television, no radio, and no reading	**10.** Same as 9
11. Visitors are limited to immediate family and then only two at one time.	**11.** Visitors are restricted to keep the patient as quiet as possible. Even this limitation is contingent on the patient's response to the visitors. A sign limiting visitors should be posted at the patient's door. A simple explanation, both to the patient and the family, is in order.
12. *No* enemas are given.	**12.** Enemas would greatly increase intra-abdominal pressure and subsequently increase intracranial pressure. They are contraindicated.
13. Stool softeners and/or mild laxatives are prescribed.	**13.** Stool softeners and mild cathartics prevent constipation, which would cause an increase in intracranial pressure.

CHART 24–1. (continued)

NURSING RESPONSIBILITY	RATIONALE
14. Headache medications are prescribed.	**14.** The patient should be medicated for headache because the pain could cause restlessness, with a resultant increase in intracranial pressure.
15. Elastic stockings should be worn at all times.	**15.** Elastic stockings are applied to improve blood return to the heart and to prevent the development of thrombophlebitis on this bed patient. The stockings are removed daily and the legs inspected for any signs of thrombophlebitis or skin breakdown. The stockings are then reapplied.
16. The physician may modify precautions, if deemed advisable.	**16.** The problem of maintaining a patient on complete bed rest may be managed easily for a comatose patient but becomes more complex when the patient is conscious, despite sedation. In accordance with the patient's condition, the degree of complete bed rest may be altered slightly in order to decrease whatever anxiety he might experience from having the nurse perform his basic daily care for him. Therefore, the doctor may allow selected patients to bathe and feed themselves and to use a bedside commode.

* Because of the concerns of possible seizure activity and a lowered level of consciousness, rectal rather than oral temperatures may be taken. The crux of the issue surrounds the concern of vasovagal stimulation as a result of the rectal thermometer. It is known that vasovagal stimulation does increase intracranial pressure. However, some authors state that it is minimal and of little clinical consequence. The concern for the safety of the patient who may go into seizure or who has an altered level of consciousness should be of primary importance. Axillary temperatures take too long to obtain and are not always accurate. Still others state that no rectal temperatures should be taken. At our hospital, rectal temperatures are taken. The best policy for the nurse to follow is to check with the physician if she is not sure of his routines.

Anticonvulsants

The purpose of anticonvulsant drugs is to prevent seizure activity. Although phenytoin (Dilantin) is the most frequently used drug, it is a drug that can potentiate or be potentiated by other drugs concurrently prescribed for the patient. Therefore, a drug profile should be maintained with careful attention to drug interactions. The hospital formulary can serve as a reference in this regard. Side-effects of rash, tremors, ataxia, and nystagmus might occur and require reevaluation of the drugs presently ordered for the patient.

Although phenytoin (Dilantin) can be administered orally or parenterally, it is poorly absorbed by the intramuscular route. Intravenous administration must be slow to prevent hypotension. The very high alkalinity of phenytoin (Dilantin) is very irritating to the veins. This drug is contraindicated in patients with complete heart block or bradycardia.

Analgesics

The patient who is experiencing pain must be evaluated in order to determine the severity of the pain. If the pain is mild, acetaminophen (Tylenol) or propoxyphene (Darvon) might be sufficient to keep the patient comfortable. If the patient complains of severe pain or severe headache, codeine is considered a good choice because it does not mask the neurological signs. The side-effect of codeine is constipation, but administration of stool softeners and a bowel regimen with mild cathartics will usually counteract this problem.

Sedatives

The drug of choice is phenobarbital. Restlessness and irritability may be problems, particularly if the patient has meningeal irritation caused by blood in the subarachnoid space. Thrashing in the bed will only increase blood pressure. Phenobarbital is a mild and safe sedative, which also has a slightly hypotensive effect on the arterial blood pressure.

Drugs to Control Cerebral Vasospasms

As mentioned in the section on vasospasms, this is an area of controversy and investigation. Various drug protocals are in use. Among these are Isuprel, serotonin antagonists, and calcium blocking agents.

Aminophylline–Isoproterenol (Isuprel). One protocol used to modify and control cerebral vasospasms following an initial bleed is the aminophylline–Isoproterenol (Isuprel) regime, which acts on enzymes active in vasomotor contraction.[3] An initial dose of 350 mg of aminophylline may be given intravenously, followed by continuous intravenous administration of 125 mg/hour of aminophylline and 125 mg/hour of Isoproterenol (Isuprel). This treatment can be continued for 2 weeks or until there is evidence of the cessation of vasospasms.

- While the patient is receiving these drugs the vital signs are checked hourly. Because tachycardia is a side-effect, the patient should be placed on a cardiac monitor to observe for premature ventricular contractions or a pulse rate of 140 per minute or greater.

Upon achievement of the therapeutic effect, the drugs are gradually tapered and discontinued over a period of 3 days.

Serotonin Antagonists. Finally, for those who subscribe to the hypothesis that elevated serotonin levels cause vasospasms, serotonin antagonists can be administered to prevent vasospasms. Once vasospasms have developed, drug therapy with serotonin antagonists would be discontinued.

One drug used is reserpine (Serpasil), of which 0.1 mg is given four times daily by the subcutaneous route. Normally, serotonin is stored in the platelets. The pharmacological effect of reserpine is to interfere with the platelet's ability to store serotonin.

Another drug that has been used is kanamycin sulfate (Kantrex), 1 gm three times daily, administered by the oral route only. Kanamycin is believed to decrease the production of serotonin in the gastrointestinal tract.

The nurse should be aware of the side-effects of each drug. The major side-effect of reserpine is hypotension, while diarrhea is the most common concern with kanamycin.

Calcium-Blocking Agents. The major drug administered from this group at this time is nifedipine (Procardia). It was briefly discussed in the section on Cerebral Vasospasms.

NURSING MANAGEMENT OF THE PATIENT WITH A CEREBRAL ANEURYSM

The patient who has sustained a rupture of a cerebral aneurysm is acutely ill and requires ongoing assessment, supportive care, implementation of the protocols specific for a cerebral aneurysmal patient (e.g., subarachnoid precautions, drug therapy), and management of increased intracranial pressure. If surgery is planned, the nurse will also need to care for the patient after the craniotomy.

ASSESSMENT

The initial assessment of the patient must include the following:

- Level of consciousness
- Size and reaction of pupils to light
- Motor and sensory function
- Presence of headache
- Cranial nerve dysfunction (ptosis of eyelid, difficulty in moving the eyeball in all directions, facial weakness)
- Blurred vision
- Aphasia
- Other neurological deficits
- Increased intracranial pressure
- Nuchal rigidity

Frequent neurological assessments should be conducted periodically. The frequency of the assessment will depend on the acuity and stability of the patient. The assessment may be necessary every 15 minutes or every 4 hours. Any changes in the patient's condition require neurological assessment and documentation.

Upon diagnosis of a cerebral aneurysm, the patient is assigned to a grade classification based on presenting symptoms. He is placed on strict bed rest with a controlled and quiet environment. Monitoring and support devices also physically immobilize the patient. Most patients have an altered level of consciousness, pain caused by nuchal rigidity and headache, paresis and/or plegia, visual problems caused by photophobia and cranial nerve dysfunction, and other neurological deficits based on the specific areas involved.

The altered level of consciousness negates or diminishes the patient's ability to comprehend the significance and implications of events around him. Environmental information is reduced by alteration or blockage of sensory receptors due to central nervous system injury. Sensory loss is usually multimodal, that is, visual, auditory, and tactile. Motor deficits reduce or prevent any voluntary movement.

It is very difficult to determine the cause of a deteriorating level of consciousness in a patient. It may be due to rebleeding, cellular hypoxia, subdural hematoma, or hydrocephalus, or it may be due to behavioral changes resulting from psychological immobility, sensory deprivation, powerlessness, or any other behavioral response experienced by the patient. There really is no assessment tool that is clear-cut in identifying the cause.

Because the nurses have continuous contact with the patient, they have the responsibility of making a baseline assessment and detecting any subtle or acute changes from the initial data. Accurate intershift reporting is essential in providing for continuity of care.

The common nursing diagnoses made in the acute phase of management for the patient with a ruptured cerebral aneurysm are included in Chart 24–2. The patient usually has an elevation in intracranial pressure; nursing management of this problem is discussed in Chapter 12.

SUBARACHNOID PRECAUTIONS

General nursing care must be modified to incorporate the points of subarachnoid precautions. These precautions, along with the accompanying rationale, are described in Chart 24–2.

ADDITIONAL POINTS OF NURSING MANAGEMENT

1. Fluid Restriction

The practice of fluid restriction is being abandoned by many physicians because it is thought that vasospasms and cerebral ischemia are increased with hemoconcentration.

CHART 24-2. SUMMARY OF NURSING DIAGNOSES ASSOCIATED WITH CEREBRAL ANEURYSMS

NURSING DIAGNOSIS	EXPECTED OUTCOMES	NURSING INTERVENTIONS
Altered neurological function due to hemorrhage from the cerebral aneurysm	• Evidence of neurological alterations will be identified. • Based on an assessment of deficits, any signs of deterioration will be noted and definitive action taken immediately.	• Monitor neurological and vital signs at frequent intervals and note any changes. • Document findings and compare them with previous assessment to denote change.
Pain (headache) due to cerebral hemorrhage	• The characteristics of the headache will be noted and recorded. • Analgesics and comfort measures will be administered. • The patient will provide objective evidence that the pain has been relieved.	• Assess the type, location, and specific characteristics of the headache. • Document your findings. • Note any change in the character of the pain. • Administer analgesics. • Stay with the patient; reposition patient. • Be supportive. • Evaluate response to the analgesic in a reasonable amount of time. • Report lack of response to analgesic.
Stiff neck and pain in the neck due to meningeal irritation	• Patient will be moved carefully, avoiding unnecessary movement of the head. • Patient will be made as comfortable as possible.	• Assess for pain and other signs and symptoms of meningeal irritation. • Reposition patient gently, avoiding any unnecessary movement of the neck or head. • Administer analgesics as ordered.
Sensory input distortion: photophobia due to meningeal irritation	• Photophobia will be controlled by maintaining a darkened room.	• Note evidence of discomfort when assessing direct light response of the pupils. • Maintain a darkened room by drawing the blinds or shades and avoiding direct light.
Potential for seizure activity due to cerebral irritation	• Seizure activity will be prevented. • If a seizure does occur, the patient will not be injured.	• Maintain on seizure precautions. • Monitor patient for any signs of seizure activity and document in the chart. • Administer anticonvulsant drugs prophylactically, as ordered.
Anxiety (mild, moderate or severe) due to illness and/or restrictions of subarachnoid precautions	• Depending on the patient's level of consciousness, he will understand the purpose of the subarachnoid precautions. • The patient will be informed of the plan of care and reassured. • Specific cause of anxiety will be identified. • Anxiety will be minimized or controlled.	• Assess patient for objective and subjective evidence of anxiety. • If anxiety is present, try to identify the specific cause(s). • Attempt to clarify, control, or change the circumstances surrounding the anxiety. • Make appropriate referral, if necessary. • Reassure the patient. • Continue to assess the level of anxiety and stress response in the patient. • Depending on the patient's level of consciousness, use imagery, relaxation technique, and so forth to control anxiety. • Administer sedatives if ordered.
Sensory deprivation due to restrictions of subarachnoid precautions	• Depending on the patient's level of consciousness, he will receive enough reality orientation to understand who he is, where he is, and the time.	• In a calm, soothing manner, provide enough verbal cues to help the patient stay oriented.

(continued)

CHART 24–2. (continued)

NURSING DIAGNOSIS	EXPECTED OUTCOMES	NURSING INTERVENTIONS
Potential of neurological deterioration due to rebleeding or cerebral vasospasms	• Patient will be carefully monitored so that any signs or symptoms of neurological deterioration will be quickly identified. • If evidence of deterioration develops, the physician will be immediately notified. • Nursing interventions and standing orders will be quickly implemented.	• Assess neurological signs frequently for evidence of neurological deterioration. • Report immediately any significant changes in patient's condition. • Recognize the peak times of occurrence of rebleeding and vasospasms. • If deterioration occurs, implement nursing protocols and standing orders so that ischemic response is treated.
Fluid and electrolyte imbalance due to fluid restriction	• Fluid and electrolyte parameters will be monitored. • Significant alterations that can lead to complications, such as a low potassium blood level, will be reported and documented.	• Maintain an intake and output record. • Monitor blood electrolytes, osmolarities of blood and urine, and other parameters. • Report significant alterations in parameters to the physician.

(See the discussion of fluid restriction in the section on Cerebral Vasospasms earlier in this chapter.) If the physician chooses to restrict the patient's fluid intake, he will order the number of milliliters of fluid the patient may be given in a 24-hour period. For example, the patient may be restricted to a 1800-ml daily intake. This means that regardless of the route of administration, the total intake in the 24-hour period should not exceed 1800 ml. The nurse is responsible for maintaining an accurate intake and output record.

- A large sign placed over the head of the bed indicating that the patient is on a fluid restriction is helpful in reminding the entire staff and the family that the patient is not allowed fluids as desired.

A simple explanation will help the family to understand the rationale and importance of this restriction.

2. Seizure Precautions

As a precaution in the event of seizure activity, aspiration, or deterioration of the patient's condition, a standby suction setup is kept in readiness at the bedside, along with a padded tongue blade and oral airway. Padded siderails are also in place to protect the patient from injury.

3. Restraints

The use of wrist and ankle restraints is avoided as much as possible, since the patient may be inclined to strain against them. Should restraining measures become necessary to protect the patient from injury, a vest or jacket restraint is usually effective in keeping the patient in bed. Full siderails at the top and bottom of the bed should be pulled up at all times and the bed should be kept low when the nurse is not at the bedside. At times, to prevent a confused patient from pulling on his tubes or his intravenous line, it may be necessary to apply wrist restraints. The wrist must be properly padded to prevent skin irritation and must be inspected daily.

4. Support Equipment

Use of monitoring devices, a cooling blanket, and respiratory equipment may be ordered for the patient.

5. Drug Therapy

In addition to the nursing care outlined, the nurse is responsible for administering the drug therapy prescribed by the physician and for being aware of the action, toxicity, and interactions of the various drugs used. In this way, pertinent observations can be made in assessing the patient's response to the drug therapy.

PSYCHOLOGICAL SUPPORT

Considering the restrictions placed on the patient's activity, it is important to evaluate and make nursing judgments to meet the patient's psychological and emotional needs. A calm and reassuring approach to the patient is most therapeutic.

The following are general suggestions to prevent adverse behavioral or psychological responses from immobility, sensory deprivation, and powerlessness:

1. Orient the patient often to time, place, and person.
2. Familiarize the patient with his environment.
3. Be alert for cues from the patient indicating areas of concern.
4. Provide information to clarify his concerns in a simple manner. Clarify any misconceptions and quickly reorient him.
5. As his condition improves, allow the patient to make simple decisions (e.g., "Which way is it easiest to turn?")

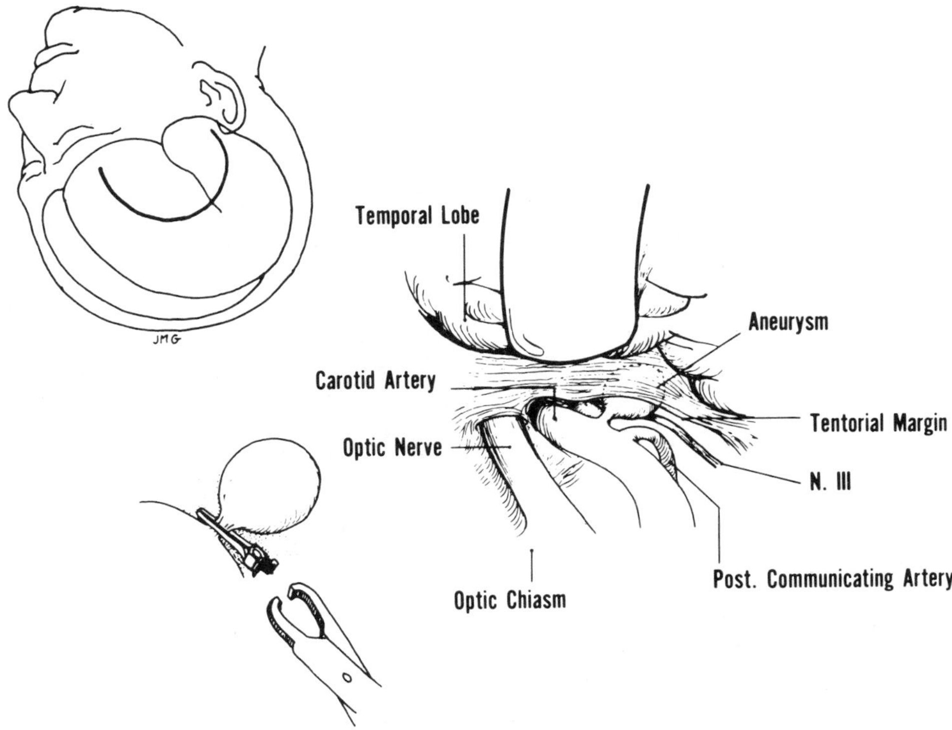

FIG. 24–4. Clipping or a ligation of the aneurysmal neck provides the best protection against rebleeding, although the initial risk may be slightly higher. (Smith RR: Essentials of Neurosurgery. Philadelphia, JB Lippincott, 1980)

6. Report any severe responses to the patient's restrictions that might indicate the need for modification by the physician.
7. Be supportive and helpful to the family throughout the hospitalization period.

SURGICAL INTERVENTION FOR CEREBRAL ANEURYSMS

The physician usually outlines the proposed plan of care to the patient and family to help them understand the seriousness of the patient's problem. If the patient is relatively alert and shows signs of improving, he and his family may not be able to accept the idea of his undergoing an operation as serious as a craniotomy. It is equally difficult for some to understand that at any moment the patient could have a catastrophic rebleed with very serious consequences, including death. The patient and his family, therefore, need a realistic assessment of the consequences of refusing surgery.

For those patients for whom surgery is indicated, new surgical techniques, better anesthetic agents, and sophisticated equipment provide good surgical outcomes. The greatest development has been the use of a special microscope that provides increased visualization. Intracranial aneurysmal surgery is usually accomplished with microsurgical techniques. Controlled systemic hypotension during the actual 5 or 10 minutes of the dissection of the aneurysm may be used to provide a bloodless surgical field. The hypotensive effect on the aneurysmal sac causes it to collapse slightly and allows for easier dissection. A drug that causes peripheral vasodilation such as nitroprusside (Nipride) is administered at the moment of clipping.

Self-closing spring clips are used on aneurysms that can be clipped (Fig. 24–4). Those aneurysms that cannot be clipped are wrapped in a special gauze material and coated with an acrylic substance to provide added support. Aneurysms of the vertebral–basilar system present a more difficult problem of surgical accessibility, but the same principles as those outlined above are generally used. Cerebral angiography at the time of clipping ensures that the bleeding aneurysm is indeed the one that was clipped.

After surgery, the care of the patient is the same as for any other craniotomy patient (see Chap 14), with special adaptation based on the site on the surgical incision. A postoperative cerebral angiography can be used to check the integrity of the surgical procedure. Patients who have preexisting disease, heart disease, and other conditions are more apt to have postoperative problems relating to their preexisting illness. Postoperative problems similar to those anticipated with other craniotomy patients may occur. Hydrocephalus is more common in the aneurysm patient because the free blood may obstruct the reabsorption of cerebrospinal fluid from the arachnoid villi. There is also the possibility of diabetes insipidus, since the pituitary gland is so close to the operative site.

MICROSURGERY

Microvascular neurosurgery has been one of the most important applications of microsurgery in neurosurgery. Giant aneurysms that are not accessible by other operative procedures may be managed by extracranial–intracranial bypass procedures. The superficial temporal artery to middle cerebral artery anastomosis as well as the new occipital artery to posterior–inferior cerebellar artery and superficial temporal artery to superior cerebellar artery anastomoses are also gaining wider application for patients who need occlusion of a proximal artery such as for a giant aneurysm or neoplastic process.[11]

REFERENCES

1. Rhoton A et al: Congenital and traumatic intracranial aneurysms. Clin Symp 29(4): entire issue, 1977
2. Heros RC, Zervas NT, Makoto N: Cerebral vasospasm. Surg Neurol 5:354, June 1976
3. Sundt TM: Cerebral vasospasm following subarachnoid hemorrhage: Evolution, management, and relationship to timing of surgery. Clin Neurosurg 24:228, 1976
4. Farrar JK, Roach MR: The effects of increased intracranial pressure on flow through major cerebral arteries in vitro. Stroke 4:795, 1973
5. Persaud D: Nursing implications: Cerebral vasospasms—Rx: Aminophylline–Isuprel regime. J Neurosurg Nurs 10(2):63, June 1978
6. Amibielli M: Drug stop: Calcium ion antagonists in the treatment of cerebral arterial vasospasm. J Neurosurg Nurs 15(2):119, April 1983
7. Brandt L et al: Effects of a calcium antagonist on cerebral–vascular smooth muscle in vitro and in vivo. In Wilkins RH (ed): Cerebral Arterial Spasm, pp 604–607. Baltimore, Williams & Wilkins, 1980
8. Kassell PF et al: Treatment of ischemic deficits from vasospasm with intravascular volume expansion and induced arterial hypertension. Neurosurgery 11(3):337, 1982
9. Rosenwasser RH et al: Control of hypertension and prophylaxis against vasospasm cases of subarachnoid hemorrhage: A preliminary report. Neurosurgery 12(6):658, 1983
10. Emerg Med 16(17):231, September 15, 1983
11. Camp PE: The newer microsurgical techniques in neurosurgery. Head Neck Surg, p 514, July/August 1982

BIBLIOGRAPHY

Books

Bigger JT: A Primer on Calcium Ion Antagonists. Knoll Pharmaceutical Co, March 1980

Brackett CE, Morantz RA: Special problems associated with subarachnoid hemorrhage. In Youmans JR: Neurological Surgery, 2nd ed, pp 1807–1820. Philadelphia, WB Saunders, 1982

Guyton A: Textbook of Medical Physiology, 6th ed. Philadelphia, WB Saunders, 1981

Howe JR: Manual of Patient Care in Neurosurgery, 2nd ed, pp 89–104. Boston, Little, Brown & Co, 1983

Peerless SJ, Drake CG: Management of aneurysms of posterior Circulation. In Youmans JR: Neurological Surgery, 2nd ed, pp 1715–1763. Philadelphia, WB Saunders, 1982

Pickard J et al: Autoregulation of cerebral blood flow and the prediction of late morbidity and mortality after cerebral aneurysm surgery. In Wilkins RH (ed): Cerebral Arterial Spasm. Baltimore, William & Wilkins, 1980

Roberts S: Behavioral Concepts and the Critically Ill Patient. Englewood Cliffs, NJ, Prentice–Hall, 1976

Ropper AH, Kennedy SK, Zervas NT (eds): Neurological and Neurosurgical Intensive Care, pp 175–189. Baltimore, University Park Press, 1983

Sah A et al (eds): Intracranial Aneurysms and Subarachnoid Hemorrhage: A Cooperative Study. Philadelphia, JB Lippincott, 1969

Smith RR: Nonoperative Treatment of Subarachnoid Hemorrhage. In Youmans JR: Neurological Surgery, 2nd ed, pp 1645–1662. Philadelphia, WB Saunders, 1982

Smith RR: Pathophysiology and clinical evaluation of subarachnoid hemorrhage. In Youmans JR: Neurological Surgery, 2nd ed, pp 1627–1644. Philadelphia, WB Saunders, 1982

Smith RR: Essentials of Neurosurgery, pp 199–219. Philadelphia, JB Lippincott, 1980

Wilkins RH (ed): Cerebral Arterial Spasm. Baltimore, Williams & Wilkins, 1980

Yasargil MG, Smith RD: Management of aneurysms of anterior circulation by intracranial procedures. In Youmans JR: Neurological Surgery, 2nd ed, pp 1663–1696. Philadelphia, WB Saunders, 1982

Periodicals

Bader D: Microsurgical treatment of intracranial aneurysms. J Neurosurg Nurs 7(1):25, July 1975

Chase M, Whelan–Decker E: Nursing management to a patient with a subarachnoid hemorrhage. J Neurosurg Nurs 16(1):23, February 1984

Drake CG: Progress in cerebrovascular disease: Management of cerebral aneurysms. Stroke 12:273, 1981

Fairbanks D: Identifying cavernous sinus syndrome. Hosp Med 25, March 1982

Farrar JK et al: Effects of profound hypotension on cerebral blood flow during surgery for intracranial aneurysms. J Neurosurg 55:857, 1981

Ferguson G et al: Serial measurements of CBF as a guide to surgery in patients with ruptured intracranial aneurysms. J Cereb Blood Flow Metab 1 (Suppl 1):518, 1981

Finch K: Vasospasm secondary to subarachnoid hemorrhage: The current controversy, research, and nursing dilemmas. J Neurosurg Nurs 12(4):199, December 1980

Gary R: Cerebral vasospasm: Process, trends and interventions. J Neurosurg Nurs 13(5):256, October 1981

Gerk MK, Kassell N: Cerebral vasospasm: Update and implications. J Neurosurg Nurs 12(2):66, June 1980

Goldman M et al: Subarachnoid hemorrhage associated with unusual electrocardiographic changes. JAMA 234:957, 1975

Guidetti B, Spallone A: The role of antifibrinolytic therapy in the preoperative management of recently ruptured intracranial aneurysms. Surg Neurol 15:239, 1981

Hartshorn J: Administering calcium-channel blocking agents. Dimens Crit Care Nurs 2(2):70, 1983

Hartshorn J: Intracranial aneurysms. RN 47(1):30, 1983

Houston CS: Hypothermia and cardiac arrest in the treatment of giant aneursyms. J Neurosurg Nurs 16(2):15, February 1984

Hudson C, Raaf J: Timing of angiography and operation in patients with ruptured intracranial aneurysm. J Neurosurg 29:37, 1968

Hunter C: Nursing problems of patients undergoing aminocaproic acid treatment for subarachnoid hemorrhage due to aneurysm. J Neurosurg Nurs 11(3):160, September 1979

McFadden EA, Zaloga GP: Calcium regulation. Crit Care Q 6(3):12, December 1983

Merory J et al: Cerebral blood flow after surgery for recent subarachnoid hemorrhage. J Neurol Neurosurg Psychiatry 43:214, 1980

Morris D: Intra-operative aneurysm clipping. J Neurosurg Nurs 14(3):150, June 1982

Oertel LB: The dilemma of cerebral vasospasm treatment. J Neurosurg Nurs 17(1):7, February 1985

Osaka K: Prolonged vasospasm produced by the breakdown products of erythrocytes. J Neurosurg 47:403, September 1977

Peck S: Calcium blocking agents for treatment of cerebral vasospasms. J Neurosurg Nurs 15(3):123, June 1983

Spetzler RF, Schuster H, Roski RA: Elective extracranial–intracranial arterial bypass in the treatment of inoperable giant aneurysms of the internal carotid artery. J Neurosurg 53:22, 1980

Spielman G: Cerebral vasospasm following subarachnoid hemorrhage. Crit Care Q 2(1):77, June 1979

Sundt TM, Szurszewski J, Sharbrough F: Physiological considerations important for the management of vasospasm. Surg Neurol 7(5):259, May 1977

Tanaka S et al: Gastrointestinal bleeding in cases of ruptured cerebral aneurysm. Acta Neurochir 48:233, 1979

Yamamoto M et al: Noninvasive measurements of cerebral vasospasm in patients with subarachnoid hemorrhage. J Neurol Sci 43:301, 1979

chapter 25

Arteriovenous Malformations and Other Cerebrovascular Anomalies

TRUE ARTERIOVENOUS MALFORMATIONS OF THE BRAIN

An arteriovenous malformation (AVM) is composed of a tangled array of dilated vessels that form an abnormal communication network between the arterial and venous systems (Fig. 25–1). The arterial blood is shunted directly into the venous system without the usual connecting capillary network. The malformation may be small and focal, or it may be a large lesion encompassing an entire hemisphere. The general appearance of the brain is one of many tortuous blood vessels of varying diameters that extend like cones or wedges into the subcortical region of the brain. Arteriovenous malformations are often cone-shaped, with the apex pointing inward and the base toward the surface of the cerebral cortex of the brain. The lesion may be so deep that the ventricular area and choroid plexus may be involved, resulting in hydrocephalus. Calcification may be found in a large number of arteriovenous malformations.

The feeder arteries supplying the lesion initially are normal anatomical structures, but they become tortuous, thick- or thin-walled, and dilated as the demands for a blood supply are increased by the lesion. As the vessels of the arteriovenous malformation descend into the subcortical area, they become thin-walled and connect directly with the veins without any intervening capillaries. The vessels connecting the arterial and venous blood systems are exceptionally thin, without the normal characteristics of arteries or veins being evident. The venous vessels of the arteriovenous malformation form huge, dilated, pulsating channels that carry away the oxygenated arterial blood. If only one vein is responsible for drainage of the malformation, the vessel can develop into an aneurysmal sac because of the increased pressure.

The arteriovenous malformation can be fed by one artery (usually the middle cerebral artery) or other major arteries. Some authorities believe that an arteriovenous malformation is static, while others contend that it can enlarge with time. Viewing it as an enlarging entity, it is suggested that collateral circulation develops by means of naturally occurring pia anastomosis and that eventually it is being supplied by two, three, or more major arteries. The vessels supplying the malformation continue to enlarge, shunting blood from surrounding areas so that the blood flow through the malformation is increased by 50% to 100%.

As a result of the shunting of blood to the malformation, other cerebral areas are deprived of adequate perfusion of blood. Chronic ischemia occurs with cerebral atrophy and focal infarction evident. The overlying meninges may form thick scar tissue. There is usually degeneration of the parenchymal tissue, both proximal and within the lesion. Hemosiderin deposits are often noted in and around the arteriovenous malformation because of minor hemorrhage. Venous vessel enlargement is noted to be greater and more extensive than arterial vessel enlargement.

ARTERIOVENOUS MALFORMATIONS OF THE DURA, FALX, AND/OR TENTORIUM

An arteriovenous malformation may involve any portion of the dura, including the falx cerebri and/or tentorium, with or without brain involvement. Lesions of the dura or tentorium are often associated with a bruit.

The feeder vessels supplying a dural arteriovenous malformation vary in number, size, and source. The blood is often contributed by so many vessels that surgical obliteration may be impossible. The venous sinuses draining the lesion are usually dilated.

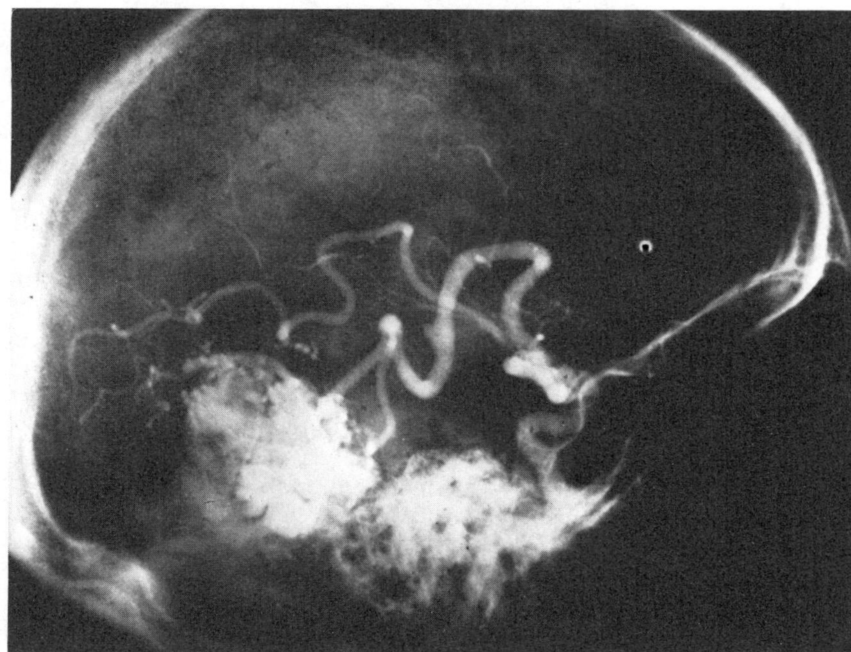

FIG. 25-1. Arteriovenous (AV) malformations consist of dilated arterial and venous channels with the apex pointing toward the lateral ventricle. They cause headaches, seizures, subarachnoid hemorrhage, increased ICP, and strokelike syndromes. (Smith RR: Essentials of Neurosurgery. Philadelphia, JB Lippincott, 1980)

PATHOPHYSIOLOGY OF CEREBRAL ANTERIOVENOUS MALFORMATIONS

The neurological deficits that develop from an arteriovenous malformation or vascular anomaly will depend on the size and location of the lesion. Signs and symptoms will occur as a result of any one or combination of the following mechanisms: ischemia, gliosis, dysgenesis, compression, hemorrhage, noncommunicating hydrocephalus, and occasional cardiac decompensation.

Ischemia. With true arteriovenous malformations, so much blood may be shunted through the lesion that adjacent cerebral tissue may be temporarily or permanently deprived of an adequate blood supply. Irreversible neuronal changes with infarction can occur if the oxygen deprivation is prolonged. Signs or symptoms of a clinical thrombotic stroke or seizure activity may be observed.

Gliosis. Gliosis is stimulated by prolonged ischemia or focal hemorrhage. Because the tissue is structurally abnormal in development, one would expect that there would be interference with normal cerebral function. In the description of many vascular anomalies, it has been noted that gliotic changes develop in adjacent tissue.

Dysgenesis. Dysgenesis describes abnormal tissue resulting from an atypical developmental pattern. For example, shunting of blood away from a portion of the brain by an arteriovenous malformation interferes with normal development of the tissue in the deprived area. Deprivation of normal nutrients contributes to the abnormal cellular development.

Compression. Both arteriovenous malformations and vascular anomalies can interfere with cerebral tissue by direct compression. This is the same mechanism by which a space-occupying lesion produces neurological dysfunction. The type of neurological deficits incurred will depend on the area compressed and the degree of cerebral irritation created. Seizure activity, hemiparesis, and cerebral atrophy are possible consequences of compression.

Hemorrhage. The major concern and complication of arteriovenous malformation and vascular anomalies is hemorrhage. The fragility of the thin-walled blood vessels makes hemorrhage a very real possibility. Bleeding can be very minor with no neurological deficits. Evidence of previous minor bleeding may be noted by hemosiderin deposits. Major bleeding can also result in an intracerebral or subdural hematoma, or it may cause blood to enter the subarachnoid space. Neurological deficits will depend on the location of the hemorrhage. Cerebral edema and increased intracranial pressure develop as a result of bleeding.

With arteriovenous malformations, a large intracerebral hematoma can develop proximally to the site of bleeding. If the dura is the site of the arteriovenous malformation, bleeding will probably be evident in the cerebrospinal fluid.

Noncommunicating Hydrocephalus. Particularly with a vein of Galen anomaly, downward pressure from the tortuous vein can obstruct the ventricular system (aqueduct of Sylvius), thereby preventing normal flow of cerebrospinal fluid. Arteriovenous malformations can extend into the choroid plexus, resulting in hydrocephalus.

Cardiac Decompensation. Large quantities of blood passing through a vein of Galen anomaly can produce cardiac hypertrophy and congestive heart failure. This is due to the demands exerted upon the cardiovascular system which exceed its capability, particularly in the infant or young child. Immediate management of congestive heart failure is necessary.

Other Presenting Symptoms. Some patients experience transient episodes of syncope, fainting, dizziness, motor weakness, sensory deficits or tingling, aphasia, dysarthria, visual deficits (usually hemianopsia), and mental confusion. Others develop dementia or intellectual impairment as a result of chronic ischemia of the frontal lobes.

SIGNS AND SYMPTOMS OF CEREBRAL ARTERIOVENOUS MALFORMATIONS

While some vascular lesions may continue to be asymptomatic throughout life, arteriovenous malformations usually become symptomatic between the ages of 10 and 30 years.

The most important signs and symptoms of arteriovenous malformation include hemorrhage, seizure activity, headache, bruit, syncope, motor deficits and sensory deficits, visual deficits, and mental changes.

Hemorrhage. *Hemorrhage and seizure activity are the most frequent initial symptoms of arteriovenous malformations.* In approximately 50% of patients admitted with arteriovenous malformations, the anomaly has bled sometime before admission. Studies show that this occurs before the age of 30 years in about 50% of patients. By the age of 40 years, 72% have bled. The possibility of bleeding does not appear to be directly related to size, site, age, or sex.[1]

An arteriovenous malformation that has bled once has a 1:4 chance of bleeding again within 4 years. One that has bled more than once has a 1:4 chance of bleeding again within the year. Hemorrhage associated with arteriovenous malformation can be intracerebral, subdural, or subarachnoid.

Seizure Activity. *Seizures are one of the two most common initial symptoms of arteriovenous malformations.* Seizure activity ir 'tially may be focal or jacksonian but often becomes generalized. Psychomotor seizures are seen with temporal lobe lesions, while focal (motor and/or sensory) or generalized seizures are evident with frontal and pareital lesions.

Headache. Headache is a common complaint of patients with arteriovenous malformation; however, it is difficult to assess the significance of headache because it is common in many other avascular conditions. Some patients experience migrainelike headaches. The combination of onset of seizure activity and headache should prompt careful evaluation for the presence of arteriovenous malformation.

Bruit. Only 2% to 10% of patients with cerebral arteriovenous malformation experience bruit. The possibility of auscultation of a bruit depends on the size and location of the arteriovenous malformation and the thickness of the skull. A bruit is more apt to be heard in a child because a child's skull is thinner. A dural arteriovenous malformation, because of its peripheral position, is more likely to be auscultated than one that is located intracranially.

DIAGNOSIS OF CEREBRAL ARTERIOVENOUS MALFORMATIONS

Regardless of the circumstances prompting the patient to seek medical attention, a detailed history and physical and neurological examination are essential in establishing a definitive diagnosis of arteriovenous malformation. The following is a list and description of the common diagnostic studies ordered in diagnosing arteriovenous malformations.

Arteriography. The most essential definitive diagnostic procedure is cerebral arteriography. In addition to localizing the arteriovenous malformation, cerebral arteriography allows for visualization of large feeding arteries and large drainage veins. In true cone- or wedge-shaped arteriovenous malformations, an enlarged drainage vein frequently follows the direction of the cone. It can be a landmark in delineating the arteriovenous malformation and its arterial supply.[2]

An arteriogram will also indicate whether an intracerebral hematoma has developed from hemorrhage. At times, findings will not be observed. For example, if malformations are destroyed as a result of bleeding, the arteriogram will appear normal. Also, the presence of cerebral vasospasms will prevent the visualization of a malformation upon arteriogram.

Computed Tomography (CT) Scan. The CT scan, especially with contrast media, can allow differentiation of an arteriovenous malformation from a clot or tumor.

Brain Scan. If the scan is conducted immediately after injection of the isotopes, an uptake in the arteriovenous malformation will be noted.

Electroencephalogram (EEG). An EEG can be helpful in localizing an arteriovenous malformation. However, cerebral tissue adjacent to the malformation has frequently undergone atrophic or ischemic changes, thereby producing abnormal electrical potential. These findings of the EEG can be misleading in localizing the lesion.

Skull Films. Frequently, the walls of cortical vessels are atypically embedded with areas of calcification. In such instances skull films will reveal a suspicious area that requires further investigation. Certain brain tumors can also have areas of calcification within their boundaries. Therefore, calcified areas are abnormal but not indicative of a specific diagnosis.

Lumbar Puncture. Clinical evidence of increased intracranial pressure would contraindicate a lumbar puncture. If no such clinical signs are present and a lumbar puncture is done, the pressure may be normal or elevated. Red blood cells and xanthochromia are evident with bleeding into the subarachnoid space.

Laboratory Values. The white blood cell count and protein are also elevated if bleeding has occurred. The glucose level is usually within normal limits. (Normal values: white blood count — a few lymphocytes; protein — 15 mg to 45 mg/100 ml; glucose — 45 mg to 85 mg/100 ml)

Chest Radiography. Cardiomegaly or cardiac hypertrophy, which is possible in infants and young children with a vein of Galen anomaly, can be evidenced by chest radiography.

Electrocardiogram (ECG). A vein of Galen anomaly can also produce cardiac decompensation and congestive heart failure (Fig. 25-2). Evidence of such abnormality can be noted on ECG, allowing definite treatment of the congestive heart failure to be instituted.

Blood Flow Studies. Blood flow studies can measure regional blood flow before and after surgical intervention. Blood flow studies provide data on improvement of regional blood supply.

Nursing Implications During the Diagnostic Work-up. The patient requires much emotional support during the diagnostic work-up. He should be given an explanation of the procedure, preparation, and postprocedural management.

FIG. 25-2. Aneurysm of the vein of Galen, causing heart failure in the newborn. (Hardy J: Rhoads Textbook of Surgery. Philadelphia, JB Lippincott, 1977)

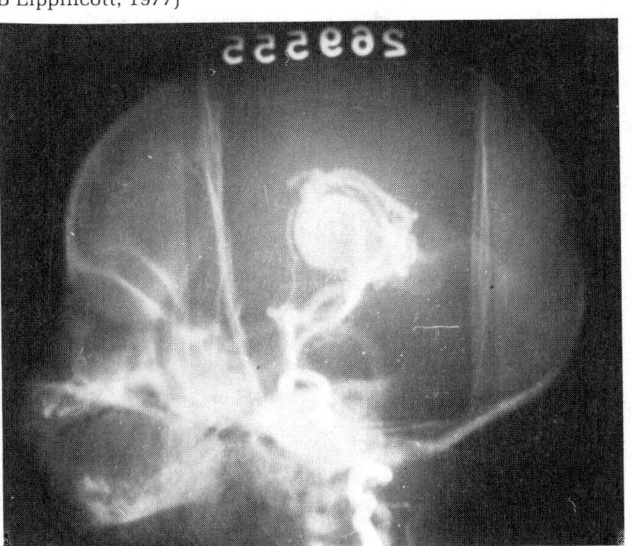

TREATMENT OF CEREBRAL ARTERIOVENOUS MALFORMATIONS

Various methods of treating arteriovenous malformations are in current use. The choice of treatment depends on the size and location of the arteriovenous malformation, feeder vessels supplying it, age and condition of the patient, and cerebral dominance. The availability of particular treatment modalities at the facility to which the patient has been admitted is another consideration. The methods used to treat arteriovenous malformations include: conservative medical management, embolization, proton-beam radiation, Nd:YAG, surgical excision, and a combination of embolization and surgery. Each method will be discussed briefly.

Conservative Medical Management

If a patient is first seen after hemorrhage that has resulted from an arteriovenous malformation, he is managed as a candidate for potential rebleeding. He is conservatively managed on subarachnoid precautions until a definitive plan of care has been developed. (See Chap. 24 for subarachnoid precautions.) The major concerns in the posthemorrhagic period are rebleeding and vasospasms.

If surgery is considered, it is usually postponed until the patient has been well stabilized after the hemorrhage (about 2 to 3 weeks). The patient is managed like the patient with bleeding from a cerebral aneurysm. The patient treated with conservative, symptomatic management should have a nursing care plan that implements the principles and goals of conservative management for subarachnoid precautions (see Chap. 24.) The patient will need an explanation and reinforcement of the goals of care. Because the patient diagnosed with an arteriovenous malformation tends to be young and often is very active, the enforced bed rest and limitation of activity needs to be reinforced frequently.

Cerebrovascular lesions, other than arteriovenous malformations, are often asymptomatic. Problems most often arise because of hemorrhage and require careful medical management. If bleeding and a hematoma develop, surgical evacuation of the clot may be necessary. Vein of Galen anomalies are always treated surgically.

Embolization

Embolization may be elected for surgically inaccessible arteriovenous malformations. The embolization technique was pioneered by Luessenhop in the early 1960s.[4] This procedure involves introducing small Silastic beads into the internal carotid artery by means of a catheter, which enters the malformation (Fig. 25-3). The results are thrombosis and destruction of the lesion.

Embolization is most effective for arteriovenous malformations supplied by the middle cerebral artery because the Silastic beads tend to follow the flow pattern of the middle cerebral artery. Therefore, malformations supplied by anterior or posterior cerebral arteries will most likely not respond to embolization.

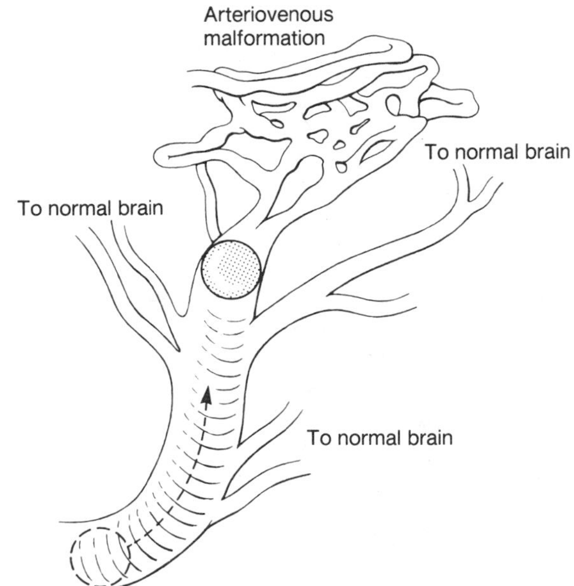

FIG. 25-3. Small Silastic beads or spheres are introduced into artery to block blood flow to the AV malformation.

The usual preparation of the patient is similar to that for any surgical patient (nothing given orally, skin prep, and so forth). The area of the skin shave will depend on whether the catheter is to be introduced into the femoral or carotid area. After an arteriogram is performed to verify anatomical consideration of the malformation, the catheter is positioned in the cervical portion of the internal carotid artery. The Silastic spheres are introduced through the catheter one at a time and are carried by the increased blood flow to the lesion. The spheres range in size from 1.0 mm to 6.0 mm. The size selected is based on estimation of the lumen of the artery. A size slightly smaller than the feeder vessel is chosen. The most common sizes used are 2.0 mm and 2.5 mm.

Serial arteriograms are taken throughout the procedure to verify the position of the beads. The beads can be introduced two or three at a time after the first few singular ones have been lodged in position. When the vessel is almost filled with spheres, the introduction of additional spheres, once again, is reduced to one at a time. The procedure is concluded when the arteriovenous malformation is occluded, the circulatory time of the blood through the lesion is reduced, visualization of normal proximal vessels is noted, or a normal vessel has been occluded.[5]

Occasionally, a bead may escape from the lesion and lodge in the capillaries of the lung. Lodging in the lung usually produces minor difficulties. However, if a normal cerebral vessel has been inadvertently occluded, neurological deficits can result.

Upon conclusion of the procedure, another arteriogram is taken. Although arteriovenous malformations may be occluded temporarily, leptomeningeal collateral circulation often provides a new vascular supply that tends to activate the lesion again.

The postprocedural management includes close monitoring of vital and neurological signs. If the femoral approach is used, routine precautions and observations for a femoral puncture are followed (check pedal pulse, immobilize upper leg, observe pressure dressing in groin for bleeding).

If embolization is to be followed by surgical excision of the lesion, the surgery may be postponed for about 4 weeks. The patient may be discharged to his home for the interim.

Proton-Beam Radiation

For surgically inaccessible arteriovenous malformations, proton-beam radiation is an option to be used as an ablative procedure to shrink the arteriovenous malformation. This is a noninvasive procedure that utilizes the radiation emitted by protons that have been accelerated in a cyclotron.[6] The procedure is conducted by using stereotaxic technique to direct the beam to the target area.

The major advantages of this approach are that hospitalization is very short and there is limited risk to the patient. The full effect of the treatment may not be apparent immediately. It may take up to 2 years for the optimal effects of the treatment to be realized. A disadvantage of proton-beam radiation is that it is available in very few facilities.

Laser Nd: YAG

A laser is a light beam that can be focused on an area to destroy or shrink selected tissue and coagulate blood vessels, while having no negative effects on surrounding structures. The Nd: YAG laser is a laser beam of a particular wave length. A discussion of lasers is included in Chapters 14 and 21. Laser therapy uses stereotaxis to accurately locate the target tissue. Laser therapy is appropriate for inaccessible arteriovenous malformations in delicate areas of the brain.

Surgical Excision

Complete surgical excision is the treatment of choice, but unfortunately, about half of arteriovenous malformations are surgically inaccessible for various reasons. The decision for surgical intervention is based on an assessment of the following criteria: location of the lesion, anatomy of the lesion, surgical accessibility, age and condition of the patient, previous history of hemorrhage, and the presence of neurological deficits. Patients who have bled once have an increased risk of bleeding again, as has been previously mentioned. A history of previous bleeding is therefore an additional reason for considering surgery rather than risk the very real possibility of another hemorrhage.

Surgical excision of an arteriovenous malformation requires a craniotomy, a major surgical procedure. The management of the patient is consistent with that of any other craniotomy patient. If the successful removal of the entire arteriovenous malformation is not possible, ligation of the feeder vessels may be attempted so that a thrombosis of the lesion will result, thereby obliterating the blood flow through the vessel. Partial or complete destruction or removal of an arteriovenous malformation is demonstrated by cerebral arteriography.

Combined Embolization and Surgery

With some large arteriovenous malformations, embolization is first scheduled to decrease the size of the lesion. Once the size has been decreased, surgical removal is planned.

NURSING MANAGEMENT OF THE PATIENT WITH A CEREBRAL ARTERIOVENOUS MALFORMATION

The patient who is suspected of having a cerebral arteriovenous malformation is at risk for hemorrhage. If hemorrhage has not occurred, patient management will be directed at preventing bleeding and includes controlling hypertension, seizure activity, and any other activity or stress that could elevate the systemic blood pressure. The patient is managed in the same manner as a patient with a cerebral aneurysm would be managed before rupture:

- Maintain a quiet therapeutic environment by placing the patient on subarachnoid precautions (see Chap. 24).
- Monitor and control associated hypertension with drug therapy, as ordered by the physician.
- Conduct baseline and ongoing neurological assessments.
- Monitor vital signs frequently.
- Assess and monitor characteristics of headache, if present.
- Assess and monitor presence of seizure activity.
- Assess and monitor bruit, if present.
- Provide emotional and psychological support.

If the arteriovenous malformation has ruptured, the patient will be managed in the same manner as the patient with a ruptured cerebral aneurysm. This includes the same principles as those outlined for before rupture of a cerebral aneurysm as discussed in Chapter 24, but with the addition of nursing management directed at the control of elevated intracranial pressure and intracranial hemorrhage. Management of the patient with increased intracranial pressure is included in Chapter 12. The patient with a ruptured arteriovenous malformation will have bleeding into the subarachnoid, subdural, or epidural space or into the brain itself (intracerebral hemorrhage). The rupture from the malformation usually causes a concurrent elevation in intracranial pressure.

For the patient undergoing surgery, the nurse plays a major role in patient teaching. The specifics of preparation and postsurgical management will depend on the specific procedure selected by the surgeon. Regardless of the procedure, the nurse will assess and monitor vital and neurological signs, as well as maintain body functions and prevent complications. Rehabilitative principles will be incorporated into the plan of care to help the patient achieve the highest level of independence possible.

PROGNOSIS FOR CEREBRAL ARTERIOVENOUS MALFORMATIONS

The prognosis for all vascular lesions depends on many factors such as location, size, surgical accessibility, and results of treatment. The major concern with an arteriovenous malformation is bleeding. Even after treatment, if complete excision of the lesion has not been possible, there is the ever-present risk of bleeding.

ARTERIOVENOUS MALFORMATIONS OF THE SPINAL CORD

An arteriovenous malformation can arise anywhere on the spinal cord, although it usually occurs on the posterior surface of the cord. Symptoms associated with the arteriovenous malformation tend to appear more often in the fourth or fifth decade of life although they may appear at any time. The spinal cord arteriovenous malformation has the same description as a cerebral malformation.

PATHOPHYSIOLOGY

As a result of the shunting of blood away from the spinal cord, ischemia and infarction of a portion of the spinal cord can develop and lead to myelopathy and/or thrombosis. The malformation can also rupture. Infarction, thrombosis, or hemorrhage can precipitate edema of the cord. The altered blood supply and/or cord edema will result in loss of spinal cord function.

SIGNS AND SYMPTOMS

The specific signs and symptoms will depend on the level of cord involvement. The patient may experience particular signs and symptoms in the early stages such as easy fatigability of muscles, particularly the legs; leg cramps; gait disturbances; spastic ataxia; sexual dysfunction; and bowel and bladder dysfunction. There may also be radicular pain at the level of the malformation and back pain. An acute episode caused by infarction or hemorrhage will result in loss of dissociated sensory function (loss of selected sensory modalities), paraplegia or quadriplegia, and loss of bowel and bladder sphincter control. These signs and symptoms develop immediately or within a few hours.[7]

DIAGNOSIS

The major diagnostic tool for spinal cord arteriovenous malformations is spinal angiography. Specific information is collected on the size, location, and number of feeder vessels; the overall size and location of the arteriovenous malformation; and the size, location, and number of the draining vessels. Based on this information, the physician can make a decision about appropriate treatment.

TREATMENT

Infarction of the cord is treated symptomatically. An arteriovenous malformation of the spinal cord consists of reducing the amount of blood shunted from the cord or excising the malformation, if possible. If the arteriovenous malformation has feeders located entirely on the posterior surface of the spinal cord, surgical resection is usually the treatment approach selected.

Another treatment protocol, in selected patients, is gluing of the spinal cord arteriovenous malformation. This new procedure may be elected when the arteriovenous malformation is located either totally or partially on the anterior surface of the cord.[7] The gluing procedure may be used alone or in conjunction with a resection. With the assistance of fluoroscopy, the procedure consists of insertion of a French catheter into an individual intercostal artery supplying the arteriovenous malformation and injecting a glue. The glue used is a FDA-approved material called isobutylcyanoacrylate (IBC), which is a liquid bioadhesive that polymerizes immediately upon contact with blood. It acts within 1 to 4 seconds, forming a matrix in which fibrin forms.[8] The major complication of the procedure is infarction of the proximal blood vessels.

NURSING MANAGEMENT OF THE PATIENT WITH A SPINAL CORD ARTERIOVENOUS MALFORMATION

Regardless of the treatment selected for the patient, the nurse will need to include the following points in the plan of care:

- Initial and ongoing neurological assessment including evaluation of motor and sensory function of the extremities and sphincter control
- Control of pain
- Patient teaching in the preoperative phase
- Emotional and psychological support
- Rehabilitation of the neurological deficits present

CAROTID–CAVERNOUS FISTULA

A carotid–cavernous fistula is a rare complication described as a direct communication between the high-pressure arterial blood of the internal carotid artery and the low venous pressure of the cavernous sinus. The internal carotid artery passes through the cavernous sinus. A fistula develops most often from a laceration of the carotid artery caused by head trauma, especially a basal skull fracture. Less frequently, it occurs as a result of a ruptured intracavernous carotid artery aneurysm.

PATHOPHYSIOLOGY

The cavernous sinuses are located at the base of the skull on either side of the body of the sphenoid bone. In this venous channel are located portions of the internal carotid artery and several of its branches, the oculomotor nerve, the trochlear nerve, two divisions of the trigeminal nerve, and the abducens nerve.

The high-pressure arterial blood is pumped into the low-pressure orbital veins that normally empty into the cavernous sinus, causing distention of the veins, proptosis, and pain in the affected orbit. The pressure within the cavernous sinus causes decreased motion or opthalmoplegia of the extraocular muscles (III, IV, and VI). There may be pain in the face because of pressure on the two divisions of the trigeminal nerve.

SIGNS AND SYMPTOMS

The most consistent features of a carotid–cavernous fistula noted on the affected side are bruit heard over the orbit of the eye, pulsating proptosis, conjuctival edema, orbital pain and chemosis, limitation of ocular movement, headache, and visual deficits (diplopia, photophobia, decreased visual acuity that can lead to blindness).

DIAGNOSIS

The definitive diagnostic procedure is carotid angiography. The size, characteristics, circulatory pattern and drainage, and collateral circulation are outlined so that treatment can be planned.

TREATMENT

Although spontaneous resolution may occur in a few patients, surgery will be necessary for most. Surgical procedures include surgical ligation and trapping procedures (e.g., ligation of the internal carotid artery above and below the fistula), embolization procedures (e.g., balloon occlusion, and electrothrombosis.

NURSING MANAGEMENT

The nurse will be responsible for conducting an initial and ongoing assessment of the patient that includes neurological and vital signs, visual deficits, extraocular movement, auscultation of the bruit, presence of headache, position of the eyeball, presence of orbital pain, and conjunctival edema. In addition to basic nursing management, the nurse should provide special eye care, control pain (headache and/or orbital pain), prevent injury to the eye (e.g., corneal ulcerations), and provide psychological support.

REFERENCES

1. Sah A et al (eds): Intracranial Aneurysms and Subarachnoid Hemorrhage: A Cooperative Study. Philadelphia, JB Lippincott, 1969
2. Kahn E et al: Correlative Neurosurgery, 2nd ed, pp 247–249. Springfield, IL, Charles C Thomas, 1969

3. Foster D et al: Arteriovenous malformations of the brain. J Neurosurg 37:562, 1972
4. Luessenhop A et al: Clinical evaluation of artificial embolization in management of large cerebral arteriovenous malformations. J Neurosurg 23:400, 1965
5. Wolpert S, Stein B: Catheter embolization of intracranial arteriovenous malformations as an aid to surgical excision. Neuroradiology 10:73, 1975
6. D'Agostino J, Pelczynski L: An overview of cyclotron treatment, Bragg Peak proton hypophysectomy, and Bragg Peak radiosurgery for arteriovenous malformation on the brain. J Neurosurg Nurs 11(4):208, December 1979
7. Adams RD, Victor M: Principles of Neurology, 2nd ed, pp 631–633. New York, McGraw-Hill, 1981
8. Stewart DJ: Gluing spinal cord AVMs. J Neurosurg Nurs 15(1):5, February 1983

BIBLIOGRAPHY

Books

Bebin J, Smith E: Vascular malformations of the brain. In Smith R, Haerer AF, Russell W (eds): Seminars in Neurological Surgery, pp 13–29. New York, Raven Press, 1982

Day AL, Rhoton AL: Aneurysm and arteriovenous fistulae of the intracavernous carotid artery and its branches. In Youmans JR (ed): Neurological Surgery, 2nd ed, pp 1764–1785. Philadelphia, WB Saunders, 1982

Haerer AF: Arteriovenous malformations of the brain: Some comments on their natural history. In Smith R, Haerer AF, Russell W (eds): Seminars in Neurological Surgery, pp 1–12. New York, Raven Press, 1982

Jennett B, Teasdale G: Management of Head Injuries, pp 279–280. Philadelphia, FA Davis, 1981

Malis LI: Arteriovenous malformations of the brain. In Youmans JR (ed): Neurological Surgery, 2nd ed, pp 1786–1806. Philadelphia, WB Saunders, 1982

Malis LI: Arteriovenous malformations of the spinal cord. In Youmans JR (ed): Neurological Surgery, 2nd ed, pp 1850–1854. Philadelphia, WB Saunders, 1982

Prolo DJ, Hanbery JW: Treatment of carotid cavernous fistula with catheter balloon. In Morley TP (ed): Current Controversies in Neurosurgery, pp 250–254. Philadelphia, WB Saunders, 1976

Smith RR: Essentials of Neurosurgery, pp 148–149. Philadelphia, JB Lippincott, 1980

Periodicals

Ambler M et al: Bilateral carotid cavernous fistulae of mixed type with unusual radiological and neuropathological findings. J Neurosurg 48(1):117, January 1978

Avman N, Ozkal E, Obken B: Aneurysm and arteriovenous malformation of the spinal cord. Surg Neurol 11:5, January 1979

Doolittle N: Arteriovenous malformations; The physiology, symptomatology, and nursing care. J Neurosurg 11(4):221, December 1979

Fode NC: Cerebral AVM's: An update for neuroscience nurses. J Neurosurg Nurs 16(6):319, December 1984

Hartshorn J: Carotid-cavernous fistula. Focus on Crit Care 10(2):32, April 1983

Kjellberg RN et al: Bragg-peak protron-beam therapy for arteriovenous malformations of the brain. New Engl J Med 309:269, August 1983

Kreber CW, Cromwell LD, Sheptak PE: Intraarterial cyanoacrylate: An adjunct in the treatment of spinal/paraspinal arteriovenous malformations. Am J Radiol 130:99, January 1978

Leslie DJ, Kammer KS: Carotid cavernous fistula: A case study and subject review. J Neurosurg Nurs 16(2):68, April 1984

Manuel S, Nolt S: Cerebral arteriovenous malformations and the role of embolization in treatment. J Neurosurg Nurs 9(4):152, December 1977

McDonald L: Carotid cavernous sinus fistula. J Neurosurg Nurs 8(1):23, July 1976

Sawitzke S, Teter A: Arteriovenous malformations of the brain: General review including role of embolization. J Neurosurg Nurs 8(2):132, December 1976

Stein BM, Wolpert SM: Arteriovenous malformations of the brain. I. Current concepts and treatment. Arch Neurol 37:1, 1980

Stein BM, Wolpert SM: Arteriovenous malformations of the brain. II. Current concepts and treatment. Arch Neurol 37:69, 1980

Sundt TM, Piepgras DG: The surgical approach to arteriovenous malformation of the lateral and sigmoid dural sinuses. J Neurosurg 59:32, July 1983

Williams MH: Arteriovenous malformations, complications of surgical intervention, and implications for nursing care. J Neurosurg Nurs 17(1):14, February 1985

part eight

Special Problems of the Neurological System

chapter 26

Headaches

HEADACHES

Headache, perhaps the most common and distressing human ailment, is experienced in varying degrees by most individuals at one time or another. Approximately 42 million Americans consult a physician each year for relief of headache. Headache is a symptom and not a specific disease. The symptoms of headache may indicate: (1) organic disease (intracranial, extracranial, or other disease), (2) physiological response to stress, (3) vasodilation, (4) skeletal muscle tension, or (5) a combination of these factors. Much more is known now than in the past about the nature and management of headaches because of extensive research on headaches in recent years.

CLASSIFICATION OF HEADACHE

Because the indications of headache are broad and varied, one would rightly expect an extensive classification system. The following classification of headache prepared by the *Ad Hoc* Committee of the National Institute of Neurological Diseases and Blindness has been a worthwhile system for categorizing headaches and is useful today.

1. Vascular Headache of Migraine Type

Vascular migraine-type headaches are a major classification of recurrent attacks that includes headaches of varied intensity, frequency, and duration. Commonly of unilateral onset, the headaches are usually associated with anorexia and sometimes with nausea and vomiting. There may be prodromal sensory, motor, or mood changes associated with the headache. Migraine-type headaches are often familial, more often affecting females.

The basic physiological alteration with migraine-type headaches is distention and dilation of cranial arteries in the painful phase. However, no permanent changes have been noted in the involved vessels.

Under the broad heading of migraine-type headaches are several subdivisions that are variations of the general description provided above. They include the classic migraine, common migraine, cluster headache, hemiplegic migraine, and ophthalmoplegic migraine. These variations will be discussed later in this chapter.

2. Muscle-Contraction Headache

Muscle-contraction headache is associated with prolonged contraction of skeletal muscles without structural damage as a result of a person's reaction to the stresses of living. The so-called "tension" or "nervous" headache is synonymous with this group.

The person experiences a sensation of aching, tightness, or pressure around his head. The frequency, duration, and location vary, although the suboccipital region is a common site. Treatment is directed toward developing coping mechanisms and using mild analgesics during an attack. This headache type will be discussed further in this chapter.

3. Combined Headache: Vascular and Muscle-Contraction

Features of both the vascular headache of the migraine type and muscle-contraction headache are concurrently present during the attack.

4. Headache of Nasal Vasomotor Reaction

Nasal vasomotor reaction headache is precipitated by stress rather than allergens, infections, or anatomical defects. The headache is predominantly anterior in location and is usually mild or moderate in intensity. The characteristic headache and nasal discomfort of stuffiness, rhinorrhea, tightness, and burning occur as a result of congestion and edema of nasal and paranasal mucous membranes.

5. Headache of Psychogenic Origin

The outstanding clinical features of this type of headache are depressive, delusional, conversional, or hypochondrial states that are experienced as headache by the patient. Treatment is directed toward diagnosis and management of the underlying problem.

6. Nonmigrainous Vascular Headache

Nonmigrainous vascular headaches are associated with incidental, nonrecurrent dilation of cranial arteries because of specific exposures to physiological and environmental factors. The list of common disorders includes

- Systemic infections, particularly with fever
- Other toxic systemic reactions such as "hangover" reaction, carbon monoxide poisoning, caffeine withdrawal, and foreign protein
- Metabolic conditions such as hypoxia, hypoglycemia, and hypercapnia
- Vasodilator drugs such as histamines and nitrites
- Acute cerebrovascular insufficiency
- Acute pressor reactions such as those seen in autonomic hyperreflexia and pheochromocytoma
- Early morning headache of hypertension
- Postconvulsive headache

Treatment of headaches in this category would be directed toward diagnosis and treatment of the underlying cause.

7. Traction Headache

Traction headache is due to traction on intracranial structures, usually vascular, by an intracerebral or extracerebral mass. Common causative agents include

- Primary and metastatic tumors of the meninges, blood vessels, and brain
- Hematomas such as extradural, subdural, or intracerebral
- Abscesses involving the meninges or brain
- Increased intracranial pressure from hydrocephalus, superior sagittal or lateral sinus thrombosis, cerebral edema, and pseudotumor cerebri
- Decreased intracranial pressure from leakage of cerebrospinal fluid (as from a lumbar puncture)

Control of the symptom of headache is associated with treatment of the underlying problem. Once that pathophysiology is corrected, the symptoms, including headache, will subside.

8. Headache of Cranial Infections

Headache of cranial infections is usually a symptom of a nonrecurrent inflammation or infection.

- Intracranial disorders that cause meningeal irritation such as meningitis, encephalitis, subarachnoid hemorrhage, postpneumoencephalographic reaction, arteritis, and phlebitis
- Extracranial disorders such as arteritis and cellulitis

Management of the symptoms of headache includes the administration of mild analgesics. Successful treatment of the underlying cause will eventually eliminate the symptom of headache.

9. Headache Caused by Referred Pain

The symptom of headache caused by referred pain is the result of trauma, new growth, inflammation, and occasionally allergens. Noxious impulses stimulate the involved dermatomal area, thereby causing referral of pain to the head.

- Ocular structures cause pain from increased intracoular pressure, excessive contraction of ocular muscles, trauma, inflammation, or a mass.
- Nasal and paranasal structures cause referred pain from nasal trauma or neoplasms and sinusitus from infections and allergens
- Structures of the ear can generate noxious stimuli from trauma and ear infections (middle ear infections).
- Neck and throat structures can cause headache from cervical spondylosis, cervical roots, periosteum, and ligaments of the neck. Carcinoma or trauma of the throat can cause headache.
- Dental structures can precipitate the symptoms of headache from caries, abscesses, and gum inflammation.

The symptom of this type of headache can be controlled by nonnarcotic or narcotic analgesics, depending on the severity of the pain. The underlying problem can be very diverse and treatment may require a referral to medical specialists in several other fields. For example, excessive contraction of the extraocular muscles without evidence of an intracranial mass would probably be treated by an ophthalmologist who would consequently suggest strengthening exercises or possibly surgery.

Headache caused by allergic sinusitis would probably be managed by the ear, nose, and throat specialist with possible referral to the allergist. Desensitizing injections, antihistamines, decongestants, analgesics, nasal sprays, and irrigations are all commonly prescribed protocols for management of sinusitis and associated headache.

Infections of ear, nose, throat, dental structures, or neck will most likely be treated with antibiotics. Trauma to any of the structures may require surgical repair or possible traction, followed by surgery in the case of neck injuries. Neoplasms will most likely require surgical removal or radiation therapy.

It is obvious from this brief discussion of headache from referred pain that it is important to identify and treat the underlying cause that makes its presence known by many signs and symptoms including headache.

10. Headache Caused by Local Cranial Disorders

The stretching of the periosteum from expanding lesions of the cranial bone or inflammation of the cranium or scalp causes headaches.

11. Headache Caused by Cranial Nerve Disorders

The most common cranial nerve disorders are trigeminal neuralgia and glossopharyngeal neuralgia. Both will be discussed in Chapter 30.

12. Headache of Posttraumatic Nervous Instability

Headache is a prominent feature of the syndrome of posttraumatic nervous instability. The pain varies from day to day and is very individualized. It is intensified by mental or physical exertion. Headache is very common in patients who have experienced unconsciousness. The intensity and duration of the head injury has no relationship to the severity of the headache. Mild head injury may be followed by severe headache. The intensity of the headache gradually subsides with time.

Treatment consists of analgesics to alleviate the headache. Nonnarcotic drugs should be ordered to prevent addiction to the drug, since headaches often last for an extended period.

SUMMARY

Some of the headache types described above relate to disorders discussed in other chapters in this book and will, therefore, be treated as symptoms in the appropriate chapters. Because 90% of patients seeking help for headaches experience vascular, migraine, or muscle-contraction headaches or a combination of them, these particular types will be discussed in greater detail.

APPROACH TO MANAGEMENT OF HEADACHES

GENERAL CONSIDERATIONS

The management of headaches in the patient is directed toward identification of the underlying cause. If the underlying cause is treatable, then the symptoms of headache will improve or disappear. For example, if the patient with headache is found to have a cerebral aneurysm or brain tumor that is surgically treatable, then clipping the aneurysm or removing the brain tumor will treat the underlying cause, and the symptom of headache will disappear. The patient with fever caused by a systemic infection may have headache as a symptom associated with the process. Controlling the fever will often control the headache. It is important for the physician to make an accurate diagnosis of the etiology of the headache. When headache is diagnosed as a vascular or muscle-tension headache, management is directed at treating the episodes of headache, and if they are frequent, preventing recurrent headache. The prevention aspect may entail patient teaching to control precipitating factors, change in lifesytle or health habits, drug therapy, or a combination of all three.

NURSE'S ROLE

The nurse's role in managing the patient with headache complements the role of the physician in that the nursing actions are directed at controlling the pain and discomfort of the headache episode and helping the patient to develop strategies to prevent recurrent episodes.

Assessment

A detailed nursing assessment and nursing history are the foundations for beginning the nursing process. Chart 26–1 is a sample of an assessment and history that can be conducted to collect necessary data. A quiet environment, unhurried manner, and adequate time are necessary to collect sufficient data. In order to gather all of the details necessary for planning care, one must establish a good rapport with the patient who will supply the information. The nurse must also interpret and adapt the questions to an appropriate level of understanding for the patient. Based on the information gathered in the history, indications for further assessment in particular areas may be evident.

Nursing Intervention

Once the diagnosis of the specific type of headache has been established, the nurse can help the patient to learn how to limit the number of attacks and minimize the effects, should the headache occur, by developing a patient teaching plan. With some types of headache such as migraine headaches, abortive drug therapy may prevent a headache from occurring if the specific medication and other measures are taken before the headache develops. In the instance of migraine headaches, early administration of Cafergot, a combination of 100 mg of caffeine and 1 mg of ergotamine, can completely abolish or significantly reduce the severity of the headache in 90% of patients.

Regardless of the type of headache, headaches are most apt to occur when the patient is physically ill, overworked, tired, or under stress. Stress is the major initiating factor in migraines. Therefore, the nurse should encourage proper diet, adequate rest and exercise, and effective coping mechanisms to deal with stress. If the patient is able to identify circumstances that tend to precipitate headache, the nurse may be able to explore alternatives and adjustments in lifestyle that can be made to minimize these triggering circumstances. Sometimes just helping a patient to learn to pace himself can be most beneficial.

Patients should be encouraged to keep a headache diary for reference. See Chart 26–2 for a sample diary. The purposes of headache diaries are to (1) collect data for analysis

CHART 26–1. ASSESSMENT OF HEADACHE

General History

1. Were any birth injuries noted?
2. Did you have encephalitis or meningitis either as a complication of childhood disease or as a separate entity?
3. Any history of abnormal nervous system development such as bed wetting, sleep disturbances, anxiety reactions (nail biting, fear, and so forth), or fainting?
4. Have you had middle ear infections, sinusitis, or surgical procedures to the ears or sinuses?
5. Have you had any injuries to the head, neck, or upper spine?
6. Is there evidence now or in the past of cardiovascular disease such as hypertension, heart disease, or orthostatic hypotension?
7. Have you ever had kidney disease, phenochromocytoma, tuberculosis, or tropical infections?
8. Have you ever had visual problems such as astigmatism, dysconjugate gaze, or eye strain? Have you had any eye surgery?
9. Have you ever had nervous system disease, such as a seizure disorder, vertigo, visual disturbances (diplopia), or psychiatric or emotional problems?
10. Do you see the dentist periodically? Have you had any dental problems?
11. Have you ever had arthritis or arthropathies of the neck, shoulder, or upper back?
12. Do you have any difficulty with chewing?
13. Do you use alcohol, tobacco, or any drugs? What kind? How much?
14. Do you have any food, drug, or environmental allergies?
15. (With women) Are there any particular symptoms associated with menstruation, pregnancy, childbirth, or menopause that are troublesome?

Familial History

1. Does anyone in your family suffer from headaches? If so, describe the headaches.
2. Is there a history of seizure disorders, allergies, emotional problems, or depression in your family?

Occupational History

1. What kind of work do you do?
2. What kind of work would you like to be doing? Why?
3. Describe the physical environment in which you work.
4. Are chemicals or fumes present? What kind?
5. Are other workers in your work area plagued by complaints of headaches?

Personal and Family Relationships

1. What kinds of things in your life are concerning you? (Most often anxiety is associated with loss—death, divorce, separation, independence, and so forth.)
2. Describe your overall emotional makeup.
3. What do you do to relax? Hobbies? Sports?
4. Describe how you react to stress. What body signals tell you that you are in a stressful state?
5. How do you get along with family members?
6. Are you able to discuss problems with family members?
7. What would you most like to change about your life?

Specific Headache History

1. At what age did the headaches start?
2. Where is the headache located (generalized, focal, unilateral, bilateral, frontal, occipital)?
3. Describe the type of pain (severe, mild, throbbing, aching, constant or intermittent, and so forth).
4. How frequent are the attacks?
5. How long do they last?
6. What factors are associated with the onset of headache (emotions, intoxication, specific foods, temperature, trigger points, menstruation, stress)?
7. What factors relieve the headache?
8. What factors aggravate the headache?
9. What is the usual course of events with the headache?
10. What symptoms accompany the headache (nausea, vomiting, visual disturbances, vertigo, watering eyes, flushing, sweating, hemiparesis, numbness, fainting, facial tic)?
11. How incapacitating is the headache in terms of your normal routines?

CHART 26–2. SAMPLE HEADACHE DIARY

Instructions: The purpose of the headache diary is to help us understand the circumstances and type of headaches that you have. This form should be completed every time that you have a headache and then shared with the nurse or physician.

Duration

- When did the headache start? Time: Date: Day of the week:
- When did the headache end? Time: Date: Day of the week:

Onset

- Does the headache come on suddenly or gradually?
- Are there any warning signs that a headache is about to occur such as
  —Changes in vision?
  —Numbness or strange sensations? What kind? Where?
  —Swelling?
  —Stuffy nose?
  —Fullness of the head?
  —Feeling of uneasiness?
  —Other? Please describe.
- What were you doing when the headache started?
- Did anything unusual happen recently?
- During the 24 hours before the attack did you have any special worries or shock, or were you overtired? Please describe.

Location

- Where is the pain located? Underline the terms that apply: frontal, occipital, temporal, unilateral, bilateral, generalized
- Where is the headache located when it begins?
- Does the headache move or extend as it develops?
- Does the headache involve the neck and shoulders?

Menstruation

- What was the date of the first day of your last period?
- When do you expect your next period?
- Do you have fluid retention, bloating, fatigue, or other unusual signs and symptoms associated with your periods?

Other

- When you have a headache do you have any other physical signs or symptoms (nausea, vomiting, dizziness, sensitive scalp, other)?
- What makes you feel better when you have a headache?
- What makes you feel worse?
- What do you think caused this headache? Is that different from other headaches that you have had?
- Is there anything else that you want to tell me about your headaches?

to demonstrate relationships between diet, drugs, physiological activities, emotional responses/states, and/or lifestyle and the occurrence of headache; (2) identify characteristics of the headaches experienced; (3) document the individual headache pattern; (4) provide a tool to document and alert the patient to the overall circumstances and characteristics of his headaches; and (5) provide the health professional with data for diagnosis and patient teaching. This diary can be very enlightening to the patient. For example, the chart may reveal that headaches seem to occur mostly on weekends when the entire family is home. Or, headaches may be noted to occur around the time of menstruation. It is most important to identify any rhythm or pattern in the occurrence of headaches.

For patients who tend to have weight gain and fluid retention around menstruation, a salt-restricted diet 1 week prior to menstruation should be encouraged. If this is not helpful, the physician may wish to prescribe diuretics. Other types of elimination diets should be encouraged for those patients who have identified relationships between the ingestion of certain foods and beverages and the occurrence of headaches. The major nursing diagnoses associated with headaches are found in Chart 26–3.

Patient Teaching

The last major responsibility assumed by the nurse is that of patient teaching in the area of drug therapy. The patient must be well versed on when to take his medication and what precautions should be taken (see Table 26–1 and Chart 26–4).

CHART 26–3. COMMON NURSING DIAGNOSES ASSOCIATED WITH HEADACHE

NURSING DIAGNOSES (actual or potential)	EXPECTED OUTCOMES	NURSING INTERVENTIONS
Alterations in comfort	• Reduce or abolish the pain. • Identify and reduce factors that precipitate headache.	• Document the characteristics and circumstances of the painful experience. • Help the patient identify factors that precipitate headache. • Manipulate the environment to control or prevent headache.
Ineffective individual coping	• Identify the causes of ineffective coping. • The patient will gain insight into the effects of ineffective coping. • Effective adaptive coping skills will be developed.	• Develop techniques to identify the causes of ineffective coping. • Establish therapeutic nurse–patient interpersonal relationships. • Assist the patient to gain insight into the cause–effect relationship of ineffective coping. • Assist the patient to develop adaptive coping skills.
Fluid volume excess: fluid retention	• Fluid retention will be eliminated or controlled.	• Help the patient to understand why fluid retention can contribute to the onset of headaches. • Identify signs and symptoms of fluid retention. • Identify dietary intake that contributes to fluid retention. • Discuss the purpose and need to take medications as ordered.
Noncompliance	• Patient will comply with the treatment protocol.	• Identify reasons for noncompliance. • Develop a teaching plan to provide appropriate information. • Develop a contract for compliance including techniques that help the patient to become compliant.
Sensory–perceptual alterations	• Sensory–perceptual alterations will be identified and controlled or eliminated. • Precautions to prevent injury will be implemented.	• Document type and characteristics of sensory–perceptual alterations. • Develop strategies to control or eliminate these signs and symptoms, if possible. • Institute measures to prevent injury. • Collaborate with physician to provide therapeutic protocol to treat the problem.
Sleep-pattern disturbance	• A satisfactory sleep–wakefulness pattern will be established.	• Document the sleep–wakefulness pattern. • Identify factors that prevent adequate sleep. • Develop stategies to overcome the obstacles to adequate sleep.
Knowledge deficit	• Patient will be knowledgeable about his headache type, precipitating factors, and treatment.	• Identify the specific areas of knowledge deficits or misinformation. • Develop a teaching plan to correct these deficits. • Evaluate the acquisition of new knowledge by the patient.
Anxiety	• Anxiety related to headache or potential of headache onset will be reduced or eliminated.	• Assess the reason for the anxiety caused by headache onset. • Help the patient to set realistic goals. • Develop anxiety and stress reduction strategies.

CHART 26–4. PATIENT TEACHING FOR MIGRAINE HEADACHES

The following are known to precipitate migraine headaches in the susceptible person and should be avoided:

1. Coffee, tea, cola, strong cheeses, chocolate, alcohol, red wine, citrus fruits, chicken livers, pickled herring, canned figs, broad beans, monosodium glutamate, and cured meats
2. Bright lights, sleep deprivation, fatigue, fever, and especially stress
3. A reduction in estrogen levels such as occurs just before menstruation or after the last oral contraceptive pill is taken; patients prone to migraine headaches should avoid oral contraceptives

The following should be included in the teaching plan for patients taking ergot preparations to abort a migraine attack:

1. The drug should be taken at the earliest sign of the headache, such as when the prodromal neurological signs appear.
2. If the medication is taken within 30 to 60 minutes of the onset of headache, 90% of patients will be relieved of the headache.
3. The earlier the drug is taken, the less of the drug is necessary to be effective.
4. Once the headache is full-blown, ergot preparations are of no therapeutic value.
5. Taking more than 10 mg of ergotamine per week can lead to a cumulative reaction with signs and symptoms of ergotism, which includes numbness and tingling of the fingers and toes, muscle pain and weakness, gangrene of the distal extremities, and possible blindness.
6. The patient should lie down in a quiet, darkened room after taking medication. (Photophobia appears to be associated with the pain of migraine headaches.)

DIAGNOSIS OF HEADACHE

The patient with frequent or severe headaches will usually consult his family doctor. If the family physician cannot identify the type of headache or underlying cause based on the history and physical examination, the patient may be referred to a neurologist or headache clinic. In this setting there will be a review of the referral summary followed by a complete physical, family, and headache history. A complete physical and neurological examination will be conducted to rule out any underlying disease. Based on the findings, referrals to other specialists may be made or diagnostic procedures may be scheduled. Typical diagnostic procedures may include a computed tomography (CT) scan, electroencelphalogram (EEG), and cerebral angiogram, among others.

Once the underlying etiology or diagnosis of headache type is made, the appropriate treatment can be instituted. The specific treatment protocols will be discussed under the type of headache.

VASCULAR HEADACHES

Vascular headaches, as the term implies, are associated with distention and dilation of cranial arteries in the early phase of the episode. Arteries of the brain are structures that are sensitive to stimulation and produce pain. The major subdivisions of vascular headaches include the classic migraine, common migraine, cluster headache, hemiplegic migraine, and ophthalmoplegic migraine.

CLASSIC MIGRAINE HEADACHE

The classic migraine headache is periodic and recurrent, beginning in childhood, adolescence, or early adult life and occurring less frequently with advancing age. It is more prevalent in women than in men and has a familial tendency. Most often, the headache begins after awakening although it can occur at any time. An attack of classic migraine is divided into three phases: the aura phase, the headache phase, and the postheadache phase.

The aura phase lasts between 15 and 30 minutes and is characterized by sensory manifestations, most commonly, visual disturbances (bright spots, dazzling zigzag lines). Other possible sensory symptoms include unilateral or bilateral numbness or tingling of the lips, face, or hand; slight difficulty in cerebration; paresis of an arm or leg; mild aphasia; slight incoordination of gait; confusion; and drowsiness. The neurological deficits last 5 to 15 minutes. In addition to the aura, some patients will experience a premonition of the forthcoming attack the day before it occurs. This feeling can be accompanied by nervousness or other alterations of mood. The period of the aura corresponds to the painless vasoconstriction that is the initial physiological change characteristic of the classic migraine headache. An associated increase in serotonin is noted.

The headache phase begins with vasodilation, a drop in serotonin, and the onset of a throbbing headache. The headache is often unilateral at onset but may involve both sides as the episode intensifies in the next 1 to several hours. Nausea and vomiting are common. The headache can last from 4 to 6 hours or sometimes as long as a day or two. The headache is very incapacitating. The walls of the cerebral arteries are dilated and stretched. Local tenderness of the scalp and periarterial edema develop. The walls of the vessels become edematous and rigid. This event is concurrent with a change in the character of the headache from a throbbing headache to one that is a dull ache.

In the postheadache phase, there may be a prolonged period of muscle contraction of the scalp or neck, resulting in deep aching and sensitivity to touch. The patient may feel exhausted. Any attempt at physical activity or bending may cause throbbing head pain.

The severe forms of classic migraine headache are hemiplegic migraine and ophthalmoplegic migraine headache.

HEMIPLEGIC MIGRAINE HEADACHE

In hemiplegic migraine headaches, the mechanism causing the headache may produce cerebral ischemia and subsequent hemiparesis or hemiplegia that lasts less than an hour. This type of migraine headache runs in families, a fact that is helpful in establishing the diagnosis of hemiplegic migraine headaches. A complete neurological work-up is necessary to rule out other possible intracranial disease processes.

OPHTHALMOPLEGIC MIGRAINE HEADACHE

Recurrent unilateral vascular headaches that are associated with extraocular muscle palsies have been termed *ophthalmoplegic migraines.* This rare form of migraine occurs most often in young adults. The discomfort from the headaches is moderate. The headache is accompanied by a transient oculomotor nerve (III) palsy often associated with ptosis on the same side as the headache. If the abducens nerve is affected, lateral movement is impaired; however, the abducens is rarely involved. It is not uncommon for some patients to also experience hemiparesis and sensory deficit along with the headache. The neurological deficits persist during the headache as well as days after the pain has terminated. On occasion, a mild nerve (III) palsy may become permanent, as evidenced by dilated pupil.

Psychic disturbances such as irritability, depression, or slight confusion may be noted with the headache. The headache is usually unilateral—frontal or temporal—but may occasionally be bilateral. Unlike other migrainous headache types, ophthalmoplegic migraine headaches may begin in adult or middle life. These headaches may also increase in intensity and frequency during menopause or with the onset of hypertension and vascular disease.

COMMON MIGRAINE HEADACHE

The common migraine headache may begin gradually at any age. There is a high hereditary correlation. Episodes occur at various times and are frequently associated with developmental life crises. Headaches also have a tendency to occur during periods of premenstrual tension and fluid retention. The incidence often decreases during pregnancy. The common migraine bears some resemblance to the classic migraine headache. With common migraines, the prodromal or preheadache phase is usually absent, although some patients do experience an awareness of a forthcoming headache hours or days before its occurrence. This may be accompanied by slight nausea, anorexia, or psychic disturbances.

The headache, which develops gradually, may last several hours to days. The pain is described as constant and throbbing. There may be accompanying chills, feverishness, fatigue, nasal congestion, nausea, vomiting, or depression.

CLUSTER HEADACHES (ATYPICAL MIGRAINE HEADACHES)

Cluster headaches are also called paroxysmal nocturnal cephalalgia, migrainous neuralgia, and (Horton's) histamine cephalalgia. The cluster headache is a vascular headache most often seen in older men. The headache begins without prodromal signs approximately 2 to 3 hours after falling asleep. The patient is awakened from sleep with intense unilateral pain of the orbitotemporal area, accompanied by rhinorrhea, possible miosis or ptosis, and unilateral or bilateral flushing, sweating, or edema of the face. The attack lasts between 30 minutes and 3 hours, ceasing as quickly as it began.

The term *cluster* is descriptive in that the attacks tend to occur frequently in clusters for weeks or a few months which are then followed by an extended period of remission. The same side of the head is usually involved in each cluster of attacks.

SPECIAL CONSIDERATIONS IN VASCULAR HEADACHE

Migraine Equivalents

Of the vascular migraine headaches described, it is important to be alert to the fact that several variations or "migraine equivalents" may be seen clinically. *Migraine equivalents* are migrainous headaches or other physical disturbances of decreased severity that have some correlation to specific migraine manifestations. These are often seen in patients who have been treated with antimigraine drugs. Patients who suffer from migraine headache may also have a history of headache interlaced with muscle-contraction headaches.

Food Cause

Another interesting point to consider is the association of certain foods, which are precipitating factors, with migraine headaches. Allergic reactions leading to headache have developed in some people from the ingestion of foods such as wheat, corn, apples, chocolate, nuts, and milk. Skin testing has confirmed this relationship in some individuals.

Foods may contain substances that trigger a headache

episode on a nonimmunological basis. For example, tyramine, a vasoactive substance that has been demonstrated to aggravate preexisting EEG abnormalities in individuals susceptible to migraine, is found in foods such as chocolate, wine, and certain cheeses.[1] As a prophylactic measure against migraine headaches, it has been recommended that the ingestion of the following be avoided: alcohol, strong cheeses, citrus fruit, chicken livers, pickled herring, canned figs, broad beans, monosodium glutamate, and cured meats containing nitrites.[2] The so-called "hot dog" headache has been associated with nitrites found in this processed meat.[3] The "Chinese restaurant syndrome" results in headache from the monosodium glutamate found in Chinese food.[4]

Patients should be carefully questioned in order to identify existing relationships between ingestion of certain substances and headache. If such a relationship can be identified, the patient can be encouraged to eliminate these substances from his diet.

Personality Factors

Stress is the major initiating factor in migraine headaches although the headache occurs after the stress is removed. Some texts discuss the *migraine personality* as a person who is intelligent, compulsive, and a perfectionist and copes poorly with stress. Although some authors question the validity of behavior profiles of patients who suffer from migraine headaches, certain tendencies in the individual's personality are acknowledged by most authorities to be contributing factors to migraine headaches. The patient tends to come from families placing a high priority on achievement. Aggressive and hostile feelings are repressed. Should the patient openly express such feelings or scorn achievement, he would be subtly punished by the family group. This leads to deep-seated hostility. The dilemma the patient faces concerns the anxiety created by emerging hostility that needs to be expressed and the pressure to conform to family standards. The migraine headaches are said to be a natural result of the conflict.

TREATMENT OF MIGRAINE HEADACHES

The treatment of migraine headaches involves a combination of patient teaching, control of contributing factors, and drug therapy. Patient teaching requires knowledge of precipitating factors, appropriate use of drug therapy, and other specific approaches such as stress management or biofeedback. The specific protocol depends on the type of migraine headache.

Drug Therapy

Drug therapy for migraine headache is usually divided into abortive and prophylactic treatment. Abortive therapy is directed at abolishing or significantly limiting a headache that is just beginning or is in progress. With migraine headaches, ergotamine tartrate administered orally, sublingually, rectally, subcutaneously, or intramuscularly at the first sign of a migraine headache is frequently effective in aborting the headache. With rectal administration, 2 mg of ergotamine is administered at the onset followed in 45 minutes and 90 minutes by the same dose until a maximum dose of three suppositories is reached. Cafergot tablets, a combination of 100 mg of caffeine and 1 mg of ergotamine, can be taken at the onset of the headache and again in 30 minutes. Rectal suppositories can be used if nausea or vomiting occur. Many patients are given medication such as Phenergan to control nausea and vomiting. Once the migraine headache is fully developed, the ergot derivatives are not helpful. The ergot preparations are therapeutic in two ways: first, they are alpha-adrenergic agonists and antagonists causing vasoconstriction or vasodilation depending on the state of the vessel; and second, they block the uptake of serotonin by platelets, which is known to reduce the precipitous drop of serotonin, a mechanism triggering a migraine attack.[5] One side-effect from ergot preparations is that of rebound headache, which results if the drug is administered for 2 consecutive days or if a certain dosage is exceeded. Ergotism is also a result of drug overdose.

For the patient who has frequent headaches, prophylactic drug treatment is instituted. The following drugs are used for this purpose:

- Methysergide (Sansert)—a serotonin agonist that acts by preventing serotonin release from platelets
- Propranolol (Inderal)—a beta blocker that prevents the dilation of blood vessels; it also inhibits serotonin uptake
- Clonidine hydrochloride (Catapres)—especially useful in migraines precipitated by dietary factors; acts by a central effect on the vessels making them less responsive to vasoconstriction or vasodilation
- Amitriptyline (Elavil)—tricyclic antidepressant drug that acts by blocking the uptake of serotonin and catecholamines centrally and peripherally; it is most effective for migraine headache associated with muscle-contraction headaches

The drugs commonly used in the management of migraine headaches are listed in Table 26-1. When a migraine headache is fully developed, the use of codeine sulfate or meperidine is useful to control the pain.

Patient Teaching

Points to be included in a patient teaching plan are included in Chart 26-4.

NURSING MANAGEMENT OF THE PATIENT WITH MIGRAINE HEADACHES

Nursing management is directed toward treatment of the acute attack and prevention. If the patient appears to be developing a migraine headache, abortive drug therapy should be instituted immediately. If the migraine headache becomes fully developed before abortive therapy is instituted, nursing intervention is directed toward keeping the patient comfortable. This includes

- Providing a darkened quiet environment
- Elevating the head
- Administering analgesic and antiemetic medication

TABLE 26–1. *Drugs Used in the Treatment of Vascular Migraine Headaches*

Drug	Use	Dose	Action	Side-Effects
Ergotamine tartrate (Gynergen)	Abortive treatment of vascular migraine headaches A single dose of ergotamine, 1 mg or 3 mg by injection at bedtime, is effective for cluster headaches	2 mg orally 2 mg sublingually, initially to be followed by 2 mg every 30 minutes until the headache subsides, or until 6 mg have been taken 0.25 mg to 0.5 mg subcutaneously or intramuscularly at onset; dose may be repeated hourly up to 1.0 mg in 24 hours 0.25 mg intravenously at onset; no more than 0.5 mg/24 hours; rarely given intravenously 2 mg to 4 mg by rectal suppository at onset; 2 mg may be repeated hourly, up to 6 mg to 8 mg	Ergot alkaloids result in cerebral vasoconstriction, which decreases the amplitude of the pulsations of the cranial arteries. In addition to its powerful vasconstrictive property, it also constricts the smooth muscles of the uterus. However, the major use of ergot alkaloids is for the treatment of migraine headaches.	Has a cumulative action, so that it must be taken sparingly and as ordered or ergotism will develop. (*Ergotism:* Numbness and tingling of fingers and toes, muscle pain and weakness, gangrene, and blindness) *Contraindications:* Diabetes mellitus, sepsis, hepatorenal disease, peripheral and coronary disease, hypertension, and pregnancy
Dihydroergotamine (DHE 45)	Treatment of migraine headaches that tend to be severe	1 mg intramuscularly or intravenously at onset; repeat in 1 hour	Action is not clear, but a majority of patients receive relief in 15 minutes to 2 hours after administration.	Less toxic and fewer side-effects than ergotamine; less likely to cause vomiting than ergotamine
Ergotamine with caffeine (Cafergot)	Same as ergotamine	Each tablet contains 1 mg of ergotamine tartrate and 100 mg of caffeine. Usual dose is 1 or 2 tablets at onset and another tablet in 30 minutes, not to exceed 6 tablets per attack (also available in suppositories if vomiting occurs)	The caffeine increases the effectiveness of the ergotamine by its vasoconstrictive action.	Same as ergotamine
{ *Ergotamine tartrate, 0.3 mg* *Phenobarbital, 20 mg* *Belladonna alkaloid, 0.1 mg* (*Bellergal*) }	Phophylactic, reduces the number of attacks in patients who have one or more weekly	Give two or three times daily for a few weeks.	Vasoconstriction, sedation, and reduction of spasm	Same as ergotamine, along with dryness of mucous membrane and drowsiness *Contraindications:* In addition to those of ergotamine, do not give to patients with glaucoma.
Methysergide maleate (Sansert)	For prophylactic treatment of vascular headaches such as migraine, cluster, and others that have been difficult to control; not effective for an acute attack; a serotonin antagonist *Alert:* Patient must be under medical supervision because this drug has such serious side-effects.	2 mg orally three times a day with meals; after taking drug for 5 months, it should be discontinued for 3 to 4 weeks to reduce the incidence of serious side-effects; dosage should be reduced gradually to prevent rebound headache.	The action is not clear, but it decreases the frequency of headache in patients who have a few headaches weekly that are difficult to control with other drugs.	Fibrotic changes in the retroperitoneal and pleuropulmonary tissue and in the mitral and aortic valves are the most serious complications. Any of the following symptoms should be reported at once: urinary tract obstruction; dysuria; back pain; peripheral vascular insufficiency;

TABLE 26–1. *(continued)*

Drug	Use	Dose	Action	Side-Effects
				cold, numb, or painful extremities and diminished pulse; dyspnea; and chest pain. *Contraindications:* Cardiac conditions, severe hypertension, pregnancy, peripheral vascular disease, and atherosclerosis
Propranolol (Inderal)	Prophylactic treatment for frequent migraine headache	20 mg to 40 mg three times a day	Beta blocker that inhibits the vasodilation of blood vessels Inhibits serotonin uptake	Fatigue, insomnia, nausea
Clonidine (Catapres)	Same as propranolol	0.1 mg two or three times a day	Direct effect on blood vessels causing diminished responsiveness	Drowsiness, dry mouth, weight gain, orthostatic hypotension, rebound hypertension if discontinued abruptly
Amitriptyline (Elavil)	Same as propranolol	50 mg to 75 mg daily	Blocks the uptake of catecholamines and serotonin centrally and peripherally A tricyclic antidepressant	Drowsiness, dry mouth, dizziness, weight gain
Others				
Analgesics				
Codeine sulfate, 30 mg or Meperidine (Demerol), 50 mg		Either drug may be given for severe pain once the headache has become full-blown. Narcotics are avoided unless the pain is very severe; precautions should be taken to avoid addiction.		
Aspirin, 0.6 gm Propoxyphene (Darvon), 65 mg Butalbital (Fiorinal), 2 tablets		These drugs may be tried for less severe pain.		
Diuretics				
Hydrochlorothiazide (Esidrix) or acetazolamide (Diamox)		These drugs are given 1 week before menstruation if premenstrual tension predisposes the individual to headaches. In addition, mild tranquilizers and analgesics such as aspirin may be given.		
Antihistamines				
Diphenhydramine (Benadryl) and others		May be helpful in cluster headaches		
Calcium channel blockers				
Verapamil (Isoptin)		May be helpful for migraine headaches		

Migraine headache is prevented by using a patient teaching plan that stresses avoiding precipitating factors and following the medication protocol prescribed by the physician. In addition, since stress is the major precipitating factor for migraine headaches, stress management is a necessary part of patient management. The specific plan for stress management will depend on the types of stresses experienced by the patient and the development of appropriate coping mechanisms. Referrals may be necessary to meet these needs.

MUSCLE-CONTRACTION HEADACHES (TENSION HEADACHE)

The *muscle-contraction headache* is defined as a sensation of aching tightness, pressure, constriction, or a viselike feeling around the head. The headache is usually bilateral and often poorly localized. The bilateral areas of the neck and the occipital and frontal regions are common sites. Onset is gradual, sometimes associated with slight anxiety, nausea, or dizziness. The intensity, frequency, and duration vary widely, sometimes lasting for a prolonged period. With prolonged headaches, there is often tenderness of the scalp. Muscle-contraction headaches are associated with a state of extended contraction of muscles with no structural change in the involved muscles. Other terms used synonomously for muscle-contraction headache are tension headache or nervous headache.

In some patients only slight muscle contraction will result in pain and headache if, concurrently with muscle contraction, there is also vasoconstriction of arteries supplying the area. Muscle contraction can be reflexly induced, secondary to noxious stimuli from diseases of the eyes, ears, paranasal sinuses, or cervical vertebrae. Anxiety and psychic tension are often common causes of muscle contraction that plague every person living in this complex society to a greater or lesser degree.

Exploring common, prolonged postures assumed by the patient throughout the day can often uncover sources of prolonged muscle contraction that can lead to headache. People engaged in occupations that require peering over a desk are prime candidates for headaches. Such workers include typists, office workers, auditors, and students. Knitting or slouching while reading or watching television can also lead to muscle contraction. Abnormal posture, muscle contraction, and spasms can be caused by sequelae from previous injury. So-called "trigger areas," resulting from previous injury elsewhere in the body, can relay impulses to the central system to produce referred pain to the head.

Diagnosis of muscle-contraction headache is made based on a history and negative findings in both the physical and neurological examinations. Laboratory examinations are also negative.

TREATMENT OF MUSCLE-CONTRACTION HEADACHES

Treatment of the headache is directed at prophylactic measures to prevent or reduce the occurrence of headaches and management of the individual attack. Prophylactic therapy is usually difficult because, most often, it requires behavioral changes for the patient. Most muscle-contraction headaches are caused by anxiety and psychic tension. Less often, headache can be attributed to the effects of former injury or poor posture. Developing new ways of coping with stress requires the unraveling of behavior patterns that have been learned and reinforced throughout life. However, some patients will have improvement of their headaches simply as a result of a thorough physical and neurological examination. The deep-seated fear of serious neurological disease is dispelled by the examination as well as by the reassurance of the physician.

Treatment of the acute headache is achieved by physical therapy and drugs. Gentle head massage and special placement of pillows to support the head and neck are of value.

Drug Therapy

Relief of pain with the use of drugs is best accomplished by a combination of analgesics and sedatives to relieve anxiety. Phenobarbital, meprobamate, and diazepam are commonly used sedatives. Diazapam has the added property of being a muscle relaxant. For control of pain, aspirin, propoxyphene (Darvon), butalbital (Fiorinal), and possibly oxycodone (Percodan) can be used. Narcotics should be avoided, if at all possible, because of the concern for habituation. Psychotherapy is usually of no benefit in controlling muscle-contraction headaches.

Other Approaches

Depending on the patient, biofeedback and relaxation techniques may be very helpful in controlling headaches.

NURSING MANAGEMENT OF THE PATIENT WITH MUSCLE-CONTRACTION HEADACHES

Many of the same principles suggested for migraine headaches can be applied to this patient. Proper diet, rest, exercise, and relaxation should be encouraged. Many people either do not have time in their busy schedules for relaxation or do not know how to relax. The patient needs to be helped to understand that the marvelous machine called the human body has limits of physical and emotional endurance. Exceeding these limits results in danger signals such as irritability, fatigue, gastrointestinal upset, or headache.

Another substantial area that needs to be explored is that of dealing with stress with effective reality perception, coping mechanisms, and problem-solving skills. These methods require honest evaluation by the patient, as well as much hard work, to alter previous ways of dealing with stress. This is indeed a gradual process. The patient can begin by keeping a headache history to note associations of stress and headache. Even the patient who is certain that no correlations exist can be surprised to be confronted by indisputable facts. The patient should be encouraged to start with one situation that leads to headache and develop alternatives to avoid the usual outcome.

Enrolling in adult education or college courses on self-awareness, self-assertiveness, and stress adaptation is just one means that can help the patient develop support systems for behavioral change. There are also many popular books addressing similar subjects.

In summary, the role of the nurse is to prod the patient to look at areas of his life and lifestyle and help him reflect on what he reveals to help him decrease the stress and tension that lead to muscle contraction and headache. The nurse should also encourage the judicious use of physical therapy and drugs to treat the acute headache episodes. Use of biofeedback and relaxation techniques should be considered.

REFERENCES

1. Moffett A et al: Effects of tyramine in migraine: A double-blind study. J Neurol Neurosurg Psychiatry 35:496, 1972
2. Current concepts of headache. Postgrad Med 56: entire issue, September 1974
3. Henderson W, Raskin N: Hot dog headache: Individual susceptibility to nitrite. Nurs Digest 1:55, 1973
4. Schaumberg H et al: Monosodium L-glutamate: Its pharmacology and role in the Chinese restaurant syndrome. Science 163:826, 1969
5. Ambielle M: Drug stop: Migraine headache: Current therapy. J Neurosurg Nurs 14(3):203, June 1982

BIBLIOGRAPHY

Books

Adams R, Victor M: Principles of Neurology, 2nd ed. New York, McGraw–Hill, 1981

Bogin M: The path to Pain Control. Boston, Houghton Mifflin, 1982

Brena SF, Chapman SL (eds): Management of Patients With Chronic Pain. New York, SP Medical & Scientific Books, 1983

Diamond S, Dalessio DJ: The Practicing Physician's Approach to Headache, 3rd ed. Baltimore, Williams & Wilkins, 1982

Meinhart NT, McCaffery M: Pain: A Nursing Approach to Assessment and Analysis. New York, Appleton–Century–Crofts, 1983

Saper JR: Headache Disorders: Current Concepts and Treatment Strategies. Boston, Wright-PSG, 1983

Van Meter MJ (ed): Neurological Care: A Guide for Patient Education, pp 92–109. New York, Appleton–Century–Crofts, 1982

Periodicals

Asher SW: Headache and facial pain. Hosp Med 33, November 1980

Barnett D, Hair B: Use and effectiveness of transcutaneous electrical nerve stimulation in pain management. J Neurosurg Nurs 13(6):323, December 1981

Barrett–Griesemer P et al: A guide to headaches and how to relieve their pain. Nurs81 11(4):50, April 1980

Basmajian JV: Biofeedback in rehabilitation: A review of principles and practices. Arch Phys Med Rehabil 62:469, October 1981

Beyerman K: Flawed perceptions about pain. Am J Nurs 82:302, February 1982

Booker JE: Pain: It's all in your patient's head (or is it?). Nurs82 12(3):47, March 1982

Bourbonnais F: Pain assessment: Development of a tool for the nurse and the patient. J Adv Nurs 6:277, July 1981

Dalessio D: Headache: Clinical guide to identifying the cause. Hosp Med 10, September 1979

Diamond S, Medina Jose: Headache. Clin Symp 33(2): entire issue, 1981

Friedman A et al: Ad hoc committee on classification of headache of the National Institute of Neurological Disease and Blindness. JAMA 179:127, 1962

Goldberg–Sklar C: Chronic pain management: A research focus. J Neurosurg Nurs 16(1):10, February 1984

Hanington E et al: A symposium on migraine. Nurs Mirror 13, August 11, 1977

Harvey P: Biofeedback: Trick or treatment. Nurs Mirror 15, April 27, 1978

Kozody R, Murphy T: Chronic pain: Current concepts in evaluation and management. Hosp Med 70, December 1982

Krieger DT: Endorphins and enkephalins. Disease of the Month 28(10): entire issue, July 1982

Lamb S: Cerebellar stimulation. J Neurosurg Nurs 12(1):32, March 1980

Lamb S: Neuroaugmentation for the chronic pain patient. J Neurosurg Nurs 11(4):215, December 1979

Leicht M: Non-traumatic headache in the emergency department. Ann Emerg Med 9:404, August 1980

Mason DJ: An investigation of the influences of selected factors on the nurses' inferences of patient suffering. Int J Nurs Stud 18(4):251, 1981

McDonald D: TENS in treating chronic pain. AORN J 32(3):401, September 1980

Meyer J: Diagnosis: Headache. Hosp Med 19, August 1981

Pawlicki RE: The pain clinic: A unique new prospect for nurses. Rehabil Nurs, pp 23–25, 29, May–June 1982

Piper M: Commissurotomy: Revival of surgery for the relief of central and bilateral pain. J Neurosurg Nurs 13(3):150, June 1981

Robb D, Ongkiko C: The differential diagnosis of headache and its nursing management. J Neurosurg Nurs 12(4):214, December 1980

Shealy CN: Holistic management of chronic pain. Top Clin Nurs 2(1):1, April 1980

Stein JM et al: The pain clinic. Hosp Pract 17:166, April 1982

Stieg R, Williams R, Gallagher L: Multidisciplinary pain treatment centers. J Occup Med 23(2):94, February 1981

Terzian MP: Neurosurgical interventions for the management of chronic intractable pain. Top Clin Nurs 2(1):75, April 1980

Wallace KG, Hays J: Nursing management of chronic pain. J Neurosurg Nurs 14(4):185, August 1982

Williams AE: Deep brain stimulation: A contemporary methodology for chronic pain. J Neurosurg Nurs 16(1):1, February 1984

Wilson RW et al: Endorphins. Am J Nurs 81:722, April 1981

Wolf ZR: Pain theories: An overview. Top Clin Nurs 2(1):9, April 1980

chapter 27

Seizures

The word *epilepsy* is of Greek origin and means "to be seized by a force from without." To the Greeks, epilepsy was a sacred disease; to Hippocrates it was a disease of the brain. In later ages it became known as "the falling sickness" or "falling evil" and was viewed as a form of mental illness, with victims being consigned to asylums for the insane.

The first steps toward understanding epilepsy were taken by Jackson in the 1870s. He theorized that seizures originated from a localized discharging focus in the brain. He also defined epilepsy as an "occasional, sudden, excessive, rapid, and local discharge of gray matter of some part of the brain."*

The introduction of the electroencephalogram (EEG) by Berger in 1929 provided the first recordings of epileptic discharge from the brain. Further work along this line by Gibbs and his colleagues in the 1930s correlated the clinical evidence of epilepsy with EEG findings. As a result of these studies, the EEG has become the primary tool in the diagnosis of epilepsy.

Regardless of the insights gained into epilepsy, stigma and fear are still associated with this problem. Because the word "epilepsy" has many negative connotations, the term "seizure disorders" has been adopted by many clinicians and writers. (In this chapter the terms epilepsy, seizures, and seizure disorders are used interchangeably.)

It is apparent that even though most legal restraints against epileptics have been removed, the social barriers still remain. Public awareness of the true nature of epilepsy is needed to dispel misconceptions and fears associated with this health problem.

DEFINITION AND DESCRIPTION

Epilepsy is a chronic syndrome that is peculiar to cerebral tissue and is characterized by recurrent paroxysmal episodes in which there is a disturbance in skeletal motor function, sensation, autonomic visceral function, behavior, or consciousness.

Because of the discontinuity of symptoms, epilepsy is categorized as a paroxysmal disorder. Periods between seizures can vary widely and can be measured in minutes, hours, days, weeks, months, or even years. However, there is repetition of seizure activity at some time in the future, regardless of the interval.

Epilepsy is a symptom of central nervous system irritation, the dysfunction being produced by excessive and abnormal neuronal discharge. In approximately 50 diseases, epilepsy or seizure activity may be one manifestation of the disease. Epilepsy is therefore considered a syndrome rather than a singular disease.

At one time, incidences of epilepsy that occurred without any identifiable central nervous system lesion or contributing extracerebral disease were called true epilepsy or idiopathic epilepsy. The term idiopathic epilepsy was reserved for seizure activity of unknown etiology. This concept has fallen out of vogue because it is now thought that the reason we cannot identify the etiology of certain forms of epilepsy is our lack of knowledge about some facets of central nervous system function. With the growing body of knowledge about neurological function, it is believed that other discrete etiologies will be identified.

* Penfield W: Ictus Epilepticus. Reprint No. 422, Vols 34, 35. Montreal Neurological Institute, 1953.

EPIDEMIOLOGY

Accurate figures concerning the incidence of epilepsy are not available, both because it is generally not a reportable problem and because patients are not apt to admit that they are epileptic. It is estimated that there are about 2 to 4 million Americans who suffer from epilepsy, many of them children.

Epilepsy varies in its clinical presentation according to the age of the patient and the maturation of the brain. In other words, the type of seizure varies with different age groups. The three most common age groups for the onset of epilepsy in childhood are (1) 0 to 2 years, (2) 5 to 7 years, and (3) early puberty, particularly in girls. About 90% of all epileptic patients experience the onset of their seizure before the age of 20 years.

ETIOLOGY

Given the right circumstances (created by physical or chemical stressors), anyone can be subject to seizures; however, some individuals have inborn genetic predisposition to seizure activity. In these instances, the seizure threshold of the brain is lower than normal, so that certain stimuli, benign for most other people, will precipitate seizures.

There appears to be a genetic tendency toward cerebral dysrhythmia in families with an incidence of epilepsy. However, not all people with cerebral dysrhythmia as noted on EEG will develop clinical symptoms of epilepsy. Nonetheless, the incidence of epilepsy in this population is greater than in families without cerebral dysrhythmia.

Epilepsy may also be caused by pathological processes that produce epileptogenic lesions in those areas of the cerebral cortex associated with recurrent seizures. In such instances, the epilepsy is said to be acquired, as would be the case with epilepsy that results from cerebral injury or insult, even when the correlation between the injury and the seizures is not initially apparent. Although cerebral injury is sustained, the onset of seizure activity may not be apparent for months or years. Sometimes the incident of injury is so insignificant that it is not noted at the time or recalled by the patient. The delay in onset is probably due to the gradual development of the metabolic and structural alterations of the involved cellular focus.

In general, epileptogenic categories may be described as cerebral, biochemical, posttraumatic, or idiopathic.

Cerebral lesions account for a large category of factors that may lead to seizure activity. They include (1) birth injuries such as trauma, anoxia, perinatal jaundice, and antenatal factors (infections or drugs); (2) infectious disorders such as meningitis, encephalitis, abscesses, or high fever; (3) cerebral circulatory disturbances such as subarachnoid hemorrhage, stroke, hypertensive encephalopathy, vasospasms, and vascular anomalies; (4) cerebral trauma such as epidural, subdural, or intracerebral hematoma, as well as cerebral laceration; and (5) neoplasms of the brain and metastic lesions to the brain.

Biochemical disorders often include epilepsy as a clinical feature. Some disorders are identifiable disease entities associated with genetic causes, such as Wilson's disease. Most conditions, however, are devoid of genetic cause. Examples of biochemical disorders that may produce seizures include (1) alcohol injection, (2) drug overdose, (3) seizure-inducing drugs such as pentylenetetrazol (Metrazol), (4) inorganic substances, (5) electrolyte imbalance, (6) vitamin deficiency, (7) diabetes mellitus and other carbohydrate metabolic disorders, and (8) endocrine disorders caused by pregnancy and menstruation.

Posttraumatic epilepsy results from previously sustained cerebral trauma. Common examples include craniocerebral trauma, birth injuries, and cerebral infections. The Epilepsy Foundation of America states that 8,000 new cases of posttraumatic epilepsy occur every year as a result of head injury.

Seizures can occur at any time following a head injury. However, there appears to be a definite pattern of onset. Few people develop seizures before 2 months or later than 5 years posttrauma. The highest incidence of onset of seizures is between 6 months and 2 years posttrauma.

Idiopathic epilepsy is epilepsy resulting without an identifiable cause. It is considered an acquired epilepsy because it is thought that the cause escapes current knowledge or diagnostic methods. The basis of this epilepsy is probably a biochemical imbalance.

The conditions and diseases mentioned are by no means all-inclusive of disorders associated with seizures. Any condition that causes cerebral irritation, either directly or by altering the biochemical milieu of the neurons, may precipitate seizure activity.

PRECIPITATING FACTORS

In patients with epilepsy, seizures can be triggered by a variety of stimuli. Sometimes the precipitating factor is very specific for a particular person. One of the most common precipitating events in children is a poorly adjusted television. Other precipitating stimuli include particular odors, certain types of music, loud noises, or simply being startled.

Other situations that appear to trigger seizure activity in epileptic patients are fatigue, hypoglycemia, lack of sleep, emotional stress, electrical shock, febrile illness, alcohol consumption, drinking too much water, constipation, menstruation, and hyperventilation.

If a stimulus can be identified, then the seizure is called *reflex epilepsy*.

GENERAL SIGNS AND SYMPTOMS ASSOCIATED WITH SEIZURES

The clinical manifestations of epilepsy can assume any number of forms. The epileptic attack may be characterized by a momentary cessation of activity or it may involve complex alterations of activity in which consciousness may or may not be lost.

A few terms that define or describe general signs and

symptoms are encountered repeatedly when considering seizures.

Tonus refers to a state of muscle contraction in which there is excessive muscle tone. A phase of the generalized seizure, also called a grand mal seizure, is composed of a tonic phase and clonic phase. In the tonic phase all of the voluntary muscles of the body are in a state of contraction.

Clonus is a term used to describe spasms in which a continuous pattern of rigidity and relaxation is repeated. In the second phase of a grand mal seizure, called the clonic phase, rhythmic movements are followed by muscle relaxation (Fig. 27–1). In the clonic phase, the process is repeated again and again.

Aura refers to a peculiar sensation immediately preceding the definite symptoms of a seizure. An aura can take the form of a gustatory, visual, or auditory experience, or it can be a feeling of dizziness or numbness of a body part.

Prodromal is a term that pertains to early manifestations or symptoms of a disease, such as a headache or feeling of depression, hours or a few days before the onset of seizures.

Ictus refers to an acute seizure attack such as a grand mal seizure.

The word *postictal* refers to the period immediately after a seizure has occurred.

PATHOPHYSIOLOGY

Most epileptic seizures are believed to arise from a few abnormally hyperactive and hypersensitive neurons that form an epileptogenic focus. (It is important to realize that the epileptogenic cells are abnormal in many physical, physiological, and chemical respects when compared to the so-called normal neuron.) The epileptogenic focus is largely autonomous and emits an excessively large number of paroxysmal discharges, often in bursts. Even when epileptogenic cells are relatively quiet (with no EEG evidence of seizure activity), they are hyperactive as compared with normal neurons.

CELLULAR MECHANISM OF SEIZURES

The exact cellular mechanism that initiates seizure activity is not clear. However, the involved neurons generate an autonomous paroxysmal discharge that can be enhanced or minimized depending on the neurotransmitter that is active on the postsynaptic membrane. The alterations on the synaptic membrane during seizures are not clear. It is known, however, that an epileptogenic focus has the ability to induce secondary epileptogenic foci in a synaptically related area and that there are connecting pathways between the same anatomical areas in opposite cerebral hemispheres. For reasons unknown, the normal cells sometimes undergo epileptic transformation, probably because of the continuous excitation from the epileptogenic lesion. This phenomenon is called a *mirror focus*.

The common denominator in epilepsy is rapid, repetitive depolarization of the abnormal epileptogenic focus. The frequency of cell firing can reach 300 to 1000 per second during a seizure through rapid depolarization of the resting membrane potential. Depolarization is associated with an intracellular accumulation of sodium as well as a depletion of intracellular potassium. It is in repolarization that the cell membrane returns to its normal resting potential. The sodium pump actively pumps sodium out of the cell when there is a concurrent intracellular influx of potassium.

As stated above, the cellular mechanism that initiates cellular activity leading to a seizure is unknown. At the onset of neuronal stimulation, depolarization is followed by a period of hyperpolarization, which is probably caused by an inhibitory postsynaptic potential. The hyperpolarization is soon replaced by depolarization, which rapidly increases in amplitude. The cell begins to fire repeatedly, thereby producing sustained membrane depolarization and seizure activity.

Tonic Phase

As the hyperexcitation spreads to the subcortical, thalamic, and upper brain stem, consciousness is lost and the tonic phase of the seizure commences. There are also con-

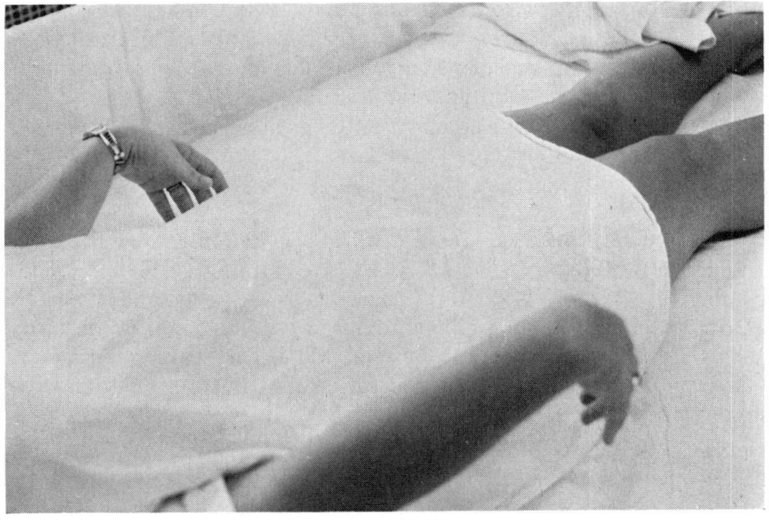

FIG. 27–1. Seizures are characterized by a continuous pattern of rigidity and relaxation.

current signs of autonomic nervous system overactivity such as salivation, pupillary dilation, tachycardia, and increased blood pressure. Apnea is possible, but it usually lasts for only a few seconds. Occasionally, death can ensue from the apnea and associated cardiac malfunction.

Clonic Phase

Inhibitory neurons of the cortex, anterior thalamus, and basal ganglion nuclei become active and intermittently interrupt the tonic seizure discharge with clonic activity. The clonic bursts gradually subside until they cease altogether. The involved cells are left exhausted.[1]

Posticital Period

Termination of seizure activity is associated with major membrane hyperpolarization, possibly initiated by the electrical potential generated by the sodium pump. On EEG, the high voltage spikes and waves (Fig. 27–2) gradually decrease. The involved cells cease firing, which, in turn, suppresses the abnormal firing of surface cells. In the postictal period the patient may initially be in a deep sleep, which is followed by confusion and lethargy. There may also be temporary paresis, aphasia, or hemianopsia.

Adenosine Triphosphate

During a seizure there is a drastic demand and consequent increase in the production of adenosine triphosphate (ATP). ATP is the major direct source of energy for the brain. The brain relies chiefly upon the metabolism of glucose for the production of the phosphate bonds necessary for ATP. During a seizure the demand for ATP is increased approximately 250%. The ATP provides energy for the sodium pump, synthesis of neurotransmitters, axoplasmic transport, and other basic cellular processes.

Cerebral Blood Flow

Cerebral blood flow to the brain is increased approximately 250% during a seizure in order to provide increased oxygen and remove carbon dioxide, a by-product of cellular metabolism. Cerebral oxygen consumption is increased by approximately 60%.

The cerebral blood flow can respond to the metabolic demands created by a seizure as long as hypoxemia, hypoglycemia, and cardiac irregularities do not develop. Increased metabolic activity in contracting skeletal muscles and apnea can result in hypoxemia and hypoglycemia, particularly if the patient experiences repeated seizures as in status epilepticus. The brain may require more energy than it can produce from the limited oxygen and glucose supply in the blood. A rapid decrease in ATP, phosphocreatine, and glucose occurs concurrently with increased levels of lactate, so that an energy debt occurs. Cellular exhaustion and some cellular destruction are the usual serious consequences.

THE ELECTROENCEPHALOGRAM AND SEIZURES

The *electroencephalogram* (EEG) is a diagnostic tool in which the amplified electrical potential of the brain is recorded by placing 14 to 21 electrodes on the patient's scalp. The electrical potential must be amplified because the average cortical potentials are about 30 millionths of a volt and would be too minute to be picked up without amplification. The tracings of electrical activity reflect the combined electrical activity of several neurons rather than only one. The basic resting electrical pattern of the brain is altered by opening the eyes or focusing attention on a problem, or by hyperventilation, photic stimulation, drugs, and sleep. In order to collect valid data on the EEG, the patient must be quiet, relaxed, cooperative, and seated comfortably in a chair with his eyes closed, although he is not asleep. He must follow instructions carefully, such as when he is asked to hyperventilate or open his eyes. The room in which the test is conducted must be shielded from extraneous electrical interference and noise.

Even though the EEG appears to have the greatest value in diagnosing seizures, it must be considered in conjunction with other information, including the history, physical examination, and other laboratory studies. Normal EEGs have been recorded in patients who have various types of seizure disorders between seizures. Conversely, nonspecific abnormalities have been found on the EEGs of 10% to 15% of the population who have never experienced seizures. In addition, EEGs considered "borderline" by one interpreter have been read as "normal" by another, indicating subjectivity and the fact that various criteria are applied in the interpretation of data.

The tracings for the EEG are made with special ink on electromagnetic paper. The recorded tracings signify the electrical potential difference from the scalp to the ear electrodes, and from the scalp to the scalp electrodes. The average EEG consists of 150 to 300 or more pages of recordings, with each page accounting for 10 seconds of tracings.

The frequency of EEG waves varies from 1 per 3 seconds to 50 per second. In the normal adult the most characteristic normal tracings noted at rest are (Fig. 27–2, *top*)

- Alpha waves—8½ Hz to 12 Hz (cycles/minute) seen best in the occipital and parietal areas
- Beta waves—18 Hz to 30 Hz, a faster wave, seen in the anterior areas of the brain

Both the alpha and beta waves are normally bilaterally symmetrical with their own characteristic shapes and amplitudes. Changes occur in the EEG pattern normally with various activities such as

- When eyes are opened, there is an immediate decrease in the amplitude of the brain waves.
- In early stages of sleep, the waves slow (lower voltage).
- In later stages of sleep, 14 to 16/second "sleep spindles" occur with subsequent high voltage and slow waves (½ to 3/second).

Abnormal EEG waves include (Fig. 27–2, *bottom*)

- Delta waves—less than 4/second with high amplitude
- Theta waves—4 to 7/second (not always abnormal)

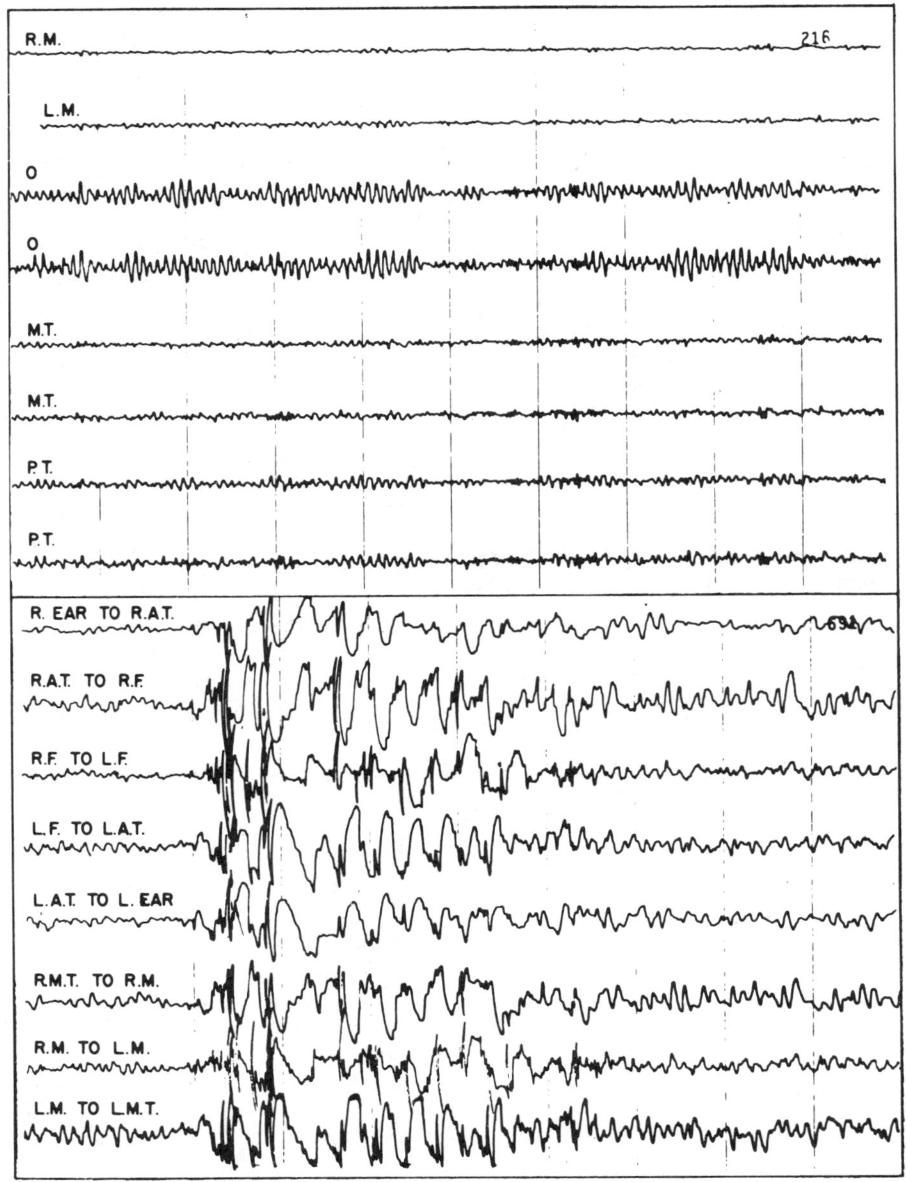

FIG. 27-2. Contrast of a normal electroencephalogram (EEG) *(top)* with that of an epileptic patient during a grand mal seizure *(bottom)*. Note the sharp, spiky waves recorded during the seizure. (Smith DW, Germain CP: Care of the Adult Patient: Medical-Surgical Nursing, 4th ed. Philadelphia, JB Lippincott, 1975)

- Spikes or sharp waves—high voltage, faster waves
- Asymmetry of frequency and amplitude from one side to the other

On an abnormal EEG, slow and fast waves may be combined in paroxysmal runs, thereby interrupting the normal pattern. These paroxysmal waves are highly suggestive of epilepsy. Recordings taken between seizures in the epileptic patient often include isolated spikes without evidence of a clinical seizure.

Abnormalities on EEG Noted in Specific Seizure Disorders (Fig. 27-3)

- Petit mal—3/second, rounded spike wave complex observed in all leads
- Grand mal—fast, high voltage spikes seen in all leads
- Temporal lobe seizures (psychomotor seizures)—spike complexes over the involved temporal lobe that can be square-topped 4 to 6/second waves (found particularly during sleep)
- Delta waves—often associated with destruction of brain tis-

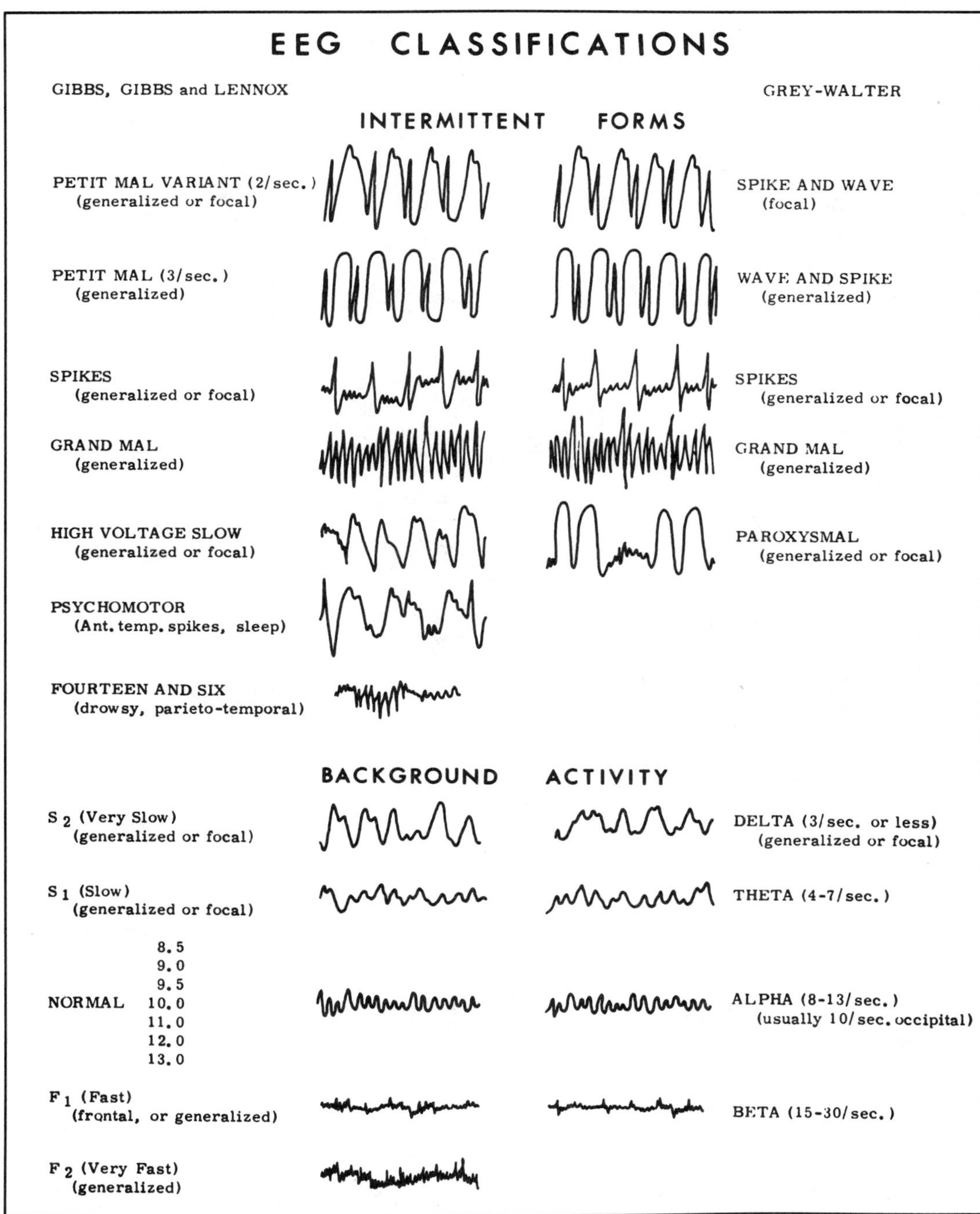

FIG. 27-3. EEG classifications.

sue such as infarction, tumor, or abscess (localized over abnormal area)

- Theta waves—not always abnormal

DIFFERENCES BETWEEN PARTIAL AND GENERALIZED SEIZURES

A clinical seizure will not necessarily occur each time a few epileptogenic cells become hyperactive. Much more seizure activity is noted on EEG than ever develops into clinical seizures. There are a few possible outcomes that might occur from the hyperactivity of an epileptogenic focus. The first possibility is that the hyperactivity will remain confined to the focus and eventually stop. Secondly, the hyperactivity may spread to other neurons within the general area, but the spread is local and does not involve the entire brain. The firing of the cells does not continue to spread because the cells come in contact with a resistance strong enough to cause the firing to stop. The third possibility is that the epileptic discharges will spread throughout the entire central nervous system. The first two situations are termed *partial seizures* because only part of the brain is involved, while the last situation describes a *generalized seizure* because the entire brain is involved.

There are times when a patient who usually experiences generalized seizure, such as grand mal seizure, may experience only a part of the usual manifestations of a seizure. This form of a partial seizure is termed *abortive epilepsy*. Following treatment with an anticonvulsant drug such as phenobarbital, a grand mal seizure may be observed or experienced as only a momentary loss of consciousness. The introduction of the anticonvulsant drug will afford some, although not complete, control of the seizure activity.

Partial (Focal) Seizures

The signs and symptoms of a partial seizure depend on the area of the brain involved. Consciousness is usually maintained as long as the seizure activity is restricted to one hemisphere. If the midline structures of the midbrain, thalamus, and hypothalamus are involved, unconsciousness results. This is particularly true if the reticular formation and thalamic nuclei are involved.

Generalized (Unlocalized) Seizures

With generalized seizures, both cerebral hemispheres and connections with the subcortical nuclei (thalamus, basal ganglia, upper brain stem) are involved. Consciousness is always impaired or lost with generalized seizures.

Some texts differentiate between primary and secondary generalized seizures. *Primary generalized seizures* involve the cerebral hemispheres and subcortical nuclei with immediate loss of consciousness. *Secondary generalized seizures* begin with a focal or partial seizure, which then spreads to involve both cerebral hemispheres and subcortical nuclei. In this variety of seizure the patient is initially conscious and experiences some focal manifestation. As the seizure spreads and converts to a generalized seizure, consciousness is lost and the other characteristics of a generalized seizure also become evident.

CLASSIFICATION OF SEIZURES

Attempts to classify seizures date back to Hippocrates (400 BC). New classification systems have been developed as new knowledge and techniques have been proposed. Bases for classification have been derived from the following categories: symptomatology, electrophysiology, anatomical origins, etiology, and response to treatment. Most authorities cite the International Classification of Epileptic Seizures, which was revised in 1969 by Gastaut, as the most practical and usable system currently available. It is based on the clinical nature of the onset of the seizure. The following classification for this discussion is adapted from Gastaut.[2]

- **I.** Partial seizures (seizures with a local origin)
  - **A.** Simple (elemental symptoms)
    - **1.** Focal motor (without jacksonian march)
    - **2.** Jacksonian
    - **3.** Adversive
    - **4.** Focal sensory (somatic sensory, visual, auditory, gustatory, and vertiginous)
    - **5.** *Epilepsia partialis continua*
  - **B.** Complex (symptoms usually include loss of consciousness)—temporal lobe seizures (psychomotor seizures)
  - **C.** With secondary generalized seizure
- **II.** General seizures (generalized bilateral without focal onset)
  - **A.** Tonic–clonic seizures (grand mal)
  - **B.** Absences (petit mal)
  - **C.** Myoclonic seizures
  - **D.** Infantile spasms
  - **E.** Tonic seizures
  - **F.** Atonic seizures
  - **G.** Akinetic seizures
- **III.** Unclassified epileptic seizures (including all seizures that cannot be classified because of inadequate or incomplete data)

The descriptions presented on the following pages will be limited to simple focal seizures, jacksonian seizures, and general seizures of the grand mal and petit mal variety. The remaining seizures are outlined in Tables 27–1 and 27–2.

I. PARTIAL SEIZURES

A. Simple Focal Seizures

1. Simple Motor Seizures (Focal Motor Seizures). Focal motor seizures, with or without a jacksonian-type march, originate from an irritative focus located in the motor cortex of the frontal lobe. The nature of the motor activity is usually clonic. The convulsive movement elicited by the seizure will depend on the specific anatomical–physiological portion of the irritated cortex. The particular convulsive movements are significant in locating the site of the lesion. The irritative focus is located in the hemisphere opposite the convulsive movement. In humans, a large area of the motor strip represents the face and hand movements. Not surprisingly, motor seizures most often begin in the face and hands.

2. Jacksonian Seizures. If the convulsive movements do not extend into the adjacent areas, the seizure is described as a focal motor seizure (without march). If the seizure activity spreads in an orderly fashion to adjacent areas, the seizure is termed a focal motor seizure with jacksonian march, or simply jacksonian seizure. The seizure is named for Hughlings Jackson, the English neurologist who first described the attack. With a jacksonian seizure, convulsive movements that begin in the fingers of one side, for example, spread to the hand, wrist, forearm, arm, face, and finally the lower extremity on the same side of the body.

A focal seizure begins with slow, repetitive jerking of a body part that increases in strength and rate over a period of 5 to 15 seconds. The seizure can cease spontaneously, with a gradual decrease in clonic movement. The other possibility is that the seizure activity could spread to adjacent areas after the momentum of the initial clonic movement increases. After spreading, the jerking movements in

TABLE 27-1. ***Partial Seizures (Seizures With a Local Origin)***

Type	*Description*	*Site*
Simple (elemental symptoms)		
Focal motor seizure (without jacksonian march)	See discussion on page 562.	Motor strip
Jacksonian seizure	See discussion on page 562.	Motor strip
Adversive seizure (any age affected)	• Turning of head and eyes to the side opposite the irritative lesion • Often associated with contractions of the trunk and extremities • May remain local or develop into a generalized seizure	Frontal lobe anterior to the motor strip
Focal sensory seizures (any age affected)	• Less common than focal motor seizures • Sensory experience is subjective and confined to the primary sensory modalities (somesthetic, visual, auditory-vestibular, or olfactory) • If sensory seizure begins in the hand area of the sensory cortex, the patient experiences numbness, tingling, or "pins and needles" phenomena. Other sensory experiences include burning, a crawling sensation, or a feeling of movement of the body part. • Areas most frequently affected include lips, fingers, and toes • May remain local or develop into a generalized seizure	Postcentral gyrus (parietal lobe), with involvement of the sensory motor strip
Epilepsia partialis continua	• A form of focal status epilepticus characterized by repetitive clonic movements in face and upper extremities • May continue for minutes, days, or weeks without spreading to other parts of the body • Consciousness not impaired but a postictal motor weakness is often seen • Often associated with a cerebral lesion	Varied

TABLE 27-2. ***Generalized Bilateral Seizures Without Focal Onset***

Type	*Description*	*Site*
Tonic-clonic seizures (grand mal)	See page 564.	Generalized
Absence seizures (petit mal)	See page 565.	Generalized
Myoclonic seizures Affect both adults and children but are most often seen in children	• Characterized by sudden, uncontrollable jerking movements of one or more extremities or the entire body • Seizure usually occurs in morning • Usually momentary loss of consciousness is followed by postictal confusion. • Patient often violently flung to the ground so that injury is a real possibility • Myoclonic seizures can occur in clusters. • If the frequency and amplitude of the seizures are severe, mental retardation can result.	Generalized
Infantile spasms Affect 3-month to 2-year age group	• Characterized by flexor spasms of the extremities and the head that have been described as jackknife seizures • Seizures last a few seconds and often appear in clusters with several clusters occurring daily. • Infantile spasms associated with metabolic, degenerative, or structural illness in 50% of cases; in other 50% no correlation is noted • Majority of victims are mentally retarded.	
Tonic seizures Affect infants and children	• Loss of postural tone without evidence of clonicity, with flexion of the upper limbs and extension of the lower limbs. • Patient assumes an abnormal posture for seconds or minutes without losing consciousness.	
Atomic seizures Affect infants and children	• Loss of postural tone with alterations of consciousness • Postictal period follows attack	Generalized
Akinetic seizures	• Characterized by sudden loss of postural muscle tone; "drop attacks"	Generalized

all areas would spontaneously stop. A jacksonian seizure can involve the subcortical structures, which would lead to unconsciousness and a generalized seizure.

3. Other Simple Seizures. Adversive, focal sensory, and *epilepsia partialis continua* are described in Table 27–1.

B. Partial Complex Seizures; Temporal Lobe Epilepsy (Psychomotor Seizures)

Temporal lobe seizures are partial complex seizures often associated with loss of consciousness. This form of seizure activity is common in both children and adults; however, the onset occurs before the age of 20 years in most patients. The characteristic EEG pattern has 4 Hz to 6 Hz, 50 to 100 microvolts, and flat-topped waves throughout the cortex.

The epileptogenic focus is located within the temporal lobe and its connections (limbic system). The attack is described as a seizure of altered behavior for which the patient is amnesic. He is able to interact with the environment with purposeful, although inappropriate, movements. A wide variety of sensory experiences are often reported by the patient. These experiences precede the automatism and include illusions, hallucinations, and primitive visceral, olfactory, and gustatory sensations. However, the most characteristic event of the temporal lobe seizure is the automatism.

Common examples of automatism are lip-smacking, chewing, facial grimacing, swallowing movements, and patting, picking, or rubbing oneself or one's clothing. Although the body muscles stiffen, the patient does not fall. He appears "wild-eyed" and might attempt to speak in jumbled, repetitive phrases, if addressed. Although it is less common, the patient may continue complex activity, such as driving, in which he was involved at the time of seizure onset. Temporal lobe seizures generally last from 1 to 4 minutes and are followed by several minutes of postictal confusion.

Common Subjective Symptoms of Temporal Lobe Seizures. The following subjective phenomena commonly precede the automatism seen in temporal lobe seizures; any may occur:

- Olfactory hallucinations may occur in the form of foul or disagreeable odors of an indefinable nature.
- Gustatory experiences, although rare, are described as acidic, metallic, or bitter.
- Common auditory experiences include sensations of buzzing, ringing, hissing, or machinelike noises. Vertigo, associated with tinnitus, is also present.
- Vague visceral sensations of the thorax, epigastric region, and abdomen are very common.
- Frequent autonomic experiences include hypertension, tachycardia, "gooseflesh," and increased esophageal peristalsis.
- Common illusory and hallucinatory experiences include feelings of déjà vu (a sense of familiarity with a seemingly unfamiliar environment), jamais vu (a feeling of unfamiliarity with a known environment), depersonalization, a sense of unreality, sudden changes in the perception of the size of objects, feelings of being in a dreamy or twilight state, and a sensation of time standing still.
- Affective or emotional experiences may occur, including feelings of fear, anger, paranoia, and anxiety, as well as sexual feelings. Less frequently, feelings of pleasure or laughter may be the predominant emotional theme. Rage reactions are rare.

C. Partial Seizures With Secondary Generalized Seizures

Partial seizures that become secondary generalized seizures arise from the spread of a focal seizure to the central structures, which causes unconsciousness and generalized symptoms. This is possible with any of the partial seizures discussed. Whether or not a focal seizure will extend into a generalized seizure will depend on the intensity of the epileptogenic focus and the general threshold and resistance of the brain.

Certain parts of the brain, such as the parietal lobe, are more resistant to seizure activity than other parts of the brain. The underlying physiology of this resistance is unknown. In contrast, the temporal lobe, with its well-established pathways, appears to have less resistance to the spread of seizure activity.

Following a seizure of any kind (partial or partial with secondary generalization), the patient may experience focal weakness lasting up to 24 hours. This postictal deficit is called *Todd's paralysis*. The weakness is significant in that it indicates a focal cortical lesion even though the seizure appears to be generalized from the onset. Physiologically, the basis for the temporary paralysis is probably because of neuronal exhaustion temporary depletion of oxygen and/or glucose supply. Todd's paralysis is commonly seen following a jacksonian seizure.[3]

II. GENERALIZED BILATERAL SEIZURES WITHOUT FOCAL ONSET

A. Tonic–Clonic Seizures (Grand Mal Seizures)

The grand mal seizure affects both children and adults and is a common variety of seizure activity. A prodromal period of irritability and tension may precede a grand mal seizure by several hours or days. In a majority of patients, however, the seizure begins without warning. Characteristically, the grand mal seizure begins with a sudden loss of consciousness and generalized tonic convulsion, later alternating with clonic convulsions.

With the sudden onset of unconsciousness, there is a major tonic contraction of the musculature (tonic phase). The body stiffens in the opisthotonos position, and the patient falls to the ground with legs and usually arms extended. The jaw snaps shut and the tongue may be bitten in the process. A shrill cry may be heard because of the forcible exhalation of air through the closed vocal cords as the thoracic muscles initially contract. The bladder and, less often, the bowel may empty. During the tonic phase the patient is apneic with subsequent cyanosis. The pupils dilate and are unresponsive to light. The tonic phase lasts less than 1 minute (average of 15 seconds).

The clonic phase begins with a gradual transition from the tonicity of the tonic phase. The clonic phase is characterized by violent, rhythmic, muscular contractions accompanied by strenuous hyperventilation. The face is contorted, the eyes roll, and there is excessive salivation with frothing from the mouth. Profuse sweating and a rapid pulse are also evident. The clonic jerking gradually subsides in frequency and amplitude over a period of about 30 seconds. The attack lasts from 2 to 5 minutes.

After the clonic phase, the patient is in a stupor or coma for about 5 minutes. The extremities are limp, breathing is quiet, and the pupils, which may be equal or unequal, begin to respond to the light reflex. When the patient awakes he may be confused and disoriented. He often complains of headache, generalized muscle aching, and fatigue. There is no recollection of the attack. If undisturbed, the patient may fall into a deep sleep for several hours.

Because the seizure frequently occurs without warning, it is possible for injury to be sustained when the patient falls to the ground. Head injury, fracture of the limbs or vertebral column, and burns are examples of serious injuries that may be sustained.

Grand mal seizures generally occur singularly or in groups of two or three. If the patient experiences another grand mal seizure without fully regaining consciousness between them, the term *status epilepticus* applies. Immediate medical management is necessary to prevent permanent brain damage.

Grand mal seizures may occur at any time of the day or night, whether the patient is awake or asleep. The frequency of recurrence can vary from hours to weeks, months, or years.

The typical pattern during a grand mal seizure is characterized by long runs of rapidly repeating spikes in the tonic phase and spikes of slow wave discharges in the clonic phase. An EEG taken during an actual seizure would probably have the typical pattern obscured by artifacts from muscle contractions. After the seizure is terminated, there is depression and slowing of the EEG pattern. A typical EEG tracing during a grand mal seizure is shown in Figure 27–2, *bottom*.

B. Absences Seizures (Petit Mal Seizures)

Petit mal seizures are almost always restricted to children over the age of 4 years who have not yet reached puberty. The attack is characterized by an abrupt cessation of activity with a momentary arrest of consciousness lasting about 5 to 10 seconds, although a few last 30 seconds. If the child were lifting a spoonful of food to his mouth, the activity stops. If he were walking, he stands absolutely motionless. He does not fall to the floor, and his normal breathing continues. The eyes become vacant and may roll, or the child may stare straight ahead. The lids may droop or twitch. The child is unresponsive if spoken to during an attack. He resumes his previous activity after the seizure. If he was talking, he will have lost the thread of the conversation, which may draw attention to the pause because of his lack of knowledge of what was said just moments ago. Many times, petit mal seizures go unnoticed by others. The victim is also unaware of the attack.

Some forms of petit mal seizures may be more complex. The most complex variety is more common in seizures lasting longer than 5 to 10 seconds. The complex components can be either automatism or clonic contractions. Automatism is of two types: perseveration and de novo. In the perseveration type, the patient continues in the activity in which he was involved, although his movements are distorted. In the latter type, new movements initiated after the seizure onset are observed. These activities might include smacking the lips, sticking out the tongue, or rubbing the face. Petit mal seizures with the clonic contracture component may be characterized by jerky muscle contractions around the eyelids, mouth, or other muscle groups. Another manifestation may be increased or decreased postural tone.

Petit mal seizures can occur a few times to hundreds of times daily. Patients who have several attacks daily most often have difficulty in learning, because of inattention in school. Petit mal seizures may be the only seizures experienced by the child in his childhood years. They often disappear at adolescence, or grand mal seizures may replace the petit mal seizures at adolescence. Hypoglycemia or photic stimulation can precipitate petit mal seizures in the susceptible child.

On EEGs, petit mal seizures are characterized by symmetrical, three-cycles-per-second spikes and wave patterns with abrupt starts and stops.

III. UNCLASSIFIED EPILEPTIC SEIZURES

The last major category of seizures is unclassified epileptic seizures. This group includes all seizures that cannot be classified because of inadequate or incomplete data. This self-explanatory category is a catch-all for seizures that do not conform to any of the other headings.

DIAGNOSIS

Because epilepsy is a syndrome associated with several conditions and diseases, it is important that an aggressive search be made for the underlying cause of seizure activity. This is no small task because the cause-and-effect relationship between underlying etiology and symptoms of epilepsy is not always apparent, expecially when there is an extensive interlude before seizures commence. For example, birth injuries that pass unnoticed in the neonatal and childhood periods may result in seizures in early adolescence, or posttraumatic epilepsy following head injuries may not develop until 2 to 4 years after injury.

Diagnosing epilepsy and any underlying causes requires a careful history as well as a physical and neurological examination. Questions about the details of the seizures should be asked to collect the following information: (1) age of onset, (2) progression of the seizure, (3) loss of consciousness, (4) subjective and objective details of the attack, (5) time intervals and frequency, (6) prodroma or aura experienced by patient, (7) precipitating factors, (8) postseizure behavior, and (9) any injuries associated with seizures.

Additional helpful data are gathered from the following studies: complete blood count (CBC), urinalysis, blood chemistries such as fasting blood sugar (FBS), Ca^+, P^+, blood urea nitrogen (BUN), and electrolytes; liver studies; blood and urine amino acids in infants and children; skull films; EEG; lumbar puncture, if not contraindicated; CT scan; and cerebral arteriogram.

Some patients will not require all of the procedures listed, while others may require additional studies. The objective of the studies is to identify systemic or central nervous system disease that is manifested, in part, by seizure activity. For many patients an extensive search for underlying etiology will be negative.

The EEG is perhaps the most indispensable procedure of all because it identifies patterns of electrical activity that can be correlated with particular types of seizures. An EEG can aid in localizing an epileptogenic focus in the brain that is in a trigger area for seizure activity.

DIFFERENTIAL DIAGNOSIS

With the plethora of causes of seizure activity, diagnosis can become a very complex problem. Brain tumor, cerebral aneurysm, cerebral arteriovenous malformation, drug toxicity, metabolic disorders, and psychogenic problems are but a few of the possibilities that must be ruled out. Many of the common conditions associated with seizure activity are discussed in this text. However, a condition referred to as pseudoseizure should be mentioned briefly because it is not covered elsewhere in this text.

Pseudoseizure has also been called hysterical epilepsy. The clinical picture has many similarities to that of an epileptic seizure, but there is no epileptogenic origin. The behavior is triggered by psychogenic internal or external factors. The diagnosis of pseudoseizure is difficult to make except with simultaneous EEG tracings and audiovisual monitoring. The nurse can focus observations on the patient to differentiate the specific characteristics of the event. With pseudoseizures, the onset is often dramatic, bizarre, gradual, and in the presence of witnesses. By comparison, epileptic seizures are sudden, paroxysmal, and orderly. Emotional upset usually precipitates pseudoseizure, and the episode lasts longer than a true seizure. The dramatic, violent flinging of the extremities, wiry movements, and inconsistent pattern of development are a sharp contrast to the tonic–clonic, orderly, repetitive movements of true seizures. If a scream is heard with a true seizure, it is at the onset of the event. With pseudoseizures, screams are heard throughout the course of the episode. Although incontinence, tongue biting, and postictal sequelae are common with epileptic activity, these same findings are absent with pseudoseizures. Observing the features, development, and finale of seizure activity can be most helpful in differentiating between true seizures and pseudoseizures.[4,5]

TREATMENT

The underlying condition responsible for the seizure will determine the type of treatment instituted. For example, if the diagnostic work-up has revealed a brain tumor as being the cause of the seizures, treatment is directed toward management of the brain tumor. Often, however, no underlying cause is identified, and treatment is directed toward management of the seizures.

About 75% of patients with seizures can be medically managed with drugs satisfactorily. For a small group of patients, surgery is considered if an epileptogenic focus can be identified or if seizures are intractable even with drug therapy. The most significant progress in surgical management of seizures has been with temporal lobe epilepsy.

Dietary therapy using a ketogenic diet has been given to some patients, particularly children, in an attempt to control seizures. A ketogenic diet is high in fat, producing acidosis. The ratio of fat : carbohydrates is 3 : 1, while the fat : protein ratio is 4 : 1. It is such an unpalatable diet that most patients refuse it. It cannot be considered a modern, accepted treatment protocol.

Another method of managing seizures is with the use of cerebellar stimulation. This method is still experimental, but is being more widely used and accepted. Biofeedback is also being used.

SURGICAL MANAGEMENT

About 5% of patients with epilepsy may be good candidates for surgery. Patients are carefully selected for surgical management of epilepsy. Patients who have not responded to medical management of seizure, who have a unilateral focus that will not cause a major neurological deficit if excised, and who have had a significant alteration in the quality of life are good candidates for possible surgery.[6] An extensive diagnostic work-up precedes surgery. The purpose of surgery is to locate and excise as much of the epileptogenic area as possible without extension of existing neurological deficits or the development of new ones. Local anesthesia is used for adolescents and adults unless they have behavior problems. In that case a light, general anesthetic is given. The patient *must* be able to follow commands and answer questions during the EEG and cortical stimulation portion of the lengthy surgical procedure.[2] After surgical exposure of the brain surface and depth, electrodes are applied so that an EEG can be taken to identify the epileptogenic focus. Cortical stimulation is used to identify sensory, motor, and speech areas. Stimulation is also used in an attempt to precipitate the particular aura experienced by the patient.

Once the tissue to be excised has been identified, the cortical resection is undertaken. Following excision, the electrodes are reattached to determine the presence of any other epileptogenic activity that would require further resection. If the EEG pattern is satisfactory, the patient is anesthetized so that the incision can be closed.

Postoperatively, the patient is managed as is any craniotomy patient (see Chap. 14), with the addition of high doses of anticonvulsant drugs. If the seizure pattern is reduced to the desired levels, the anticonvulsant drug is also reduced. Under the supervision of the physician, the patient usually continues the drug for the first year postoperatively. Routine EEG recordings are also taken to determine the presence of seizure activity. The average dose of phenytoin (Dilantin) for this first year is 200 mg daily, but the dose must be individualized based on the needs of the patient. The decision to discontinue drug therapy after 3 or more years is based on an individual evaluation of the patient.

One study indicated that in about 50% of patients with intractable seizures, control of or a substantial decrease in seizure activity is obtained from surgery. Another 25% of patients derive some benefit, while the remaining group shows little change in seizure activity.[7]

DRUG MANAGEMENT

In the vast majority of epileptic patients (75%), seizure activity can be reduced or controlled satisfactorily with anticonvulsant therapy. It should be emphasized that drugs are not a cure for epilepsy but a chemical means of managing a symptom that can seriously affect daily living.

Certain drugs are more effective for particular seizure types, making proper selection of the drug most important (Table 27–3). The drug is introduced and the dose increased until therapeutic levels have been reached, as determined by assessing blood drug levels. A reasonable trial period should be allowed for valid evaluation of the drug's effectiveness.

If desired results are not obtained, then another drug should be tried. The drug is introduced in gradually increasing doses until the optimal level is reached while, concurrently, the first drug is gradually tapered and finally discontinued. This practice is necessary because the sudden withdrawal of a drug can cause status epilepticus, even though a new drug has been introduced in its place.

Some patients do best on a combination of two drugs such as phenytoin (Dilantin) and phenobarbital. Use of more than two drugs is not recommended. The need for a combination of drugs could be prompted by the development of toxicity from a primary drug with seizure activity developing if the dose is lowered. Introduction of a second drug could allow for lowering of the dose of the primary drug without sacrificing control of seizure activity.

Drug Toxicity

The therapeutic dose for a patient is ascertained by trial and error. Some patients will develop signs of drug toxicity much sooner than others. Monitoring the blood for drug levels is helpful in evaluating toxicity in conjunction with clinical examination of the patient.

Time Element in Prophylactic Therapy

Once prophylactic anticonvulsant therapy has begun, it should be continued until 2 to 3 years have elapsed without any seizures.

TABLE 27–3. ***Summary of Drugs Often Given for the Treatment of Particular Types of Epilepsy***

Seizure Type	*Drugs Given (Generic Name)*	*Trade Name*
Grand mal, focal motor, and focal sensory	Phenytoin	Dilantin
	Phenobarbital	Luminal
	Primidone	Mysoline
	Mephenytoin	Mesantoin
Temporal lobe epilepsy (psychomotor seizures)	Phenytoin	Dilantin
	Phenobarbital	Luminal
	Primidone	Mysoline
	Carbamazepine	Tegretol
	Mephenytoin	Mesantoin
	Phenacemide	Phenurone
Petit mal seizures	Ethosuximide	Zarontin
	Trimethadione	Tridione
	Methsuximide	Celontin
	Valproic acid	Depakene
	Paramethadione	Paradione
	Phensuximide	Milontin
Myoclonic and akinetic epilepsy	Nitrazepam	Mogadon
Infantile spasms	Prednisone	
	Corticotropin	ACTH
	Nitrazepam	Mogadon
Neonatal epilepsy, febrile convulsions	Phenobarbital	Luminal
	Phenytoin	Dilantin
Major status epilepticus	Diazepam	Valium
	Paraldehyde	
	Thiopentone	
	Phenobarbital	Luminal
Minor forms of status epilepticus (petit mal, status, minor epileptic status, and epilepsia partialis continua)	Diazepam	Valium
	Corticotropin	ACTH
	Ethosuximide	Zarontin
Epilepsy related to menstruation	Hydrochlorothiazide	Hydrodiuril
	Acetazolamide	Diamox

Choice of Drug

When drug therapy is a major part of patient management, it is vital to know the usual dosage, methods of administration, side-effects, drug half-life, therapeutic serum levels, toxicity, and drug interactions. The drug half-life is important to note because drugs of long duration (phenytoin, phenobarbital) may be taken once a day in some circumstances.[1] The physician attempts to limit the number of various drugs taken by the patient in order to decrease the chances of drug interaction.

Although Table 27–4 has been developed to consolidate pertinent data about drugs administered in seizure disorders, a few drugs of choice will be discussed to emphasize nursing management. These drugs include phenytoin (Dilantin) and phenobarbital.

Phenytoin (Dilantin). Phenytoin (Dilantin), introduced in 1938, is a synthetic drug chemically classified as a hydantoin. It is an anticonvulsant drug that inhibits the spread of seizure discharges within the nervous system. Because it is

TABLE 27–4. *Pertinent Data Concerning Drugs Administered in Seizure Disorders**

Drug	Description	Use	Average Adult Daily Dose in mg (Range)
Barbiturates			
Phenobarbital (Luminal)	Most widely used anticonvulsant; often given in combination with phenytoin	Tonic–clonic and all forms of partial seizures	60 to 200
Mephobarbital (Mebaral)		Tonic–clonic seizures	400 to 600
Metharbital (Gemonil)		Tonic–clonic seizures	100 to 400
Primidone (Mysoline)	Frequent drug of choice for tonic–clonic seizures	Tonic–clonic seizures, temporal lobe epilepsy, and other forms of partial seizures	750 to 1500
Hydantoins			
Phenytoin; formerly called diphenylhydantoin (Dilantin)	Often used in combination with phenobarbital or primidone; frequent drug of choice for tonic–clonic seizures	Tonic–clonic seizures, temporal lobe epilepsy, and other forms of partial seizures	300 to 400
Mephenytoin (Mesantoin)		Tonic–clonic seizures, temporal lobe epilepsy, all other forms of partial seizures	200 to 600
Ethotoin (Peganone)		Tonic–clonic seizures	2000 to 3000
Phenacemide (Phenurone)		Temporal lobe epilepsy	1500 to 5000
Oxazolidinediones			
Trimethadione (Tridione)		Absence (petit mal) seizures	900 to 2400
Paramethadione (Paradione)		Absence (petit mal) seizures	900 to 2400
Succinimides			
Phensuximide (Milontin)		Absence (petit mal) seizures	1000 to 3000
Methsuximide (Celontin)	Used for absence seizures that are refractory to other drugs	Absence (petit mal) seizures	300 to 1200
Ethosuximide (Zarontin)	Drug of choice for petit mal seizures; effective within 24 hours of first dose	Absence (petit mal) seizures	750 to 1500
Other			
Carbamazepine (Tegretol)	Adjunct drug to drug regimen when seizures not well controlled by phenytoin, phenobarbital, or primidone	Grand mal seizures, temporal lobe epilepsy	600 (200 to 1200)
Valproic acid (Depakene)	Increases the brain's concentration of gamma-aminobutyric acid (GABA; inhibitory synaptic agent)	Simple (petit mal) and complex absence seizures	800 to 2000
Diazepam (Valium)	Considered drug of choice for status epilepticus	Status epilepticus	5 to 10 intravenously initially; may be repeated at 10- to 15-minute interval to a maximum of 30 (10 to 150)
Clonazepam (Clonopin)	May be useful for patients with absence seizures (petit mal) who have not responded to succinimides	Akinetic myoclonic, and Lennox–Gastaut syndrome (petit mal variant)	0.5 to 1.0 every 3 days until seizures controlled
Paraldehyde	Give deep intramuscular injection in glass syringe because plastic may be dissolved by the drug.	Status epilepticus	5 ml to 10 ml intramuscularly; 3 ml to 6 ml intravenously over 30 to 60 minutes
Corticotropin (ACTH)		Infantile spasms	
Prednisone		Infantile spasms	
Hydrochlorothiazide (Hydrodiuril)		Used only for seizures related to menstruation	50 (25 to 100)
Acetazolamide (Diamox)	Rapidly absorbed; not metabolized in body (excreted in urine)	Used for seizures related to menstruation	750

* There are wide variations in drug therapy prescribed by physicians. Dosages provided in Table 27–4 are the average ranges provided in standard texts and are subject to change.

Average Child Daily Dose (Range)	*Serum Half-Life in Hours*	*Therapeutic Serum Levels mcg/ml*	*Major Side-Effects and Toxicity*
3 mg to 5 mg/kg	96 ± 12	15 to 40	Drowsiness, dizziness, fever, irritability, rash, ataxia, anemia
6 mg to 12 mg/kg			Drowsiness, dizziness, rash
5 mg to 15 mg/kg			Gastric distress, dizziness, irritability, rash
10 mg to 25 mg/kg	12 ± 6	5 to 15	Drowsiness, dizziness, gastric distress, irritability, ataxia, rash, diplopia, nystagmus, anemia
4 mg to 7 mg/kg	24 ± 12	15 average; 10 to 20 range	Drowsiness, gastric distress, megaloblastic anemia, rash, ataxia, nystagmus, diplopia, fever, hirsutism, gingival hyperplasia
100 mg to 400 mg			Drowsiness, rash, blood dyscrasia, ataxia, nystagmus, dizziness, gastric distress
500 mg to 1000 mg	3 to 9	15 to 50	Dizziness, diplopia, rash, blood dyscrasias, nystagmus, gastric distress, lymphadenopathy
Age 5 to 10 years; 750 mg to 1500 mg			Rash, blood dyscrasias, hepatotoxicity, drowsiness, dizziness, nephritis, psychic changes
300 mg to 900 mg		600 to 800	Drowsiness, gastric distress, dizziness, photophobia, diplopia, hemeralopia, blood dyscrasias, nephrosis
300 mg to 900 mg			Same as Tridione
1000 mg to 3000 mg			Nausea, rash, ataxia, dizziness, hematuria, gastric distress, drowsiness
10 mg to 20 mg/kg	30 ± 6	40 to 100	Drowsiness, headache, anorexia, blood dyscrasia, ataxia
20 mg to 30 mg/kg	30 ±	40 to 100	Drowsiness, dizziness, blood dyscrasia, nausea, vomiting, anorexia, rash
20 mg to 30 mg/kg	12 ± 3	4 to 12	Dizziness, ataxia, diplopia, nystagmus, skin eruptions, and psychotic behavior
20 mg to 60 mg/kg	10 ± 2	50 to 100	Do not use in pregnancy; liver toxicity, nausea, vomiting, sedation, skin rash muscle weakness, thrombocytopenia
0.15 mg to 2 mg/kg intravenously			Fatigue, drowsiness, ataxia
0.01 mg to 0.2 mg/kg	20 to 40	0.01 to 0.07	Drowsiness, ataxia
			Local irritation can cause sterile absecesses and tissue sloughing.
20 u to 30 u intramuscularly for 3 to 4 weeks, then reduce dose			Usual steroid side-effects and toxicity
2 mg/kg			Usual steroid side-effects and toxicity
			Nausea, vomiting, dizziness, paresthesia, skin eruptions, photosensitivity; prolonged treatment can lead to hypokalemia, hyponatremia, diabetes mellitus, and gout
			Drowsiness and paresthesia

devoid of hypnotic effect, it is considered a safe and effective drug. Phenytoin is alleged to affect the sodium pump mechanism by stabilizing it.

Use. Phenytoin has been very effective in reducing and controlling the number of grand mal and psychomotor seizures. It is not effective against petit mal epilepsy and can actually increase the number of these attacks. Partial seizures have also responded well to phenytoin. The drug is often given prophylactically after intracranial surgery to prevent seizure activity. Phenytoin may be given in combination with phenobarbitol or primidone (Mysoline). This may be ordered when phenobarbital alone has failed to control seizures. By adding phenytoin, drug toxicity is decreased while a synchronous therapeutic effect is achieved. Phenobarbital reduces the plasma level of phenytoin when given in combination.

Administration. Administration is by the oral or parenteral route. If taken orally, it is slowly absorbed from the gastrointestinal tract over a 4- to 8-hour period. Slow absorption allows the drug to be taken twice daily rather than three or four times. It takes from 7 to 10 days for therapeutic levels to be reached, if standard doses are given. Phenytoin is also supplied as a suspension.

An interesting problem surrounds the administration of phenytoin suspension to patients who are also receiving entereal feedings via nasogastric, gastrostomy, or jejunostomy tube. By monitoring patients, it has been found that patients receiving phenytoin suspension and enteral feedings have a lower blood phenytoin level than patients receiving phenytoin and no enteral feeding. Although the problem continues to be studied, patients receiving phenytoin suspension and enteral feedings appear to require an increased dosage of phenytoin. Once the enteral feeding is discontinued, the dosage of phenytoin must be decreased. Monitoring phenytoin blood levels provides a guide for adjusting drug dosage of phenytoin.[8,9,10]

Although the drug literature states that phenytoin can be administered by the intramuscular route, the absorption rate is unpredictable and the drug is irritating to the tissue. The pH of phenytoin is approximately 12, which is indeed irritating to the tissue at the injection site. Frequent administration by this route causes discomfort for the patient. If the drug is administered parenterally, the intravenous route is preferred. Therapeutic blood levels of 10 mg to 20 mg/ml can be achieved rapidly by the intravenous route. Intravenous phenytoin (Dilantin) must be administered slowly at a rate no faster than 50 mg/minute in a solution of normal saline. If given in another solution such as 5% dextrose in water, the drug will precipitate into crystals in the solution. Proper administration is very important to remember because rapid administration depresses the myocardium and can cause cardiac arrhythmias and cardiac arrest.

Phenytoin is not given by intravenous push because the high pH of the drug is very irritating to the veins and the effect of rapid administration on the myocardium is very dangerous. Patients receiving intravenous phenytoin should be observed for the development of phlebitis.

Drug Interactions. Various drugs in common use can enter into drug interactions with phenytoin.[11]

Drugs that potentiate the action of phenytoin include aspirin, phenylbutazone, chloramphenicol, cycloserine, isoniazid, estrogens, disulfiram (Antabuse), chlordiazepoxide (Librium), sulfonamides, and anticoagulants (especially Dicumarol).

Drugs that inhibit the action of phenytoin include alcohol, antihistamines, barbiturates, glutethimide (Doriden), hypnotics, and sedatives.

Phenytoin potentiates the action of the following drugs: antihypertensives, folic acid antagonists, methotrexate, propranolol (Inderal), quinidine, and tubocurarine.

Phenytoin inhibits the action of corticosteroids and digitalis.

Toxicity. Acute overdose can produce nystagmus, ataxia, slurred speech, diplopia, lethargy, and disturbance in coordination. Chronic overdose causes confusion that can appear as dementia. Peripheral neuropathy is common. Some authors suggest that choreoathetosis and incoordination (cerebellar fits) can result from a reduction of the cerebellar Purkinje cells from chronically high doses of phenytoin; however, this has not been satisfactorily proven.

Side-Effects. A morbilliform rash may occur 10 to 14 days after beginning the drug in some patients. The appearance of such a rash indicates that the drug should be discontinued. A lupuslike syndrome has also been reported and is reversible when phenytoin is withdrawn.

Patients on long-term phenytoin therapy are subject to megaloblastic anemia, blood dyscrasias, and low serum folate concentrations. The patient should be monitored with periodic routine CBC counts to assess the development of anemia or dyscrasias. The low folic acid levels respond to folic acid therapy.

Gingival hyperplasia occurs in approximately 40% of patients on phenytoin therapy within 2 to 3 months after therapy is begun. The gums may even grow over the teeth. Gingival hyperplasia most often occurs in children and is rare in adults. Good oral hygiene, frequent brushing and flossing, and gum massage are highly recommended to prevent this problem. In some patients oral surgery is required.

Hypertrichosis (increased body hair on the face, arms, and body) may occur in a number of patients receiving phenytoin, particularly in young girls. This symptom is very distressing to the the patient and is irreversible after the drug is withdrawn.

Other reported problems include hypocalcemia, rickets, and osteomalacia. Coagulation deficits, depression of T_4 and protein-bound iodine, and increased formation of blood cortisol has also been reported. Phenytoin should be given cautiously during pregnancy, because evidence appears to indicate that it causes a higher incidence of birth defects.

Phenobarbital (Luminal). Phenobarbital introduced in 1912, was one of the first drugs for the control of seizures and is still widely used. It depresses repetitive electrical activity of the multineuronal networks. There is a sedative–hypnotic effect from the drug. The routes of administration are oral and parenteral. Phenobarbital is absorbed slowly from the gastrointestinal tract. It takes 10 to

12 hours to achieve peak blood concentration when administered orally and 20 minutes when given intravenously.

Toxicity. Dose-related toxicity includes sedation, nystagmus, ataxia, and learning difficulties. *Drug rash* is common. Periodic routine CBC should be monitored to detect anemia, another side-effect of long-term phenobarbital therapy.

Summary of Drug Therapy. In summary, any patient on long-term drug therapy should be watched carefully for the development of side-effects or toxicity. Routine periodic drug blood levels should be assessed. If anemia or blood dyscrasias are side-effects common to the drug that the patient is receiving, a CBC should be done routinely.

Patient Teaching. It is imperative to provide adequate information to the patient and/or a responsible family member about epilepsy and the drug therapy. Side-effects and signs of toxicity should be provided. The patient must understand that the drug must be taken as ordered *every day*. The most common cause of seizures in a patient whose seizures have previously been controlled by drugs is failure to take the medication. The patient should be asked to maintain a chart of the drug and the amount taken, along with a record of the frequency and characteristics of the seizures.

Because seizures are a chronic condition that is rarely arrested, the patient must understand the nature of his problem, the precipitating factors, and adaptation in lifestyle that is required.

The following is an outline of the major points of a drug-teaching plan:

1. The drug must be taken as ordered even if there is no seizure activity. A therapeutic blood level must be maintained for the drug to be effective.
2. Anticonvulsant drugs will probably to necessary for life.
3. Discontinuation of drugs on the patient's part is the most common cause of seizure activity. This should *never* be done.
4. The patient should know the *signs* of toxicity of the drugs that he is taking. He should promptly report symptoms of toxicity to the physician.
5. Because the side-effects of anemia and blood dyscrasia are common, the patient should report for routine blood work as ordered.
6. Because phenytoin is absorbed slowly from the gastrointestinal tract, daily drug schedules can be adjusted for the convenience of the patient. Missed doses can be "made up" safely when the forgotten dose is remembered.
7. Some patients can enjoy seizure control with the use of extended-release phenytoin, while other patients will require divided doses of prompt-release phenytoin.
8. Many patients refuse to wear a Medic Alert bracelet or tag or carry a card. If so, they should be encouraged to carry a card that indicates that they are being treated by a particular physician. If the patient is found unconscious or injured, the physician can be notified.
9. Patients should be followed by a physician and reevaluated periodically.
10. Status epilepticus can be precipitated by abrupt withdrawal of anticonvulsant drugs.

GENERAL CONSIDERATIONS IN LONG-TERM MANAGEMENT

Long-term management and periodic reevaluation are necessary with any chronic condition. All drugs have side-effects and toxicity, so the patient must be monitored for signs of toxicity. Medication may need to be adjusted or changed. Periodic reevaluation provides the opportunity for assessment of emotional, psychological, social, and vocational problems that are apt to develop as the patient adjusts to living with a seizure disorder.

NURSING MANAGEMENT OF THE PATIENT WITH SEIZURES

The objective of nursing management for the patient with seizures is directed toward providing accurate data based on observation of the patient, protecting the patient from injury during a seizure, controlling seizures, and rehabilitating and teaching the patient.

PROVIDING DATA

Collecting data about the events of a seizure requires highly developed observation skills and an understanding of what to look for and how to record the observations. It may be helpful to softly verbalize the observations as they occur. This technique can serve a secondary purpose by helping to control the fear experienced by observing the seizure. The verbal reinforcement also provides for better recall.

Nursing Assessment

The following list identifies the points that should be considered when observing a seizure:

1. Were there any warning signs or was there an aura?
2. Where did the seizure begin and how did it proceed? (If the beginning of the attack was observed, this should be recorded.)
3. What type of movement was noted and what parts of the body were involved?
4. Were there any changes in the size of the pupils or conjugate gaze position?
5. Was there urinary or bowel incontinence?
6. What was the duration of the entire attack and of each phase?
7. Was the patient unconscious throughout the attack?
8. What was the behavior of the patient after the attack?
9. Was there any weakness or paralysis of the extremities after the attack?
10. Did the patient sleep after the attack?

The observations can be recorded in narrative form in the nurse's notes or on a separate seizure activity sheet (Fig. 27–4), which becomes a part of the patient's permanent record.

SEIZURE ACTIVITY SHEET

Patient's Name ______________________
Room No. ______________________ *Age* ________
Physician ______________________

Date	Time	Before		During		Duration of each Phase				Other	After				Nurse's Initials
		Warning Signs	Part of Body Where Seizure Began	General or Localized	Type of Movement	Tonic	Clonic	Level of Consciousness	Pupils		Behavior	Paralysis	Location of Paralysis	Sleep	

FIG. 27–4. An example of a seizure activity chart.

MANAGING THE PATIENT DURING A SEIZURE

Protecting the patient from injury requires that any patient subject to seizure activity be placed on seizure precautions (Fig. 27–5). This means that (1) the siderails of the bed are up and padded, (2) a padded tongue depressor and an airway are conspicuously taped to the top of the bed (the padded tongue depressor can be used with special precautions to prevent injury from splinters or aspiration if an airway is not available), (3) a suction setup is available at the bedside, and (4) the bed is kept low.

Management of the patient during a seizure is directed toward prevention of injury. The following points should be followed:

1. Provide for privacy by pulling the bed curtains or screen or closing the door. (This protects the patient from embarrassment and curious onlookers.)
2. If the patient experiences an aura prior to a convulsion, have him lie down in order to prevent injury that might occur if he fell to the ground.
3. Insert a padded tongue depressor between the teeth, provided that the teeth are not clenched. Do not try to pry the mouth open when the teeth are clenched. (Inserting a tongue blade between the teeth will prevent the patient from biting his tongue or chipping his teeth.)
4. Loosen any constricting clothing around the neck to improve respiration.
5. Guide the patient's movements so that he will not be injured; do not restrain him.
6. Provide for adequate ventilation by maintaining a patent airway. The patient may need to be suctioned to prevent aspiration (Fig. 27–6).
7. After the seizure, place the patient on his side to facilitate the drainage of secretions.
8. Allow the patient to sleep after the seizure.
9. Reorient the patient when he awakes since he may be amnesic after the attack.
10. Stay with the patient throughout the seizure to ensure his safety.
11. If the patient is in a chair when a major seizure occurs
    - Ease the patient to the floor immediately, if possible.
    - Guide the patient's movements to prevent injury from banging his head and hands on the floor.

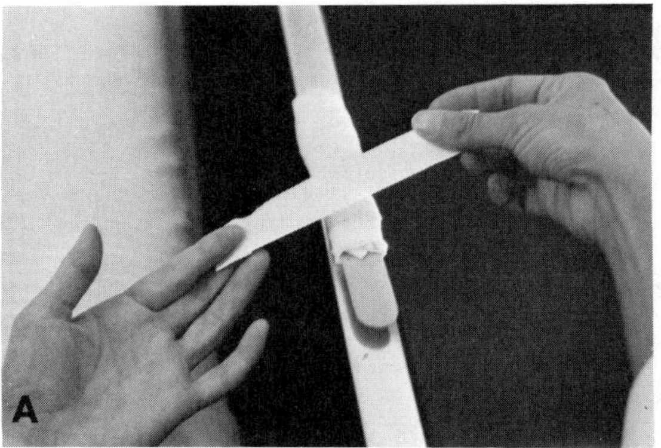

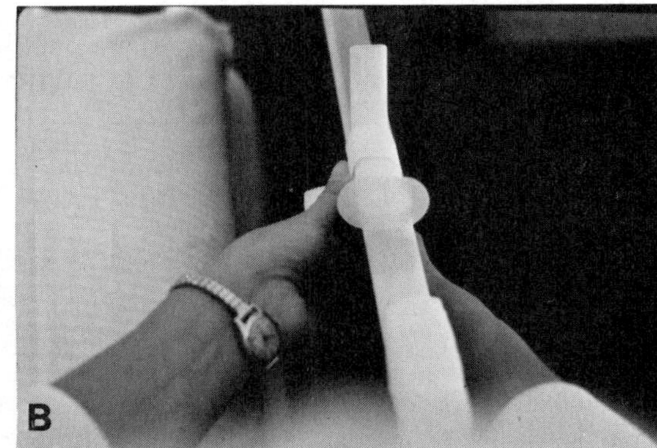

FIG. 27-5. Part of seizure precautions includes taping a padded tongue depressor (*A*) and an oropharyngeal tube (*B*) to the top of the bed. (Decision Audiovisual Media. Neurological Care Series. Philadelphia, JB Lippincott. 1972)

CONTROLLING SEIZURES

The following precautions may be taken to control seizures:

1. Administer medications as ordered to maintain a therapeutic blood level.
2. Avoid precipitating factors that could lead to a seizure.
3. Assess the effectiveness of the drug and observe any reactions to the anticonvulsant drugs that may indicate seizure activity.
4. Observe for any signs of toxicity to the drug and report them immediately.

STATUS EPILEPTICUS

Status epilepticus has been defined as "recurrent generalized convulsions at a frequency which does not allow consciousness to be regained between seizures (tonic–clonic status)."[1] About 10% of patients will develop status epilepticus, which is said to result from untreated or inadequately treated seizures. The most common cause, however, is abrupt discontinuation of anticonvulsant drugs. Status epilepticus is a serious medical emergency because the systemic and cerebral anoxia caused by the impairment of respirations will produce brain damage, mental

FIG. 27-6. Following a seizure, an oropharyngeal tube may have to be inserted (*A* and *B*) and suctioning initiated (*C* and *D*) to maintain a patent airway.

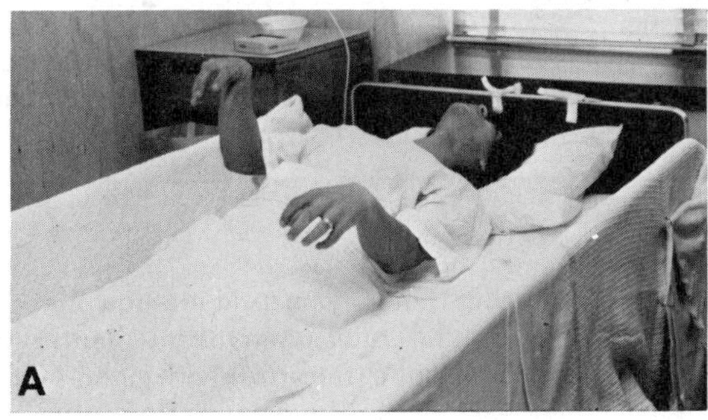

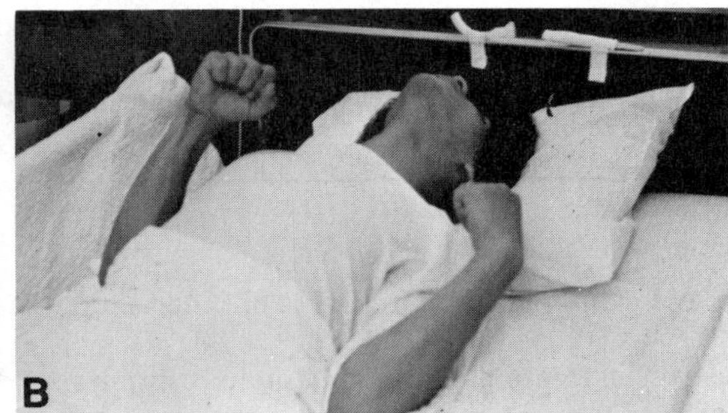

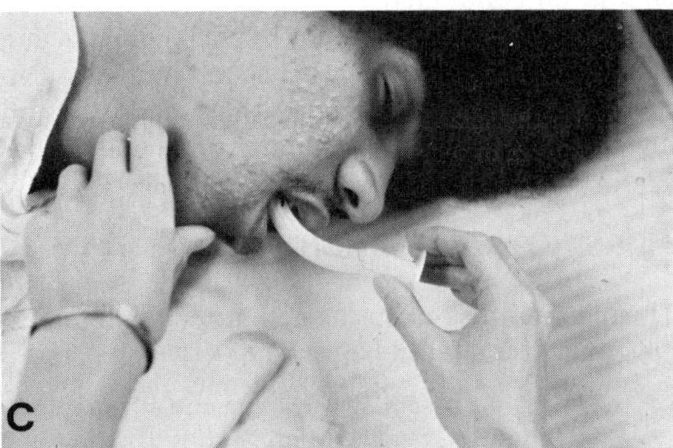

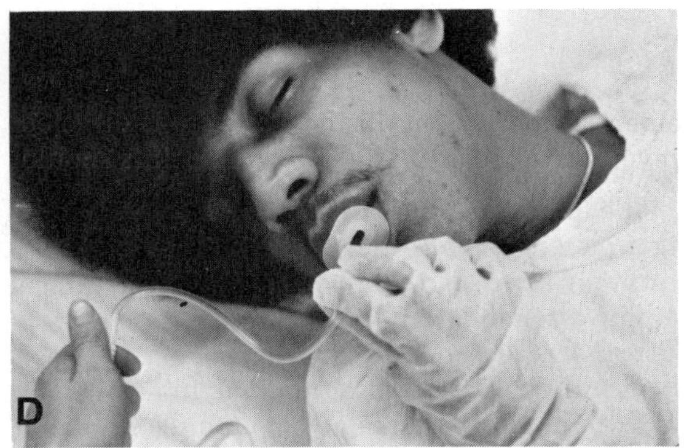

CHART 27-1. INFORMATION APPLICABLE TO THE PATIENT WITH A SEIZURE DISORDER (POINTS THAT SHOULD BE KNOWN AND FOLLOWED BY THE PATIENT TO DECREASE SEIZURES)

Diet

1. Alcoholic beverages in any form should be avoided.
2. Coffee should be limited to a moderate amount.
3. Fluid intake should be restricted to 1000 ml to 1500 ml daily.

General Health

1. Constipation should be avoided.
2. Seizures are most apt to occur around the time of menstruation.
3. Fatigue should be avoided (8 hours of sleep are needed).
4. Excessive stress should be avoided.
5. Electrical shocks increase the possibility of an attack.
6. Febrile illness increases the possibility of a seizure.
7. A poorly adjusted television should not be watched.
8. Showers should be taken rather than tub baths.

Physical Activity

1. Normal activity is encouraged. Activity tends to inhibit rather than increase seizures.
2. Activities that could harm the patient should be avoided (*e.g.,* mountain climbing, parachute jumping, and so forth). Other activities do not necessarily have to be eliminated, but precautions should be taken. A patient may swim if he is accompanied by a friend who would know what to do if a seizure occurred. He should stay in shallower water so that he could be managed more easily if a seizure occurred.

Occupational Factors

1. The patient should not take a job where he could be injured or cause injury to others. Working around power machinery could cause an injury if a seizure occurred, while being an aviator could jeopardize the lives of others as well as his own life.
2. Legislation prohibits discrimination against the handicapped in employment by firms receiving any amount of federal funds.
3. Because some employers fear increased workmen's compensation premiums from hiring epileptic individuals, most states have legislated "subsequent injury funds." Provisions of the law may vary from state to state and must be explored for the particular state in question.

Other

1. A driver's license is granted in all states with evidence of a seizure-free period of 1 to 3 years, depending on the state.
2. There are no restrictions concerning the marriage of epileptic patients.
3. Antidiscrimination laws require that all buildings, programs, or facilities funded in part by the federal government provide access for the handicapped. Persons with epilepsy cannot be denied access to recreational, educational, on other activities because they are victims of epilepsy.

retardation, or even death. Aspiration is another serious concern.

The objectives of treatment are to maintain respirations and oxygenation, prevent complications, and control the seizures.

PRINCIPLES OF MANAGEMENT

Principles of management for the patient with status epilepticus include quickly establishing an adequate airway, maintaining a patent airway by frequent suctioning, administering oxygen by nasal catheter or endotracheal tube, and maintaining a reliable route for administration of intravenous drugs. The drug of choice is diazepam (Valium) because, given intravenously, it is a rapid-acting anticonvulsant drug with much less tendency to produce respiratory depression or hypotension, common with barbiturates. Other drugs that may be used include phenobarbital, amobarbital (Amytal), and phenytoin (Dilantin). Steroids such as dexamethasone (Decadron) are given to treat cerebral edema. As long as the seizure continues, a search should be conducted to determine the underlying cause (e.g., analyze blood sugar for hypoglycemia, echoencephalogram for space-occupying lesions such as a cerebral hematoma, and so forth). Note that sudden withdrawal of anticonvulsants can precipitate status epilepticus.

NURSING MANAGEMENT

During an attack of status epilepticus, the following nursing measures should be taken:

- Maintain a patent airway to ensure adequate ventilation.
- Suction as necessary to prevent obstruction of the airway and possible aspiration.

CHART 27-2. SUMMARY OF NURSING DIAGNOSES ASSOCIATED WITH SEIZURES

NURSING DIAGNOSES	EXPECTED OUTCOMES	NURSING INTERVENTIONS
Potential of physical injury due to epilepsy	• Patient will not sustain any injury due to seizure activity.	• If the patient has an aura, teach him to lie down as soon as he feels the aura beginning. • Discuss safety precautions with patients, such as taking showers instead of tub baths, avoiding swimming alone, and other points included in Chart 27-1. • Teach family members what to do if a seizure develops.
Potential of noncompliance to drug and overall treatment program due to nonacceptance of the diagnosis of seizures	• Patient will comply to comprehensive individualize treatment plan.	• Teach the patient about his drugs, toxic signs and symptoms, need for routine periodic CBC, and other points. • Allow the patient to express his feelings about his diagnosis. Misinformation will be clarified. • If epilepsy support groups are available, referral may be made. • Acquaint patient with the services of the Epilepsy Foundation of America. • Help the patient to understand the consequences of noncompliance.
Knowledge deficit concerning diagnosis and individual treatment plan for epilepsy	• Patient will be able to demonstrate a clear understanding of his specific type of epilepsy and treatment plan.	• Develop an individualized, comprehensive teaching plan. • Encourage the patient to be actively involved in the teaching-learning process. • Be sure that the patient can explain how his lifestyle and schedule will be adjusted to conform to the parameters necessary.
Potential of anemia due to use of certain anticonvulsant drugs	• Patient will not develop anemia or any other nutritional deficiency.	• Discuss the need for a periodic CBC. • Principles of good nutrition will be discussed.
Potential of diversional activity deficit due to fear of seizure activity	• Patient will be able to participate in diversional activities that he enjoys and that are not contraindicated based on his diagnosis.	• Assess what the patient likes to do for diversion. • Identify with the patient those activities that he will be able to continue to enjoy. • Identify with the patient those activities that should be avoided. • Identify new activities that the patient may wish to develop that are acceptable.
Potential of anxiety due to diagnosis and its impact on his life	• Cause of anxiety will be identified. • Anxiety will be reduced to a manageable level.	• Assess for verbal and nonverbal cues indicating anxiety. • Try to help the patient identify cause(s) of anxiety. • Correct misinformation. Help the patient develop specific methods of dealing with identified problems. • Identify stress reduction techniques that the patient may try. • Discuss with the patient the need to control anxiety.

(continued)

CHART 27.2. (continued)

NURSING DIAGNOSES	EXPECTED OUTCOMES	NURSING INTERVENTIONS
Social isolation due to stigmatization and/or withdrawal from social contacts due to diagnosis	• Patient will continue to engage in social interactions without feeling stigmatized or uncomfortable.	• Encourage patient to discuss how he views social interactions now. • Correct misinformation. • Assess patient for feeling of stigmatization. • Encourage social interactions. • Refer to support groups, if available.
Disturbance in self-esteem due to diagnosis	• Self-esteem will be maintained.	• Assess patient's self-concept (verbal and nonverbal data). • Support a positive self-concept and self-esteem. • Help the patient to see himself realistically.

- Provide oxygen as ordered.
- If drugs are being administered intravenously, protect the intravenous site so that the flow is maintained.
- Maintain seizure precautions to protect the patient from injury (see p. 572).

REHABILITATION AND PATIENT TEACHING

Patient rehabilitation and teaching are treated together because rehabilitation requires a comprehensive teaching plan to help the patient adjust to his problem.

Family teaching cannot be excluded, because the family needs help to adjust to a chronic condition that can be frightening by its very nature. The family must be instructed in what to do if a seizure occurs.

A teaching plan is based on a systematic assessment of patient needs. Social, psychological, vocational, and physical needs should be considered in addition to a drug-teaching plan.

Each teaching plan is individualized to the needs of the patient. A patient who is followed over time will face problems that will require help from the nurse or physician. Some of the major points of information which should be presented to the patient are outlined in Chart 27–1. These points must be expanded so that the patient understands the implications as they apply to his lifestyle.

The patient may express concerns about how he will cope with certain aspects of his life. One common concern most adult patients face is whether or not they should reveal their ailment when applying for a job. Many report that they are discriminated against by employers when they reveal their condition. Those who choose to conceal this information often feel guilty and live in fear that they will experience a seizure on the job or that their seizures will become known to the employer. Information that is deliberately concealed is cause for immediate dismissal in most places of employment. It is the patient's decision to determine if he will disclose his epileptic condition. Regardless of which alternative is selected, the consequences are serious.

The major nursing diagnoses often made for a newly diagnosed patient with a seizure disorder are included in Chart 27–2.

REFERENCES

1. Adams R, Victor M: Principles of Neurology, 2nd ed, pp. 211–229. New York, McGraw–Hill, 1981
2. Gastaut H: Clinical and electroencephalographical classifications of epileptic seizures. Epilepsia 11:102, 1970.
3. Vinken P, Bruyn G (eds): Handbook of Clinical Neurology, Vol 15. New York, American Elsevier, 1974
4. Konikow NS: Hysterical seizures or pseudoseizures. J Neurosurg Nurs 15(1):22, February 1983
5. Barry K, Teixeria S: The role of the nurse in the diagnostic classification and management of epileptic seizures. J Neurosurg Nurs 15(4):243, August 1983
6. Norman SE: Surgical treatment of epilepsy. Am J Nurs 994, May 1981
7. Hawken M: Seizures: Etiology, classification, intervention. J Neurosurg Nurs 11(3):166, September 1979
8. Ozuna J, Friel P: Effect of enteral tube feeding on serum phenytoin levels. J Neurosurg Nurs 16(6):289, December 1984
9. Bauer LA: Interference of oral phenytoin absorption by continuous nasogastric feedings. Neurology 32:570, 1982
10. Bauer LA et al: Importance of unbound phenytoin serum levels in head trauma patients. J Trauma 23:1058, 1983
11. Physicians' Desk Reference, pp 1478–1484. Oradell, NJ, Medical Economics, 1983

BIBLIOGRAPHY

Books

Block RB et al: Nursing Management of Epilepsy. Rockville, MD, Aspen Systems, 1982

Browne TR, Feldman RG (eds): Epilepsy: Diagnosis and Management. Boston, Little, Brown & Co, 1983

Eliasson S et al (eds): Neurological Pathophysiology, 2nd ed, pp 173–197. New York, Oxford University Press, 1978

Guyton A: Textbook of Medical Physiology, 5th ed, pp 736–738. Philadelphia, WB Saunders, 1976
Hermann B (ed): A Multidisciplinary Handbook of Epilepsy. Springfield, IL, Charles C Thomas, 1981
Howe J: Patient Care in Neurosurgery, 2nd ed, pp 14–15, 186–189. Boston, Little, Brown & Co, 1983
Laidlaw JB, Richens A: A Textbook of Epilepsy, 2nd ed. New York, Churchill–Livingstone, 1982
Middleton AH et al: Epilepsy. Boston, Little, Brown, & Co, 1982
Penry JK: Intensive monitoring of epileptic patients. In Advances in Epileptology. The Tenth Epilepsy International Symposium. New York, Raven Press, 1980
Penry JK: Epilepsy: The Eighth International Symposium. New York, Raven Press, 1977
Plum F, Posner J: The Diagnosis of Stupor and Coma, 3rd ed, pp 348–349. Philadelphia, FA Davis, 1980
Sands H, Minters F: The Epilepsy Fact Book. Philadelphia, FA Davis, 1977
Strub R, Black F: The Mental Status Examination in Neurology, p 34. Philadelphia, FA Davis, 1977
Tyrer JH (ed): The Treatment of Epilepsy. Philadelphia, JB Lippincott, 1980
Van Meter MJ (ed): Neurologic Care: A Guide for Patient Education, pp 133–151. New York, Appleton–Century–Crofts, 1982
Woodbury DM, Penry J, Pippenger C (eds): Antiepileptic Drugs, 2nd ed. New York, Raven Press, 1982

Periodicals

Amibielli MP: Drug stop: Valproic acid. J Neurosurg Nurs 12(3):174, September 1980
Annegers J et al: Seizures after head trauma: A population study. Neurology 30(7, Part I):683, July 1980
Beniak J: Patient education in epilepsy. J Neurosurg Nurs 14(1):19, February 1982
Bruya M, Bolin R: Epilepsy. Part I. Classification; Part II. Drug therapy and nursing care. Am J Nurs 76(3):338, March 1976
Clark A: Antileptic update. RN 43(5)
Commission on the Classification and Terminology of the International League Against Epilepsy. Proposal for the revised clinical and electroencephalographic classification of epileptic seizures. Epilepsia 22:489, 1981
DeRienzo B: Nursing care in the evaluation of the epilepsy surgery candidate. J Neurosurg Nurs 14(6):285, December 1982
Epilepsy: Hope through research. US Department of Health and Human Services, US Government Printing Office, Washington, DC, 1981
Gendelman S: Grand mal seizures. Hosp Med 37, October 1981
Isaacs N: Surgical treatment of epilepsy. J Neurosurg Nurs 8(2):155, December 1976
Lamb S: Cerebellar stimulation. J Neurosurg Nurs 12(1):32, March 1980
Lovely M: Identification and treatment of status epilepticus. J Neurosurg Nurs 12(2):93, June 1980
Norman S, Browne T: Seizure disorders. Am J Nurs 984, May 1981
Ozuna J: Psychological aspects of epilepsy. J Neurosurg Nurs 11(4):242, December 1979
Rasmussen T: Surgical treatment of patients with complex partial seizures. Adv Neurol 11:425, 1975
Snyder M: Effect of relaxation on psychosocial functioning in persons with epilepsy. J Neurosurg Nurs 15(4):250, August 1983
Tucker C: Complex partial seizures. Am J Nurs 996, August 1981
Tucker C: Nursing care of patients with temporal lobe epilepsy during phases I and II on telemetry recording. J Neurosurg Nurs 11(4):227, December 1979
Woodward E: The total patient: Implications for nursing care of the epileptic. J Neurosurg Nurs 14(4):166, August 1982

chapter

28

Central Nervous System Infections

Of the many infectious diseases that can affect the central nervous system, only the more common conditions will be covered here. These include bacterial meningitis, viral encephalitis, and the parameningeal infections of brain abscess, subdural empyema, and extradural abscess. Other selected nervous system infections are presented in tabular format. In addition, Guillain–Barré syndrome, an inflammatory process affecting the peripheral nervous system, is discussed.

ROUTE OF ENTRY FOR INVADING ORGANISMS

For any organism to affect the body, an appropriate route of entry for the specific organism must be available. In central nervous system infections the routes of entry include the (1) bloodstream, (2) direct extension from a primary site, (3) cerebrospinal fluid, (4) extension along cranial and peripheral nerves. (5) mouth and nasopharynx, and (6) *in utero.*

Bloodstream. Perhaps the most common route by which infectious microorganisms reach the central nervous system is the bloodstream. Microorganisms may enter the bloodstream as a result of insect bites, spread of infection from primary foci (middle ear infection, mastoiditis, sinusitis, cellulitis), or infection of congenital anomalies such as myelomeningocele.

Direct Extension From a Primary Site. Fracture of the frontal or facial bones may result in seepage of infectious contents, thereby causing contamination of the central nervous system. Any compound cranial fracture that creates direct communication between the sterile intracranial area and the outside environment is a prime source for infection. Thus, aggressive treatment with antibiotics is absolutely necessary to prevent infection.

Cerebrospinal Fluid. Dural tearing as a result of injury can create a connection between the cerebrospinal fluid and the ear or nose. Drainage of fluid from either of these areas is referred to as *otorrhea* and *rhinorrhea*, respectively. If microorganisms are directly extended into the cerebrospinal fluid, a major central nervous system infection develops rapidly. Poor sterile technique during a lumbar puncture or spinal surgery can also contaminate the cerebrospinal fluid.

Extension Along Cranial and Spinal Nerves. Some microorganisms reach the central nervous system by following peripheral nerves to the central nervous system. Rabies is an example of such a disease.

Mouth and Nasopharynx. Certain organisms are transmitted by oral and nasopharyngeal secretions, especially in areas where people are in close contact. An example of a central nervous system infection transmitted in this way is meningococcal meningitis.

In Utero. The fetus *in utero* is also subject to central nervous system infections from the following possible causes: (1) contaminated amniotic fluid from amniocentesis, (2) massive maternal infection that is transmitted across the placenta, (3) viruses such as rubella or other microorganisms that cross the placental barrier, and (4) microorganisms that come in contact with the fetus as it passes through the vaginal canal. The newborn infant is also subject to contamination of the postnatal environment with organisms that proliferate in the moist, warm environment of an incubator or isolette.

FACTORS CONTRIBUTING TO INFECTION

Certain deficiencies and circumstances are associated with the incidence of central nervous system infections. Such factors include

- Deficiencies in the major immunoglobulins
- Defects in polymorphonuclear leukocyte function
- Congenital asplenia
- Malignancy of the reticuloendothelial system (leukemia, lymphoma, and so forth)
- Therapy involving radiation
- Immunosuppressive agents or antimetabolites
- Debilitation (chronically ill patients and the elderly)
- Poor nutritional level (vitamin deficiency, alcoholism)
- Infections in other parts of the body
- Contacts with vectors known to carry certain microorganisms

BACTERIAL MENINGITIS

CAUSES

The causes of bacterial or pyogenic meningitis are many, but the most common organisms are *Hemophilus influenzae*, *Neisseria meningitidis*, and *Diplococcus pneumoniae*. Table 28–1 includes the disease, causative organism, and comments about the major organisms that cause bacterial meningitis.

Most bacteria capable of causing bacterial meningitis reach the meninges by way of the bloodstream or by extension from cranial structures such as paranasal sinuses or the ear. Bacteria can also enter from penetrating head wounds and skull fractures. However, the bloodstream is probably the most frequent route of entry. Many people have the three major organisms of bacterial meningitis as inhabitants of their nasopharynx.[1] Under conditions not clearly understood, these organisms can enter the bloodstream and localize themselves in the meninges. It is known that these three major causative organisms have a propensity for the meninges.

The level of incidence is fairly constant throughout the seasons with the exception of summer, at which time a decrease in incidence is noted.

PATHOPHYSIOLOGY

Bacterial meningitis is a pyogenic (purulent or suppurative) infection that involves the pia–arachnoid layers of the meninges and the subarachnoid space, including cerebrospinal fluid. Because the cerebrospinal fluid circulates around the brain and spinal cord, the inflammation spreads quickly by means of the purulent exudate. The ventricles are involved, the accumulation of exudate upon the choroid plexus causes hydrocephalus, and the arachnoid villi become plugged, causing obstruction within the ventricular communication system.

Initially, when bacteria invade the pia–arachnoid and subarachnoid spaces, the blood supply to the involved area increases rapidly. Neutrophils soon migrate into the subarachnoid space in massive numbers and engulf the bacteria. These phagocytic cells rapidly degenerate and disintegrate, combining with the exudate from tissue destruction to form purulent material within the subarachnoid space. The exudate increases, particularly over the base of the brain, extending into the sheaths of cranial and spinal nerves and even slightly into the perivascular spaces of the cortex. The introduction into the perivascular space leads to a slight encephalitis.

The cortical vessels, especially the veins, become dilated and congested. If the inflammation extends through the walls of the veins (vasculitis), thrombosis or necrosis with possible hemorrhage develops. Arterial changes within the small and medium vessels of the subarachnoid space begin to occur early in the infection. The irritation from the bacteria and toxins causes swelling and an increase in endothelial cells. Neutrophils and lymphocytes migrate between the layers of the vessel with resulting fibrotic changes.

In an acute case of meningitis, the cerebral cortex undergoes little change except for perivascular inflammation with some infiltration into the cortex. In subacute cases, there may be diffuse degenerative changes with necrosis and glial proliferation within the superficial areas of the brain, spinal cord, or cranial nerves. The optic and acoustic nerves are often affected, although the oculomotor, trochlear, abducens, and facial nerves can also be involved. With meningitis, there is often an associated encephalitis.

The resolution of the meningitis depends on how extensive the infection is and how quickly effective treatment is initiated. If the process is arrested early, resolution may be complete without any major sequelae. However, fibrotic changes of the arachnoid layer can cause fibrosis and scar tissue formation. Adhesions and effusions can develop in the subarachnoid space, thereby interfering with the normal communication of cerebrospinal fluid. Fibrotic changes in the structures responsible for the production and absorption of cerebrospinal fluid may result, contributing to the development of hydrocephalus. Some organisms may produce abscesses. Much of the outcome from bacterial meningitis depends on early and aggressive treatment to prevent the development of the various complications.

SIGNS AND SYMPTOMS

Although many different organisms are capable of producing meningitis, common signs and symptoms are shared by all. In infants and very young children many of the characteristic signs and symptoms may not be present or may be nonspecific. In such instances, diagnosis can be very difficult. Common symptoms of meningitis in young children

TABLE 28–1. *Causative Organisms of Bacterial Meningitis**

Disease	Organism	Comments
Pneumococcal meningitis	*Streptococcus pneumoniae* (gram-positive diplococci)	Found in the young and those over 40 years of age Most common meningitis in adults Predisposing conditions to pneumococcal meningitis include pneumonia, sinusitis, alcoholism, head traumat, splenectomy, and sickle cell anemia
Hemophilus influenzae meningitis	*Hemophilus influenzae* (gram-negative cocci)	Pediatric problem seen in those 3 months to 8 years of age (6 to 8 months, highest incidence) Chief cause of acquired mental retardation Often follows upper respiratory or ear infections
Meningococcal meningitis	*Neisseria meningitidis* (gram-negative diplococci)	Highest incidence in children and young adults Petechial rash, purpuric lesions, or ecchymosis develops in 50% of patients About 10% of patients develop a fulminating infection with overwhelming septicemia (meningococcemia); this can create a medical emergency due to high fever, purpuric lesions, and circulatory collapse from adrenocortical insufficiency due to hemorrhage and necrosis of the adrenals (called Waterhouse–Friderichsen syndrome); disseminated intravascular coagulation may also be evident; death can result hours after onset
Other less common diseases	*Staphylococcus aureus* *Streptococcus* group A	
	Streptococcus group B *Escherichia coli*	Common in newborns
	Escherichia coli *Klebsiella* *Proteus* *Pseudomonas*	Often introduced during neurosurgical procedures (especially shunting), lumbar puncture, spinal anesthesia; seen often in the hospitalized neurosurgical patient, head-injury patient particularly with cerebrospinal fluid rhinorrhea, or debilitated patient
	Myobacterium tuberculosis	Secondary infection due to bacterial seeding of the meninges from tuberculosis elsewhere in the body Most common in children Incidence reflects the rate of tuberculosis in a country; relatively low in the United States
	Listeria monocytogenes	Seen in newborns, the aged, and the immunosuppressed
	Salmonella *Shigella* *Clostridium* Gonococcus	Rare

* The organisms presented here are responsible for 80% to 90% of the causes of bacterial meningitis worldwide; these organisms are normally found in the nasopharynx of significant numbers in the population. The mechanism by which they cause illness in some people and not others is not clear.

include fever, refusal to eat, vomiting, diarrhea, listlessness, a shrill cry, and bulging fontanels.

In the older child and the adult, the following symptoms are noted:

- Headache
- Fever
- Deterioration in the level of consciousness
- Signs of meningeal irritation
- Generalized convulsions
- Increased intracranial pressure
- Cranial nerve dysfunction
- Endocrine disorders
- Others (hypersensitivity, hyperalgesia, muscle hypotonia)

Headache and Fever

The headache, which is usually the initial symptom, is described as very severe. This symptom is probably due to irritation of the pain-sensitive dura and traction on related vascular structures.

Fever is the rule with bacterial meningitis and can vary from 38° C to 39.5° C (101° F to 103° F) or above. The temperature remains high throughout the course of the illness, and can rise to 40.5° C (105° F) and above in the terminal stages because of decompensation of increased intracranial pressure on the brain stem.

Changes in the Level of Consciousness

In the very early stages of the illness, the patient demonstrates a shortened attention span and often misinterprets environmental stimuli. The patient becomes disoriented to time, place, and person. In addition, the patient becomes easily bewildered, has poor memory, and appears to have difficulty following commands. Other patients may demonstrate the change in the level of consciousness differently. Their behavior may be characterized by restlessness, agitation, irritability, and disorientation. The patient is often noisy, combative, and sometimes fearful of personal harm as a result of his misinterpreting environmental stimuli.

As the course of the illness progresses, a deterioration in the level of consciousness develops concurrently. The patient is in a drowsy, lethargic state and is generally unresponsive, except for repeated stimulation. If he speaks, he is not coherent. He gradually becomes unresponsive—even to painful stimuli—and there is no evidence of any spontaneous movements. As the coma deepens, reflexes are lost.

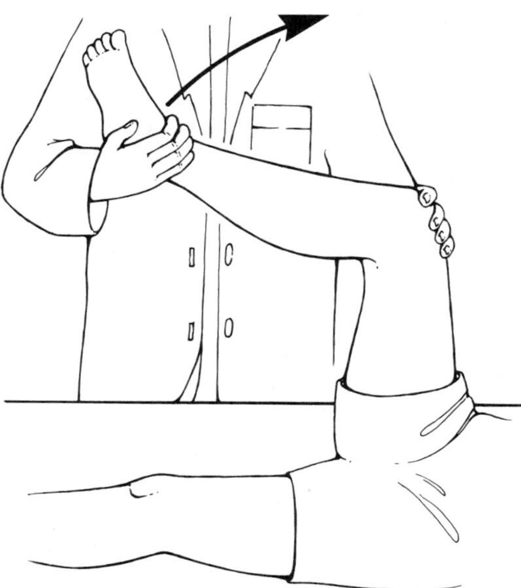

FIG. 28-1. Testing for Kernig's sign.

Signs of Meningeal Irritation

A stiff neck is an early sign of meningeal irritation. Attempts to flex the neck forward, either actively or passively upon examination, are difficult. This resistance is due to spasms of the extensor muscles of the neck. Forceful flexion produces severe pain. The extensor position may be so exaggerated that the patient may assume the opisthotonos position in bed.

Two additional signs of meningeal irritation are Kernig's and Brudzinski's signs. Kernig's sign is elicited by flexing the upper leg at the hip to a 90-degree angle and then attempting to extend the knee. In the presence of meningitis, there is pain and spasm of the hamstrings when an attempt is made to extend the knee (Fig. 28-1). The pain is caused by inflammation of the meninges and spinal roots. The spasms are a protective mechanism to deter painful flexion.

Brudzinski's sign is described as positive when both the upper legs at the hips and the lower legs at the knees are flexed in response to passive flexion of the neck and head on the chest. This reflex is caused by exudate around the roots in the lumbar region.

Photophobia, too, is a common sign of bacterial meningitis, but the pathophysiology for this symptom is not clear.

Generalized Convulsions

Development of generalized seizures (grand mal) indicates irritation of the cerebral cortex. Following a seizure, transitory paralysis may be noted. A focal motor seizure may be evident if there is an accumulation of exudate over one cortical convexity.

Increased Intracranial Pressure

Increased intracranial pressure is present with meningitis because of purulent exudate, cerebral edema, and hydrocephalus. Papilledema, a sign of increased intracranial pressure, is rare with an acute attack of meningitis. If it is apparent, it is most often associated with a brain abscess, subdural empyema, or venous sinus occlusion. Symptoms of brain stem pressure are noted in vital sign changes such as widening of pulse pressure, decreased pulse, and ataxic respirations. Vomiting is a frequent finding.

If the infection is not aggressively treated or responds poorly to treatment, the patient becomes subject to various herniation syndromes, such as cingulate, central transtentorial, or uncal, which are associated with major increased intracranial pressure caused by cerebral edema. Signs and symptoms include deterioration in the level of consciousness, pupillary dilation or constriction with alterations in the response to the light reflex, changes in vital signs (elevated blood pressure, decreased pulse, widening pulse pressure), changes in respiratory function, decreased sensory function, loss of motor function (hemiparesis or hemiplegia), headache, and vomiting. (See Chap. 12 for specific signs and symptoms of herniation syndromes.)

Cranial Nerve Dysfunction

Inflammation or vascular changes can cause cranial nerve dysfunction. The major deficits are ocular palsies (involving cranial [III, IV, VI] nerves), facial paresis (cranial [VII] nerve), and deafness and vertigo caused by involvement of the cranial (VIII) nerve.

Pupils are often unequal and sluggish to light. If the patient's condition deteriorates, the pupils will become dilated and fixed. Other eye symptoms that relate to cranial nerve dysfunction are ptosis and diplopia.

Endocrine Disorders

A small percentage of patients develop hyponatremia (a decrease in sodium in the blood) and excessive release of the antidiuretic hormone. Sodium is excreted by the kidneys while water is retained in the body. There are signs and symptoms of water intoxication along with oliguria and hypervolemia. Intracranial pressure will be further increased by this situation. Limiting fluid intake and sodium replacement are necessary.

Other Signs

Other signs and symptoms noted include hypersensitivity, hyperalgesia, and muscular hypotonia although motor function is well preserved. Sensory loss does not occur. Toxic effects on the brain or thrombosis of vascular supply to a cerebral area can cause permanent disability of cerebral function. If such pathological changes do occur, examples of deficits might include hemiparesis, dementia, and paralysis. The deficits would depend on the area of pathological changes.

One specific complication of meningococcal meningitis should be mentioned. There is a phase of meningococcemia often noted before the meningitis is evident or diagnosed. The combination of signs during this period is referred to as *Waterhouse–Friderichsen syndrome* and includes

1. Chills, fever, headache, malaise, and joint and muscle pain are possible.
2. Petechial hemorrhage or ecchymosis on the skin and mucous membrane is noted.
3. Hemorrhage can also develop in the adrenal glands and result in adrenal insufficiency.
4. Hypotension, cyanosis, respiratory distress, and circulatory collapse can quickly follow.

Immediate action with administration of adrenal corticosteroids must be taken to avoid death.

DIAGNOSIS

The diagnosis of bacterial meningitis is based on a history and physical examination, along with laboratory data. In gathering a history one would be particularly interested in recent infections such as those involving the ears, sinuses, or respiratory tract. Information about contact with individuals having meningitis would be of particular value. Signs and symptoms of the meningitis syndrome upon physical examination are also highly suggestive of meningitis, although a differential diagnosis must be considered.

Data gathered from lumbar puncture and cerebrospinal fluid analysis is vital for accurate diagnosis. Table 28–2 includes the basic cerebrospinal fluid criteria for diagnosis of bacterial meningitis and compares those findings with those found in aseptic (viral) meningitis. Methods of identification of the specific causative organisms include gram stain, smear, or culture.

Other laboratory findings that may be of diagnostic value include blood culture and nose and throat cultures. Radiographs of the patient's chest, skull, and sinuses should be taken for the purpose of noting infection, abscess formations, or fractures.

TABLE 28–2. ***Comparison of the Classic Cerebrospinal Fluid Findings in Acute Bacterial Meningitis and Acute Aseptic (Viral) Meningitis***

Characteristics	*Acute Bacterial Meningitis**	*Acute Aseptic (Viral) Meningitis*
Appearance	Turbid, cloudy	Clear; sometimes turbid
Cells	Increased white blood cells (1000 mm³ to 2000 mm³ or more; mostly polymorphonuclear neutrophils)	Increased white blood cells (300 mm³; mostly mononuclear)
Protein	Increased (100 mg to 500 mg/dl)	Normal or slightly increased
Glucose	Decreased (<40 mg/dl or about 40% of blood glucose level)	Normal
Smear and culture	Bacteria present on Gram stain and culture	No bacteria present on Gram stain or culture; may demonstrate virus by special techniques
Pressure on lumbar puncture	Elevated (>180 mm of water pressure)	Pressure varies

* All patients do not follow this classic profile; about 30% of patients with bacterial meningitis show some of the findings seen in aseptic meningitis.

TABLE 28-3. *Drug Therapy for Bacterial Meningitis*

Type of Meningitis	*Drug (usually given for 10 to 14 days*
Pneumococcal and meningococcal meningitis	Penicillin G in divided doses intravenously Adult: 12 to 15 million units/day Children: 200,000 to 300,000 units/kg/day
Hemophilus influenzae meningitis	Chloramphenicol in divided doses intravenously; given to children over 2 months of age, 100 mg/kg/day for 2 to 3 days, then 50 mg/kg/day Ampicillin may be used instead of chloramphenicol if ampicillin has been shown to be sensitive to the organism
Due to Enterobacteriaceae (*Klebsiella–Aerobacter–Serratia* group, *Salmonella, Shigella, Escherichia coli, Proteus*)	Gentamicin in divided doses intravenously, 5 mg/kg/day
Pseudomonas meningitis	Gentamicin (as above); also carbenicillin
Staphylococcus aureus meningitis	Oxacillin or nafcillin in divided doses intravenously, 10 gm to 12 gm/day
Tuberculous meningitis	Combination of drugs for 1½ to 2 years, although all three may not be necessary for the entire period Isoniazid Adults: 5 mg/kg/day Children: 10 mg/kg/day Rifampin Adults: 600 mg/day Children: 15 mg/kg/day Ethambutol, 15 mg/kg/day Corticosteroids: cautious use in life-threatening situations and only with antituberculous drugs

TREATMENT

Once the diagnosis of pyogenic bacterial meningitis is ascertained, the principles of treatment are directed toward general supportive measures, antibacterial drug therapy, and recognition and management of complications.

General supportive measures include maintaining adequate ventilation and a patent airway, establishing fluid and electrolyte balance, instituting hypothermia management, and controlling seizures and headache.

Antibacterial drug therapy requires the selection of the drug most effective against the invading organism. Dosage will depend on the age of the patient. Table 28-3 includes the specific drug therapy used for treatment of bacterial meningitis.

COMPLICATIONS

The complications relate to the type of causative organism and the severity of the illness. Postmeningitis sequelae include visual impairment, optic neuritis, deafness, personality change, headache, seizure activity, paresis or paralysis, hydrocephalus, pneumonia, and endocarditis.

PREVENTION

Often, bacterial meningitis could be prevented if the following principles were observed:

1. Adequate treatment of infections such as sinusitis, mastoiditis, ear infections, pneumonias, and so forth
2. Use of strict aseptic technique during all intracranial, intraspinal, mastoid, and sinus operations
3. Use of strict aseptic technique in changing the dressing for the procedures cited above
4. Prophylactic antibiotics after procedures cited above
5. Prophylactic antibiotics with head injuries, especially with basal skull fractures, compound skull fractures, dural tear, and injuries with drainage from the ear or nose

VIRAL MENINGITIS

Viral meningitis is also known as acute benign lymphocytic meningitis and acute aseptic meningitis. Any number of viruses, such as mumps, can cause symptoms that correspond to those of meningitis caused by bacteria and other organisms. Viral meningitis is not usually fatal and occurs sporadically or as small epidemics. All age groups are susceptible, but children are most often affected.

SIGNS AND SYMPTOMS

Symptoms of viral meningitis include those of the meningitis syndrome such as headache, fever, and signs of meningeal irritation. A major elevation in lymphocytes in the cerebrospinal fluid is noted, as well as lymphocytic infiltration of the pia–arachnoid layers. Often perivascular infiltration of the brain and spinal cord develops. Because of the similarities in symptoms, a clear-cut distinction between encephalitis and meningitis is not always possible.

DIAGNOSIS

Diagnosis corresponds to that of other meningitis. Lymphocytes are the predominant cell in the cerebrospinal fluid. The glucose content is also normal, unlike in bacterial meningitis. The protein level is elevated and the cerebrospinal fluid is turbid.

TREATMENT

Treatment of viral meningitis is symptomatic and supportive. No drug therapy is effective against the virus. Complete recovery is usual, although some paralysis and arachnoiditis have been reported.

NEED FOR ISOLATION

The need to place the patient on isolation precautions to prevent the spreading of the disease depends on the type of invading organism and the stage of the illness. For example, in the acute phase of meningococcal meningitis it is possible to infect others with secretions from the nasopharynx and droplets from the respiratory tract. Meningococci usually disappear within 24 hours of administration of appropriate antimicrobial drugs. Therefore, isolation of the patient to protect the nursing and health care personnel, visitors, and other patients should be maintained until cultures are negative.

The hospital infectious control department is the best source of information for the conditions requiring isolation. The type and duration of the isolation can also be ascertained from the personnel of this department.

NURSING MANAGEMENT IN MENINGITIS

The nursing management of the patient with meningitis, regardless of etiology, is directed toward assessing the patient's condition, providing supportive care and specific protocols, preventing complications, and enhancing rehabilitation. Within this framework, care can be divided into the acute and convalescent phases, with special nursing management being the most important.

ASSESSMENT

In the acute stage of meningitis, the patient appears to be seriously ill. The nurse should frequently assess the vital signs, comparing them with previous recordings in order to detect changes. Rectal temperatures should be taken because the level of consciousness is usually diminished, making an oral thermometer dangerous to the patient. It is not uncommon for the temperature to go as high as 40.5° C (105° F). The pulse and respiratory rate may also be high in response to the fever. If the patient has signs and symptoms of increased intracranial pressure, however, the pulse may be decreased, blood pressure elevated, and pulse pressure widened.

The neurological signs should also be assessed frequently and compared with previous recordings in order to determine trends.

Assessment would include

- Level of consciousness
- Size and reaction to light of each pupil
- Conjugate eye movement
- Visual fields
- Other cranial nerves, especially VIII
- Motor function
- Sensory function
- Signs of meningeal irritation

The level of consciousness characteristically deteriorates from confusion to restlessness, lethargy, stupor, and finally coma. The behavioral manifestations apparent with each level of consciousness have been described. As the level of consciousness deteriorates, the nurse should take special precautions to prevent injury, such as raising the siderails, padding the siderails, keeping the bed in the low position, and restraining the arm with an intravenous line if it appears that the patient may inadvertently disturb the infusion site. Often, the patient is restless and thrashes in the bed, vulnerable to injury unless special precautions are taken.

If the meningitis has caused increased intracranial pressure, one or both pupils may be dilated, with a sluggish or nonresponsive reaction to light. Checking the pupillary size and reaction to light can help in determining the presence of increased intracranial pressure.

The conjugate movement of the eyes should be observed as they follow the six cardinal positions of movement of the orbits. In meningitis, a common finding is ocular paralysis of one or all three of the ocular nerves (III, IV, and VI). In addition, the visual fields should be checked to determine the presence of visual deficits in half of the visual fields. Another cranial nerve frequently affected is the cranial (VIII) nerve. Therefore, the patient's ability to hear should also be evaluated by assessing his ability to follow commands or to hear a whisper. Of course, if the patient is unconscious it will not be possible to assess hearing.

Assessment of sensory and motor functions rounds out the neurological assessment. Hemiparesis or hemiplegia is possible with meningitis. Sensory function may be heightened in that the patient hyperreacts to even the most minimal stimulation.

The patient should be maintained on an accurate intake and output record so that his hydration level and urinary tract function can be assessed. A patient with an elevated temperature can easily become dehydrated. If the patient perspires profusely, there can be a substantial loss of fluid from the skin accompanied by oliguria. Profuse perspiration, oliguria, and dry skin indicate dehydration requiring fluid replacement by the intravenous route.

Blood electrolytes should be monitored daily to identify electrolyte imbalances such as hyponatremia. Replacement of sodium would be necessary to correct this deficit.

Note anything in the nursing history or clinical evidence that indicates a primary pyogenic focus such as infected incision, intravenous site, or decubitus ulcer. This information can be of value in identifying the cause of the meningitis.

Check the patient for any signs of nuchal rigidity (meningeal irritation) such as (1) stiff neck, (2) photophobia, (3) pain upon neck flexion, (4) flexion of the neck anteriorly resulting in flexion of the knees and thighs, or (5) flexion of the upper leg on the abdomen and extension of the lower leg producing pain and resistance.

Because hydrocephalus is a common complication with meningitis, observe for signs and symptoms that include (1) rapid deterioration in the level of consciousness, (2) rapid increase in intracranial pressure, (3) incontinence, (4) dementia, and (5) gait disturbances. The signs and symptoms of hydrocephalus are more apt to occur after the acute phase of the illness has subsided.

NURSING PROTOCOLS

Nursing management protocols for the patient with meningitis are included in Chart 28–1.

REHABILITATION

The specific rehabilitative needs of the patient depend on the degree of disability resulting from the meningitis. Minor disabilities may not require any special intervention because they will reverse themselves with time. Others require an aggressive rehabilitation plan. A team approach with periodic team conferences is the best means of setting realistic goals. The nurse plays an active role in these conferences and is instrumental in helping the patient to regain the skills of activities of daily living when the acute phase of illness subsides.

ENCEPHALITIS

Encephalitis is an inflammation of the brain caused by viruses, bacteria, fungi, or parasites, although viruses are the most common offending organism. Several of the viruses are endemic to particular geographic areas as well as to seasons of the year. The list of specific viruses known to cause viral encephalitis is lengthy, but there are only a few that appear with any appreciable frequency in the United States. Table 18–4 includes a list and description of the major viruses capable of causing viral encephalitis. Other less frequent causes of encephalitis include toxic substances such as ingested lead or arsenic or inhaled carbon monoxide; vaccines for measles, mumps, and rabies, which cause postvaccination encephalitis; and viral infections such as measles, mumps, infectious mononucleosis, and others.

This section will address encephalitis caused by viruses because viruses are the most common cause of encephalitis in the United States.

SIGNS AND SYMPTOMS

The list of signs and symptoms of viral encephalitis is long and varies depending on the particular invading organisms and the area of the brain involved. The basic syndrome of viral encephalitis is characterized by fever, headache, seizures, stiff neck, and a change in the level of consciousness, which varies from disorientation, agitation, restlessness, and short attention span to lethargy or drowsiness. As the condition of the patient deteriorates he no longer responds to the environment, either voluntarily or reflexly. He is said to be in a coma.

In addition to the wide diversity of levels of consciousness that may be present, the patient may exhibit any combination of the following symptoms:

- Aphasia or mutism
- Hemiparesis
- Alterations in motor activity such as involuntary movements, ataxia, myoclonic movements, nystagmus, ocular paralysis
- Facial weakness
- Generalized seizures
- A positive Babinski sign and changes in tendon reflexes on the affected side associated with the hemiparesis

Although the basic components of an acute viral encephalitis have been outlined, variations of signs and symptoms are noted with specific groupings of viral organisms that produce encephalitis. The following is a general summary of specific encephalitis-causing syndromes.

VIRAL ENCEPHALITIS CAUSED BY ARTHROPOD-BORNE VIRUSES

The effects on the brain include degenerative changes in the nerve cells with scattered areas of inflammation and necrosis. There is also some inflammation of the meninges.

Signs and Symptoms

The clinical picture presented by all arthropod-borne viruses in the United States is essentially the same. In infants, viral encephalitis begins with an acute onset of febrile ill-

CHART 28-1. SUMMARY OF THE NURSING MANAGEMENT OF PATIENTS WITH ACUTE MENINGITIS

NURSING RESPONSIBILITIES	RATIONALE
Assessment	
1. Assess vital signs at frequent intervals.	1. Establishes a baseline and provides ongoing data to denote stability, improvement, or deterioration in overall conditions
2. Assess neurological signs at frequent intervals.	2. Establishes a baseline and provides ongoing data for comparison to determine change
3. Assess for signs of meningeal irritation (nuchal rigidity, hyperirritability, hyperalgesia, photophobia).	3. Indicates irritation of the covering of the brain and the need for special nursing intervention
4. Assess respiratory function (auscultate chest, observe chest movement).	4. Alerts the nurse to support respirations if necessary
Basic Supportive Care	
1. Maintain a patent airway. • Position to facilitate drainage. • Suction as necessary.	1. Provides for adequate drainage of oral and nasal secretions and oxygen intake; also important in the patient with increased intracranial pressure because obstruction of the airway causes elevation of carbon dioxide, which leads to vasodilation of the cerebral vessels and a further increase or spike in intracranial pressure
2. Maintain adequate oxygenation. • Monitor blood gases. • Administer oxygen therapy, as ordered. • Assess for signs and symptoms of dyspnea and cyanosis.	2. Provides adequate oxygen for the body's needs
3. Administer basic hygienic care to the patient (bedbath).	3. Keeps the patient clean and comfortable especially when patient is diaphoretic
4. Provide for mouth care every 2 hours.	4. Refreshes and moistens the patient's oral cavity, particularly when his temperature is elevated
5. Protect the patient from injury by • Putting siderails up; if patient is very restless, bottom siderails should be added • Keeping bed low when patient is left alone • Observing the patient frequently • Protecting the intravenous site or any tubes by restraining the extremity	5. Prevents physical injury to a patient who has a deteriorated level of consciousness and who is often extremely restless
6. If the temperature is elevated, measures should be taken to control the elevated temperature, which include • Administering antipyretic drugs such as acetaminophen (Tylenol), 650 mg orally or rectally • Removing excess bedclothes • Maintaining a cool room temperature (68° F or 20° C) • Giving tepid or alcohol sponge baths • Using a hypothermia blanket	6. An increase in temperature increases the need for oxygen to support the increased metabolism. An elevated temperature also increases intracranial pressure.
7. Control pain of headache, if present, by measures that include • Elevating the head 30 degrees • Applying an ice cap as necessary • Maintaining a quiet, darkened room • Administering analgesics as necessary (acetaminophen [Tylenol], 650 mg, or codeine, 325 mg to 650 mg, is a common choice of analgesic)	7. Provides for patient's comfort and removes a major source of restlessness
8. Provide for adequate nutrition. If the patient is not able to tolerate oral intake because of reduced level of consciousness, or if his intake is not sufficient, the intravenous route will be necessary. • Maintain an intake and output record.	8. A patient with an infection and a fever requires additional carbohydrates, fluid, and calories.

CHART 28–1. (continued)

NURSING RESPONSIBILITIES	RATIONALE
9. Monitor parameters (intake and output record, arterial blood gases, electrolytes, creatinine, osmolarities).	**9.** Provides evidence of the development of complications or maintenance of homeostasis
10. Provide emotional and psychological support to the patient and family.	**10.** The patient and family need emotional support throughout the illness to decrease anxiety and improve their coping skills.
Specific Protocols	
1. Provide a quiet environment in a private darkened room where the patient is maintained on strict bed rest.	**1.** Because the meningitis patient may be hypersensitive to environmental stimuli such as noise, a quiet environment eliminates the sensory overload produced by normal environmental noise. The darkened room is necessary to provide a soothing environment, because most patients experience photophobia.
2. In the acute stage of meningitis the patient is hyperirritable and experiences hyperalgesia. The hyperirritability intensifies the perception of environmental stimuli to such a degree that the sound of running water in the sink is perceived as the noise of Niagara Falls. Touching the patient slightly initiates a startle response. Even the weight of the bed linen on the patient is irritating. • Avoid needless stimulation of the patient by consolidating nursing activities. • Be careful when touching the patient; the intensity of the stimuli should be reduced to the minimum amount necessary to accomplish the required activity. • Loosen any constricting bedclothing (do not restrain patient unless absolutely necessary). • Adjust tone of voice so that it is soft and calm. Communication should be simple and direct. • Control environmental noise. • Control direct light (many patients experience photophobia, making indirect light more comfortable for them).	**2.** Minimizes the effects of hyperirritability and hyperalgesia
3. Maintain the patient on seizure precautions, which include • Padded siderails • Padded tongue blade • Oral airway • Oropharyngeal suction (Prophylactic anticonvulsant drugs are routinely ordered.)	**3.** Seizure activity is common in patients with central nervous system infections.
4. If seizure activity occurs, a seizure chart should be maintained (see Chap. 27).	**4.** Provides documentation of frequency, type, and characteristics of seizure activity
5. Incorporate nursing protocols to manage the increased intracranial pressure that has resulted from cerebral edema, which should include • Elevating the head to a 30-degree angle • Administering anti-inflammatory steroids, such as dexamethasone (Decadron), to control the cerebral edema with the usual precautions (give magnesium hydroxide [Maalox] to control gastric irritation, check stools for occult blood, taper dose of drug when it is discontinued) • Preventing the initiation of the Valsalva maneuver by preventing straining at stool; administering stool softeners such as docusate sodium (Colace), 100 mg three times a day as ordered • Maintaining 24-hour fluid restriction, if ordered, to control cerebral edema • Noting any signs that correlate with an increase in intracranial pressure due to herniation syndromes such as vomiting or changes in neurological or vital signs	**5.** Managing increased intracranial pressure is a major responsibility in caring for the patient.

(continued)

CHART 28–1. (continued)

NURSING RESPONSIBILITIES	RATIONALE
6. Administer antimicrobial drugs as ordered.	**6.** Because antimicrobial drugs are ordered specifically for an infection such as meningitis, adhere carefully to the times of administration so that therapeutic blood levels of the drug will be maintained.
Prevention of Complications	
The duration of the acute and chronic phase of meningitis depends on many variables. However, specific nursing protocols are followed to prevent complications.	
1. Provide for skin care every 2 to 4 hours. • If the feverish patient perspires profusely, he may need to have his linen changed to prevent irritation of the skin. • Give special attention to bony prominences.	**1.** Prevents skin breakdown. In a patient who is unable to change his position, lubrication and inspection of the skin are necessary.
2. If the patient is not able to turn spontaneously, turn him every 2 hours. • If the patient can follow instructions, have him do deep breathing exercises every 2 hours.	**2.** Prevents lung congestion, atelectasis, and pneumonia
3. Apply elastic stockings for the patient on bed rest.	**3.** Improves blood return to the heart and decreases the chances of thrombophlebitis
4. Position carefully in good body alignment.	**4.** Prevents development of orthopedic deformities
5. Administer range-of-motion exercises.	**5.** Prevents contractures and shortening of muscles
6. Observe for signs of adrenal insufficiency in the patient with meningococcal meningitis (hypotension, respiratory collapse, petichiae).	**6.** Immediate intervention is necessary to preserve the patient's life.

ness and convulsions. In older children and adults, the onset is gradual with a febrile illness, headache, listlessness, drowsiness, and nausea and vomiting for several days. Convulsions, confusion and stupor, stiff neck, muscle pain, ataxia, photophobia, and tremors then become apparent. Reflexes are abnormal and hemiparesis may be present.

Residual effects after acute arbovirus encephalitis include mental retardation, epilepsy, personality changes with psychosis, dementia, paresis or paralysis, deafness, and blindness.

The mortality rate and residual effects caused by viral encephalitis from arboviruses vary greatly. Eastern equine encephalitis has a higher mortality rate than the western variety. Approximately 80% to 90% of patients with eastern equine encephalitis develop complications, as opposed to only 5% to 10% of patients with western equine infections.

Diagnosis

Diagnosis is based on the clinical picture and findings of cerebrospinal fluid analysis from lumbar puncture.

Laboratory findings often found with arboviruses include

- Elevated white blood cells in the cerebrospinal fluid, with mononuclear cells
- Small increase in cerebrospinal fluid protein
- Normal glucose of cerebrospinal fluid

Treatment

There is no definitive treatment or drug therapy available for the patient with viral encephalitis. Treatment is supportive and symptomatic. Drugs often administered include steroids to control cerebral edema; anticonvulsants to prevent seizures; analgesics for headache; and antipyretics to control hyperthermia.

Nursing Management

The nursing management for all patients with viral encephalitis is supportive. The basic points of care are outlined in Chart 28–2.

HERPES SIMPLEX ENCEPHALITIS

The most important nonepidemic encephalitis in the United States that affects all age groups is herpes simplex encephalitis. It is caused by herpes simplex virus type 1. Recall that there are two types of herpes simplex virus: type 1, which is associated with the common cold sore and is present in most people in the dormant state, and type 2, which is associated with the sexually transmitted genital disease. The type 2 herpes virus can also cause encephalitis in the newborn but only if it passes through the birth canal of a mother with a genital herpes infection. Herpex simplex virus type 1, which is responsible for the common herpetic

TABLE 28-4. *Major Viruses Responsible for Viral Encephalitis*

Type of Virus or Disorder	*Specific Disorder or Causative Organism*	*Comments*
Arboviruses (arthropod borne)	Eastern equine encephalitis*	Early autumn outbreak in eastern states; year-round incidence throughout country
	Western equine encephalitis	
Altered cycle of infection of mosquito and host	St. Louis encephalitis	Late summer outbreak throughout US, except on the west coast
Mosquito bites infect host thus becoming infected	California virus encephalitis	
	Venezuelan equine encephalitis	Early autumn outbreak in midwest
Infected mosquito infects host (including humans)	Japanese B encephalitis	Year-round incidence in southwestern US, South and Central America
	Murray Valley (Australian X) encephalitis	Not in US
? of type of virus	von Economo disease, also called encephalitis lethargica and sleeping sickness	Epidemic in US following influenza epidemic of 1918; has not recurred sine 1926
Postviral disease resulting in CNS infection	Measles	
	Mumps	
	Chickenpox	
Postvaccination encephalitis	Develops within a week after vaccination for measles, rubella, mumps, or rabies	Appears to be an immune reaction
Other viral infections	Poliomyelitis	
	Rabies	
	Herpes simplex	
	Herpes zoster	
	Coxsackievirus	
	Infectious mononucleosis	

* Most serious of the arboviruses in the US; significant mortality rate and serious deficits in many that survive (e.g., retardation, seizures, personality changes, hemiplegia); least frequent arbovirus.

lesions on the oral mucosa, is also capable of producing acute encephalitis in the adult. The reason the latent virus becomes activated is not known, although fever, emotional stress, and infectious diseases may be responsible. It is also unclear how the virus enters the central nervous system although it is postulated that it may enter through the bloodstream or peripheral nerves.

Herpes simplex encephalitis is a severe, life-threatening illness. Death occurs in 70% to 80% of patients if treatment is not begun before the patient becomes comatose. The mortality rate is reduced to 28% if treatment with vidarabine is begun before coma occurs. Morbidity varies from moderate to severe neurological deficits for those who survive.

Pathophysiology

The virus attacks the brain and has a particular propensity for the frontal and temporal lobes. The brain, or more specifically, the temporal lobes become edematous, and necrotic areas with or without hemorrhage develop. The cerebral edema, once developed, is pronounced, and intracranial pressure is increased, with temporal lobe herniation. The pathophysiology is associated with the cerebral edema and subsequent increased intracranial pressure.

Signs and Symptoms

Symptoms, whose onset evolves over a few days, include fever, nausea and vomiting, headache, confusion, stupor, hemiparesis, focal neurological deficits, and seizures. Some patients also experience symptoms of temporal lobe–limbic system deficits such as olfactory and/or gustatory hallucinations, anosmia, temporal lobe seizures, periodic bizarre behavior manifestations, and aphasia. If the disease is allowed to progress, temporal lobe herniation of one or both lobes develops, leading to deep coma, respiratory arrest, and death.

The cerebral edema and hemorrhagic areas of the brain cause an abrupt increase in intracranial pressure. Temporal and/or brain stem herniation can result. The marked increase in intracranial pressure produces coma, causes changes in vital signs, and affects the respiratory patterns.

CHART 28–2. SUMMARY OF THE MAJOR NURSING DIAGNOSES ASSOCIATED WITH ENCEPHALITIS

Note: Some points of nursing management are similar to those outlined for meningitis. Areas of difference focus on the wide variations in the level of consciousness, behavior disturbances, sleep–wakefulness pattern, and tolerance to stress.

NURSING DIAGNOSES	EXPECTED OUTCOMES	NURSING INTERVENTIONS
Altered level of consciousness (can vary widely in a short period) due to the disease process	• Alterations in consciousness will be expected, and the patient will be well managed and safe at all times.	• Assess the patient's level of consciousness at frequent intervals and document findings. • Institute safety measures to protect the patient from injury. • Expect wide variation in alertness and consciousness throughout the day.
Altered cognitive and behavioral functions (dementia) due to the disease process	• The optimum level of cognitive and behavioral function will be supported.	• Assess cognitive function and behavioral responses of patient. • Support the highest level of function possible. • Individualize plan of care to provide supervision and support as necessary. • Work collaboratively with other health professionals on cognitive and behavioral retraining.
Sleep pattern disturbance due to disease process	• Patient will have sufficient sleep. • His altered sleep pattern will be minimally disruptive to others.	• Assess sleep–wakefulness cycle. • Try to structure day so that patient is not sleeping most of day; manipulate schedule as much as possible to conform to normal activities. • When patient is awake at night, provide for his safety.
Ineffective coping when dealing with minimal stress due to disease process	• Stress will be kept to a minimum. • Patient will be protected from unnecessary stress, as much as possible.	• Assess the major sources of stress. • Control the environment. • Be as nonauthoritative as possible in interacting with the patient. • Set limits as gently as possible. • Use a calm, soothing approach. • Provide supervision as necessary. • Structure the patient's day.

Death is most apt to occur in the first 72 hours when the cerebral edema is most pronounced. As mentioned earlier, for patients who progress to a comatose state, the mortality rate is very high.

Diagnosis

The diagnosis of herpes simplex encephalitis is difficult to establish in its early state. By the time a diagnosis is established, it may be too late to benefit the patient; therefore, an aggressive approach to diagnosis is essential.

The usual diagnostic work-up includes the history and neurological examination, cerebrospinal fluid analysis from lumbar puncture, computed tomography (CT) scan, electroencephalogram, and brain biopsy. The history and examination reveals an acutely ill patient who demonstrates some of the early signs and symptoms noted earlier. If the patient has been vomiting, confusion may be attributed to fluid and electrolyte imbalance. In an older patient who demonstrates hemiparesis, an altered level of consciousness, and focal signs, a cerebral vascular accident may be suspected. Other possible diagnoses may also be considered in the early course of the illness.

A lumbar puncture to measure pressure and to collect cerebrospinal fluid for laboratory analysis is often ordered. Analysis of the cerebrospinal fluid may reveal

- Increase in lymphocytes (possibly in polymorphonuclear cells in the early stage)
- Increase in protein
- Possible increase in cerebrospinal fluid pressure in the early stages; increased pressure as the intracranial pressure rises markedly
- Possible xanthochromia, if hemorrhagic cerebral lesions are present
- Usually normal glucose
- Herpes simplex virus is difficult to isolate early; a fourfold elevation in antibody titer may be seen in the convalescent serum, but this is of no help in crucial early diagnosis and may be misleading (other diseases can activate the virus).

A CT scan is a basic diagnostic tool that may be ordered.

Early in the illness it may be normal but later, hemorrhagic areas in the inferior frontal–temporal region with surrounding edema will be evident on the CT scan. The electroencephalogram may show focal or generalized slowing. Often there is evidence of seizure activity in the temporal region.

The brain biopsy is the only definitive method for establishing the diagnosis of herpes simplex encephalitis. A burr hole must be made to collect a specimen for biopsy. The specimen is subjected to fluorescent antibody study and culture to identify the viral organism.

Treatment

A controversial treatment for herpes simplex encephalitis is the use of the drug vidarabine (ara-A, Vira-A, adenine arabinoside). The drug must be given *before* coma occurs. Once coma occurs, treatment is ineffective. The controversy surrounding the use of the drug centers on when to begin administering the drug. Some experts believe that a positive brain biopsy *must* be obtained before vidarabine is begun. Others say that a biopsy is *not necessary* in every case. If the diagnosis is reasonably clear, the drug should be given at once. Dangers of drug toxicity must be weighed against dangers of delay in initiating treatment. See Chart 28–3 for drug description.

Other drugs that are commonly administered include

- Dexamethasone (Decadron) in tapering doses to reduce cerebral edema
- Cimetidine (Tagamet) to decrease gastric secretion and prevent development of gastric hemorrhage associated with the use of steroids
- Furosemide (Lasix) or mannitol for diuresis
- Phenytoin (Dilantin) to prevent or control seizures
- Acetaminophen (Tylenol) to control hyperthermia and headache

In addition to the drug therapy, treatment is supportive and symptomatic and includes support of respiratory function and an adequate oxygen supply, support of fluid and electrolyte balance, nutritional support, and management of increased intracranial pressure.

Nursing Management

See Chart 28–2 for basic principles of management. Management is also similar in some instances to the care rendered to the patient with meningitis (see Chart 28–1). Additional nursing interventions include the following:

- Observations should be made to detect deterioration in consciousness; coma indicates a poor prognosis.
- Isolation of the patient is *not necessary;* however, good handwashing technique should be followed.
- Control of a rapidly rising intracranial pressure with subsequent herniation syndromes becomes a main focus of nursing management.

Prognosis

If the patient survives the acute episode, neurological deficits are common and may include cognitive deficits (e.g., memory, reasoning), personality changes with dementia, seizure disorders, motor deficits, and dysphagia.

EPIDEMIC ENCEPHALITIS LETHARGICA (VON ECONOMO'S DISEASE, SLEEPING SICKNESS)

An epidemic disease of viral origin that affects all age groups, encephalitis lethargica was first noted at the beginning of World War I (1914). After persisting for the next 10

CHART 28–3. INFORMATION ON VIDARABINE IN THE TREATMENT OF HERPES SIMPLEX ENCEPHALITIS

Vidarabine (ara-A, Vira-A, adenine arabinoside)

- *Type:* antiviral durg
- *Action:* unclear
- *Use:* approved by Food and Drug Administration in 1979 to treat herpes simplex encephalitis
- *Dosage:* 15 mg/kg/day for 10 days
- *Route:* by intravenous route only (administer by an intravenous volume pump such as an IVAC)
- *Administration:* each milligram of drug must be dissolved in 2.22 ml of intravenous fluid
- *Excretion of drug:* mainly through kidneys
- *Side-effects:* anorexia, nausea, vomiting, bone marrow depression, elevation in liver function test for serum glutamic oxaloacetic transaminase (SGOT)

Nursing Implications:

1. Monitor blood studies (hemoglobin, hematocrit, white blood cells, and platelets).
2. Monitor SGOT.
3. Monitor kidney function studies.
4. Monitor flow rate carefully.
5. Note that to dissolve drug in 2.22 ml of fluid, substantial intravenous fluid will be given to the patient, who probably has an elevated intracranial pressure; provide nursing intervention to control the rising intracranial pressure.

years, it then practically disappeared. Although the virus evaded all attempts to be isolated, it is clear that the etiology is viral.

Signs and Symptoms

Encephalitis lethargica is characterized by an acute, subacute, or gradual onset of symptoms that last for several weeks. In the early epidemics, symptoms were often explosive and included headache, dizziness, delirium, facial weakness, and severe pain in the lower extremities. Later, the characteristic symptoms become headache, disturbances in the sleep–wakefulness pattern, and ophthalmoplegia. The disturbance in the sleep pattern is described as lethargy during daytime hours with nighttime insomnia and restlessness. Hemiparesis, sensory loss, aphasia, and hearing and visual loss are not part of the clinical picture.

Clinical Course

Approximately 38% of the victims of encephalitis lethargica die within a few weeks. Those who survive often develop various deficits or a parkinsonian syndrome. Several years can elapse between the initial illness and the development of parkinsonism.

Other chronic symptoms that may persist include sleep pattern disturbances; mental symptoms such as dementia, inability to concentrate, depression, and psychopathic disorders in children; ocular abnormalities; myoclonic movements or bradykinesias; and metabolic and endocrine disorders involving the hypothalamus that result in obesity. Only about 25% of these patients completely recover from encephalitis lethargica to resume normal lives.

Diagnosis

Diagnosis is made by observing signs and symptoms and noting the course of the illness. An elevated lymphocytic white blood cell (WBC) count is noted in the cerebrospinal fluid of half of the patients, while the protein level is elevated in most.

Treatment

Treatment is symptomatic because there is no definitive treatment. Children with behavior disorders need special treatment and may need to be placed in an extended care facility. The antiparkinsonism drugs such as levodopa are given to patients who develop the parkinsonian syndrome.

Nursing Management

Nursing management is supportive and symptomatic. See Chart 28–2 for major nursing diagnoses.

OTHER VIRAL ORGANISMS THAT ATTACK THE CENTRAL NERVOUS SYSTEM

A few selected uncommon diseases caused by viruses are presented in Table 28–5.

PARAMENINGEAL INFECTIONS: BRAIN ABSCESS

Parameningeal infections are infectious processes that occur around the meninges. The three major localized, suppurative lesions are cerebral abscesses, subdural empyema, and extradural abscesses.

CEREBRAL OR BRAIN ABSCESS

A brain abscess is caused by an infectious process extending into the cerebral tissue or by organisms carried from other sites in the body.

The major sources of primary infections that extend directly into the brain are infections of the middle ear, mastoid, and sinus. Approximately 40% of all brain abscesses result from middle ear and mastoid infections. Sinus infections (frontal and sphenoid) are responsible for another 10%. A few abscesses occur as a result of intracranial surgery or compound skull fractures. Those remaining (approximately 50%) are carried by the blood throughout the body from infectious sites such as lung infections, lung abscess, bronchiectasis, empyema, skin infections, acute bacterial endocarditis, and congenital heart disease with a right-to-left shunt. These abscesses are sometimes called metastatic abscesses.

The location of the abscess depends on the source and method of the spread of the infection. Those infections that spread directly from a primary focus create an abscess directly adjacent to the primary site. Infections around the face spread in retrograde fashion through venous sinuses and can be located at some distance from the primary focus. The so-called metastatic abscesses are most often found along the distribution of the middle cerebral artery.

Pathophysiology

Initially, the infected tissue is soft, edematous, congested, and infiltrated with polymorphonuclear leukocytes. The lesion is poorly delineated and may represent a localized, suppurative encephalitis. Within the next 2 weeks the necrotic tissue liquefies. The abscess becomes encapsulated by a zone of fibroblasts that surround the site and progressively thicken. This wall of granulated tissue is replaced by collagenous connective tissue. The wall is not of uniform thickness and tends to be thinner in its deepest portion. The abscess, which can vary in size and shape, usually lies in the white matter. The deepest thin-walled portion of the abscess lying in the white matter can eventually rupture into the ventricles with catastrophic results. One or more poorly encapsulated daughter abscesses may surround the major abscess with direct communication possible between the two.

Signs and Symptoms

The signs and symptoms of brain abscess can be considered in two stages: (1) the initial acute invasion, and (2) the enlarging lesion.

TABLE 28-5. *Other Selected Nervous System Infections*

Disease/Organism	*Comments*	*Description*
Creutzfeldt-Jakob; slow virus	Three years average incubation period Usually occurs in fifth or sixth decade Vacuole spongelike appearance of brain tissue	Spongiform encephalopathy chacterized by progressive dementia, dysarthria, spastic weakness of the limbs, myoclonic jerks, and seizures Diagnosis confirmed by brain biopsy Death is the final outcome
Herpes zoster (shingles) (herpesvirus-varicella zoster)	Latent virus from an attack of chickenpox that remains latent in the sensory ganglia Four people of every 1000 have an attack each year When the host defenses fail, virus multiplies within the sensory ganglia Virus is then transported down the sensory nerve and released to the vesicles at the nerve endings Isolation is not necessary	Involves the dorsal root ganglia, follows sensory distribution of dermatome A *painful* affliction in which a rash (vesicles and large irregular bullae on the erythematous base) develops; rash develops from papules → vesicles pustules → scabs Some patients may develop postherpetic neuralgia after an attack
Poliomyelitis (caused by one of three polioviruses): type 1, 2, or 3	Enters by way of gastrointestinal tract Spread through contact with feces and pharyngeal secretions from infected person Need to be on isolation precautions for a period of time With the advent of effective Salk vaccine, incidence virtually eliminated because of mass immunization	Attacks the motor cells of the anterior horn cells of the spinal cord Severity varies from mild to paralysis with death from paralysis of respiratory muscle
Rabies (Rhabdovirus)	Transmitted to humans from saliva of infected animals through bite or contact with saliva Spread from wound to central nervous system by the peripheral nerves One to five cases annually in United States Negri bodies found in nerve cells of infected host Incubation period varies depending on distance of wound from head Isolation is necessary	An acute encephalomyelitis infection *Early phase:* mimics vague flulike symptoms (headache, malaise, vomiting, fever, drowsiness) *Second phase:* exhibits extreme excitement and salivation, deranged behavior, convulsions, severe and painful spasms of the pharyngeal and laryngeal muscles from slight stimuli or sight of food (lasts 2 to 7 days) *Final phase:* onset of coma followed by cardiac and respiratory arrest Treatment with vaccine (causes serious side-effects)
Tetanus (*Clostridium tetani*)	Spread through horse and cattle feces that contaminate soil Contaminates soil, dust, and objects in soil Enters human from penetrating and crush wounds Immunization is available: Tetanus toxoid Tetanus immune globulin	Produces three exotoxins that attack the spinal cord and cranial nerves Causes severe muscle spasms, extreme sensitivity to stimuli, and convulsions Death may occur from asphyxia

Initial Acute Invasion. The initial acute invasion corresponds to the initial formation of the abscess. The patient may encounter the following symptoms:

- Headache
- Chills and fever
- Malaise
- Elevated white blood cells in the blood
- Neurological signs
  - —Confusion and drowsiness
  - —Focal or generalized seizures
  - —Motor or sensory deficits
  - —Speech disorders

Some patients may be asymptomatic during this period. There may be a history of reactivation of an infectious process in a patient who has had a previous ear, sinus, or lung infection. Symptoms of this earlier recurring infection may be superimposed on the symptoms of the brain abscess formation. Symptoms associated with the initial stage may subside for a period in response to drug therapy.

The Enlarging Lesion. In the second stage, the formalized abscess behaves as a rapidly growing space-occupying lesion. Within a few weeks, depending on the size of the abscess, the following signs and symptoms may be observed:

- Recurrent headache that becomes increasingly severe
- Confusion, drowsiness, and stupor
- Focal or generalized seizures
- Localized symptoms (deficits)
- Signs of increased intracranial pressure
  - —Central herniation syndrome
  - —Lateral (uncal) herniation syndrome

Symptoms According to Abscess Location. Abscesses in particular areas have characteristic signs and symptoms. The following are three common areas of abscess formation with a list of related symptoms:

- Frontal lobe abscess—contralateral hemiparesis, expressive aphasia (if dominant hemisphere is involved), focal or jacksonian seizure, and frontal headache
- Temporal lobe abscess—localized headache, upper quadrant deficit, contralateral facial weakness, and minimal aphasia
- Cerebellar abscess—postauricular (below the ear) or postoccipital headache, ipsilateral ataxia and limb paresis, nystagmus and weakness of gaze to the side of the lesion

Diagnosis

The diagnosis of brain abscess is based on the following criteria:

1. Identification of a primary infection, such as middle ear, sinus, or lung infection, will help pinpoint the source of the problem. Chest, skull, and sinus radiographs may be necessary to identify the primary focus of infection.
2. Focal cerebral and cerebellar deficits can be observed by clinical inspection.
3. There is evidence of increased intracranial pressure with signs and symptoms of the herniation syndromes (see Chap. 12).
4. Cerebrospinal fluid changes can be obtained by a lumbar puncture and laboratory analysis. The cerebrospinal fluid pressure will be elevated to 200 mm to 300 mm of water pressure or higher. The white blood cell count in the cerebrospinal fluid will be elevated from a few to several thousand, with lymphocytes the predominant cell. (An abrupt onset of coma with a white blood cell count of 50,000 in the cerebrospinal fluid should make one highly suspicious of rupture of an abscess into the ventricles.)

   The glucose levels in the cerebrospinal fluid will be normal, but the protein will be substantially elevated.
5. Other laboratory data will include
   - Electroencephalogram to localize the lesion (area of high voltage over the abscess)
   - CT scan, brain scan, or arteriogram to localize the lesion
   - Possible ventriculogram to disclose deformity of the ventricles

Treatment

Drug Therapy. Early diagnosis and prompt antimicrobial treatment are essential. Because anaerobic streptococci and bacteroides are the predominant causative organisms, penicillin G (20 million units) and chloramphenicol (4 gm to 6 gm daily in divided doses) are given intravenously. In addition, management of the rapidly rising intracranial pressure is contained with intravenous mannitol, followed by a course of dexamethasone (Decadron, 6 mg to 12 mg every 6 hours). If this is not effective, surgery will be necessary to remove or aspirate the abscess.

Surgery. If the abscess is well encapsulated, attempts are made to totally excise both the abscess and membrane. If this is not possible, the abscess is aspirated and drained. Injection of the sac with antimicrobial drugs follows. It may be necessary at some future time to once again drain the sac because of a buildup of suppurative material.

Prognosis. The use of drugs has greatly reduced the mortality rate from brain abscess. The aggressive treatment of infections that can lead to the formation of brain abscesses has also been a prophylactic aid. The cause of death from brain abscess is the massive increase in intracranial pressure and rupture of the abscess into the ventricles. Of the patients who survive, approximately 30% develop neurological deficits, of which focal seizures are most common.

Subdural Empyema

Subdural empyema (less accurately called a subdural abscess) refers to a collection of suppurative material between the dura and arachnoid layers. Infection develops by direct extension from the sinuses and, less often, the middle ear and mastoids. It is rarely a result of metastatic infection.

Pathophysiology

Pus, ranging from a few milliliters to 100 ml to 200 ml, accumulates within the subdural space over the cerebral hemisphere. The underlying cerebral tissue is depressed, with signs of ischemia and necrosis. Various polymorphonuclear leukocytes and some mononuclear leukocytes are noted in the arachnoid and subdural membrane. Thrombosis of meningeal veins may also occur in the affected area.

Signs and Symptoms

There is usually a history of chronic sinusitis or mastoiditis with a recent acute episode. The patient experiences the localized pain associated with sinus infections (over brow and between eyes), with tenderness and possible swelling in these areas. With mastoid infections there is pain and possible swelling around the mastoid area. Purulent drainage is noted from the nose or ear. Spread to the subdural area is indicated by the onset of malaise, fever, headache, and vomiting. The severity of the headache increases from localized pain to pain that is generalized and severe. Focal symptoms of neurological deficit also appear. These symptoms include focal seizures, hemiplegia, sensory loss, aphasia, and lateral conjugate gaze paralysis. Leukocytosis accompanies the fever.

Diagnosis

Skull films, CT scan, and an arteriogram aid in the diagnosis. If a lumbar puncture is done, the following will be present:

1. Increased pressure
2. Elevated white blood cell count (50 to 1000 per cubic millimeter)
3. Polymorphonuclear cells are the predominant cell
4. Elevated protein
5. Normal glucose

Treatment

Treatment consists of immediate surgical drainage and antimicrobial therapy.

EXTRADURAL ABSCESS

Extradural abscesses may be caused by osteomyelitis of a cranial bone, and they may be associated with an infection of the sinuses or the ear or a surgical procedure in which the frontal sinus or mastoid has been opened. A pus pocket accumulates between the bone and dura.

Symptoms include localized pain, fever, tenderness, and purulent discharge. Stiffness of the neck is possible. Localized neurological signs are often absent. If they occur, focal seizures, cranial (VI) nerve palsy, and decreased sensory perception of the face are the most common symptoms. The only abnormalities in the cerebrospinal fluid are the presence of a few lymphocytes and neutrophils and a slightly elevated protein.

Treatment consists of antibiotics and surgery for removal of the diseased bone at a future date.

NURSING MANAGEMENT IN PARAMENINGEAL INFECTIONS

The nursing management of the patient with a brain abscess can be viewed in two stages: the acute initial invasion when the infection organizes into an abscess and the second stage when the abscess behaves like a space-occupying lesion.

During the initial stage, the patient experiences symptoms that correspond to a general systemic infection. If neurological symptoms are present, they can be important in localizing the lesion. Often symptoms are so general that the physician is in the process of making a differential diagnosis.

Nursing management during this period would include assessing the patient's condition, managing any presenting symptoms, providing supportive care, and carrying out drug treatment.

- If the patient shows signs of increased intracranial pressure, the basic regimen to follow would be to elevate the head of the bed, restrict fluid intake, and prevent the Valsalva maneuver by preventing the patient from straining.
- Seizure precautions must be maintained to prevent injury to the patient. Noting how seizure activity progresses can be a diagnostic aid by providing the information needed to localize the lesion.
- Motor and sensory deficits are to be noted.
- The patient should be evaluated for signs and symptoms of meningitis, which is a common complication:
  - —Nuchal rigidity
  - —Headache
  - —Irritability
  - —Fever
- The medication ordered is given intravenously. The intravenous site must be protected from injury and asepsis maintained. As with meningitis, adherence to the administration time table is imperative for maintaining therapeutic blood levels. Because the drugs used are potent, the patient must be observed for both the drugs' side-effects and the development of secondary infections, which can flourish when antimicrobial therapy is used.
- If surgery is necessary to remove or drain the abscess, the nursing management pertaining to the craniotomy patient should be implemented (see Chap. 14).

GUILLAIN–BARRÉ SYNDROME

Guillain–Barré syndrome (GBS) is a postinfectious polyneuritis of unknown etiology. It is one of the most common diseases of the peripheral nervous system, with an incidence of 1.7 in 100,000. The disease is thought to be an inflammatory disorder caused by an allergic or hypersensitive reaction or an autoimmune response of the body. Others suggest that has a viral origin.

PATHOPHYSIOLOGY

About 50% of patients with Guillain–Barré syndrome give a history of a mild febrile illness 1 to 3 weeks before the onset of signs and symptoms. The predisposing febrile infection is usually a respiratory or gastrointestinal infection.

Guillain–Barré syndrome is a disease of the peripheral nerves. The peripheral nervous system is composed of the sensory, motor, and autonomic components of the cranial and spinal nerves. The peripheral nervous system is attached to the central nervous system (brain and spinal cord) but anatomically is outside the central nervous system. A nerve has an axon that carries the impulse toward the cell body. Many nerves have a myelin sheath surrounding the axon to increase the speed by which an impulse is carried. There are variations in the amount of myelin surrounding a nerve. Some axons are heavily myelinated while others are lightly myelinated. In Guillain–Barré syndrome, the more heavily myelinated peripheral nerves are affected more than the lightly myelinated fibers.

The major pathological finding with Guillain–Barré syndrome is segmental demyelination of the peripheral nerves.[1] This means that there is destruction of myelin between the nodes of Ranvier without concurrent axonal destruction although there may be secondary damage to the axon. Under microscopic examination, aggregates of lymphocytes are noted at the point of the myelin breakdown. It has been noted that the more thinly myelinated axons supply sensations of cutaneous pain, touch, and temperature. These fibers are less involved in Guillain–Barré syndrome, which explains the sparing of these sensations early in the disease.[2] The more highly myelinated cranial nerves are affected to a greater degree in Guillain–Barré syndrome; those cranial nerves affected most frequently are the oculomotor, facial, glossopharyngeal, vagus, sensory accessory, and hypoglossal nerves.

Guillain–Barré syndrome is an immune reaction disease. Immune reactions, mediated through T-lymphocytes (T-cells) and B-lymphocytes (B-cells) of the lymphatic system, are the bases of the disease. T-lymphocytes, thymocyte-derived cells, are long-lived cells surviving for month to years that are responsible for delayed (cell-mediated) sensitivity. The B-cells are nonthymus-dependent short-lived cells of the immunological system. They are responsible for the production of immunoglobulins, which combine with antigens and prevent the organisms from having a harmful effect.

The patient who develops Guillain–Barré syndrome often gives a history of an acute illness or immunization prior to the onset of signs and symptoms. It is believed that the acute illness or immunological event was the stimulus that caused the T-cells to have a deleterious effect on the myelin sheaths of the patient's peripheral nerves. This abnormal response is considered a temporary malfunction of the immunological system.[2]

Myelin sheaths and axons are able to regenerate after injury. However, in some instances severe secondary injury to the underlying axon postpones recovery or causes permanent deficits. On microscopic examination of the involved peripheral nerves, varying degrees of wallerian degeneration and regeneration are noted.

SIGNS AND SYMPTOMS

Because there are frequent variations in the clinical picture, it has been necessary to qualify descriptions with terms such as "often" and "usually." However, the reader must bear in mind that variations in the typical clinical picture are common. For example, in milder forms only the legs may be affected, with the arms being completely spared or affected only slightly.

The onset of neurological symptoms is usually abrupt. Symptoms can be summarized as muscle weakness, paresthesia, other sensory changes, and sometimes autonomic dysfunction.

The motor weakness usually begins in the lower extremities and is most often symmetrical. The flaccid ascending weakness evolves over a period of hours to several (1 to 10) days. Both proximal and distal muscles of the extremities are equally involved, contrary to what is noted in other types of polyneuritis. In some patients the trunk and cranial nerves become involved. Death can result if the respiratory muscles are affected, because of respiratory insufficiency. Slight urinary retention occurs rarely, necessitating temporary catheterization. Because the flaccid paralysis develops so rapidly, there is no apparent muscle wasting. Hypotonia is noted. Superficial and deep reflexes are usually lost. Some patients experience tenderness and pain on deep pressure or movement of the muscles. Occasionally, a patient may have a stiff neck.

If the cranial nerves are involved, the facial (VII) nerve is most often affected. Other cranial nerves that are less often affected are the glossopharyngeal (IX), vagus (X), spinal accessory (XI), and hypoglossal (XII). Signs and symptoms of facial nerve dysfunction include inability to smile, frown, whistle, or drink with a straw. Dysphagia and laryngeal paralysis can develop from the cranial (IX and X) nerve paralysis. Vagus nerve deficit, if present, is thought to be responsible for the autonomic dysfunction noted in some patients. Autonomic dysfunction is characterized by hypotension, hypertension, and sinus tachycardia. The hypertension has been noted in the acute phase and is associated with an abnormal release of catecholamines. Interruption of the autonomic reflex arcs that control the circulation usually results in hypotension. The duration and extent of the hypotensive episode can be mild or can continue to severe circulatory collapse. These patients are particularly susceptible to sudden postural changes. Use of vasopressor drugs may be necessary to maintain blood pressure. Slight changes in the electrocardiographic pattern are common. Autonomic dysfunction is not considered a common symptom.

Sensory symptoms in the peripheral segments include paresthesia and pain. The paresthesia is frequent and temporary and may tingle, feel like "pins and needles," or be numb. Pain may begin as cramping and progress to frank pain in the arms, legs, back, or buttocks. Analgesics are often necessary to keep the patient comfortable. Guillain–Barré syndrome does not affect the level of consciousness, pupillary signs, or cerebral function.

CLINICAL COURSE

There are three stages in the acute courses of Guillain–Barré syndrome: (1) acute onset, which begins with the onset of the first definitive symptom and ends when no further symptoms or deterioration is noted (lasts from 1 to 3 weeks); (2) the plateau period, which lasts for several days to 2 weeks; and (3) the recovery phase, which is synonymous with the remyelination and axonal regeneration process. In some patients who have sustained secondary axonal injury, recovery may take up to 2 years for maximum improvement even though permanent deficits may result.

PROGNOSIS

Mortality rates from respiratory paralysis in Guillain–Barré syndrome are approximately 10% to 20%. The rate of recovery depends on the extent and degree of neurological deficit. About 95% of surviving patients recover completely within weeks or months. Motor function returns in

CHART 28-4. NURSING MANAGEMENT OF THE PATIENT WITH GUILLAIN-BARRÉ SYNDROME

NURSING RESPONSIBILITY	RATIONALE
Assessment of Condition and Function	
1. Carry out frequent evaluation of vital signs (every 2 hours; more often in the acute phase).	1. Autonomic dysfunction, such as hypertension or hypotension, is common.
2. Assess neurological function frequently.	2. This provides baseline assessment to which subsequent assessments can be compared.
3. Assess cranial (VII, IX, X, XI, and XII) nerves. • VII—whistling, smiling, frowning, closing the eyes, and so forth • IX and X—gag, cough, and swallow reflex • XI—shrug shoulders • XII—deviation or paralysis of tongue	3. These cranial nerves are frequently involved.
4. Assess respiratory function frequently. • Check for confusion, dyspnea, air hunger, abdominal breathing, color of nail beds, and so forth • Assess arterial blood gases taken periodically for hypoxia. • Assess tidal volume and vital capacity for respiratory failure.	4. Check for signs of respiratory failure, a common problem in Guillain-Barré syndrome. In evaluating confusion, the nurse must decide if it is due to hypoxia, sensory deprivation, hyperthermia, and so forth.
5. Place a tracheostomy set and respirator on standby.	5. It will be available if arrest occurs.
6. Place patient on cardiac monitor and assess frequently.	6. Cardiac arrhythmia occurs occasionally.
7. Give oxygen by way of nasal cannula, as ordered. (Other methods may be used.)	7. This provides oxygenation.
8. Assess for presence of stiff neck.	8. This is a common symptom in Guillain-Barré syndrome.
Basic Hygienic and Maintenance Care	
1. Provide routine, basic hygienic care such as bedbath, as necessary.	1. Helps to maintain cleanliness and self-esteem
2. Have patient cough and deep breathe every 2 hours.	2. Improves respiratory function
3. Give eye care as necessary. Administer artificial tears, cleanse twice daily, apply shields, or tape the eyes closed.	3. Provides lubrication and protection from drying and corneal abrasion
4. Apply elastic stockings.	4. Prevents development of thrombophlebitis
5. Turn every 2 hours. • Position carefully in proper body alignment. • Change position gradually.	5. Do not interfere with breathing when patient is positioned on side. Handle extremities carefully because often they are painful when touched. • Helps to avoid orthostatic hypotension
6. Maintain an accurate intake and output record.	6. Enables assessment of fluid intake and output to be made
7. Suction as necessary if patient is unable to manage own secretions	7. Aids in maintaining a patent airway and prevents aspiration
8. Carry out range-of-motion exercises four times daily.	8. Helps to maintain muscle tone and prevents contractures
9. Administer analgesics as necessary (acetaminophen [Tylenol], codeine).	9. Provides relief of pain in muscles
10. Provide diet as tolerated (soft, tube feeding, and so forth).	10. If patient is unable to swallow, oral intake is contraindicated. If swallowing is impaired, he may be able to manage a soft diet.
Management of Tracheostomy and Respirator, If Present	
1. Give tracheostomy care every 4 hours.	1. Maintains patency of tube
2. Suction every hour and as necessary (hyperaerate with 100% oxygen for 1 minute before and after suctioning, unless contraindicated by physician).	
3. Deflate tracheostomy cuff for 5 minutes every hour. Ambu and suction well.	3. Helps to prevent development of necrosis on trachea due to vascular impairment from pressure of cuff
4. Instill 5 ml of normal saline if secretions are tenacious (with approval of physician).	4. Stimulates coughing

(continued)

CHART 28–4. *(continued)*

NURSING RESPONSIBILITY	RATIONALE
5. Maintain aseptic technique with all procedures.	5. Decreases possibility of infection
6. Give intermittent positive pressure breathing (IPPB) treatment and carry out pulmonary physiotherapy as ordered.	6. Improves respiratory function
7. Raise head of bed 30 degrees.	7. Facilitates respirations and removal of secretions
Prevention of Complications	
1. Give antibiotics as ordered to prevent infections.	1. This is a prophylactic measure.
2. Check stools for occult blood.	2. Indicates if there is presence of gastrointestinal bleeding
3. Check routine complete blood count, urinalysis, and arterial blood gases.	3. Provides assessment data
4. Administer anticoagulation therapy as ordered.	4. Thrombophlebitis is a frequent complication.

a descending pattern. Once respiratory complications are overcome, complete recovery can occur. If the nerves have degenerated, nerve regeneration will require 6 to 18 months before motor function is regained. A few patients may suffer a relapse.

DIAGNOSIS

The diagnosis of the Guillain–Barré syndrome is distinguished from other forms of polyneuritis by the clinical picture. The course of the illness is as follows: (1) acute onset, (2) rapid development of weakness and paralysis, (3) involvement of both the proximal and distal limbs, and (4) absence of, or slight, muscle atrophy.

Laboratory findings include

1. Albuminocytologic dissociation is most characteristic, as noted by an increase in cerebrospinal fluid protein without an increase, or only a slight to moderate increase, in the cell count. These changes are not noted initially, but develop several days after the onset of symptoms, reaching a peak in 4 to 6 weeks.
2. There may be a moderate leukocytosis in the peripheral blood early in the illness, but it soon returns to normal unless a concurrent illness or complication develops.
3. The sedimentation rate is normal.
4. Nerve conduction velocities are slowed soon after paralysis develops. If denerved potentials (fibrillations) develop, they will occur later in the illness.

MEDICAL TREATMENT AND NURSING MANAGEMENT

There is no specific treatment for Guillain–Barré syndrome other than supportive therapy. A mild controversy surrounds the use of prednisone and ACTH during the illness. The decision to use the drug will depend on the preference of the physician. However, if it is used, the usual precautions and procedures of steroid therapy should be recognized (low-salt diet, measures to alleviate fluid retention and gastrointestinal irritation, tapering of doses, and potassium replacement).

The patient should be managed in the hospital because of the possible development of respiratory paralysis and, less frequently, cardiovascular complications. A cardiac monitor is often used to detect cardiac abnormalities. The high incidence of respiratory insufficiency (50%) is caused by the involvement of the trunk muscles and possible vagal dysfunction, which diminishes or prevents bronchial constriction or dilation. The patient must be carefully observed and monitored by laboratory methods to note the development of respiratory insufficiency. Arterial blood gases are evaluated routinely for signs of hypoxia. If hypoxia develops, it will be necessary to perform a tracheostomy and attach a ventilator. The tracheostomy is done when dyspnea occurs (vital capacity below 800 cc). Oxygen is regulated in conjunction with arterial blood gases. Patients on positive pressure ventilators are prone to the development of syndrome of inappropriate secretion of antidiuretic hormone (SIADH). The patient should be monitored for the development of this disorder (see Chap. 13).

Once a tracheostomy is done, an aggressive program of tracheal care, chest physiotherapy, and prophylactic antibiotics must be instituted to prevent infection. Weaning from the respirator is cautiously attempted as the paralysis begins to recede and there is evidence of return of respiratory function. The process gradually proceeds, following the usual steps of weaning until the respirator and, later, the tracheostomy can be completely discontinued.

Other supportive care includes maintenance of proper nutrition by the intravenous, nasogastric, or gastrostomy tube if the oral route cannot be used; special eye care if the eyelids are not closed properly; physiotherapy program as soon as the patient's condition has stabilized; and maintenance of other body systems.

The details of nursing management are outlined in Chart 28–4.

Plasma Exchange in Guillain–Barré Syndrome

The serum of a patient in the acute stage of Guillain–Barré syndrome contains antibodies to peripheral nervous system tissue. This is the basis for understanding plasmapheresis as an experimental treatment protocol in this disease. Plasma exchange is thought to be most effective if begun within 2 weeks of the onset of the illness. The usual protocol involves three to five exchanges. Each exchange takes from 2 to 4 hours. Patients treated with plasmapheresis have either markedly improved, partially improved, or not improved. In some patients improvement is not immediately noted. A multicenter study is presently investigating the use of plasma exchange for Guillain–Barré syndrome.

There are potential complications from the treatment that include hypotension, arrhythmias, infection, phlebitis, clotting disorders, and hypocalcemia. The nurse caring for the patient must monitor the patient for potential complications. The potential of such complications added to the signs and symptoms already present for acute Guillain–Barré syndrome increase the risk to the patient.

REHABILITATION

The type of rehabilitation any patient will need depends on a systematic assessment by the health team members. The major areas in which the patient usually will need help are relearning the activities of daily living and retraining muscles because of deficits of the motor system. However, the specific rehabilitation plan of physiotherapy and other therapies will be individualized for the patient.

REFERENCES

1. Asbury AK, Arnason BG, Adams RD: The inflammatory lesion in idiopathic polyneuritis. Medicine 48:173, 1969
2. Griswold K, Guanci MM, Ropper AH: An approach to the care of patients with Guillain–Barré syndrome. Heart Lung 13(1):66, January 1984

BIBLIOGRAPHY

Books

Adams R, Victor M: Principles of Neurology, 2nd ed, pp 475–523. New York, McGraw–Hill, 1981

Bannister R: Brain's Clinical Neurology, 5th ed, pp 347–350, 369–370, 397–441. New York, Oxford University Press, 1978

Coxe WS: Viral encephalitis. In Youmans JR: Neurological Surgery, 2nd ed, pp 3358–3367. Philadelphia, WB Saunders, 1982

Goodman SJ, Stern WE: Cranial and intracranial bacterial infections. In Youmans JR: Neurological Surgery, 2nd ed, pp 3323–3357. Philadelphia, WB Saunders, 1982

Ropper AH, Kennedy SK, Zervas NT (eds): Neurological and Neurosurgical Intensive Care, pp 163–174. Baltimore, University Press, 1983

Rowe FA et al: Parasitic and fungal diseases of the central nervous system. In Youmans JR: Neurological Surgery, 2nd ed, pp 3366–3440. Philadelphia, WB Saunders, 1982

Walton J: Brain's Diseases of the Nervous System, 8th ed. New York, Oxford University Press, 1977

Wehmaker SL, Wintermute J: Case Studies in Neurological Nursing, pp 77–90. Boston, Little, Brown & Company, 1978

Periodicals

Angelo NP: Acute transverse myelitis: Dilemma of diagnosis but not of nursing care. J Neurosurg Nurs 16(2):74, April 1984

Belshe RB: Commonly misdiagnosed viral infections. Hosp Med 29, October 1980

Blanco AK, Cuomo N: A personal experience with Guillain–Barré syndrome. J Neurosurg Nurs 15(6):355, December 1983

Bolton R: Creutzfeldt–Jakob disease. J Neurosurg Nurs 14(1):1, February 1982

Cobert B: Identifying Reye's syndrome. Hosp Med 69, August 1982

Ferguson CK, Roll LJ: Human rabies. Am J Nurs 81(6):1175, June 1981

Fuller E (ed): Herpesvirus: Agent of many ills. Patient Care 15(19):200, November 15, 1981

Giesser B: Landry–Guillain–Barré syndrome. Resident & Staff Physician 29(8):45, August 1983

Heerema MS: Diagnosis: Meningitis. Hosp Med 13, May 1982

Kealy S: Respiratory care in Guillain–Barré syndrome. Am J Nurs 58, January 1977

Lavigne J: Respiratory care of the patient with neuromuscular disease. Nurs Clin North Am 14(1):133, March 1979

McKinney A: Brain abcesses. Hosp Med 13, February 1983

Mills N, Plasterer H: Guillain–Barré syndrome: A framework for nursing care. Nurs Clin North Am 15(2):257, June 1980

Overturf GD: Meningitis. Top Emerg Med 4:16, April 1982

Polk B: Cardiopulmonary complications of Guillain–Barré syndrome. Heart Lung 5(6):967, November–December 1976

Powers LL, Schiro A: Tetanus: A challenge to nursing. Crit Care Nurs 62, March/April 1983

Prydun M: Guillain–Barré syndrome: Disease process. J Neurosurg Nurs 15(1):27, February 1983

Rodnitzky RL: Complications of plasma exchange in neurological patients. Arch Neurol 39:350, June 1982

Swisher C, Williams A: Herpes encephalitis: A nursing challenge. J Neurosurg Nurs 13(1):34, February 1981

Tikkanen P: Landry–Guillain–Barré–Strohl syndrome. J Neurosurg Nurs 14(2):74, April 1982

Vedeler C, Nyland H, Fagius J et al: The clinical effect and the effect on serum IgG antibodies to peripheral nerve tissue of plasma exchange in patients with Guillain–Barré syndrome. J Neurol 228:59, 1982

Wahlquist G: A great nursing challenge: Recognition and effective management of the patient with herpes simplex encephalitis. J Neurosurg Nurs 13(5):220, October 1981

Wing S: Brain abscess. J Neurosurg Nurs 13(3):123, June 1981

chapter 29

Nervous System Degenerative Diseases

While there are several degenerative diseases of the nervous system, only a few of the more common disorders will be discussed in this chapter, namely, acute brain syndrome and dementia, Alzheimer's disease, multiple sclerosis, amyotrophic lateral sclerosis, myasthenia gravis, and Parkinson's disease.

A similar philosophy of care can be applied to most degenerative diseases; that is, the patient is kept as independent as possible for as long as possible. This goal is achieved by an integration of physical, psychological, educational, vocational, and recreational therapies.

The patient and family must be actively involved in the process of planning care. Management is based on a systematic assessment to evaluate assets and needs. Through a team approach, a care plan is developed to meet the individual needs of the patient, help him to accept his illness, and set realistic goals.

PSYCHOSOCIAL CONSIDERATIONS

The very nature of a degenerative disease indicates a process of loss. How quickly deterioration occurs depends on the particular disease, its medical management, and the adaptations made by the patient. The adjustments and ability to cope will depend on how the patient perceives the loss of function. Loss of mobility and control of body functions creates various deprivation syndromes and changes in body image and day-to-day living. Some patients become apathetic, while others become hostile and angry.

Degenerative diseases most often deprive the individual of degrees of independence. Patients need help to cope with this loss, which can take the form of accentuating the positive and identifying those activities in which independence can be maintained. At the same time it is important to realistically accept those areas of dependency that exist.

The educational needs of the patient and family are met by developing a teaching plan, the objectives of which include knowledge of the illness and therapies used, precautions to be taken, and accentuation of the positive aspects of the condition. The patient is helped to modify his environment, lifestyle, and routines to allow for maximum independence. Occupational and vocational counseling should be available to help in the adjustments necessary for gainful employment and life roles such as homemaking. Recreational activities, hobbies, and interests enjoyed by the patient are encouraged.

Physiotherapy provides a major contribution in the management of degenerative diseases. Based on a systematic assessment and ongoing evaluation, specific exercises and therapies are selected for the patient. They may include any of the following: (1) passive range-of-motion exercises as well as active, resistive, and stretching exercises to strengthen muscles, reduce spasticity, and control the development of contractures; (2) massage; (3) relaxing baths and whirlpool treatment; (4) gait retraining; (5) exercises to improve coordination; (6) prescription of specific exercises such as swimming or walking barefooted; and (7) selection of helping devices such as braces, splints, canes, and feeding equipment.

In summary, the challenge of managing patients with nervous system degenerative diseases concerns high stakes—the quality of life and independence.

ACUTE BRAIN SYNDROME AND DEMENTIA

Acute brain syndrome is a clinical diagnosis that is made when disorientation or recent memory deficits are present. According to Taylor, the diagnosis is made when either symptom is noted on the mental status examination.[1] A variety of organic problems can be the cause of the syndrome, some of which are reversible. Drug toxicity, metabolic disorders, neurological conditions, and dysfunction in other body systems are common underlying causes. The most important aspect of patient management is identification of the specific underlying etiology. At times, acute brain syndrome is difficult to distinguish from a functional psychotic state of acute onset, particularly when the signs and symptoms of irritability, hallucinations, delusions, depression, and lability are present. These features may be present in either acute brain syndrome or functional psychotic states.

A term closely associated with acute brain syndrome is *dementia*. Dementia is characterized by the loss or reduction in general mental capacity.[2] There is a generalized slowing in all cognitive functions, and the patient loses his ability to acquire and store new information along with his ability to retrieve stored information from memory. The causes of progressive dementia are numerous and varied and include head trauma, normal-pressure hydrocephalus, degenerative diseases, cerebrovascular disorders, hypoxic and anoxic states, metabolic disorders, neoplasms, infections, and toxin- or drug-induced conditions, among others. Regardless of the cause, the effects on the brain are the same — nerve cell degeneration. If a significant number of neurons are affected, the condition is irreversible. In some instances the dementia can be arrested, if the underlying etiology can be controlled. Oftentimes the dementia is a chronic condition resulting in progressive loss of cognitive function.

Management of the patient can be difficult. A stable and controlled environment is helpful for minimizing confusion, frustration, and agitation. Disorientation can lead to hallucinations, delusions, and combative behavior. The patient must be controlled to ensure that he will not sustain personal injury or inflict injury on others. If the patient is at home, his behavior, which is often exaggerated at night, can be a tremendous burden on the family. His agitation and wandering can prevent other family members from sleeping. Using medication to control unacceptable behavior may have a detrimental effect on the patient. Management of the patient with dementia is consequently difficult.

One important disease that has dementia as its primary clinical symptom is Alzheimer's disease. This condition will be discussed in some detail because of its prevalence and its profound impact on the victim, family, and health care system.

ALZHEIMER'S DISEASE

Alzheimer's disease is a chronic neurodegenerative disorder with progressive profound impairment of cognitive functions. It is characterized by premature, severe, diffuse cerebral atrophy, particularly of the frontal lobes, with destruction of cerebral cortex neurons. The onset is gradual, progressing from forgetfulness to severe dementia. Women are affected more often than men. It can affect people at any age, but it usually involves people 45 years old and older.

The disease was first identified in 1907 by Alois Alzheimer, a German physician who was treating a 51-year-old woman with senility. The diagnosis was based on findings at autopsy that included cerebral atrophy, neurofibrillary tangles, and senile plaques in the brain. There was little interest in Alzheimer's disease from the identification of the disorder until the 1950s. It is now recognized that more than 50% of nursing home beds in the United States are occupied by patients with a form of dementia.[3] The major cause of dementing disease is Alzheimer's disease. Because of the ever-increasing population of the elderly, the number of patients will undoubtedly increase, taxing the limits of the health care system.

Two terms, Alzheimer's disease and senile dementia of the Alzheimer's type, need clarification. Alzheimer's disease is applied to dementia occurring in patients under the age of 65 years while senile dementia of Alzheimer's type is used to classify patients with dementia who are 65 years old and older. It is now generally accepted that, in most cases, Alzheimer's disease and senile dementia of the Alzheimer's type are one and the same.

CAUSES

The cause of Alzheimer's disease is unknown although several etiologies have been proposed, including arteriosclerotic changes, heredity, slow viruses, an autoimmune response, and increased aluminum in the body tissue.

SIGNS AND SYMPTOMS

Three stages of Alzheimer's disease are described in the literature.[4] Mental changes usually begin with forgetfulness that can be so sublime that it can be dismissed easily by the patient. The patient can try to conceal his forgetfulness with excuses and compensate with notes and reminders to himself. The progressive course of the illness continues until the patient's loss of cognitive functions becomes obvious and the patient becomes unable to do the simplest of calculations, reasoning, or recall. Alzheimer's disease robs a patient of his personality and humanism; he can no longer interact as an adult and be responsible for his own behavior. In the terminal stage, the patient is bedridden, emaciated, agnosic, aphasic, and apraxic and lacks control of his body, including sphincters. All cognitive functions and emotional responses are lost. Death is caused by infection such as aspiration pneumonia. Chart 29–1 summarizes the time span and behavior associated with each of the three stages of Alzheimer's disease.

DIAGNOSIS

The diagnosis is usually not established until the second stage of the illness. The neurological examination in association with a mental status examination or neuropsycholog-

CHART 29-1. STAGES OF ALZHEIMER'S DISEASE

The stages of Alzheimer's disease vary from patient to patient, but a few time approximations as well as characteristic behaviors can be identified.

Stage 1. Early Stage (2 to 4 years)

- Forgetfulness — may be very subtle and patient may try to cover up by using lists and notes
- Declining interest in environment, people, and present affairs
- Vague uncertainty and hesitancy in initiating actions
- Poor performance at work by end of this stage; may be dismissed from his job

Stage 2. Middle Stage (2 to 12 years)*

- Progressive memory loss
- Hesitates in response to questions; shows signs of aphasia
- Has difficulty following simple instructions or doing simple calculations
- Has episodic bouts of irritability
- Becomes evasive, anxious, and physically active
- Becomes more active at night because of disturbance of the sleep-wakefulness cycle
- Wanders, particularly at night
- Becomes apraxic for many basic activities
- Loses important papers
- Loses way home in familiar surroundings or loses way in his own home
- Forgets to pay bills; lets household chores slip and newspapers pile up; does not dispose of garbage; does not take medications
- Loses possessions and then claims that they were stolen
- Neglects personal hygiene (bathing, shaving, dressing)
- Loses social graces; his behavior can be a major embarrassment to family and friends; this usually ends in social isolation of the family and patient

Stage 3. Final Stage (up to a year)

- Marked loss of weight because of lack of eating; becomes emaciated
- Unable to communicate verbally or in writing
- Does not recognize family
- Incontinence of urine and feces
- Possibility of major seizures
- Grasping, snout, and sucking reflexes are readily elicited
- Finally loses the ability to stand and walk and becomes bedridden
- Death is usually caused by aspiration pneumonia

* Diagnosis is frequently made in this stage.

ical testing points to the diagnosis. The CT scan is the most helpful of diagnostic procedures because it demonstrates the cerebral atrophy. In the later stages there is diffuse slowing of the waves on the electroencephalogram.

Other possible causes of the presenting signs and symptoms, such as frontal lobe brain tumor, normal-pressure hydrocephalus, and reversible causes of dementia (e.g., metabolic disorders, drug toxicity) must be ruled out.

TREATMENT

Unfortunately, there is no treatment for Alzheimer's disease. The physician must prepare the patient and family for what lies ahead. This includes making the patient and family aware of the support services available, and encouraging and supporting them in the difficult decisions that must be made about home or institutional care, financial arrangements, and other matters.

NURSING MANAGEMENT

The number of patients diagnosed as having Alzheimer's disease is steadily rising, giving nurses increased opportunity to care for these patients. A poignant article, "Another Name for Madness," describes the perils of a patient and family as they face the diagnosis and impact of Alzheimer's disease.[5] It is recommended reading for the health professional to gain insight into the impact of the disease on the family.

Although there is no specific treatment, the patient and family need much sensitivity and emotional support during the process of this devastating disease. Several principles can guide the nurse in working with the patient and family of a victim with Alzheimer's disease; these include the following:

- Provide supervision to protect the patient from becoming injured, humiliated, or lost.

- Encourage the patient to participate in the activities of daily living for as long as possible.
- Provide for the patient's nutritional needs.
- Provide the family and patient with specific information about the disease.
- Make the patient and family aware of resources such as the Alzheimer's Disease and Related Disorders Association, which has chapters in many states and several family support groups.
- Encourage the family to seek legal advice on financial and legal measures to be taken to protect the patient and family. The Alzheimer's Disease and Related Disorders Association may be of some guidance.
- Make referrals to social services and community resources that may assist the patient and family.
- Encourage the development of realistic short- and long-term planning.
- Encourage the patient to stay under medical supervision for the management of other health problems that may arise and for periodic reassessment of cognitive abilities.
- Help the patient and family develop coping skills. Referral for counseling may be appropriate.
- Help the family or caregiver to develop strategies to deal with the specific problems of patient management.
- Help family in the decision concerning institutionalization.

The nurse is in a position to support the patient and family and assist them in dealing with the various painful and monumental decisions that will need attention as the disease develops. See Chart 29–2 for a summary of major nursing diagnoses associated with Alzheimer's disease.

MULTIPLE SCLEROSIS (MS)

Multiple sclerosis or disseminated sclerosis is a chronic, progressive, degenerative disease that affects the myelin sheath and conduction pathways of the central nervous system. The illness is characterized by periods of remissions and exacerbations. Early in the disease, the periods between exacerbations tend to be longer than at later stages. As the illness progresses, the periods of exacerbation are closer together, with the severity and duration of each exacerbation increasing.

ETIOLOGY AND EPIDEMIOLOGY

The etiology of multiple sclerosis is unknown; however, theories of causation include viral infections and a possible autoimmune response.

Many studies have ascertained that multiple sclerosis is more prevalent in the colder northern latitudes and that it is more common in the northern Atlantic states, the Great Lakes region, and the Pacific Northwest than in southern parts of the United States. In Europe, high-incidence areas include Scandinavia, Northern Germany, and Great Britain. However, moving to a warmer climate after diagnosis does not produce an arrest of the disease.

Multiple sclerosis has been called the disease of young adults because the highest rate of incidence is between the

CHART 29–2. SUMMARY OF MAJOR NURSING DIAGNOSES ASSOCIATED WITH ALZHEIMER'S DISEASE

NURSING DIAGNOSES (actual or potential)	EXPECTED OUTCOMES	NURSING INTERVENTIONS
Self-care deficits	• Self-care needs will be provided by patient under supervision, or, when this is no longer possible, self-care needs will be provided by caregiver.	• Provide for ongoing assessment of self-care needs and the patient's ability to participate in this activity. • Provide direct care to the patient as needed.
Sleep pattern disturbance	• An adequate sleep–wakefulness pattern will be established. • The pattern will not be disruptive to others living in the environment.	• Control the patient's activity so that he will stay awake during the daytime. • Provide measures to facilitate sleep at night. • Manipulate the environment to provide an environment conducive to sleep. • Administer medications as ordered.
Impaired verbal communications	• An alternate method of communications will be established. • Patient's needs will be anticipated.	• Develop alternate methods of communication. • Anticipate patient needs.
Impaired cognitive function	• The patient will be protected from being required to participate in cognitive functions beyond his ability. • Protect the patient from stress that leads to behavioral outbursts.	• Do not ask patient to perform cognitive skills beyond his ability. • Control patient's stressors. • Develop a daily routine for the patient to follow. • Provide for continuity of care.
Potential of injury	• The patient will not be injured.	• Recognize that the patient's impaired cognitive functions can lead to injury. • Provide a safe environment. • Provide for frequent supervision.

ages of 20 and 40 years, with about 20% of patients experiencing first symptoms in their 40s and 50s. The socioeconomic impact from loss of gainful productivity is considered major.

There are approximately 500,000 cases of multiple sclerosis in the United States, with women affected slightly more frequently than men. It has been noted that the incidence of the disease in first-degree relatives of persons with multiple sclerosis is 15 times greater than that of the general population.

PATHOPHYSIOLOGY

Multiple sclerosis affects the white matter of the brain and spinal cord by causing scattered demyelinated lesions of the long conduction pathways of the central nervous system. The destruction or demyelination of the fatty substance, called the myelin sheath, that surrounds the axons leaves patches of sclerotic tissue. Eventually, the nerve fibers degenerate, so that disabilities increase and become permanent. Upon autopsy, multiple sclerotic plaques are scattered throughout the white matter of the brain and cord. The scattering differs from patient to patient, accounting for the various presenting symptoms experienced by the individual patient. Neurological deficits are apparent during periods of exacerbation and can completely disappear during remission.

The remission of symptoms is due to the healing of the demyelinated areas by sclerotic tissue. Eventually, symptoms become permanent because of the nerve fiber degeneration.

SIGNS AND SYMPTOMS

The signs and symptoms of multiple sclerosis are widely varied and may be vague. Initial symptoms can occur alone or in any combination. Signs and symptoms include the following:

- Sensory symptoms—numbness, anesthesia, paresthesia (burning, prickling, tingling), pain, decreased proprioception and sense of temperature, depth, and vibration
- Motor symptoms—paresis, paralysis, dragging of foot; spasticity; diplopia; bladder and bowel dysfunction (incontinence or retention)
- Cerebellar symptoms—ataxia, staggering, loss of balance and coordination; nystagmus; speech disturbances (dysarthria, dystonia, scanning speech, slurred speech); tremors (intentional tremors described as tremors that increase when a purposeful act is initiated); vertigo
- Other symptoms—optic neuritis; impotence or decreased genital sensation, sexual dysfunction; depression or euphoria; fatigue or decreased energy level

Other symptoms that are seen in fewer than 5% of patients include hemiplegia, trigeminal neuralgia, facial paralysis, and deafness.[6]

In summary, a multiplicity of symptoms is the hallmark of multiple sclerosis. Characteristically, the disease strikes different areas of the central nervous system. The presenting symptoms of an episode can be very different from the symptoms noted in other episodes.

Motor Symptoms

Motor symptoms often begin with weakness in the lower extremities. The patient complains of a feeling of heaviness or uselessness of the involved limb. Although complaints initially center on one limb, both limbs are usually involved to varying degrees. Spastic paralysis eventually develops.

The decline in motor function may last from minutes to hours and is, therefore, not always observed by the physician. Motor function can worsen spontaneously, after strenuous exercise, or after a hot shower or hot tub bath. Decline in motor function after exposure to a hot shower or tub bath is known as *Uhthoff's phenomenon*. It can be of diagnostic significance in the determination of multiple sclerosis.

Incoordination is another frequent symptom. Intentional tremors are noted in the upper extremities. An *intentional tremor* is defined as a tremor occurring when a voluntary act is initiated. The finer the required movement, the greater the tremor. In the lower extremities, the incoordination appears as ataxia. Head tremors are not evident until the terminal stages when the cerebellum is involved.

Spastic weakness or ataxia of the muscles of speech is responsible for the dysarthria common in multiple sclerosis. Speech, in the early stages, is often slurred. Later, it becomes explosive or staccato and unintelligible. Scanning speech, sometimes said to be characteristic of this disease, is seen only in the later stages, if cerebellar ataxia is prominent.[7] *Scanning speech* is defined as speech that is slow and measured, with pauses between syllables.

Sensory Symptoms

Numbness and tingling are often experienced on the face or involved extremities. Loss of proprioception and joint sensation is frequently accompanied by edema of the limb or feelings of constriction. Fifty percent of patients develop objective sensory loss (position, vibration, shape, texture). Pain is uncommon except with flexor spasms of the limbs.

Ocular Symptoms

Optic neuritis, a common early symptom, is evidenced by visual clouding, loss of vision in part of the visual field (often central), and pain upon movement of the eye. There may be pallor of the optic discs. Nystagmus is noted in approximately 70% of patients. Diplopia is most common without ocular paralysis, but a palsy of one or more ocular muscles is possible. Internuclear ophthalmoplegia of lateral gaze strongly suggests multiple sclerosis. The Marcus Gunn phenomenon may be noted in one eye because of retrobulbar neuritis. This is a response to the reduced light perception in the affected eye.

Auditory and Vestibular Symptoms

Vertigo is a common early symptom usually noted as a mild instability. Vomiting and nystagmus can accompany the vertigo. Deafness is a rare finding.

Paroxysmal Symptoms

Paroxysmal symptoms, which are less common but can occur in multiple sclerosis, include focal or generalized epilepsy, tonic seizures, and occasionally tetanic spasms in advanced illness, although a few patients experience the spasms in the early stages. The spasms are described as contractions of the hands or feet into a dystonic, sustained, abnormal position. The spasms can be very painful and last from about 30 seconds to a few minutes.

Mental and Behavioral Changes

Euphoria, mild depression, irritability, apathy, inattentiveness, poor judgment, and emotional lability are common. Later, depression, memory deficits, confusion, and disorientation are common.

Other Symptoms

Loss or impairment of sphincter control is common. Retention or reflex emptying of the bladder is seen in later stages. Impotence is common in the male. Reflexes of the limbs are hyperactive and the Babinski sign is present. About 50% of patients have ankle clonus. Eighty percent of patients lose the abdominal reflexes. *Lhermitte's phenomenon* is seen in a small percentage of patients afflicted with multiple sclerosis. It is described as an electric or shocklike sensation that extends down the arms, back, or lower trunk bilaterally upon flexion of the neck. It is believed that the abnormal sensation results from the buckling effect on the dorsal roots of the posterior columns upon stimulation of this area by sclerotic plaques. (Unilateral Lhermitte's phenomenon has been noted in such conditions as cervical spondylosis and narrowing of the cervical spinal canal.) As with other symptoms of multiple sclerosis, Lhermitte's phenomenon may be present for a while and then disappear.

COURSE OF THE ILLNESS

The course of multiple sclerosis is unpredictable. According to Hallpike and colleagues, a few categories of progression can be identified that include:[8]

- Benign form (20%)—The patient has a few mild early attacks with complete or nearly complete clearing of signs and symptoms. There is minimal or no disability.
- Exacerbating-remitting form (25%)—The patient has more frequent attacks that begin earlier in the illness. There is less complete clearing of signs and symptoms than in the benign form although there are longer periods of stability when the same signs and symptoms are present.
- Chronic-relapsing form (40%)—The remissions are fewer and less complete after an exacerbation of symptoms than in the exacerbating-remitting form. The disease is cumulative, with a greater number of symptoms seen in each episode.
- Chronic-progressive form (15%)—This is similar to the chronic-relapsing form except that the onset is more insidious, and the course is slowly progressive without remissions.

Certain symptoms have been found in a cluster when a certain area of the brain is involved. For example, *Charcot triad*, which includes nystagmus, intentional tremors and staccato speech, occurs in multiple sclerosis when the brain stem is involved. However, the disease is not usually confined to only one area, so it is not a particularly useful classification.

Early periods of exacerbation develop over days or hours. An attack that produces a measurable deficit rarely lasts less than a few days. Many periods of exacerbation last approximately 2 weeks with incomplete reversal of symptoms. Deficits present after 3 months are usually permanent. It is impossible to predict when the next episode will occur. Some patients may experience another attack in a few weeks while others may be spared for many years. The frequency of the attacks in the first 1 or 2 years appears to have a direct relationship to the course of the illness. The more frequent the attacks during this period, the more ominous the outlook. Patients live an average of 35 years after diagnosis.

Multiple sclerosis can be a very benign disease. Upon autopsy, characteristic sclerotic lesions may be found in patients who never noticed neurological deficits. The number of sclerotic plaques can be surprisingly high and the patient can still be asymptomatic.

PRECIPITATING FACTORS

A few of the factors that may precipitate the onset of multiple sclerosis or a relapse of the disease include infections, trauma, and pregnancy. With trauma, the site of injury bears a relationship to the first symptom of the disease. For example, extraction of teeth will correlate with jaw symptoms, while injury to a limb would be followed by paresis or paresthesia of the involved limb.

Other events that may precipitate an attack in a diagnosed patient are menstruation, emotional stress, cold or humid weather, hot baths, overheating, and fatigue.

DIAGNOSIS

The diagnosis of multiple sclerosis is difficult to make because various symptoms that are evident during exacerbation may completely disappear during remission. The physician becomes suspicious when neurological deficits are noted in an exacerbation-remission cycle. Other suspicious circumstances are a familial history and worsening of symptoms during exposure to heat. When the body temperature is raised even slightly by exposure to dry heat, moist heat (as created by soaking in a hot bath), or fever, the affected nerves may stop transmitting impulses. Thus, symptoms would be exaggerated. Additional signs include abnormal reflex reactions.

There is no single reliable diagnostic test for multiple sclerosis. Certain laboratory tests may help to establish the diagnosis, but no test is definitive. The total protein in the cerebrospinal fluid may be elevated to 45 mg to 75 mg/dl (normal, 15 mg to 45 mg/dl). Cerebrospinal fluid immunoglobin G (IgG, a protein fraction of gamma globulin) is elevated in two thirds of patients, and oligoclonal bands are seen in the gamma globulin region on electrophoresis in 80% to 90% of the patients. In addition, myelin basic protein, the major protein in the myelin sheath, is liberated from the sheath in an acute attack.

The diagnosis is made by exclusion of all other neurological disorders that have similar presenting symptoms and the following criteria:

- Neurological examination must reveal objective abnormalities attributable to the central nervous system.
- Two or more parts of the white matter of the brain or spinal cord must be involved.
- Involvement must follow one of two possible patterns:
  - —Two or more exacerbations, each lasting at least 24 hours and each 1 month or more apart
  - —Slow, stepwise progression for at least 6 months
- At onset, the patient must be 10 to 50 years old.

The use of positron emission transaxial tomography (PETT) is being considered as a new tool in the diagnoses of multiple sclerosis.

TREATMENT

The treatment of multiple sclerosis is symptomatic and supportive. There is no specific treatment.

Drug Therapy

Drug therapy for periods of exacerbation is somewhat controversial, with some authorities giving ACTH (Acthar), 40 to 50 units twice a day for 7 to 10 days. Others prefer to give intravenous infusion of 500 ml of D/W with 80 units of ACTH for 3 days, followed by 40 units intramuscularly every 12 hours for 7 days. A potassium supplement is necessary because of potassium depletion when this steroid is administered. The usual steroid precautions should be followed. The use of steroids during a period of exacerbation is said to hasten remission. Another drug that has been administered to precipitate a remission is prednisone (Meticorten), 10 mg four times a day. Other oral steroids are now widely used in multiple sclerosis clinics. A drug used frequently to control spasticity is baclofen (Lioresal). Other drugs used for this purpose are diazepam (Valium) and dantrolene sodium (Dantrium).

A controversial drug protocol is the use of immunosuppressive agent, azathioprine (Imuran) or cyclophosphamide (Cytoxan). The basis for this protocol is that it suppresses the immune system of the body. In some clinics the drug Cytoxan is given once a month on an outpatient basis. This is sufficient, in many instances, to control signs and symptoms of multiple sclerosis. The risk of bone marrow suppression and the increased risk of infection are the major side-effects of the treatment. Periodic blood studies and monitoring for infection are necessary for patients receiving this drug protocol.

Diet

The role of *diet* has stimulated great interest as an effective management protocol. A low-fat diet has been endorsed by some experts as therapeutic. Others propose a diet rich in linoleic acid because some patients with multiple sclerosis have reduced levels of serum linoleic acid. Neither proposal can be considered to be a widely accepted treatment.

Physiotherapy

The symptomatic management will vary depending on the needs of the patient. The goal of care is to keep the patient as independent as possible for as long as possible. A physiotherapy progam is designed to postpone the ultimate bedridden phase for as long as possible. Methods and devices can be employed to allow for ambulation, self-feeding, dressing, and other activities of daily living.

Although lost motor power cannot be regained, muscles that are not being used can be prevented from becoming weak by strengthening exercises. The physiotherapist can prescribe a brace or support device (cane, walker) to maintain ambulation and independence.

If the patient develops spasticity of the legs, gait retraining may be instituted by developing alternate muscles and stretching exercises. Stretching exercises are effective for spastic arms also. With severe spasticity drugs such as baclofen (Lioresal), diazepam (Valium), and dantrolene sodium (Dantrium) may be beneficial in improving muscle function. However, these drugs have serious side-effects and should be used cautiously.

Should irreversible shortening of the muscles or joint contractures develop, passive range-of-motion exercises are begun to maintain function. The patient who is ataxic may be helped by means of gait training to widen the base of support and by using a weighted cane or walker. Weighted bracelets on either extremity are also of value. Speech deficits can be improved by initiating progressive resistive exercises to the muscles of phonation, accessory respiratory muscles, and tongue and facial muscles.

Patients with sensory loss must be taught to protect themselves from injury by using their eyes to locate the extremities. The body must also be protected from trauma, heat, cold, and pressure. The key in helping the patient to maintain independence is planning by the health care team based on an individualized assessment of the patient's needs.

PROGNOSIS

The course of the illness is nearly impossible to predict. Some patients will live a fairly normal life. Life expectancy and cause of death will be similar to those of the population at-large. Those patients who die of illness associated with multiple sclerosis succumb from infections of the urinary or respiratory system. Rarely will patients die in a matter of weeks or months after diagnosis. If this does occur, the underlying etiology is damage to the vital centers of the brain stem.

NURSING MANAGEMENT OF THE PATIENT WITH MULTIPLE SCLEROSIS

Many patients with multiple sclerosis live normal lifestyles between periods of exacerbation. When exacerbations occur, most patients are managed at home. Patients who have permanent disabilities can often live independently with the aid of a community health nurse and adaptation of the physical environment of the home. Other patients need family members to help care for them. Some patients with advanced disease are managed in nursing homes.

Patients with multiple sclerosis are seen in the acute-care setting when exacerbations or complications occur. In other instances, the nurse may have contact with the patient in the multiple sclerosis clinic or outpatient department. Regardless of the setting in which the nurse comes in contact with the multiple sclerosis patient, it is important for the nurse to assess the patient's understanding of his illness, factors that cause exacerbation of signs and symptoms (Chart 29–3), and adaptation of his lifestyle to live as independently and normally as possible. A teaching plan should be developed based on the patient's needs.

The major nursing diagnoses associated with multiple sclerosis and the appropriate nursing interventions are contained in Chart 29–4. As permanent disabilities develop, the amount of support necessary from the nurse and other health care professionals increases. Many patients will note a decreased energy level, urinary tract problems, motor deficits, sexual dysfunction, changes in their social and recreational activities, and concerns about roles and employment. Most patients need support in their adjustment process. Some patients need counselling and psychotherapy. Patients should also be made aware of the purposes and services offered by the National Multiple Sclerosis Society. Many patients and family members benefit from special multiple sclerosis support groups.

For the patient with advanced disease, the use of braces and canes and finally confinement to a wheelchair may be a reality. These patients need instruction and help in modifying their lifestyles to maintain the greatest level of independence possible. In some instances the patient will be bedridden. In addition to considering all of the nursing diagnoses listed in Chart 29–4, the nurse will need to incorporate measures to control the potential problems of immobility.

CHART 29–3. AGGRAVATING FACTORS IN MULTIPLE SCLEROSIS

The following factors are known to increase exacerbation of symptoms and should be avoided:

- Undue fatigue or excessive exertion
- Overheating or excessive chilling or cold
- Infections
- Hot baths
- Fever
- Emotional stress
- Pregnancy (should be discussed with the physician to weigh the problems before a decision is made to become pregnant)

AMYOTROPHIC LATERAL SCLEROSIS (ALS)

Amyotrophic lateral sclerosis, also known as Lou Gehrig's disease, is a rapidly progressing, fatal, degenerative disease characterized by destruction of motor cells in the anterior gray horns of the spinal cord along with degeneration of the pyramidal tracts, resulting in wasting of the muscles of the body. The disease involves the upper and lower motor neurons and may attack the motor neurons of the spinal cord, brain stem, or both. Sensory changes are not a part of the disease. Some muscles become weak and atrophy while spasticity and hyperreflexia are noted in others. Various patterns of involvement can develop, but the classic pattern begins with weakness, atrophy, and fasciculations of the muscles of the hands and arms. Later, this converts to spastic paralysis of the limbs.

The etiology of amyotrophic lateral sclerosis is unknown. It has been noted that there is a high incidence of the disease in the natives of Guam. In the United States the incidence of amyotrophic lateral sclerosis is 1.4 per 100,000 people. Men are affected approximately three times more frequently than women. The average amount of time from the onset of the first symptoms until death is about 3 years.

PATHOPHYSIOLOGY

There are marked degenerative changes in the following structures: anterior horn cells of the spinal cord; motor nuclei of the brain stem (especially cranial nuclei VII [facial] and XII [hypoglossal] nerves); corticospinal tracts; and Betz cells and precentral cells of the frontal cortex. Involvement of the upper motor neurons results in spasticity and reduced muscle strength while lower motor neuron involvement results in flaccidity, paralysis, and muscle atrophy. Functions that are not affected include intellectual ability, sensory function, vision, and hearing.

SIGNS AND SYMPTOMS

The signs and symptoms of amyotrophic lateral sclerosis can vary from patient to patient. The initial symptoms are usually weakness and wasting of the upper extremities. A

CHART 29-4. SUMMARY OF THE MAJOR NURSING DIAGNOSES ASSOCIATED WITH MULTIPLE SCLEROSIS

NURSING DIAGNOSES	EXPECTED OUTCOMES	NURSING INTERVENTIONS
Decreased energy level due to disease process	• Patient will develop a realistic daily schedule with rest periods so that he will not feel unduly tired.	• Assess sleep patterns, periods of day when patient feels most tired, length and frequency of rest periods, daily energy requirements, and circadian rhythms. • With the patient, develop a realistic schedule with sufficient rest periods. • Have the patient keep an hourly accounting of his energy level. A graph may be devised to display this.
Control of body temperature to prevent exacerbation	• Patient will avoid hot baths; overexertion; hot weather; high humidity; getting too warm, cold, or chilled; and fever.	• Alert patient to the role of heat and cold in exacerbation of signs and symptoms of multiple sclerosis. • Teach patient the factors that aggravate multiple sclerosis. • Help patient to plan schedule and environment to control for extremes in temperature. • Teach the patient to control fever if it exists.
Musculoskeletal deformities and spasticity	• Patient will participate in an exercise program to maintain motor function. • Spasticity, if present, will be controlled.	• Teach the patient the importance of physical activity and physical therapy in maintaining motor function. • Encourage the greatest degree of physical independence possible. • Control spasticity with drugs and prevention of noxious stimuli (cold, immobility). • Encourage mobility for as long as possible.
Sexual dysfunction	• The patient will maintain or regain maximum sexual function possible. • Sexual integrity will be maintained; patient will express satisfaction with his sexuality.	• Assess patient's satisfaction with his sexuality. • Allow patient to express his feelings. • Make appropriate referrals to other health professionals as necessary. • Encourage the patient to identify ways to maintain his sexual integrity.
Potential of impairment of skin integrity from spasticity, impaired sensation, or development of decubitus ulcers	• Integrity of skin will be maintained.	• Assess skin integrity at frequent intervals. • Keep patient off reddened areas; massage these areas. • Reposition frequently. • Have the patient check position of extremities visually if there is sensory impairment. • Protect the patient from injury (mechanical, thermal).
Potential of social isolation due to physical limitations of illness	• Patient will maintain or regain satisfying social interactions.	• Assess patient's social interactions and his satisfaction with these interactions. • Help the patient develop appropriate strategies for satisfying social interactions. • Help him assess physical barriers that will impede social interactions and develop effective ways of coping.

CHART 29–4. (continued)

NURSING DIAGNOSES	EXPECTED OUTCOMES	NURSING INTERVENTIONS
Role disturbance	• Patient will accept necessary role changes.	• Assess impact of illness on roles. • Help the patient to adjust to necessary changes.
Disturbance in self-concept	• An integrated positive self-concept will be maintained or supported.	• Assess patient's self-concept. • Allow the patient to verbalize concerns. • Correct misconceptions. • Support a positive self-concept.
Bladder dysfunction (urgency, frequency, incontinence, hesitancy, nocturia)	• Urinary continence and adequate bladder elimination will be maintained.	• Assess bladder function and voiding pattern. • Maintain an intake and output record. • Develop an appropriate bladder program (may include self-catherization).
Urinary tract infection	• Urinary tract infection will be prevented.	• Monitor periodic urinalyses and urine cultures. • Encourage an adequate fluid intake.
Bowel dysfunction	• Normal bowel evacuation pattern will be maintained or reestablished.	• Assess bowel function and evacuation pattern. • Provide for an adequate diet and fluid intake. • Develop an appropriate bowel program.

summary of the signs and symptoms includes the following:

- Muscle weakness, wasting, and atrophy; the muscles most commonly affected are the intrinsic muscles of the hand, as evidenced by clumsiness. The next-most-commonly affected muscles are the shoulder and upper arm muscles. The lower limbs are affected last and characteristically feel heavy and are subject to fatigue and easy cramping.
- Muscle spasticity and hyperreflexia
- Fasciculations
- Brain stem signs, which are evidenced by atrophy of the tongue causing dysarthria. The muscles of speech, chewing, and swallowing may be affected so that dysarthria and dysphagia occur.
- Dyspnea will result if the respiratory muscles are involved.
- Fatigue

DIAGNOSIS

The diagnosis of amyotrophic lateral sclerosis is made primarily on the basis of the history and neurological examination. An electromyogram will demonstrate fibrillations, which are indicative of denervation, muscle wasting, and atrophy. The blood creatine phosphokinase (CPK) level is elevated. A myelogram may be ordered to rule out other diseases.

TREATMENT

There is no known treatment to cure or arrest this fatal disease. Management is symptomatic and includes the following:

- Physical therapy—range-of-motion exercises to control or improve the weakness or spasticity. Support devices such as a cervical collar, foot brace, splints, or slings may be ordered. A cane, walker, gait training, or wheelchair may be prescribed to assist the patient in ambulation. Even though the disease is progressive and fatal, the patient is allowed to be as independent as possible for as long as possible.
- Occupational therapy—useful in selecting equipment such as special eating utensils and electronic equipment for alternate ways of accomplishing activities of daily living
- Speech therapy—helpful in giving the patient instruction on projection of the voice
- Gastrostomy tube—if the patient's ability to chew and swallow are severely limited, a gastrostomy tube may be inserted to facilitate nutrition.
- Ongoing counseling and patient and family teaching—the patient and family need support and help in coping with the problems associated with this debilitating, fatal disease.
- Management of any other health problems or complications precipitated by the disease
- Drug therapy for the various problems
  - —Spasticity: diazepam (Valium) or dantrolene sodium (Dantrium)
  - —Cramps: quinidine
  - —Sialorrhea, increased salivation: trihexyphenidyl hydrochloride (Artane), clonidine hydrochloride (Catapres), or amitriptyline hydrochloride (Elavil)

COURSE OF THE ILLNESS

Because the onset of amyotrophic lateral sclerosis is insidious, the early signs and symptoms may be overlooked. Diverse muscle groups gradually become involved, and then weakness, atrophy, muscle wasting, and fasciculations are noted. As the disease progresses, the arms and legs become severely impaired, and spasticity and hyperreflexia are noted. If the frontal lobe cells are involved, emotional lability may be apparent even though intellectual function is not affected. In the advanced stages when the brain stem is involved, the muscles of speech and swallowing are affected. Speech is thick and hard to understand, and chewing, swallowing, and managing secretions become very difficult. At the terminal stage, the patient has dyspnea and shortness of breath. Speaking may no longer be possible. Death usually occurs as a result of aspiration, infection, or respiratory failure.

NURSING MANAGEMENT OF THE PATIENT WITH AMYOTROPHIC LATERAL SCLEROSIS

Although nothing can be done to arrest the fatal disease called amyotrophic lateral sclerosis, the nurse's role is directed toward

- Assisting the patient to be as independent and comfortable as possible for as long as possible by managing presenting patient problems
- Limiting the development of complications
- Assisting the patient to prepare for discharge and crisis
- Providing emotional and psychological support for the patient and family
- Developing and implementing an individualized teaching plan
- Making appropriate referrals to other health professionals and community resources

Nursing Management of Presenting Problems

Patient problems are numerous in this rapidly developing disease. The major nursing diagnoses and interventions are included in Chart 29–5.

Preparation for Discharge and Crisis

The patient and family should be included in planning for discharge from the hospital. If the patient is to go home at least temporarily, plans must be made that include

- Collection of necessary home management equipment (e.g., suction, oxygen, walker)
- Adjustment in household routines
- Arrangement for outpatient services and community resources
- Special therapies such as physical therapy, speech therapy, and occupational therapy
- Awareness of the services offered by the National Amyotrophic Lateral Sclerosis Foundation

The patient and family need to know what lies ahead so that tentative plans can be made to deal with the inevitable.

Providing Emotional and Psychological Support for the Patient and Family

The stresses of coping with the fatal diagnosis and its effect on roles, relationships, self-concept, self-esteem, and body image are overwhelming. The patient and family need a tremendous amount of support. The nurse can contribute to these needs, but other support groups, persons, and resources must be identified depending on the particular needs of the patient and family.

Developing and Implementing an Individualized Teaching Plan

What the patient and family need to learn must be systematically assessed and an individualized teaching plan developed and implemented.

Referrals

Since the needs of the patient and family are many and change as the disease progresses, it is important for the nurse to suggest and make referrals, as necessary.

MYASTHENIA GRAVIS

Myasthenia gravis is a chronic, progressive disease of muscular weakness that is caused by a defect at the myoneural junction. The hallmarks of the disease are

- Increased weakness of certain voluntary muscles, particularly those of chewing, swallowing, and speaking, as well as the facial and extraocular muscles
- Partial improvement of muscle strength with rest
- Dramatic improvement in muscle strength with anticholinesterase drugs

The disease is not hereditary, although in approximately 15% of infants born to myasthenic mothers, symptoms of myasthenia gravis are apparent (weak muscles, weak cry, difficulty in sucking, ptosis, and respiratory difficulty). With treatment with neostigmine (Prostigmin), 7.5 mg to 15 mg daily, the transient illness disappears completely and permanently in about 8 to 12 weeks. The incidence of transient neonatal myasthenia gravis appears to offer support to the theory of toxic factors in the blood from the thymus gland causing the illness.

PATHOPHYSIOLOGY

Studies of normal muscles indicate that the compound action potential remains constant when maximum stimulation is applied. In myasthenic muscles the action potential begins to fall off quickly. As previously noted, the pathophysiology of myasthenia gravis is due to a defect at the myoneural junction. As an impulse travels down the peripheral nerve, it relies on the release of acetylcholine to transmit the impulse across the myoneural junction to the innervated muscle for a contraction to take place. In myasthenia gravis, the amount of acetylcholine in the presynaptic membrane is reduced. One hypothesis suggests that a defect in the presynaptic membrane causes a reduced amount of acetylcholine. There is also evidence that the

CHART 29-5. SUMMARY OF THE MAJOR NURSING DIAGNOSES ASSOCIATED WITH AMYOTROPHIC LATERAL SCLEROSIS

NURSING DIAGNOSES	EXPECTED OUTCOMES	NURSING INTERVENTIONS
Loss of motor function due to muscle weakness and wasting	• Motor function and tone will be maintained for as long as possible.	• Administer or supervise a moderate exercise program as selected by the physiotherapist. • Apply necessary support equipment, teaching patient to apply equipment correctly. • Teach the patient how to use ambulatory aids. • Protect the patient from injury.
Spasticity due to cord involvement	• Spasticity will be controlled as well as possible.	• Administer drugs as ordered. • Control noxious stimuli that are known to increase spasticity (cold, maintaining same position for too long).
Deficit in fluid intake and nutrition due to difficulty in swallowing	• Adequate fluid and nutrition intake will be consumed. • Patient will not aspirate.	• Provide a soft diet. • Provide small frequent feedings. • Encourage the patient to eat slowly. • Have suction equipment accessible. • If a gastrostomy tube is in place, provide for feedings. • Teach patient and family correct procedure in tube feedings.
Speech difficulty due to brain stem involvement	• A method of communication will be developed.	• Suggest speech therapy if necessary. • Develop an alternate method of communication if speech is incomprehensible.
Respiratory insufficiency	• Respiratory function will be supported.	• Assess for signs and symptoms of respiratory insufficiency. • Elevate head of bed. • Provide for proper body alignment. • Administer oxygen as necessary. • Maintain a patent airway. • Suction as necessary.
Bowel and bladder dysfunction	• Elimination from bowel and bladder will be supported.	• Assess bowel and bladder function. • Provide a bowel and bladder program based on the patient's needs. • Monitor urinalysis and urine culture and sensitivity for signs of infection.
Depression due to having a chronic degenerative disease	• A positive body image will be supported.	• Focus on the positive (the functions that remain intact). • Allow patient to express feelings. • Correct misconceptions. • Refer for counseling if necessary.

postsynaptic membrane lacks sufficient receptor sites to use acetylcholine.* Both of these reasons contribute to the fact that the muscle is not able to contract fully or normally. With repeated stimulation, the muscle becomes exhausted and cannot contract at all.

The prognosis without treatment is grave. Until the advent of anticholinesterase therapy, most patients died from respiratory insufficiency and, less frequently, from aspiration.

The onset is usually gradual, although rapid onsets have been reported in association with respiratory infections or emotional upset. The course of the illness is extremely variable. In some patients the disease is unchanged for months before progressing, while in others there is rapid spread from one muscle group to others. The greatest incidence of death from myasthenia gravis is in the first year after the onset of the disease. Another critical period occurs during the time from 4 to 7 years after onset. After this time the disease tends to stabilize, greatly diminishing the danger of severe relapses.

* There is another popular theory that proposes an autoimmune basis for myasthenia gravis. This theory appears to correlate with certain thymic changes noted. Whatever the etiology, research continues into the causes of myasthenia gravis.

An interesting correlation noted is that 80% of myasthenic patients are said to have thymic hyperplasia. Fifteen percent have thymic tumors. There is some evidence to suggest that toxic substances are produced by the hyperplasic thymus, which influence the development of myasthenia gravis.

EPIDEMIOLOGY

The prevalence of myasthenia gravis is estimated at from 1 in 10,000 to 1 in 50,000 of the population.[9] The peak incidence is between 20 and 30 years of age. Incidence in the first decade or after the age of 70 years is rare. Up to the age of 40 years, women are affected two to three times as frequently as men. After the age of 40 years, the frequency in men and women is about equal.

SIGNS AND SYMPTOMS

Usually the muscles of the eyes are affected first. In most patients the levator palpebrae and extracular muscles are involved. Ptosis, ocular palsy, and diplopia are common symptoms. Ptosis may be unilateral or bilateral and becomes intensified when the patient attempts to look upward. There is often difficulty in closing the eyelids (orbicularis oculi innervated by the facial nerve). Pupillary response to light and accommodation remain normal.

The next series of muscles to be affected are the facial, masticatory, speech, and neck muscles. When chewing food, the patient becomes tired and must rest. After a few moments of rest he is able to resume chewing but quickly becomes fatigued again. Because the facial muscle is affected, the mobility and expression of the face are altered. Any attempt to smile looks like a snarl. The jaw may hang open loosely and may need to be closed by the hand. The voice becomes weak and fades after conversation, frequently diminishing to a whisper. There may be problems in managing saliva because of the swallowing difficulty. Food must be taken very slowly to prevent aspiration.

The muscles of flexion and extension of the neck, the muscles of the shoulder girdle, and the flexors of the hip are less often involved. Weakness of the neck muscles tends to cause the head to fall forward. If the shoulder girdle is involved, the patient has difficulty keeping his arms above his head when reaching for an object or combing or fixing the hair.

The muscles for fine hand movements may be affected early, with or without concurrent involvement of coarse shoulder movement. If the hand movements are involved, sewing, writing, and other fine movements will be impaired. In severe cases with upper arm involvement, there may be great difficulty in lifting the hands to the mouth. While the patient may carry out this movement initially, the muscles quickly become fatigued, making any further action of this type impossible.

The most life-threatening situation exists when the intercostal muscles and/or diaphragm become affected. Breathlessness is often an early sign of this involvement. Respiratory weakness can develop rapidly and cause death. Sudden respiratory failure is often due to the development of a myasthenic crisis.

Involved muscles do not usually atrophy, which is noted in only 10% of females and 20% of males.[9] Tendon reflexes almost always remain brisk, even when paresis is severe and cardiac and smooth muscles are spared.

In summary, the muscle groups affected tend to be weaker after use or toward the end of the day when the patient is fatigued. As the disease progresses, muscle fatigue is noted with less exertion and earlier in the day. See Chart 29–6 for the clinical classification of myasthenia gravis.

DIAGNOSIS

The diagnosis of myasthenia gravis is based on a history of weakness in certain muscle groups, particularly those with motor nuclei located in the brain stem. A period of rest improves the motor function, but the muscle becomes fatigued again quickly.

The most useful and highly reliable diagnostic test is the edrophonium chloride (Tensilon) test. The test is performed by drawing 10 mg of Tensilon into a syringe and administering 2 mg. If no symptoms appear, the remaining 8 mg are injected. Within 30 to 60 seconds of the first dose, most patients with myasthenia gravis will demonstrate a marked, objective improvement in muscle tone, lasting for 4 to 5 minutes. A few myasthenic patients will respond only to the larger dose. This test is also a valid tool for differentiating between myasthenic and cholinergic crises.

The neostigmine (Prostigmin) test is a much less frequently used test for diagnosing myasthenia gravis. One to 2 mg of neostigmine is injected intramuscularly. In about 30 minutes improvement of muscle tone should be noted in the myasthenic patient.

TREATMENT

Once the diagnosis of myasthenia gravis has been established, the physician must propose a management plan that is based on drug therapy. Drug protocols are the major management approach used for the management of signs and symptoms in patients with myasthenia gravis. Other approaches used with selected patients in addition to drug therapy are thymectomy and plasmapheresis.

Drug Protocols

Because the best medication protocol for a patient is highly individualized, the cooperation of the patient must be gained to evaluate the effects. The pharmacological treatment of myasthenia gravis uses two groups of drugs: anticholinesterase drugs and sometimes corticosteroids. With proper medication most patients can lead virtually normal lives. For some patients, a thymectomy is effective in controlling the disease.

CHART 29-6. CLINICAL CLASSIFICATION OF MYASTHENIA GRAVIS*

Ocular Myasthenia

- Involves ocular muscles only with the symptoms of ptosis and diplopia
- Very mild
- Usually responds poorly to medication
- No mortality; high rate of spontaneous remission

Generalized Myasthenia

Mild

- Slow onset, usually ocular; gradually spreads to bulbar and skeletal muscles but spares respiratory system
- Responds well to medication
- Remission possible
- Low mortality rate

Moderate

- Gradual onset, usually ocular; progresses to more severe bulbar symptoms and generalized involvement of skeletal muscles
- Responds to medication less satisfactorily than other types
- Restricts activities of daily living
- Remission possible
- Low mortality rate

Acute Fulminating

- Rapid onset of generalized skeletal weakness and severe bulbar symptoms; involves respiratory system early
- Rapid deterioration
- Frequent crises (myasthenic and cholinergic)
- High mortality rate

Late Severe

- Severe symptoms develop at last 2 years after onset of ocular or generalized myasthenia
- Marked bulbar involvement
- Progresses gradually or with sudden deterioration
- Responds poorly to medication
- High mortality rate

* Adapted from Osserman KE: Myasthenia Gravis, p 80. New York, Grune & Stratton, 1968

Anticholinesterase Drugs. Two drugs in this group have been particularly valuable in managing the disease: neostigmine (Prostigmin) and pyridostigmine (Mestinon).

Neostigmine (Prostigmin). Neostigmine enhances cholinergic action by facilitating the transmission of impulses across the neuromuscular junction. As a parasympathetic stimulant, it inhibits the destruction of acetylcholine by cholinesterase, thus enhancing the transmission of impulses across the myoneural junction.

Neostigmine taken orally has an onset within 20 minutes, with the peak effect in about 2½ hours. The usual oral dose is 7.5 mg to 45.0 mg every 2 to 6 hours. This is a wide range, but the optimal dosage and drug schedule must be determined by trial and error. Neostigmine tablets are supplied in 15-mg scored tablets.

The side-effects of neostigmine are of the muscarinic and nicotinic types as follows:

Muscarinic Type

- Gastrointestinal tract — heartburn, belching, epigastric distress, abdominal cramps, increased peristalsis, diarrhea, nausea, and vomiting
- Genitourinary tract — involuntary micturition, increased tone and motility of uterus
- Cardiovascular — bradycardia and hypotension, or tachycardia and hypertension
- Vision — blurred vision, constricted pupils, photophobia, myopia, and so forth
- Respiratory tract — bronchoconstriction, increased mucus secretions, wheezing cough, chest pain and tightness
- Other — profuse sweating and salivation

Nicotinic Type

- Skeletal muscle fasciculations, followed by muscle twitching and cramping, followed by fatigue, weakness, and paralysis of all voluntary muscles including the diaphragm

Pyridostigmine (Mestinon). Like neostigmine, pyridostigmine inhibits the destruction of cholinesterase. The daily dosage of this drug is approximately 15 mg to 90 mg orally. Its action is longer and smoother than that of neostigmine. Pyridostigmine is also supplied in 180-mg timesspan tablets that are particularly effective in maintaining the patient overnight. Side-effects are of the muscarinic and nicotinic types.

Ambenonium (Mytelase). Ambenonium is another drug of this group used less frequently. The usual dosage is 5 mg to 25 mg three to four times daily. Its side-effects are similar to those of pyridostigmine.

Summary of Drug Protocols. Often, neostigmine and pyridostigmine are used in combination for maintenance therapy. The drug dosages are carefully manipulated to produce maximal muscle strength with minimal side-effects. All patients not achieve therapeutic control of their symptoms with the anticholinesterase drugs.

Atropine is the antidote for anticholinesterase drugs and must be available for any patient on anticholinesterase therapy.

Corticosteroids. For those who do not respond well to anticholinesterase drugs, corticosteroids may be tried. ACTH and prednisone are the drugs selected. When interest in this protocol was first developed, 100 to 160 units of ACTH daily for 10 days was suggested. The patient temporarily worsened but then improved progressively after the course was completed. The remission lasted 3 to 6 months with ACTH, requiring that the treatment be repeated periodically. Current practices suggest the administration of 100 mg of prednisone every other day. Because the symptoms worsen in the first 7 to 10 days, the patient should be hospitalized and observed carefully so that definitive action can be taken if respiratory difficulty develops. The prednisone is administered concurrently with the anticholinesterase drugs. As symptoms improve, the prednisone can be gradually reduced to the lowest level of effectiveness. The usual steroid precautions of giving potassium supplements, tapering dosage, and giving antacids should be followed. Corticosteroids appear to cause a remission in the severity of the disease.

Thymectomy

In cases in which a tumor of the thymus is related to the myasthenia gravis, surgical removal is indicated unless contraindicated for other reasons. Thymectomy for hyperplasia, which is apparent in 80% of patients, is often recommended for many patients. This procedure induces a remission of symptoms in approximately 40% of patients if the procedure is done early in the disease (within the first 2 years). Women seem to achieve the greatest benefit from thymectomy.

Surgery must be planned well by the surgeon and anesthesiologist because the myasthenic patient is prone to have unpredictable responses to drugs and the possibility of respiratory failure is ever present. The surgical site is close to the lungs and can also result in a pneumothorax. The surgeon has two possible surgical approaches: the suprasternal and the transsternal. The suprasternal approach results in less postoperative pain and morbidity. Its disadvantage is that less of the thymus gland can be removed because of the difficulty of accessibility. The transsternal approach continues to be selected by many surgeons because it allows better access to the thymus gland, making complete removal possible. The disadvantage to this approach is that the sternum is split for surgical access, thereby causing more postoperative discomfort and requiring a longer convalescence.

Plasmapheresis

The newest treatment for myasthenia gravis, called plasmapheresis, is a process of washing the plasma of circulating antibodies that allegedly interfere with the acetylcholine receptors. The washing is done by way of an antecubital vein or shunt and takes between 2 and 5 hours to complete. The patient may need less medication after the procedure. Improvement is not noted for 2 to 3 days after the treatment in some patients.

Other Therapies

Cyclophosphamide (Cytoxan) and azathioprine (Imuran) are also being used in some institutions. The exact mechanism by which these drugs affect the disease process is not clear.

CHOLINERGIC CRISIS *VERSUS* MYASTHENIC CRISIS

Cholinergic crisis is caused by overmedication with cholinergic (anticholinesterase) drugs. The signs and symptoms include nausea, vomiting, miosis, pallor, sweating, salivation, gastrointestinal hyperirritability, severe cramps, diarrhea, and bradycardia. In addition, there is acute exacerbation of the myasthenic muscle weakness. The patient often experiences acute respiratory distress and has difficulty managing his own saliva. Without immediate help he can quickly aspirate, suffer respiratory arrest, and die. Clinically, the patient appears acutely ill and in need of immediate respiratory support. His muscles are so weak that he cannot utter even a few words or move any part of his body.

Myasthenic crisis refers to an exacerbation of the myasthenic motor weakness because of undermedication or no medication at all with cholinergic drugs. Acute respiratory difficulty may also be identical to the acute respiratory distress seen in cholinergic crisis. In addition, the acute motor weakness of the voluntary muscles, including those for swallowing, speaking, and moving other body parts, is the same as that described for cholinergic crisis.

Because muscle weakness is a prominent feature of both crises, there is often difficulty in diagnosing by clinical observation whether the crisis is cholinergic or myasthenic. Use of the Tensilon test, as previously described, is an important procedure for making that differentiation. If the patient becomes worse upon injection of Tensilon, he is in cholinergic crisis. The Tensilon is discontinued and atropine sulfate, 0.6 mg, may be given cautiously by the intravenous route. If the patient's muscle tone improves with the Tensilon test, he must be started on cholinergic (anticholinesterase) drugs because he is in myasthenic crisis.

Management of the myasthenic patient during complications depends on the specific presenting symptoms. In the case of cholinergic or myasthenic crisis, nursing care is directed at early detection of the type of crisis and having the necessary equipment available, such as a suctioning apparatus to maintain a patent airway. A tracheostomy set, endotracheal tube, and respirator should be present if respiratory distress occurs. The acutely ill patient needs constant nursing care to carefully monitor his condition and maintain his body functions.

Once the appropriate medication is administered there should be dramatic improvement in the patient's condition. Provided that respiratory complications such as aspiration or pneumonia have not developed, there will most likely be rapid improvement.

If an endotracheal or tracheostomy tube with or without respirator is present, nursing standards will be followed to promote respiratory function. The patient will need complete care. As he begins to respond to treatment, he will require much help because he tires so easily with minimal exertion.

NURSING MANAGEMENT

The patient with myasthenia gravis is usually managed at home. The more the patient knows about his disease and the drug treatment program, the less apt he is to develop complications. Family members must also be knowledgeable so that they will know what to do in the event of respiratory difficulty or the development of crisis. The need for hospitalization may be necessary during the evaluation and diagnostic process, myasthenic or cholinergic crisis, respiratory failure, and periods of exacerbation when respiratory function is threatened regardless of cause (e.g., pneumonia, heat exhaustion, and so forth). During these times an endotracheal or tracheostomy tube may be necessary and may be used in conjunction with a respirator.

Management of the myasthenic patient during complications will depend on the specific presenting complications. However, assessment of muscle weakness and drug therapy are major concerns when complications occur. See Chart 29–7 for major nursing diagnoses associated with myasthenia gravis.

Patient Teaching

While the patient is undergoing diagnostic tests for myasthenia gravis or making adjustments in lifestyle because of the disease, a teaching plan should be devised as part of nursing management. The patient should be encouraged to live as normal a life as possible.

The patient should be generally familiar with his disease. Determine what information the physician has conveyed to the patient. Clarify and reinforce this information and allow the patient to ask questions.

The patient and a responsible family member should be familiar with any drugs being taken as well as dosage and side-effects. They should also know the signs, symptoms, and differences between cholinergic and myasthenic crises. An Ambu bag and portable suction device should be available at home for patients prone to crisis. The patient should be familiar with the Myasthenia Gravis Foundation and its publications.

The following points should be included in the teaching plan:

- Wear a Medic Alert bracelet to identify self as having myasthenia gravis and carry a card stating the name of your attending physician.
- Take medication with bread or a cracker to reduce nausea and gastric irritation.
- Take medication 30 minutes before eating for maximal strength of muscles for chewing and swallowing.
- Do not take any over-the-counter medication without your doctor's permission.
- Eat slowly and select a soft diet if you have difficulty in swallowing.
- Exacerbations of symptoms can be caused by menstruation, infections, extremes in temperature, extensive exposure to sunlight (ultraviolet light), and emotional stress.
- Provide for adequate rest periods during the day.
- Set priorities and plan ahead so that undue fatigue will not develop. Pace yourself.
- Wear sensible shoes to minimize weakness and loss of balance.
- Evaluate respiratory function by auscultation and observation and by evaluating respiratory tests for vital capacity and tidal volume.
- Observe for symptoms of pneumothorax. (This complication may be due to the surgical approach used.)
  - —Restlessness
  - —Perspiration
  - —Cyanosis
  - —Tachycardia
  - —Respiratory distress
- If patient has chest tubes, provide proper care by milking the tubes when necessary and assuring proper function.
- Observe for unpredictable responses to any drugs used; for example, excessive sedation, decreased respirations, or agitation.
- Evaluate degree of strength or weakness of all muscles involved:
  - —*Respirations*—rate, rhythm, quality (labored or smooth), evidence of abdominal breathing
  - —*Voice*—quality of voice (whisper, monotone, moderate loudness, full range of quality)
  - —*Hand grasps*—strength and equality of both hands (ability to hold or pick up objects)
  - —*Leg movement*—ability to move legs freely in bed
  - —*Extraocular muscles*—the patient should follow your finger through the six cardinal positions. (Note the presence of ptosis of the upper eyelid.)
  - —*Head*—ability to hold up head

(See Chapter 5 for assessment of neurological function.)

CHART 29-7. SUMMARY OF THE MAJOR NURSING DIAGNOSES ASSOCIATED WITH MYASTHENIA GRAVIS

NURSING DIAGNOSES (ACTUAL OR POTENTIAL)	EXPECTED OUTCOMES	NURSING INTERVENTIONS
Impaired physical mobility due to voluntary motor weakness.	• Voluntary motor function will be supported for optimum physical mobility.	• Assess effect of drug program in supporting motor function. • Note times of day when patient is weakest. • Consult with physician and patient to adjust drug program. • Help patient plan a schedule that allows for periods of rest. • Help patient pace himself so that he has realistic goals.
Potential of injury	• Physical injury will be avoided.	• Suggest wearing sensible shoes. • If there is noted weakness, use assistive devices as necessary (*e.g.,* walker, hand rails). • Do not allow patient to lift heavy loads. • Practice good body mechanics.
Easy fatigability and decreased energy level	• The patient will follow a daily schedule that will provide for periods of rest and activity. • An adequate energy level will be maintained. • Undue fatigue will be avoided.	• Develop a daily schedule that allows for periods of rest and activities. • Assess adequacy of drug program. • Teach patient about activities or circumstances that cause increased fatigue.
Ineffective breathing pattern	• An adequate, effective breathing pattern will be maintained.	• Assess the breathing pattern. Note any abnormalities. • If breathing pattern is not adequate, assess reasons for the problems. • Take definitive action to support an adequate breathing pattern.
Potential of aspiration	• Patient will not aspirate.	• Develop a teaching plan to include practices to decrease the possibility of aspiration (*e.g.,* encourage small bites and swallowing frequently, provide a soft diet). • Provide for emergency management measures to be observed if aspiration occurs.
Disturbance of self-concept	• A realistic and positive self-concept will be maintained.	• Teach the patient about his illness and how to adapt his lifestyle to live with the problem. • Support a positive self-concept. • Encourage the patient to live as normal a life as possible.

Nursing Management After a Thymectomy

The patient will be managed as any patient with chest surgery. Chest tubes and a tracheostomy will probably be in place. Special considerations of nursing care include the following:

- Maintain a patent airway by suctioning, giving tracheostomy care, and encouraging the patient to cough. These measures decrease stress on the respiratory muscles and provide for adequate oxygenation.
- Provide chest physiotherapy, turn the patient every 2 hours, and encourage deep breathing exercises to prevent pulmonary infection.

PARKINSON'S DISEASE

Parkinson's disease, also called paralysis agitans, is a chronic degenerative disorder of the basal ganglia. The disease usually begins insidiously, often unilaterally, with only a few apparent symptoms. Because the onset is insidious and the population affected is elderly, symptoms are frequently disregarded as consequences of the aging process.

The following classification of Parkinson's disease is helpful in evaluating disability and charting progression of the disease:

- Stage I: Unilateral involvement only
- Stage II: Bilateral involvement only
- Stage III: Impaired postural and righting reflexes; mild to moderate disability
- Stage IV: Fully developed, severe disease; marked disability
- Stage V: Confinement to bed or wheelchair[10]

ETIOLOGY AND EPIDEMIOLOGY

The etiology of Parkinson's disease is unknown. The epidemiological profile of Parkinson's disease indicates that (1) it is a disease of the elderly, (2) first symptoms are usually noted in the 60s, although a few patients may experience symptoms in the 50s, and (3) men are affected slightly more often than women. There are approximately 1 to 1.5 million patients with Parkinson's disease in the United States. The number of patients is growing and will continue to grow as people live longer and the overall population of the elderly increases.

PATHOPHYSIOLOGY

Basal ganglia is a collective term that includes the subcortical motor nuclei of the cerebrum. The structures that compose the basal ganglia include the striatum, globus pallidum, subthalamic nucleus, substantia nigra, and red nucleus. In Parkinson's disease pigmented cells in the substantia nigra are lost because of degenerative changes. The motor cells of the motor cortex and pyramidal tracts are not affected. The cell degeneration does create impairment of the extrapyramidal tracts, semiautomatic functions, and coordinated movements.

It has been noted that the dopamine normally stored in the cells of the substantia nigra is greatly depleted in Parkinson's disease. The reason for this is unclear.

SIGNS AND SYMPTOMS

Because symptoms may develop slowly, years may pass before diagnosis is made. The disease is progressive, so that eventually the patient's ability to perform the activities of daily living and other independent functions are reduced. Some patients become confined to bed.

The signs and symptoms of Parkinson's disease include the following:

- Muscle rigidity
- Masklike face
- Tremors
- Restlessness
- Disturbance in free-flowing movement
- General weakness and muscular fatigue
- Muscle cramps
- Loss of postural reflexes
- Mental depression
- Autonomic manifestations

Muscular Rigidity. Muscular rigidity is associated with slowness of voluntary movement (bradykinesia). The muscle feels stiff and requires much effort to move. Because muscle position does not change when the patient is sitting, edema of the feet and legs may develop. The trunk of the body tends to stoop forward. The forearms are semiflexed while the fingers are flexed at the metacarpophalangeal joints. The characteristic appearance and posture of the patient with Parkinson's disease are illustrated in Figure 29–1.

Masklike Face. The patient appears to stare straight ahead and assumes an expressionless look on his face. His eyes tend to blink less frequently than normal—5 to 10 times per second rather than the normal 15 to 20 times.

Tremors. Tremors occur most often in the upper extremities, particularly in the distal portions of the limbs and in the hands. The so-called "pill-rolling" motion of the hands is noted. The tremors are present when the hand is motionless and thus are termed "resting tremors" (see Fig. 29–2). At complete rest the tremors are absent or greatly diminished. They are completely absent when the patient is asleep.

Other areas where tremors are seen include the foot, lip, tongue, and jaw. The *cogwheel phenomenon* is noted, especially in the arms. This term refers to the rigidity or rhythmic contractions noted upon passive stretching of the muscles in Parkinson's disease.

Restlessness (Motor Restlessness, Akathisia). Some patients experience *akathisia*, a condition of compelling need to walk about constantly.

FIG. 29–1. The clinical features of Parkinson's disease. (Smith R: Essentials of Neurosurgery. Philadelphia, JB Lippincott, 1980)

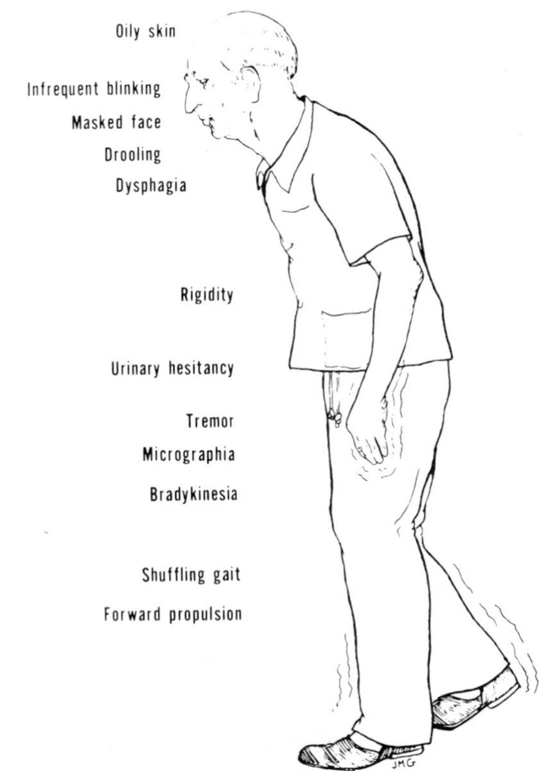

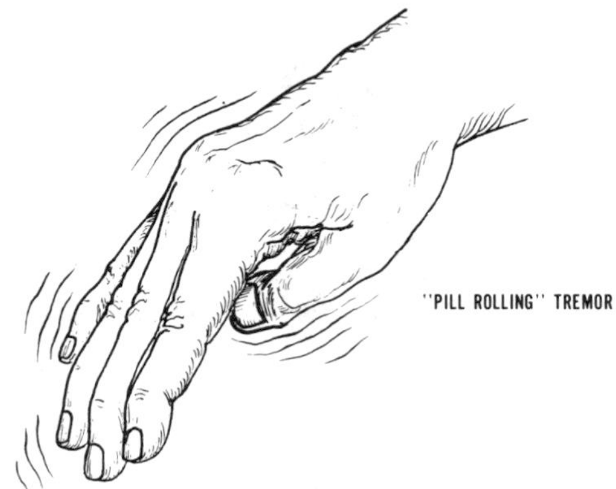

FIG. 29-2. The tremor in Parkinson's disease is exaggerated by the resting posture, is often relieved by movement, and usually disappears during sleep. The movement of the thumb across the palm gives it a "pill-rolling" character. (Smith R: Essentials of Neurosurgery. Philadelphia, JB Lippincott, 1980)

Disturbance in Free-flowing Movement (Dyskinesia). Movements are jerky and uncoordinated. Handwriting becomes progressively smaller, choppier, and jerkier. Some patients experience upward and lateral rotation of the eyes, which become fixed. The patient is unable to move them and appears pained. The term used to describe this occurrence is *oculogyric crisis.*

General Weakness and Muscular Fatigue. Initiation of movement for purposeful acts is slow. During the movement the patient may become momentarily frozen. Fatigue is a common complaint when a patient tries to conduct the activities of daily living. Muscle cramps of the legs, neck, and trunk occur frequently. The voice may be so weak that the patient speaks in a monotonic whisper.

Loss of Postural Reflexes. The patient has difficulty in maintaining balance and cannot sit erect. He usually walks in a stooped-over position with small shuffling steps. Movement, once begun, frequently accelerates almost to a trot. If the patient is pushed, he makes no attempt to brace himself or to reach out and stop his movement.

Mental Depression. Mental depression is common because of a generally abnormal physical appearance, a weakened voice that affects communication, and a frequent tendency to withdraw from normal interaction because of self-consciousness and embarrassment. The isolation further increases his depression.

Common Autonomic Manifestations. Additional signs and symptoms associated with the autonomic system include the following:

- Drooling—due to decreased frequency of swallowing. When the patient awakens, his pillow is wet.
- Seborrhea (oily, greasy skin)—probably due to hypothalamic dysfunction, which causes an increased amount of sebotrophic hormone to be released
- Dysphagia—due to the neuromuscular inccordination of the hypopharyngeal musculature. This problem can interfere with normal fluid and dietary intake.
- Excessive perspiration—probably due to a disorder of the hypothalamic heat regulator mechanism as well as impairment of perspiration controls. The patient may be diaphoretic even in cold weather and have a fever in warmer weather.
- Constipation—due to hypomotility of the gastrointestinal tract, associated with prolonged gastric emptying time. The decreased fluid intake, lack of roughage, and decreased activity contribute to the development of constipation.
- Orthostatic hypotension—possibly due to peripheral autonomic failure noted in parkinsonism. It may also be a side-effect of L-dopa therapy.
- Urinary hesitation and frequency—due to autonomic dysfunction. A catheter will rarely be necessary.

TREATMENT

Drug Therapy

Although there is no known treatment that will either temporarily or permanently stop the degeneration of the basal ganglia, drug therapy offers an effective method for relieving the many symptoms of Parkinson's disease. The need for surgery is rare because drug control is adequate.

L-Dopa. The most important drug in current use is L-dihydroxyphenylalanine (L-dopa). The basic therapeutic principle is based on the knowledge that the level of dopamine in the basal ganglia is decreased in the patient with Parkinson's disease. L-dopa converts to dopamine in the basal ganglia, thereby relieving the symptoms of rigidity and bradykinesia. This drug is effective for long-term management of the disease.

Dopa Decarboxylase Inhibitors. One might wonder why dopamine is not given forthright rather than its precursor, L-dopa. If dopamine were given orally, it would be metabolized before reaching the brain. L-dopa, however, is able to cross the blood-brain barrier and then become converted into dopamine. For this chemical reaction to take place, the enzyme dopa decarboxylase must be present. In the presence of this enzyme, L-dopa converts to dopamine and carbon dioxide, both in peripheral tissue and in the brain.

For the symptoms of Parkinson's disease to be controlled, L-dopa must be converted to dopamine within the brain. If the reaction occurs in peripheral tissue, side-effects of nausea, vomiting, cardiac arrhythmia, and other symptoms occur. Inhibitors are given to prevent the conversion of L-dopa to dopamine in peripheral tissue. The inhibitors selected to block the dopa decarboxylase enzyme do not cross the blood-brain barrier and allow for production of dopamine mainly in the brain. By using L-dopa in combination with dopa decarboxylase inhibitors, the dosage of L-dopa can be reduced and side-effects eliminated or greatly diminished. The inhibitor most often used is carbidopa (Sinemet). When used in combination, the dosage often used is carbidopa (Sinemet), 10 mg to 25 mg, and L-dopa, 100 mg to 250 mg three or four times daily. The therapeutic level is reached faster when used in combination.

Contraindications in L-Dopa Use. Most patients should be given a trial period on the drug. Those who probably should not be given the drug include people with severe cerebral or cardiovascular disease, psychosis, and severe medical problems.

Side-Effects. Side-effects include nausea and vomiting, orthostatic hypotension, dry mouth, gastrointestinal bleeding, constipation, dizziness, anemia, hypertension, cough, dark red urine retention, cardiac arrhythmias, and the "on–off" phenomenon (episodic loss of symptomatic control). When choreiform movements occur, the level of optimal drug therapy has been surpassed. Reducing the dose slightly helps to eliminate the choreiform movements.

Patient Teaching Precautions for L-Dopa. The patient should be made aware of the following limits when taking L-dopa:

- Pyridoxine (vitamin B_6) is a cofactor of the enzyme dopa decarboxylase. It increases the decarboxylation of L-dopa in the liver, thereby decreasing the amount available to be converted to dopamine in the brain. Therefore, patients on L-dopa therapy should not take vitamin B_6 or multivitamin preparations that include vitamin B_6.
- Large amounts of alcohol antagonize the effects of L-dopa and should be avoided.
- High-protein meals block the effect of L-dopa when given alone or in combination. Therefore, intake of the following foods should be controlled: milk, meat, fish, poultry, cheese, eggs, peanuts, nuts, sunflower seeds, whole grain, and soybean products.
- L-dopa should be taken with meals to decrease the side-effect of nausea.
- Dryness of the mouth can be combated by chewing gum or sucking on hard candy.
- Wearing elastic stockings will help to avoid orthostatic hypotension. Changing positions slowly is also helpful.
- Depression is common and may develop into severe depression with suicidal overtones. The physician should be advised if the patient feels depressed.

Anticholinergic Drugs. Anticholinergic drugs are used in conjunction with L-dopa or singularly if the patient cannot tolerate L-dopa or his symptoms are mild. The drugs of this classification include (1) trihexyphenidyl (Artane), (2) cyrimine (Pagitane), (3) procyclidine (Kemadrin), (4) biperiden (Akineton), and (5) benztropine mesylate (Cogentin). These drugs are effective in managing cramps, tremors, and rigidity. Trihexyphenidyl (Artane) is usually the drug of choice in initial management of moderate to severe parkinsonism. A patient may respond better to one drug rather than another in this group. Side-effects include blurred vision, drowsiness, nausea and vomiting, and dryness of the mouth. It is the physician's responsibility to choose the most effective drug, often by the trial-and-error method. Dosage ranges are as follows:

Drug	*Average Dosage*
Artane	2 mg to 5 mg tid or qid
Pagitane	1.25 mg to 5 mg tid or qid
Kemadrin	5 mg to 10 mg tid or qid
Akineton	1 mg to 2 mg tid or qid
Cogentin	0.5 mg to 6.0 mg daily

Antihistamines and Antiparkinsonism Drugs. This group of drugs includes diphenhydramine hydrochloride (Benadryl) and orphenadrine hydrochloride (Disipal). Antihistamines may be used alone for initial treatment of mild parkinsonism or for patients who cannot tolerate other drug protocols. It is effective when given in combination with the anticholinergic drugs.

Diphenhydramine hydrochloride (Benadryl) is used for its central cholinergic blocking action. It decreases rigidity and improves voluntary movement and speech. Dosage is 10 mg to 50 mg, not to exceed 400 mg daily.

Chlorphenoxamine hydrochloride (Phenoxene) has an action similar to diphenhydramine hydrochloride (Benadryl). Dosage is 50 mg three times a day to 100 mg two to four times a day.

Orphenadrine hydrochloride (Disipal) is helpful in controlling rigidity, depression, and fatigue. Its anticholinergic action helps to control the increased salivation, diaphoresis, and oculogyria. The dose is 50 mg three times a day, not to exceed 250 mg daily. The side-effects of drowsiness, nausea, headache, vertigo, dry mouth, rash, blurred vision, and hypotension are common with diphenhydramine hydrochloride and chlorphenoxamine hydrochloride. Disipal has few side-effects, and they are considered mild.

Amantadine Hydrochloride (Symmetrel). This drug is a synthetic antiviral compound used in the treatment of parkinsonism. Its exact mechanism is not clear. It is suggested that amantadine hydrochloride releases dopamine and other catecholamines from neuronal storage sites. It may also delay the re-uptake of these neurotransmitters into the synaptic vesicles. This drug is often used in combination with other antiparkinsonism drugs discussed. Amantadine hydrochloride is rapid-acting and improves most of the symptoms of Parkinson's disease. Dosage is 100 mg daily for 5 to 7 days. Another 100 mg daily may be added if side-effects do not develop. Side-effects include nervousness, depression, slurred speech, ataxia, and other symptoms of central nervous system dysfunction.

Ethopropazine Hydrochloride (Parsidol). This is a phenothiazine derivative that improves tremors, rigidity, posture, gait, and speech in the parkinsonian patient. Its main side-effect is depression. Dosage varies greatly, from 20 mg to 400 mg daily. Severe cases may require 500 mg to 600 mg daily.This drug is often given in combination with other antiparkinsonism drugs.

Surgery

The successful management of most patients with drugs has eliminated the need for surgery. The type of surgery used is stereotaxis, whereby parts of the basal ganglia are destroyed. Only one side can be operated upon at a given time. If symptoms are bilateral, an interval of approximately 6 months should elapse before the other side is operated upon. This surgical procedure is beneficial in eliminating tremors and rigidity.

MEDICAL MANAGEMENT

The management of the patient with Parkinson's disease is directed toward (1) control of the symptoms of the disease with drug therapy, (2) supportive therapy and maintenance, (3) physiotherapy program, and (4) psychotherapy referral, if necessary.

Although the disease cannot be cured or arrested, symptoms can usually be controlled well by drugs, as indicated in the preceding section. It takes time to select and adjust the drug schedule for optimal results. The patient must know the side-effects of and precautions to be taken with the drugs.

Supportive therapy is directed toward managing other symptoms common with parkinsonian patients such as constipation, perspiration, urinary dysfunction, and so forth. Advising the patient on adjustments in lifestyle and prevention of complications and injuries is also important. Speech therapy may be recommended for some patients.

A comprehensive physiotherapy program can be most helpful in retarding the rate of disability. Gait retraining, balance maintenance, heat, massage, and exercise programs can be developed.

As mentioned earlier, depression is not uncommon. It can become so severe that suicidal tendencies develop. In such instances, psychotherapy may be necessary. However, intellectual deterioration is not considered to be part of the disease.

Most patients are managed nicely at home. An effective drug program often allows the patient to maintain his normal lifestyle. In the advanced stages, the patient may be managed in a nursing home if adequate arrangements cannot be made at home. Admission to the acute-care facility may be necessary for special problems in drug adjustment, stereotactic surgery, and treatment of complications or injuries sustained as a result of the disease. Such complications include pneumonia, urinary tract infection, and fluid and electrolyte imbalance from excessive vomiting or diarrhea. Another possible cause for admission to a hospital is injuries sustained in falls. Parkinsonian patients are accident-prone because of incoordination, loss of postural reflexes, and rigidity; therefore, falls are not uncommon, and a patient may be admitted with a fractured hip, head injury, or spinal fracture.

NURSING MANAGEMENT OF THE PATIENT WITH PARKINSON'S DISEASE

Parkinson's disease is a slowly progressing disease. Drug therapy and effective methods of dealing with the signs and symptoms can prolong independence and provide for basic

CHART 29–8. SUMMARY OF MAJOR NURSING DIAGNOSES ASSOCIATED WITH PARKINSON'S DISEASE

NURSING DIAGNOSES (ACTUAL OR POTENTIAL)	EXPECTED OUTCOMES	NURSING INTERVENTIONS
Altered mobility	• Optimal level of mobility will be supported.	• Provide for range-of-motion exercises to extremities four times a day. • Evaluate the effectiveness of drug program and adjust as necessary. • Suggest a physical therapy referral to assist the patient in mobility.
Potential of injury	• Physical injury will be avoided.	• Provide assistive devices to support the patient in mobility. • Remove objects in the environment that could cause the patient to fall.
Altered self-concept	• A realistic positive self-concept will be supported. • Patient will demonstrate adaption of a positive altered body image.	• Develop a trusting nurse–patient relationship. • Provide a positive attitude toward the patient. • Promote social interaction. • Provide patient with necessary information to adjust to changes brought about by the disease.
Altered communications: verbal and written	• Methods of communication will be supported and adapted as necessary.	• Accept the patient's attempt to communicate. • Suggest speech therapy evaluation for the patient with a verbal deficit. • For writing difficulty, develop an alternate method of communication. • Evaluate the patient's drug therapy program to determine whether adjustments are necessary.

needs. A teaching plan in which the patient and family are involved should be developed. The teaching needs of the patient will depend on the stage of the illness and the present symptoms. General considerations in developing a teaching plan should include the following:

- The patient and family member should have a realistic concept of the disease. Determine what the physician has told the patient so that you can clarify and reinforce those facts.
- The patient and family member should know what drugs (and dosage) are being taken. They should be well aware of the side-effects and precautions. (See section on Patient Teaching Precautions for L-Dopa.)
- Discuss accident prevention by identifying symptoms that contribute to falls. Help family to evaluate home environment for potential dangers (scatter rugs, poor lighting, and so forth).
- Advise the patient to maintain a weight chart. Weight loss can develop from lack of nutrition because of vomiting and dysphagia. Obesity would also be a problem, particularly with ambulation.
- Dietary alterations for dysphagia should be a soft, ground diet and small feedings.
- Constipation can be managed with the use of stool softeners.
- Urinary problems should be evaluated carefully. Incontinence may be caused by an inability to get to the bathroom fast enough, rather than neurogenic changes. Offer suggestions (urinal at bedside at night and so forth).
- A bath should be taken daily to remove perspiration and oil from the skin.
- Orthostatic hypotension can be controlled by wearing elastic stockings and changing position slowly.
- If the patient is confined to bed for any period, his position should be changed every 2 hours to prevent contractures and pulmonary complications. Deep breathing should also be carried out to avoid lung congestion and pneumonia.
- Range-of-motion exercises prevent stiffness and development of contractures.
- Speech can be improved by reading aloud, singing, and raising the voice. (A consultation with a speech therapist may be beneficial.)
- Patients tend to be hypersensitive to heat and develop a fever in hot weather.
- Using a wide-based (12 to 15 inches) stance helps to maintain balance and improves walking. It may also help to practice getting into and out of a chair.
- The National Parkinson Foundation provides educational material and help to patients.

See Chart 29–8 for summary of nursing diagnoses associated with Parkinson's disease.

REFERENCES

1. Taylor JR: Identifying acute brain syndrome. Hosp Med 34, June 1981
2. Boss BJ: The dementias. J Neurosurg Nurs 15(2):87, April 1983
3. News update. J Gerontol Nurs 9(2):119, February 1982
4. Hayter J: Patients who have Alzheimer's disease. Am J Nurs 74(8):1460, August 1974
5. Roach M: Another name for madness. New York Times, January 16, 1983
6. McAlpine D, Lumsden C, Acheson E: Multiple Sclerosis: A Reappraisal. Baltimore, Williams & Wilkins, 1972
7. Walton J: Brain's Diseases of the Nervous System, 8th ed. Oxford, Oxford University Press, 1977
8. Hallpike JF, Adams CWM, Tourtellotte WW (eds): Multiple Sclerosis, pp 41–42. Chapman & Hall, 1983.
9. Adams R, Victor M: Principles of Neurology. New York, McGraw–Hill, 1977
10. Hoehn M, Yahr M: Parkinsonism: Onset, progression, and mortality. Neurology 17:427, May 1967

BIBLIOGRAPHY

Books

Adams R, Victor M: Principles of Neurology, 2nd ed, pp. 647–663, 795–832. New York, McGraw–Hill, 1981

Eliasson SG, Prensky AL, Hardin WB (eds): Neurological pathophysiology, 2nd ed, pp 71–82, 373–393. New York, Oxford University Press, 1978

Hallpike JF, Adams CWM, Tourtellotte W (eds): Muliple Sclerosis: Pathology, Diagnoses, and Management. Baltimore, Williams & Wilkins, 1983

Osserman K: Myasthenia Gravis. New York, Grune & Stratton, 1968

Scheinberg LC (ed): Multiple Sclerosis: A Guide for Patients and Their Families. New York, Raven Press, 1983

Vick N: Grinker's Neurology, 7th ed. Springfield, IL, Charles C Thomas, 1976

Wells CE: Dementias. Philadelphia, FA Davis, 1977

Periodicals

Beam IM: Alzheimer's disease: Helping families survive. Am J Nurs 84(2):229, February 1984

Blount M et al: Plasma exchange in the management of myasthenia gravis. Nurs Clin North Am 14(1):173, March 1979

Brand K: Multiple sclerosis, adrenocorticotropic hormone, and nursing implications. J Neurosurg Nurs 12(2):62, June 1980

Cantanzaro M: Nursing care of the MS patient (Part II). Neurology 30(7):44, July 1980

Coyle J, Price D, DeLong M: Alzheimer's disease: A disorder of cortical cholinergic innervation. Science 219:1184, March 11, 1983

Evans RL, Becker V, Stone BW: Identifying social needs of patients with neuromuscular disorders. Rehabil Nurs 7(5):21–25, 45, September–October 1982

Fischbach F: Easing adjustment to Parkinson's disease. Am J Nurs 66, January 1978

Gresh C: Helpful tips you can give your patients with Parkinson's disease. Nurs80 10(1):26, January 1980

Gould MT: Nursing diagnosis concurrent with multiple sclerosis. J Neurosurg Nurs 15(6):339, December 1983

Guze S: Acute brain syndrome. Hosp Med 63, April 1977

Hartley F: A nurse's view: Amyotrophic lateral sclerosis. J Neurosurg Nurs 13(2):89, April 1981

Hauser SL et al: Intensive immunosuppression in progressive multiple sclerosis. N Engl J Med 308:173, 1983

Holland NJ, McDonnell M, Wiesel–Levison P: Overview of multiple sclerosis and nursing care of the MS patient. J Neurosurg Nurs 13(1):28, February 1981

Holland NJ, Wiesel–Levison P, Schwedelson ES: Survey of neurogenic bladder in multiple sclerosis. J Neurosurg Nurs 13(6):337, December 1981

Kinley A: MS: From shock to acceptance. Am J Nurs 80(2):277, February 1980

Kolata GB: Clues to the cause of senile dementia. Science 211:1032, March 6, 1981

Kruger L: Normal pressure hydrocephalus in the parkinsonian patient. J Neurosurg Nurs 14(5):299, October 1982

Lavigne J: Respiratory care of the patient with neuromuscular disease. Nurs Clin North Am 14(1):133, March 1979

Lewis SM: Viral and immunopathology in multiple sclerosis. J Neurosurg Nurs 15(6):346, December 1983
Mackey AM: OBS and nursing care. J Gerontol Nurs 9(2):74, February 1983
McDonnell M et al: MS: Problem-oriented nursing care plans. Am J Nurs 80(2):292, February 1980
McFarlin DE, McFarland HF: Multiple sclerosis. New Engl J Med 307:1183, 1246, 1982
Olsen B: Motor neuron disease: Amyotrophic lateral sclerosis. J Neurosurg Nurs 13(2):83, April 1981
Pajk M: Alzheimer's disease: Inpatient care. Am J Nurs 84(2):216, February 1984
Palmer MH: Alzheimer's disease and critical care. J Gerontol Nurs 9(2):86, February 1983
Paulson G: Multiple sclerosis: The great imitator. Hosp Med 48, August 1980
Price G: MS: The challenge to the family. Am J Nurs 80(2):283, February 1980
Rabins PV, Mace NL, Lucas MJ: The impact of dementia on the family. JAMA 248(3):333, July 16, 1982
Reisberg B: Stages of cognitive decline. Am J Nurs 84(2):225, February 1984
Rasmussen D: Amyotrophic lateral sclerosis. Am J Nurs 80(2):2050, November 1980
Richardson K: Hope and flexibility: Your keys to helping OBS patients. Nurs82 12:65, June 1982
Slater R, Yearwood A: MS: Facts, faith, and hope. Am J Nurs 80(2):276, February 1980
Stewart C: Age-related changes in the nervous system. J Neurosurg Nurs 14(2):69, April 1982
Stipe J, White D, Van Arsdale E: Huntington's disease. Am J Nurs 79(8):1428, August 1979
Weldon PR, Murray TJ, Quine DB: Hearing changes in multiple sclerosis. J Neurosurg Nurs 15(2):98, April 1983
Winter A: Clinical highlights: Some important clinical features of the tremors of parkinsonism. Hosp Med 98, April 1978
Yearwood A: Being disabled doesn't mean being handicapped. Am J Nurs 80(2):299, February 1980
Zaretsky S: The extrapyramidal nervous system. J Neurosurg Nurs 14(5):295, October 1982

chapter 30

Cranial Nerve Diseases

Certain cranial nerves are especially vulnerable to injury because of their location within the cranial vault. About half of the twelve cranial nerves are subject to specific disease processes, mainly cranial nerves V, VII, IX, and X. Major diseases included in this chapter are trigeminal neuralgia, facial paralysis, Meniere's disease, and glossopharyngeal neuralgia.

TRIGEMINAL NEURALGIA (TIC DOULOUREUX)

Trigeminal neuralgia, also known as tic douloureux, is a fifth cranial nerve disease characterized by intense paroxysmal pain in the distribution of one or more branches of the trigeminal nerve. The term *tic*, as used in relation to the disease, refers to the contortions of the face in response to the pain. The pain is usually abrupt in onset, unilateral, and lasts from a few seconds to a few minutes. There are no motor or sensory deficits with trigeminal neuralgia. Terms commonly used to describe the pain are paroxysmal, sharp, piercing, shooting, burning, and lighteninglike jabs.

Most patients are able to identify trigger zones that initiate a bout of pain when stimulated. The trigger zone is usually a small area on the cheek, lip, gum, or forehead. These trigger zones are sensitive to the simplest of stimuli —touch, cold, pressure, or a blast of air. Chewing, talking, smiling, shaving, brushing the teeth, or going out of doors on a windy day are common activities of daily living that may result in an attack of pain.

ETIOLOGY

The etiology of trigeminal neuralgia is unknown, although many contributing factors have been identified. It has been suggested that trauma and infection of the teeth or jaw, as well as flulike illnesses, may be contributing causes of the disorder. Pressure on the cranial (V) nerve by an aneurysm, compression or arteriosclerotic changes of a small artery proximal to the nerve, a neoplasm, or arachnoiditis can cause sensory compression and produce symptoms of trigeminal neuralgia. In making a diagnosis, the physician must rule out cerebellopontine-angle tumors, acoustic neuromas, and meningiomas.

Trigeminal neuralgia may occur at any age, although it is most common in middle and later life. Women are affected more frequently than men, at a ratio of 3:2, respectively. If a young person complains of facial pain, multiple sclerosis should be considered.

DIAGNOSIS

The diagnosis of trigeminal neuralgia is based on the history. The neurological examination is entirely negative. The pain is precipitated by stimulation of trigger points; it is also unilateral, paroxysmal, and confined to the distribution of the fifth cranial nerve.

COURSE OF THE DISEASE

Many patients with trigeminal neuralgia experience bouts of pain for several weeks or months, followed by a spontaneous cessation of symptoms and remission. The length of the remission varies from days to years. With aging, there is a tendency for these remissions to be shorter.

The pain from the disease causes much suffering and limitation of the activities of daily living. Because of the fear of pain, patients may not talk, eat, or attend to personal hygiene such as washing the face, brushing the teeth, or shaving. Some individuals have become emaciated from not eating in their attempts to keep the face immobilized so that bouts of pain will be averted.

ANATOMICAL CONSIDERATIONS

The trigeminal nerve emerges from the pons, passing across the petrous ridge to become the gasserian ganglion, which, in turn, separates into the ophthalmic, maxillary, and mandibular divisions (Fig. 30–1). It is the largest of the cranial nerves, possessing both motor and sensory components. The following areas are supplied by each branch:

- Ophthalmic—forehead, eyes (including cornea), nose, temples, meninges, paranasal sinuses, and part of the nasal mucosa
- Maxillary—upper jaw, teeth, lip, cheeks, hard palate, maxillary sinus, and part of the nasal mucosa
- Mandibular—lower jaw, teeth, lip, buccal mucosa, tongue, part of the external ear, auditory meatus, and meninges.

The sensory fibers relay touch, pain, and temperature sensations. The motor component innervates the temporal and masseter muscles used for chewing, jaw-clenching, and lateral movement.

In trigeminal neuralgia, the second and third branches of the trigeminal nerve are about equally affected. Fortunately, involvement of the first branch is rare (about 10%). When the ophthalmic or first branch is involved, the corneal reflex, a very important protective mechanism, may be lost.

TREATMENT

Many treatments such as drugs, local nerve blocking, and surgical procedures have been developed to treat trigeminal neuralgia.

Medical Management

Drugs. The two most commonly used drugs to control the pain of trigeminal neuralgia are phenytoin (Dilantin) and carbamazepine (Tegretol). Although some patients derive benefits from these drugs, the side-effects are both numerous and serious.

Phenytoin (Dilantin), an anticonvulsant, may be given intravenously to abort an acute attack. Daily oral doses of 200 mg to 400 mg of phenytoin may be prophylactic in controlling pain. It is believed that the action of phenytoin decreases the paroxysmal afferent impulses, a reaction that is similar to that when this drug is used in the treatment of epilepsy. The side-effects of phenytoin include gastrointestinal upset, ataxia, skin rash, drowsiness, aplastic anemia, and leukopenia.

Carbamazepine (Tegretol) is another anticonvulsant drug than has been more effective than phenytoin. Many

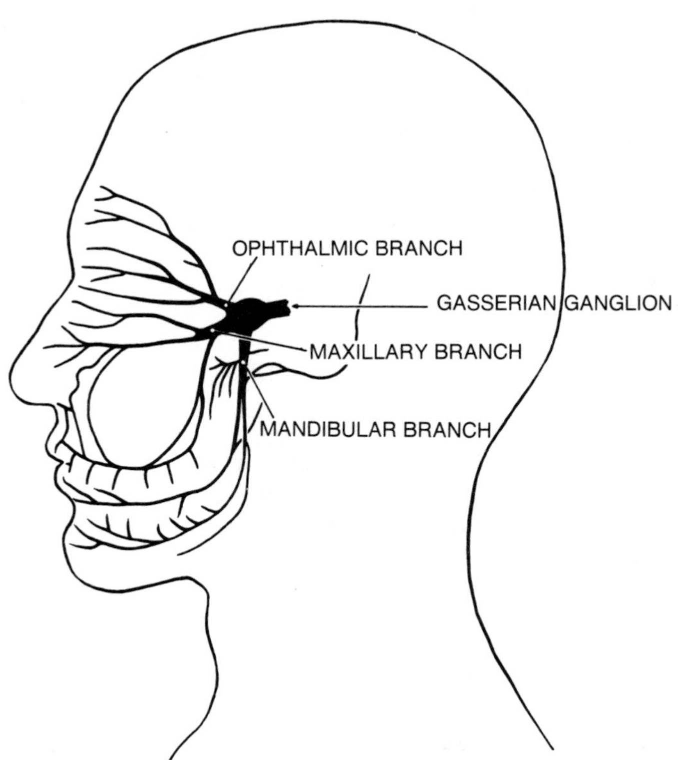

FIG. 30–1. The main divisions of the trigeminal nerve are ophthalmic, maxillary, and mandibular. Sensory root fibers arise in the gasserian ganglion. (Brunner LS, Suddarth DS: Textbook of Medical–Surgical Nursing, 5th ed. Philadelphia, JB Lippincott, 1984)

patients have had complete remission of symptoms. The action of this drug is similar to that of phenytoin, although more prolonged. The average dose is 200 mg to 1200 mg daily. The side-effects include headache, nausea and vomiting, rash, vertigo, ataxia, drowsiness, aplastic anemia, leukopenia, urinary dysfunction, paresthesia, and speech disturbance.

Both drugs require routine complete blood count studies to detect the development of blood abnormalities. Because of the high dosage often required to control the pain of trigeminal neuralgia, the precipitation of side-effects at the therapeutic level makes use of these drugs inappropriate for some patients. For those patients in whom drugs are effective, there is a tendency for either drug to lose its effectiveness in time. Therefore, drug therapy is not a permanent solution to the control of pain.

Alcohol Block. Injection of alcohol into one or more branches of the trigeminal nerve for the temporary relief of pain has been used with less frequency (Fig. 30–2). The relief of pain usually lasts from 8 to 16 months, with complete anesthesia to the areas supplied by the injected branches. The first and second branches are rarely injected because avulsion of these branches is easy to accomplish, thereby providing a better and longer period of pain relief. Even with avulsion of a cranial nerve, there is usually regeneration of the nerve because it is a peripheral nerve capable of regeneration. Pain recurs with regeneration. Recurrent injections can lead to scar tissue formation and more pain.

Blocking of the gasserian ganglion provides more permanent control of pain, but the possibility of extraocular palsies, keratitis, blindness, masticatory paralysis, and lack of selective cell destruction makes it an unattractive alternative. With both blocking procedures, the complete anesthesia to a portion of the face can be most distressing to the patient.

Glycerol Injection. Hakanson of Stockholm has found that percutaneous injection of small amounts of glycerol into the subarachnoid spaces surrounding the gasserian ganglion provides relief of trigeminal neuralgia comparable to that achieved from percutaneous trigeminal radiofrequency coagulation. There appear to be fewer side-effects with glycerol injection than with the other procedure.[1]

Surgical Management

Open Surgical Retrogasserian Rhizotomy. The gasserian ganglion is located in the middle fossa. Access can be gained by the subtemporal intradural or extradural route. However, if the middle fossa approach is used, the temporal lobe may be injured. On the other hand, the extradural approach could result in facial injury. The posterior craniotomy approach presents the possibility of both facial and acoustic nerve injury, along with the usual hazards of suboccipital craniotomy with retraction of the cerebellum and brain stem. The best attempts to prevent injury to the motor components of the trigeminal nerve may fail. The corneal sensation is preserved by sparing a few sensory fibers, but this, too, is not always successful.

Regardless of the approach, the complications of direct surgical retrogasserian rhizotomy include paresthesias, anesthesia dolorosa (a burning, itching, or scratching sensation in the anesthetized area), facial paralysis, corneal ulceration, keratitis, extraocular palsies, hemiparesis, and aphasia.

Postoperative Care. The nursing care follows the principles of care outlined for a craniotomy, in which there is frequent neurological assessment. In addition, the nurse would evaluate the corneal reflex, the extraocular muscles, and the facial nerve at frequent intervals.

- The corneal reflex is checked by lightly touching the cornea with a wisp of cotton. If the corneal reflex is intact, the patient will blink.

FIG. 30–2. Infraorbital *(A)* and supraorbital *(B)* nerve blocks may relieve the pain of tic douloureux when these two divisions are affected. After a few drops of local anesthetic are injected, the sensory loss is confirmed. Then 1 ml of absolute alcohol is injected into the nerve without disturbing the location of the needle. (Hardy J: Rhoads Textbook of Surgery. Philadelphia, JB Lippincott, 1977)

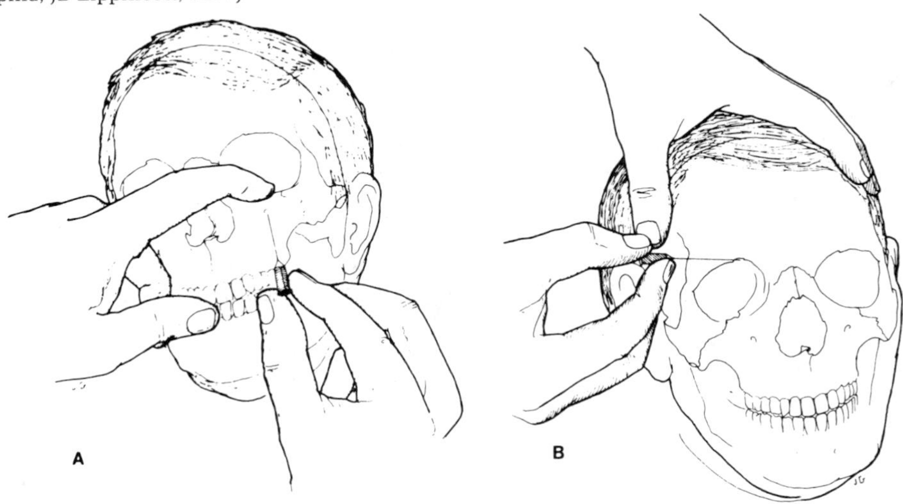

- The extraocular muscles are evaluated by asking the patient to follow the finger as it directs the eyes through the six cardinal positions of vision on the axis. Movements should be conjugate.
- The facial nerve is tested by asking the patient to wrinkle his forehead, frown, wink, close his eyes tightly, wrinkle his nose, whistle, and blow air out of his cheeks. Any weakness is readily detectable by lack of or limited movement on the involved side of the face. In addition, the anterior two thirds of the tongue is innervated by the facial nerve. Taste is checked by placing sugar, salt, and a bitter substance (e.g., quinine) on the tongue (one at a time) and asking the patient to identify the taste.

It is also advisable to evaluate the presence of abnormal sensations and pain along the distribution of the trigeminal nerve, as well as injury to the muscle of chewing.

- Touch, pain, and temperature sensations are evaluated on the forehead, cheek, and jaw areas.
- The motor component of the trigeminal nerve is evaluated by asking the patient to clench his teeth. The contracted masseter and temporal muscles are then palpated to feel the bulk and tightness of the contracted muscles. To test the pterygoid muscles, the patient is directed to open his mouth slightly and press the examiner's finger laterally with his jaw. Weakness of the muscle will result in deviation of the jaw toward the weak side.

Since hemiparesis and aphasia are other possible complications, attention to these aspects of the neurological assessment should be carefully evaluated. Abnormal findings should be documented and reported to the physician.

Decompression of the Sensory Root. Taarnhop's procedure of decompression of the roots was based on the premise that trigeminal neuralgia resulted from pressure on the sensory root as it crossed near the apex of the petrous bone. Following a middle fossa approach, the dural sheath surrounding the gasserian ganglion and root is cut, thereby producing a decompression of the intact nerve. The result is relief of pain without anesthesia or paresthesia. Unfortunately, there is a high incidence of recurrent pain. Other hazards of surgery include facial nerve or temporal lobe injury.

Postoperative Care. The nursing management follows principles of supratentorial surgery as discussed in Chapter 14. Periodic neurological assessment is an important part of nursing management. Special attention should be directed toward evaluation of the sensory and motor components of the trigeminal nerve as well as the facial nerve, both of which can be injured inadvertently. Methods of evaluation of both nerves have been outlined above under Postoperative Care.

Vascular Decompression of the Trigeminal Nerve. Many patients have been found to have a small artery compressing the trigeminal nerve as it enters the pons. Relocating the artery away from the trigeminal nerve produces immediate or delayed (by a few days) relief of the pain associated with trigeminal neuralgia without compromising facial sensation. A posterior fossa craniotomy is performed using microsurgery. The procedure as refined by Jannetta involves displacement of the vascular loop from the nerve and placement of a small Silastic sponge between the vessel and the nerve.[2] Complications include headache, persistent facial pain, and those complications associated with posterior fossa surgery.

Postoperative Care. The nursing management includes the principles of care outlined previously for posterior fossa surgery (Chap. 14). As soon as the patient is awake, an assessment of his trigeminal neuralgia pain is conducted and compared with the preoperative assessment. Cranial (V) nerve is checked in order to note any deficits, with special attention directed toward evaluating the corneal reflex. The diet and ambulation are advanced as tolerated by the patient.

Electrocoagulation. Radiofrequency percutaneous electrocoagulation is a recently developed method of providing lasting relief of pain with limited destruction of the trigeminal nerve. The basic principle is that small, poorly myelinated fibers that carry pain impulses are more sensitive to thermal lesions. With a heat-controlled electrocoagulation instrument, the sensory fibers are sufficiently destroyed to relieve pain without compromising touch or motor function.

The procedure is best done in the operating room, where fluoroscopical, radiological, and emergency equipment is available. A state of neuroleptoanalgesia is achieved by administering small doses of diazepam (Valium) and fentanyl (Sublimaze) intravenously during the procedure.[3] The patient is comfortable but still able to verbally respond to questions. After each lesion is made, the corneal and ciliary reflexes, as well as facial sensation, are checked. Access to the foramen ovale, an opening from which the third branch of the trigeminal emerges, is gained through the cheek (Fig. 30–3). The needle is advanced until cerebrospinal fluid is obtained. Radiographic verification of the location within the foramen ovale follows. The electrode is inserted so that the selective electrocoagulation can proceed.[4]

The advantages of the procedure are many, and include (1) long, if not permanent, relief of pain; (2) short-term hospitalization (may be discharged the day after the procedure); (3) good toleration by the elderly; (4) no facial paralysis; and (5) intactness of the sensation of touch. Disadvantages include the possibility of puncturing the internal carotid artery and the occurrence of anesthesia dolorosa.

Postoperative Care. Nursing management immediately after surgery includes application of an ice pack to the operative site on the jaw for 4 hours. Methylcellulose drops are instilled into the eyes on the affected side. The patient is not allowed to chew on the operative side until the paresthesia has diminished. A soft diet is ordered.[3]

Patient Teaching. After surgery, the affected side of the face is insensitive to pain permanently. The patient must be cautioned against rubbing the eye because the protective mechanism of pain, which warns of injury, is lost. The eye should also be inspected for redness and conjunctival erythema, which should be reported to the physician immediately. Blurred vision is another reportable

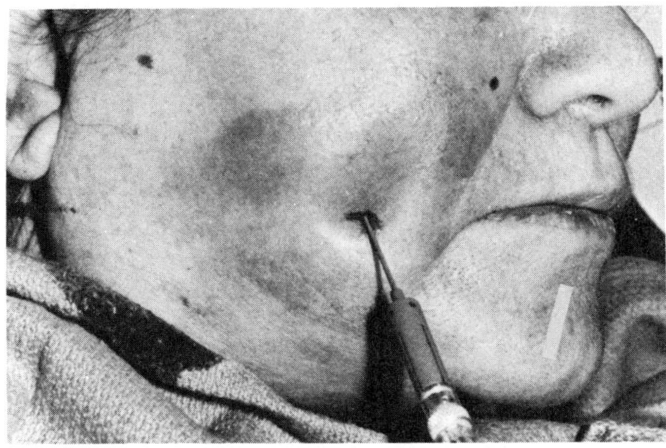

FIG. 30-3. Percutaneous radiofrequency rhizotomy for relief of pain from trigeminal neuralgia. The needle electrode has been inserted so that it may be advanced under radiographic control to the area where the heat lesion will be made. This procedure requires only a brief hospital stay without the time, expense, and hazards of an open cranial procedure. (Silverberg GD: Percutaneous radio-frequency rhizotomy in the treatment of trigeminal neuralgia. Western J Med, August, 1978)

problem. Because pain sensation is lost on the affected side, routine visits to the dentist should be scheduled so that caries can be detected.[3]

NURSING MANAGEMENT

The major nursing diagnoses for patients with trigeminal neuralgia who are being managed medically are listed in Chart 30-1. Specific nursing management after surgery is included under Postoperative Care for each procedure.

Psychological Considerations of Treatment Protocols. As indicated, the major methods of treatment that have been available include drugs, alcohol blocking, and various surgical procedures. If drugs are ineffective in the control of pain, other treatment methods will be suggested by the physician. In addition to phenytoin (Dilantin) and carbamazepine (Tegretol) for pain control, analgesics and tranquilizers are frequently prescribed. However, prolonged use of such drugs can often result in habituation. Poor control of pain may also be a disappointing outcome of surgery.

Drug habituation, disappointment from ineffective drug therapy or surgery, and fear that pain will be initiated by any activity all contribute to the anxiety of a patient who may be difficult for the nurse to manage. In collecting a nursing history, the nurse should carefully question the patient about his use of drugs. At the same time, an effort should be made to gain the patient's confidence. The nurse accomplishes this by indicating that she understands his illness and the mechanism by which pain can be triggered. The patient may not speak or move his face in an attempt to prevent pain. However, his behavior may be interpreted as withdrawal or antisocialness. The goal of nursing care is to help the patient control pain so that it is at least tolerable.

FACIAL PARALYSIS (BELL'S PALSY)

Sir Charles Bell of England first described acute paralysis of cranial (VII) nerve (facial nerve) in 1821. Because of Bell's interest in this cranial nerve disorder, the disease has been called facial paralysis or Bell's palsy.

SIGNS AND SYMPTOMS

The disorder may be preceded by symptoms of pain behind the ear or on the face for a few hours or days prior to the onset of paralysis. Facial paralysis is characterized by a drawing sensation on the affected side of the face, followed by paralysis of all ipsilateral facial muscles. The eye does not close and the forehead does not wrinkle (Fig. 30-4). The patient cannot smile, whistle, or grimace. The affected side of the face is masklike and sags, with constant tearing of the eye and possible drooling. The sense of taste on the anterior two thirds of the tongue may be affected.

DIAGNOSIS

The diagnosis is based on the history and clinical picture of seventh cranial nerve deficits that are unilateral.

COURSE AND PROGNOSIS

Bell's palsy can occur at any age but is most frequent in the 20- to 60-year age group. The sexes are affected about equally. The onset of the disorder may evolve gradually over 24 to 36 hours or may be completed upon awaking. Complete paralysis may never develop in some patients. Eighty percent of patients will completely recover from an attack within a few weeks or a few months. Electromyographic studies conducted 10 days after the onset on symptoms can indicate denervation and a prolonged recovery, which may never be complete. Recovery in this instance depends on nerve regeneration. Although the etiology of Bell's palsy is unknown, it is believed to be caused by an inflammatory reaction. It may be also secondary to other diseases such as Guillain-Barré syndrome or the mass effect of a tumor.

Cranial (VII) nerve, or the facial nerve, originates in the pons and emerges from the stylomastoid foramen. It is composed mostly of motor nerves, which supply all the muscles associated with expression on one side of the face. The sensory component innervates the anterior two thirds of the ipsilateral half of the tongue.

TREATMENT

Prednisone, 60 mg daily, is helpful for the first week after the onset of symptoms. Analgesics are given to relieve pain. Gentle massage, warm moist heat, and electrical stimulation of the nerve are common methods of treatment. Spe-

CHART 30-1. SUMMARY OF NURSING DIAGNOSES ASSOCIATED WITH TRIGEMINAL NEURALGIA

NURSING DIAGNOSES	EXPECTED OUTCOMES	NURSING INTERVENTIONS
Altered comfort: pain due to paroxysmal bouts	• Patient will not experience pain, or if he does, it will be controlled, brief, and not incapacitating.	• Assess the patient to identify those activities and circumstances that trigger pain. • Develop strategies with the patient to control the precipitating factors. • Discuss with patient common precipitating factors. • Administer pain medication at the first indication of paroxysmal bouts of pain. • Assess effectiveness of pain medication. • Assess and document characteristics, frequency, and intensity of pain.
Altered self-care: bathing, oral hygiene due to precipitating or fear of precipitating pain	• Bathing, oral hygiene, and, for male patients, shaving will be continued.	• Encourage the patient to take care of hygiene between bouts of pain. • Teach the patient to avoid trigger points and precipitating factors such as extremes in temperature. • Provide necessary equipment appropriate for the activities. • Discuss need for semi-annual visits to the dentist for examination and care of teeth.
Altered nutrition: less than adequate due to fear of precipitating a bout of pain from eating	• Adequate nutrition will be maintained.	• Assess the patient's diet for the proper consistency and temperature of appropriate food. • Consult with the dietitian in planning for nutrition. • Teach the patient to chew on the unaffected side. • Develop a written nutritional plan with the patient. • Discuss alterations in diet with the person who will be responsible for the patient's food preparation on discharge. • If adequate nutrition cannot be consumed orally, a nasogastric feeding tube will be necessary. Teach the patient and family techniques for feeding using this route. • Teach the patient to maintain a written weekly record of his weight.
Physical and social isolation due to fear of precipitating pain	• Patient will engage in satisfying activities to meet his physical and social needs.	• Assess physical and social activities in which the patient engages. • Assess patient's level of satisfaction with these activities. • Develop specific strategies to deal with the identified problems.
Potential of eye injury: involvement of opthalmic branch of trigeminal nerve due to rubbing or irritating the eye	• The eyes will not sustain injury.	• Assess presence of corneal reflex. • Inspect cornea periodically for signs of irritation. • Alert patient to avoid rubbing his eye.
Potential for lack of knowledge about drug therapy program	• Patient will adhere to drug protocol and be aware of side-effects and toxic signs. • Patient will be monitored to prevent toxicity from developing.	• Develop and implement a drug teaching program. • Alert the patient to the need for periodic complete blood counts if he is receiving phenytoin or carbamazepine. • Provide patient with written material on drug, dosage, side-effects, toxicity, and so forth. • Discuss with patient the need to be monitored by his physician.

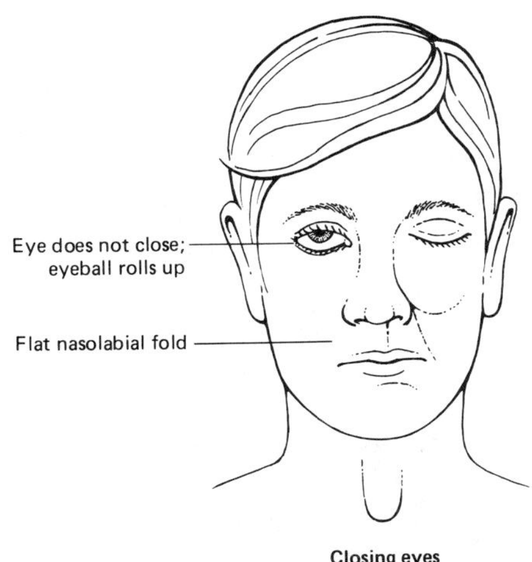

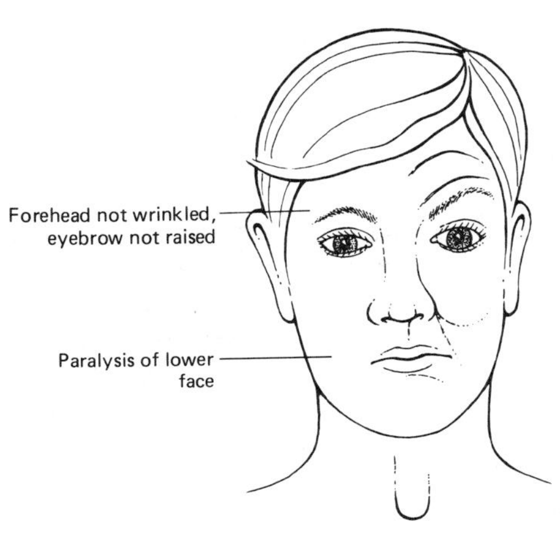

FIG. 30-4. Manifestations of Bell's palsy.

cial facial slings have been developed to support the sagging face. Such a device may be suggested for selected patients. As muscle tone improves, grimacing, wrinkling the brow, forcing the eyes closed, whistling, and blowing air out of the cheeks should be practiced three or four times daily for 5 minutes in front of a mirror.

NURSING MANAGEMENT

The nursing management is directed toward the major deficits and need to provide psychological and emotional support.

Eye Care

Because the eye does not close, the cornea must be protected from injury and from drying to prevent corneal ulceration and blindness. The patient should be instructed to manually close the eyelid at intervals. Artificial tears should be instilled four times daily for lubrication. The eyelids may be taped closed, or an eye patch may be worn for protection. Eye strain and sunlight are other stresses that may be avoided by wearing sunglasses.

Nutrition

Eating becomes a problem because the patient is unable to sip through a straw, chew, or control his saliva on the affected side. Frequent small feedings of soft food can best be managed by the patient. The problems associated with eating are major sources of anxiety and embarrassment to the patient. Mealtime, a time of relaxation and socialization for many, becomes a nightmare unless the patient is helped to cope and adapt to the situation.

Physiotherapy

The simple techniques of moist heat application, massage, and facial exercise can easily be taught to the patient at home. A patient who develops Bell's palsy without other disorders will probably be treated at home. If electrostimulation therapy is ordered, it will be provided on an outpatient basis. The patient who is managed at home must have a teaching care plan developed for him that will outline eye care and protection, mechanical adjustments of the diet, and a simple physiotherapy and exercise program.

Psychosocial Considerations

All patients with Bell's palsy need much emotional support in order to cope with the radical change in self-concept and body image. Fortunately, most patients (80%) will recover completely, but that is of little comfort when the patient views the distorted reflection of himself in the mirror.

MENIERE'S DISEASE

The most common cause of true vertigo is labyrinthine lesions, of which Meniere's disease is a classic variety. The disorder affects cranial (VIII) nerve, involving both the vestibular and cochlear branches.

SIGNS AND SYMPTOMS

Meniere's disease is characterized by recurrent attacks of vertigo associated with tinnitus and deafness. Tinnitus and deafness may not be evident initially but will gradually become apparent with increased severity as the attacks continue.

The vertigo is of the rotational or whirling variety, lasting from minutes to hours and becoming so severe that the patient is unable to stand or walk. Accompanying symptoms include nausea and vomiting, a feeling of fullness in the ears, tinnitus, and rotational or horizontal nystagmus with the slow movement on the ipsilateral side. In most patients, vertigo ceases with complete deafness, although there are exceptions. The attacks vary in frequency and severity, with a possibility of remissions between a series of bouts. Patients with recurrent attacks are apt to be anxious and in a mild state of disequilibrium.

The hearing loss associated with Meniere's disease may begin as early as before the onset of vertigo. Hearing loss occurs gradually until there is complete unilateral deafness. In 10% of patients, the disorder is bilateral. Both sexes are affected with equal frequency. The fifth decade of life is the most frequent time of onset.

Diagnosis is by caloric testing and audiometry. The audiometric studies reveal depression of the air and bone conduction.

DIAGNOSIS

The diagnosis of Meniere's disease is based on the history and clinical picture of fluctuating progressive hearing loss leading to deafness, episodes of vertigo, and significant tinnitus. The disease is usually unilateral and is characterized by periods of remission and exacerbation.

TREATMENT

During an attack, bed rest is most effective. The patient should be encouraged to try different recumbent positions until he finds one that minimizes the vertigo. Drugs are of value in controlling the vertigo and include dimenhydrinate (Dramamine), cyclizine (Marezine), or meclizine (Bonine, Antivert) in dosages of 25 mg to 50 mg every 4 hours during acute attacks. Mild sedatives and hypnotics are worthwhile in controlling anxiety in the anxious individual.

If the attacks are frequent and disabling, surgical labyrinthine destruction for the patient with unilateral disease and complete deafness is possible. In patients with bilateral disease or incomplete hearing loss, the vestibular portion of cranial (VIII) nerve can be resected intracranially, or the labyrinth can be selectively destroyed with cryotherapy.

NURSING MANAGEMENT

Most patients with Meniere's disease are treated at home unless they are admitted for surgery or other conditions. A major concern to the nurse is the prevention of accidents from falls as a result of the vertigo. Suggestions should be made to the patient concerning the prevention of injury, based on an assessment of his home environment and vertigo pattern.

The nurse should also help the patient to evaluate the control of the symptoms achieved from drugs. The patient needs much emotional support throughout the illness.

GLOSSOPHARYNGEAL NEURALGIA

Glossopharyngeal neuralgia is a much rarer syndrome than trigeminal neuralgia. The syndromes resemble each other in many respects. Similar aspects include (1) attacks of intense paroxysmal pain, (2) certain activities triggering bouts of pain, (3) no sensory or motor loss of the cranial nerve, and (4) unclear etiology.

SIGNS AND SYMPTOMS

In glossopharyngeal neuralgia the paroxysmal pain originates in the throat around the tonsillar area. Pain may also be localized in the ear or radiate to the ear from the throat. The pain in the ear implicates the auricular branch of the vagus nerve.

The paroxysmal pain described may be initiated most commonly by swallowing, talking, chewing, yawning, laughing, sneezing, coughing, or blowing the nose. With time, more and more activities of this type (requiring less stimulation) will become trigger mechanisms. After an attack, the trigger area is insensitive for a time, but gradually builds up to a state of hypersensitivity.

DIAGNOSIS

The diagnosis of glossopharyngeal neuralgia is based on the history and clinical picture.

TREATMENT

Using phenytoin (Dilantin) or carbamazepine (Tegretol) or spraying the throat with a topical anesthetic may be of some benefit to the patient. If this is unsuccessful, an intracranial surgical procedure might be indicated. The surgery would include division of the glossopharyngeal nerve and upper rootlets of the vagus nerve near the medulla. This posterior fossa procedure carries the risk of cerebellar and brain stem injury as well as injury to cranial nerves located in the area.

NURSING MANAGEMENT

The nursing management is directed toward helping the patient evaluate the response to drug therapy in relation to pain control and development of side-effects. If proven drug therapy is unsuccessful, the patient will probably need surgery for it is unlikely that the patient can function for long if swallowing, blowing the nose, and so forth create pain. These basic activities are necessary to maintain nutrition, control saliva, and maintain patency of the upper respiratory tract.

If surgery is performed, the nursing management follows the principles outlined for posterior fossa surgery (see Chap. 14). Cranial (IX and X) nerves are impossible to evaluate soon after surgery because of edema and irritation of the pharynx and trachea from the intubation of anesthesia.

REFERENCES

1. Camp PE: The newer microsurgical techniques in neurosurgery. Head Neck Surg 514, July/August 1982
2. Jannetta PJ: Treatment of trigeminal neuralgia by suboccipital and transtentorial cranial operations. Clin Neurosurg 24:538, 1977
3. Coleman P: Diagnosis and treatment with special reference to

percutaneous radiofrequency rhizotomy. J Neurosurg Nurs 7(2):91, December 1975

4. Poole M: Percutaneous electrocoagulation for tic douloureux. AORN J 24(5):87, November 1976

BIBLIOGRAPHY

Books

Adams R, Victor M: Principles of Neurology, 2nd ed, pp 929–939. New York, McGraw–Hill, 1981

Deparis M: Glossopharyngeal neuralgia. In Vinken P, Bruyn G (eds): Handbook of Clinical Neurology, vol 5, pp 350–361. Amsterdam, North Holland Publishing, 1968

Jannetta PJ: Treatment of trigeminal neuralgia by micro-operative decompression. In Youmans JR: Neurological Surgery, 2nd ed, pp 3589–3603. Philadelphia, WB Saunders, 1982

Penman J: Trigeminal neuralgia. In Vinken P, Bruyn G (eds): Handbook of Clinical Neurology, vol 5, pp 296–322. Amsterdam, North Holland Publishing, 1968

Smith RR: Essentials of Neurosurgery, pp 171–174. Philadelphia, JB Lippincott, 1980

Tew JM: Treatment of pain of glossopharyngeal and vagus nerves by percutaneous rhizotomy. In Youmans JR: Neurological Surgery, 2nd ed, pp 3609–3612. Philadelphia, WB Saunders, 1982

Tew JM: Treatment of trigeminal neuralgia by percutaneous rhizotomy. In Youmans JR: Neurological Surgery, 2nd ed, pp 3564–3579. Philadelphia, WB Saunders, 1982

Tytus JS: General considerations, medical therapy, and minor operative procedures for trigeminal neuralgia. In Youmans JR: Neurological Surgery, 2nd ed, pp 3554–3563. Philadelphia, WB Saunders, 1982

Tytus JS: Glossopharyngeal and geniculate neuralgia. In Youmans JR: Neurological Surgey, 2nd ed, pp 3604–3608. Philadelphia, WB Saunders, 1982

Tytus JS: Treatment of trigeminal neuralgia through temporal craniotomy. In Youmans JR (ed): Neurological Surgery, 2nd ed, pp 3580–3585. Philadelphia, WB Saunders, 1982

Welch K: Treatment of trigeminal neuralgia by section on the sensory root in the posterior fossa. In Youmans JR: Neurological Surgery, 2nd ed, pp 3586–3588. Philadelphia, WB Saunders, 1982

White J, Sweet W: Pain and the Neurosurgeon. Springfield, IL, Charles C Thomas, 1969

Periodicals

Apfelbaum R, Kirk M, Terra AM: Microvascular decompression of the trigeminal nerve for the treatment of trigeminal neuralgia. J Neurosurg Nurs 10(2):77, June 1978

Bayer D, Stenger T: Trigeminal neuralgia: An overview. Oral Surg 48(5):393, November 1979

Glasscook M: Meniere's disease. Hosp Med 48, December 1979

Graham M: Surgery for facial paralysis. AORN J 23(5):772, April 1976

Keane J: Vertigo as a vestibular symptom. Hosp Med 76, December 1978

Kirkland J, Williams A: Trigeminal neuralgia: Approaches to nursing care. J Neurosurg Nurs 15(3):149, June 1983

Mancall E: Diagnosis: Facial pain. Hosp Med 38, October 1982

Rovit R: Trigeminal neuralgia: Guidelines for the practitioner. Hosp Med 58, November 1979

Sell S: The treatment of tic douloureux by vascular decompression of the trigeminal nerve. J Neurosurg Nurs 9(1):19, March 1977

Index

Page numbers in *italics* indicate illustrations. Page numbers followed by the letter "c" indicate charts. Page numbers followed by the letter "n" indicate footnotes. Page numbers followed by the letter "t" indicate tabular material.